The Lippincott Manual of Nursing Practice

LILLIAN SHOLTIS BRUNNER,
R.N., B.S., M.S.

Consultant, Medical and Surgical Nursing, Project Director, Curriculum Studies, Bryn Mawr Hospital School of Nursing; formerly Assistant Professor of Surgical Nursing, Yale University School of Nursing.

DORIS SMITH SUDDARTH,
R.N., B.S.N.E., M.S.N.

Consultant in Health Occupations, Job Corps Health Office, U. S. Department of Labor; formerly Coordinator of the Curriculum, Alexandria Hospital School of Nursing.

Bette Bonine Faries, R.N., M.S.
Maternal and Infant Health, Professor of Department of Nursing, Montgomery Community College, Takoma Park, Maryland.

Kathleen A. Galligan, R.N., M.S.N.
Cardiovascular Nurse Clinician, Children's Hospital National Medical Center, Washington, D.C.

Donnajeanne Bigos Lavoie, R.N., M.S.N.
Neonatalogy Nurse Clinician, Children's Hospital National Medical Center, Washington, D.C.

Anne C. Schwalenstocker, R.N., M.S.N.
Clinical Unit Coordinator, Children's Hospital National Medical Center, Washington, D.C.

CONTRIBUTORS

Herbert H. Butler, M.D.
Emergency Department Physician, Underwood-Memorial Hospital, Woodbury, New Jersey; Immediate Past President, New Jersey Chapter American College of Emergency Physicians.

James F. Elam, PH.D.
Clinical Biochemist, Pathology Department, Alexandria Hospital, Alexandria, Virginia.

Richard E. Palmer, M.D., F.A.C.P.
Pathologist, Alexandria Hospital, Alexandria, Virginia; Clinical Associate Professor, George Washington University School of Medicine, Washington, D.C.; formerly President, American Society of Clinical Pathologists.

The
Lippincott
Manual
of
Nursing
Practice

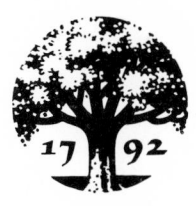

J. B. LIPPINCOTT COMPANY

PHILADELPHIA
TORONTO

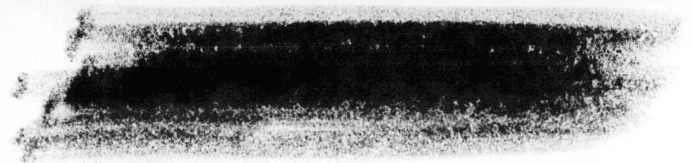

Distributed in Great Britain by
Blackwell Scientific Publications
Oxford, London, and Edinburgh

ISBN 0-397-54150-3

Printed in the United States of America

  5 7 9 8 6

Library of Congress Cataloging in Publication Data

Brunner, Lillian Sholtis.
    The Lippincott manual of nursing practice.

    Includes bibliographies.
    1. Nurses and nursing.   2. Medicine—Practice.
I. Suddarth, Doris Smith, joint author.   II. Title.
[DNLM: 1. Nursing care. WY100 B897L 1974]
RT65.B78   610.73   74-832
ISBN 0-397-54150-3

NOTE ON DRUGS: Because medicine and nursing are continually changing, the reader is advised to review the product information sheet included in the package of each drug administered.

Preface

Into the mind of every nurse caring for a suffering human being comes the question, "Have I done everything possible for *this* patient?" This Manual contains the principles of nursing practice written in a concise manner so that practitioners can be guided in caring for persons with various clinical problems. Included are underlying facts essential for the development of clinical logic necessary in assessing patients and developing plans of patient care.

The writers have endeavored in most instances to present the material in a logical fashion, beginning with a definition of the disorder and progressing to a presentation of the clinical manifestations, the diagnostic evaluation and the objectives and modalities of treatment and nursing management. The therapeutic rationale is given whenever it is felt that it will aid the nurse in clarifying the problems pertinent to the condition being considered. The authors believe that therapeutic and nursing management cannot be separated since each complements and is essential to the other. The information thus presented can be incorporated into a plan of nursing care adapted to specific individual patient requirements. Principles and suggestions for patient education are also included.

Throughout the volume are Guidelines to nursing and medical techniques and procedures frequently (and not so frequently) encountered. There must be an understanding of *method* of treatment before any nursing action can be initiated. Although equipment and techniques may vary in health agencies, there are certain underlying principles that form the basis for nursing action. The Guidelines are divided into three phases: preparatory, performance and follow-up, with appropriate rationale and amplification. By reviewing the Guidelines, the nurse will be able to engage in anticipatory nursing—*what* is to be done, *why* it is done and the expected patient reactions. With these Guidelines, complications can be prevented or managed, should they occur.

Because we work with and for people, there can be no absolutes in nursing. The broad field of medicine changes daily. Clinical discussions, therefore, are as varied as the patients for whom we care. Emphasis is on current concepts of therapy. The authors recognize the importance of a therapeutic relationship based on knowledge and application of psychosocial principles. Whenever possible the emotional components of an illness are identified. The reader is referred to specialized books on these subjects for more complete discussion.

A book such as this has some arbitrary restrictions. It cannot present all modalities of treatment. The clinical problems selected are those most frequently seen. Since repetition is a law of learning, it is used whenever it is necessary for emphasis or amplification, especially in areas where there is overlapping or where the material is used in a different context. To further enhance the usefulness of this volume, there is wide cross-referencing besides a complete index. A separate listing of Guidelines is also included. An authoritative, useful and up-to-date bibliography is placed where pertinent. The line drawings and illustrations should be studied carefully for they explain, demonstrate and clarify many facets of patient care.

Inasmuch as this Manual is designed primarily for the practitioner, it will be of value to the nursing student, a returning-nurse in need of refresher information, an instructor or a seasoned practitioner. The Manual presents and emphasizes clinical problems. It is intended to provide *instant information necessary for immediate use.*

Preface

In the Maternity Nursing section, the complications of pregnancy, delivery and the postpartum period are discussed in depth as these problems present the greatest challenges in terms of nursing assessment, clinical judgment and performance. In the section on Pediatric Nursing the objectives and components of nursing are presented in *detail* since so many of the children entering health care facilities have acute problems that require broad understanding and clinical nursing expertise. Emotional support and inclusion of the parents in the therapeutic and teaching program are spelled out.

The student of nursing is advised to take the Manual to the clinical unit for optimum usefulness. After reading the individual patient's record, the clinical problem can be reviewed in the Manual. This will help the student to anticipate the patient's problems, define the nursing objectives and initiate the plan of care. It is hoped that this will help to ease a problem that has proved difficult for many students, i.e., writing and implementing nursing care plans. Reviewing the Manual before the initial patient contact, will help the student to observe with seeing eyes, to listen with hearing ears and to perform nursing activities with the intellect as well as with the hands. As a unit of study is completed in the classroom, the same unit can be reviewed in the Manual. It is by this method that the integration of nursing knowledge will take place within the learner.

Because the art is long, the subject matter vast and the value of human life immeasurable, the study of nursing is the task of a lifetime. We offer this volume in the hope that it will increase understanding and clinical expertise as the nurse engages in the most challenging and rewarding of tasks, that of caring for patients.

Acknowledgments

The authors wish to express their appreciation for the assistance and efforts offered by the following groups of people.

Consultants in Medicine and Surgery:

Kenneth Balls, M.D.
Thomas E. Bressi, Jr., M.D.
Kjell H. Christiansen, M.D.
Edward V. Dillon, M.D.
Robert D. Dripps, Jr., M.D.
Jeffrey Frank, M.D.
Gilman E. Heggestad, M.D.
Stephen Levin, M.D.
Joseph D. Mashburn, M.D.
James Mills, M.D.
Thomas F. McGough, M.D.

Ernest L. McKenna, Jr., M.D.
James W. Preuss, M.D.
Robert L. Ravel, M.D.
Richard Rhame, M.D.
Rita C. Rigor, M.D.
Harold G. Scheie, M.D.
Abigail A. Silvers, M.D.
H. Millard Smith, M.D., Ph.D.
William C. Stainback, M.D.
Howard Sullivan, M.D.
Kirkley R. Williams, M.D.

Nursing and Allied Fields:

Eliza St. Clair Aiken, R.N.
Loretta Call Boyle, R.N.
Jean DeVries, R.N.
Cecil P. Greene, Biomedical Engineer
Pamela Humphrey, R.P.T.

Raymond S. Meck, ARIT
Kristin Pfeiffer, R.N.
Barry Stimmel, R.P.T.
John Vought, ARIT
Alice Cullis Weeming, R.N.

Photography—Art:

Neil O. Hardy
Barbara Mathews
John O'Connor, M.D.

Leslie H. Pitton
Robert Stamper
Janice Wojcik

Research/Library Assistance:

Alvin Barnes
Edith Blair
Evelyn F. Bowling
Leslie D. Gundry

Charlotte Moulton
Alice Sheridan
Gaston St. Dennis

The authors are also grateful to David T. Miller, Managing Editor, Nursing Department, for his inspiration, guidance, support and encouragement through all phases of the development of this book.

Special commendation is given to Diana Intenzo, editor, for her complete dedication to the manual, for painstaking attention to detail, for patience with and understanding of the authors' intent, and for a most pleasant and delightful working relationship.

Contents

Contents

LIST OF GUIDELINES

MATERNITY NURSING

PEDIATRIC NURSING

PART I

Medical-Surgical Nursing

Rehabilitation Concepts

REHABILITATION NURSING

Rehabilitation is an active and dynamic program which enables an ill or disabled person to achieve the greatest possible efficiency in his physical, emotional, social and economic functions.

Objective of Rehabilitation

To achieve optimal functioning by the use of an individualized approach.

Rehabilitation Team

Rehabilitation is a creative process requiring a team of persons working together and contributing those specialized services that may be required to assist the patient to become as functional as possible. In group sessions the team members evaluate the patient's progress and make necessary program changes.

1. *Physician*—makes the diagnosis so that therapy can be directed toward realistic goals; directs the patient's therapeutic program.
2. *Physiatrist*—a physician who is a specialist in physical medicine and rehabilitation.
   a. Tests the patient's physical functioning.
   b. Supervises the patient's rehabilitation program.
3. *Psychologist*—assesses the patient's motivation, values and attitudes towards his disability.
4. *Vocational counselor*—tests patient to determine his interests and aptitudes so that vocational training can be instituted.
5. *Physical therapist*—teaches and supervises the patient during his prescribed exercise program and gait training; uses physical agents and materials in restoration of bodily function after illness or injury.
6. *Occupational therapist*—develops those skills which can be transferred to home and work situations.
7. *Social worker*—investigates patient's background and socioeconomic status and assists patient and family in his adjustment to home and social environment.
8. *Nurse*—supports the therapy initiated by other members of the rehabilitation team.

Rehabilitative Nursing Functions

1. Develop a plan for nursing care services based upon nursing assessment of patient needs.
2. Provide direct nursing care services that will maintain optimum physical and mental health for the patient and will meet his medical treatment needs.
3. Apply nursing measures that prevent crippling and superimposed infections and ensure the safety and comfort of the patient in his environment.
4. Establish a sustained supporting relationship with the patient.
5. Participate in the retraining of the patient in self-care activities.
6. Provide health teaching and training that will meet the needs of the individual patient and his family.
7. Record and report nursing observations of the patient's condition, progress and personal needs, and the action taken to meet the patient's nursing needs.
8. Assist with patient discharge plans and provide for nursing referral of the patient for continued nursing services where needed.
9. Evaluate the nursing care in terms of the overall goals in patient care.

CAUSES OF DISABILITY*

Primary Disability—the result of a pathologic process, including congenital disorders, disease or injury.

Secondary Disability—the result either of inactivity or contraindicated and injurious activity.

Disuse Syndrome—disabilities from inactivity.

DISABILITIES FROM INACTIVITY

Disability	Cause	Prevention
1. Muscle atrophy (diminution in muscle strength and size)	Lack of exercise	Exercise
2. Joint contracture (limited range of motion)	Lack of joint motion	Passive range of motion; splinting; proper positioning
3. Metabolic disturbances Osteoporosis	Lack of weight-bearing	Tilt table (p. 33) and stand-up exercises
Urinary tract stones	Demineralization of bone Immobilization Dehydration/urine concentration Hypercalcemia Urinary tract infection	Mobilization High fluid intake No excess vitamins or minerals Prompt treatment of urinary infections; minimal use of catheter
4. Circulatory disturbances Orthostatic hypotension Venous thrombosis	Recumbent position Slowing of venous return	Tilt table and stand-up exercises Change of position; exercise; elastic stockings
Hypostatic pneumonia	Lack of chest expansion Poor position	Change of position Prone position to drain bronchial tree; exercise and deep breathing
Decubitus ulcers	Pressure	Change of position (p. 5)
5. Sphincter disturbances Urinary incontinence	Lack of opportunity	Urinal or bedpan instead of indwelling catheter Increased sensory input (p. 36)
Bowel incontinence/constipation	Improper diet Lack of activity Lack of opportunity	Regular bowel routine (p. 38)
6. Psychological deterioration	Inactivity Isolation Separation from accustomed environment Institutional routine	Maximal activity Active participation in planning own care Participation in decision making Increase sensory input; build self-esteem with meaningful activity

* Adapted from Hirschberg, G. G., Lewis, L., and Thomas, D.: Rehabilitation. Philadelphia, J. B. Lippincott, 1964.

PSYCHOLOGICAL IMPLICATIONS OF A DISABILITY

Disability has a tremendous impact upon the patient's body image (physical appearance, bodily sensations, beliefs and emotions about the body).

Nursing Objectives

1. To be aware of the factors influencing the patient's behavior.
2. To help the patient feel worthwhile.

Nursing Insight

The mode of the patient's interpersonal relations will be altered by the changes he makes concerning his body image.

Emotional Reactions of the Patient to Newly Acquired Disability

A. *Period of Confusion, Disorganization and Denial*
1. Is in a state of conflict; has to cope with problems of forced dependence, loss of self-esteem and feelings of threat to self and family integrity.
2. Uses mechanism of denial by refusing to accept new limitations.
   a. May have false hopes for a speedy and complete recovery.
   b. Likely to be self-centered and child-like.
   c. May attempt to remain "normal" and nondisabled.
   d. Denial is the mechanism used by those who have placed great value on strength and attractive appearance.

B. *Period of Depression and Grief; a Period of Situational Reaction*
1. Appears to mourn for his lost function or missing body part.
2. May have body-image distortions.
3. Depression is also due to sensory deprivation and restricted environmental stimulation.
4. Limited mobility and sensory stimulation may produce behavioral disruptions.

C. *Period of Adaptation and Adjustment*
1. Energies are redirected into channels concerning physical functioning, etc.
2. Revises his body image and modifies his former picture of himself; has a reorientation of values.
3. Accepts a degree of dependency.
4. Accepts limitations imposed by the disability.
5. Begins to develop realistic goals for the future.

PREVENTING COMPLICATIONS AND DEFORMITIES

Deformities and complications of illness or injury often can be prevented by *frequent changes of position, proper positioning in bed* and *exercise.*

Positioning

Purposes for Changing Positions

1. To prevent contractures.
2. To stimulate circulation and to help prevent thrombophlebitis, decubiti and edema of the extremities.

3. To promote lung expansion and drainage of respiratory secretions.
4. To relieve pressure on a body area.

Principles of Body Alignment in Body Positioning

A. *Dorsal or Supine Position*
   1. The head is in line with the spine, both laterally and anteroposteriorly.
   2. The trunk is positioned so that flexion of the hips is minimized.
   3. The arms are flexed at the elbow with the hands resting against the lateral abdomen.
   4. The legs are extended with a small firm support under the popliteal area.
   5. The heels are suspended in a space between the mattress and the footboard.
   6. The toes are pointed straight up.
   7. Small towel rolls are placed under the greater trochanters in the hip-joint areas.

B. *Side-lying or Lateral Position*
   1. The head is in line with the spine.
   2. The body is in alignment and is not twisted.
   3. The uppermost hip joint is slightly forward and supported by a pillow in a position of slight abduction.
   4. A pillow supports the arm, which is flexed at both the elbow and shoulder joints.

C. *Prone Position*
   1. The head is turned laterally and is in alignment with the rest of the body.
   2. The arms are abducted and externally rotated at the shoulder joint; the elbows are flexed.
   3. A small flat support is placed under the pelvis, extending from the level of the umbilicus to the upper third of the thigh.
   4. The lower extremities remain in a neutral position.
   5. The toes are suspended over the edge of the mattress.

Therapeutic Exercises

Exercise involves the function of muscles, nerves, bones and joints. The return of function is dependent upon the strength of the musculature that controls the joint.

Objectives
   1. To develop and retrain deficient muscles.
   2. To restore as much normal movement as possible.
   3. To stimulate the functions of various organs and body systems.

Accomplishments of Exercise Programs
   1. Maintain and build muscle strength
   2. Maintain joint function
   3. Prevent deformity
   4. Stimulate circulation
   5. Build tolerance and endurance

Types of Exercises
   1. Passive
   2. Active assistive
   3. Active
   4. Resistive
   5. Isometric or muscle-setting

A. *Passive*—an exercise carried out by the therapist or the nurse without assistance from the patient.
1. Purpose: to retain as much joint range of motion as possible.
    to maintain circulation.
2. Action
    a. Stabilize the proximal joint and support the distal part.
    b. Move the joint smoothly, slowly and gently through its full range of motion (pp. 8–18).
    c. Avoid producing pain.

B. *Active Assistive*—an exercise carried out by the patient with the assistance of the therapist or the nurse.
1. Purpose: to encourage normal muscle function.
2. Action
    a. Support the distal part and encourage the patient to take the joint actively through its range of motion.
    b. Give as little assistance as is necessary to accomplish the action.
    c. Short periods of activity should be followed by adequate rest periods.

C. *Active*—an exercise accomplished by the patient without assistance.
1. Purpose: to increase muscle strength.
2. Action
    a. Active exercise when possible should be done against gravity.
    b. The joint is moved through full range of motion without assistance.
    c. The patient should not substitute another joint movement for the one intended.
    d. Other active forms of exercise include turning from side to side, turning from back to abdomen and moving up and down in bed.

D. *Resistive*—an active exercise carried out by the patient working against resistance produced by either manual or mechanical means.
1. Purpose: to provide resistance in order to increase muscle power.
2. Action
    a. The patient moves the joint through its range of motion while the therapist provides slight resistance at first and then progressively increases resistance.
    b. Sandbags and weights can be used and are supplied at the distal point of the involved joint.
    c. The movements should be done smoothly.

E. *Isometric or Muscle-Setting*—an exercise performed by the patient.
1. Purpose: to maintain strength when a joint is immobilized.
2. Action
    a. The patient contracts or tightens the muscle as much as possible without moving the joint.
    b. He holds for several seconds, then "lets go" and relaxes.
    c. He breathes deeply during the contraction of muscles.

Range of Motion Exercises

Range of motion is the movement of a joint through its full range in all appropriate planes. It may be passive, active or resistive.

Objectives

1. To maintain function and prevent deterioration.
2. To maintain or increase the maximal motion of a joint.

Underlying Principles

1. Range of motion testing is done by the physician to determine the movement that exists at the joint areas. Testing helps set realistic and positive goals.
2. The patient's range of motion is affected by his physical condition, the disease process and his genetic makeup.
3. Each joint of the body has a normal range of motion (Table 1-1).
4. Joints may lose their normal range of motion, stiffen and produce a permanent disability—frequently seen in muscular conditions, hemiplegia.
5. Range of motion exercises are individually planned as there is a wide variation in the degrees of motion among patients of varying body builds and age groups.
6. Range of motion exercises should be carried out whenever there is physical inactivity provided the patient's clinical status allows such activity.

Techniques of Range of Motion

1. Place the patient in a supine position with his arms to the side and the knees extended.
2. Hold the extremity at the joint, e.g., elbow, wrist and knee, and move the joint smoothly, slowly and gently through its range. If the joint is painful (as in arthritis) hold the muscle "belly" to support the extremity.
3. Move each joint through its range of motion about 3 times.
4. Avoid moving a joint beyond its free range of motion; avoid forcing movement and causing pain.
5. Refer to Table 1-1 to review the normal movement of each joint and to know the part to be stabilized and the part to be moved.
6. Refer to the figures in Table 1-2 for pictorial review of range of motion exercises.

Definitions

Adduction—movement of a limb toward the body's center.

Abduction—movement away from midline of the body; turning outward.

Extension—when referring to an extremity means straightening out the joint.

Hyperextension—extension beyond the ordinary range.

Pronation—turning downward.

Supination—turning upward.

Flexion—bending the various joints, such as the knee or the elbow, or the thigh on the trunk.

Dorsiflexion—bending backward.

Rotation—turning or movement of a part around its axis.

Internal: turning inward toward the center.

External: turning outward away from the center.

TABLE 1-1. PASSIVE RANGE OF MOTION EXERCISES ADAPTED FOR NURSING

Joint	Normal Movement of Joint	Part to be Stabilized	Part to be Moved
Shoulder	Flexion Extension Abduction Adduction Internal rotation External rotation Hyperextension (done in prone position)	Shoulder girdle	Arm
	Forward flexion · Extension · Hyperextension · Abduction · Adduction		
Elbow	Flexion Extension Supination Pronation	Arm	Forearm
	Flexion · Extension · Pronation · Supination		

TABLE 1-1.   PASSIVE RANGE OF MOTION EXERCISES ADAPTED FOR NURSING (continued)

Joint	Normal Movement of Joint	Part to be Stabilized	Part to be Moved
Joints of fingers Metacarpophalangeal joints	Flexion Extension Abduction Adduction	Metacarpals of hand	Fingers
Interphalangeal joints	Flexion Extension	Proximal or middle phalanx	Middle and distal phalanx
Toe Interphalangeal joints	Flexion Extension	Proximal or middle joint phalanx	Middle and distal phalanx
Metacarpophalangeal joints	Flexion Extension Abduction Adduction	Metatarsal	Proximal phalanx

Flexion

Extension

Abduction

Adduction

Flexion

Extension

Abduction

Adduction

Joint	Normal Movement of Joint	Part to be Stabilized	Part to be Moved
Ankle	Dorsiflexion Plantar flexion Eversion Inversion	Leg	Foot
Wrist	Flexion Extension Ulnar deviation Radial deviation	Forearm	Hand

Dorsal flexion

Plantar flexion

Eversion

Inversion

Flexion

Extension

Hyperextension

Radial deviation   Ulnar deviation

TABLE 1-1. PASSIVE RANGE OF MOTION EXERCISES ADAPTED FOR NURSING (continued)

Joint	Normal Movement of Joint	Part to be Stabilized	Part to be Moved
Thumb	Flexion Extension Abduction Adduction Opposition	Metacarpals and wrist	Metacarpophalangeal joint of thumb
	Flexion Extension	Proximal phalanx of thumb	Distal phalanx of thumb
Knee	Flexion Extension	Thigh	Leg

Flexion — Extension — Abduction — Adduction — Opposition

Flexion — Extension

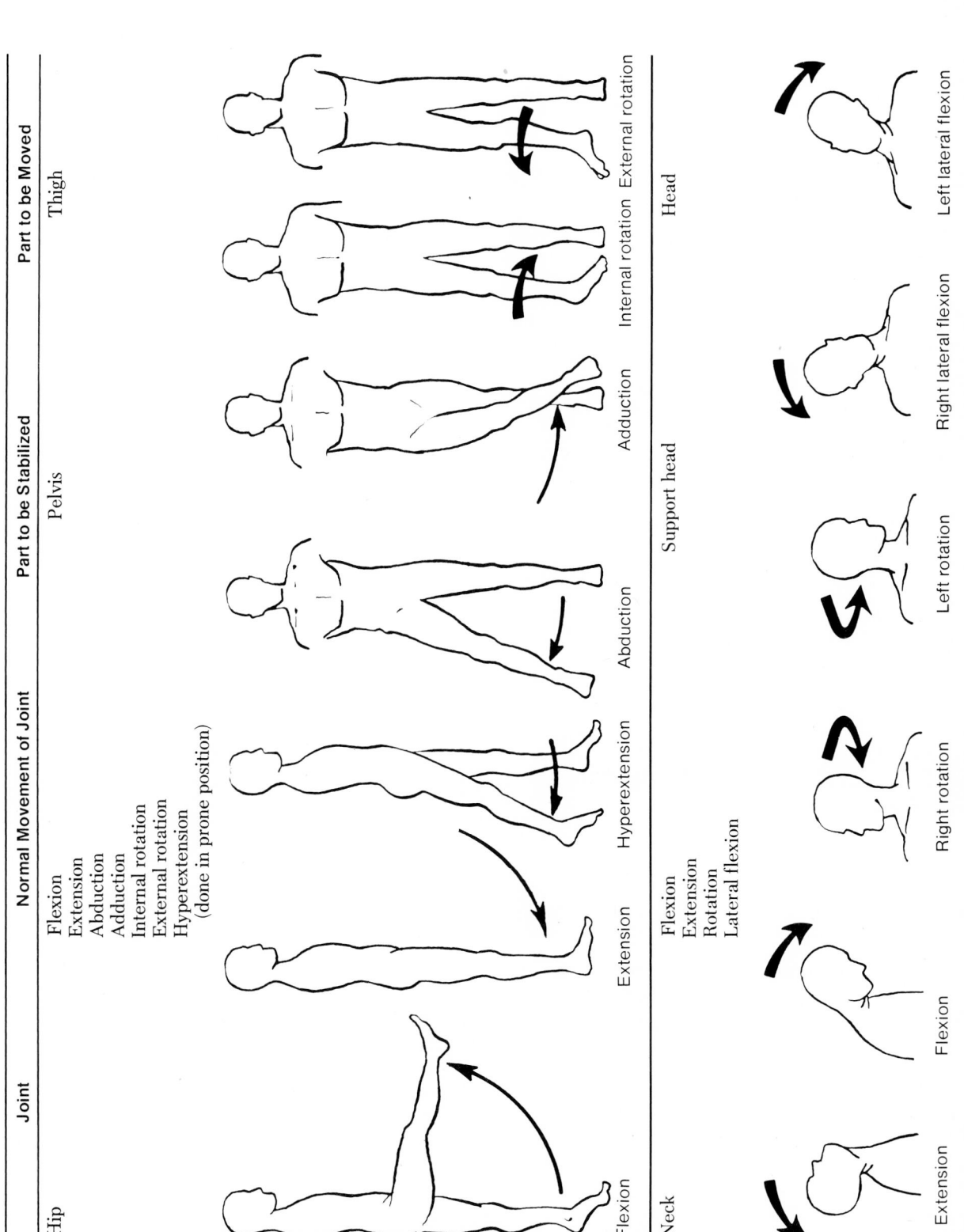

Joint	Normal Movement of Joint	Part to be Stabilized	Part to be Moved
Hip	Flexion Extension Abduction Adduction Internal rotation External rotation Hyperextension (done in prone position)	Pelvis	Thigh
Neck	Flexion Extension Rotation Lateral flexion	Support head	Head

Flexion   Extension   Hyperextension   Abduction   Adduction   Internal rotation   External rotation

Extension   Flexion   Right rotation   Left rotation   Right lateral flexion   Left lateral flexion

TABLE 1-2.   RANGE OF MOTION EXERCISES*

SHOULDER: Flexion and Extension

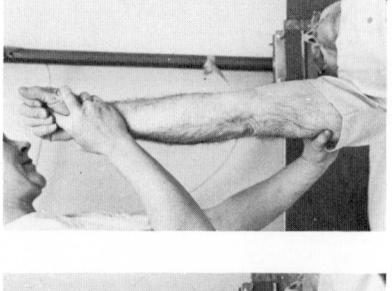 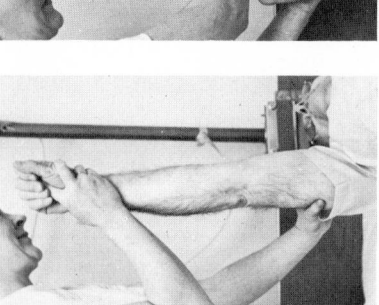 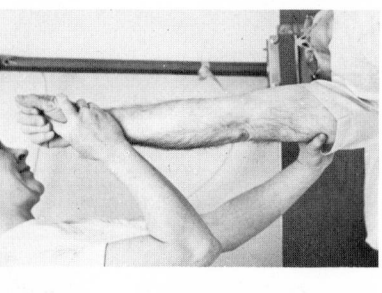 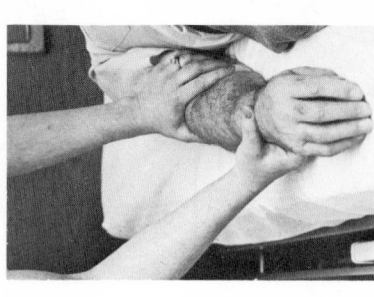

1. Start by placing one hand above the patient's elbow. Hold the patient's hand with your other hand.

2. Lift his arm up from the side of his body.

3. Move the arm slowly and gently toward his head as far as possible without causing pain.

4. If the bedboard prevents full forward flexion, bend the arm at the elbow.

5. Lift arm again before returning to side or neutral position. Repeat the exercise.

SHOULDER: Abduction and Adduction

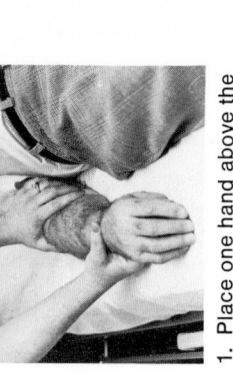 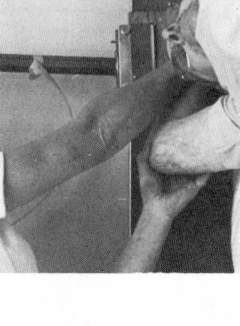 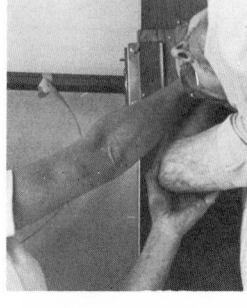 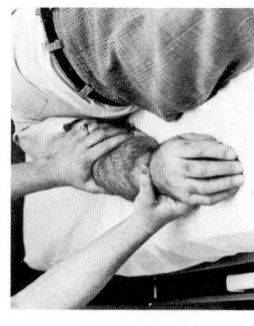

1. Place one hand above the patient's elbow. Hold his hand with your other hand.

2. Keeping his arm straight, move it sideways away from his body.

3. Bend and move the arm slowly around toward the patient's head. Move his arm back as far as possible without pain.

4. Return the arm to the side or neutral position. Repeat the exercise.

* From Nursing '72, April, 1972.

SHOULDER: Internal and External Rotation

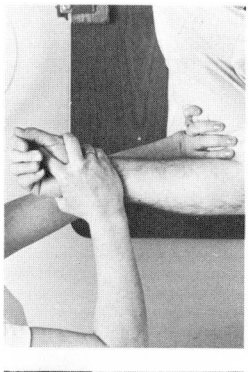

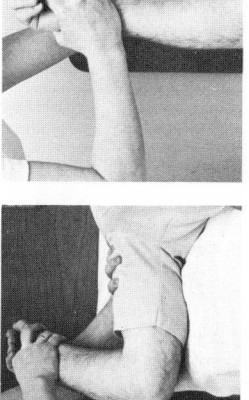

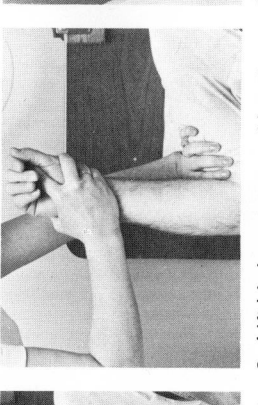

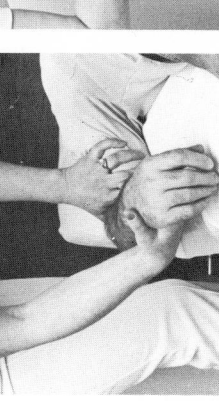

1. Place the patient's arm pointed away from his body, elbow bent. Hold his upper arm against the mattress.

2. Lift his lower arm and hand.

3. Move his lower arm and hand slowly and gently back toward his head, as far as possible without causing pain.

4. Return his arm to the starting position. Repeat exercise.

SHOULDER: Cross Adduction

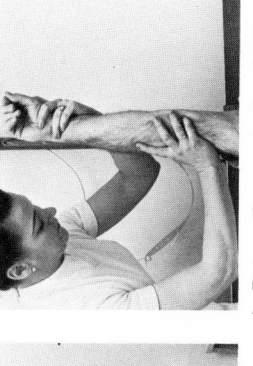

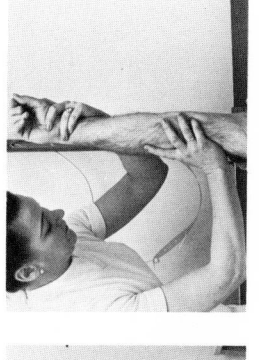

1. Place one hand on the patient's arm above his elbow. Hold his hand with your other hand.

2. Lift his arm.

3. With arm at shoulder height move arm across the body as far as possible toward the other shoulder.

4. Return the arm to the starting position. Repeat the exercise.

FOREARM: Supination and Pronation

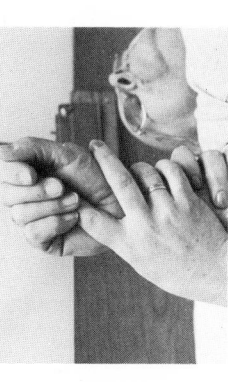

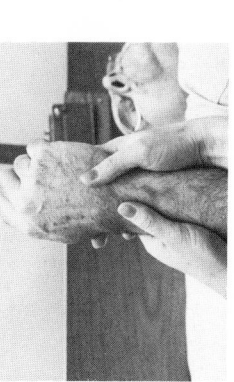

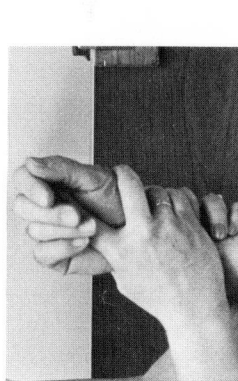

1. Starting position: Note the position of the patient's hands and the nurse's hands.

2. Twist the palm of the patient's hand toward his face.

3. Then, twist the palm of his hand back toward his feet. Repeat.

TABLE 1-2 (continued)

WRIST AND FINGER: Flexion and Extension

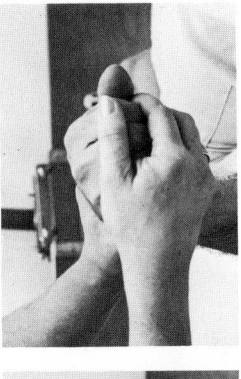
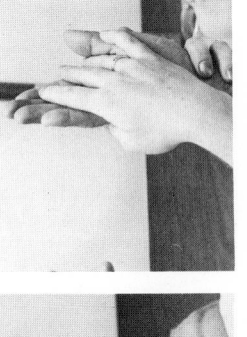
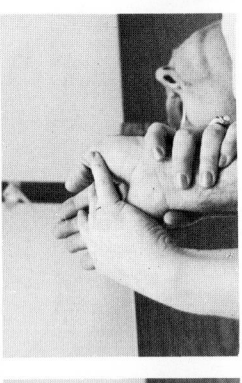
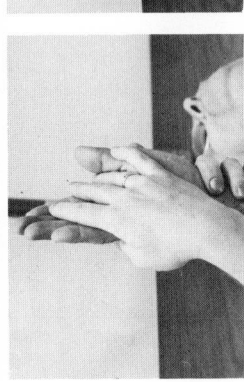

1. Hold the patient's wrist with one hand and his hand with your other hand.

2. Bend his hand backward while keeping his fingers straight.

3. Straighten the hand.

4. Bend his hand forward, closing his fingers to make a fist. Open his hand and repeat the exercise.

THUMB: Flexion and Extension

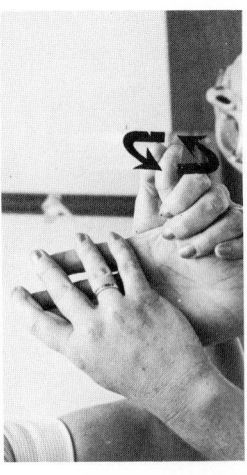
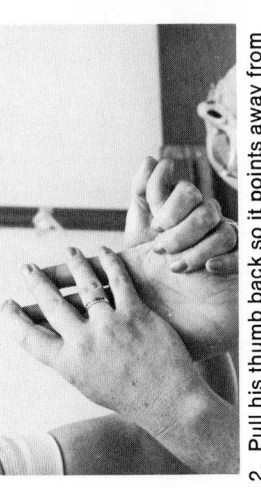
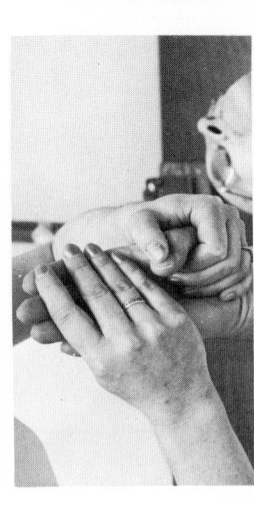

1. Hold the patient's fingers straight within one of your hands. Bend the patient's thumb into the palm of his hand with your other hand.

2. Pull his thumb back so it points away from his palm. Repeat the exercise.

3. Move his thumb around in a circle.

KNEE AND HIP: Flexion and Extension

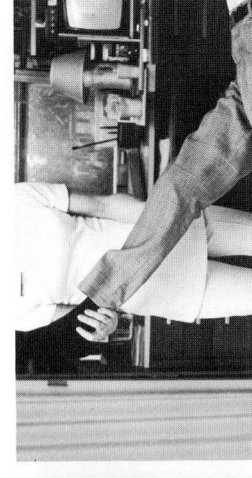
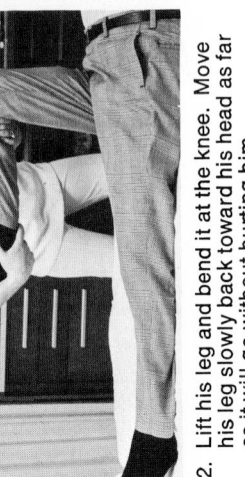
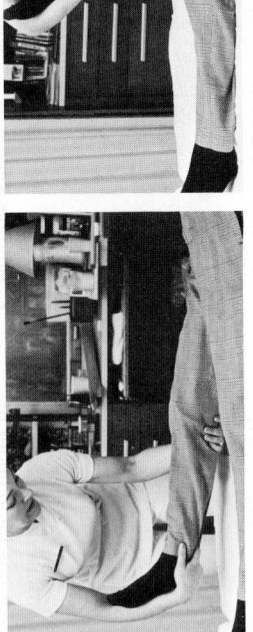

1. Place one of your hands under the patient's knee. Place your other hand on the heel of his foot.

2. Lift his leg and bend it at the knee. Move his leg slowly back toward his head as far as it will go without hurting him.

3. Then straighten his knee by lifting the foot upward. Lower his leg to the starting position and repeat the exercise.

HIP: Internal and External Rotation

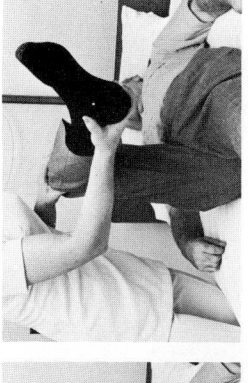

4. Then push his foot away from you. Move his foot back to the starting position and repeat the exercise.

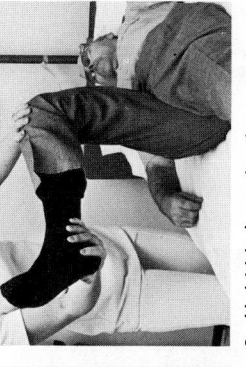

3. Move his foot back to the starting position.

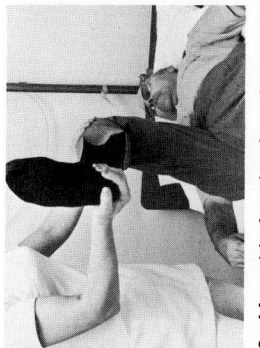

2. Hold his knee in place and pull his foot toward you.

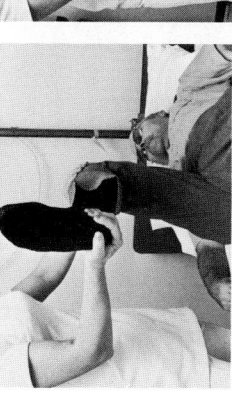

1. Place one hand under the patient's knee and your other hand on the heel of his foot. Lift his leg and bend it to a right angle at the knee.

HIP: Abduction and Adduction

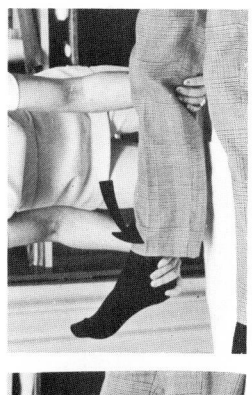

3. Push the leg back to the starting position (adduction). Repeat the exercise.

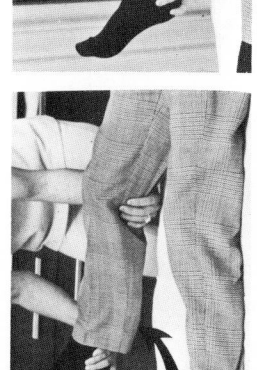

2. Pull the leg out toward you (abduction).

1. Place one hand under the patient's knee. Place your other hand under his heel. Hold the leg straight and then lift it up about 2 inches from the mattress.

ANKLE: Dorsiflexion and Plantar Flexion

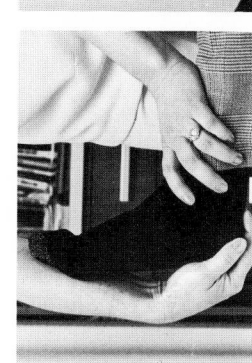

4. Move your hand up to the top of the foot, below the toes. Push down on the foot to point the toes and at the same time, push up against the heel (plantar flexion).

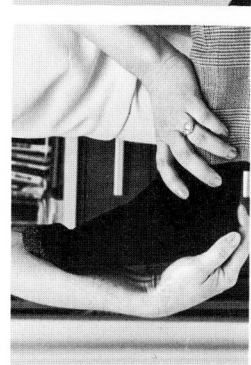

3. Move your arm back to the starting position.

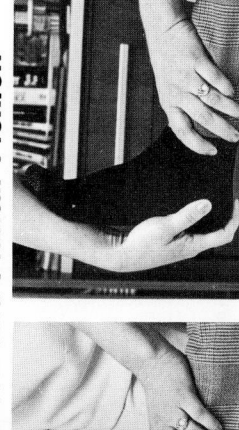

2. Press your arm against the bottom of the foot, moving it back toward the leg (dorsiflexion). At the same time, pull on the heel.

1. Hold the patient's heel with your hand, letting the sole of his foot rest against your arm.

TABLE 1-2 (continued)

FOOT: Inversion and Eversion

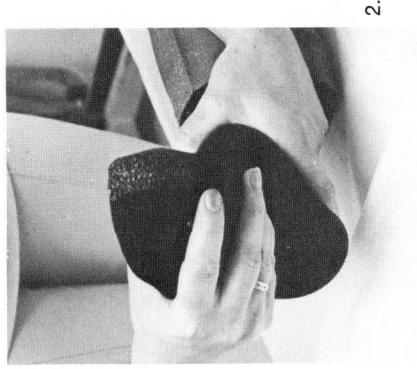

1. Start by turning the whole foot so that the sole is facing outward (eversion).

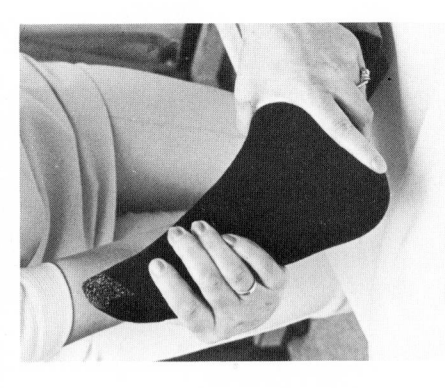

2. Then turn the foot so that the sole is facing inward (inversion).

TOE: Flexion and Extension

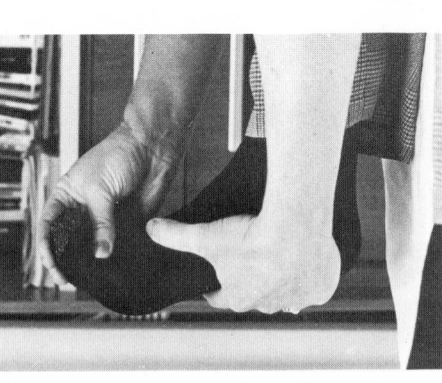

1. Start by pulling up on the toes (flexion).

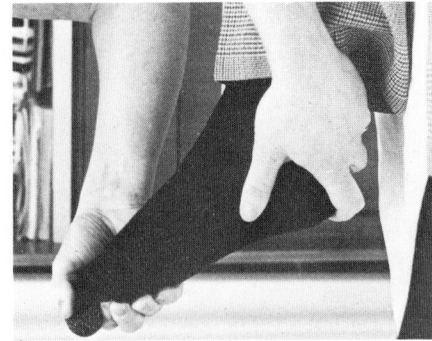

2. Then push down on the toes (extension).

Preventing External Rotation of Hip

Patients on prolonged bedrest may develop external rotation deformity of the hip. The hip (being a ball-and-socket joint) has a tendency to rotate outwardly when the patient lies on his back.

Nursing Management

1. To prevent this deformity use a trochanter roll extending from the crest of the ilium to the midthigh when the patient is lying on his back. A trochanter roll serves as a mechanical wedge under the projection of the greater trochanter.

2. Use a footboard when the patient is in the dorsal position.

3. To make a trochanter roll (Fig. 1-1):

   a. Take both ends of the towel (A) and bring them to the center. The towel is now folded in half with the edges at the center.

   b. Turn the towel over so that the ends (A) are facing downward.

   c. Turn the patient on his side with his upper leg flexed.

   d. Place one side (B) of the towel in the midline of the buttock. The towel should extend from the crest of the ilium to the midthigh.

   e. Then place the patient in a dorsal position with his leg extended.

   f. Grasp the remaining side (B) of the towel and roll inward in an underneath fashion until the entire roll is well under the patient's buttocks. The roll should be taut and smooth.

   g. For the larger patient, a drawsheet or a bath blanket may be used.

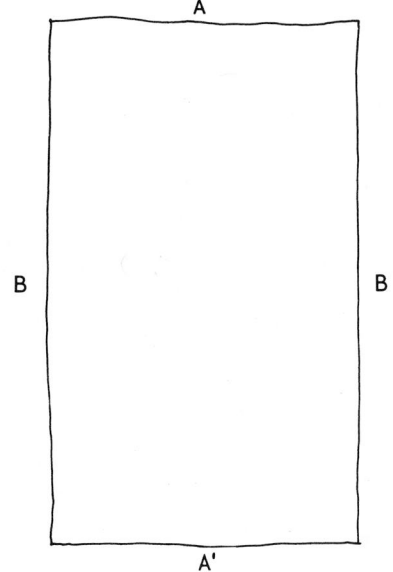

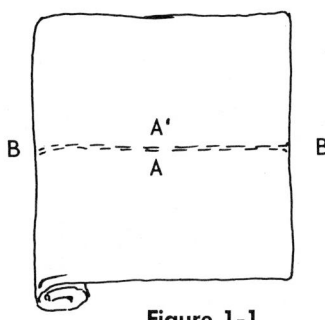

Figure 1-1

Preventing Footdrop

Footdrop (plantar flexion) is a deformity caused by contraction of both the gastrocnemius and the soleus muscles.

Causes

1. Prolonged bedrest and lack of exercise
2. Incorrect positioning in bed
3. Weight of bedding forcing the toes into plantar flexion

Clinical Problem

If footdrop continues without correction, the patient will walk on his toes without the heel of his foot touching the ground.

Nursing Management

1. Use a footboard to keep feet at right angles to the legs when the patient is lying on his back.
   a. Position the feet with the entire plantar surface firmly against the footboard.
   b. Maintain the legs in a neutral position. Use a trochanter roll.
2. Encourage the patient to flex and extend (curl and stretch) his feet and toes frequently.
3. Have the patient rotate ankles clockwise and counter-clockwise several times each hour.

Preventing and Treating Decubitus Ulcers

Decubitus ulcers (bedsores) are localized areas of necrosis of skin and subcutaneous tissues produced by pressure.

Altered Physiology

Pressure → tissue anoxia and ischemia → necrosis of tissue cells → sloughing and ulceration → infection → sepsis → involvement of underlying body structure → rapidly irreversible condition.

Causes

A. *Pressure*—exerted on skin and subcutaneous tissues by bony prominences and the object on which the body part rests (mattress, cast, etc.).

B. *Contributing Factors*
1. Poor nutrition—negative nitrogen, phosphorus, sulfur and calcium balance will produce wasting of tissue, osteoporosis and loss of weight.
   a. Anemia—may determine whether cellular hypoxia and necrosis will occur.
   b. Hypoproteinemia
   c. Vitamin deficiencies
2. Motor paralysis with associated muscular atrophy—causes reduction of padding between overlying skin and underlying bone.
3. Sensory loss—produces absence of awareness of pain and pressure.
4. Edema—interferes with supply of nutrients to the cell.
5. Friction and moisture.
6. Shearing force (when bed is raised over 30 degrees).

Sites

A. Weight-bearing bony prominences covered only by skin and small amounts of subcutaneous fat—75% of all decubiti located here
1. Sacrum
2. Greater trochanter
3. Ischial tuberosities—especially in patients who sit for prolonged periods.

B. Other bony promontories—knees, malleoli, heels and elbows.

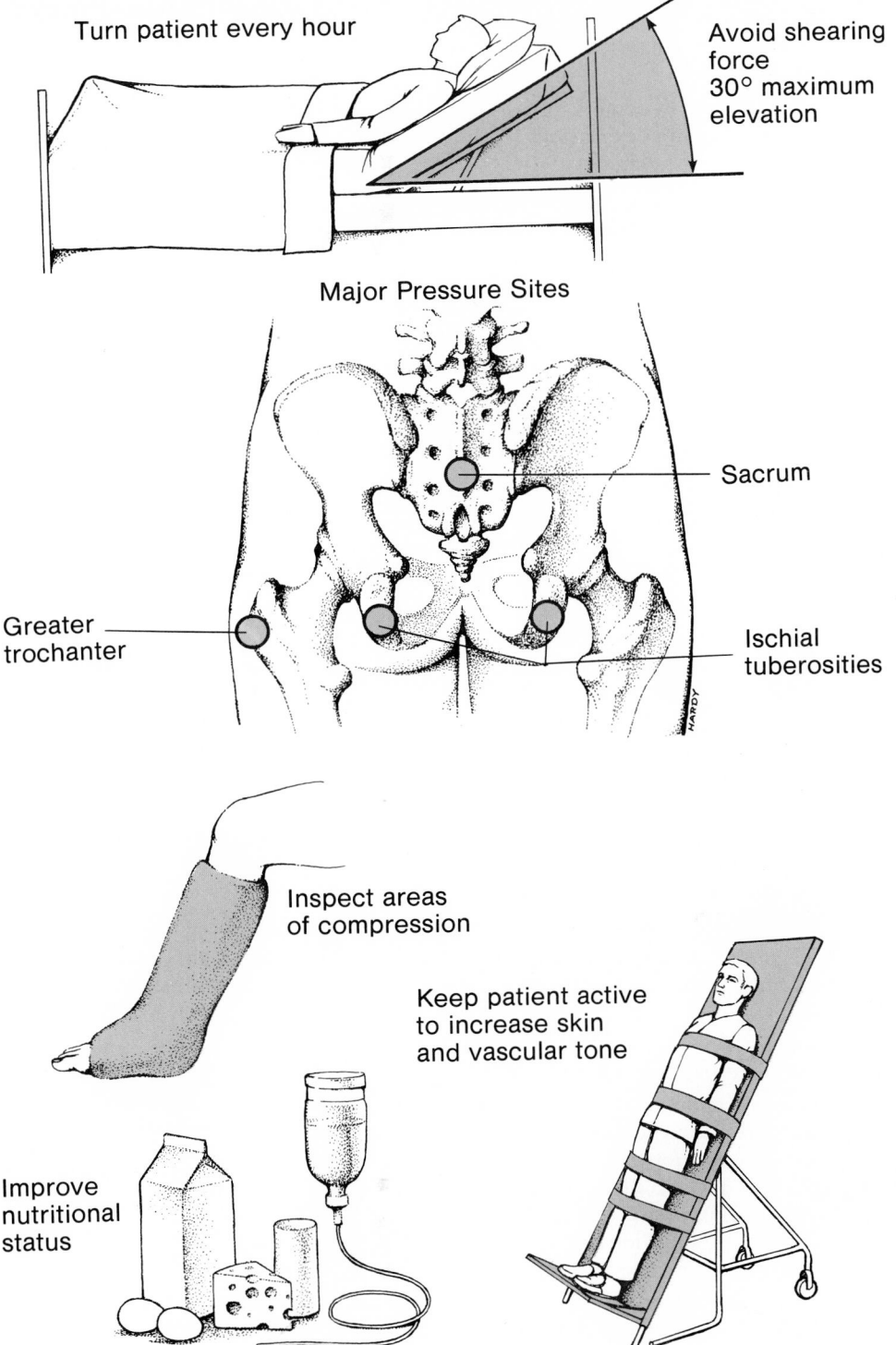

Turn patient every hour

Avoid shearing force 30° maximum elevation

Major Pressure Sites

Sacrum

Greater trochanter

Ischial tuberosities

Inspect areas of compression

Keep patient active to increase skin and vascular tone

Improve nutritional status

Figure 1-2. Prevention of decubitus ulcers.

Preventive Measures

Objectives: to relieve or remove pressure.
to stimulate circulation.
to keep the skin dry.

1. Relieve pressure by encouraging the patient to keep active.
   a. Turn the patient hourly or at 2-hour intervals.
   b. Position patient with pillows, pads, etc. to relieve pressure.
   c. Avoid elevating head of bed more than 30 degrees.
   d. Avoid the use of rubber rings or doughnuts—they merely increase pressure around bony prominences.
   e. Keep foundation sheet dry and tightly stretched to prevent wrinkles.
2. Maintain meticulous skin hygiene.
   a. Wash skin with mild soap, rinse and *blot* dry with soft towel.
   b. Lubricate skin with emollient lotion—keeps skin soft and pliable.
3. Employ active and passive exercises—increases muscular, skin and vascular tone.
4. Ambulate or use tilt table whenever possible—the level of mobility is an important criterion for prognosis and treatment.
5. Use alternating pressure mattress or alternating pressure chair—changes pressure against skin thereby improving circulation.
6. Employ sheepskin padding—softness and resilience of padding results in even distribution of pressure, freedom from wrinkles and friction and dissipation and absorption of moisture.
7. Inspect the skin frequently for signs of pressure.
   a. Teach the patient to use a mirror and inspect posterior areas if he is paraplegic or has another neuromuscular disorder.
   b. Massage and stroke lightly around bony prominences—promotes venous return, reduces edema and increases vascular tone.
8. Use antiseptic plastic spray dressing—protects susceptible areas with an antiseptic dry barrier.
9. Inspect, adjust and pad casts, braces, splints and compression bandages.
10. Use fluid-supported mattresses (waterbeds) and fluid-supported seats—eliminates all pressure points; as the body sinks into the fluid, additional surface area becomes available for weightbearing thereby further decreasing body weight per unit area.
11. Relieve pressure on those patients sitting in wheelchairs for prolonged periods—use foam-padded seat boards that are cut out posteriorly over ischial areas.
12. Improve nutritional status and maintain a positive nitrogen balance—decubitus ulcers develop more quickly and are more resistant to treatment in patients suffering from nutritional disorders.
    a. High protein diet
    b. Vitamins and protein supplements
    c. Iron preparations and transfusions of whole blood—hemoglobin level a critical criterion for the development of decubiti.
13. Carry out frequent hemoglobin, hematocrit and blood sugar determinations.
    a. Keep hemoglobin level above 12 gm.
    b. An elevated blood sugar level is a poor prognostic sign.

Treatment

Objectives: to continue with preventive measures on a more vigorous level.
to encourage restoration of circulation and cellular function.
to prevent necrosis of deeper structures.

1. Continue preventive measures (see p. 22) on a more vigorous level.
2. Employ daily mechanical cleansing of ulcer—clears up sepsis and stimulates regeneration of epithelium.
3. Débride ulcer.
4. Utilize physical modalities of treatment.
    a. Expose ulcer to air and sunlight.
    b. Employ light stroking around lesion—promotes venous return and reduces edema.
    c. Use ultraviolet irradiation—prevents growth of contaminating organisms.
        (1) Clean discharges from surface of ulcer.
        (2) Cover normal skin surrounding ulcer during irradiation.
    d. Use oxygen under pressure applied directly on ulcer (hyperbaric oxygen therapy) —directs more oxygen to tissues, hastens metabolic processes and reduces healing time.
5. Utilize topical applications as directed.
    a. Antibiotics
    b. Tincture of benzoin
    c. Antiseptic plastic sprays
    d. Aerosol spray containing a corticosteroid and an antibiotic—prednisolone with neomycin (Meti-Derm)
    e. Absorbable gelatin sponges—placed at base of ulcer
6. Prepare patient for surgical intervention—radical excision of skin and underlying bone and full-thickness skin-graft closure.

SUPPORTING THE PATIENT IN DAILY SELF-CARE

Activities of Daily Living

Activities of daily living are those self-care activities which must be accomplished each day in order for the patient to care for his own needs and participate in modern society. They include:

1. Getting in and out of bed (transfers)
2. Personal hygiene
3. Dressing
4. Eating
5. Using a wheelchair (if necessary)
6. Ambulating (when possible)
7. Performing manual tasks

Patient Objective

To care for himself in his daily routine without depending on others.

Role of Nurse

To teach and support and supervise patient while he does these activities.

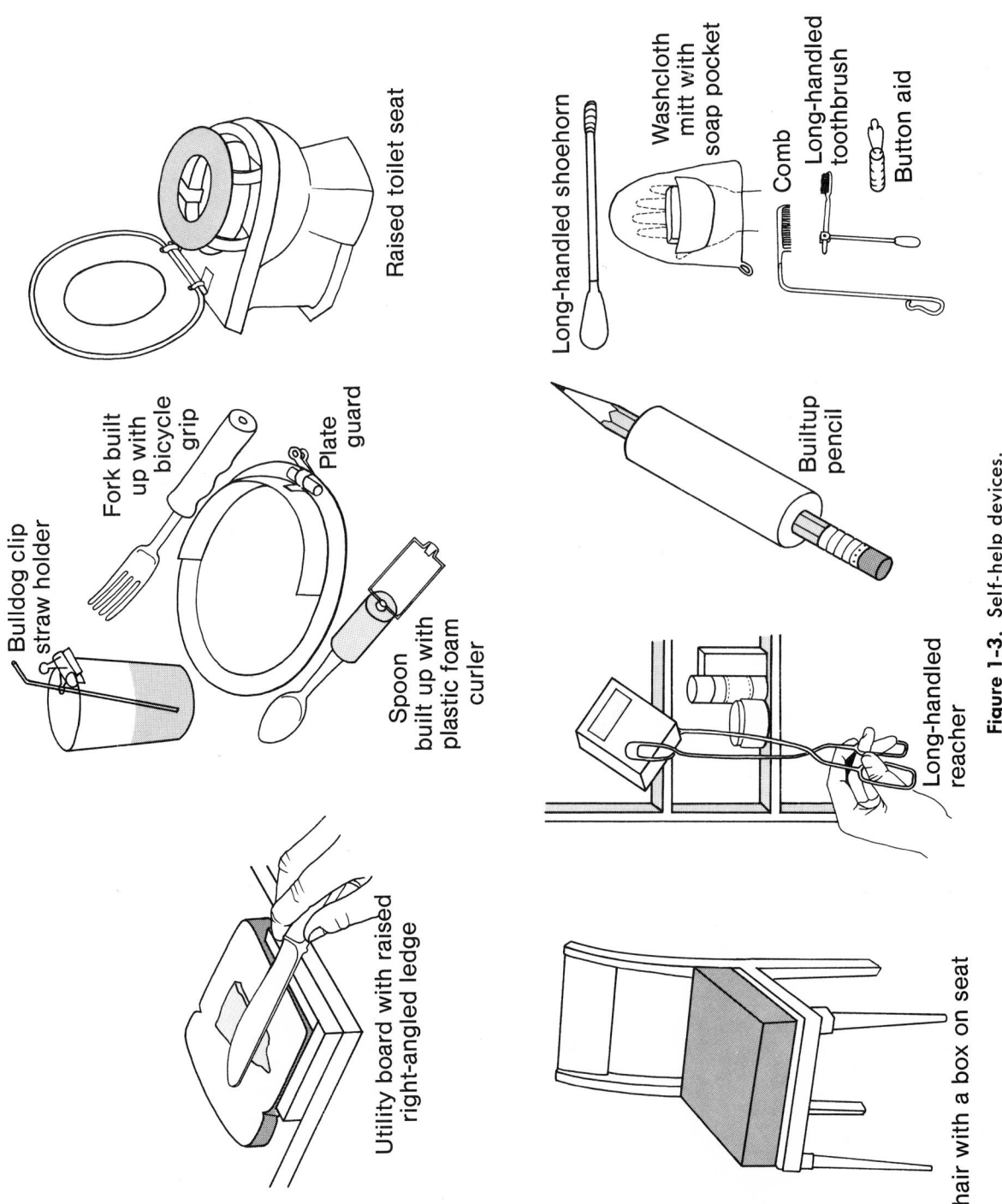

Raised toilet seat

Long-handled shoehorn

Washcloth mitt with soap pocket

Comb

Long-handled toothbrush

Button aid

Fork built up with bicycle grip

Plate guard

Bulldog clip straw holder

Spoon built up with plastic foam curler

Builtup pencil

Long-handled reacher

Utility board with raised right-angled ledge

Chair with a box on seat

Figure 1-3. Self-help devices.

Patient Teaching

1. Study each component motion of the desired activity.
2. Ascertain what methods can be used to accomplish the task. (Example: There are several ways of putting on a given garment.)
3. Determine what the patient can do by watching him perform.
4. Encourage the patient to exercise the muscles necessary to perform the motions involved in the activity.
5. Select activities that encourage gross functional movements of the upper and lower extremities (e.g., bathing, holding larger objects).
6. Gradually include activities that use finer motions, e.g., buttoning clothes, eating with a spoon.
7. Increase the period of activity as rapidly as the patient can tolerate.
8. Have the patient perform and practice the activity in a real-life situation.
9. Encourage the patient to do every activity up to his maximal capabilities within the framework of his disability.
10. Support the patient by giving justifiable praise for effort put forth and for acts accomplished.

The Activities of Daily Living (ADL) Sheet

This is an information sheet for those who are caring for the patient. It is a guide to the assessment of the functions of the patient. (See p. 26.)

Purposes: to inform each member of the rehabilitation team what activities the patient can do.
to serve as an index of progress.

Nurse's Responsibility in Using ADL Sheet
1. Review the ADL sheet each morning to know what the patient is capable of doing and what activities he is learning.
2. Avoid doing for the patient what he can do for himself.

Self-help Devices

Self-help devices are adaptive equipment that assist a patient to do his daily activities (Fig. 1-3). They may be devised and made by the patient, nurse or family or purchased ready-made. Publications are available offering extensive information on self-help devices.*

ASSISTING THE PATIENT WITH AMBULATION

Transfer Activities

A *transfer* is the movement of the patient from one piece of furniture or equipment to another (from bed to chair, bed to commode, bed to wheelchair).

Weight-bearing Transfers—carried out by patients who have at least one stable lower extremity (hemiplegics, unilateral lower extremity amputees, patients with hip fractures).

Nonweight-bearing Transfers—done by double lower-extremity amputees, or paraplegics who are not wearing braces (Fig. 1-4).

---

* See Bibliography.

ACTIVITIES OF DAILY LIVING (ADL) SHEET

	Total Assistance	Partial Assistance	Independent

Prescribed Activities:

Range of Motion

Positioning

Use of Tilt Table

  Degree

  How long

Exercises

  Breathing

  Balancing

  Crutch Training

  Parallel Bars

  Steps

Other Information:

Appliances or Prosthesis

Ambulation

Time Permitted Up

Bladder/Bowel Program

Bathing/Grooming Schedule

Speech Problems

Activities Being Learned

Name:

Diagnosis:

Doctor:

Functional Capabilities:

1. Flexes neck

2. Raises hand to head

3. Raises hand behind head

4. Reaches out at shoulder level to side (laterally)

5. Pronates/supinates forearm

6. Grasps objects

7. Begins grasp ability

8. Closes fist

9. Opens fist

10. Flexes and extends knee joint

11. Touches floor while seated

12. Crosses leg over opposite knee while sitting (with or without help of hands)

13. Transfers from sitting to standing (with or without holding to support)

14. Walks

Preparation for Transfers

Objective: to develop ability to raise and move the body in different positions.

A. *Exercises to Strengthen Arm and Shoulder Extensors*

1. Have the patient sit upright in bed.
2. Place a book under each hand.
3. Instruct the patient to push down on the book thus raising his body weight.

B. *Technique for Moving the Patient to the Edge of the Bed*

1. Move the patient's head and shoulders toward the edge of the bed.
2. Move his feet and legs to the edge of bed. (The patient is now in a crescent position giving good range of motion to the lateral trunk muscles.)
3. Place both of your arms well under the patient's hips. (Before the next maneuver tighten or set the muscles of your back.)
4. Straighten your back while moving the patient toward you.

C. *Technique for Sitting the Patient on the Edge of the Bed*

1. Place one hand under the patient's shoulders.
2. Instruct the patient to push his elbow into the bed while you lift his shoulders with one arm and swing his legs over the edge of the bed with the other. (Gravity pulls the legs downward, which aids in raising the patient's trunk.)

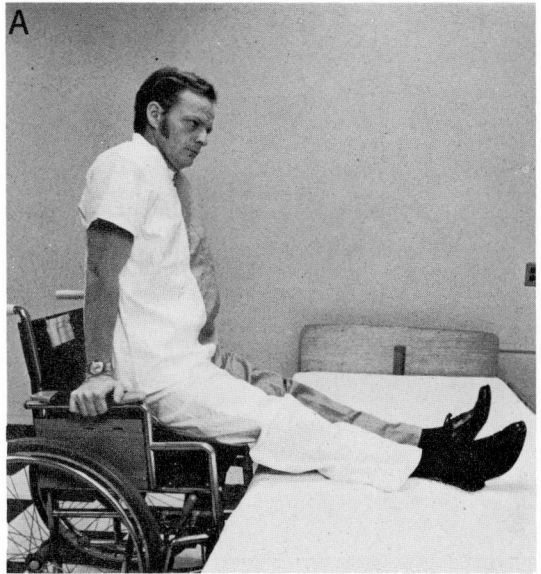 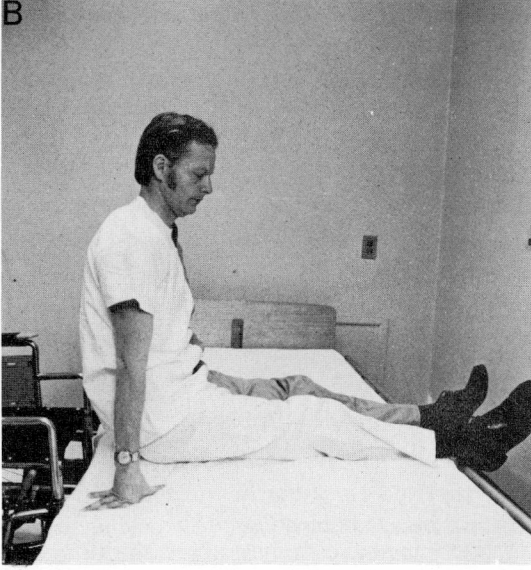

Figure 1-4. Vertical transfer of a paraplegic patient. A. Place the wheelchair facing the bed as close to the bed as possible. Lock brakes. Instruct the patient to push up on his hands and arms and slide his body forward onto the bed. B. This is a nonweight-bearing transfer in which the patient learns to transfer on the same level. Later this type of nonweight-bearing transfer can be done to a higher and lower level by the push-up method.

D. *Technique for Assisting the Patient to Stand*
   1. Place the patient's feet well under him.
   2. Face the patient and firmly grasp each side of his rib cage.
   3. Push your knee against one of the patient's knees.
   4. Rock the patient forward as he comes to a standing position. (Your knee is pushed against the patient's knee as he comes to the standing position.)
   5. Ensure that the patient's knees are "locked" (full extension) while he is standing. (Locking the patient's knees is a safety measure for those patients who are weak or have been in bed for a period of time.)
   6. Pivot the patient, positioning him to sit in the chair.

E. *Technique for Transfer by Sliding Board*
   1. A *sliding board* (or transfer board) is a polished light-weight board that is used to bridge the gap between the bed and the chair (or chair to tub, etc.).
   2. When the muscles that the patient uses to lift himself off the bed are not strong enough to overcome the resistance of body weight, use the following maneuver:
      a. Place one side of the sliding board under the patient's buttocks and the other side on the surface of the chair, bed, toilet, etc., to which the transfer is being made.
      b. Instruct the patient to push up with his hands to shift his buttocks and slide across the board to the other surface.

Cane Use

Purposes

A cane is used for balance and support:
   1. To assist the patient to walk with greater stability and speed and less fatigue.
   2. To compensate for deficiencies of function normally performed by the neuromuscular skeletal system.
   3. To relieve pressure on weight-bearing joints.
   4. To provide forces to push or pull the body forward or to restrain the forward motion of the patient while walking.

Underlying Principles

   1. An adjustable aluminum cane, fitted with a 1½-inch rubber suction tip to provide traction while walking, gives optimum stability to the patient.
   2. The cane handle should be approximately level with the greater trochanter (Fig. 1-5).
   3. The patient's elbow should be flexed 25 to 30 degrees when the cane is the proper length.

Technique for Walking with a Cane

Instruct the patient as follows:
   1. Hold the cane in the hand opposite to the affected extremity, i.e., the cane should be used on the good side.
   2. Move the cane at the same time the affected leg is moved (Fig. 1-5).
   3. Keep the cane fairly close to the body to prevent leaning.
   4. When climbing steps
      a. Step up on *unaffected* extremity.
      b. Then place cane and affected extremity on the step.
      c. Reverse this procedure for descending steps.

Crutch Walking

Crutches are artificial supports which assist patients needing aid in walking because of disease, injury or a birth defect.

Preparation for Crutch Walking

Objective: to develop power in the shoulder girdle and upper extremities which bear the patient's weight in crutch walking.

A. *To Strengthen the Muscles Needed for Ambulation*

    Instruct the patient as follows:

    1. For *quadriceps setting*

        a. Contract the quadriceps muscle while attempting to push the popliteal area against the mattress and raise the heel.

        b. Maintain the muscle contracture for the count of 5.

        c. Relax for the count of 5.

        d. Repeat this exercise 10 to 15 times hourly.

    2. For *gluteal setting*

        a. Contract or pinch the buttocks together for the count of 5.

        b. Relax for the count of 5. Repeat.

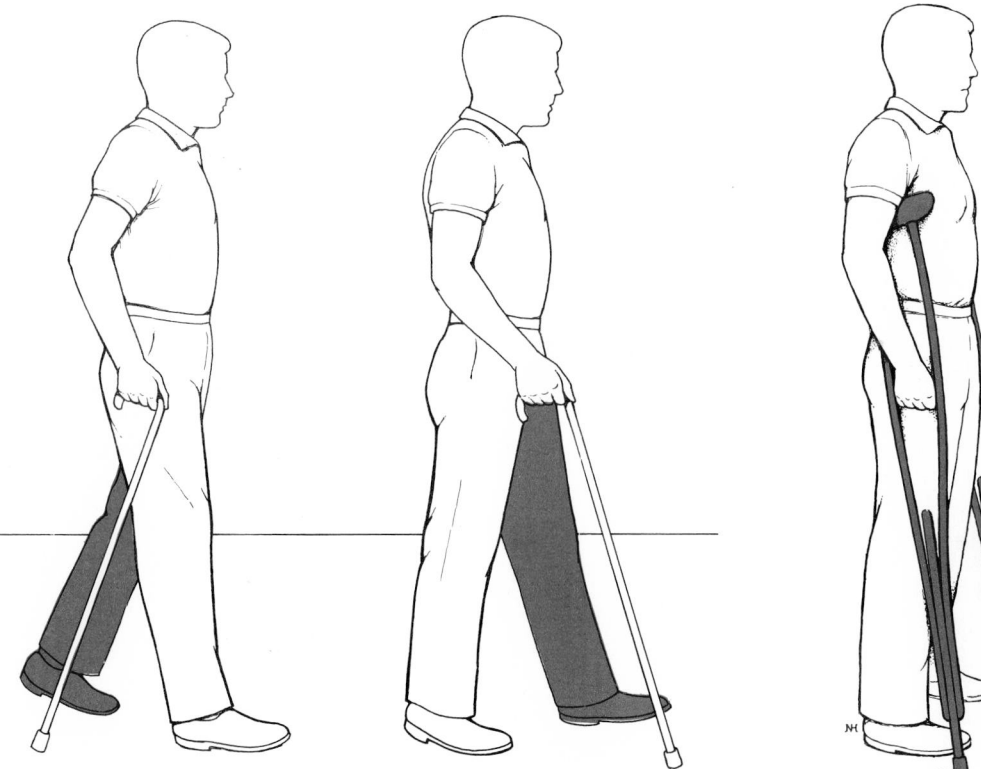
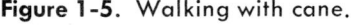
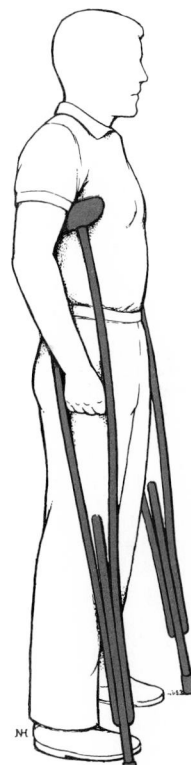

Figure 1-5. Walking with cane.   **Figure 1-6.** Crutch stance.

B. *To Strengthen the Muscles of the Upper Extremities*

Instruct the patient as follows:

1. Flex and extend arms slowly while holding traction weights; gradually increase poundage of weight.
2. Do push-ups while lying in a prone position.
3. Squeeze rubber ball—increases grasping strength.
4. Raise head and shoulders from bed; stretch hands forward as far as possible.
5. Sit up on bed or chair.
   a. Raise body from chair by pushing the hands against the chair seat (or mattress).
   b. Raise body out of seat. Hold. Relax.

C. *To Measure for Crutches*

1. When the patient is lying down
   a. Measure from the anterior fold of the axilla to the sole of the foot. Then add 5 cm. (2 inches).
   b. Or subtract 40 cm. (16 inches) from the patient's height.
2. When the patient is standing erect (most desirable)
   Measure 3.75 cm. (1½ inches) from the axillary fold to a position on the floor 10 cm. (4 inches) in front of the patient and 15 cm. (6 inches) to the side of his toes.

D. *Crutch Stance*

1. Have the patient wear well-fitting shoes with firm soles.
2. The crutches should be fitted with large rubber suction tips.
3. Have the patient stand by a chair on the unaffected leg to achieve balance.
4. Position the patient against a wall with his head in a neutral position.
5. Place crutches 10 cm. (4 inches) in front of patient and 10 cm. (4 inches) to the side (Fig. 1-6).
   a. The hand piece should be adjusted to allow a 30-degree elbow flexion.
   b. There should be a 2-finger-width insertion between the axillary fold and the arm piece.
   c. A foam-rubber pad on the underarm piece will relieve pressure on the upper arm and thoracic cage.

Teaching the Crutch Gait

1. The selection of the crutch gait depends on the type and severity of the disability and the patient's physical condition, arm and trunk strength and/or body balance.
2. Teach the patient at least 2 gaits; a faster gait to be used for making speed, and a slower one to be used in crowded places.
3. Instruct the patient to change from one gait to another—relieves fatigue as a different combination of muscles is used.
4. Make sure the patient is bearing weight on his hands—If the weight is borne on the axilla, the pressure of the crutch can damage the brachial plexus and produce crutch paralysis.

Crutch Gaits

4-Point Gait (4-point alternate crutch gait)

Crutch-foot sequence (Fig. 1-7)
1. Right crutch
2. Left foot
3. Left crutch
4. Right foot

1. This is a slow but stable gait; the patient's weight is constantly being shifted.
2. 4-point gait can be used only by patients who can move each leg separately and bear a considerable amount of weight on each of them.

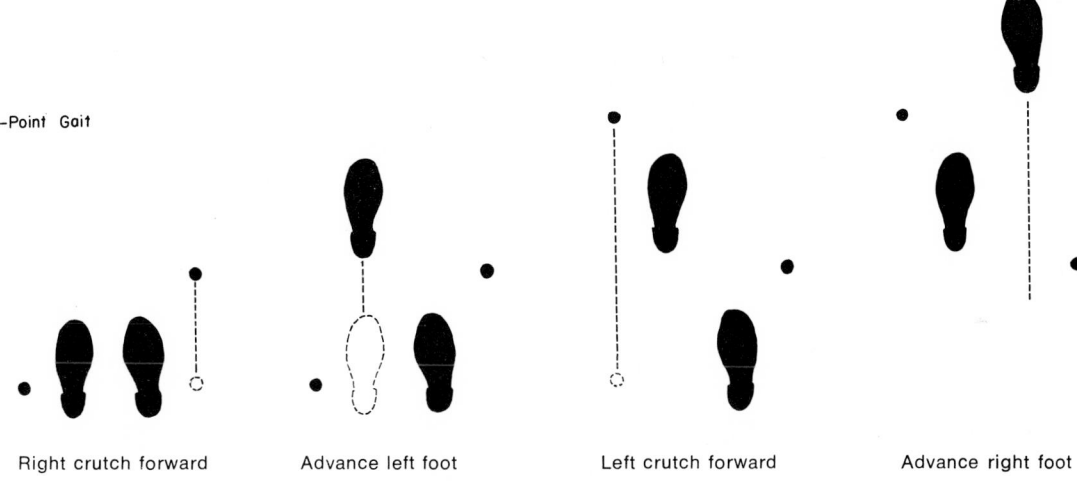

Four—Point Gait

| Right crutch forward | Advance left foot | Left crutch forward | Advance right foot |

Figure 1-7. Four-point gait.

2-Point Gait (2-point alternate crutch gait)

Crutch-foot sequence (Fig. 1-8)
1. Right crutch and left foot
2. Left crutch and right foot simultaneously

1. This is a faster gait but requires more balance since there are only 2 points of contact with the floor.

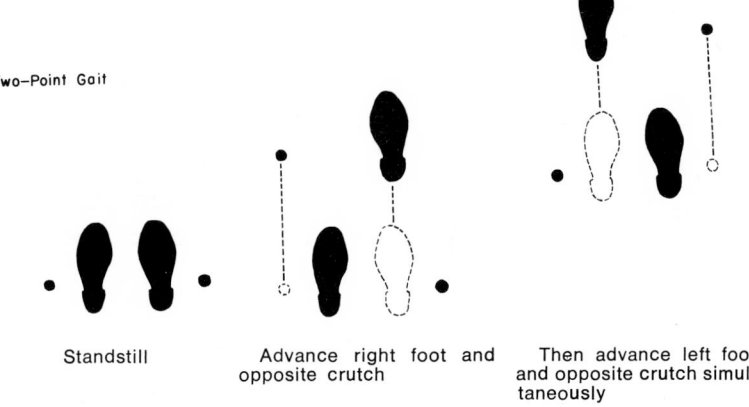

Two—Point Gait

| Standstill | Advance right foot and opposite crutch | Then advance left foot and opposite crutch simultaneously |

Figure 1-8. Two-point gait.

3-Point Gait

Crutch-foot sequence (Fig. 1-9)
1. Both crutches and the weaker lower extremity simultaneously
2. Then the stronger lower extremity

1. This is a fairly rapid gait but requires more strength and balance.
2. The patient's arms must be strong enough to support his entire body weight.

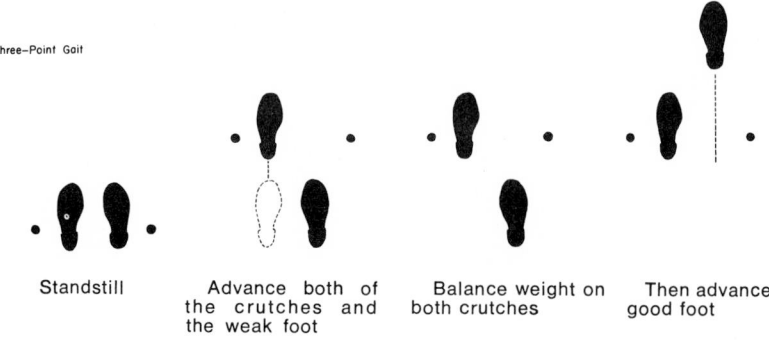

Three–Point Gait

Standstill   Advance both of the crutches and the weak foot   Balance weight on both crutches   Then advance good foot

Figure 1-9. Three-point gait.

Tripod Crutch Gaits

TRIPOD ALTERNATE CRUTCH GAIT
Crutch-foot sequence
1. Right crutch
2. Left crutch
3. Drag body and legs forward.

TRIPOD SIMULTANEOUS CRUTCH GAIT
Crutch-foot sequence (Fig. 1-10)
1. Both crutches
2. Drag body and legs forward.

1. The patient constantly maintains a tripod position.
2. At the start, both crutches are held fairly widespread out front while both feet are held together in the back.
3. These gaits are slow and labored.

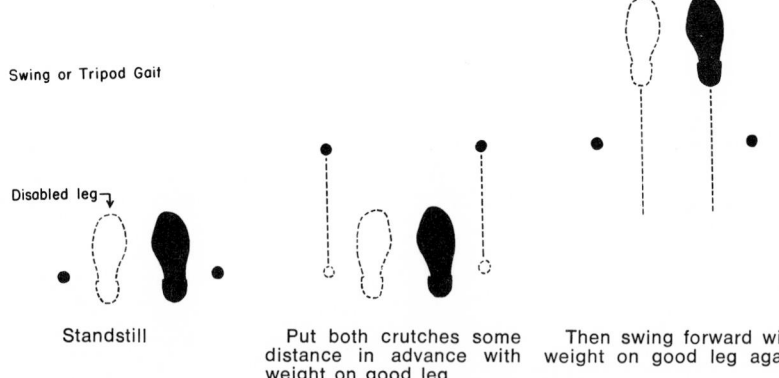

Swing or Tripod Gait

Disabled leg

Standstill   Put both crutches some distance in advance with weight on good leg   Then swing forward with weight on good leg again

Figure 1-10. Tripod simultaneous crutch gait.

Swinging Crutch Gaits

SWINGING-TO GAIT

Crutch-foot sequence
1. Both crutches forward
2. Then lift and swing body *to* crutches.
3. Place crutches in front of body and continue.

SWINGING-THROUGH GAIT

Crutch-foot sequence
1. Both crutches forward
2. Lift and swing body *beyond* crutches.
3. Place crutches in front of body and continue.

1. In the swinging crutch gaits, both legs are lifted off the ground simultaneously and swung forward while the patient pushes up on the crutches.

GUIDELINES: *Using a Tilt Table*

A *tilt table* is a board or table that can be tilted gradually from a horizontal to a vertical (upright) position.

Purposes

1. To help patient gradually adjust to varying degrees of the upright posture and ultimately to complete upright position.
2. To help patient start weight-bearing activities.
3. To increase standing tolerance.
4. To prevent disuse syndrome.
5. To prevent demineralization of bone and development of urinary tract stones.
6. To condition the vascular system.

Clinical Usefulness

Orthostatic hypotension
Brain damage

Spinal cord injuries
Plastic repair of decubitus ulcers

Equipment

Tilt table with footboard
Straps
Sphygmomanometer and stethoscope
Abdominal binder, elastic stockings or venous pressure gradient leotard*

Procedure

Nursing Action	Rationale / Amplification
Preparatory Phase	
1. Apply snug-fitting abdominal binder, elastic compression bandages from toes to groin on both legs or a leotard (waist-high venous pressure gradient support*).	1. Compression on the abdomen prevents pooling of blood in splanchnic area and subsequent postural hypotension and inadequate cerebral circulation. Compression to the legs restricts the vascular walls of the blood vessels and prevents pooling of blood in the legs with development of edema.

* Jobst Venous Pressure Gradient Support.

Nursing Action	Rationale/Amplification

Performance Phase

1. Transfer the patient to tilt table by 3-man carry method. Place the patient in a dorsal position with his feet placed firmly against the footboard. Position the body in correct alignment (p. 6).
2. Fasten the straps across the pelvis, knees, chest and abdomen.
3. Apply the blood pressure cuff to the arm and take and record the blood pressure while the patient is lying flat.
4. Tilt the table 15–30 degrees. Take the blood pressure every 3–5 minutes.
5. Evaluate patient constantly and assess for a drop in blood pressure. If the patient feels dizzy and the blood pressure drops, return him to a flat position.
6. Observe for pallor, diaphoresis, tachycardia and nausea.
7. Increase the standing tolerance by 5- to 10-degree increments.

8. Continue the procedure until the patient tolerates the desired tilt; usually between 45–80 degrees.
9. Avoid allowing the patient to stand for prolonged periods.
10. Do not leave patient unattended.

3. This serves as a base-line recording for future comparisons.

4. Tilting the patient from a supine to upright position causes a decrease in systolic pressure.

6. These are signs and symptoms of insufficient cerebral circulation.
7. The angle of tilt will be determined by the patient's tolerance and the desired amount of weight-bearing.

9. Prolonged standing may cause pressure ulceration on plantar surfaces of feet.

Follow-up Phase

1. Place the patient back in bed at the end of the prescribed period or when his condition indicates.
2. Record degree of tilt, amount of time on tilt table and reaction of patient.

Prosthetic and Orthotic Devices

A *prosthesis* is an artificial replacement for a missing portion of the body.

An *orthosis* is a device commonly known as a brace.

A *brace* is a support that protects weakened muscles, prevents and corrects anatomic deformities, aids in controlling involuntary muscle movements and immobilizes and protects a diseased or injured joint (Fig. 1-11).

Preprosthetic Nursing Management

1. Help the patient to develop an attitude of realistic hopefulness.
2. *Prevent deformities*—to limit the time between the healing of tissues and the fitting of a prosthesis.
3. Bandage an extremity stump correctly so that proper shrinkage and shaping of the stump occurs.

Figure 1-11. VAPC Dropfoot brace. This is a new type of brace that is particularly useful for a patient following a stroke. The brace provides a positioning force to hold the foot in a neutral or slightly dorsiflexed position during the swing phase of walking and provides mild resistance to inversion or eversion of the ankle joint. The brace has a clip which fits on the counter of the shoe allowing it to be clipped on any stiff-counter shoe without special attachment. (Courtesy Veterans Administration Prosthetics Center.)

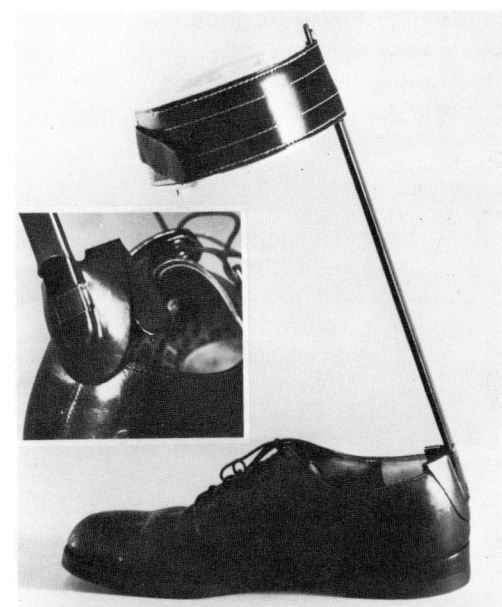

The Care of Braces

The patient himself should care for his brace when he is able.

1. All locks should be opened once a week and cleaned with fine wire or a hairpin; place a drop of machine oil in each joint.
2. Repair leather when necessary. Little can be done about perspiration stains; however, washing the leather in lukewarm water with saddle soap helps to preserve leather.
3. When the brace is not being used place it on a table or the floor in good alignment; hanging may distort its position.
4. Twisting of the brace may occur with use; check alignment frequently. The joints should coincide with the body joints.
5. Before putting a brace on, check carefully for worn areas, missing or loose screws and the condition of straps and buckles.
6. Pressure areas may occur if metal or plastic rubs the skin. After removing a brace, check the skin immediately for reddened areas.
7. Have the brace checked periodically by the prosthetist.

OVERCOMING ELIMINATION PROBLEMS
Bladder Training

Objectives

1. To keep the patient dry and free from odor.
2. To prevent urinary tract infections and preserve renal function.
3. To help the patient maintain social acceptance.

Neurogenic Bladder

See pages 764–766 for discussion of neurogenic bladder.

Bladder Training Regimen

1. Set up a schedule of definite times for patient to try to empty his bladder using a toilet or commode.
2. Give patient a measured amount of fluid to drink.
3. Have patient wait 30 minutes and then ask him to attempt to void; *regularity is the key to success.*
   a. Position patient with thighs flexed and feet and back supported.
   b. Instruct him to press or massage over bladder area or increase intra-abdominal pressure by leaning forward—helps to initiate evacuation of bladder.
   c. Have patient try to void every 2 hours; interval may be lengthened as control is gained.
      (1) Set alarm clock at 2-hour intervals during the daytime.
      (2) Set alarm clock 2 times during night.
      (3) Curtail or limit fluids after 5 p.m.
4. Have patient keep a voiding calendar—a continuous record of time and amount of fluid ingested and time and amount of each voiding.
5. Encourage the patient to hold his urine until specified voiding time if possible.
6. Assess for signs of urinary retention; test (catheterize) for residual urine as directed.
7. Encourage patient to continue self-care and exercise programs; encourage patient to wear his own clothing.

Management of Incontinent Patient

(Not due to neurogenic bladder impairment)

1. Assist patient to bathroom at a regularly scheduled time—delay in responding to call for bedpan or urinal or for assistance to toilet is a common cause of incontinence.
2. Encourage patient to do self-care activities—boredom and frustration lead to incontinence.
3. Give adequate amounts of fluids.
4. Avoid overt encouragement of incontinence such as the routine use of pads, diapers, and other depersonalizing procedures.
5. Create an environment which keeps sensory monotony to a minimum.
   a. Have wall clock and calendar to orient patient to time and place.
   b. Hang wall posters, pictures, etc. for visual stimulus.
   c. Use telephone, radio and television selectively.
   d. Encourage patient to make decisions (menu selection, keeping intake/output chart)—improves self-esteem.
   e. Have patient do meaningful tasks (sort mail, straighten his bureau drawers, etc.).
   f. Extend patient's environment beyond the confines of his room.
   g. Increase patient's social contacts.
6. Encourage patient to wear his own clothes—enhances his self-esteem and dignity and is a strong deterrent to regressive behavior.

GUIDELINES: *Using a Condom Urine Collecting Appliance*

A *condom urine collecting appliance* (Fig. 1-12) is an external device made of latex worn by incontinent male patients who do not have urinary tract infections, obstruction or ureteral reflux. It may be used for short-term or long-term therapy.

Figure 1-12. Condom urine-collecting appliance. The elastic foam strap comfortably holds the catheter in place and prevents backflow. The drainage tubing is attached to the connector and then to a drainage bag or receptacle. (Courtesy Chesebrough-Pond's Inc.)

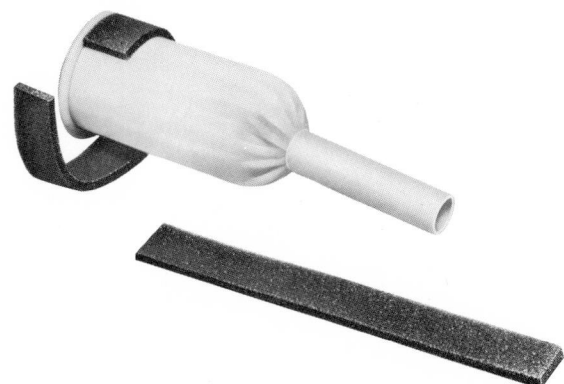

Advantages

1. It is an external device—no indwelling catheter is required.
2. It funnels urine away from the skin thereby avoiding pressure sores and ulcerations.

Equipment

Texas catheter and collecting device.*

Procedure

Nursing Action	*Rationale / Amplification*

Performance Phase

Instruct (or assist) the patient to do the following:

1. Cleanse the shaft of the penis with warm soap and water. Dry thoroughly.

    1. Cleansing is for hygienic purposes.

2. Roll the condom catheter over the penis to approximately 5 cm. (2 inches) behind the head of the penis if possible.

3. Leave about 1.75-cm. (½-inch) slack at the connecting end.

    3. This slack prevents rubbing or chafing with the connecting device.

4. Remove paper backing from foam adhesive strip.

5. Apply the adhesive strip around the penis on the outside of the catheter 2.5 cm. (1 inch) behind the head of the penis.

    If the patient requires additional security (child, elderly male, paraplegic or quadraplegic patient), surgical cement may be applied to the penis before the catheter is applied.

    5. The adhesive should be snug enough to prevent catheter slippage and retrograde urine flow but not so tight as to restrict circulation. A paraplegic or quadraplegic patient may have periodic involuntary erections. The foam adhesive expands and contracts with a minimum of pressure that compensates for the physiologic change during involuntary erection.

6. Connect the adapter to latex or plastic tubing of sufficient length to attach to a urine receptacle. Ambulatory patients may use a leg-drainage bag.

    6. The drainage tubing should be of adequate diameter to provide sufficient capillary action to keep condom empty.

7. Instruct the patient to remove the catheter daily for skin care and cleansing.

    7. The catheter may be used up to 2 days prior to disposal.

* Manufactured by Chesebrough-Pond's Inc., 485 Lexington Ave., New York 10017.

Bowel Training

Objectives

1. To develop regular bowel habits.
2. To prevent fecal incontinence, impaction, irregularity.

Bowel Training Program

1. Establish a *specific and definite time* for the bowel movement; *regularity is necessary to establish reflex assistance.*
   a. The exact time period depends on the patient's schedule.
   b. Attempts at evacuation should be done within 15 minutes of this same time daily.
   c. Establish bowel evacuation after a regularly scheduled meal—utilizes the stimulation of peristalsis and the gastrocolic reflex.
   d. Stimulate anorectal reflex if necessary.
      Insert a glycerine suppository into the rectum 30 minutes before the scheduled bowel time.
   e. Have patient use a normal posture for defecation—a toilet seat or commode approximates most nearly the physiologic position for defecation.
      (1) Instruct patient to bear down and contract the abdominal muscles.
      (2) Have patient lean forward to increase intra-abdominal pressure by compression against the thighs.
2. Ensure adequate roughage and fluid intake (2000–4000 ml.) daily.
   Give 120 ml. of prune or fig juice at the same time daily (i.e., 30 minutes before breakfast)—helps establish regularity.
3. Encourage patient to exercise—muscular activity is helpful in bowel training.

REFERRAL FOR FOLLOW-UP CARE

1. Plan for care at home as soon after hospital admission as possible.
2. Gather information about the home situation (from patient, social worker, community health nurse).
3. Estimate the patient's functional potential; make plans with this in mind.
4. Plan, with the patient, ways and methods to cope with problems that may arise.
5. Teach the family as much about the patient's condition as possible, so that they will not fear his return home.
   a. Encourage family to ask questions.
   b. Assess family's attitude toward patient, his disability and his return home.
6. Send referral form to local community health agency so nurse can evaluate the home environment.
   a. Review patient's ADL sheet with community health or visiting nurse—so community nurses will know exactly what activities patient can perform.
   b. Determine what modifications will be necessary in the home (for wheelchair, for self-care activities).
   c. Inquire how patient expects to be transported for clinic visits, special therapy, etc.
   d. Send referral to State Division of Vocational Rehabilitation if patient will require additional educational or job training.

7. Assist with transfer of patient to extended-care facility if he is unable to return to home situation.

Send ADL sheet with patient to help orient staff to activities that patient can perform independently.

BIBLIOGRAPHY

Books

Brunner, L., et al.: Textbook of Medical-Surgical Nursing, 2nd ed. Philadelphia, J. B. Lippincott, 1970, pp. 158–178.

Coles, C. H., and Bergstrom, D.: Basic Positioning Procedures. Minneapolis, Kenny Rehabilitation Institute, 1969.

Downer, A. H.: Physical Therapy Procedures. Springfield, Charles C Thomas, 1970.

Downey, J. A., and Darling, R. C.: Physiological Basis of Rehabilitation Medicine. Philadelphia, W. B. Saunders, 1971.

Jurkovich, S., and Flaherty, P.: Transfers for Patients with Acute and Chronic Conditions. Minneapolis, Kenny Rehabilitation Institute, 1970.

Kamenetz, H. L.: The Wheelchair Book. Springfield, Charles C Thomas, 1969.

Krusen, F. H. (ed.): Handbook of Physical Medicine and Rehabilitation. Philadelphia, W. B. Saunders, 1971.

Lowman, E. W., and Klinger, J.: Aids to Independent Living: Self Help for the Handicapped. New York, McGraw Hill, 1969.

McDaniel, J. W.: Physical Disability and Human Behavior. New York, Pergamon Press, 1969.

Rusk, H. A.: Rehabilitation Medicine. St. Louis, C. V. Mosby, 1971.

Safilios-Rothschild, C.: The Sociology and Social Psychology of Disability and Rehabilitation. New York, Random House, 1970.

Stryker, R. B.: Rehabilitative Aspects of Acute and Chronic Nursing Care. Philadelphia, W. B. Saunders, 1972.

Willard, H. S., and Spackman, C. S.: Occupational Therapy. Philadelphia, J. B. Lippincott, 1971.

Yates, J. A.: Moving and Lifting Patients: Principles and Techniques. Minneapolis, Kenny Rehabilitation Institute, 1970.

Articles

Abramson, A. S., and Kutner, B.: A bill of rights for the disabled. Archives Phys. Med. and Rehab., 53:99–100, March 1972.

Brower, P., and Hicks, D.: Maintaining muscle function in patients on bed rest. Amer. J. Nurs., 72:1250–1253, July 1972.

Carnevali, D., and Brueckner, S.: Immobilization—reassessment of a concept. Amer. J. Nurs., 70:1502–1507, July 1970.

Griffin, W., et al.: Group exercise for patients with limited motion. Amer. J. Nurs., 71:1742–1743, Sept. 1971.

Harvin, J. S., and Hargist, T. X.: The air-fluidized bed: a new concept in the treatment of decubitus ulcers. Nurs. Clin. N. Amer., 5:181–187, March 1970.

Lohman, E. W. (ed.): Symposium on rehabilitation. Med. Clin. N. Amer., 53:487–733, May 1969.

Martin, N., et al.: The nurse therapist in a rehabilitation setting. Amer. J. Nurs., 70:1674–1697, Aug. 1970.

O'Connor, J. R.: Traumatic quadriplegia—A comprehensive review. J. Rehab., 37:14–20, May-June 1971.

Welch, Sister R.: Tilt-table therapy in rehabilitation of the trauma patient with brain damage and spinal injury. Nurs. Clin. N. Amer., 5:621–630, Dec. 1970.

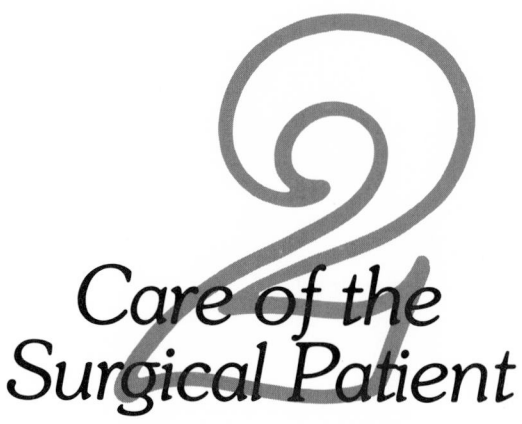

Care of the Surgical Patient

TYPES OF SURGERY

1. *Optional*
   Surgery is scheduled completely at the preference of the patient, e.g., cosmetic surgery.
2. *Elective*
   The approximate time for surgery is at the convenience of the patient; failure to have surgery is not catastrophic, e.g., superficial cyst.
3. *Required*
   The condition requires surgery within a few weeks, e.g., eye cataract.
4. *Urgent*
   Surgical problem requires attention within 24 to 48 hours, e.g., cancer.
5. *Emergency*
   Requires immediate surgical attention without delay, e.g., intestinal obstruction.

REGIONS AND INCISIONS OF THE ABDOMEN

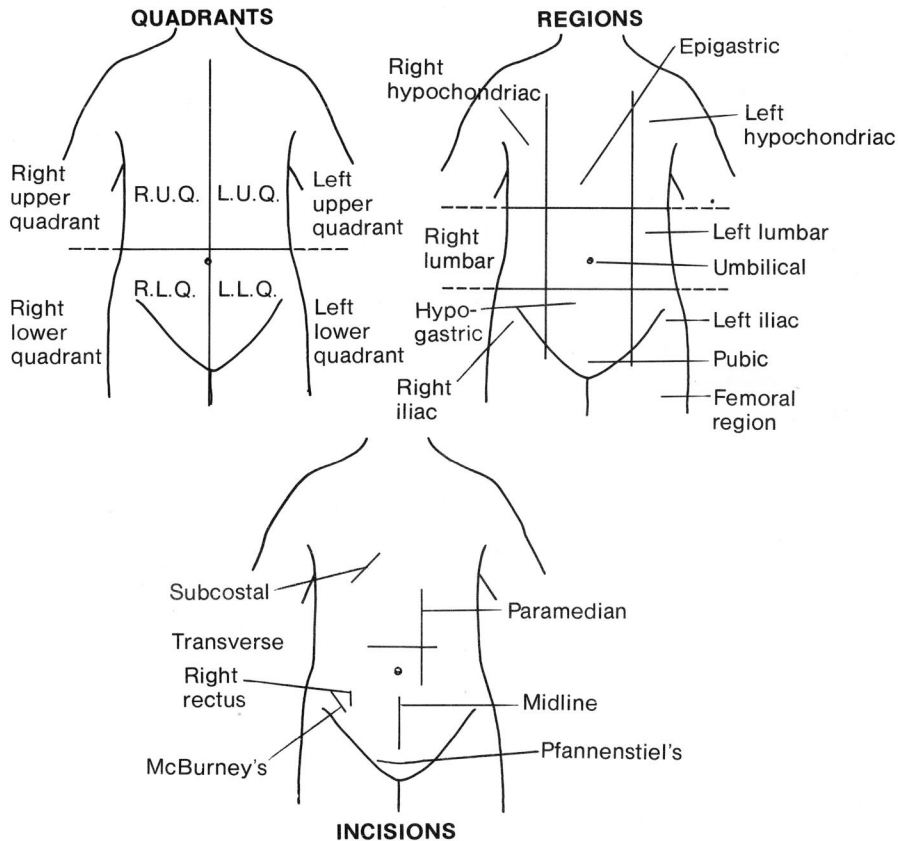

Figure 2-1. Regions and incisions of the abdomen.

INITIAL ASSESSMENT AND EARLY PHYSICAL PREPARATION OF THE SURGICAL PATIENT

General Physical Examination and Diagnostic Determinations

1. Observe the patient for skin lesions, rashes, decubitus ulcers and other abnormalities.
2. Engage the patient in conversation to determine his reaction and concerns about hospitalization and the forthcoming operation.
3. Prepare him for various diagnostic tests by telling him why and how they are done and how he may contribute to the success of the test.
4. Record his reactions to tests as well as the outcome of such tests.

Specific Conditions and Their Effect on Surgery

A. *Obesity*
   1. Danger
      a. Increases the difficulty in the technical aspects of performing surgery (e.g., sutures are difficult to tie because of fatty secretions); wound dehiscence is greater.
      b. Increases the likelihood of infection because of lessened resistance.
      c. Postoperatively, more difficult to turn and ventilate the patient when he is lying on his side. This leads to hypoventilation, pneumonia, and other pulmonary problems.
      d. Increases demands on the heart leading to cardiovascular embarrassment.
      e. Increases possibility of renal, biliary, hepatic and endocrine disorders.
   2. Therapeutic Approach
      Encourage weight reduction if time permits.

B. *Fluid, Electrolyte and Nutritional Status*
   1. Danger
      Dehydration and malnutrition have adverse effects in terms of a general anesthetic, the shock of surgery and postoperative recovery—can disturb fluid and electrolyte balance and lead to shock.
   2. Therapeutic Approach
      a. Administer fluids (parenteral) as prescribed.
      b. Keep a detailed input and output record.
      c. Provide high calorie diet to alleviate malnutrition; supplement with protein and vitamin C—helps repair tissue and serves as a deterrent to infection.
      d. Recommend repair of dental caries and proper mouth hygiene to prevent respiratory tract infection.
      e. Assist with administration (and surveillance) of blood transfusion, protein hydrolysates or blood plasma if there is a protein deficiency.

C. *Aging*
   1. Danger
      a. Recognize that reactions to injury are not as obvious and are slower in appearing.
      b. Be alert to the more cumulative effect of medications in the older person than is true of younger people.
      c. Note that such medications as morphine, scopolamine and barbiturates in the usual dosages may cause confusion and disorientation.
   2. Therapeutic Approach
      a. Give consideration to lesser doses for desired effect.

      b. Anticipate problems from long-standing chronic disorders such as anemia, obesity, diabetes, hypoproteinemia.
      c. Adjust nutritional intake to conform to the higher protein and vitamin needs.
      d. When possible cater to set patterns in older patients such as sleeping and eating patterns, use of alcohol and laxatives.

D. *Presence of Disease*
  1. *Cardiovascular*
      a. Requires increased diligence when surgical problem is complicated by a cardiovascular problem.
      b. Avoid overloading the body with fluids (oral, parenteral, blood) because of possible congestive failure and pulmonary edema.
      c. Prevent prolonged immobilization, which results in stasis of circulating fluids.
      d. Encourage change of position but avoid sudden exertion.
      e. Note evidence of hypoxia and initiate therapy.
  2. *Diabetes*
      a. Be aware that hypoglycemia due to inadequate carbohydrate intake or insulin overdosage is life-threatening in uncontrolled diabetes.
      b. Recognize the signs and symptoms of ketoacidosis and glycosuria (p. 639) which can be a threat to a smooth surgical experience.
      c. Reassure the diabetic patient that when his disease is controlled, the surgical risk is no greater than it is with the nondiabetic person.
  3. *Alcoholism*
      a. Anticipate the additional problem of malnutrition in the presurgical alcoholic patient.
      b. Recognize that the acutely intoxicated person is susceptible to injury and may receive serious injuries without being aware of them.
      c. Be prepared to perform gastric lavage on the intoxicated patient if surgery cannot be postponed; this may lessen the chance of vomiting and aspiration during anesthesia induction.
      d. Note that the risk from surgery is increased for the individual who is a chronic alcoholic.
  4. *Pulmonary and Upper Respiratory Disease*
      a. Surgery may be contraindicated in the patient who has an upper respiratory infection because an acute upper respiratory infection may be the forerunner of more serious illness, such as pneumonia.
      b. Patients with chronic pulmonary problems such as emphysema, bronchiectasis, etc. should be treated for several days preoperatively with bronchodilators, aerosol medications, postural drainage, conscientious mouth care.
  5. *Concurrent or Prior Pharmacotherapy*
      a. Hazards exist when certain medications are given concomitantly with others; therefore, an awareness of prior drug therapy is essential. (Example: interaction of some drugs with anesthetics can lead to arterial hypotension and circulatory collapse.)
      b. Notify anesthesiologist if the patient is taking any of the following drugs:
         (1) Certain antibiotics*—many, when combined with a curariform muscle relaxant, interrupt nerve transmission, causing respiratory paralysis and apnea.

---

* Neomycin, streptomycin, dihydrostreptomycin, polymyxin A and B, colistin, viomycin, paromomycin, and kanamycin.

(2) Antidepressants, particularly monoamine oxidase inhibitors (MAO), increase hypotensive effects of anesthesia.

(3) Phenothiazines increase hypotensive action of anesthetics.

(4) Diuretics, particularly thiazides, cause electrolyte imbalance and respiratory depression during anesthesia.

OPERATIVE PERMIT (Informed Consent)

An *operative permit* is a form signed by the patient (and witnessed), granting permission to have the operation performed as described by the patient's physician; this is a medicolegal requirement.

Purposes

1. To protect the patient against unauthorized procedures.
2. To protect the surgeon and hospital against legal action by a patient who claims that an unauthorized procedure was performed.

Circumstances Requiring a Permit

1. Any surgical procedure where scalpel, scissors, suture, hemostats or electrocoagulation may be used.
2. For entrance into a body cavity—paracentesis, bronchoscopy, cystoscopy.
3. For general anesthesia, local infiltration and regional block—i.e., reduction of a fracture.

Obtaining Operative Permit

1. *Written* permission is best and is legally acceptable.
2. Signature is obtained with the patient's complete understanding of what is to occur; it is obtained before he receives sedation and is secured without pressure or duress.
3. A witness is desirable—nurse, physician or other authorized person.
4. In emergency, permission via telephone or telegram is acceptable.
5. For a minor (or one who is unconscious or irresponsible), permission is required from a responsible member of the family—parent or legal guardian.
6. For a married minor, permission from the husband or wife is acceptable.
7. If the patient is unable to write, an "X" to indicate his sign is acceptable if there are 2 signed witnesses to his mark.

PREPARATION OF SPECIFIC OPERATIVE AREAS

1. Head surgery	Obtain specific instructions from surgeon as to the extent of shaving.
2. Neck and thyroid	Anterior—neck under chin down to nipple line Bedline to bedline with patient lying supine Up to hair line.
3. Chest (Fig. 2-2*B*)	Affected side Spine posteriorly to midline anteriorly Above clavicle to umbilicus

4. Breast amputation (Fig. 2-2A)   Affected side
    Axilla
    Above clavicle to umbilicus
    Beyond midline anteriorly to beyond midline posteriorly
    Special attention to fold below breast.

5. Nephrectomy (Fig. 2-2D)   Affected side
    Anterior midline to posterior midline.

6. Abdomen (Fig. 2-2C)   Males: Nipple to and including pubic area.
    Females: Below breast to and including pubic area.
    Bedline to bedline as patient lies supine.
    Special attention to umbilicus and inguinal folds.

7. Inguinal hernia   Lower abdomen—umbilicus down through suprapubic region
    Approximately 15 cm. (6 inches) of upper thigh on affected side
    Special attention to groin area.

8. Anal operations (Fig. 2-2E)   25 cm. (10 inches) around anus
    Special attention to folds

9. Spinal surgery   Approximately 30 cm. (12 inches) above and below incision site
    Bedline to bedline as patient lies prone

10. Amputation   Ascertain proposed site of amputation
    Approximately 30 cm. (12 inches) above and below proposed site of amputation.

GUIDELINES: *Preparing the Patient's Skin for Surgery*

Purpose

To cleanse the skin and reduce the number of organisms on the skin so as to eliminate as much as possible the transference of such organisms into the incision site.

> NURSING ALERT: Unless contraindicated, it may be desirable for the nonemergency patient to bathe with a bacteriostatic soap for several days prior to surgery.

Pharmacophysiologic Emphasis

1. By nature human skin harbors transient and resident bacterial flora, some of which are pathogenic.
2. Skin cannot be sterilized without destroying skin cells.
3. Friction enhances the action of detergent antiseptics.
4. No existing antiseptic produces instant skin disinfection.

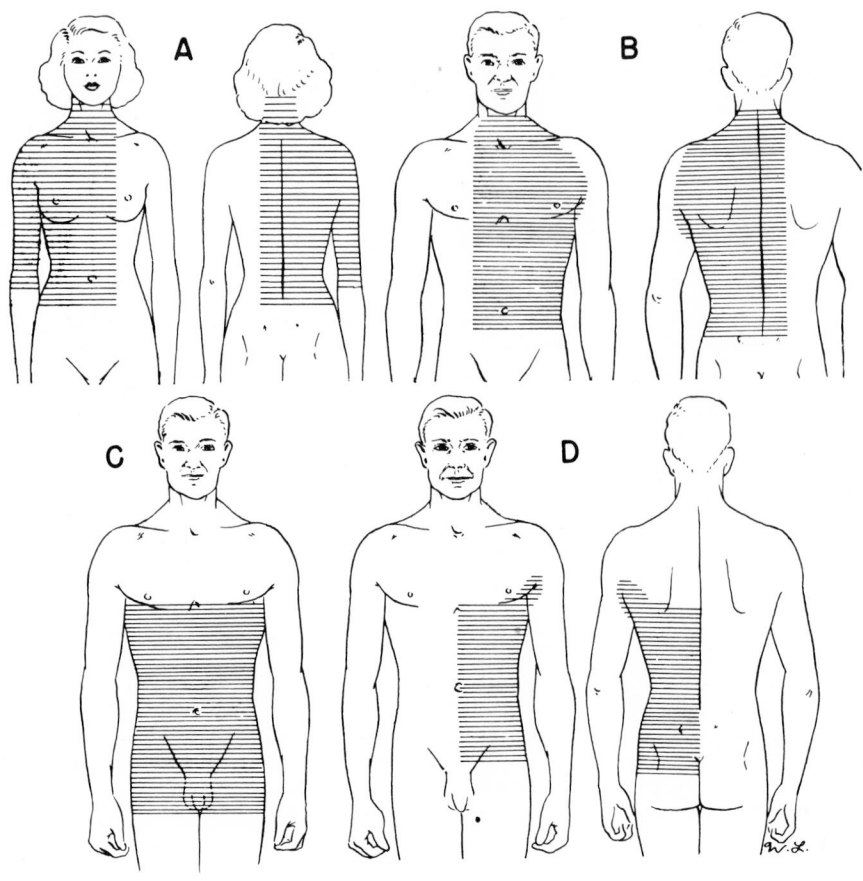

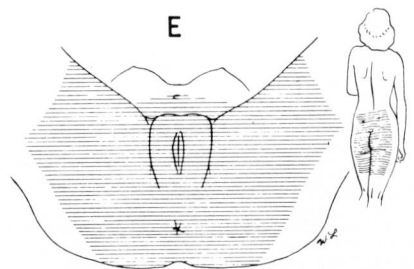

Figure 2-2. Areas to be prepared for operation. The shaded areas are those to be shaved. (A) Preparation for amputation of breast. Note that the area to be prepared includes the front and the back of the trunk and extends from the neck to the umbilicus. The axilla and the upper portion of the arm also are included. (B) Area of preparation for operation on the thorax. (C) Area of preparation for operation upon the abdomen (laparotomy) and for hernia. The preparation should extend from the nipple line to well below the crest of the ilium. For herniorrhaphy the upper limit of preparation may be the area of the umbilicus. (D) Area to be prepared for nephrectomy. Note that the preparation should be on both the anterior and the posterior sides of the trunk. (E) Area to be prepared for operations on the perineum. These areas should be shaved completely for all gynecologic operations, for operations around the anus and for such combined operations as an abdominoperineal resection of the rectum.

Equipment

Disposable tray with essentials, or a tray containing

2 bowls for detergent-germicide	6 or 8 4 × 4-inch gauze squares
1 emesis basin	Razor and blades
2 applicator sticks	Scissors for cutting long hair, if required

Procedure

Preparatory Phase

1. Explain to the patient the purpose of the activity.
2. Instruct the patient to assume the most comfortable and satisfactory position for the required skin preparation.
3. Cover him with a bath blanket, protect bedding, and expose the area to be shaved.

Nursing Action	**Rationale / Amplification**

Performance Phase

1. Apply warm detergent-germicide with gauze pledgets and cleanse area using light friction; begin at incision site and, in a circular manner, work outward from the center.

1. Oils, soil, and organisms are removed from skin surface. Working away from incision site prevents the clean area from becoming recontaminated.

2. Cut long hairs with scissors.

2. Much easier and quicker than with a razor.

3. Provide extra attention to areas where there are folds of skin, e.g., axillae, pubic area, umbilicus. Draw loose skin taut. Use cotton-tipped applicators where necessary.

3. Greater numbers of organisms are harbored in folds of skin, requiring extra effort to remove.

4. If the operative area includes calloused areas or the nails, use a brush.

4. Facilitates cleansing in out-of-the-way areas.

5. With free hand, apply smooth traction in opposite direction; with other hand shave the lathered hair using firm steady strokes.

5. Traction provides a smoother surface and allows the hairs to assume a more upright position; this facilitates cutting.

6. Use a disposable or sterilized razor and a sharp new blade.

6. Avoids infectious hepatitis from contaminated razor.

7. For denuded or sensitive areas, soak gently with detergent and flush thoroughly with saline or sterile water.

7. Prevents additional trauma.

8. Avoid nicking the skin; report any skin abrasions.

8. An opening in the skin increases the hazard of infection.

9. Scrub the skin area after the shaving is completed; rinse carefully and blot dry.

9. Prevents irritation and chapping.

Follow-up Phase

1. Remove all equipment and dispose of expendable materials according to local policy.
2. Remind the patient of the necessity for keeping the prepared area clean for surgery; provide for his comfort.

IMMEDIATE PRESURGICAL PREPARATION OF THE PATIENT

Physical and Psychological Attention to the Patient

1. Provide patient with a short gown to be worn to the operating room.
2. Remove hairpins; braid women's long hair; cover hair with a cap.
3. Remove dentures or plates (unless anesthesiologist orders these left to reduce respiratory tract obstruction) and inspect mouth for foreign material such as chewing gum.

4. Remove jewelry, identify properly, and place in the hospital safe; if wedding ring cannot be removed, tie with gauze bandage fastened around wrist.
5. Remove contact lens; have patient place them in properly marked receptacle (left and right), identify properly, and deposit in the hospital safe.
6. Have patient void immediately before leaving for the operating room; measure amount and note time of voiding; record.
7. Continue to support the patient emotionally and correct any misconceptions he may have.

Preanesthetic Medication
(prescribed to meet individual needs)

Purposes
1. To facilitate the administration of any anesthetic and to relax the patient.
2. To minimize respiratory tract secretions and changes in heart rate and to reduce anxiety.

NURSING ALERT: Administer preanesthetic medication precisely at the time it is ordered. If given too early, the maximum potency will have passed before it is needed; if given too late, the action will not have begun before anesthesia is to begin.

"On Call" Medications
1. Have medication ready and administer as soon as call is received.
2. Proceed with remaining preparation activities.
3. Indicate on the chart or preoperative check list the time when medication was administered.

Transporting Patient to the Operating Room
1. Adhere to the principle of maintaining the comfort and safety of the patient.
2. Accompany operating room attendants to patient's bedside for introduction and proper identification.
3. Assist in transferring patient from bed to stretcher.
4. Complete chart and preoperative check list; include laboratory reports and x-rays as may be required in the operating room.
5. Recognize importance of coordinating team effort to ensure arrival of the patient in the operating room at the proper time.

The Patient's Family
1. Direct patient's family to the proper waiting room where magazines, television and coffee may be available.
2. Inform them that the surgeon will probably come to this room immediately after surgery to inform them of the operation.
3. Acquaint the family with the fact that length of time does not mean the patient is in the operating room all the while; anesthesia preparation and induction take time; and after surgery, the patient is taken to the recovery room.
4. Tell the family what to expect postoperatively when they see the patient—tubes, monitoring equipment, and blood transfusion, suctioning, and oxygen equipment.

IMMEDIATE POSTSURGICAL NURSING CARE

Objective

To assist the patient in recovering from operation and from the effects of the anesthetic agent as quickly, safely, and comfortably as possible.

NURSING ALERT: This phase of nursing care is geared to *recognizing* the significance of signs and *anticipating* and *preventing* postoperative difficulties.

Remain in attendance and carefully *observe* the patient coming out of anesthesia until:
1. Vital signs are stable.
2. He is breathing easily.
3. Reflexes have returned to normal.
4. He is out of anesthesia and fully awake.

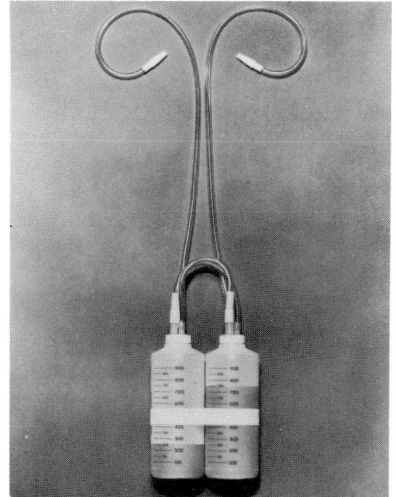

Figure 2-3. Blow bottles are an inexpensive, nonmechanical device for respiratory stimulation. They provide the most effective and most commonly used forced-expiration exercise. Water in the bottles provides resistance, gives the patient the benefit of prolonged expiration and helps to bring the relatively unused muscles of the abdomen into play—all vital in providing maximum ventilatory effort for the patient. (Chesebrough-Pond's Inc.)

HOW TO USE BLOW BOTTLES

1. Remove contents from package. Fill 1 bottle with water. Remove coloring tablet from foil packet and drop into water-filled bottle.

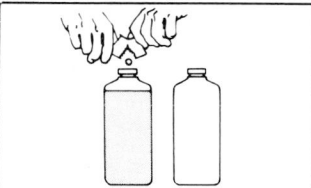

2. Insert rigid tubing from caps into each bottle and screw caps firmly onto bottles.

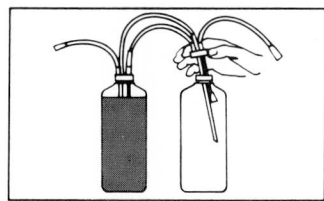

3. Join the 2 bottles with elastic strap.

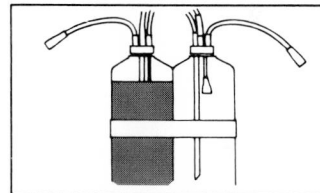

4. Patient blows into mouth-piece on water-filled bottle to transfer water into 2nd bottle. Process can be reversed by blowing into tubing connected to 2nd bottle and can be repeated as often as desired.

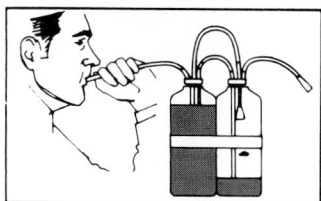

Nursing Management

A. *Ensure the Maintenance of a Patent Airway*
1. Place the patient in the lateral position with neck hyperextended—this permits the best possible expansion of the lungs.
2. Allow metal, rubber or plastic airway to remain in place until the patient begins to waken and is trying to eject the airway.
   a. The airway keeps the passage open and prevents the tongue from falling backward and obstructing the airway.
   b. Leaving the airway in after the pharyngeal reflex has returned may cause the patient to gag and vomit.

   > NOTE: Many seriously ill patients return from the operating room with a tracheal tube in place; this may be left in place for hours or days and requires special management.

3. When patient is partially awake and the airway is removed, he may show signs of gagging, nausea or vomiting; place him in the lateral position with the upper arm supported on a pillow.
   a. This will promote chest expansion.
   b. Turn the patient every hour or two to facilitate breathing and ventilation.
4. Aspirate excessive secretions when they are heard in the nasopharynx and oropharynx.
   a. Using a Y-connecting tube with catheter, turn suction machine on, insert catheter into pharynx (15–20 cm.; 6–8 inches), then close Y-tube outlet with finger to activate suction; withdraw slowly as catheter is rotated.
   b. If secretions are lower in the tracheobronchial tree, intratracheal suctioning may be necessary (Fig. 3-3).
5. Encourage patient to take deep breaths to aerate lungs fully and prevent hypostatic pneumonia; use blow bottles to facilitate this function (Fig. 2-3).
6. Administer humidified oxygen if required.
   a. Heat and moisture are normally lost during exhalation.
   b. Dehydrated patients may require oxygen and humidity because of higher incidence of irritated respiratory passages in these patients.
   c. Secretions can be kept soft to facilitate removal.
7. Employ mechanical ventilation to maintain adequate pulmonary ventilation if required (see p. 137).

B. *Assess Status of Circulatory System*
1. Take vital signs (blood pressure, pulse and respiration) frequently as clinical condition indicates until patient is well stabilized. Then check every 4 hours thereafter.
   a. Know patient's preoperative blood pressure in order to make significant comparisons.
   b. Report immediately a falling systolic pressure.
   c. Variations in blood pressure or cardiac arrhythmias are reportable.
   d. Respirations over 30 should be reported.
2. Recognize the variety of factors which may alter circulating blood volume.
   a. Reactions to anesthesia and medications
   b. Blood loss and organ manipulation during surgery
   c. Moving the patient from one position on the operating table to another on the stretcher

3. Monitor temperature hourly to avoid malignant hyperthermia (more significant in pediatrics).

Over 37.7°C. (100°F.) or under 36.1°C. (97°F.) is reportable.

4. Be cognizant of early symptoms of shock or hemorrhage.
   a. Rapid, thready pulse and a falling blood pressure may indicate hemorrhage, leading to a decrease in blood volume.
   b. Initiate oxygen therapy to increase oxygen availability from the circulating blood.
   c. Place patient in shock position with feet elevated (unless contraindicated).
   d. See page 76 for more detailed consideration of shock.

C. *Promote Comfort and Maintain Safety*
   1. Provide a therapeutic environment with proper temperature and humidity; remove unnecessary blanket which might cause loss of body fluid.
   2. Place side-rails in protecting position until patient is fully awake.
   3. Protect extremity into which intravenous fluids are running so that needle will not become accidentally dislodged.
   4. Turn patient frequently and maintain good body alignment.
   5. Avoid nerve damage and muscle strain by properly supporting and padding pressure areas.

D. *Continue Constant Surveillance of the Patient Until he is Completely Out of Anesthesia*
   1. Be aware of the fact that the patient cannot complain of injury, such as the pricking of an open safety pin, a clamp that is exerting pressure, a burn from a hot-water bottle.
   2. Examine dressings for unexpected drainage or bleeding.
   3. Check dressings for constriction.
   4. Observe drainage tubes for proper connection and patency.
   5. Note proper functioning of monitoring and suctioning devices, oxygen therapy equipment, etc.
   6. Inspect skin and tissue surrounding intravenous needles to detect early infiltration.
   7. Evaluate periodically the patient's status of orientation—how he responds to being addressed by his name or performs simple movements upon receiving a command.
   8. Determine return of motor control following spinal anesthesia as indicated by how the patient responds to a pinprick or a request to move a part.

THE PATIENT RECEIVING INTRAVENOUS THERAPY

Objectives
1. To maintain or replace body stores of water, electrolytes, vitamins, proteins, calories, and nitrogen in the patient who cannot maintain an adequate intake by mouth.
2. To restore acid-base balance.
3. To replenish blood volume.
4. To provide avenues for the administration of medications.

Physiological Assimilation of Intravenous Solutions

A. *Principles*
   1. Blood cells (erythrocytes, etc.), are surrounded by a semipermeable membrane.
   2. Osmotic pressure is the pressure demonstrated when a solvent moves through the semipermeable membrane from weaker to stronger concentrations.

   3. Osmotic characteristics of different solutions are often determined by the way they affect red blood cells in the blood.

B. *Types of Fluids*
   1. *Isotonic*—a solution which has the same osmotic pressure externally as that found across the semipermeable membrane within the cell.
      a. Normal saline 0.9%   c. Lactated Ringers
      b. Dextrose 5% in water   d. Normosol-R
   2. *Hypotonic*—a solution which has less osmotic pressure than that of blood serum causing the cells to expand or swell.
         Sodium chloride 0.45%
   3. *Hypertonic*—a solution which has higher osmotic pressure than that of blood serum causing the cells to shrink.
      a. Dextrose 5% in saline   d. Dextrose 5% in ½ strength saline
      b. Dextrose 10% in saline   e. Dextrose 20% in water
      c. Dextrose 10% in water

C. *Composition of Fluids*
   1. Saline solution—fluids and electrolytes (Na^+ Cl^-)
   2. Dextrose—fluid and calories
   3. Lactated Ringers—fluid, electrolytes (Na^+, K^+, Cl^-, Ca^{++}, Lactate)
   4. Normosol-R—fluid, electrolytes, some calories (Na^+, K^+, Mg^{++}, Cl^-, HCO_3^-, gluconate)
   5. Blood related fluids
      a. Whole blood
         (1) Approximately 45% cellular—red cells, white cells, blood platelets
         (2) Approximately 55% plasma
            (a) 90% water
            (b) 7% protein (albumin, globulin, fibrinogen)
            (c) 2% lipids, vitamins, carbohydrates, inorganic salts
         (3) Whole blood is used to replace blood lost in acute hemorrhage.
      b. Packed cells—red blood cells obtained by centrifuging whole blood and drawing off the plasma
            Packed cells are used in treatment of anemia or for the patient in whom there is a risk of circulatory overload (congestive heart failure).
      c. Fresh frozen plasma
         (1) To restore blood volume in shock
         (2) To correct hypoproteinemia
         (3) To treat coagulation disorders
            (see p. 227 also)
   6. Plasma expanders: albumin, dextran, plasminate
         To improve circulating blood volume
   7. Parenteral hyperalimentation.

Nursing Assessment

A. *Diagnosis*
      Know the major and minor medical problems of the patient as indicated by the physician in his diagnostic evaluation and the nurse in her assessment of the patient.

B. *Fluids*
   1. Can the patient's illness affect his fluid balance?
   2. What medication or treatment is he receiving that can affect fluid components? How?
   3. What is the relation of his fluid intake to fluid output?
   4. Does he have dietary restrictions?
   5. Is he taking adequate fluids by mouth?
   6. What is the physician's plan of treatment?

C. *Evidence of Fluid Imbalance*
   1. Determine body temperature—febrile conditions suggest loss of body fluids through perspiration.
   2. Is he thirsty? Possible dehydration.
   3. Observe for dry warm skin, cracked lips—signs of dehydration.
   4. Check skin for elasticity—lightly pull up a pinch-fold of skin, release it. Does it rapidly resume its normal position?
   5. Note color and amount of urine—concentrated, scanty urine indicates lack of fluids.
   6. Compare present weight with admission weight—it may indicate fluid change.

Criteria for Selecting a Suitable Vein for Venipuncture

   1. Choose largest convenient vein just distal to venous junction; *however,* if the patient needs repeated venipunctures, use distal branches of a large vein rather than the best sites—these then are available for emergencies.
   2. Select if possible the antecubital fossa—median basilic and median cephalic for relatively short-term infusion.
      a. They are large and easily accessible.
      b. Note, however, that it precludes arm movement.
      c. Choose site below elbow crease for patient's comfort.
   3. Otherwise, select other available veins
      a. Hand—metacarpal and dorsal venous network
      b. Forearm—accessory cephalic and median antebrachial
      c. Thigh—great saphenous and femoral veins
      d. Ankle—great saphenous
      e. Foot—venous plexus of dorsum, dorsal venous arch, medial marginal vein

---

NURSING ALERT: Avoid leg veins if there are marked degrees of varicosity at or above proposed site of injection. Otherwise, injected solutions may stagnate along varicosed vessels.

---

   4. Use a small needle (see p. 54). (see p. 54)

Distending a Vein Prior to Insertion of an Infusion Needle

   1. Apply manual compression above site of needle to be inserted.
   2. Have patient periodically clench his fist (if arm is used).
   3. Massage area in direction of venous flow.
   4. Apply sphygmomanometer cuff (keep pressure just below systolic pressure).
   5. Fasten soft rubber tubing with a hemostat.
   6. Tie soft rubber tubing as a slip knot.
   7. Lightly slap at vein site or over wrist.

8. Allow extremity to be dependent for a few minutes.
9. Apply moist heat by wringing out turkish towel and wrapping the part.
   Apply water-resistant wrapper externally and place a warm-water bottle or two along extremity. Leave in place from 10 to 20 minutes.
10. Apply external heat to extremity using a thermostatically controlled electric blanket. Hand-operated hair dryer can be used to direct heat to a possible needle site.
    NOTE: Should the above measures fail, it may be necessary to perform a "cutdown"— this is a surgical procedure exposing the vein for venipuncture; the incision site is treated as a surgical wound.

Stabilizing the Upper Extremity with a Padded Armboard

1. Fasten wrist by first applying a doubled 4 × 4-inch gauze dressing; use 1-inch adhesive or 2-inch gauze bandage.
2. Prevent compression of nerves or blood vessels; check pulse and ask patient if pressure is too great.
3. Secure upper end of splint to arm for stabilization.

Providing Local Anesthesia for Infants or Unusually Sensitive Patients

1. Raise a wheal in the skin just over the vein by injecting 0.5 ml. procaine hydrochloride 1.0% solution.
2. Advance the needle close to the wall of the vein so that this area is also anesthetized.

Equipment

A. *Needle*
  1. Usually an 18-, 19- or 20-gauge needle which is 2½–4 cm. long (1 or 1½ inches long) is used.
  2. For rapid infusion, use a 15-gauge needle.
  3. Use a *sharp* needle; if the needle is not disposable, check its sharpness by passing the needle back and forth through sterile gauze (any hook or broken tip will pull a snag of thread).

B. *Bevel*
  To facilitate entering a vein with least injury to skin, the bevel should face—
  a. Upward—when entering a vein lumen which is larger than the needle (Fig. 2-4A).
  b. Downward—when entering a small vein and lumen which approaches the size of the needle (Fig. 2-4B).

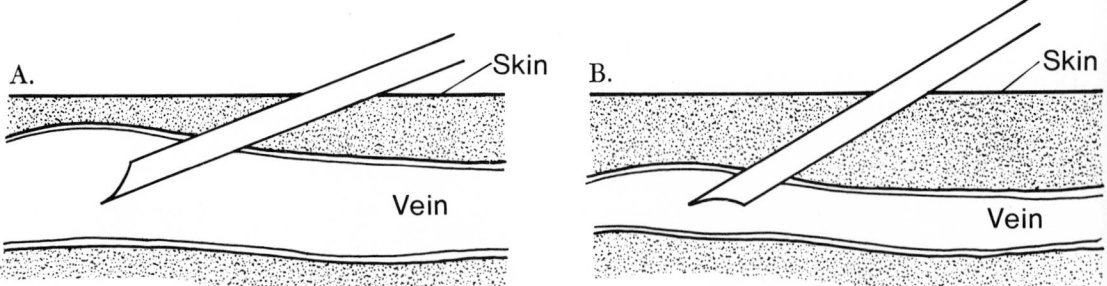

Figure 2-4.

C. *Catheter Needle* (Cannula)
1. Usually they are color-coded to indicate needle gauge.
2. Tapered sheath covers and protects needle.
3. A catheter needle has a wide (tapered) top or hub so that it will not be drawn into vein.
4. Some are radiopaque.

D. *Catheter-Over-Needle Units and Catheter-Inside-Needle Units* (Intra-cath, Medi-cath)

Depending upon unit, the needle is removed either immediately after venipuncture is performed or when therapy is to be discontinued.

Rate of Flow of Fluid Therapy

Physician will prescribe flow rate.

A. *Factors Affecting Rate of Flow*
1. Pressure gradient—the difference between 2 levels in a fluid system
2. Friction—the interaction between fluid molecules and surfaces of inner wall of tubing
3. Diameter and length of tubing
4. Height of column of fluid
5. Size of opening through which fluid leaves receptacle
6. Fluid viscosity—the thicker the fluid, the slower the flow

B. *A Rule-of-Thumb Guide for Rate of Administration of Fluids**
1. Isotonic solutions—not faster than 600 ml./hr.
2. Hypotonic solutions—not faster than 400 ml./hr.
3. Hypertonic solutions—not faster than 200 ml./hr.
4. Average rate—60 drops/min.
   For dehydrated patients, the rate is increased.
   For elderly or cardiac patients, the rate is decreased.

C. *Calculation of Flow Rate†*
1. Drops per milliliter vary with commercial parenteral sets. (Check directions on set or calculate by timing for 1 minute.)
2. Utilize the following formula:

$$\text{Drops/min.} = \frac{\text{Total volume infused} \times \text{drops/ml.}}{\text{Total time for infusion in minutes}}$$

Example:

Infuse 1000 ml. of 5% D/W in 2½ hours
(Set indicates 10 drops in 1 ml.)

$$\frac{1000 \times 10}{150 \text{ min.}} = 60 \text{ drops/min.}$$

* Davis, H. A.: Principles of Surgical Physiology. New York, Paul B. Hoeber, Inc., 1957.

† Metheney, N. M., and Snively, W. D., Jr.: Nurse's Handbook of Fluid Balance. Philadelphia, J. B. Lippincott, 1967, p. 119.

GUIDELINES: *Administering an Intravenous Infusion Using the Cubital Fossa*

Procedure

Nursing Action	Rationale / Amplification
Preparatory Phase	
1. Place patient in bed in semi-Fowler's position. Inform him of the procedure and its purpose.	1. This is comfortable for the patient and permits arm to assume a flexed comfortable position. To solicit his understanding and cooperation.
2. Remove sleeve of patient's garment.	2. To permit removal of gown or pajama top if necessary while infusion is in progress (without cutting sleeve).
3. Position (but do not tighten) tourniquet under lower end of upper arm (5 cm. above joint).	3. To immobilize arm while needle or catheter is in vein; this will prevent dislodging of needle and injury to vein.
4. Place padded splint under arm; fix arm to splint by bandaging firmly.	4. Padding will prevent constriction of nerves or blood vessels.
5. Connect intravenous materials; hang fluid receptacle after checking label for proper solution.	5. Intravenous fluids are considered as medications; labeling needs to be verified.
6. Allow fluid to flow through the system; tighten the clamp; lay sterile needle in or on sterile surface until arm is prepared.	6. To eliminate air bubbles which could cause air emboli in the circulatory system.
Performance Phase	
1. Tighten tourniquet. Ends of tubing should be opposite or away from infusion site.	1. To distend veins (for better visualization) because of preventing blood flow back to heart. To prevent contamination of injection area by tubing ends.
2. Request patient to open and close his fist. Palpate and note suitable vein for injection.	2. By contracting muscles of lower arm, blood is forced into veins thereby distending them further.
3. Cleanse skin thoroughly, using an antiseptic (of room temperature) on a cotton ball; apply friction in a circular motion outward from injection site.	3. To remove skin pathogens and sebum which might otherwise be drawn into the subcutaneous tissue or vein as the needle is advanced. Avoid application of cold antiseptic solution particularly if patient has very small veins; cold application would further constrict the vessels.
4. Use thumb to apply tension down on tissue and vein about 5 cm. (2 inches) distal to injection site.	4. To aid in anchoring the vein as the needle is introduced.
5. Hold the needle at a 45-degree angle alongside the wall of the vein in the direction and near the intended site of injection; pierce skin.	5. This angle permits greatest ease and accuracy in entering the vein.
6. Decrease angle of needle until it is nearly parallel with the skin and slightly to one side of the vein; apply pressure in same direction to puncture and enter the vein.	
7. If there is a backflow of blood through the needle, the vein has been entered; advance the needle slowly about 2½ cm. (1 inch) while lifting the vein.	7. To prevent the needle from becoming dislodged and puncturing the posterior wall of the vein.

Nursing Action	**Rationale/Amplification**
8. Release tourniquet.	8. To permit infusion solution to enter circulatory system.
9. Release clamp on infusion tubing and relax skin tension.	9. To allow flow of solution and to prevent blood from clotting in the needle.
10. Slip a sterile gauze square (3 x 3-inch) under the needle (double if necessary) to anchor it in the proper position.	10. To prevent needle orifice from pressing against vein wall and the needle from piercing vein wall.
11. Anchor needle in position using adhesive strips (Fig. 2-5); fasten a loop of tubing to prevent pull on needle (Figs. 2-6 and 2-7).	11. Effective taping allows some mobility for the patient and retains safe inflow of solution.
12. Regulate flow rate of solution.	12. Proper monitoring of solution will prevent overloading of the circulatory system.

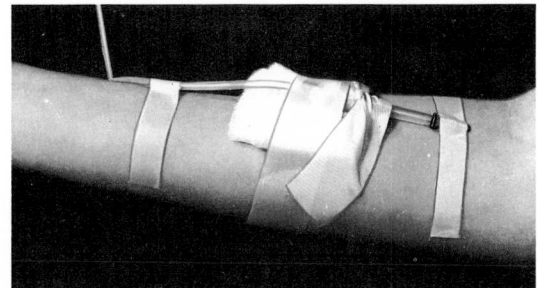

Figure 2-5. Method for securing needle and tubing for I.V. infusion or blood transfusion. Needle is inserted into antecubital vein with arm secured to padded board. After the needle is inserted it is secured with ½-inch wide strips of tape. A sterile gauze pad may be used to build up the angle of insertion.

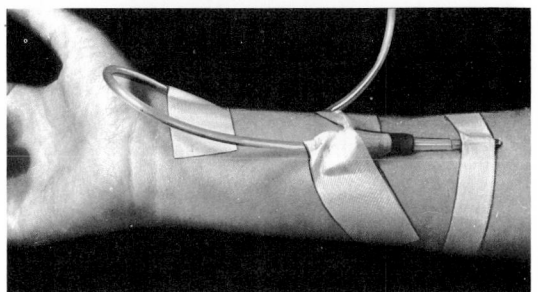

Figure 2-6. Simple method of holding needle and tubing in forearm vein with tape to prevent traction on needle.

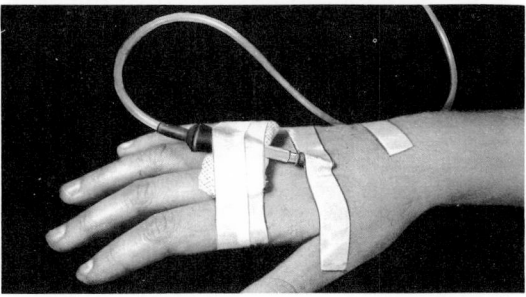

Figure 2-7. Method of securing vein on back of hand with tape.

(Figures 2-5–2-7: © Johnson & Johnson, 1972. Used by special permission of Johnson & Johnson, the copyright owners, and not to be reproduced for any purpose without Johnson & Johnson's permission.)

Follow-up Phase

1. Gently loosen adhesive taping and fixation near injection site.
2. Place a sterile gauze square over needle or cannula where it enters vein; withdraw needle (or cannula) and *exert pressure at site.* If bleeding persists, apply a gauze square or band-aid and elevate part.
3. Remove adhesive marks with solvent.
4. Record:
   a. Nature of therapy and time given   d. Any problems
   b. Type of solution and rate of flow   e. Patient's reaction
   c. Total amount of solution

Complications of Intravenous Therapy

Mechanical Failures
(solution flow slowing down or stopping, etc.)

1. Causes
   a. Needle may be lying against the side of the vein, cutting off fluid flow. (Patient may have moved his arm.)
   b. Level of intravenous receptacle may change rate of flow (gravity):
      (1) Higher—more rapid
      (2) Lower—less rapid
   c. Needle may be clogged due to clotting.
   d. Regulator of flow rate may be faulty; the clamp with a tapered v-shaped groove seems to provide greater dependability than the regular clamp.

2. Nursing Assessment and Approach
   a. Note whether there is swelling at needle site; if edema is present, it suggests infiltration (p. 59).
   b. Remove tape and check for kinking of tubing.
   c. Rotate needle slightly—the bevel of the needle may be lying against wall of vein.
   d. Move the arm of the patient to a new position.
   e. Elevate or lower needle to prevent occlusion of bevel of needle; if necessary, to maintain a slightly different position use a gauze pad or cotton ball as a prop and maintain position by placing a few adhesive straps.
   f. Try pulling back the needle or catheter a short distance since it may be occluded at a bifurcation.
   g. Check patency of needle by lowering the receptacle below level of needle; a flashback of blood from the patient into the intravenous tubing indicates patency.
   h. Flush out cannula or needle by injecting sterile saline with a sterile syringe and needle directly into tubing; pinch off tubing leading to receptacle.
   i. If none of the preceding steps produces the desired flow, remove needle and restart infusion.

NURSING ALERT: Sterile distilled water is never added to an intravenous set-up because it is hypotonic.

Pyrogenic Reaction

A generalized reaction due to contaminated equipment or solutions (less apparent with disposable equipment).

1. Symptoms (occur about 30 minutes to 1 hour after start of infusion)
   a. Abrupt temperature elevation, chills
   b. Face flushing, sudden pulse rate change
   c. Complaints of backache, headache
   d. Nausea and vomiting
   e. Hypotension—vascular collapse
   f. Cyanosis—vascular collapse

2. Preventive Nursing Measures
   a. Apply antibiotic ointment to skin where needle or catheter enters.
   b. Use indwelling catheters only when absolutely necessary; infection increases significantly with the length of venous catheterization.
   c. For long-term infusions, change infusion site every 48 hours; mark catheter to indicate when it is to be changed.
   d. For long-term catheterization, a larger needle (i.e., a No. 14 needle with No. 16 catheter 20 cm. or 8 inches long) in external jugular or subclavian vein directed to superior vena cava seems to minimize complications.
      (1) Less disparity in diameters of tube and vessel
      (2) Rapid dilution of irritating fluids

3. Nursing Treatment Measures
   a. Discontinue infusion.
   b. Check vital signs; reassure patient.
   c. Notify physician.
   d. Save equipment for further laboratory study.
   e. Record name, lot number and information—i.e., manufacturer of solution and any medications that have been added.

Infiltration

Dislodging of needle will cause fluid to infiltrate tissues.

1. Symptoms at Site
   a. Edema, blanching of skin
   b. Discomfort depending upon nature of solution
   c. Fluid flows more slowly or stops
   d. With a vasoconstrictor, such as norepinephrine (Levophed), infiltration can cause serious injury leading to necrosis and sloughing of tissues.

2. Preventive Nursing Measures
   a. Fasten needle securely.
   b. Limit arm movement by properly splinting.

3. Nursing Treatment Measures
   a. Stop infusion.
   b. Notify intravenous therapist, physician, etc.
   c. Place a sterile 3 x 3-inch gauze pad over needle and vein; withdraw needle and apply firm pressure over venipuncture site for several minutes.

   d. Apply warm compresses to increase fluid absorption.
   e. Restart infusion elsewhere.
   f. Use plastic cannula to reduce trauma when site is moved.

Circulatory Overload

Patient receives an excessive amount of solution (happens more frequently in elderly patients or in infants).
   1. Symptoms
      a. Headache, flushed skin, rapid pulse
      b. Venous distention
      c. Increased blood pressure
      d. Increased venous pressure
      e. Coughing, shortness of breath, increased respirations
      f. Syncope, shock
      g. Pulmonary edema leading to dyspnea and cyanosis
   2. Preventive Nursing Measures
      a. Know whether patient has existing heart condition—more prone to develop acute pulmonary edema.
      b. Monitor solution flow.
      c. Place patient in semi-sitting position during infusion.
      d. Be especially attentive to the elderly or the infant.
   3. Nursing Treatment Measures
      a. Stop the infusion; notify physician.
      b. Raise patient to sitting position—will ease the breathing problem.
      c. If norepinephrine (Levophed) was used:
         (1) Notify physician of infiltration.
         (2) Prepare antidote—phentolamine (Regitine). When this is injected liberally into site, tissue necrosis and sloughing may be prevented.

Drug Overload

Patient receives an excessive amount of fluid containing drugs.
   1. Toxic concentrations of drug are collected in main organs, brain and heart.
   2. Symptoms
      a. Dizziness, fainting leading to shock
      b. Specific symptoms related to the offending drug
   3. Preventive Nursing Measures
      Monitor flow rate carefully.
   4. Nursing Treatment
      Related to the nature of the medication

Thrombophlebitis

   1. Causes
      a. Overuse of a vein which may cause vasospasm; this may lead to inflammatory process
      b. Irritating infusion solution (strong acids or alkalies)
      c. Clot formation in an inflamed vein.

2. Symptoms
   a. Tenderness at first, then pain along course of the vein
   b. Edema and redness at injection site
   c. Arm feels warmer than other arm
3. Preventive Nursing Measures
   a. When cephalothin is to be given for several days, via infusion, change veins used.
   b. Add a small volume (20 ml.) of sterile 1% sodium bicarbonate* immediately prior to infusion to raise pH level to an acceptable level (on physician's prescription).
4. Nursing Treatment Measures
   a. Apply cold compresses immediately to relieve pain and inflammation.
   b. Later follow with moist warm compresses to stimulate circulation and promote absorption.

Air Embolism

Air manages to get into the circulatory system.

> NURSING ALERT: Recognize the high possibility of this problem when physicians pump in blood (such as 500 ml.—1 pint in 10 minutes) since this builds high pressure in blood receptacle.

1. Symptoms
   a. Hypotension, cyanosis, tachycardia
   b. Increased venous pressure, loss of consciousness
2. Nursing Preventive Measures
   a. Replace initial bottle before it is completely empty with a fresh full bottle; check attachment to be certain it is tight.
   b. In "Y" type sets, tightly clamp the nearly empty bottle to prevent air from being sucked into the tubing.
   c. Allow fluid to flow through tubing and needle or catheter to force air out—before starting infusion.
3. Nursing Treatment Measures
   a. Turn patient on left side with head down—air will rise into right ventricle and allow blood to pass into the lungs. The trapped air will be slowly dissipated through pulmonary system.
   b. Administer oxygen.

Nerve Damage

May be the result of tying the arm too tightly to the splint.
1. Symptoms
      Numbness of fingers or hands
2. Nursing Preventive Measures
      Place padding around arm where bandage is to be applied.
3. Nursing Treatment Measures
   a. Massage arm and move shoulder through its range of motion.
   b. Instruct patient to open and close hand several times each hour.
   c. Physical therapy may be required.

* Pederson, B. M.: A solution for post-infusion thrombophlebitis. Amer. J. Nurs., 70:325, Feb. 1970.

CARE OF THE WOUND

A *wound* is an injury to the tissues of the body causing disruption of the normal tissue pattern; such an injury is caused by physical means.

Classification

According to the manner in which it is made

Incised—made by a clean cut with a sharp instrument, e.g., a surgeon's incision with a scalpel.

Contused—made by blunt force, which does not break through the skin but causes considerable soft tissue damage, e.g., a rock when thrown bruises a person.

Lacerated—made by an object which tears tissues, producing jagged irregular edges, e.g., blunt knife, jagged wire, glass.

Puncture—made by a pointed instrument, such as an ice pick, bullet, knife stab, nail.

Surgical Classification

Clean—an aseptically made wound, as in surgery, in which all bleeding vessels have been ligated (tied).

Infected—a wound which may not be closed may contain devitalized or infected material.

Debridement—the process whereby devitalized or necrotic tissue is cut out and flushed clean with saline solution.

Physiology of Wound Healing

A. *First Intention Healing (Primary Union)*

Healing which takes place aseptically with a minimum of tissue damage and tissue reaction; this is the ideal sought by the surgical staff.

B. *Second Intention Healing (Granulation)*
1. Pus has formed due to infection; drainage is accomplished by incision and perhaps insertion of drains.
2. Necrotic material disintegrates and sloughs off.
3. Cavity fills with a red, soft, sensitive tissue which bleeds easily.
4. Buds, called granulation tissue, enlarge to fill area formerly destroyed thereby forming a scar (cicatrix).

C. *Third Intention Healing (Secondary Suture)*
1. Occurs when a wound breaks down and is resutured or when a wound has been kept open and fills with granulation tissue and then is closed with sutures (2 faces of granulation tissue are brought together in apposition).
2. Scar tissue formation is deeper, wider and more pronounced.

Factors Affecting Wound Healing

1. Adequate nutrition through proper diet.
   Protein and vitamin C are particularly effective in promoting healing.
2. Administration of whole blood—to maintain adequate levels of red blood cells.
3. Edema—interferes with healing process.
4. Age
   Tissues of younger individuals heal more rapidly than those of older persons.

Figure 2-8. Laparotomy dressings. Laparotomy dressings are of many types, depending, of course, upon the nature of the operation; the most frequent use of adhesive tape on the abdomen is in the application of postoperative dressings.

For the ordinary laparotomy, 2″ or 3″ wide strips of adhesive tape are usually applied transversely in close arrangement over the dressing; the ends of such strips should extend at least to the midaxillary line in order to provide good support and fixation. The illustration shows an effective method of securing a standard abdominal dressing.

Some surgeons cover the dressing solidly with adhesive tape, but others question this practice on the grounds that it interferes with transpiration of water vapor from the area around the wound and thus may produce maceration and aid in the development of infection. (© Johnson & Johnson, 1972. Used by special permission of Johnson & Johnson, the copyright owners, and not to be reproduced for any purpose without Johnson & Johnson's permission.)

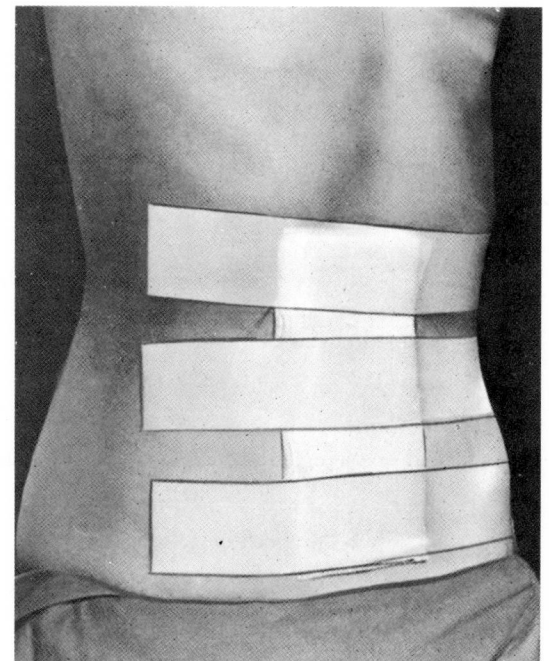

The Purposes of Dressings

1. To protect the wound from mechanical injury.
2. To splint or immobilize the wound (Fig. 2-8).
3. To absorb drainage and fluid wastes.
4. To promote homeostasis as in a pressure dressing.
5. To prevent contamination from bodily discharges.
6. To provide physical and psychological comfort for the patient.

Wound Healing Without Dressings

Preferred by some surgeons and may be desirable in a simple, clean wound.

A. *Advantages*
1. Permits better observation and early detection of problems.
2. Promotes cleanliness and facilitates bathing.
3. Eliminates conditions necessary for organism growth.
   a. Warmth   b. Moisture   c. Darkness
4. Avoids adhesive tape reaction.
5. Facilitates patient activity.
6. Is economical.

B. *Disadvantages*
1. Psychologically, a patient may object to an exposed wound.
2. Wound is more vulnerable to injury.
3. Bedding and clothing may catch on stitches.

GUIDELINES: *Assisting with a Change of Surgical Dressings*

Surgical Dressing Technique

The procedure of changing dressings, examining and cleansing the wound, utilizing principles of asepsis.

1. A team works together to change a patient's dressing—nurse with surgeon or nurse with a colleague.
2. The condition of the wound is noted in order to better understand the nature of the patient's surgical recovery.
3. The healing process is facilitated by keeping the wound clean.
4. Stitches or clips are removed after the 5th or 6th day since wound edges have begun to knit together.

Procedure

Preparatory Phase

1. Inform the patient that his dressing is to be changed. Have him lie in his bed.
2. Avoid changing dressings at mealtime.
3. Ensure his privacy by drawing the curtains or closing the door; expose the dressing site.
4. If the dressings have a foul odor, perhaps the dressings can be changed in a separate treatment area adequately ventilated.
5. Prevent undue exposure of the patient; respect his modesty and prevent him from becoming chilled.

Nursing Action	Rationale/Amplification
Removing Adhesive Tape	
1. Remove tape along longitudinal axis.	1. Removing tape in same plane is less injurious and less painful.
2. Peel back edges by holding skin taut and pulling away from skin.	2. It is less traumatic to push skin away from tape than to pull tape from skin.
3. Remove tape near a wound by pulling toward the wound.	3. To pull away from a wound may tear some of the delicate newly formed tissues.
4. Use a suitable solvent such as baby oil if the tape does not pull away easily.	4. Oil is safe, works as well as true solvents and, in addition, lubricates and soothes the sensitive skin beneath.
Removing Old Dressing	
1. Use an unsterile forceps to remove soiled dressings.	1. Dressings are not to be handled by ungloved hands because of the possibility of transmitting pathogenic organisms.
2. Deposit dressings in a disposable bag which can be closed easily and destroyed by burning.	
3. Place unsterile instrument in a paper bag or wrap in a towel.	3. Such placement prevents contamination of a clean area. This instrument will be cleansed later.

Assistant Nurse	Nurse or Surgeon	Rationale
Cleaning the Simple Wound		
1. Use aseptic technique.		1. To prevent contamination of a clean wound or to prevent further contamination of a "dirty" wound. Also to prevent transmission of pathogenic organisms to clean areas.
2. Open sterile package of gloves.	2. Don rubber gloves.	

Assistant Nurse	Nurse or Surgeon	Rationale
3. Open a sterile pack containing a scissors, forceps, a grooved director, cotton balls, dressings and solution container.	3. Pick up cotton ball with forceps and hold ball over emesis basin.	
4. Pour antiseptic solution over cotton ball.	4. Clean wound gently but thoroughly.	
	5. Use forceps to pick up each stitch, cut with scissors and pull stitch out (Fig. 2-9). Deposit in emesis basin or on a sterile gauze square.	5. After 5th or 6th day, stitches serve no useful purpose. If they remain in place, they can act as a wick in carrying pathogenic organisms from the skin.

Completion of Dressing

1. Select proper size and type of adhesive for securing dressing; rubber-based or acrylate adhesive.	1. Place minimal dressing over wound.	1. *Rubber-based* (cloth-backed or plastic-backed) dressing used principally for heavy support and where a high level of adhesion is required. *Acrylate* (nonwoven or fabric backing) usually used for surgical taping because of hypoallergenic quality.
2. Apply minimum amount of taping necessary to keep dressing in place (Fig. 2-10).	2. Remove gloves and complete dressing fixation with adhesive.	

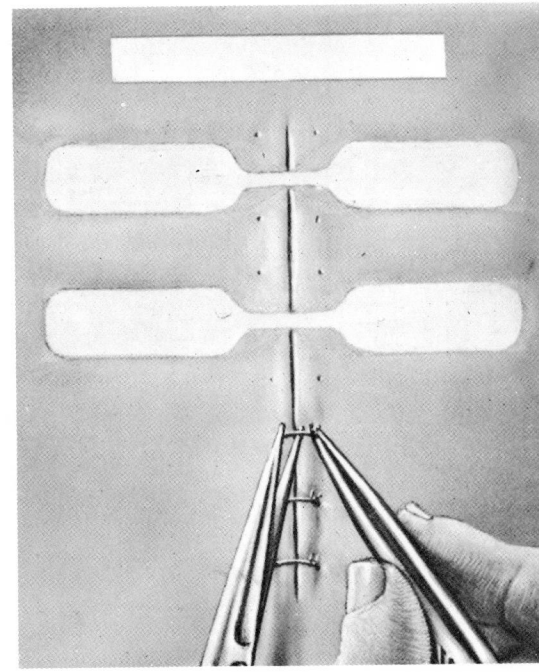

Figure 2-9. Suture removal. It is always well to use butterfly strips after stitches are removed to prevent separation of the edges and the possible formation of a wide scar due to lateral traction of the tissues. The strips should be left on for at least one week, covered by a protective gauze dressing kept in place only by long, narrow strips of tape. The strips shown on this page are butterfly closures, which are sterile, waterproof, and ready to use. (© Johnson & Johnson 1972. Used by special permission of Johnson & Johnson, the copyright owners, and not to be reproduced for any purpose without Johnson & Johnson's permission.)

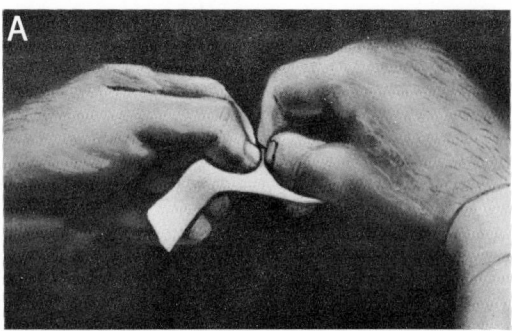
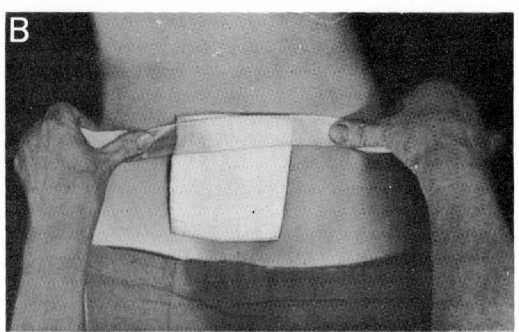

Figure 2-10. Applying tape. *A.* When scissors are not at hand, adhesive tape can readily be torn by holding the strip of tape between the thumbnail and forefingers, as illustrated. Tearing is started by a quick rotary twist of the hands in opposite directions.

   B. To avoid undue traction on the skin beneath adhesive tape, thus lessening trauma and reducing the possibility of irritation, place tape on the dressing and affix to the skin on either side so that tension is applied evenly away from the midline of the dressing. (© Johnson & Johnson 1972. Used by special permission of Johnson & Johnson, the copyright owners, and not to be reproduced for any purpose without Johnson & Johnson's permission.)

Nursing Action	Rationale/Amplification
Follow-up Care	
1. Make patient comfortable.	
2. Remove emesis basin and dispose of soiled dressings in proper receptacle. Discard disposable items and clean equipment which is to be reused.	2. To prevent transmission of pathogenic organisms.
3. Record nature of procedure and condition of wound as well as patient reaction.	

GUIDELINES: *Dressing a Draining Wound*

Reinforcement of Dressings

Draining wounds may require frequent changes of dressings.

   Outer layers may be removed and fresh dressings applied without disturbing wound site.
   a. Saturated dressings cause discomfort to the patient.
   b. Dressing edges may become dry, hard and scratchy.
   c. Odor may be unpleasant.

Auxiliary Aids to Facilitate Dressing Changes

A. *Montgomery Straps*

   Strips of adhesive tape, the ends of which have been folded back for a short distance with a small hole cut in the folded portion and threaded with gauze strips or cotton tape. Two opposing strips are brought together and the tapes tied (Fig. 2-11).

B. *Scultetus Binder*

   A many-tailed binder which when applied snugly (starting at the lower end) produces a comfortable and conforming support for the patient (Fig. 2-12).

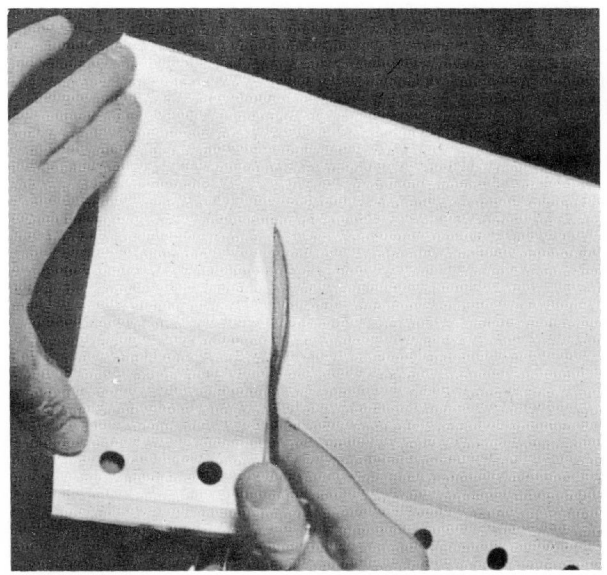
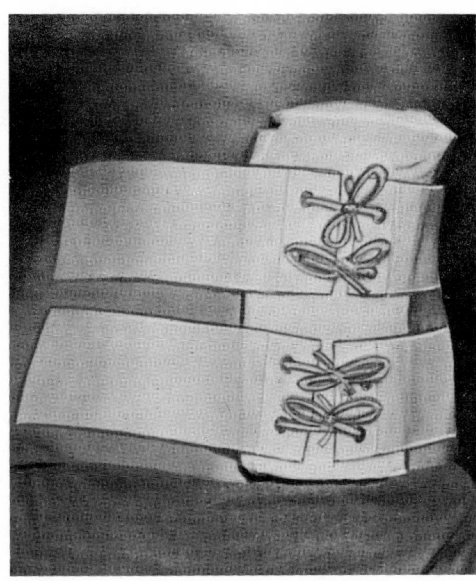

Figure 2-11. Use of Montgomery straps. Montgomery straps consist of strips of adhesive tape, the ends of which have been folded back for a short distance, with a small hole cut in the folded portion and threaded with gauze strips of cotton tape. Two opposing strips are brought together and the tapes tied. This type of tie obviates the need of new adhesive strips at each change and is especially useful when dressings must be changed frequently. These are now available ready-prepared in convenient form, providing the advantage of a hyporeactive acrylic mass and permeable cloth backing.

Instead of tied strips, another method frequently used to join Montgomery straps is to place safety pins through holes on each side and then hook a strong rubber band into the opposing pins. The rubber allows a slight "give" with body movement and the dressings are readily changed by merely unsnapping the safety pins on one side. (© Johnson & Johnson 1972. Used by special permission of Johnson & Johnson, the copyright owners, and not to be reprinted for any purpose without Johnson & Johnson's permission.)

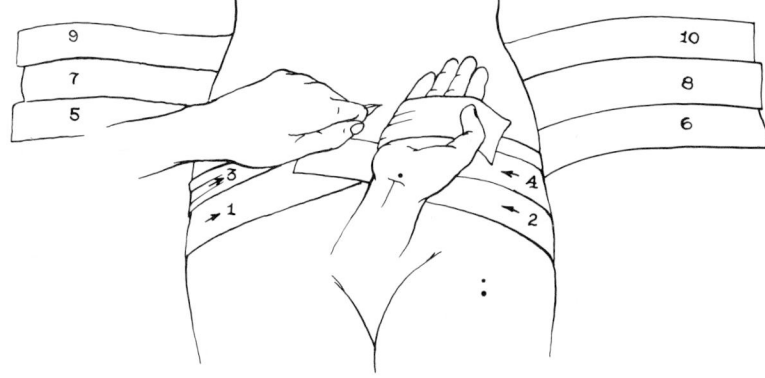

Figure 2-12. Procedure for applying a many-tailed binder. (From Fuerst, E. V., and Wolff, L.: Fundamentals of Nursing, 5th ed. Philadelphia, J. B. Lippincott, 1974.)

Removal of Adherent Dressings

1. To prevent the discomfort of removing dry sticking dressings, moisten the dressing with peroxide of hydrogen using an asepto-bulb syringe.
2. Provide an emesis basin to catch excess fluid.

Anchoring and Gradual Withdrawal of Drainage Tubes

1. With each dressing change, the drainage tube is often pulled out of the wound a few centimeters and the excess tube is cut.
2. Hollow hard rubber or polyethylene tubes are used occasionally to drain a cavity. After the tube is anchored with a suture, the tube is taped to the skin.
   a. Cut a 5-cm. (2-inch) length of adhesive tape; trifurcate the tape lengthwise to the middle.
   b. Place right half of tape on skin up to emerging rubber drain; allow 2 end tails to straddle tube and neatly fasten middle tail around drain in a spiral fashion.
   c. Repeat process in opposite direction. Then place 2 cross strips of 5-cm. (2-inch) adhesive tape on either side of drain.

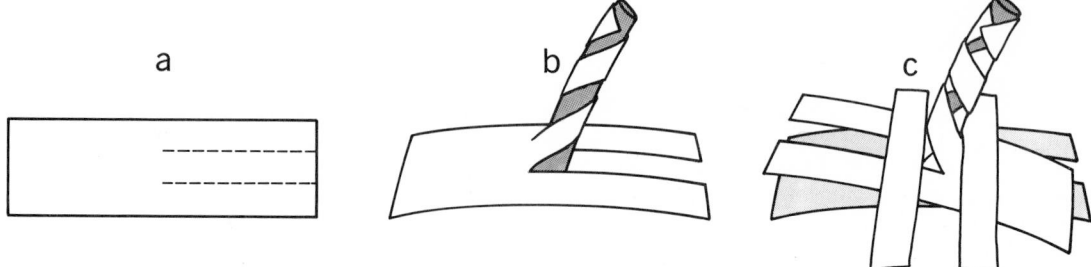

3. Penrose tube with a safety pin or a Taut "Safety Klip".
   For the drain, such as a penrose, which is drawn out of the wound a few centimeters each day, a safety pin or Taut "Safety Klip" is positioned to prevent the drainage tube from slipping back into the wound (see Fig. 2-13).

Skin Care

1. Drainage is often irritating to surrounding skin tissues.
2. Apply protective ointment.
   a. Petrolatum gauze
   b. Zinc oxide ointment
3. Recognize value of portable wound suction in maintaining cleanliness of surrounding tissues (p. 70).
4. Attach drainage tubing to suction bottle.
   Check tubing frequently for kinking or looping which would restrict flow of drainage.

GUIDELINES: *Using Portable Wound Suction*
(HemoVac, Porto-Vac)

Portable wound suction is a suction system (approximately 30 mm. Hg) which gently removes adventitious fluid and debris from a wound by means of a perforated catheter connected to a portable suction apparatus.

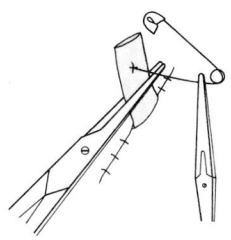

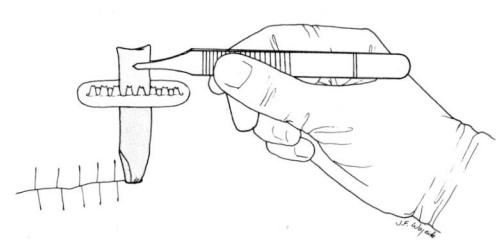

1.
Grasp pin with a hemostat, and the drain with a dressings forceps or another hemostat. Insert pin into drain distal to where it is being held by forceps.

4.
Advance drain with a dressing forceps.

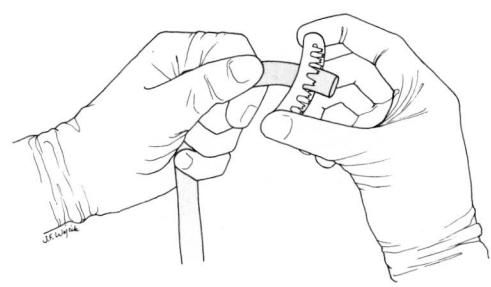

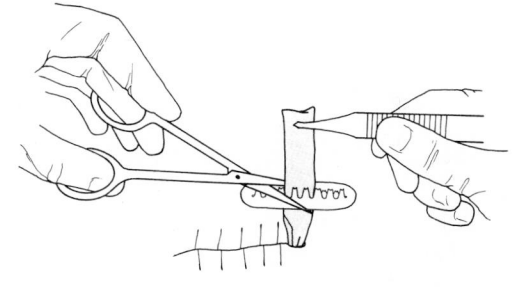

2.
Bend Taut sterile "Safety Klip" to spread teeth. Push drain through opened teeth.

5.
Using opened surgical scissors, slide down "Safety Klip." A dressing can be placed between "Klip" and wound.

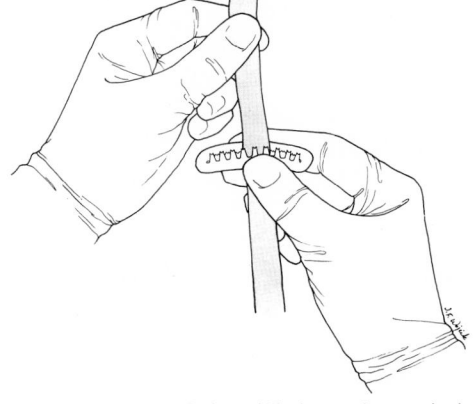

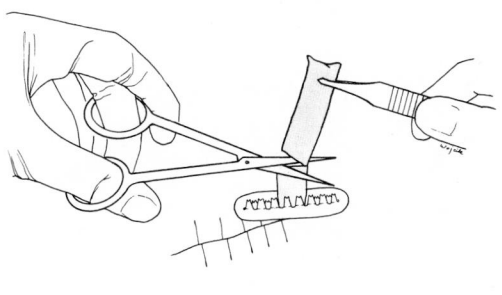

3.
Pull drain through "Safety Klip" evenly to desired position.

6.
Cut excess drain.

Figure 2-13. Anchoring a drainage tube with a Taut "Safety Klip." (Courtesy Taut Inc. for American Hospital Supply.)

Equipment

1. A long (⅛–¼ inch) (0.25–0.5 cm.) malleable stainless steel introducing needle with a cutting edge on one end and a fine screw thread at the other.
2. A long 0.25 cm. (⅛ inch) calibre, siliconized, noncollapsible, polyethylene catheter with many small perforations in the center.
3. A noncollapsible, siliconized, polyethylene connecting tube. The wound catheter fits snugly into the lumen of this tube.
4. A vacuum source (evacuator) consisting of an unbreakable plastic container with rigid ends and collapsible sides (may be a size to collect 200, 400 or 800 ml. of fluid).
   Box has 1 cuffed hole into which the connecting tube fits snugly and an airhole

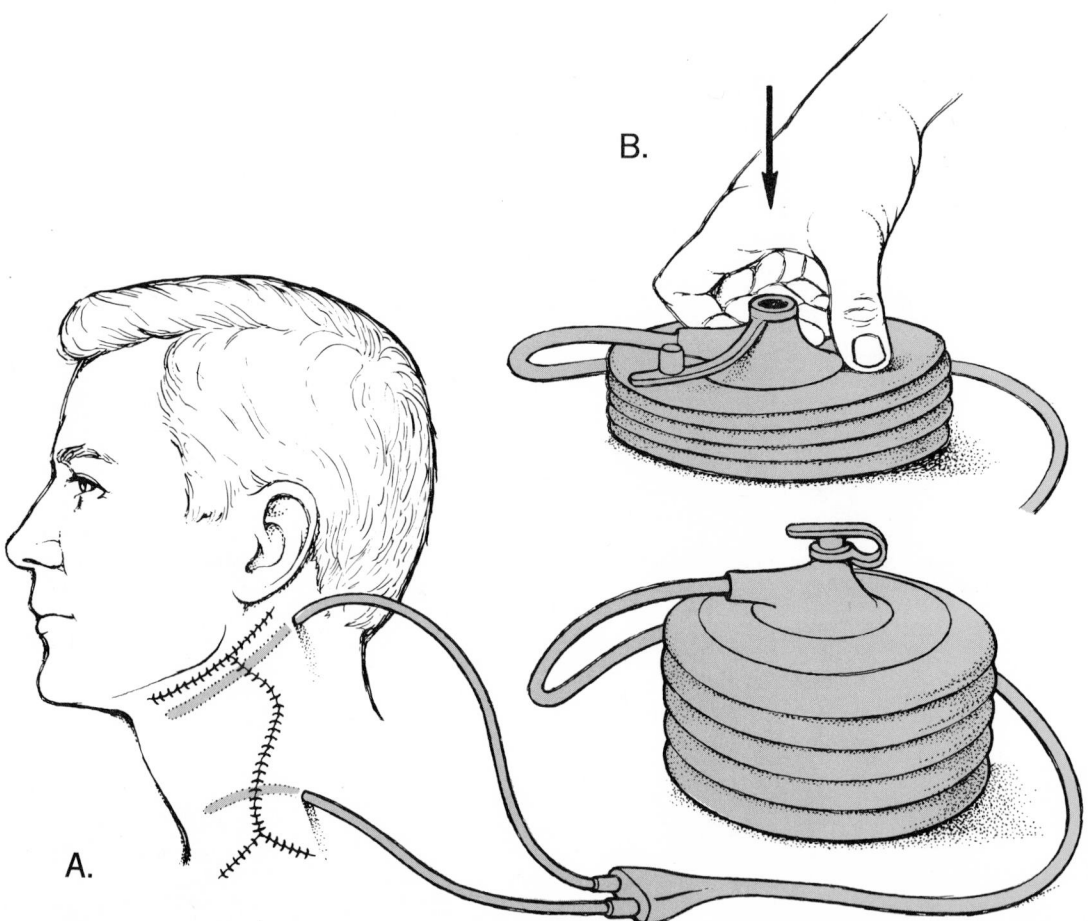

Figure 2-14. A. Two perforated catheters are draining the incisional area following a radical neck dissection. By means of a Y-tube, drainage is drawn into a portable wound suction receptacle. When full, open top plug of receptacle and empty.

B. To re-establish negative pressure, compress receptacle as indicated and replace plug; suction drainage will resume.

supplied with a plug. This box may be accordion-like collapsible plastic or it may have steel coil springs on the inside to hold the ends of the box apart.
5. A plastic Y-connector which fits between wound catheters and connecting tube and allows 2 wound tubes to be connected to 1 evacuator if desired.

Method of Inserting Drainage Tube(s)

1. In the operating room, the surgeon places the perforated drainage tubing in the desired wound area.
2. A stab wound is made with the needle end and excess tubing is drawn through the wound (stab wound is preferred because a more seal-tight porthole is created; if the wound opening is used, drainage may seep through the incision line).
3. Needle is cut off and tubing is attached via adaptor to evacuator tubing (Fig. 2-14).

Method of Initiating Suction

Nursing Action	*Rationale / Amplification*
1. Connect tubes to evacuator.	
2. Squeeze ends of box together.	2. This will expel air.
3. Plug air hole.	3. To create a negative pressure.
4. As spring expands, a negative pressure of approximately 45 mm. Hg is produced.	4. Any fluid and blood in tissues is sucked into evacuator. Negative pressure is not great enough to suck the soft tissues into the holes of the catheters.
5. When evacuator is full (200, 400, or 800 ml.— depending upon size of evacuator), it is time to empty.	5. Negative pressure has been fully dissipated.

Emptying Evacuator

1. Carefully remove plug, maintaining its sterility.	
2. Empty contents of evacuator into calibrated container.	2. Measure drainage.
3. Place evacuator on flat surface.	3. To permit adequate compression.
4. Cleanse opening as well as plug with an alcohol sponge.	4. To maintain cleanliness of outlet.
5. Compress evacuator completely (Fig. 2-14).	5. To remove air.
6. Replace plug while evacuator is compressed.	6. To re-establish negative pressure (suction).
7. Check system for proper operation.	7. Look for fluid entering receptacle.
8. Record character and amount of drainage.	

Wound Irrigation Combined with Portable Wound Suction

1. Perforated wound tubes are placed side to side in wound (Fig. 2-15A); One is connected to irrigating fluid (or antibiotic solution), the other to portable wound suction.
2. At least 30% of the perforated section of one tube should be positioned to the perforated area of the other.
3. If tubes are to remain for some time, a suture (usually stainless steel wire) is used (note arrow in Fig. 2-15B).
4. By having the drainage tube exit through a stab wound (away from main incision line) it is convenient to manipulate, inspect and remove the drainage tube without disturbing the wound dressing.
5. After drip fluid has been stopped, all remaining tubes should have suction applied for at least 48 hours.

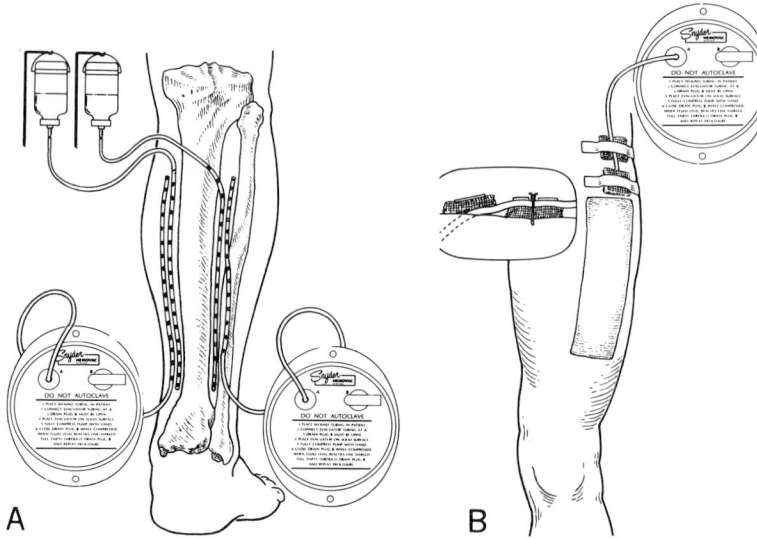

Figure 2-15. A. An example of an efficient antibiotic drip and suction system. Note that the perforated wound tubes lie parallel to each other (intake and output).

B. When drainage of long duration is anticipated, the wound-drainage tubing can be fixed (so that it won't slip out of the wound) by a stainless steel wire suture (size 40 or 50) as the magnified drawing indicates. The drainage tubing is cushioned on a pad of gauze. (Courtesy Zimmer, U.S.A., Warsaw, Ind.)

Tube Removal

1. At conclusion of use, discard tubing and evacuator by placing in a paper bag and depositing in trash container for incineration.
2. See Guideline: Assisting with a Change of Surgical Dressings (p. 64).

POSTOPERATIVE DISCOMFORTS

Vomiting

Incidence

1. Occurs in many postoperative patients.
2. Results from an accumulation of fluid or food in the stomach before peristalsis returns.
3. May occur as a result of abdominal distention which follows manipulation of abdominal organs.
4. Induced during anesthesia from inadequate ventilation.
5. Likely to occur if the patient believes preoperatively that he will vomit (psychological induction).

Preventive Measures

1. Insert nasogastric tube preoperatively for operations on gastrointestinal tract to prevent abdominal distention which triggers vomiting.
2. Determine whether patient is susceptible to morphine and meperidine (Demerol) since they may induce vomiting in some patients.
3. Be alert for any significant comment such as "I just know I will vomit under anesthesia." Report such a comment to the anesthesiologist who may prescribe an antiemetic drug and also talk to the patient before the operation.

Treatment and Nursing Management

1. Support the wound during retching and vomiting.
2. Discard vomitus and refresh patient with mouthwash, clean linens, etc.
3. Suspect idiosyncracy to a drug if vomiting is worse when a medication is given (but diminishes thereafter).
4. Administer antiemetic medication such as prochlorperazine (Compazine).
5. Offer hot tea with lemon or small sips of a carbonated beverage such as ginger ale, if tolerated.
6. Report excessive or prolonged vomiting so that the cause may be investigated.

Restlessness and Sleeplessness

Promoting Factors	*Relief Measures*
1. Discomfort such as back pain, headache and thirst	1. Massage the back gently using an emollient lotion. Administer acetylsalicylic acid as prescribed.
2. Tight dressings or drainage-soaked dressings.	2. Change dressings and check for tightness.
3. Urinary retention	3. Utilize nursing measures to initiate voiding (see p. 82).
4. Abdominal distention	4. Insert rectal tube to relieve flatus—stimulates peristalsis and propels gas to rectum.
5. Noise and environmental stimuli	5. Keep noise level at a minimum. Limit visitors. For rest periods, provide privacy, darkness and quiet.
6. Worry and anxiety	6. Attempt to find cause of concern. Provide time to talk with the patient and permit him to vent his feelings. Seek advice of spiritual counselor or psychologist if necessary. Offer sedatives or hypnotics as required.

Thirst

Causes

1. Inhibition of secretions by preoperative medication of atropine.
2. Fluid lost via perspiration, blood loss.

Nursing Management

1. Administer fluids by vein or by mouth if tolerated.
2. Offer sips of hot tea with lemon juice to dissolve mucus.
3. Apply a moistened gauze square over lips occasionally to humidify inspired air.
4. Allow patient to rinse mouth with mouthwash; lemon juice and glycerin swabbing of the mouth is also refreshing.
5. Obtain hard candies or chewing gum to help in stimulating saliva flow and keeping the mouth moist.

Constipation

Causes
1. Trauma and irritation to the bowel during surgery.
2. Local inflammation, peritonitis or abscess.
3. Long-standing bowel problem: This may lead to fecal impaction.

Preventive Measures
1. Early ambulation to aid in promoting peristalsis.
2. Adequate fluid intake to keep stool soft.
3. Proper diet to promote peristalsis and maintain adequate fluid balance.

Treatment (Fecal Impaction)
1. Administer an oil enema of 180–200 ml. to assist in softening the mass and helping in its evacuation.
2. Inject 30–60 ml. of peroxide of hydrogen into rectum; the foaming action may break up the fecal masses.
3. Insert a gloved finger and break up the impaction manually.

Pain

Pain is a subjective symptom in which the patient exhibits a feeling of distress caused by stimulation of certain nerve endings; usually it indicates that the beginning of tissue damage is taking place.

Clinical Manifestations
1. Autonomic
   a. Outpouring of epinephrine
   b. Elevation of blood pressure
   c. Increase in heart and pulse rate
   d. Rapid and irregular respiration
   e. Increase in perspiration
2. Skeletal muscle
   Increase in muscle tension or activity
3. Psychological
   a. Increase in irritability
   b. Increase in apprehension
   c. Increase in anxiety
   d. Attention focused on pain
   e. Complaints of pain

Patient's reaction depends upon:
1. Previous experience
2. Anxiety or tension
3. State of health
4. His ability to concentrate away from the problem or be distracted

Physiological and Psychological Observations
1. Pain is one of the earliest symptoms which the patient expresses upon return to consciousness.
2. Maximal postoperative pain occurs between 12 and 36 hours and usually disappears by 48 hours.
3. Anesthetic agents which are soluble are slow to leave the body and therefore control pain for a longer time than agents which are insoluble; the latter produce rapid recovery, but the patient is more restless and complains more of pain.

4. Older persons seem to have a higher tolerance for pain than younger or middle-aged persons.
5. There is no documented proof that one sex tolerates pain better than the other.
6. Psychological conditioning of the patient affects pain tolerance.
7. The quality of nurse-patient interaction may have a greater influence on relief from pain than does the medication.
8. The nurse may reduce the patient's need for pain relief by making him more comfortable physically; frequent change of position, back rubs, talking to him and letting him express his concern can help lower his anxiety level.
9. Patients who have had abdominal or chest surgery are more likely to need narcotics. The exchange of respiratory gases can be reduced by pain that causes reflex chest-muscle contraction.
10. Potent drugs such as morphine may produce depression of the patient's respiratory center thereby reducing rate and depth of breathing; also such drugs tend to constrict bronchiolar smooth muscles and increase tracheal bronchial secretions leading to atelectasis and pneumonia.

Nursing Management

1. Assess the nature, location, quality, intensity and duration of pain and record such evaluation.
   a. Ask the patient to point to the pain center.
   b. Find out what the patient *means* by pain.
   c. Determine whether the pain is associated with an activity, such as turning or taking a deep breath.
   d. Encourage the patient to describe the pain in his own words, e.g., stabbing, consistent, dull.
   e. Investigate possible causes of pain such as bandage or adhesive which is too tight or cast which is too snug.
2. Evaluate the patient's response to his pain.
   a. Observe the patient's facial expression and bodily movements as he experiences the pain.
   b. Is he pain-free when distracted by visitors or television?
   c. Does he appear to complain in anticipation of the next dose of medication?
   d. Help patient to express his angry feelings about pain and discomfort.
3. Employ comfort measures in caring for the patient.
   a. Provide therapeutic environment—proper temperature and humidity, ventilation, visitors.
   b. Determine patient's bodily comfort by adding blanket if he is cold, and vice versa.
   c. Massage his back in soothing strokes—move him easily and gently.
   d. Offer diversional activities, soft radio music, or favorite quiet television program.
   e. Provide for fluid needs by giving a cool drink, offering a bedpan.
4. Initiate measures to reduce the likelihood of pain.
   a. Encourage the patient to turn frequently.
   b. Massage pressure areas; support vulnerable areas—strategic placement of pillow, anchoring a footboard, placing a pillow between legs in the Sims's lateral position.
   c. Determine patient's need to void and need for relief from intestinal distention.
   d. Loosen constricting dressings.
   e. Keep bedding clean, dry and free from crumbs.
   f. Maintain the patient in correct physiological position.

    g. Encourage patient's verbalization to help reduce pain reaction and threshhold.

    h. Give analgesic drugs as prophylaxis to prevent pain.

5. Relieve localized pain.

    a. Carefully support the painful area and elevate painful extremities.

    b. Apply medications or counterirritants gently; use heat or cold applications as prescribed.

    c. Encourage and assist the patient to follow prescribed exercise program.

6. Recognize the power of suggestion that relief of pain will take place when a "reasonable" method is selected and used.

    a. Combine chosen method of pain-relief with verbal assurance that it will help.

    b. Explain why the method chosen will help in relieving pain—positive assurance has been recognized as enhancing the effect of the "reasonable" action.

    c. Indicate to the patient that you understand that he has pain, that you have time to listen and to help him and that you care.

7. Be selective in administering pain-relieving agents.

    a. Administer tranquilizers to relieve anxiety.

    b. Use narcotic analgesics where postoperative pain justifies such medication.

    c. Provide soporifics for sleep induction.

    d. Administer muscle-relaxant and antispasmodic medications for uncontrolled muscle tension.

    e. Utilize specific medications for specific conditions such as relief of nausea, relief of undesirable coughing, relief of headache.

8. Recognize desired effects and untoward reactions of all medications given.

    a. Observe patient for desired effect of medication.

    b. Be alert to toxic manifestations and hypersensitivity reactions.

    c. Be knowledgeable regarding drug interactions.

    d. Note signs of respiratory embarrassment, adverse vital signs, rashes.

POSTOPERATIVE COMPLICATIONS

Shock

Shock is a response of the body to a decreased circulating volume of blood.

Classification

1. *Oligemic* (hematogenic)—shock resulting from loss of plasma or whole blood; this may be external or internal. When 10% of the blood volume is lost, *hypovolemic* shock occurs.

2. *Bacteremic* (septic or toxic shock)—characterized by a change in the capillary endothelium, permitting loss of blood and plasma through capillary walls into surrounding tissues; no actual fluid volume is lost from the body.

3. *Cardiogenic*—observed when there is an interference of heart pumping action as might occur in myocardial infarction, cardiac tamponade, which results in inadequate vascular circulation.

4. *Neurogenic* (vasogenic)—marked vasodilation and reflex inhibition which results in sluggish circulating system, depriving vital centers of proper blood supply.

5. *Psychic*—results from extreme pain or deep fear.

Altered Physiology and Clinical Manifestations

1. Loss of effective circulating blood volume—initiates metabolic and physiologic reactions resulting in poor tissue perfusion.
2. Pituitary hormones are released
   ACTH (adrenocorticotropic)—stimulates the adrenal cortex to secrete glucocorticoids.
   ADH (antidiuretic)—stimulates kidney tubules to absorb more fluid.
   ASH (aldosterone-stimulating)—stimulates potassium excretion by kidney, stimulates sodium chloride retention and water retention.
3. Epinephrine and nonepinephrine promote capillary vasoconstriction—increases flow through vital organs but diminishes through peripheral tissues. Later, peripheral vasoconstriction produces *pale, cold, clammy skin.*
4. Acidemia causes lung to compensate—increased rate (tachypnea) and volume.
5. Heart rate accelerates; diastole lessened.
   Coronary perfusion occurs during diastole; with lessened perfusion, cardiac output falls resulting in *reduced systolic pressure* and *lowered pulse pressure* and generalized vasoconstriction.
6. Weak, thready pulse and subnormal temperature.
7. Lip cyanosis, circumoral pallor.
8. At first patient appears *nervous* and *apprehensive;* later, *apathy develops* and *sensations are dulled.*

Effects of Shock

1. Anoxia—lack of oxygen in the body
2. Anoxemia—decreased amount of oxygen in the blood
3. Hyperpyrexia—an excessive fever, about 42.2 to 42.8°C. (108–109°F.) which occurs shortly before death
4. Oliguria—decreased kidney secretion and urinary output
5. Anuria—absence of urinary secretion
6. Thrombosis with subsequent emboli due to blood stasis

Treatment and Nursing Management

Chief Objective: to restore circulating blood volume.

A. *Prophylactic Approach*
1. Prepare adequately the mental as well as physical condition of the patient.
2. Anticipate any complications that may arise during and after surgery.
3. Have blood available if there is any indication that it may be needed.
4. Measure accurately any blood loss.
5. Keep operative trauma to a minimum; minimize postoperative disturbance of the patient.
6. Anticipate progression of symptoms upon earliest manifestation.
7. Monitor vital signs frequently until they are stable.
8. Assess vital sign deviations; evaluate blood pressure in relation to other parameters.
9. Institute therapy immediately following an injury, etc., which is likely to lead to shock.
10. Recognize that blood pressure limits vary with individuals; in some patient 90/60 may be normal whereas in others it may indicate severe shock.

B. *Definitive Management*
1. Keep the airway patent!
   a. Use an airway or place an endotracheal tube.
   b. Remove oral and tracheal secretions.
   c. Institute resuscitative measures if necessary.
2. Arrest hemorrhage.
   Ascertain where hemorrhage is occurring; if external, utilize pressure control.
3. Place patient in most physiologically desirable position in shock (Fig. 2-16).
   a. Elevate the head on a pillow.
   b. Keep trunk horizontal.
   c. Elevate lower extremities about 20 to 30 degrees, keeping knees straight.

NURSING ALERT: Do not use Trendelenburg head-low position because (1) after initial increase of blood to the head, a reflex compensatory action takes place causing vasoconstriction thereby decreasing blood supply to the brain and (2) viscera tend to fall against the diaphragm causing increased resistance to breathing and inadequate ventilation.

---

4. Ensure an adequate venous return.
   a. Insert intravenous catheter for infusion in upper extremities; 2 may be required.
   b. Place a central venous pressure (C.V.P.) catheter in or near right atrium (see Fig. 5-3).
      (1) Note direction and degree of change from initial reading.
      (2) Utilize route established by C.V.P. catheter for emergency fluid volume replacement.
   c. Start plasma expanders if needed until whole blood is available.
   d. Begin blood transfusion when blood is available.
5. Obtain blood for determinations of pH, pO_2, pCO_2 and hematocrit.
   a. pH—may indicate acidosis resulting from anaerobic metabolism.
   b. pCO_2—assesses function of pulmonary alveolar membrane.

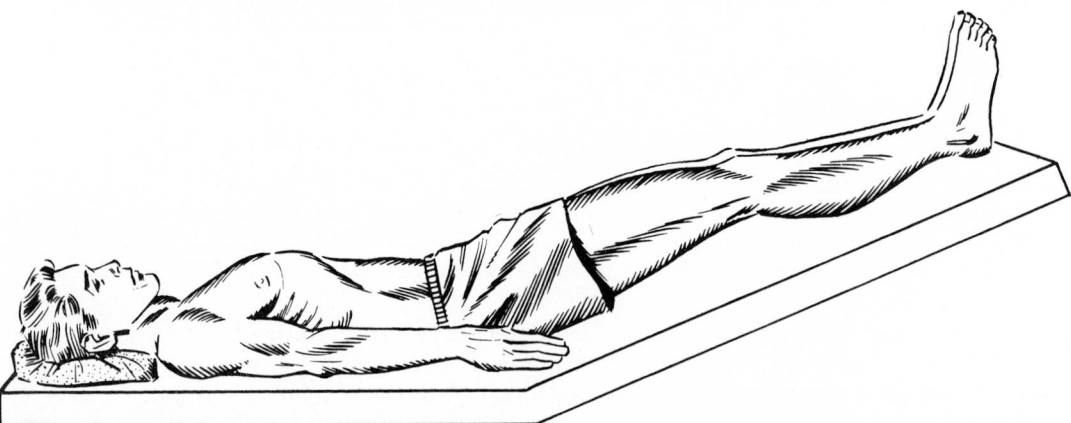

Figure 2-16. Proper positioning of the patient who shows signs of shock is to elevate the lower extremities about 20 degrees keeping the knees straight, trunk horizontal and head slightly elevated.

      c. pO_2—determines level of oxygen tension.

      d. Hematocrit—reveals losses due to obstruction or peritonitis.

  6. Insert a urinary catheter to monitor hourly urinary output.

      Objective is to maintain a 1 ml./kg./hr. urinary volume output to ensure adequate kidney perfusion.

  7. Administer antibiotics in order to offset infection which can occur due to stagnant hypoxia in wounds and in peripheral tissues.

      Utilize large doses of penicillin, streptomycin or broad-spectrum chemotherapeutic agents.

  8. Support the defense mechanisms of the patient.

      a. Comfort and reassure patient if he is conscious.

      b. Resort to sedation and analgesia with discriminating judgment.

      c. Keep the patient warm but do not apply too much external covering which will produce unnecessary vasodilation resulting in more fluid loss.

  9. Recognize signs of impending cardiac failure—increasing C.V.P., distended neck veins, pulmonary rales, etc.

      Initiate prophylactic digitalization

          Use rapid-acting medications in the very young and very old (digoxin, Cedilanid).

Hemorrhage

Hemorrhage is copious escape of blood from a blood vessel.

Classification

A. *General*

  1. *Primary*—occurs at the time of operation.

  2. *Intermediary*—occurs within the first few hours of surgery.

      Blood pressure returns to normal and causes loosening of poorly tied vessels and flushing out of weak clots from untied vessels.

  3. *Secondary*—occurs some time after surgery.

      a. Ligature slips from blood vessel.

      b. Erosion of blood vessel.

B. *According to Blood Vessels*

  1. *Capillary*—slow general oozing from capillaries.

  2. *Venous*—bleeding which is dark in color and bubbles out.

  3. *Arterial*—bleeding which spurts and is bright red in color.

C. *According to Location*

  1. *Evident or External*—visible bleeding on the surface.

  2. *Concealed or Internal*—bleeding which cannot be seen.

Clinical Manifestations

  1. Apprehension, restlessness, thirst; cold, moist, pale skin.

  2. Pulse increases, respirations become rapid and deep ("air hunger"), temperature drops.

  3. With progression of hemorrhage

      a. Decrease in cardiac output.

      b. Rapidly decreasing arterial and venous blood pressure as well as hemoglobin.

    c. Circumoral pallor, spots appear before the eyes, ringing in the ears.

    d. Patient grows weaker until death occurs.

Treatment and Nursing Management

1. Treat the patient as described for shock (p. 76).
2. Inspect the wound as a possible site of bleeding.
   If an extremity is bleeding, apply a gauze-pad pressure dressing.
3. Administer blood (typed) or blood substitute until blood is available.

NURSING ALERT: In giving fluids by vein recognize that, in the case of hemorrhage, giving too large a quantity or administering fluids too rapidly may elevate the blood pressure sufficiently to recycle the hemorrhaging process.

Femoral Phlebitis or Thrombophlebitis

Phlebitis often occurs after operations upon the lower abdomen or during the course of septic conditions such as ruptured ulcer or peritonitis.

Causes

1. Injury
   a. Damage to vein resulting from tight straps or leg holders during surgery.
   b. Compression of a blanket roll under the knees.
2. Fluid loss or dehydration leading to concentration of blood.
3. Lowered metabolism and circulatory depression after surgery leading to slowing of blood flow.
4. Combinations of the above.

Clinical Manifestations

1. Left leg appears to be affected more frequently than right.
2. Pain or cramp in the calf, progressing to painful swelling of entire leg.
3. Slight fever, chills, perspiration.
4. Marked tenderness over anteromedial surface of thigh.
5. Intravascular clotting without marked inflammation may develop leading to phlebothrombosis.

NURSING ALERT: A complaint of slight soreness of the calf is never ignored. The danger from femoral thrombosis is that a clot may be dislodged and produce an embolus.

Treatment and Nursing Management

A. *Prophylaxis*

1. Hydrate the patient adequately postoperatively to prevent blood concentration.
2. Encourage leg exercises and ambulate the patient as soon as permitted by the surgeon. (Exercises can be taught preoperatively—see pp. 15–16.)
3. Avoid any restricting devices such as tight straps that can constrict and impair circulation.
4. Prevent the use of bed rolls, knee gatches, even "dangling" over the side of the bed because there is danger of constricting the vessels under the knee.

B. *Active Therapy*
  1. Initiate anticoagulant therapy whether intravenously, intramuscularly or by mouth (see p. 323).
  2. Prevent swelling and stagnation of venous blood by wrapping the legs from the toes to the groin with elastic bandage or elastic stockings.
  3. Control pain in the extremities by bandaging.

Pulmonary Complications

Preventive Measures
  1. Report any evidence of upper respiratory infection to the surgeon.
  2. Postoperatively, initiate measures to prevent chilling.
  3. Aspirate secretions that might cause respiratory embarrassment.
  4. Recognize the predisposing causes of pulmonary complications:
      a. Infections—mouth, nose, throat
      b. Aspiration of vomitus
      c. History of heavy smoking, chronic respiratory disease
      d. Obesity
      e. Irritating effect of ether on mucous membranes.

Complications
  1. *Atelectasis*—collapse of pulmonary alveoli caused by a mucous plug closing a bronchus.
  2. *Bronchitis*—inflammation of bronchi causing a cough with considerable mucopus secretion.
  3. *Bronchopneumonia*—a chest complication with elevated temperature, pulse and respiratory rate plus a productive cough.
  4. *Lobar pneumonia*—onset of a chill followed by a high temperature, pulse and respiration elevation, flushed cheeks, respiratory embarrassment.
  5. *Hypostatic pulmonary congestion*—more common in the debilitated or elderly patient whose weakened heart and vascular system permit a stagnation of secretions at base of lungs.
  6. *Pleurisy*—knife-like pain in the chest on the affected side, particularly on intake of a deep breath, and elevated temperature, pulse and respirations.
  (For greater detail see Chapter 3, Conditions of the Respiratory System.)

Treatment and Nursing Management
  1. Appraise the patient's progress very carefully on a daily basis for the first postoperative week to detect early signs and symptoms of respiratory difficulties.
      a. Slight temperature, pulse and respiration elevations
      b. Apprehension and restlessness
      c. Complaints of chest pain, signs of dyspnea or cough
  2. Promote full aeration of the lungs
      a. Turn the patient frequently.
      b. Encourage the patient to take 10 deep breaths hourly.
      c. Utilize a spirometer or any device which encourages the patient to ventilate (blowing bubbles into a water bottle).
      d. Assist the patient in coughing in an effort to bring up mucous secretions.
      e. Permit the patient to ambulate as early as the physician will allow.

3. Initiate specific measures for particular pulmonary problems.
   a. Provide cool mist or steam (electric vaporizer) for the patient who exhibits signs of bronchitis.
   b. Encourage the patient to take fluids and expectorants if he appears to be developing pneumonia.
   c. Administer antibiotics for patients with pulmonary infections.
   d. Prevent distention since this causes pulmonary and circulatory embarrassment.
   e. Provide a tight adhesive strapping to cope with the knife-like chest pain or pleurisy. Make sure patient is breathing deeply every hour.
   f. Note that the patient having pleurisy with effusion may need chest aspiration; have a thoracentesis tray ready and be prepared to assist.
   g. Be prepared to administer oxygen to assist in aeration of the lungs for oxygenation of blood.

Pulmonary Embolism

An *embolus* is a foreign body in the bloodstream—usually a blood clot that has become dislodged from the original site. When such a clot is carried to the heart, it is forced into the pulmonary artery or one of its branches. (See also p. 155.)

Clinical Manifestations

1. Sharp, stabbing pains in the chest
2. Anxiousness and cyanosis
3. Pupillary dilatation, profuse perspiration
4. Rapid and irregular pulse becoming imperceptible—leads rapidly to death.

Immediate Treatment

1. Administer oxygen and inhalations with the patient in an upright sitting position.
2. Reassure and quiet the patient.
3. Administer morphine to control panic.

Urinary Difficulties

Retention of Urine

1. *Incidence*—occurs most frequently after operations on the rectum, anus, vagina, or lower abdomen, and is due to spasm of bladder sphincter.
2. *Nursing Measures*
   a. Assist patient to sit or even stand up (if permissible) since many patients are unable to void in bed.
   b. Provide the patient with privacy.
   c. Utilize the psychological aid of running the tap water—frequently the sound or sight of running water relaxes the spasm of the bladder sphincter.
   d. Catheterize only when all other measures are unsuccessful.
      (1) May lead to possible bladder infection.
      (2) Subsequent catheterizations are often required.

NURSING ALERT: Recognize that when a patient voids very small amounts (30–60 ml. every 15–30 minutes) this may be a sign of overdistended bladder ("overflow of retention").

Urinary Incontinence

1. *Cause*—loss of tone of the bladder sphincter.
2. *Incidence*—occurs as a complication in the aged after surgery or shocking injury.
3. *Recovery*—disappears as patient gains strength and muscle tone.
4. *Management*
   a. Offer a bedpan hourly (see p. 765 for management of neurogenic bladder).
   b. Provide extra padding under patient; use special disposable pants.
   c. Initiate a consistent plan for special care of the skin to avoid skin breakdown.

Intestinal Obstruction

Causes

1. May occur following surgery on lower abdomen and pelvis, especially when there is drainage.
2. A loop of intestine may kink because of inflammatory adhesions.
3. A loop of intestine may become involved in the drainage tract.

Clinical Manifestations

1. Most commonly occurs between the 3rd and 5th postoperative day.
2. Sharp colicky abdominal pains with pain-free intervals.
3. Pain is localized and should be noted since it may become more generalized later; locale may pinpoint source of difficulty.
4. Peristaltic activity can be assessed by listening to the abdomen with a stethoscope.
5. Pain-free intervals grow shorter as time advances.
6. With completion of obstruction, intestinal contents back up into stomach causing vomiting.
7. Abdominal distention and perhaps hiccups occur, but no bowel movements.
8. Following simple enema, returns are clear indicating very little of intestinal contents have reached large intestines.
9. If obstruction is not relieved, vomiting continues, distention becomes more pronounced, pulse increases, shock develops and death occurs.

Treatment

1. Relieve abdominal distention by passing a nasoenteric suction tube.
2. Administer body-deficient electrolytes per intravenous infusion.
3. Consider surgical intervention if obstruction continues unresolved (see p. 407).

Hiccup (Singultus)

Hiccups are intermittent spasms of the diaphragm causing a sound ('hic') that results from the vibration of closed vocal cords as air rushes suddenly into the lungs.

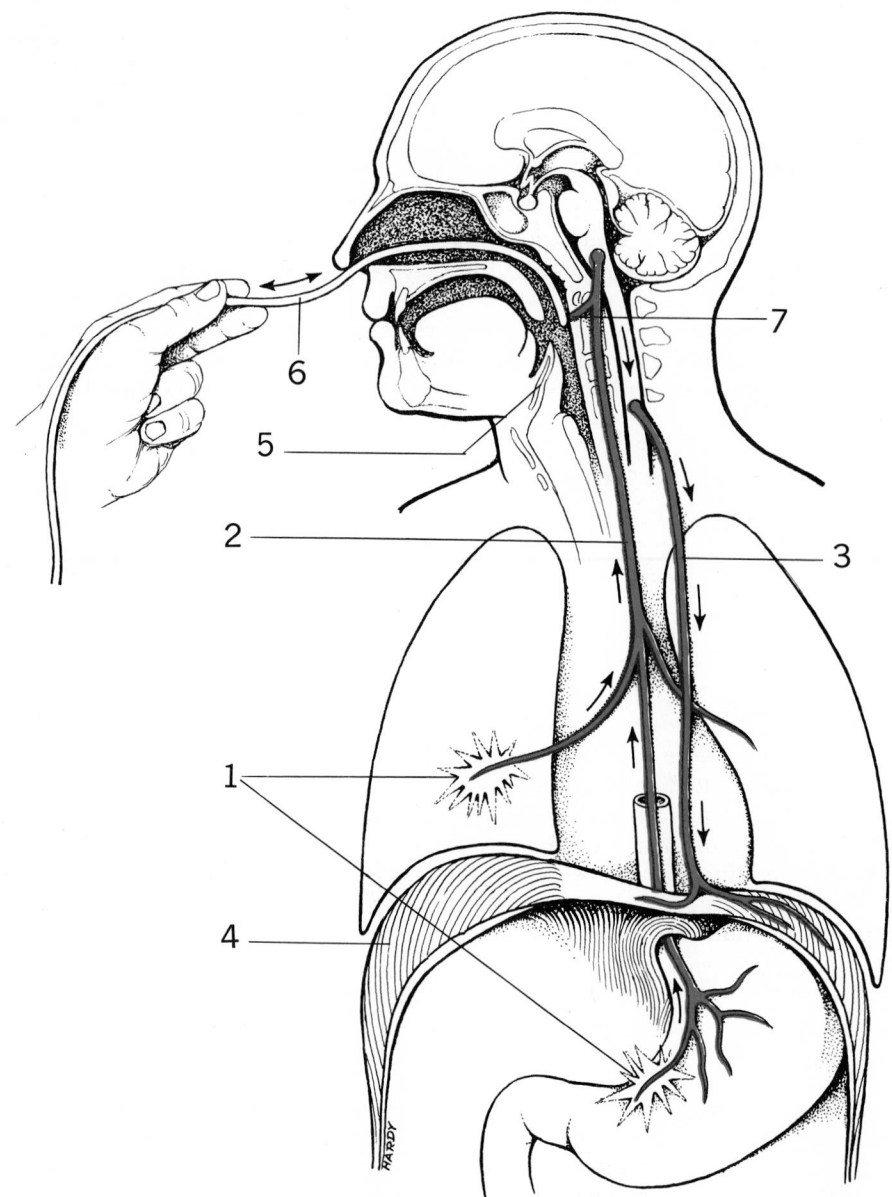

Figure 2-17. Controlling hiccups. Irritations in chest or abdomen (1) are transmitted by the vagus nerve (2). The reflex arc is completed by the transmission of the impulses to the diaphragm by the phrenic nerve (3). This causes contraction of the diaphragm (4) resulting in sudden intake of breath, which in turn is suddenly interrupted by rapid closure of the glottis (5). This is the hiccup.

Introduction of the No. 16 F catheter into the nasopharynx about 7.5–10 cm. (3 to 4 inches) (6) stimulates the pharyngeal branches of the vagus nerve (7) and interrupts the reflex arc stopping the hiccups.

Cause

Irritation of phrenic nerve between spinal cord and terminal ramifications on under-surface of diaphragm.

    a. *Direct*—distended stomach, peritonitis, abdominal distention, chest pleurisy or tumors pressing on nerves

    b. *Indirect*—toxemia, uremia

    c. *Reflex*—exposure to cold, drinking very hot or very cold liquids, intestinal obstruction

Treatment

1. Remove the cause if possible.
   a. Gastric lavage for gastric distention
   b. Adhesive strapping in pleurisy
   c. Removal of drainage tubes causing irritation
2. When removal of cause is not possible, simple favorite remedies may be tried.
   a. Holding breath while taking large swallow of water.
   b. Applying finger pressure on the eyeballs through closed lids for several minutes.
   c. Inhaling carbon dioxide (breathing in and out of a paper bag).
3. Introduce a catheter (No. 16 F.) into the patient's pharynx about 7–10 cm. (3–4 inches); rotate gently and jiggle back and forth; this action interrupts impulses from vagus nerve and hiccups stop (Fig. 2-17).

Wound Complications

Hemorrhage and Hematoma

A. *Manifestations*
1. Inspect dressings frequently during first 24 hours postoperatively.
   a. Note evidence of bright red blood on dressings.
   b. Look for bulging which may indicate bleeding and clot formation (hematoma) under the skin.
   c. Examine bedding directly underneath incision site for evidence of trickling ooze.
   d. Check drainage bottle for undue amount of red drainage.
2. Check vital signs for evidence of bleeding—elevated pulse, apprehension, air hunger (see p. 79).

B. *Treatment*
1. Notify physician.
2. If bleeding continues, it may be necessary for the patient to return to surgery to have bleeding vessel ligated, to remove large hematoma, to resuture wound.

Infection

A. *Causative Organisms*
1. *Staphylococcus aureus*
2. *Escherichia coli*
3. *Proteus vulgaris*
4. *Pseudomonas aeruginosa*

B. *Prophylaxis*
  1. Strict asepsis when wound is made and later during wound management.
  2. Housekeeping cleanliness and pertinent patient instruction concerning dressings.
C. *Clinical Manifestations*
  1. Wound tenderness and swelling—apparent in 36 to 48 hours
  2. Elevated pulse and temperature
D. *Treatment*
  1. Surgeon removes one or more stitches, separates wound edges and examines for infection using a hemostat as a probe.
  2. A culture is taken and sent to the bacteriology laboratory.
  3. Wound irrigation may be done; have asepto syringe and saline available.
  4. A drain (rubber or gauze) may be inserted.
  5. Antibiotics are prescribed.
  6. Hot wet dressings may be suggested.

Rupture (Dehiscence, Disruption, Evisceration)
A. *Causes*
  1. The wounds of elderly patients do not heal as readily as those in younger patients.
  2. Pulmonary and cardiovascular diseases contribute to wound breakdown since there is impairment in getting nutritional essentials to the wound (circulatory and pulmonary difficulties).
B. *Prophylaxis*
  1. Apply a scultetus binder for heavy or elderly patients or those with weak or pendulous abdominal walls.
  2. Encourage proper nutrition with emphasis on adequate amounts of protein and vitamin C.
C. *Clinical Manifestations*
  1. Patient complains that something suddenly gave way in his wound.
  2. In an intestinal wound, the edges of the wound may part and the intestines may gradually push out—observe for drainage of peritoneal fluid on dressings.
D. *Treatment*
  1. Notify surgeon immediately.
  2. If intestines are exposed, cover with sterile dressings.
  3. Instruct patient to bend his knees—relieves tension on abdomen.
  4. Assure the patient that his wound will be properly cared for; keep him quiet and relaxed.
  5. Prepare patient for surgery and repair of the wound.

Postoperative Psychological Disturbances

Delirium is a mental aberration which occurs only occasionally in some postoperative patients.

Classification
A. *Toxic*
  1. *Incidence*—occurs in combination with symptoms of general toxemia, e.g., peritonitis, sepsis.

2. *Symptoms*—acutely ill, restless patient with elevated temperature and pulse, flushed face, bright and roving eyes—indicates mental confusion.
3. *Treatment*
   a. Administer fluids to aid in elimination of toxins.
      NOTE: Not all delirious patients can tolerate fluids. It is also inappropriate to administer fluids if it may lead to cerebral fluid retention and delirium; treatment in this instance is fluid restriction.
   b. Control infection by giving the proper antibiotics.

B. *Traumatic*
   1. *Incidence*—develops following sudden trauma, particularly in the highly nervous person.
   2. *Symptoms*—manifests itself by wild excitement, hallucinations, delusions or melancholic depression.
   3. *Treatment*
      a. Administer tranquilizing medications; chlorate hydrate, paraldehyde.
      b. This state of delirium begins and ends abruptly.

C. *Delirium Tremens*
   1. *Incidence*—patients who have used alcohol excessively are poor surgical risks and take anesthetic agents poorly.
   2. *Symptoms*—postoperatively, after continued abstinence from alcohol, patient shows signs of delirium tremens.
      a. Restless, nervous, easily irritated.
      b. Sleeps poorly, disturbed by unreal dreams, momentarily appears to be in a strange place and does not know nursing or medical staff.
      c. Later, loses control of mental functions; his mind is filled with haunting hallucinations that torment him constantly.
      d. Additional symptoms include sleeplessness, excessive perspiration and a marked tremor of the limbs. Patient eventually becomes stuporous.
   3. *Medical and Nursing Management*
      a. Administer sedatives to keep the patient quiet and comfortable; stimulation may be required by older alcoholics in the form of whisky or strychnine.
      b. Give glucose intravenously and concentrated vitamins by mouth to control nutritional deficiencies.
      c. Recommend that the patient remain in bed; it may be necessary to restrain him so that injuries are minimized. (Bear in mind that restraining should be a last resort since this often makes such a patient quite rebellious.)
      d. Encourage ambulation as soon as the surgical condition permits.

BIBLIOGRAPHY

Books

Ballinger, W. F., et al.: Alexander's Care of the Patient in Surgery, 5th ed. St. Louis, C. V. Mosby, 1972.

Brunner, L. S., et al.: Textbook of Medical and Surgical Nursing, 2nd ed. Philadelphia, J. B. Lippincott, 1970, pp. 99–157.

Kinney, J. M. (ed.): Manual of Preoperative and Postoperative Care, 2nd ed. Philadelphia, W. B. Saunders, 1971.

McCaffery, M.: Nursing Management of the Patient with Pain. Philadelphia, J. B. Lippincott, 1970.

McGurn, W. C.: Mechanisms of shock: Pathophysiology, therapeutic measures and nursing intervention. *In* Kintzel, K. C. (ed.): Advanced Concepts in Clinical Nursing. Philadelphia, J. B. Lippincott, 1971, pp. 181–201.

Metheney, N. M., and Snively, W. D.: Nurse's Handbook of Fluid Balance. Philadelphia, J. B. Lippincott, 1974.

Nardi, G. L., and Zuidema, G. D.: Surgery, 3rd ed. Boston, Little Brown & Co., 1972.

Nealon, T. F., Jr.: Fundamental Skills in Surgery, 2nd ed. Philadelphia, W. B. Saunders, 1971.

Parenteral Administration. Published by Abbott Laboratories.

Peacock, E. E.: Wound healing and care of the wound. *In* Kinney, J. M. (ed.): Manual of Preoperative and Postoperative Care, 2nd ed. Philadelphia, W. B. Saunders, 1971, Chapter 1.

Randall, H. T., and Dudrick, S. J.: Surgical nutrition: parenteral and oral. *In* Kinney, J. M. (ed.): Manual of Preoperative and Postoperative Care, 2nd ed. Philadelphia, W. B. Saunders, 1971, Chapter 4.

Rhoads, J. E., et al.: Surgery—Principles and Practice, 4th ed. Philadelphia, J. B. Lippincott, 1970.

Snively, W. D., Jr., and Beshear, D. R.: Water and electrolytes in health and disease. *In* Kintzel, K. C. (ed.): Advanced Concepts in Clinical Nursing. Philadelphia, J. B. Lippincott, 1971, Chapter 12.

Articles

Auld, M. E., et al.: Wound healing. Nursing '72, 2:36–40, 1972.

Bergstrom, N. I.: Ice application to induce voiding. Amer. J. Nurs., 69:283–285, Feb. 1969.

Berry, M. A., and Kerlin, C. B.: The drops of life: Fluids and electrolytes. RN, 34:35–44, Sept. 1970.

Billars, K. S.: You have pain? I think this will help. Amer. J. Nurs., 70:2143–2145, Oct. 1970.

Cashatt, B.: Pain: a patient's view. Amer. J. Nurs., 72:281, Feb. 1972.

Duma, R. J., et al.: Septicemia from intravenous infusion. N. Eng. J. Med., 284:257–260, Feb. 4, 1971.

Ferguson, D. J.: Advances in the management of surgical wounds. Surg. Clin. N. Amer., 51:49–59, Feb. 1971.

Grooved clamp may cut slack on I.V. tubing (News). Med. World News, 11:16–17, Aug. 28, 1970.

Hills, N. H., and Calnan, J. S.: Deep vein thrombosis after surgery. Nurs. Mirror, 135:29–30, July 21, 1972.

Levine, D. C., and Fiedler, J.: Fears, facts, fantasies about pre- and postoperative care. Nurs. Outlook, 18:26–28, Feb. 1970.

Lipman, M.: Informed consent and the nurse's role. RN, 35:50, Sept. 1972.

Lindeman, C. A., and Van Aeram, B.: Nursing intervention with the presurgical patient—the effects of structured and unstructured preoperative teaching. Nurs. Research, 20:319–332, July-Aug. 1971.

Lowenbraun, S., et al.: Infection from intravenous "scalp-vein" needles in a susceptible population. JAMA, 212:451–453, April 20, 1970.

McBride, M. A.: The additive to the analgesic. Amer. J. Nurs., 69:974–976, May 1969.

Mezzanotte, E. J.: Group instruction in preparation for surgery. Amer. J. Nurs., 70:89–91, Jan. 1970.

Myers, M. B.: Sutures and wound healing. Amer. J. Nurs., 71:1725–1727, Sept. 1971.

Pederson, B. M.: A solution for post-infusion thrombophlebitis. Amer. J. Nurs., 70:325, Feb. 1970.

Powell, M.: An environment for wound healing. Amer. J. Nurs., 72:1862–1865, Oct. 1972.

Rodgers, B. P.: Therapeutic conversation and posthypnotic suggestion. Amer. J. Nurs., 72:714–717, April 1972.

Scribner, B. H., et al.: Long-term total parenteral nutrition. JAMA, 212:457–463, April 20, 1970.

Wilmore, D. W., and Dudrick, S. J.: Safe long-term venous catheterization, Arch. Surg., 98:256–258, Feb. 1969.

Wilmore, D. W.: The future of intravenous therapy. Amer. J. Nurs., 71:2334–2338, Dec. 1971.

Wolfer, J., and Davis, C.: Assessment of surgical patients' preoperative emotional condition and postoperative welfare. Nurs. Research, 19:402–419, Sept.-Oct. 1970.

3

Conditions of the Respiratory Tract

1. Conditions of the Nose and Throat

PROBLEMS OF THE NOSE

Epistaxis (Nosebleed)

Causes
1. May result from injury
   a. "Picking" nose or other trauma
   b. Deviated septum, perforated septum
2. May result from disease
   a. Acute rheumatic fever
   b. Acute sinusitis
   c. Arterial hypertension and hemorrhagic diseases
   d. Cancer

Treatment
1. Elevate trunk of body so that nose is above the level of the heart.
2. Promote vasoconstriction of nasal mucous membrane.
   a. Compress softer portion of nose against midline septum for 5–10 minutes.
   b. Instill vasoconstricting drug such as Neo-Synephrine, Adrenalin, silver nitrate stick.
3. Should above measures fail, it may be necessary for the physician to apply postnasal packing; remove packing after 24 hours.

Rhinitis

Rhinitis is an inflammation of the mucous membrane of the nose.

Clinical Manifestations
1. From allergic reaction, an infection (coryza) or early stage of viral infection.
2. Congested and swollen mucous membranes; when persistent → "chronic catarrh"
3. Chronic rhinitis → abnormally large amounts of connective tissue → spurs, polyps and hypertrophies on nasal septum → atrophy of mucous membrane and cartilage → abundant foul-smelling exudate (ozena).

Caution
Instruct patient as follows:
1. Do not blow nose too frequently or too hard.
2. Blow through both nostrils at same time to equalize pressure.

Nasal Obstruction

Causes
1. Deflected septum
2. Hypertrophy of turbinate bones
3. Polyps
4. Tumors
5. Common cold
6. Foreign bodies

Co-related Problems
1. Chronic infection of nose such as nasopharyngitis
2. Sinusitis which may include pain in sinus regions

Treatment
1. Nasal obstruction should be removed.
2. Measures to curb chronic infection employed.
    a. Nasal allergy corrected.
    b. Nasal sinuses drained (may be an operating room procedure).
    c. Submucous resection performed to remove deflected bone and cartilage.
    d. Nasal polyps clipped.
    e. Hypertrophied turbinates shrunk with astringent solutions.

Nursing Management
1. Raise head of bed to promote drainage, to make the patient more comfortable, and to lessen edema.
2. Administer frequent mouth care since patient is forced to breathe through his mouth.

Fracture of the Nose

Cause

Results from direct injury

Clinical Manifestations
1. Considerable bleeding from nostrils into pharynx
2. Marked swelling, deformity

Treatment and Nursing Management
1. Control bleeding by applying cold compresses.
2. Bone displacement determined by x-ray (this can also aid in determining skull involvement).
3. Under local or intravenous anesthesia, bones may be aligned.
    a. Proper nasal passageway re-established.
    b. Disfigurement minimized.
4. Nasal packing inserted; external splints applied.
5. Control swelling with ice compresses.
6. Administer analgesics for comfort.

SPECIFIC INFECTIONS OF THE UPPER RESPIRATORY TRACT

General Considerations

A. *Predisposing Conditions*

Nasal-septum and turbinate pathology, allergy, emotional problems

B. *Preventive Hygienic Measures*
1. Intended to support body defenses and reduce infection susceptibility.
2. Patient should set up a conscientious health regimen—adequate exercise, plenty of sleep, nutritious diet, relaxing hobbies.
    a. Avoid chilling, particularly of the feet since this lowers resistance.

    b. Employ humidifying measures indoors during winter months.
    c. Avoid emotionally upsetting experiences.
    d. Minimize indulgence in alcohol, smoking, drugs.
    e. Avoid inhaling irritating substances such as hair or other sprays, dust, chemicals, smoke, etc.

Streptococcal Sore Throat

Clinical Manifestations
1. Rapid onset of sore throat, chills, temperature above 38.3°C. (101°F.), headache, general malaise.
2. Children may have (in addition to the above) acute abdominal pain, nausea, perhaps repeated vomiting.
3. Red pharynx, enlarged tonsils and tonsillar nodes below angle of the mandible, edematous uvula.
4. Tonsils and pharynx may be covered with an exudate.
5. Flush face and leukocyte count over 12,000.

Treatment
Early intervention with chemotherapeutic agents is important to prevent serious complications such as acute rheumatic fever, acute glomerulonephritis.
    a. Penicillin is drug of choice—given for 10 days.
       Alternates are erythromycin, tetracycline, chlortetracycline.
    b. Administer intramuscularly.

Nursing Management
See page 267.

Adenoviral Infections

Types
A. *Acute Respiratory Disease (ARD)*

    Symptoms

Cold	Temperature elevation
Sore throat	Malaise
Headache	

B. *Pharyngoconjunctival Fever*
1. Duration—1 to 10 days
2. Symptoms (common in summer in children who swim in pools)

Fever	Headache
Sore throat	Hoarseness
Cold	Acute conjunctivitis
Large and tender cervical lymph nodes	Malaise

C. *Rhinoviral Infections*

    Examples: Common cold, croup and bronchitis which may lead to bronchopneumonia.

Treatment
1. Symptomatic
2. No specific antibiotic or chemotherapy

Herpes Simplex Infection

This infection produces common herpes labialis (fever blisters, cold sores, cankers).

Clinical Manifestations

1. Small vesicles, single or in groups, located on lips, tongue, cheeks, or pharynx.
2. Sore ruptures and becomes shallow ulcer covered with gray membrane.
3. Signs associated with other febrile conditions: pneumococcus pneumonia, meningo-coccal meningitis, malaise.
4. Virus remains latent in cells of lips or nose and is activated by febrile illnesses.

Treatment

1. Chemotherapy and antibiotics appear to be of no value.
2. Analgesics and perhaps codeine are helpful in relieving pain.
3. Spirits of nitre or campho-phenique applied locally are helpful in drying the lesion.

SINUSITIS

Sinuses are often involved in upper respiratory tract infections. Recovery is predicted on the condition that the nasal passage is clear. If passage is obstructed (blocked by deviated septum, polyps, spurs, enlarged turbinates) sinusitis may become chronic.

Acute Sinusitis

Clinical Manifestations

1. Pain
   a. Frontal headache—related to frontal sinusitis.
   b. In and about eyes—related to ethmoidal sinusitis.
   c. Lateral to nose, upper teeth—related to maxillary sinusitis.
   d. Occipital headache—related to sphenoidal sinusitis.
2. Nasal congestion and discharge may or may not be present.
3. Mild fever
4. Acute suppurative infection
   If frontal sinus involved, this can be serious because it may rupture posteriorly and lead to brain abscess.

Treatment

1. Bedrest
2. Drainage of sinuses
   a. Instill vasoconstrictor: Neo-Synephrine ¼% spray or drops.
   b. Use penicillin to speed recovery and diminish possibility of complications.
   c. Administer an antihistaminic.

Chronic Sinusitis

Clinical Manifestations

1. Persistent nasal obstruction
2. Cough—produced by constant dripping of discharge back into nasopharynx
3. Headache—more noticeable in the morning.

Treatment

1. Administration of vasoconstricting drugs to establish drainage.
   Recognize danger of prolonged use of nasal decongestants. It may lead to rhinitis and sinusitis.
2. Repair of structural deformities.
   a. Polyps excised or cauterized.
   b. Deviated septum removed.
3. Draining of sinuses.
   a. Frontal—incision through eyebrow
   b. Maxillary—Caldwell-Luc operation in which the incision is made along the upper gum line above canine teeth

PHARYNGITIS

Acute Pharyngitis

Acute pharyngitis is an inflammation of the throat accompanied by temperature elevation.

Clinical Manifestations

1. Reddened pharyngeal membrane
2. Swollen lymphoid follicles of throat
3. Enlarged cervical lymph nodes

Clinical Course

1. Viral; uncomplicated—patient may recover in 3 to 10 days.
2. Bacterial (beta hemolytic streptococcus, hemolytic *Staphylococcus aureus*, influenza); leads to more severe illness and danger of serious complications:
   Sinusitis, otitis media, mastoiditis, rheumatic fever, nephritis

Diagnostic Evaluation

Primarily by throat culture.

Nursing Management

1. Promote rest for the patient.
   a. Keep patient in bed during febrile stage.
   b. Encourage rest periods while he is ambulant.
2. Examine skin twice a day for telltale rashes indicating onset of a communicable disease.
3. Maintain medical asepsis to prevent spread of infection.
4. Assist in diagnostic evaluation by obtaining throat cultures, nasal swabbings, blood specimens.
5. Provide warm saline gargles or irrigations which approach the limit of heat tolerance for the individual (not to exceed 48.8°C. [120°F.]) to reduce pharyngeal muscle spasm and relieve throat soreness.
6. Offer symptomatic relief.
   a. Ice collar
   b. Analgesic medications—aspirin, codeine, and/or Darvon Compound 65, (propoxyphene hydrochloride and aspirin with phenaglycodol)

    c. Antitussive medications to control cough
    d. Soporific at bedtime
  7. Provide adequate mouth care for comfort and prevention of bacterial infection.
  8. Suggest a soft diet if the patient is able to swallow comfortably.
  9. Encourage fluids up to 2500 ml. a day if possible.

Convalescent Regimen

1. Assess morning and evening temperature to detect low grade infection or advent of a complication.
2. Promote rest and gradual resumption of full activity; advise patient to avoid over-exertion, chilling, fatigue, etc. which might promote the onset of a complication such as glomerulonephritis or rheumatic fever (onset occurs 2 to 3 weeks after pharyngitis subsides if it is of streptococcal origin).
3. Recognize onset of infections adjacent to the pharynx which might indicate extention of disease to the mastoid, ear, lymph nodes, etc.

Chronic Pharyngitis

Types

1. Hypertrophic—general thickening and congestion of pharyngeal mucous membrane.
2. Atrophic—characterized by a glistening thin whitish wrinkled membrane.
3. Chronic granular—numerous swollen lymph follicles.

Clinical Manifestations

1. Sense of fullness in throat, persistent irritation
2. Collection of mucus, expelled by coughing
3. Swallowing difficulty

Treatment

1. Tobacco and alcohol should be eliminated.
2. Patient should keep voice at rest.
3. Related problems (chest or upper respiratory) that may cause coughing should be corrected.

DISEASE OF THE TONSILS AND ADENOIDS

Tonsils

Tonsils are lymphatic tissue on each side of the oropharynx which are a common site of focal infection. Occasionally they grow to such a size that normal respiration is hampered.

Clinical Manifestations

1. Throat pain, ranging from mild to severe and accompanied by difficulty in swallowing, fever and swollen lymph glands in mandibular area.
2. Muscle, joint pain and frequently headache may accompany tonsillitis.
3. Inflamed edematous tonsillar area.
4. White or yellow spots which are exudate.

Treatment

1. Analgesics, such as codeine and aspirin
2. Warm throat irrigations
3. Rest
4. Antibiotics

Indications for Removal of Tonsils

1. Frequent infections, acute and/or chronic, where the recurrence rate is uncontrolled by antibiotics.
2. Hypertrophy that causes significant obstruction.

Adenoids

Adenoids are lymphatic tissue which when enlarged may obstruct nasal passages and cause headaches. Enlarged adenoids commonly accompany tonsillitis.

Chronic Adenoiditis

Produces frequent head colds, bronchitis, tonsillitis, nasal and eustachian-tube obstruction.
a. Mouth breathing, fetid breath
b. Voice impairment, snoring
c. Earaches, draining ears, mastoid infection

Tonsillectomy and Adenoidectomy

Nursing Management

A. *Immediate Nursing Concerns*
1. Reduce the possibility of postoperative bleeding and aspiration of blood and maintain a patent airway.
   a. Assess blood clotting time before surgery to determine possible needs during and after surgery.
   b. Place the patient in the sitting position postoperatively if he has had local anesthesia.
   c. Place the patient on the side with head extended and turned to allow drainage through nose and mouth (postgeneral anesthesia).
   d. Observe vital signs and recognize the changes which might indicate bleeding. (Watch for excessive swallowing—indicates bleeding.)
   e. Keep the patient as quiet as possible; excess activity will increase blood-flow rate which may overly tax suture line.
2. Minimize secretions in the throat during and after surgery and control pain.
   a. Administer atropine preoperatively.
   b. Give aspirin, Aspergum or dextropropoxyphene (Darvon) if prescribed.
   c. Place an ice collar around neck for comfort and to constrict blood vessels.

B. *Nursing Support During Convalescence*
1. Promote healing and be alert for evidence of postoperative complications.
   a. Suggest bland diet: ices, ice cream, fruit gelatin, custards, soft boiled egg, mashed potatoes, soft milk toasts, etc.
   b. Avoid serving excessively hot or cold beverages, spices, etc.
   c. Encourage rest and quiet activities during the first week.
   d. Add cooked vegetables, ground meat, as tolerated.

   e. Report any evidence of bleeding, particularly if its occurs on the 5th or 6th post-operative day; call the physician.
   f. Note any temperature elevation and if over a degree above normal, check with the physician.
2. Maintain cleanliness of the mouth to minimize infections and odors.
   a. Have the patient use mouth rinse frequently for comfort.
   b. See that patient brushes the teeth at least 3 times daily.
3. Provide comfort as the tonsillar and adenoidal beds heal.
   a. Utilize prescriptions for analgesics since the throat will be sore for several days.
   b. Recognize that occasionally this patient may experience earache; this is a referred pain which can be controlled by analgesics.

THERAPEUTIC ENDOTRACHEAL MEASURES

Tracheostomy

A *tracheostomy* is an external opening made into the trachea.

Purposes

1. To provide and maintain a patent airway.
2. To enable the removal of tracheobronchial secretions when the patient is unable to cough productively.
3. To permit the use of positive pressure ventilation.
4. To prevent aspiration of secretions in the unconscious (or paralyzed) patient by closing off the trachea from the esophagus.
5. To replace an endotracheal tube when such an airway is needed for more than 24 hours.

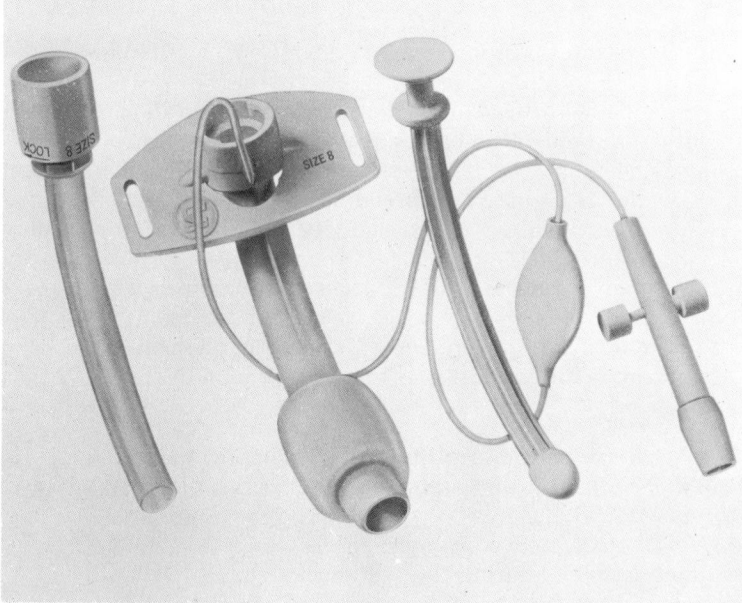

Figure 3-1. The disposable low pressure cuff tracheostomy tube consists of several parts: On the left is the translucent inner cannula that locks into the next piece, the outer cannula. Note the inflatable cuff encircling the outer cannula; this cuff is connected to an air line which emerges at the top of the tube and leads to an inflatable bag which is in turn connected to a pressure retention clamp. The clamp has a syringe connector at the extreme right of the illustration. The ribbed piece to the right of the tracheostomy tube is an obturator. (Courtesy Shiley Laboratories, Inc.)

Kinds of Tracheostomy Tubes

1. Jackson silver tracheostomy tube consisting of 3 parts: obturator (pilot), inner cannula, and outer cannula.
2. Jackson silver tracheostomy tube with Morch adaptor—similar to No. 1 with a screw-on swivel adaptor (on the inner cannula) to connect with a ventilator. Suction is permitted without disturbing respirator.
3. Endotracheal cuff may be attached to the cannula to provide a closed system (Fig. 3-1).
4. Plastic (nylon, polyvinyl chloride or silastic) tracheostomy tubes are available with or without inner tubes but usually with attached cuffs.

Performing a Tracheostomy

Done in the operating room—rarely in the patient's unit.

1. Practice sterile aseptic technique throughout.
2. Inject local anesthetic.
3. Vertical incision preferred; control bleeding before trachea is opened to prevent patient from aspirating blood.
4. Perform high tracheotomy preferably so that tip of cannula is well above carina.
5. Remove a segment of 3rd tracheal ring. (In children, ring is split but segment is not removed.)
6. Insert a dilator to permit insertion of No. 7 or No. 8 (adult) tracheostomy cannula.

Nursing Management

A. *Physical Care of Patient*

1. Provide adequate humidity since natural humidifying pathway of the oropharynx is no longer used.
2. Aspirate secretions since the patient's own cough mechanism is not as effective.
3. Suction gently to avoid injuring the epithelium; limit each suctioning time to between 10–15 seconds.
4. Introduce *sterile* aspirating tubes to prevent infection.
5. Recognize patient's ability to breathe comfortably; if he has difficulty, a mechanical ventilator (Bennett or Bird) is attached, in which case a cuff is required.
6. Elevate him to semi-Fowler or sitting position if not contraindicated inasmuch as this is usually more comfortable and makes breathing easier.
7. Observe stomal site for bleeding or irritation; when the outer tracheostomy tube is changed (by physician for first 4 or 5 days), apply small amount of antibiotic ointment before reinserting tube. Place unfrayed sterile dressing around collar of tracheostomy tube (Fig. 3-2).

B. *Psychological Care of Patient*

1. Recognize that the patient is usually apprehensive, particularly about choking, about being unable to remove secretions, and about his ability to communicate.
2. Explain and demonstrate the procedure carefully using tracheostomy equipment; proceed according to the patient's ability to absorb information and his desire; this may be divided into several sessions.

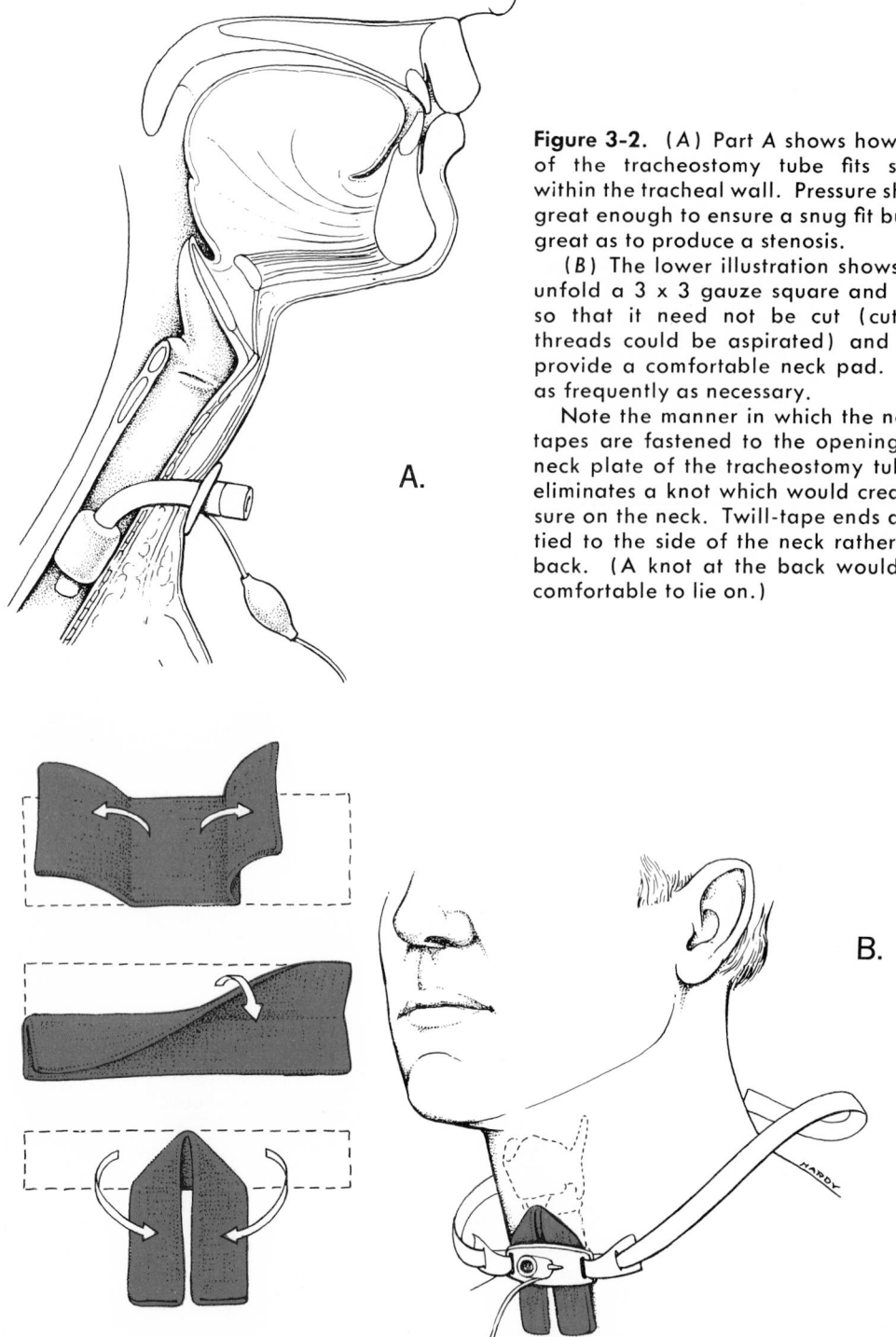

Figure 3-2. (A) Part A shows how the cuff of the tracheostomy tube fits smoothly within the tracheal wall. Pressure should be great enough to ensure a snug fit but not so great as to produce a stenosis.

(B) The lower illustration shows how to unfold a 3 x 3 gauze square and refold it so that it need not be cut (cut frayed threads could be aspirated) and yet will provide a comfortable neck pad. Change as frequently as necessary.

Note the manner in which the neck twill tapes are fastened to the openings in the neck plate of the tracheostomy tube. This eliminates a knot which would create pressure on the neck. Twill-tape ends are to be tied to the side of the neck rather than in back. (A knot at the back would not be comfortable to lie on.)

A.

B.

3. Inform the patient and his family that he will not be able to speak; determine with the patient the best method of communication, e.g., sign language, writing, etc.; supply him with note paper, pencil, "Magic slate" and call bell.
4. Anticipate some of his questions by providing the answer to "Is it permanent?" "Will it hurt to breathe?" "Will someone be with me?"
5. Provide an attendant for the first 24–48 hours, particularly if patient is fearful.

Equipment

1. Sterile gloves and duplicate sterile tracheostomy set including Trousseau dilator and 2 tracheal retractors (or hooks), 1 tissue forceps, 1 grooved director, 2 hemostats, petrolatum gauze or antibiotic ointment; sterile dressing.
2. Humidifying equipment
   a. For the room—a heated aerosol machine.
   b. For the patient—ultrasonic mist unit, ultrasonic room humidifier nebulizer attached to tracheostomy tube (Mucomyst) or a high humidity tracheal collar.
3. Suction equipment (See below, Guidelines: Aspirating the Tracheostomy Tube)
4. Communication materials: pencil, paper, etc., call bell.
5. Mirror—for use when patient is beginning self-care.

GUIDELINES: *Aspirating the Tracheostomy Tube*

NOTE: For high-risk patient, see procedure immediately following.

Purpose

To remove secretions when audible in the tracheobronchial tree so that a patent airway is maintained.

Equipment

Aseptic Technique (preferred)	Sterile gloves, individually wrapped
Sterile disposable catheter	Sterile saline
No. 14 or 16 (adult)	Sterile syringe—5 ml. and needle for
No. 8 or 10 (child)	saline instillation

General Nursing Considerations

1. Administer analgesics and sedatives with caution so that the respiratory center is not depressed.
2. Suction trachea when necessary (may be every 5 or 10 minutes for the first several postoperative hours and less frequently when need is less).

NURSING ALERT: Need for aspiration is expressed by noisy, moist respirations, increased pulse and respirations. Encourage patient to cough to bring up and expel secretions; use suction if coughing is not productive.

3. Use stethoscope to check patency of airway.
4. Avoid unnecessary suctioning which is irritating to mucosa and may initiate infection.

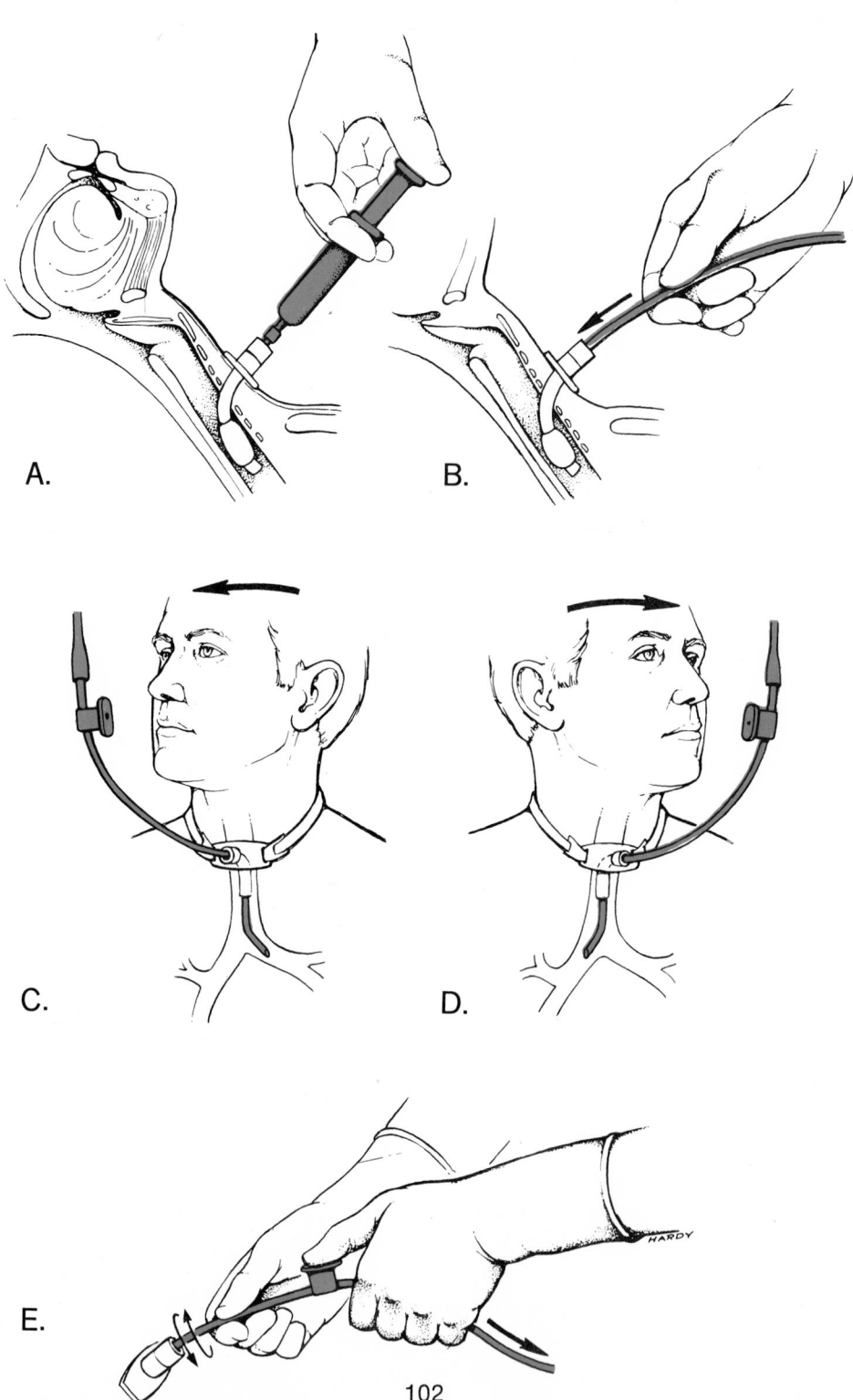

A.

B.

C.

D.

E.

102

Procedure (Fig. 3-3)

Nursing Action	Rationale/Amplification
1. Lubricate catheter with normal saline.	1. To facilitate passage of tube.
2. Insert catheter with suction turned off.	2. So as not to suction the wall of the cannula or irritate the mucous membrane wall.
3. Pass tube into bronchus from 20 to 30 cm. (8–12 inches), unless contraindicated, and then gradually open suction.	3. To stimulate coughing and to loosen secretions even beyond the cannula.
4. Remove catheter when patient coughs.	4. Catheter obstructs cannula and interferes with expulsion of secretions.
5. For tenacious secretions, instill sterile saline solution as prescribed (3–5 ml.). Use a syringe without needle attached.	5. Saline aids in dissolving mucus. It is helpful to have patient take a deep breath.
6. Have tissue ready to receive expelled secretions.	
7. To aspirate right bronchus, instruct patient to turn his head to the left, elevate the chin and tilt chest to the right (vice versa for left bronchus).	
8. Rotate catheter between thumb and forefinger; move it up and down gently as it is withdrawn with suction on.	
9. Do not suction patient more than 15 seconds at a time (rest at least 3 minutes between suctioning).	9. There is the danger of hypoxia if suctioning is prolonged.
10. Use a stethoscope along bronchial tree to detect gurgling mucous sounds.	10. Auscultation will determine effectiveness of suctioning; respiration should be quiet and essentially effortless at end of aspiration.

Aftercare of Equipment

1. When inner silver cannula is clogged with mucus, remove to clean.
2. Soak in a cold solution of half water and half hydrogen peroxide to loosen adhering particles (some prefer 2% sodium bicarbonate solution). Hot water would cause protein in mucus to coagulate.
3. A brush may be used to scrub interior of tube with soap and water. A pipe cleaner may be used for small tubes.
4. Disinfect tube by boiling for 5 minutes; cool.
5. Suction outer cannula in patient before reinserting cleaned inner cannula.

Figure 3-3. Care of the tracheostomy patient. (A) After the tracheostomy cuff is deflated (note that cuff does not touch sides of trachea), 3–5 ml. of sterile saline can be instilled into the tube to loosen secretions. (B) After donning sterile gloves, the nurse introduces a sterile catheter without applying suction. (C) To remove secretions from the right bronchus, the patient turns his head to the left. (D) To remove secretions from the left bronchus, the patient turns his head to the right. (E) Suction is applied by sealing the button outlet with the thumb; gradually withdraw the catheter in a rotating motion.

GUIDELINES: Decannulation of the Tracheostomy Tube

Purpose

To gradually wean patient away from tracheostomy tube so that eventually he may breathe without it.

Procedure

Nursing Action	Rationale/Amplification
1. Determine patient's ability to breathe deeply and cough effectively.	1. Clinical assessment of respiratory exchange over a period of time helps in determining time of weaning.
2. Check the patient's reflexes for swallowing, gagging, coughing.	2. Clinical assessment of respiratory exchange over a period of time helps in determining time of weaning.
3. Observe patient's ability to bring up tracheobronchial secretions without assistance for 24 hours.	3. Clinical assessment of respiratory exchange over a period of time helps in determining time of weaning.
4. Cork tracheostomy tube intermittently.	4. Increase the time of occlusion as much as patient can tolerate.
5. Remove tracheostomy tube as soon as safe.	5. This is determined by tolerance of the individual patient with no respiratory difficulties.
6. Tape skin edges together.	6. Tract closes spontaneously in a few days.

Nursing Management

1. Determine patient's ability to breathe deeply and cough effectively; also determine whether he can get along for 24 hours without respiratory assistance.
2. Check the patient's reflexes for swallowing, gagging, coughing.
3. Observe patient's ability to bring up tracheobronchial secretions without assistance for 24 hours.
4. Cork tracheostomy tube intermittently, increasing the time of occlusion as much as the patient can tolerate.
5. Remove tracheostomy tube as soon as safe and tolerable with no respiratory difficulties.
6. Tape skin edges together; tract closes spontaneously in a few days.

Endotracheal Intubation *(for Upper Airway Obstruction)*

In *endotracheal intubation* a tube is passed through the mouth or nose into the trachea.

Purposes

1. To provide an airway quickly and safely (done by an experienced person) when a person is having respiratory difficulty that cannot be treated by simpler methods.
2. To initiate positive pressure ventilation when a mask is ineffective.
3. To avoid aspiration by sealing off the trachea from the esophagus.
4. To remove retained tracheobronchial secretions effectively.

Treatment

1. An endotracheal tube with an 8- or 9-mm. diameter is passed by the physician usually by means of a laryngoscope.
2. A cuff around the tube is inflated to prevent leakage around the outer part of the tube.
3. Aspiration of tracheobronchial secretions is done through the tube.
4. Humidified oxygen can be introduced through the tube or it may be connected to ventilatory equipment.
5. This method is useful up to 72 hours, then a tracheostomy should be considered.

Complications

1. Vocal cord damage
2. Edema of trachea and larynx which may lead to stridor and respiratory embarrassment
3. Necrosis of tracheal wall due to prolonged inflation of cuff and impairment of tracheal circulation
4. Granuloma formation of posterior commissure of larynx

Nasotracheal Suctioning (for Lower Airway Obstruction)

Nasotracheal suctioning involves passing a catheter through the nose into the trachea.

Purposes

1. To relieve obstruction. Such a hindrance to air flow in the lower airways is caused by one or more of the following:
    a. Aspiration of blood, vomitus or other foreign material
    b. Bleeding from lacerated or damaged lung tissue
    c. Spasm of the bronchus
    d. Inhibition of cough by narcotic medications or chest pain
    e. Large amounts of mucus and transudates ("traumatic wet lung")
    f. Cessation of ciliary movement and bronchial peristaltic action
2. To facilitate air exchange. Elasticity of the lung (lung compliance) is reduced ("stiff-lung syndrome").
    a. Inability to move air in and out of lung
    b. Inability to cope with mobility of even a small quantity of obstruction.

Equipment

Small Fr. catheter, No. 14 or 16
Electric suction machine
Small gauze squares

Water-soluble lubricating jelly
Connecting Y-tube

Treatment (Fig. 3-4)

1. The catheter is introduced through the nostril.
2. Position of catheter in the nasopharynx is checked by depressing the tongue and using a flashlight.

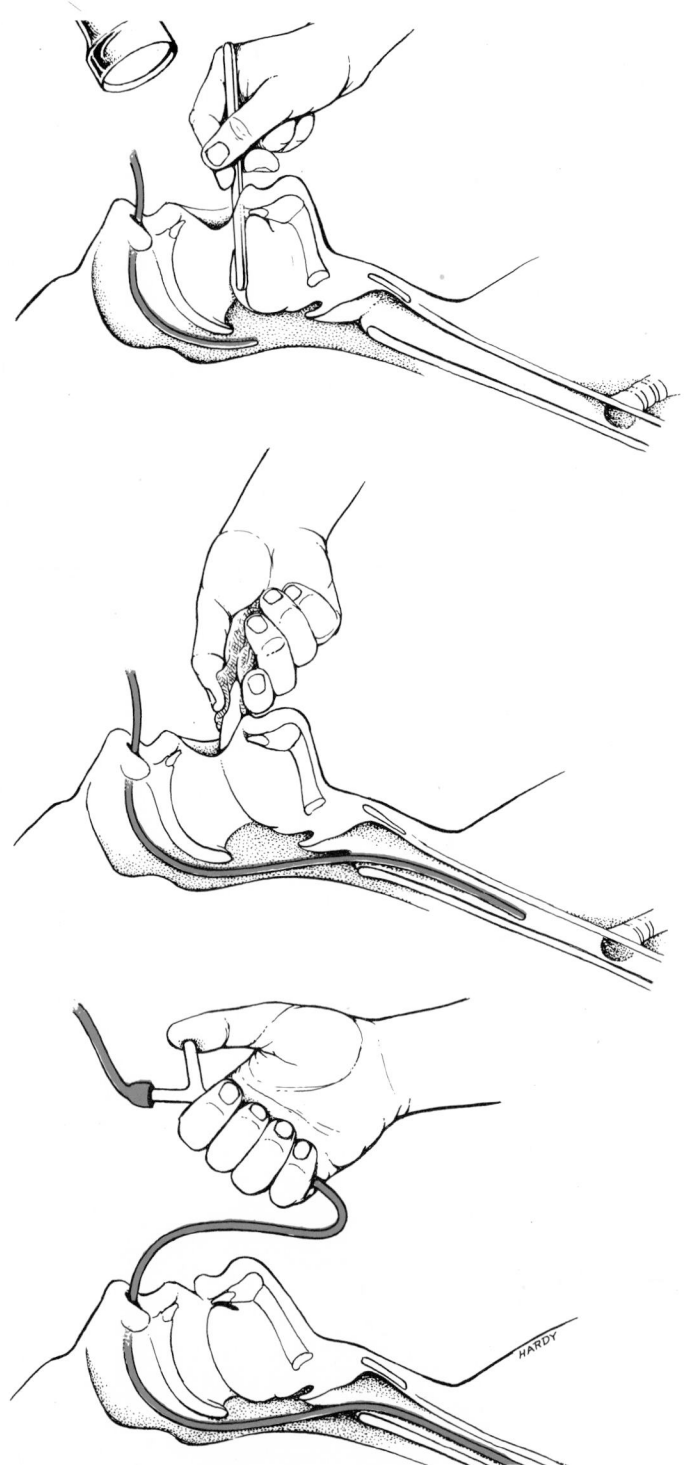

A. Introduce catheter through the nostril. Check position of catheter in pharynx by visualization, using a tongue depressor and light.

B. Grasp tongue with gauze square and hold in extension.
Request patient to take several deep breaths; advance catheter into trachea to maximal depth. Withhold suction until trachea is entered.

C. Check connection of catheter to continuous suction via Y-tube. Close Y-tube outlet with thumb for a few seconds between inspirations. Withdraw catheter gradually during suctioning.

Figure 3-4. Nasotracheal suction.

106

3. If the tongue is grasped firmly and held in extension, the catheter can be advanced into the trachea as the patient takes several deep breaths.
4. Suction is started when the catheter is at the required depth. The catheter is withdrawn gradually during suctioning.
5. Suction is closed off for a few seconds between inspirations.

GUIDELINES: *Caring for Patient With a Cuffed Tube (Tracheostomy or Endotracheal)*

A *cuffed tube* is an inflatable attachment to a tracheostomy or endotracheal tube for the purpose of providing a snug fit required for controlled or assisted ventilators. This in turn prevents leakage of air and secretions outside the tube as well as aspiration of secretions.

> NURSING ALERT: Deflate the cuff for about 3 to 5 minutes every hour or two to prevent tissue necrosis from the pressure against adjacent tissues.

General Nursing Considerations

1. Inform the patient that he will not be able to talk normally when the endotracheal cuffed tube is in place because no air passes over the larynx. (Speaking may be resumed when the tube is removed.)
   Speaking may be possible for the patient with a cuffed tracheostomy tube in place but not when the cuff is fully inflated.
2. Keep neck extended; when the patient is in sitting position, place pillows to maintain neck extension.
3. Hyperventilate patient just before, during and after the cuff is deflated and inflated to prevent the likelihood of hypoxia.
4. Recognize the importance of frequent and adequate mouth care.

Procedure

(May require a physician's order: Usually the cuff is initially inflated by the physician.)

Action	Rationale/Amplification
Deflating a Cuff	
1. Suction pharynx—oral and nasal.	1. Removes secretions which could be aspirated during the process of deflation.
2. Deflate cuff slowly.	2. On endotracheal tube, a small test balloon at end of tubing remains inflated as long as cuff is inflated.
3. Suction through the tracheostomy or endotracheal tube.	3. Removes secretions which may have been present above inflated cuff and around exterior of tube and now have seeped downward. The coughing reflex may be stimulated during deflation which helps to mobilize secretions.
4. Provide adequate ventilation while cuff is deflated.	
a. If the patient does not require assisted ventilation: provide humidified warm air.	a. Continue observation of patient: pulse, color, etc. If any signs of distress, place patient back on mechanical ventilator.

Action	***Rationale/Amplification***
b. If the patient requires assisted ventilation: provide a manually inflating breathing bag or respirator if patient has been on a mechanical ventilator.	b. If patient is apneic, cuff should not be deflated more than 30 or 45 seconds.

Inflating a Cuff (slowly)

1. Stipulations:
   a. To be done when patient requires mechanical ventilation or is being fed.

   a. To prevent aspiration of food into lungs.

      (1) Semi-Fowler's position is most comfortable if permissible and for a half hour after feeding.

      (1) Gravity assists moving food into the stomach.

      (2) On right side.

      (2) To prevent regurgitation of feeding.

   b. Inflate cuff during inspiration (positive pressure phase)

2. Method A
   a. Inject air (approximately 2–6 ml.) into cuff until complete seal is achieved. By listening with a stethoscope placed just below chin (submental) one may determine that no leak exists.

   a. The pressure-cycled respirator will turn off; air will not escape around tube or from nose or mouth. In the conscious patient, a leak-free system is present when he is aphonic.

   b. Clamp tube leading to cuff.

3. Method B (minimal leak inflation)
   a. Inject air until full seal is acquired; withdraw .5 ml. of air and clamp tube.

   a. A partial leak is purposely created so that respirator can be set to compensate for it.

   b. Note and chart amount of air required to inflate cuff.

   b. If at subsequent times, more air is required to inflate cuff, it may indicate tracheal dilation or perhaps serious difficulty i.e., erosion of a large blood vessel or tracheoesophageal diverticulum or fistula.

Suctioning (done with *sterile* equipment).

To minimize possibility of infection.

1. Tracheobronchial secretions are suctioned as frequently as necessary—5 or 10 seconds at a time and not oftener than once every 3 minutes.

1. This is a nursing judgment based on recognition of signs suggesting accumulation of secretions.

2. Via endotracheal tube
   a. Insert catheter (for an adult) approximately 45–50 cm. (18–20 inches)

   a. Tube inserted deeply since this patient has difficulty mobilizing deep secretions.

      (1) If impossible to pass suction tube this distance, it may indicate a mucous plug; inject 5 ml. saline.

      (1) Injecting saline helps in liquifying mucus.

3. Via tracheostomy tube (See Guidelines, p. 101)

4. Oropharyngeal with endotracheal tube in place
   Suction oropharynx frequently. (Patient is on nothing by mouth.)

4. Volume of secretions is greater due to irritation caused by such a tube.

5. Oropharyngeal with cuffed tracheostomy tube in place.
   (Patient is able to swallow and have a normal intake.)

Action	Rationale/Amplification
NOTE: The nurse must decide which of the following 2 methods to use: a. Cuff inflated during feeding b. Cuff deflated during feeding	Depends upon individual patient and the nurse's assessment of the situation. a. To prevent aspiration b. To prevent bulging into esophagus, which makes swallowing more difficult. If color from gelatin does not appear in aspirated material, there is little chance of aspiration during feeding, hence cuff may be deflated.
Test: Feed patient colored gelatin; if color from gelatin appears in aspirated material, inflate tube	

Maintaining Humidified Warm Inspired Air 1. Provide continuous flow of mist.	1. To prevent drying of secretions and irritation of mucous membrane.

Complications	*Means of Avoiding Complications*
1. Laryngeal irritation and damage to vocal cord due to movement of endotracheal tube.	1. Prevent movement or jarring of tube.
2. Laryngeal edema	2. Supply mist during and after extubation (may try administering adrenalin, antihistamines, steroids, immediately before extubation).
3. Tracheal stenosis	3. Proper nursing care includes humidity, suction, etc.
4. Upper airway obstruction: Restlessness, tachycardia, headache, confusion, motor incoordination and possible laryngeal stridor, chest wall retraction, and cyanosis	4. Suction secretions
5. In children: Inability to sleep and extreme fatigue may also be apparent.	

GUIDELINES: *Endotracheal Catheter Stimulation*

Purpose

To stimulate coughing when other mechanical means have failed.

Procedure

Nursing Action	Rationale/Amplification
1. Obtain permission from physician.	1. This procedure may require endotracheal suctioning; such a possibility must be anticipated and planned for.
2. Utilize sterile equipment: a. Sterile catheter No. 16 F, connecting tubing to suction equipment. b. Sterile gloves.	2. To prevent introduction of organisms into the respiratory system.
3. Pass the catheter (suction turned off) through the nose with one hand; place the other hand on the patient's forehead.	3. To stabilize the patient's head and to reassure the patient.
4. When the catheter reaches the larynx, coughing may be stimulated. Quickly advance the catheter into the trachea.	4. At this point, coughing is unproductive.

Nursing Action	Rationale/Amplification
5. Permit the patient to rest with the catheter in place; provide oxygen if nursing judgment so indicates.	5. Trachea is relatively desensitized at this time.
6. Pull catheter slightly forward; this will initiate vigorous coughing. Provide tissues for patient's expectorations.	6. Irritation of trachea triggers coughing reflex.
7. Pinch off and remove catheter gently.	
8. Comfort patient.	

CANCER OF THE LARYNX

Incidence

1. Occurs in men over 60; ratio of men to women is 10:1.
2. Greater predisposition to laryngeal cancer in some families and in people who smoke heavily or use their voices excessively.

Clinical Expectations

1. When treated early, the likelihood of cure is great.
2. When limited to the vocal cords, spread is slow because of lessened blood supply.
3. When cancer involves the epiglottis, cancer spreads more rapidly because of abundant supply of blood and lymph and soon involves the lymph nodes of the neck.

Clinical Manifestations

1. Hoarseness is usually the earliest sign; this symptom is apparent because the vocal cords are inhibited from approximating (coming close together) by the diseased tissue.
2. A feeling that there is a lump in the throat, dyspnea, dysphagia.
3. Pain in laryngeal prominence (Adam's apple), enlarged cervical nodes, cough.

Surgical Management

A. *Laryngofissure* (thyrotomy)
   1. An opening is made into the larynx through the thyroid cartilage; the involved cord and tumor are then removed. This approach is preferred if:
      a. Muscles are not affected by the tumor.
      b. Vocal cord motility is normal.
   2. Tracheostomy tube is inserted during surgery; removed when tissue edema subsides.
   3. *Nursing considerations*
      a. Administer food and fluids for the first 48 hours by nasogastric tube or intravenous methods.
      b. Gradually offer fluids by mouth.
      c. Encourage slow gradual resumption of vocal sounds; have patient begin with a whisper, until healing is complete, and then add more substantial sounds.

B. *Total Laryngectomy* (performed for advanced cancer)
   1. Removal of epiglottis, thyroid cartilage, hyoid bone, cricoid cartilage, 2 or 3 rings of trachea.
   2. Pharyngeal opening of trachea is closed; remaining trachea is brought out to the anterior neck and sutured to the skin; this is a permanent tracheostomy.

3. Breathing takes place through the tracheostomy; no breathing or smelling takes place through the nose.

C. *Radical Neck Dissection*

Performed if there is metastasis to the neck tissues and lymph nodes. (See p. 370.)

Psychosocial Preparation of the Patient for a Total Laryngectomy

1. Inform the patient that he will breathe through an opening made in his neck.
2. Apprise him of the fact that he will not have his usual speech following surgery.
3. Expect reactions of depression since the above information has a direct effect on his future.
4. Arrange for him to be visited by a laryngectomee (one who has had his larynx removed either totally or partially); such a person is able to transfer hope and encouragement to the patient.
5. Inform him of the services available for speech rehabilitation. Many patients make remarkable adjustments and pursue normal activities.

Emergency First Aid for the Laryngectomee

The Nature of the Difficulty

Clogging or obstruction of the stoma is a life-threatening problem.

NURSING ALERT: No air can get to the lungs through the mouth or nose when the stoma is clogged in a laryngectomee.

Nursing Management

1. Assess the situation.
   a. Is the victim wearing a tracheostomy or laryngectomy tube? In a laryngectomee, tube removal cannot cause immediate danger.
   b. Has he been operated on recently? If so, the tracheostomy tube cannot be removed.
   c. Check for tracheal obstruction. Clean stomal opening of mucus and encrusted matter.
2. Remove obstruction.
   a. Obtain suction equipment and pass catheter down tracheal opening while keeping catheter pinched or closed. Insert not more than 7.5 to 10 cm. (3–4 inches).
   b. Release gentle suction as the catheter is rotated and gradually withdrawn.
   c. If catheter cannot be passed, remove laryngectomy tube and clean it.
3. Initiate artificial respiration.
   a. Use same procedure as for mouth-to-mouth resuscitation; however, place your mouth over victim's stoma instead of his mouth.
   b. Provide a firm contact with the neck opening.
   c. Recognize that:
      (1) It is unnecessary to close off the nose and mouth.
      (2) Position of tongue or dentures is irrelevant.
      (3) Vomiting through stomal opening is impossible since esophagus is not open to the trachea.

2. Conditions of the Chest

MAJOR MANIFESTATIONS OF BRONCHOPULMONARY DISEASE

Cough and Expectoration

A. *General Considerations*

1. Coughing is a protective mechanism that functions to clear the airway.
2. A prolonged dry cough will eventually become productive.
    a. Thick mucopurulent sputum which is difficult to remove is more apt to cause violent coughing.
    b. Violent coughing results in spasms, bronchial obstruction and further irritation of the bronchi.
3. A severe, repeated or uncontrolled cough that is nonproductive is potentially harmful.
4. The cough-producing stimuli may be inflammatory, mechanical, chemical or thermal.
5. Clinical problems producing cough are inflammation, cardiovascular disorders, trauma, physical agents, neoplasms and allergic disorders.

B. *Nursing Management*

1. Evaluate the character of the cough.
    a. Dry and hacking—may be due to nervousness, viral infections, early congestive heart failure, bronchogenic carcinoma.
    b. Loud and harsh—irritation in larynx, trachea or main bronchi.
    c. Wheezing—associated with bronchospasm.
    d. Severe or changing—may be bronchogenic cancer (cough, chest pain, hemoptysis).
    e. Loose—indicates problems of more peripheral regions in bronchi and lung parenchyma.
    f. Painful—indicates pleural involvement, chest wall disease.
2. Note time of cough.
    a. Coughing paroxysms at night—may indicate bronchial asthma or left-sided heart failure.
    b. Cough that worsens when patient is supine—may be due to postnasal drip from sinusitis, bronchiectasis.
    c. Cough associated with food intake—results from aspiration into tracheobronchial tree.
3. Regard character and quantity of expectorated material.
    a. Clear or mucoid—stems from viral infection, chronic bronchitis.
    b. Thick yellow or green sputum—due to secondary bacterial infections, bacterial pneumonia.
    c. Rusty—may indicate bacterial pneumonia (if patient not receiving antibiotics).
    d. Malodorous—due to lung abscess, infection from fusospirochetal or anaerobic organisms.
    e. Frothy pink sputum—indicates acute pulmonary edema.

Hemoptysis (Bleeding from the Lungs)

A. *Causes*

Pulmonary infarction   Compression syndrome
Neoplasms   Blood dyscrasias
Infections

B. *Nursing Management*
　　1.　Recognize the patient's fear and apprehension to this threatening symptom and give him understanding and support.
　　2.　Ascertain if blood is coming from bronchi, lungs or gastrointestinal tract.
　　　　a.　Blood from lungs—appears bright red and frothy and is accompanied by coughing and clearing of throat.
　　　　b.　Gastrointestinal tract—appears dark red, brown or black and is usually accompanied by vomiting and retching.
　　3.　Place patient on involved side (if known).
　　4.　Save coughed up blood for inspection by physician.

Hoarseness

Types
　　1.　Acute hoarseness
　　　　When associated with febrile episode suggests viral laryngotracheobronchitis
　　2.　Persistent hoarseness
　　　　Indicates intrinsic neoplasm of vocal cord, bronchogenic cancer, mediastinal lesion.

Dyspnea

A. *Cause*
　　In lung disease, shortness of breath is due to increase in lung rigidity, airway resistance.

B. *Altered Physiology*
　　The heart will ultimately be affected by lung disease since blood flows through the lung.

C. *Nursing Management*
　　1.　Ascertain circumstances in which dyspnea occurs.
　　　　a.　How much activity provokes dyspnea?
　　　　b.　Under what circumstances does it occur?
　　　　c.　Is there associated cough?
　　　　d.　Is dyspnea related to other symptoms?
　　　　e.　Is there expiratory wheeze?
　　2.　Evaluate the nature of the shortness of breath.
　　　　a.　Acute dyspnea associated with symptoms of infection suggests pneumonia.
　　　　b.　Sudden dyspnea in ill or postoperative patient may indicate pulmonary embolism.
　　　　c.　Orthopnea—characteristic of cardiogenic pulmonary congestion.
　　　　d.　Expiratory wheeze—arising from obstructive disease in smaller airways (asthma, bronchitis, emphysema).
　　　　e.　Wheezing respirations—related to localized obstruction of major branches, tumor, foreign body.
　　　　f.　Inspiratory stridor—indicates partial obstruction at laryngeal or tracheal level.
　　　　g.　Paroxysmal wheezing unrelated to exertion—may arise from bronchial (allergic) asthma.

Chest Pain

A. *Incidence*
　　1.　Lung disease does not always produce thoracic pain since the lung and the visceral pleura covering it lack sensory nerves and are insensitive to pain stimuli.

2. Parietal pleura has rich supply of sensory nerves coming from intercostal nerves to the diaphragm. These nerve endings may be stimulated by inflammation and stretching of membrane.

B. *Clinical Manifestations*
1. Pleural pain is a common manifestation of inflammatory and malignant disease but also accompanies pneumothorax.
2. Pleural pain, usually well-localized, sharp and stabbing, occurs at end of inspiration.

C. *Constitutional Symptoms of Bronchopulmonary Disease*
1. Anorexia
2. Fever
3. Weight loss
4. Fatigue, malaise, weakness
5. Sweats
} related to duration and severity of disease

D. *Nursing Management*
1. Assess quality, intensity and radiation of pain.
2. Note factors that precipitate pain.
3. Evaluate if position of patient changes character of pain.
4. Determine the effect of inspiration and expiration on patient's pain.

DIAGNOSTIC PROCEDURES FOR RESPIRATORY CONDITIONS

Chest Auscultation and Stethoscopy

A *stethoscope* is an instrument for conveying sounds from the chest wall to the ears of the listener.

Purpose

To recognize and localize abnormalities in the lungs or pleura and heart and pericardium.

Equipment

Stethoscope—may have bell chest piece, diaphragm chest piece or both (Fig. 3-5).

Bell—transmits relatively low-pitched sounds best.
Diaphragm—transmits relatively high-pitched sounds best.

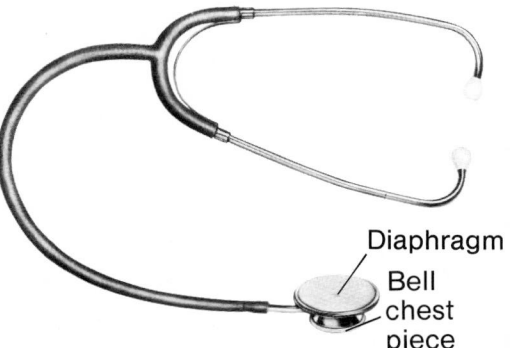

Diaphragm

Bell chest piece

Figure 3-5. Stethoscope with diaphragm and bell chest piece. (Courtesy Bard-Parker)

Underlying Principles

1. Keep the environment as quiet as possible; extraneous noises as well as contracting muscle, cloth, hair and wet skin moving beneath the diaphragm of the stethoscope can cause confusing sounds.
2. *Take time* to evaluate and correlate what is being heard. The ear has to be *trained* to differentiate the various sounds.

3. Experience in listening to a wide range of normal sounds is necessary before one can distinguish abnormal sounds.
4. Listen to one thing at a time. Develop a systematic routine of auscultation.
5. In the normal individual the only respiratory sounds heard are breath sounds; these may be barely audible unless the patient is requested to breathe deeply through the open mouth to accentuate the sounds heard.
6. Other normal sounds are the heart, bowel and muscle sounds.

Types of Sounds

A. *Breath Sounds*—sounds due to movement of air through the lungs and air passages.
    1. *Vesicular Breath Sounds*—normal sounds heard over most of the lung and principally due to movement in and out of the alveoli and finer respiratory conduits. Inspiration is longer than expiration.
    2. *Tracheal Breath Sounds*—sounds heard over side of neck in the region of the thyroid cartilage; these are harsh and high-pitched with a definite pause between inspiration and expiration; the expiratory phase is longer than the inspiratory.
    3. *Bronchial or Tubular Sounds*—sounds heard over the bronchi closely resembling tracheal breath sounds; they are less harsh but length of inspiration is still longer than expiration.

B. *Abnormal Sounds*
    1. *Rales*—abnormal respiratory sounds heard upon auscultation (simulated by rubbing the hair between the fingers near the ear) originating from the trachea, bronchi or lungs. Rales are produced by vibrations of fluid, exudate or mucus within the respiratory tract.
    2. *Crepitant Rales*—rales of crackling quality; term usually applied to moist rales. These are due to fluid in the alveoli, particularly so if they occur at the end of inspiration.
    3. *Rhonchi* (musical rales)—continuous coarse sounds arising from the trachea or bronchi produced by vibrations of thick mucus in the bronchi; indicate partial airway obstruction by fluid somewhere in respiratory tract.
       a. Small Airway Obstruction—sounds are numerous, fine and high-pitched. In asthma they typically occur in expiration; in bronchitis they occur in inspiration.
       b. Large Airway Obstruction—sounds are coarse, lower-pitched, groaning or whistling; may be abolished or altered by coughing.
    4. *Tracheal or Bronchial Breath Sounds*—heard outside of their normal chest areas are abnormal.
    5. *Bronchospasm*—wheeze or musical rales, heard predominantly during expiration; may be due to retained secretions, bronchomucosal edema, collapsing airways, muscular spasm or a combination of these problems.
    6. *Pleural Friction Rub*—low-pitched coarse grating sound heard close to the ear during both phases of respiration; disappears if patient holds his breath; indicates inflammation of the pleura.
    7. *Transmitted Sounds*—bronchial or tubular sounds or quick audible whispered or spoken sounds heard over areas of the lung typically producing vesicular sounds. These are found when the lung area becomes consolidated by inflammatory reaction.
    8. *Absent Sounds*—diminished breath sounds, occurring when air does not enter that portion of the lungs due to obstruction of the air passages or from the accumulation of pleural fluid or air between the chest wall and the adjacent lung.

GUIDELINES: *Using Auscultation and Stethoscopy*

Procedure

Nursing Action	*Rationale/Amplification*
Preparatory Phase	
1. Ask the patient to assume a sitting position leaning slightly forward (Fig. 3-6).	1. If the patient is too ill to sit up, listen to the anterior chest while he is lying supine and then turn him from side to side to listen over the lateral areas and back.
2. Make sure the room and stethoscope are warm.	2. A cold stethoscope or room may cause involuntary muscle contractions of the chest wall which can be mistaken for pulmonary abnormalities. If in doubt about muscle sounds, listen when the chest is held in deep inspiration.
3. Bare the chest.	3. A hairy chest rubbing against the stethoscope will make misleading sounds. Wetting the hair will prevent this. However wet skin (perspiration) moving beneath the diaphragm often sounds like crepitant rales.
Performance Phase	
1. Listen *systematically* to all portions of both lung fields (Fig. 3-6). a. Posteriorly—step-wise down the back. b. Laterally—under the axillae. c. Anteriorly—step-wise down the front of the chest.	1. Compare each area examined with the *symmetrical* area of the opposite thorax. Symmetrical comparison often will allow the analysis of the unknown.
2. Ask the patient to breathe a little deeper and faster than normal with his mouth open.	2. Breathing through the mouth causes more air turbulence and thus louder sound. Notice the presence of abnormal sounds especially after forced expiration.
3. Observe (inspect) the chest movements while listening.	

Diagnostic Studies

Radiography

A. *Chest Roentgenogram*
  1. Normal pulmonary tissue is radiolucent. Thus densities produced by tumors, foreign bodies, etc. can be detected.
  2. Chest x-rays may reveal extensive pathology in the lungs in the absence of symptoms.
B. *Tomography*
  1. Provides films of sections of lungs at different levels within the thorax.
  2. Useful in demonstrating presence of solid lesions, calcification or cavitation within a lesion.
C. *Angiographic Studies of Pulmonary Vessels*
  1. Contrast media injected into following blood vessels:
     a. Antecubital veins of one or both arms
     b. Superior vena cava, right atrium, right ventricle or main pulmonary artery
     c. Right or left pulmonary artery or one of its branches

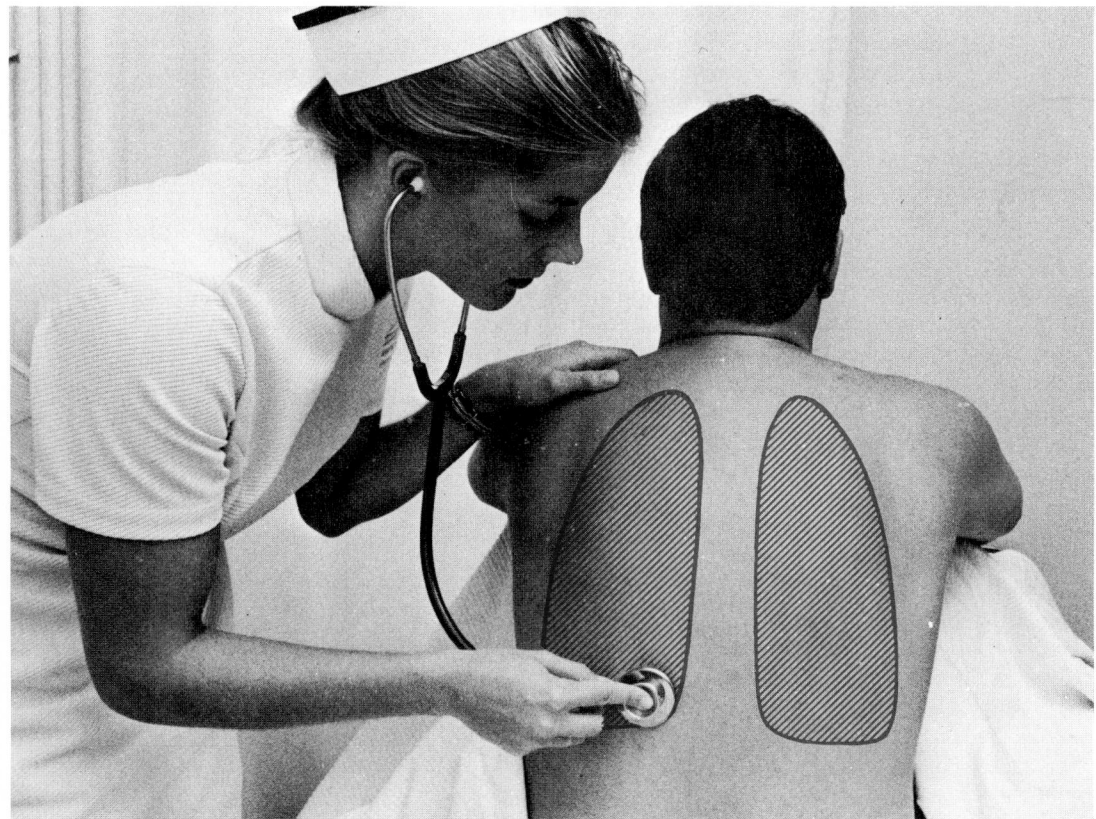

Figure 3-6. Chest auscultation. The nurse listens to one lung area and then compares it with the symmetrical area of the opposite thorax.

2. Films are taken in rapid sequence after injection.
3. Studies useful in revealing involvement of pulmonary veins, in differential diagnosis of mediastinal shadow and in diagnosis of cardiac lesions.
4. Patient should be observed for anaphylactoid reaction to contrast media (rare).

D. *Barium Swallow*

Outlines the esophagus to reveal displacement of esophagus and encroachment on its lumen.

E. *Fluoroscopy*

Enables roentgenologists to view heart, lungs and diaphragm in the dynamic state.

F. *Bronchography*

A water-soluble contrast media is instilled into various lobes of the lung to outline the smaller ramifications of the tracheobronchial tree. This study shows anomalies of bronchial tree and the presence of bronchiectasis.

1. Topical anesthesia is sprayed in the mouth, tongue and posterior pharynx.
2. Local anesthetic is injected into tracheal tree.

3. Patient is assessed for allergic reaction to anesthetic agent or contrast media.
   a. Test contraindicated in patients with respiratory insufficiency since these patients may experience temporary problems with ventilation and diffusion.
   b. Oxygen, antispasmodic agents and cortisone should be available.

Endoscopic Procedures

A. *Bronchoscopy*
   1. The introduction of a special lighted instrument into the trachea and bronchi for:
      a. Inspection of pathologic changes in the bronchial tree
      b. Removal of secretions (sputum, pleural fluid) and tissue for cytologic and bacteriologic study
      c. Removal of a foreign body
      d. Improvement of drainage
      e. Assessment of residual functional capacity of diseased lung
      f. Treatment by application of chemotherapeutic agent
   2. Local or general anesthesia is used.
      a. Patient must be relaxed before and during procedure. Administer medication to relieve anxiety and give encouragement and nursing support.
      b. Restrict food and fluid 6 hours prior to procedure. Remove dentures.
      c. After the procedure, wait until patient demonstrates he can cough before giving cracked ice.
      d. Aspirin gargle ad lib. may be ordered to relieve throat discomfort.
      e. Following bronchoscopy watch patient for:
         (1) Evidences of cardiac arrhythmia
         (2) Bleeding
         (3) Respiratory failure

Examination of Bronchial Secretions

A. *Sputum*
   1. Sputum is examined for acid-fast bacilli (tuberculosis) to rule out primary disease and to assess for hypersensitivity states (increase in eosinophils).
      a. Direct smear—shows presence of pathogenic bacteria.
      b. Sputum culture—to make diagnosis, to determine drug sensitivity and to serve as a guide for drug treatment (choice of antibiotic).
      c. Sputum cytology (exfoliative cytology)—used to identify tumor cells.
   2. Instruct the patient to *cough* and then expectorate into container.
      a. Obtain freshly expectorated sputum (not pharyngeal secretion) and see that it is transported to laboratory immediately.
      b. Avoid contaminating specimen.
      c. Give oral hygiene frequently, especially if patient has foul sputum.
   3. Patients receiving antibiotics, steroids and immunosuppressive agents for prolonged periods may have periodic sputum examinations as these agents give rise to opportunistic pulmonary infections.

B. *Pleural Fluid*
   1. Pleural fluid is obtained by aspiration (thoracentesis) (see p. 122).
   2. Pleural fluid is examined for protein content, specific gravity and presence or absence of formed elements. (Sediment may demonstrate malignant cells.)
   3. Observe and record total amount of fluid withdrawn, nature of fluids and its color and viscosity.

a. Bloody effusion—may indicate tuberculosis, inoperable cancer.
b. Purulent effusion—may indicate empyema.
c. Clear straw-colored fluid—may indicate tuberculosis (in absence of heart failure).
4. Prepare sample of fluid for laboratory evaluation if ordered.

C. *Gastric Lavage*

1. A nasogastric tube is inserted into the stomach to siphon out swallowed pulmonary secretions.
2. This test is useful for culture of tubercle bacilli. (See p. 383 for nursing implications.)

Pulmonary Function Studies (Table 3-1)

These studies assess the extent of disease and the patient's functional reserve.

TABLE 3-1. VENTILATORY FUNCTION TESTS*

Term Used	Symbol	Description	Remarks and Clinical Application
Vital capacity	VC	The largest volume measured on complete expiration after the deepest inspiration without forced or rapid effort.	This may be normal or even high in chronic obstructive pulmonary disease and is of little value by itself.
Forced vital capacity	FVC	The vital capacity performed with expiration as forceful and rapid as possible.	This volume is often significantly reduced in chronic lung disease due to air trapping, and is an important standard of measurement.
Forced expiratory volume (qualified by subscript indicating time interval in seconds)	FEV_T ($FEV_{1.0}$)	Volume of gas exhaled over a given time interval during the performance of a forced vital capacity.	If below predicted normal values, this is a valuable clue to the severity of the expiratory airway obstruction.
Percentage expired (in T seconds)	$FEV_T\%$	FEV_T expressed as a percentage of the forced vital capacity: $$\frac{FEV_T}{FVC} \times 100$$	This time-volume relationship is another way of expressing the presence or absence of airway obstruction.
Forced expiratory flow	$FEF_{200\text{-}1200}$	The average rate of flow for a specified portion of the forced expiratory volume, usually between 200 and 1200 ml.	Formerly called maximum expiration flow rate (MEFR). A slowed rate is an early manifestation of chronic obstructive pulmonary diseases.
Forced mid-expiratory flow	$FEF_{25\text{-}75\%}$	Average rate of flow during the middle half of the forced expiratory volume.	Formerly called mid-expiratory flow rate. This is slowed early in the course of ventilatory impairment.
Maximal voluntary ventilation	MVV	Volume of air which a subject can breathe with voluntary maximal effort for a given time.	Formerly called maximum breathing capacity. Another valuable test, usually correlating well with the patient's complaint of dyspnea.

* National Tuberculosis Association: Chronic Obstructive Pulmonary Disease. p. 24. 1966.

Radioisotope Diagnostic Procedure

A. *Lung Scan*

The injection of a radioactive isotope into the body followed by scanning of the lung by equipment (scanner) which detects radiation.

    1. This measures blood perfusion through the lung.
    2. It is useful in evaluating pulmonary vascularity (pulmonary embolism) and obstructive airway disorders.

Arterial Blood Gas Studies

    1. Helps measure arterial tensions of oxygen (pO_2), carbon dioxide (pCO_2) and arterial pH, oxygen saturation and bicarbonate (HCO_3) as indicators of respiratory function.
    2. Determines the state of acid-base balance, oxygen tension, carbon dioxide tension and oxygen saturation of hemoglobin.
    3. Assesses the degree to which the lungs are able to provide adequate oxygen and remove carbon dioxide.
    4. Assesses the degree to which kidneys are able to reabsorb or excrete bicarbonate ions to maintain a normal body pH.

GUIDELINES: *Assisting with Obtaining Blood for Blood Gas Analysis*

Purpose

To obtain a sample of arterial blood for blood gas analysis.

Terminology

"p"—indicates pressure   ⎫ These are referred to as partial pressures
pO_2—pressure of oxygen   ⎬ since the pressure these gases exert is a
pCO_2—pressure of carbon dioxide ⎭ part of the total atmospheric pressure.

ARTERIAL GASES

pH	Normal values: 7.35–7.45	
	below 7.35	Acidosis
	above 7.45	Alkalosis
Arterial oxygen tension (pO_2)	Normally 80–100 mm. Hg	When breathing room air
	Normally above 600 mm. Hg	When breathing 100% oxygen
	below 60 mm. Hg	Requires increase in cardiac output to maintain oxygen transport to the tissues
Arterial carbon dioxide tension (pCO_2)	Normally 35–45 mm. Hg	
	above 50 mm. Hg	Alveolar hypoventilation
	below 35 mm. Hg	Alveolar hyperventilation

Equipment

2-ml. syringe with No. 25 gauge needle
10-ml. syringe with No. 19 or 20 gauge needle (adult) (22 or 25 needle, child)
Sodium heparin (1000 units/ml. mixed with normal saline)
Stopper or cap
1% procaine
Sterile sponges and skin germicide
Basin containing ice

Clinical Indications

1. Unexpected tachypnea, dyspnea (especially in patients with cardiopulmonary disease)
2. Unexpected restlessness and anxiety in bed patients
3. Drowsiness and confusion in patients receiving oxygen therapy
4. Before thoracic surgery
5. Before and during prolonged oxygen therapy

Procedure

Nursing Action	**Rationale/Amplification**
Preparatory Phase	
1. Take patient's temperature and respiratory rate.	1. These measurements are taken into consideration when the laboratory results are evaluated.
2. Note the amount of oxygen he is receiving.	
3. Heparinize the syringe.	
a. Withdraw a sufficient amount of heparin into the syringe to wet the plunger completely.	a. This action coats the interior of the syringe with heparin to prevent the blood from clotting.
b. Hold syringe in upright position and expel excess heparin and air bubbles.	

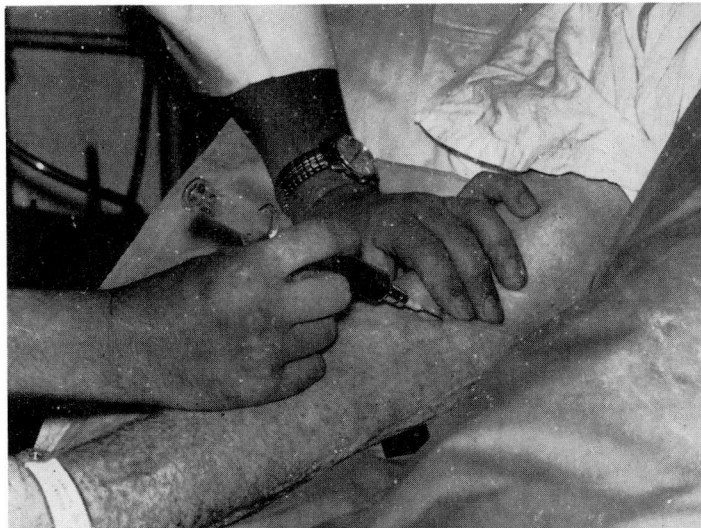

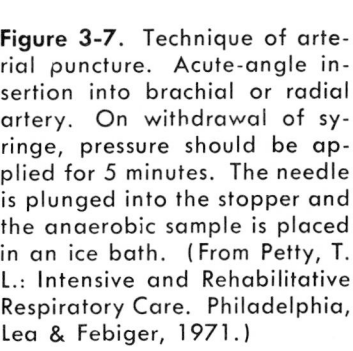

Figure 3-7. Technique of arterial puncture. Acute-angle insertion into brachial or radial artery. On withdrawal of syringe, pressure should be applied for 5 minutes. The needle is plunged into the stopper and the anaerobic sample is placed in an ice bath. (From Petty, T. L.: Intensive and Rehabilitative Respiratory Care. Philadelphia, Lea & Febiger, 1971.)

Nursing Action	**Rationale/Amplification**

Performance Phase (by physician, laboratory technician, inhalation therapist)

1. Palpate the radial, brachial or femoral artery.
2. Prepare the skin with germicide. The skin and subcutaneous tissues are infiltrated with local anesthetic agent (procaine).
3. The syringe is held at an acute angle (Fig. 3-7) and the needle is inserted into the artery.

   3. As the needle enters the artery a pulsating flow of blood will easily fill the syringe.

4. Withdraw the needle.
5. Cap the needle immediately with the needle shield. Unscrew the needle and cap the hub of the syringe.

   5. Immediate capping of the needle prevents room air from mixing with the specimen.

6. *Maintain firm pressure on the puncture site for 5 minutes.*
   a. If the patient is on anticoagulant medication, apply direct pressure over puncture site for 15 minutes and then apply a firm pressure dressing 3 to 4 hours.

   6. Firm pressure on the puncture site prevents further bleeding.

7. Place capped syringe into the container of ice.

   7. The pH of the blood will fall significantly unless the syringe containing the blood is immediately immersed in ice.

8. For patients requiring frequent monitoring of arterial blood, an arterial cannula is inserted into the brachial (preferable) or radial artery and plugged. It is unplugged when blood samples are drawn or when the tubing is flushed with heparin.

Follow-up Phase

1. Take the basin of ice with the syringe containing blood immediately to the laboratory.

   1. Blood gas determinations should be done within an hour of having the blood drawn as gas tension and pH can change rapidly.

2. Inspect the puncture site and assess the patient's condition at intervals.

   2. Hematoma, arterial thrombosis and ulnar nerve puncture are complications following this procedure.

GUIDELINES: *Assisting the Patient Undergoing Thoracentesis*

Thoracentesis is the aspiration of fluid or air from the pleural space. It may be a diagnostic or therapeutic procedure (Fig. 3-8).

Purposes

1. To remove fluid and air from the pleural cavity.
2. To obtain diagnostic aspiration of pleural fluid.

Equipment

50-ml. syringe
Aspirating needle
Stopcock and rubber tubing
Hemostat

Sterile gauze dressings
Sterile towels and drape
Sterile specimen container
Sterile gloves

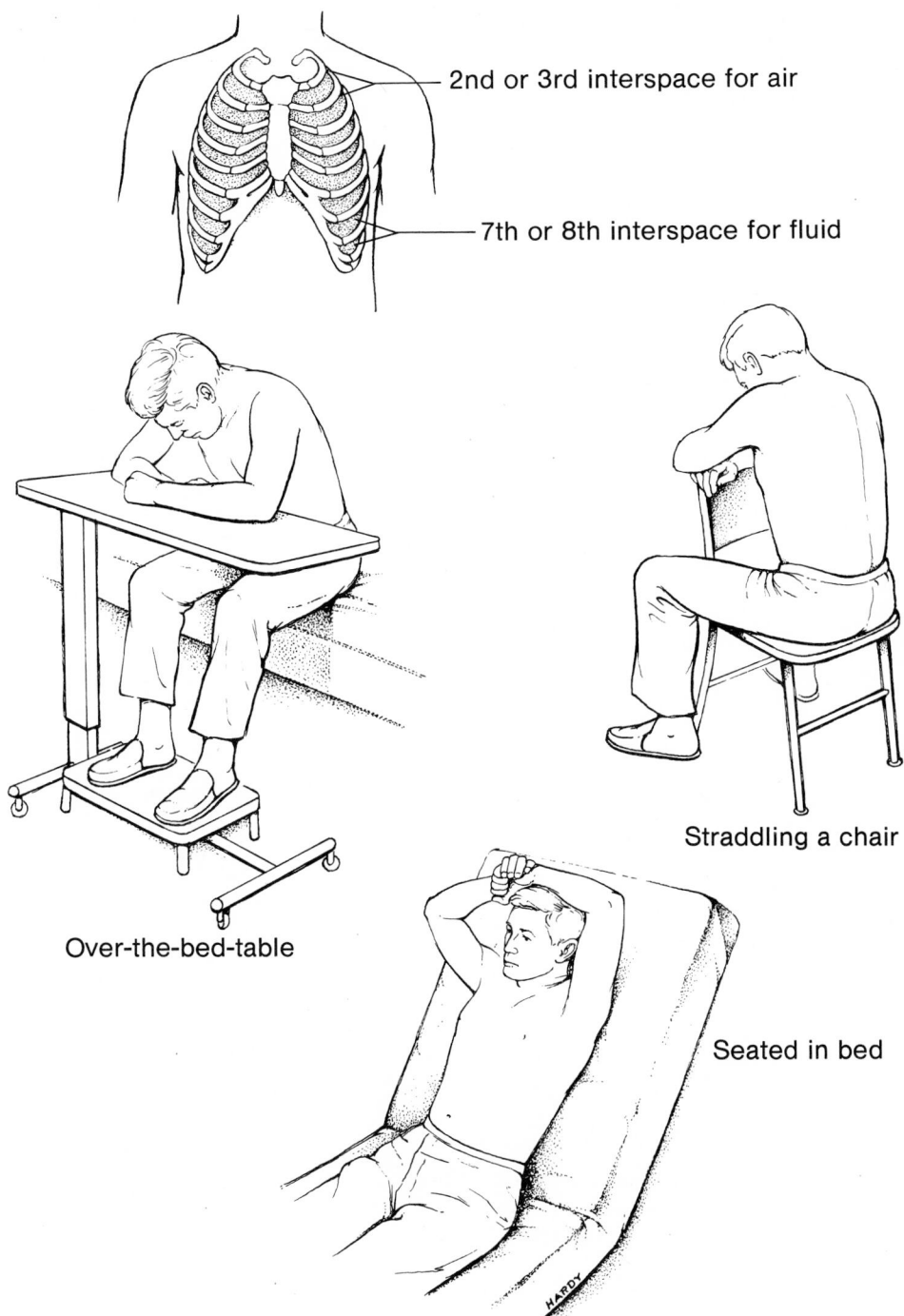

2nd or 3rd interspace for air

7th or 8th interspace for fluid

Over-the-bed-table

Straddling a chair

Seated in bed

Figure 3-8. Thoracentesis.

Procedure

Nursing Action	Rationale/Amplification
Preparatory Phase	
1. Ascertain in advance if chest roentgenograms have been ordered and completed.	1. Posteroanterior and lateral chest x-rays are used to localize fluid and air in the pleural cavity and facilitate in determining the puncture site.
2. Determine if the patient is allergic to the local anesthetic agent to be used. Give sedation if ordered.	
3. Inform the patient about the procedure and indicate how he can be helpful. Explain: a. The nature of the procedure b. The importance of remaining immobile c. Pressure sensations to be experienced d. That no discomfort is anticipated after the procedure	3. An explanation helps orient the patient to the procedure, assists him to mobilize his resources and gives him an opportunity to ask questions and verbalize anxiety.
4. Make the patient comfortable with adequate supports. If possible place him upright and in one of the following positions: a. Sitting on the edge of the bed with feet supported and head on a padded over-the-bed table. b. Straddling a chair with his arms and head resting on the back of the chair If he is unable to assume a sitting position have him lie on the unaffected side.	4. The upright position facilitates the removal of fluid that usually localizes at the base of the chest. A comfortable position assists the patient to relax.
5. Support and reassure the patient during the procedure. a. Prepare the patient for the sensations of cold and pressure from infiltration of local anesthetic agent. b. Encourage the patient to refrain from coughing.	5. Sudden and unexpected movement by the patient can cause trauma to the visceral pleura with resultant trauma to the lung.
Performance Phase	
1. Expose the entire chest.	1. If the fluid is in the pleural cavity the thoracentesis site is usually in the 7th or 8th intercostal space in the posterior axillary line. If air is in the pleural cavity, the thoracentesis site is usually in the 2nd or 3rd intercostal space in the midclavicular line. (The density of the air is much less than the density of the liquid.)
2. The procedure is done under aseptic conditions. After the skin is disinfected, the physician slowly injects a local anesthetic with a small caliber needle into the intercostal space.	2. An interdermal wheal is raised slowly; rapid interdermal injection causes pain. The parietal pleura is very sensitive and should be well-infiltrated with anesthetic before the thoracentesis needle is passed through it.
3. The physician advances the thoracentesis needle slowly and maintains constant suction on the syringe so it will be immediately apparent when the fluid pocket is reached.	

Nursing Action	**Rationale/Amplification**
a. A 50-ml. syringe with a 3-way adapter (stopcock) is attached to the needle (one end of the adapter is attached to the needle and the other to the tubing leading to a receptacle receiving the fluid being aspirated).	a. When a large quantity of fluid is withdrawn, a 3-way adapter serves to keep air from entering the pleural cavity.
b. If a considerable quantity of fluid is to be removed, the needle is held in place on the chest wall with a small hemostat.	b. The hemostat steadies the needle on the chest wall. Sudden pleuritic pain or shoulder pain may indicate that the visceral or diaphragmatic pleura are being irritated by the needle point.
4. After the needle is withdrawn, pressure is applied over the puncture site and a small sterile dressing is fixed in place.	

Follow-up Phase

1. Place the patient on his unaffected side for approximately 1 hour.	1. This permits the pleural site to seal itself and thus prevents fluid seepage from cough or from gravitational forces.
2. Record the total amount of fluid withdrawn and the nature of the fluid, its color and viscosity. If ordered, prepare samples of fluid for laboratory evaluation.	2. The fluid may be clear, serous, bloody, purulent, etc.
3. Evaluate the patient at intervals for faintness, vertigo, tightness in the chest, uncontrollable cough, blood-tinged frothy mucus and a rapid pulse.	3. Pneumothorax, tension pneumothorax, subcutaneous emphysema or pyogenic infection may result from a thoracentesis. Pulmonary edema or cardiac distress can be produced by a sudden shift in mediastinal contents when large amounts of fluid are aspirated.

OXYGEN THERAPY

General Considerations

1. Oxygen is an odorless, tasteless, colorless transparent gas that is slightly heavier than air.
2. Oxygen is given for conditions producing hypoxia, either local or generalized, to produce a higher oxygen concentration in the patient's tissues.
   a. *Hypoxia*—a state in which there is an insufficient amount of oxygen available in the tissue cells to meet the requirements of an organ or tissue at that moment.
   b. *Hypoxemia*—a decrease in oxygen content of the blood.
3. Measurement of the arterial blood gases is the best method of determining the adequacy of oxygen therapy (p. 120).
4. The clinical manifestations of oxygen deprivation depend upon the acuteness with which the condition develops.
   a. Sudden hypoxia—clinical picture resembles drunkenness. Changes in the central nervous system are important as the higher centers are more sensitive; produces impaired judgment and motor incoordination.
   b. Long-standing hypoxia—fatigue, drowsiness, apathy, inattentiveness and delayed reaction time.

TABLE 3-2. METHODS OF OXYGEN ADMINISTRATION

Method	Advantages	Disadvantages	Nursing Implications
Oropharyngeal catheter (nasal catheter)	Probably most effective method of oxygenation Allows controlled O_2 therapy Does not interfere with patient care May be used by restless patient	Can produce excoriation of the nares	Change catheter every 8 hours Use alternate nostril
Nasal cannula	Safe and simple method More comfortable and acceptable by patient Useful for patients requiring low O_2 concentrations (chronic obstructive lung disease) Allows patient to move about in bed.	Difficult to maintain in position and is easily dislodged Patient must be alert and cooperative to keep cannula in proper place	Watch for excessive flow rates—causes pain in frontal sinuses Stabilize nasal cannula when caring for restless patient
Face mask	O_2 can be given quickly for short periods of time	Lack of patient tolerance results in inadequate therapy May be uncomfortable as a tight seal must be maintained between face and mask Mask may produce a pressure necrosis of the skin Hot—confines heat radiating from face about nose and mouth Must be removed to eat or drink	Do not strap a mask on an unconscious patient Wash, dry and powder under mask every 2 hours Massage face at intervals
Face tent	Ideal for providing extra humidification for aerosols	Less reliable than face mask for maintaining high inspiration of O_2 concentration	
Tent	Able to control temperature and humidity	Limited usefulness Difficult to maintain adequate concentration Costly to maintain	Flush the tent with O_2 every time tent is opened Assess for leaks around canopy

5. Oxygen must be given with extreme caution in some patients. In certain conditions (chronic obstructive lung disease) the sudden administration of a high oxygen concentration will remove the respiratory drive that has been created largely by the patient's low oxygen tension.
   a. Ventilation becomes reduced.
   b. Acute acidosis and carbon dioxide narcosis may follow.

6. Oxygen supports combustion, and there is always danger of fire when oxygen is being used.
   a. Avoid using oil or grease around oxygen connections.
   b. Eliminate antiseptic tinctures, alcohol and ether in immediate oxygen environment.
   c. Do not permit any electrical devices (radios, heating pads, electric razors) in or near an oxygen tent.
   d. Keep the oxygen cylinder (if used) secured in an upright position away from heat.
   e. Post NO SMOKING signs on the patient's door and in view of the patient's visitors.
   f. Have fire extinguisher available.
7. Oxygen is dispensed from a cylinder or piped-in system and requires:
   a. *Reduction gauge*—reduces pressure to that of the atmosphere.
   b. *Flow meter* (flow gauge, flow control)—regulates control of oxygen in liters per minute.

Methods of Administering Oxygen

1. Oxygen may be administered by oropharyngeal catheter (nasal catheter), nasal cannula, face mask, face tent and tent (See Table 3-2).
2. The method selected depends on the concentration of oxygen required.

GUIDELINES: *Administering Oxygen by Oropharyngeal Catheter*

Purpose

To administer a low or moderate concentration of oxygen.

Equipment

Oxygen source
Flow meter
Humidifier filled with distilled
    water to appropriate mark
Oropharyngeal catheter
    No. 8–10 F for children
    No. 10–12 F for women
    No. 12–14 F for men

Connecting tubing
Tongue depressor, water-soluble
    lubricant, gauze squares
Flashlight
Hypoallergenic tape
NO SMOKING signs

Procedure

Preparatory Phase

1. Post NO SMOKING signs on door of room and in view of patient and visitors.
2. Explain the advantages of oxygen therapy to the patient.
3. Attach flowmeter to humidifier and then to wall outlet or oxygen cylinder.
4. Attach tubing to humidifier and the catheter to the connecting tube.

Nursing Action	**Rationale/Amplification**

Performance Phase

1. To measure the depth of catheter insertion:
   a. Measure the catheter from the tip of the patient's nose to the tragus (lobe) of the ear. Mark this with tape.
2. To insert oropharyngeal catheter:
   a. Lubricate the catheter with a small amount of water-soluble lubricant.
   b. Start the flow of oxygen at 2–3 liter/minute.

   c. Determine the natural droop of the catheter.
   d. Hyperextend the patient's head.
   e. Slide the lubricated catheter along the floor of either nare into the oropharynx.
   f. Inspect the oropharynx, using the tongue depressor and flashlight to see the position of the catheter.
   g. *Pull the catheter back slightly until the tip cannot be seen.*
3. Use the opposite nare if insertion is difficult.

4. Adjust flow rate to prescribed rate (6–8 liters/ minute).

5. Secure the catheter to the bridge of the nose or the side of the face with ½-inch hypoallergic tape.
6. Attach the connecting tube to the bed leaving enough slack for the patient to move about comfortably.
7. Observe and palpate the epigastrium to see if distention develops.

8. Stay with the patient for a period of time to make sure he does not swallow, gag or cough.

Follow-up Phase

1. Remove old catheter and insert a fresh catheter into opposite nostril every 8–12 hours.

2. Observe and examine the patient hourly to see if:
   a. Catheter is unobstructed and positioned correctly (use flashlight).
   b. Oropharynx is free from irritation.

---

a. This is only an approximation of the correct distance to insert the catheter.

b. This assures the patency of the catheters and its appertures. If some of the holes in the catheter become plugged the stream of oxygen flowing on a localized area of mucous membrane will cause a burning sensation.

f. The tip of the catheter should rest approximately opposite the uvula.

g. This is done to prevent aspiration of oxygen.

3. Nasal pathology (deviated septum, mucosal edema, mucous drainage, polyps) may interfere with catheter insertion.

4. A flow rate of 6–8 liters/minute should provide an inspired oxygen concentration of 30–50%.

5. Proper fixation is essential to prevent downward displacement of the catheter.

7. In patients with depressed glottal reflexes or epiglottal paralysis (coma, post stroke, etc.) the oxygen stream may be directed into the esophagus and cause gastric distention or rupture (if the catheter is positioned too deeply).

1. Frequent changes of the oropharyngeal catheter are necessary to prevent catheter encrustation and ulceration of the nasal mucosa.

Nursing Action	**Rationale/Amplification**
c. Humidifier bottle contains water.	c. Oxygen dehydrates tissues unless moistened.
d. Leaks are occurring around humidifier and tubing connections.	
e. Oxygen cylinder contains enough oxygen.	
3. Assess the patient's condition frequently.	3. Assess the patient for mental aberration, disturbed consciousness, abnormal color, perspiration, changes in blood pressure and increasing heart and temperature rates.

GUIDELINES: *Administering Oxygen by Nasal Cannula*

Purpose

To administer a low-to-medium concentration of oxygen.

Equipment

Oxygen source
Plastic nasal cannula with connecting tubing (disposable) (Fig. 3-9)
Humidifier filled with distilled water to indicated level
Flowmeter
NO SMOKING signs (2)

Procedure

Preparatory Phase

1. Post NO SMOKING signs on patient's door and in view of patient and visitors.
2. Show the nasal cannula to the patient and explain the procedure.
3. Make sure the humidifier is filled to the appropriate mark. If the humidifier bottle is too full, the bubbling water will overflow into the gauges.
4. Attach the connecting tube from the nasal cannula to the humidifier outlet.
5. Set the flow rate at 2 liters/minute. Feel to determine if oxygen is flowing through the nasal tips of the cannula.

Nursing Action	**Rationale/Amplification**
Performance Phase	
1. Place the tips of the cannula in the patient's nose.	1. Position the cannula so that the tips of the cannulae do not extend more than 2.5 cm. (1 inch) into the nares.
2. Adjust flow rate to 6–8 liters/minute (or as prescribed).	2. A flow of 6–8 liters/minute should provide an inspired oxygen concentration of 30–50%.
	Flow rates in excess of 8 liters/minute may lead to air swallowing and cause irritation to the nasal and pharyngeal mucosa.
3. Fasten tubing to the pillow and bed clothing.	
Follow-up Phase	
1. Change cannula, humidifiers, tubing and other equipment exposed to moisture daily.	1. Continuous oxygen therapy and high humidity may cause virulent infections in debilitated patients via contaminated equipment.
2. Assess patient's condition and the functioning of equipment at regular intervals.	2. Assess the patient for mental aberration, disturbed consciousness, abnormal color, perspiration, changes in blood pressure and increasing heart and temperature rates.

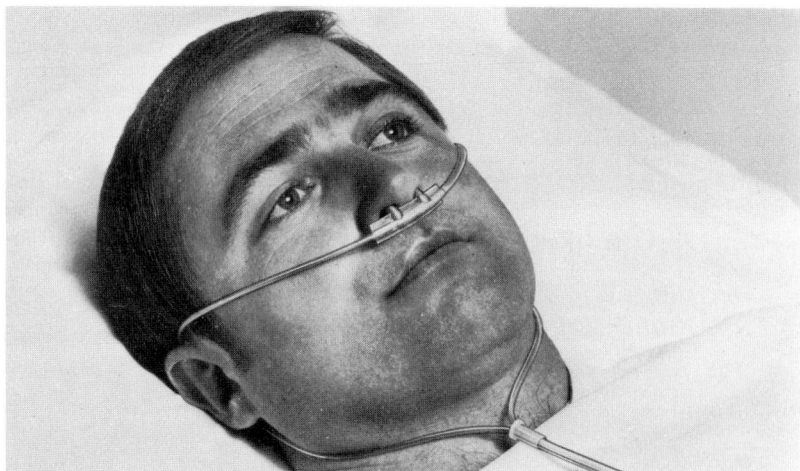

Figure 3-9. Administering oxygen by nasal cannula. (Courtesy Hudson Oxygen Therapy Sales Company.)

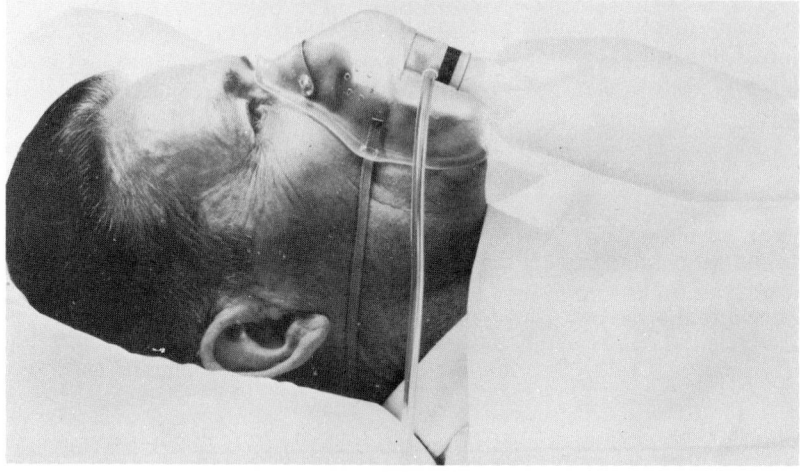

Figure 3-10. Disposable face mask which is anatomically sculptured for patient comfort. There is a flexible aluminum strip at the nose portion of the mask that prevents oxygen leakage into the patient's eyes. (Courtesy Hudson Oxygen Therapy Sales Company.)

GUIDELINES: *Administering Oxygen by Face Mask (Partial Rebreathing Type)*

A *rebreathing bag permits* the patient to inhale a high concentration of oxygen from a reservoir bag. Perforations on both sides of the mask serve as exhalation ports. High concentrations of oxygen are indicated in the acute phase of some diseases (myocardial infarction, pulmonary edema, pulmonary embolism).

Purpose

To administer a high oxygen concentration.

Equipment

Oxygen source
Plastic face mask with reservoir bag
   and tubing (Fig. 3-10)

Humidifier with distilled water
Flowmeter
NO SMOKING signs

Procedure

Preparatory Phase

1. Post NO SMOKING signs on patient's door and in view of patient and visitors.
2. Fill humidifier with sterile distilled water.
3. Attach tubing to outlet on humidifier.
4. Attach flowmeter.
5. Adjust flowmeter to 6–10 liters/minute.
6. Explain the benefits of the oxygen therapy to the patient.
7. Flush the reservoir bag with oxygen to partially inflate the bag.

Nursing Action	**Rationale/Amplification**
Performance Phase	
1. Place the mask on the patient's face and adjust liter flow so that the rebreathing bag will not collapse during the inspiratory cycle, even during deep inspiration.	1. Be sure the mask fits snugly as there must be an airtight seal between the mask and the patient's face.
	With a well-fitting rebreathing bag adjusted so that the patient's inhalation does not deflate the bag, inspired oxygen concentrations of 35–60% can be achieved at flow rates between 6–10 liters/minute.
2. Attach the tubing to the pillow and bed clothes. Keep the tubing free of kinks.	
3. Stay with the patient for a period of time to make him comfortable and observe his reactions.	3. Be sure that oxygen is not escaping from the top of the mask and blowing into the patient's eyes.
Follow-up Phase	
1. Remove mask periodically (if patient's condition permits) to dry the face around mask. Powder skin and massage face around the mask.	1. These actions reduce moisture accumulation under the mask. Massage of the face stimulates circulation and reduces pressure over the area.
2. Observe for change of condition. Assess equipment for malfunctioning and low water level in humidifier.	2. Assess the patient for mental aberration, disturbed consciousness, abnormal color, perspiration, change in blood pressure and increasing heart and temperature rates.

GUIDELINES: *Administering Oxygen by Venturi Mask*

A *venturi mask* is a face mask designed to administer precisely controlled low oxygen concentrations (Fig. 3-11). The mask is constructed so that there is a constant flow of room air mixed with a fixed concentration of oxygen. It is used primarily to increase the comfort and breathing efficiency of the patient with chronic lung disease.

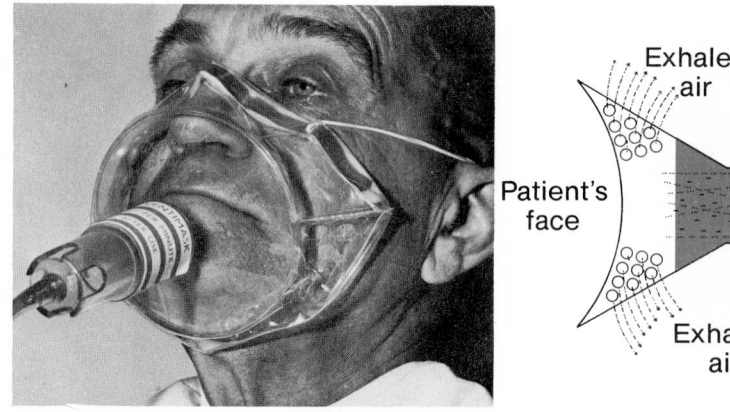

Figure 3-11. The "Ventimask" operates on the Venturi principle through which the oxygen concentration around the patient's face is precisely controlled. Rebreathing is avoided by the high airflow entering the mask. (Courtesy Bethlehem Corporation)

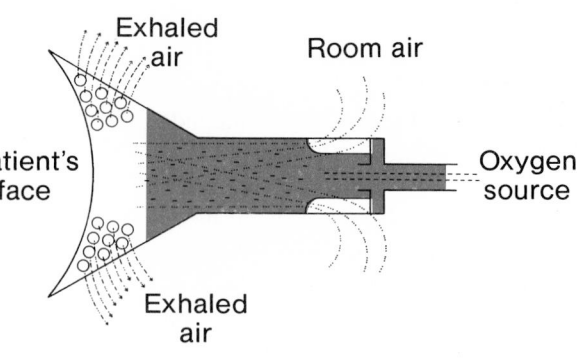

Figure 3-12. The principle of high airflow with oxygen enrichment (HAFOE).

Underlying Principles

1. The venturi mask employs the principle of air entrainment of a high air flow with oxygen enrichment (HAFOE), allowing a fixed low oxygen concentration with a flow-rate surplus according to the patient's needs (Fig. 3-12).
2. Excess gas leaves the mask through the perforated cuff carrying with it the expired carbon dioxide; this virtually eliminates rebreathing of carbon dioxide.
3. This method maintains a low oxygen concentration necessary to relieve the hypoxia of patients with chronic lung disease without inducing hypoventilation.

Equipment

Oxygen source
Venturi mask with lightweight tubing
NO SMOKING signs

Procedure

Preparatory Phase

1. Post NO SMOKING signs on the door to room and in view of patient and visitors.
2. Explain the benefits of therapy to the patient.
3. Connect the mask by lightweight tubing to the oxygen source.
4. Turn on the flowmeter and adjust to the prescribed rate (usually indicated on the mask). Check to see that oxygen is flowing out the vent holes in the flexible face piece.

Nursing Action	**Rationale/Amplification**
Performance Phase	
1. Place venturi mask over patient's nose and mouth and under the chin. Mold the mask to fit the patient's face.	

Nursing Action	**Rationale/Amplification**
2. Adjust elastic strap around the patient's head and position strap below the ears and around the neck.	

Follow-up Phase

Nursing Action	**Rationale/Amplification**
1. Assess patient's condition at frequent intervals.	1. Assess the patient for mental aberration, disturbed consciousness, abnormal color, perspiration changes in blood pressure and increasing heart and temperature rates.
2. Change mask and tubing daily.	

GUIDELINES: *Administering Oxygen by Tent**

An *oxygen tent* is a device that circulates filtered and cooled air within the environment of a plastic canopy (tent).

Purpose

To provide a low-to-moderate concentration of oxygen in a temperature-controlled environment.

Equipment

Oxygen source
Oxygen tent
Special tent call bell

Wrench
NO SMOKING signs (2)
Draw sheet

Procedure

Preparatory Phase

1. Place NO SMOKING sign on door of room and one on equipment in view of patient and visitors.
2. Explain the benefits of oxygen therapy. To allay anxiety offer this explanation before bringing the equipment into the room.
3. Place patient in a fairly high semi-Fowler's position.
4. Connect regulator to oxygen tank or wall outlet.
   a. Plug cord into wall.
   b. Turn on motor.
   c. Adjust temperature control to 18.5–22.2°C. (65–70°F.).
   d. Turn on oxygen tank and flush with high liter rate until desired concentration is reached.

Nursing Action	**Rationale/Amplification**
Performance Phase	
1. Extend the rod. Drape canopy over patient and over ½ to ⅔ of bed.	
a. Tuck top and side edges of canopy under mattress.	a. A tight seal must be made between the canopy and bed to prevent oxygen leaks.
b. Use a folded drawsheet across patient's legs to improve the seal.	
c. Tuck drawsheet under mattress.	
2. Turn flowmeter to 12–15 liters/minute.	

* Oxygen tents are used infrequently.

Nursing Action	**Rationale/Amplification**
3. Give the patient the special call bell.	3. Sparks from an electrical call bell are exceedingly dangerous as oxygen supports combustion.
4. Plan nursing care so that the patient and tent are disturbed as little as possible.	4. Oxygen is lost by displacement of incoming gas when the canopy is opened and by diffusion of gas molecules through minute leaks around the console.
a. When bathing patient slide the canopy toward the patient's neck.	
b. Flood the tent with oxygen after readjusting the canopy.	b. The oxygen environment is disrupted when the canopy is opened. The patient thereby receives only room air.
c. Wrap the patient's head and shoulders if the circulating air causes an uncomfortable draft.	
d. Take the patient's temperature via rectum.	
5. Use an oxygen analyzer to determine oxygen concentration within the tent every 4 hours.	5. An oxygen analyzer monitors oxygen concentration and permits the nurse or therapist to evaluate the operating efficiency of the tent.

Follow-up Phase

1. Assess the patient hourly to determine his condition and to check the following: a. Temperature of the tent b. Liter flow c. Amount of oxygen in the tank d. If oxygen vent is unobstructed	1. Assess the patient for mental aberration, disturbed consciousness, abnormal color, perspiration, changes in blood pressure and increasing heart and temperature rates.

GUIDELINES: *Assisting the Patient Undergoing Intermittent Positive Pressure Breathing (IPPB)*

The *intermittent positive pressure breathing* unit is a piece of equipment that supplies air or oxygen under increased pressure during inspiration (Fig. 3-13).

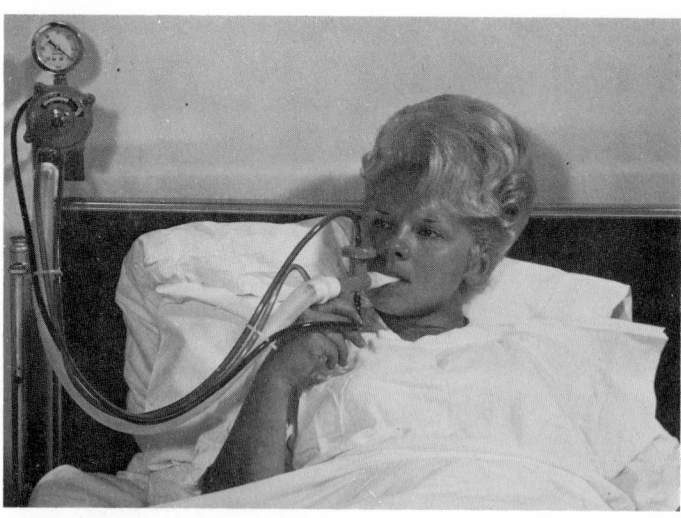

Figure 3-13. This IPPB ventilator has flow and pressure rates controlled for individual use. The patient actuates ventilator operation by inhaling. The ventilator is attached to an oxygen wall outlet. (Courtesy The Bethlehem Corporation)

Purposes

1. To increase alveolar ventilation.
2. To administer bronchodilator aerosols more effectively.
3. To aid expectoration.

Equipment

According to the type of machine used.

Procedure

Nursing Action	Rationale/Amplification
Preparatory Phase	
1. Explain the procedure to the patient.	1. Proper explanation of the procedure helps to ensure the patient's cooperation.
2. Take the blood pressure before and after the treatment for patients using bronchodilator drugs for the first time.	2. Bronchodilators accelerate cardiac action. They may produce precordial distress, palpitation, dizziness, nausea and excessive perspiration.
3. Place the patient in a comfortable sitting or semi-Fowler's position.	3. The diaphragmatic excursion is greater in this position.
4. Turn on the oxygen cylinder.	4. This is a pressure-operated machine whose source of pressure may be supplied from a cylinder of oxygen, a cylinder of compressed air, a pipe line, or a motor-driven air compressor.
5. Place the prescribed medicine in the nebulizer.	5. The volume of medication is gauged to give a treatment lasting 15 to 20 minutes. Notify the physician or inhalation therapist if medication is nebulized too quickly.
6. Select the inspiratory flow rate* according to the machine being used (usually 15 to 20 cm. H_2O). Cover the mouthpiece with a paper towel to ascertain when the predetermined pressure is reached.	6. Pressure is measured in centimeters of water pressure. Each unit should be tested to see whether the predetermined setting is accomplished before treating the patient.
7. Turn on the nebulizer control to produce a fine spray. (Some machines have a preset nebulizer.)	7. Adequate fog and particle size is essential to sufficient medication distribution.
Performance Phase	
1. Adjust the mask or mouthpiece on the patient. If the patient objects to the nose clip, instruct him to hold his nose. After several treatments, the patient can train himself to do this without the nose clip.	1. The mask or mouthpiece must constitute a closed circuit if the unit is to cycle. (If the patient exhales through the nose while using the mouthpiece, the unit will not reach the desired pressure.)
2. Have the patient place his hands on his diaphragm while breathing, concentrating on causing motion with the diaphragm rather than with the chest muscles.	2. This type of breathing encourages good diaphragmatic motion and reduces residual air volume.
3. Instruct the patient to make only a slight inspiratory effort; i.e., breathe as passively as possible.	3. A slight inspiratory effort will activate the positive pressure phase, and the lungs will be inflated with a rapid rate of flow until the predetermined pressure is reached.

* Not all IPPB machines have an inspiratory flow rate.

Nursing Action

a. Patient should take 8 to 10 respirations per minute.
b. Instruct him to hold his breath 3 to 4 seconds at the end of inspiration.
4. Remind the patient to exhale freely in a relaxed manner.

5. After several breaths, tell the patient to push all the air out, count one-two-three, and stop inhaling (on the machine) for a few seconds to assess extent of improvement.
6. Encourage the patient to continue this type of breathing until all the medication is given.

Follow-up Phase

1. Record medication used, patient's respiratory rate and effort and description of secretions expectorated.

Rationale/Amplification

b. This ensures settling of aerosol particles on bronchiolar mucosa.
4. After the lungs are inflated the flow of gas ceases and allows the patient to exhale without any assistance from the machine.

6. The medication should be completely nebulized to ensure treatment effectiveness.

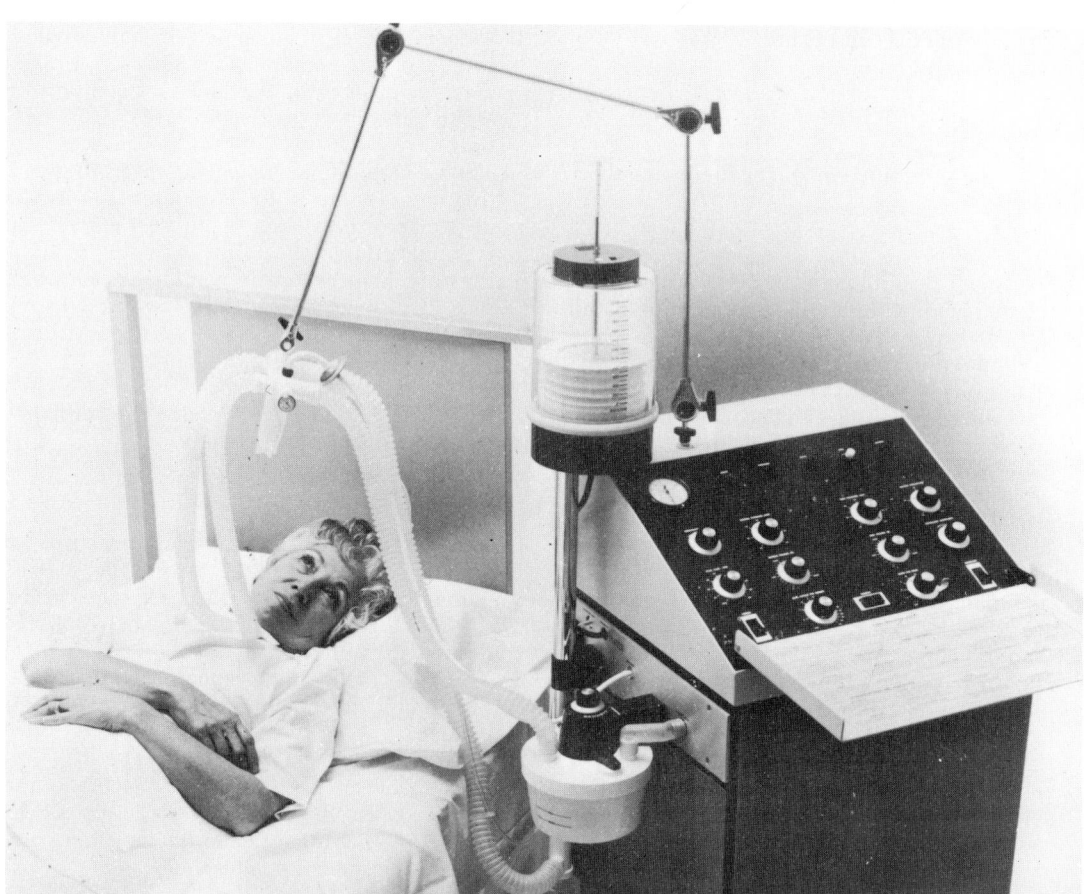

Figure 3-14. Mechanical ventilator.

MECHANICAL VENTILATION

A *mechanical ventilator* is a positive pressure breathing device which can maintain respiration automatically for prolonged periods of time (Fig. 3-14). It is indicated when the patient is unable to maintain safe levels of arterial carbon dioxide or oxygen by spontaneous breathing.

Purposes
Ventilators are used as assisters, controllers, or assister controllers:
1. The patient who is breathing by his own inspiratory effort but has inadequate ventilation is placed on the ventilator to increase his tidal volume; this is termed *assisted ventilation.*
2. The patient who has no respiratory stimulus or drive is on *controlled respiration;* the ventilator is pre-set at specific tidal volume and respiratory rate regardless of any inspiratory effort made by the patient.
3. The ventilator is capable of controlling respiratory pattern and of assisting respiration if patient makes an inspiratory effort out of phase with the ventilator; it is called *assister-controller.*

Types
1. Pressure-cycled—ventilator inflates to a pre-set pressure.
2. Volume-cycled—ventilator inflates to a pre-set volume.

Underlying Principles
1. Variables that control ventilation and oxygenation:
   a. The ventilator *rate,* measured with a watch. (Some ventilators have respiratory rate marked on respirator and adjusted by a rate knob.)
   b. The *tidal volume,* measured as expired volume with a gas meter.
   c. The *inspired oxygen concentration,* measured with an oxygen analyzer.
2. Tidal volume and rate together control the elimination of carbon dioxide.
3. The inspired oxygen concentration is controlled to produce normal arterial oxygen tension.
4. The duration of inspiration should not exceed expiration. Obstruction of venous return by prolonged inspiration lowers cardiac output and decreases the rate of oxygen transport to body tissues.
5. The inspired gas delivered to the patient must be fully saturated with water to prevent thickening of tracheobronchial secretions. Water is added by either a humidifier or nebulizer.

Clinical Indications
1. Respiratory failure
   a. Arterial pH less than 7.25; arterial blood carbon dioxide tension greater than 55 mm. Hg.
   b. Bounding pulse, small pupils, confusion, drowsiness, depressed tendon reflexes, muscular twitching, headache, coma.
2. Chronic obstructive lung disease
3. Administration of respiratory depressants
4. Neuromuscular disorders
5. Carbon monoxide poisoning or poisoning by drug intoxication
6. Cardiac arrest
7. Chest injury
8. Left ventricular failure and pulmonary edema

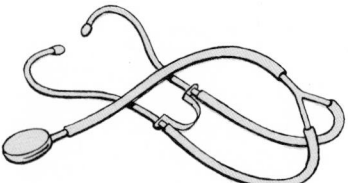

Listen to patient's chest
hourly to assess
for abnormal sounds

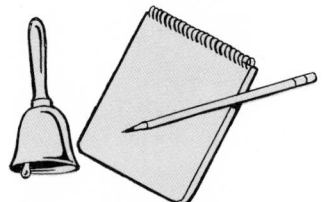

Provide means of
communication. Keep patient
in touch with reality

Assess for Complications

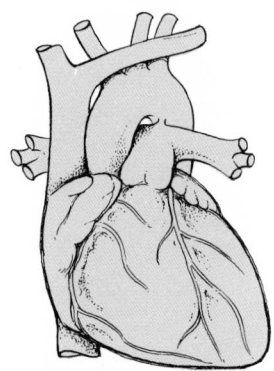

Cardiac arrhythmias
Myocardial infarction

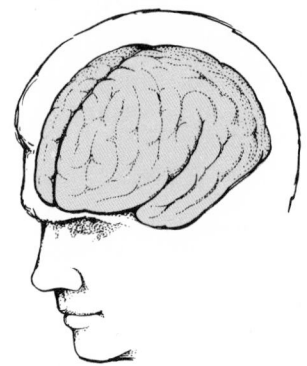

Lethargy, unconsciousness
Cerebral edema

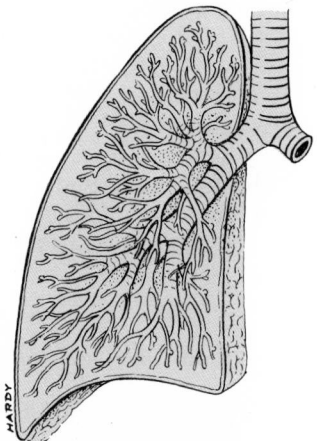

Infection, atelectasis,
pulmonary toxicity, pulmonary
emboli, damage to trachea,
pulmonary edema, tension
pneumothorax

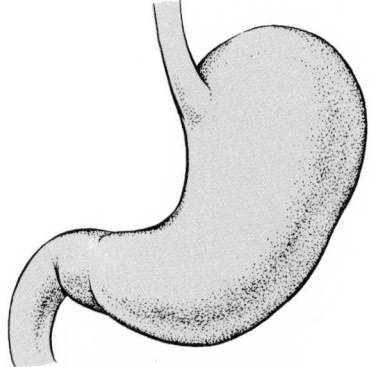

Gastrointestinal bleeding,
ileus, gastric distention,
gastric perforation. Test stool
and gastric drainage for
occult blood

Figure 3-15. Nursing support of the patient requiring mechanical ventilation.

Complications

Airway obstruction
Endobronchial intubation
Damage to the trachea
Infection
Pulmonary edema

Gastrointestinal bleeding
Tension pneumothorax
Inability to wean from ventilator
Pulmonary oxygen toxicity

GUIDELINES: Managing the Patient Requiring Mechanical Ventilation (Fig. 3-15)

Procedure

Nursing Action	Rationale/Amplification
Performance Phase	
1. Obtain base-line samples for blood gas determinations (see pp. 120–121) (pH, pO_2, pCO_2) and chest x-ray.	1. Base-line measurements serve as a guide to determine progress of therapy.
2. Give a brief explanation to the patient.	2. Emphasize that mechanical ventilation is a temporary measure.
3. Establish the airway by means of a cuffed endotracheal tube (p. 107) which is inserted by the anesthesiologist.	3. Endotracheal intubation provides access to the lower part of the airway for removal of secretions. The cuffed tube prevents leakage of air into mouth during ventilation and permits control of pressure and lung inflation.
a. Secure the tube in place with surgical adhesive. Insert a bite block (rolled gauze) between the patient's teeth if using orotracheal tube.	a. Securing the tube prevents dislodgment into the right main-stem bronchus.
4. Prepare ventilator according to manufacturer's directions:	4. Maintenance of ventilation depends on correct machine settings.
a. Turn on machine.	
b. Adjust volume control; establish tidal and minute volumes.	b. Arterial blood pH, carbon dioxide and oxygen tensions serve as a guide in adjusting the ventilator.
c. Determine oxygen concentration.	
d. Adjust respiratory rate of ventilator to 14–16 respirations/minute.	d. This setting approximates normal respiration. The patient who has respiratory stimulus will cycle machine by himself; set the control on "off." These machine settings are subject to change according to patient's condition and response and the make of the machine being used.
e. Adjust flow state (velocity of gas flow during inspiration) to 60–80 liters/minute.	
f. Couple the patient's endotracheal tube to the ventilator.	f. Be sure connections are secure. Watch for accidental disconnection between the patient's airway and the ventilator; observe for separation of ventilator tubings from nebulizer, electrical wall-plug slippage, etc.

Nursing Action	Rationale/Amplification

5. Carry out arterial blood gas determinations approximately 45 minutes after patient is on ventilator. Arterial blood sampling is carried out repeatedly during the acute period.

5. The only effective way to attain and maintain a normal oxygen tension is to measure this tention frequently in arterial blood and adjust the volume of the ventilator accordingly. Arterial blood gases are monitored to assess the effectiveness of therapy. There are no reliable physical signs of CO_2 retention and acidosis.

6. *The patient is never left unattended or unobserved.*

Positioning

1. Turn patient from side to side hourly.
2. Lateral turns of 120 degrees are desirable; from right semiprone to left semiprone.
3. Sit the patient upright at regular intervals.

3. Upright posture increases ventilation of lower lobes.

4. Position the patient in postural drainage positions as ordered (pp. 144–146).

4. Adequate postural drainage decreases the need for deep tracheobronchial catheter aspiration by preventing retention of secretions in the periphery of the lungs.

5. Carry out passive range of motion exercises of all extremities (pp. 8–18).

Deep Breaths

1. Augment the patient's spontaneous tidal volume by periodically giving him 6–8 deep breaths with a hand resuscitator bag. Provide him with adequate oxygenation during this maneuver.

1. Periodic sighing with greater than normal tidal volumes helps to prevent alveolar collapse. Provision of deep breaths by hand also helps to promote coughing and reveals the presence of retained secretions.

Aspiration of Secretions

1. Aspirate secretions from the trachea using sterile technique (p. 101).
2. Oxygenate patient for 1 to 2 minutes prior to each suctioning episode and before second passage of the catheter.
3. Note the amount, color and consistency of tracheal secretions obtained.
4. Inform the physician if there is appreciable change.

1. Ventilation and nebulization liquefy secretions causing them to rise into the upper airways.
2. Do not prolong aspiration more than 15 seconds because cardiac arrest may ensue in patients with borderline oxygenation.

Chest Auscultation

1. Listen with a stethoscope to the chest from bottom to top on both sides (hourly) (Fig. 3-6).

1. Auscultation of the chest is a means of assessing airway patency and ventilatory distribution. It also confirms the proper placement of the endotracheal or tracheostomy tube.

2. Determine whether breath sounds are present or absent, normal or abnormal, and whether a change has occurred.
3. Observe the patient's diaphragmatic excursions and changes in the use of accessory muscles of respiration.

Nursing Action	**Rationale/Amplification**
Humidification	
1. Check the water level in the humidification reservoir to ensure that the patient is never ventilated with dry gas. Empty the water condensing in the delivery tubing.	1. Water condensing in the delivery tubing may cause obstruction and sudden flooding of the trachea.
Airway Pressure	
1. Check the airway pressure gauge at frequent intervals in patients on volume-limited ventilators.	1. Since these ventilators deliver a fixed volume, a sudden drop in pressure indicates a leak in the system. A sudden rise in pressure indicates obstruction of the delivery of gas to the patient.
Tidal Volumes	
1. Measure the tidal volume with a respirometer for patients on pressure-limited ventilators.	1. An abrupt fall in tidal volume indicates increase in airway resistance (e.g., bronchospasm or other obstruction) or increase in tissue resistance (pulmonary edema).
Cuff Inflation	
1. Clean the pharynx and larynx of accumulated secretions by either suction or postural drainage.	1. If the tube becomes blocked the patient will not breathe.
2. Release air slowly from the cuff, using a syringe, while maintaining positive pressure from the ventilator or a hand resuscitator bag.	2. The cuff is deflated periodically to prevent necrosis of the tracheal mucosa.
3. Reinflate the cuff with just enough air to prevent gross leak when positive pressure is again applied to airway.	3. Too much cuff inflation may cause pressure necrosis over a period of time.
Tracheostomy	
1. Tracheostomy care should be done using sterile technique as needed (p. 98).	1. To continue ventilation while the inner cannula is removed, a substitute sterile inner cannula or adapter should be inserted into the outer cannula and connected to the ventilator.
2. The flexible connection from the tracheostomy tube to ventilator lines is cleaned or replaced by a sterile one at the same time tracheostomy care is given.	
Bacteriologic Specimens	
1. Aspirate tracheal secretions into a sterile container and send to laboratory for culture and sensitivity tests. a. This is done immediately after endotracheal intubation. b. Daily gram staining of secretions also done.	1. This technique allows the earliest detection of infection or change of infecting organisms in the tracheobronchial tree.

Nursing Action	**Rationale/Amplification**
Circulatory Measurements	
1. Monitor pulse rate and arterial blood pressure; intra-arterial pressure monitoring may be carried out.	1. To accomplish intra-arterial-pressure monitoring a catheter is introduced into an artery, usually the radial or femoral, and the pressure at the catheter tip is transmitted to a pressure transducer that converts the pressure wave into an electrical signal that is displayed for continuous visual observation on an oscilloscope.
2. Measure the central venous pressure as directed (p. 241).	2. This measurement provides a guide to the administration of blood and other intravenous fluids and also is a criterion to determine the presence of right ventricular failure.
Sedation and Muscle Relaxants	
1. Administer morphine and curare, etc. as directed.	1. Sedatives and muscle relaxants eliminate spontaneous breathing efforts between ventilator cycles and reduce oxygen consumption. Morphine and curare (or similar drugs) produce vasodilation. Measure arterial blood pressure before their administration to detect hypotension.
2. Explain procedures to patient and provide reassurance.	2. The patient may be awake although not capable of any motor response while these drugs are being given.
Fluid Balance	
1. Record intake and output precisely and obtain an accurate daily weight.	1. Positive fluid balance resulting in increase in body weight and interstitial pulmonary edema is a frequent problem in patients requiring mechanical ventilation. Prevention requires early recognition of fluid accumulation. Average adult who is dependent on parenteral nutrition can be expected to lose 0.25 kg. (½ lb.)/day; therefore, *constant body weight indicates positive fluid balance.*
Nutrition	
1. Offer patient oral fluids and food if he is able to swallow. If aspiration occurs, stop the feeding and place patient in a semiprone position with head-down; tilt and institute chest physical therapy to remove aspirated material. a. Start nasogastric feeding if oral intake is not adequate (p. 383).	1. Starvation is a frequent and serious complication of patients in respiratory failure.
Abdominal Complications	
1. Test all stools and gastric drainage for occult blood.	1. About ¼ of patients requiring mechanical ventilation develop gastrointestinal bleeding; many of these require blood transfusions.
2. Measure abdominal girth daily.	2. Abdominal distention occurs frequently with respiratory failure and further hinders respiration by elevation of the diaphragm. Measurement of abdominal girth provides objective assessment of the degree of distention.

Communication

1. Provide writing paper and pad. A patient on mechanical ventilation with tracheostomy tube is unable to talk.
2. Establish some form of nonverbal communication if patient is too sick to write. Give patient the call light.
3. Reassure patient and family that normal speech will return upon removal of tracheal tube.
4. Ensure that the patient has adequate rest and sleep.
5. Keep the patient in touch with reality; explain that mechanical ventilation is only temporary.

Recording

1. Maintain a flow sheet to record ventilation patterns, arterial blood studies, venous chemical determinations, hematocrit, status of fluid balance, weight and assessment of patient's condition.

Weaning the Patient from the Mechanical Ventilator

Weaning—permits the patient to breathe on his own for gradually increasing periods of time after mechanical ventilation is discontinued.

Stages of Weaning

1. From mechanical ventilator
2. From the tracheostomy tube cuff
3. From the tracheostomy stoma
4. From supplementary inspired air

A. *Weaning From the Ventilator*
1. Stay with the patient; try to distract him.
2. Ventilate the patient with oxygen before the weaning period.
3. Take patient off ventilator for a few minutes to ½ hour as tolerated.
4. Observe for *fatigue,* dyspnea, flaring of alae nasi, increasing pulse rate, sweating, facial pallor and cyanosis and rising blood pressure.
5. Provide him with high inspired oxygen concentration during these periods.
6. Take arterial blood samples for blood gas determinations (usually in 30 minutes and 2 and 4 hours) after weaning period to see if patient is maintaining adequate oxygenation.
7. Increase weaning time gradually.

B. *Weaning from the Tracheostomy Tube Cuff*
1. Seat patient upright and deflate tracheostomy or endotracheal cuff during periods of spontaneous breathing.
2. Test patient's ability to swallow without aspiration before cuff is deflated.
   a. Clear trachea, nasopharynx and oropharynx of secretions.
   b. Deflate the cuff.
   c. Have the patient drink dilute methylene blue solution (0.5 ml. in 60 ml. of water).
   d. Aspirate the trachea immediately; absence of blue dye in tracheal aspirate indicates the ability to swallow without aspiration.

C. *Weaning from the Tracheostomy Stoma*
1. A fenestrated tracheostomy tube (uncuffed tube with window in greater curvature to decrease resistance to air flow) may be used after mechanical ventilator has been discontinued.

2. Plug the external orifice of fenestrated tracheostomy tube.
    a. Evaluate the patient's ability to breathe spontaneously for long periods.
    b. Assess ability to cough and mobilize secretions without aid of tracheal aspiration.
3. The tube is usually removed when tracheal aspiration has been unnecessary for 24 hours.
4. Cover the stoma with a sterile dressing; stoma is allowed to close.

D. *Weaning from Supplementary Inspired Air*

Supplementary inspired oxygen by face mask may be required for an additional period until arterial oxygen tension during breathing of room air reaches safe levels.

Patient Education for Prevention of Recurrences of Respiratory Failure

Instruct the patient as follows:
1. Avoid and treat respiratory infections promptly (p. 92).
2. Avoid respiratory irritants, particularly smoking.
3. Take oral and nebulized bronchodilators on prescribed basis.
4. Ensure adequate hydration.
5. Carry out a program of gradually increasing exercise tolerance.

CHEST PHYSICAL THERAPY

Postural Drainage Exercises

Postural drainage is the use of specific positions so that the force of gravity can assist in the removal of bronchial secretions (Table 3-3).

Underlying Principles

1. The patient is positioned so that the diseased area(s) are in a vertical position, and gravity is used to assist drainage of that specific segment.
2. Postural drainage exercises are usually confined to posterior, lateral and anterior basal segments (bilaterally) of the lung.
3. The postures assumed are determined by the patient's clinical condition and diagnosis.
4. The exercises are usually performed 4 times daily, before meals and at bedtime.

Nursing Management

1. Make the patient comfortable before the procedure starts and as comfortable as possible while he assumes each position.
    a. Bronchodilator aerosol medications should be inhaled before postural drainage; this reduces bronchospasm, decreases thickness of mucus and sputum and combats edema of the bronchial walls.
    b. Flex the patient's knees and hips to assist in relaxing and lessening strain on abdominal muscles during coughing.
    c. Use a folding cot to prop up patient to desired height if his bed is not adjustable.
    d. Have an emesis basin available for draining mucus.
2. Evaluate patient's color and pulse the first few times he performs the exercises.
3. Have patient brush his teeth and use mouthwash after postural drainage.
4. Encourage patient to rest in bed ½ hour.

GUIDELINES: *Percussion and Vibration*

Percussion and vibration are manual techniques designed to promote drainage of mucus and secretions from the lungs while the patient is in the position of postural drainage indicated for his specific lung problem. The procedure requires trained personnel.

1. *Percussion*—Movement done by striking the chest wall in a rhythmical fashion with cupped hands over the chest segment to be drained. The wrists are alternately flexed and extended so that the chest is cupped or clapped in a painless manner.
2. *Vibration*—Technique of applying manual compression and tremor to the chest wall during the exhalation phase of respiration.

Purposes

1. To dislodge mucus adhering to the bronchioles and bronchi.
2. To help mobilize secretions.

Clinical Indications

Lung conditions that cause increased production of secretions
   Bronchiectasis
   Empyema
   Fibrocystic lung disease

Contraindications

1. Lung abscess or tumors
2. Pneumothorax
3. Diseases of the chest wall
4. Lung hemorrhage
5. Painful chest conditions
6. Tuberculosis

Procedure

Nursing Action	Rationale/Amplification
Performance Phase	
1. Instruct the patient to use diaphragmatic breathing (p. 149).	1. Diaphragmatic breathing helps the patient relax.
2. Position the patient in prescribed postural drainage position(s) (p. 146). The spine should be straight to promote rib-cage expansion.	2. The patient is positioned according to which area of the lung is to be drained.
3. Percuss (or clap) with cupped hands over the chest wall for 1 or 2 minutes from: a. The lower ribs to shoulders in the back. b. The lower ribs to top of chest in front.	3. This action helps to dislodge mucous plugs and mobilize secretions toward the main bronchi and trachea. The air trapped between the operator's hand and chest wall will produce a characteristic hollow sound.
4. Avoid clapping over the spine, liver, kidneys or spleen.	4. Percussion over these areas may cause injuries to the spine and internal organs.
5. Instruct the patient to inhale slowly and deeply. Vibrate the chest wall as the patient exhales slowly through pursed lips. a. Place one hand on top of the other over affected area or place one hand on each side of the rib cage.	5. This sets up a vibration that carries through the chest wall and helps free the mucus.
b. Tense the muscles of the hands and arms causing the arms to vibrate in a rapid shaking motion.	b. This maneuver is performed in the direction in which the ribs move upon expiration.

TABLE 3-3. POSTURAL DRAINAGE EXERCISES*

Begin exercise session with aerosol medication if prescribed by your doctor.

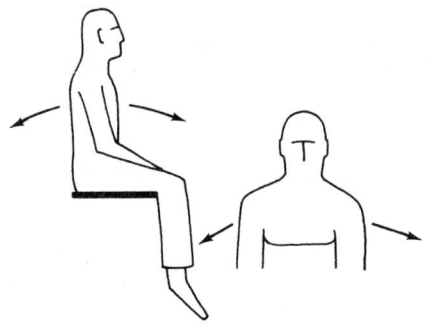

EXERCISE 1

Sit upright on edge of bed or chair, lean slightly back and forward (drains apical and lung posterior segments on the right and the posterior segments of the left lung), then lean left and right (drains upper lobe segment). Hold each position half a minute.

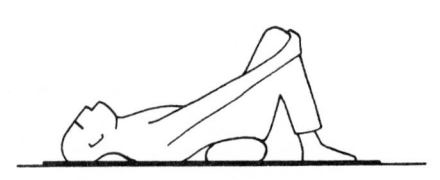

EXERCISE 2

Lie on back, with small rolled blanket or cushion under hips. Bend knees, pull thighs toward chest. Keep feet on bed. Hold position for half a minute.

Note: Foot of bed many be elevated 18 inches for greater effectiveness.

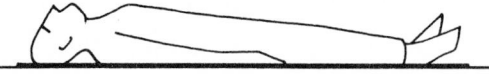

EXERCISE 3

Lie flat on back without pillow, arms at side. Hold position half a minute.

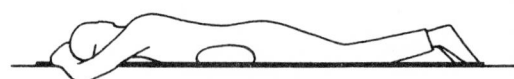

EXERCISE 4

Lie face downward, head on arms, with small rolled blanket or cushion under lower abdomen to flatten back (position for draining segments of the lower lobes). Hold position half a minute.

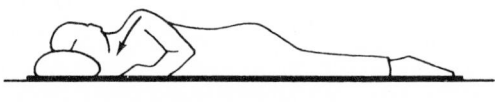

EXERCISE 5

Straight lateral position for emptying lateral segments. Lie on right side with pillow supporting head, as shown. Hold half a minute. Then swing left shoulder forward, using right shoulder as a pivot. Hold half a minute.

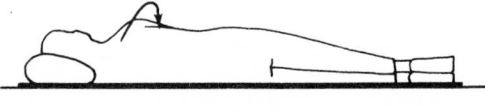

EXERCISE 6

Lie on left side with pillow supporting head, as shown. Hold half a minute. Then swing right shoulder forward, using left shoulder as a pivot. Hold half a minute. Helps drainage of right upper lobe and posterior segment of lung.

* Adapted from Breon Laboratories Inc.

TABLE 3-3. POSTURAL DRAINAGE EXERCISES (continued)

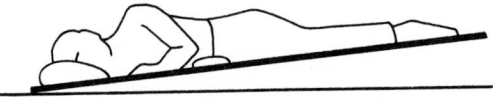

EXERCISE 7

With foot of bed elevated 18 inches, lie on right side. Place small rolled blanket or cushion between hip bone and bottom rib. Hold position half a minute. Helps drain lower lobe and lateral basal segment of lung.

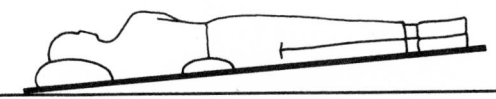

EXERCISE 8

With foot of bed elevated 18 inches, lie on left side. Place small rolled blanket or cushion between hip bone and bottom rib. Hold position half a minute.

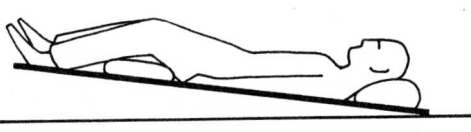

EXERCISE 9

With foot of bed elevated 18 inches, lie on back, with pillow under knees. (Pillow promotes relaxation of abdominal muscles.) Hold position half a minute. Helps drain lower lobes and anterior basal segments of lung.

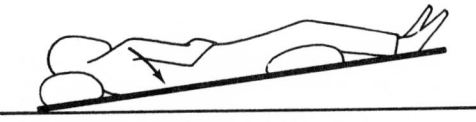

EXERCISE 10

With foot of bed elevated 18 inches, lie on back, with body turned slightly onto left side, pillow under knees. Hold half a minute. Then turn body slightly onto right side. Hold half a minute. Helps drain apical lobes of lungs.

BASIC POSITION

Use this at end of all postural drainage exercises. Lie face down across a level bed 30–60 degrees from the horizontal with hips at edge of bed. Back should be straight. Maintain a 45-degree angle for maximum drainage. (Drains lower lobes and posterior basal segments of lung.) Rest forearms on floor, forehead on upturned hands. Breathe deeply and cough gently to expel mucus and secretions raised by previous exercises. A folded towel may be used to make forehead and arms more comfortable. Have an emesis basin available to receive draining mucus.

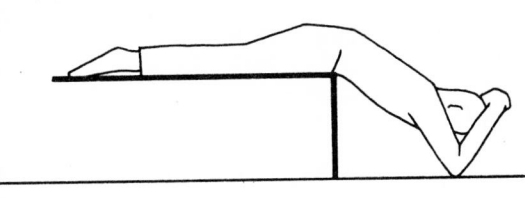

Nursing Action	**Rationale/Amplification**
c. Relieve pressure on the thorax as the patient inhales.	
d. Encourage the patient to cough using his abdominal muscles after 3 or 4 vibrations.	d. Contracting the abdominal muscles while coughing increases cough effectiveness. Coughing aids in the movement and expulsion of secretions.
6. Allow the patient to rest several minutes.	
7. Listen with a stethoscope to changes in breath sounds.	7. The appearance of moist sounds (rales, rhonchi) indicates movement of air around mucus in the bronchi.
8. Repeat the percussion and vibration cycle according to the patient's tolerance and his clinical response; usually 15 to 20 minutes.	

GUIDELINES: *Teaching the Patient Breathing Exercises*

Breathing exercises are exercises and breathing practices that are done to correct respiratory deficits and to increase efficiency in breathing.

Purposes

1. To relax muscles and relieve anxiety.
2. To eliminate useless uncoordinated patterns of respiratory muscle activity.
3. To slow the respiratory rate.
4. To decrease the work of breathing.

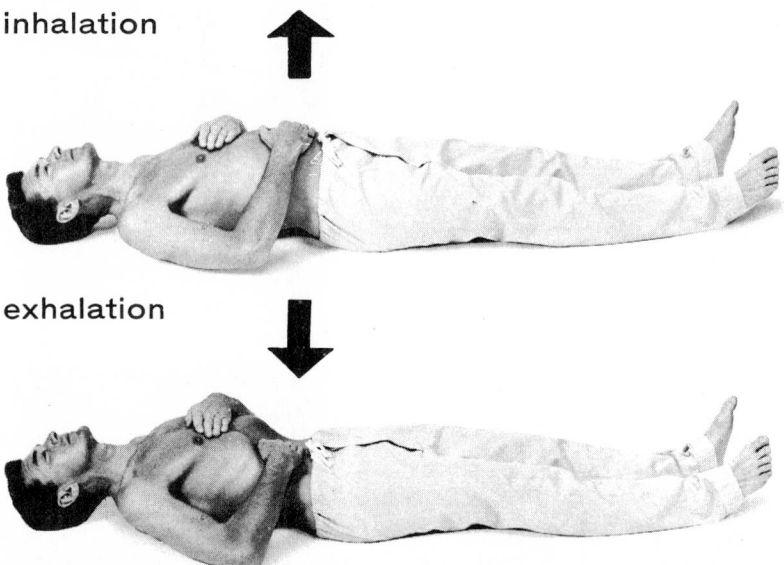

Figure 3-16. Breathing exercises for inhalation and exhalation. (From *Living with Asthma, Chronic Bronchitis, and Emphysema.* Riker Laboratories, Inc., Northridge, California.)

General Instructions

1. Breathe slowly in a rhythmical and relaxed manner—permits more complete exhalation and emptying of lungs; helps overcome anxiety associated with dyspnea and decreases oxygen requirements.
2. Clear the nasal passages before beginning breathing exercises.
3. Always inhale through the nose—permits filtration, humidification and warming of air.
4. Avoid sudden exertion.

Diaphragmatic Breathing

Purpose: To increase the use of the diaphragm during breathing.

Teaching Principles	*Rationale/Amplification*
Instruct the patient as follows:	
1. Place one hand on stomach just below the ribs and the other hand on the middle of the chest.	1. This helps the patient to become aware of the diaphragm and its function in breathing.
2. Breathe in slowly and deeply through the nose letting the abdomen protrude as far as it will (Fig. 3-16A). The abdomen enlarges during inspiration and lowers during expiration.	2. Slow inhalation provides ventilation and hyperinflation of the lungs.
3. Breathe out through pursed lips while contracting (tightening) the abdominal muscles. Press firmly inward and upward on the abdomen while breathing out (Fig. 3-16B).	3. Contracting the abdominal muscles aids the diaphragm in rising to empty the lungs.
4. The chest should move as little as possible; attention should be directed to the abdomen, not the chest.	4. Contraction of the abdominal muscles should take place during expiration.
5. Repeat for approximately 1 minute followed by a rest period of 2 minutes. Work up to 10 minutes, 4 times daily.	
6. Learn to do diaphragmatic breathing while lying, then sitting and ultimately standing and walking.	6. Diaphragmatic breathing should become automatic with sufficient practice and concentration. If the patient becomes short of breath have him stop the exercises until his breathing pattern comes under control.

Pursed-lip Breathing

Purposes

1. To train the muscles of expiration.
2. To prolong expiration and lessen amount of airway trapping and resistance.

Teaching Principles	*Rationale/Amplification*
Instruct the patient as follows:	
1. Inhale through the nose.	
2. Exhale slowly and evenly against pursed lips while contracting (tightening) the abdominal muscles.	2. Pursing the lips increases intra-alveolar pressure. The pursed-lip maneuver also prolongs the expiratory phase of breathing, makes it easier to empty the air in the lungs and promotes carbon dioxide elimination.
a. Count to 7 while prolonging expiration through pursed lips.	

Teaching Principles	Rationale/Amplification

3. Sit in a chair. Fold the arms across the abdomen.
   a. Inhale through the nose.
   b. Bend over and exhale slowly through pursed lips while counting to 7.
4. While walking:
   a. Inhale while walking 2 steps.
   b. Exhale through pursed lips while walking 4 steps.
	
	b. Leaning forward pushes the abdominal organs upward.
	4. Try any similar combinations according to breathing tolerance of patient.

Other Exercises

A. *Lower Side Rib Breathing*
1. Place hands on sides on lower ribs.
2. Inhale deeply and slowly while sides expand, moving hands outward.
3. Exhale slowly and feel the hands and ribs move in.
4. Rest.

B. *Lower Back and Rib Breathing*
1. Sit in a chair. Place hands behind back flat on lower ribs.
2. Inhale deeply and slowly while rib cage expands backward; the hands will move outward.
3. Keep hands in place. Blow out slowly; hands will move in.

C. *Segmental Breathing*
1. Place hands on sides on lower ribs.
2. Inhale deeply and slowly while concentrating on moving the right hand outward by expanding the right rib cage.
3. Ensure that the right hand moves outward more than the left hand.
4. Keeping hands in place, exhale slowly and feel the right hand and ribs moving in.
5. Repeat, concentrating on expanding left side more than the right side.
6. Rest.

WATER-SEAL CHEST DRAINAGE

In *water-seal chest drainage* an intrapleural drainage tube is used after some intrathoracic procedures. One or more chest catheters (usually No. 28 Fr. tubes) are held in the pleural space in the posterior axillary line by suture to the chest wall.

Underlying Principles

1. Breathing mechanism operates on the principle of negative pressure (pressure in chest cavity is lower than pressure of outside air, causing air to rush into chest cavity).
2. When chest has been opened, vacuum must be applied to chest to re-establish negative pressure.
3. Closed water-seal drainage is method of re-establishing negative pressure. (Open drainage system would allow air to be sucked back into chest cavity and collapse lung. Water acts as a seal and keeps the air from being drawn back into the pleural space.)
4. Closed drainage is established by placing catheter into pleural space and allowing it to drain under water. (End of drainage tube is always kept under water so air will not be drawn up through catheter into pleural space.)

Types of Water-seal Drainage

A. *The 1-bottle system*

ONE-BOTTLE WATER-SEAL SYSTEM

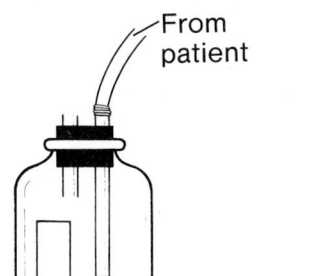

From patient

Inspiration
Expiration

Water-seal and Drainage Bottle

1. A tube extends from patient to below level of water.
2. Vent for escaping air is provided.
3. Water level fluctuates as patient breathes. (Goes up when patient breathes in and goes down when the patient breathes out.)
4. Water should *not* bubble constantly.

B. *The 2-bottle system*

TWO-BOTTLE WATER-SEAL SYSTEM

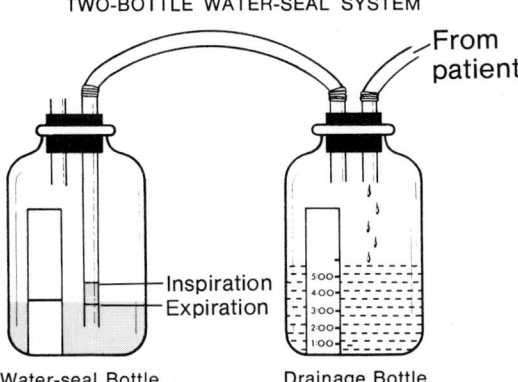

From patient

Inspiration
Expiration

Water-seal Bottle   Drainage Bottle

1. Drainage bottle
   a. A short tube extends from patient into drainage bottle (not to be below the drainage level).
   b. Drainage level is marked on outside tape.
   c. Drainage fluid can be measured accurately and its color and character observed more efficiently when drainage empties into separate bottle.
2. Water-seal bottle
   a. An under-water tube (not the patient's tube) is connected to the drainage bottle.
   b. Second tube provides air vent.
   c. Water in long tube in second bottle should go up and down as patient breathes.

C. *The 3-bottle system (Mechanical suction system)*

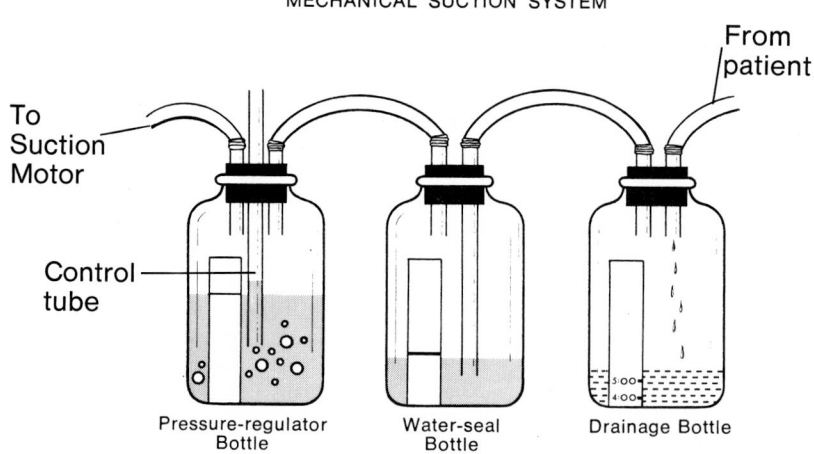

MECHANICAL SUCTION SYSTEM

From patient

To Suction Motor

Control tube

Pressure-regulator Bottle   Water-seal Bottle   Drainage Bottle

1. Mechanical suction motor creates and maintains a negative pressure throughout the closed drainage system by applying a constant amount of suction to the pleural space.
2. Drainage bottle and water-seal bottle
   Are set up as in 2-bottle system.
3. Third bottle regulates the amount of pressure in the system.
   a. Contains 3 tubes
      (1) A short tube, above water level, comes from water-seal bottle.
      (2) Another short tube leads to suction motor.
      (3) Third tube is below water level in bottle and opens to the atmosphere outside of bottle.
            Depth to which this tube is submerged in the water determines the pressure within the drainage system.
   b. When drainage system pressure becomes too low, outside air is sucked into the system which results in constant bubbling in the pressure-regulator bottle—indicates the system is functioning properly.
NOTE: Whenever the motor is off, the drainage system must be open to the atmosphere so that intrapleural air can escape from the system. Detach the tubing from the motor to provide this vent.

GUIDELINES: *Managing the Patient Undergoing Water-Seal Chest Drainage*

Purposes
1. To remove air and fluid from the thoracic cavity.
2. To facilitate re-expansion of the lung after surgery or trauma.

Equipment
Closed-chest drainage setup usually assembled in the O.R.
Holder for drainage bottle
4 hemostats or clamps taped to the head of the bed.

Procedure

Nursing Action	Rationale/Amplification

Performance Phase

1. Attach the drainage tube from the pleural cavity to the tubing that leads to a long tube that ends under sterile water.

1. Water-seal drainage provides for the escape of air and fluid into a drainage bottle. The water acts as a seal and keeps the air from being drawn back into the pleural space.

2. Tape the places where the tubing is connected.

2. Taping the connecting points of the tubing will make certain that the tubing remains airtight to re-establish negative (intrapleural) pressure.

   a. The tube should be approximately 1–2 cm. (1 inch) under the water level. The short tube is left open to the atmosphere.

   a. If the tube is submerged too deeply below the water level, a higher intrapleural pressure is required to expel air. Venting the short glass tube lets air escape from the bottle.

   b. Tape the part of the tubing entering the drainage bottle to a tongue blade.

   b. This prevents kinking of the tube and resultant obstruction of drainage.

3. Place strip of marking tape on outside of bottle (Fig. 3-17).

3. This will show the amount of blood loss and how fast fluid collects in the drainage bottle and will serve as a basis for calculating blood volume replacement.

4. Fasten the tubing to the drawsheet so flow by gravity will occur. The tubing should not loop or interfere with movements of the patient.

4. Kinking or looping or pressure on the drainage tubing can produce retrograde (back) pressure, thus forcing drainage back into the pleural cavity.

5. Encourage good body alignment. When the patient is in a lateral position, place a rolled towel under the tubing to protect it from the weight of the patient's body (Fig. 3-18).

5. The patient's position should be changed frequently to promote drainage, and the body kept in good alignment to prevent postural deformities and contractures.

   a. Encourage the patient to lie on his affected side.

   a. Drainage is facilitated when the patient lies on his affected side.

6. Put the arm and shoulder on the affected side through range-of-motion exercises several times daily.

6. Exercise helps to avoid ankylosis of the shoulder and assists in minimizing postoperative pain and discomfort.

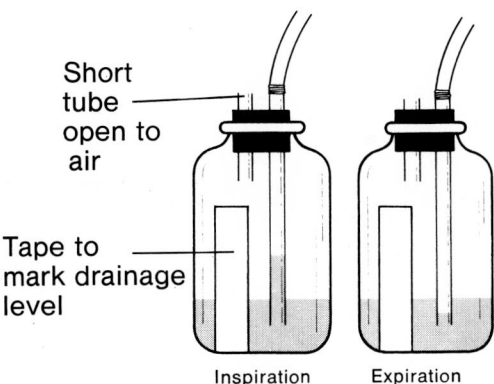

Short tube open to air

Tape to mark drainage level

Inspiration   Expiration

Figure 3-17. There is an up and down movement (fluctuation) of water in the long tube, showing the rise and fall of the patient's intrapleural pressure during inspiration and expiration. The short tube is opened to the atmosphere to permit evacuation of intrapleural air from the drainage bottle.

Nursing Action	**Rationale/Amplification**
7. "Milk" in the direction of the drainage bottle hourly.	7. "Milking" the tubes prevents them from becoming plugged with clots and fibrin. Constant attention to maintain the patency of the tube will facilitate prompt expansion of the lung and minimize later complications.
8. Make sure there is oscillation (fluctuation) of fluid level in the long glass tube:	8. Oscillation of the water level in the glass tube shows that there is effective communication between the pleural cavity and the drainage bottle.
a. The oscillation of the fluid level in the tube will stop when the lung has re-expanded.	a. Oscillation of water in the long glass tube is related to inspiration and expiration and indicates proper functioning of the apparatus.
b. Oscillation may cease before re-expansion due to blood clots and fibrin sealing off the tube.	
9. Watch for leaks of air in the drainage system as indicated by constant bubbling in the water-seal bottle.	9. Leaking and trapping of air in the pleural space can result in tension pneumothorax.
10. Observe and report immediately signs of rapid, shallow breathing, cyanosis, pressure in the chest, subcutaneous emphysema and symptoms of hemorrhage.	10. Tension pneumothorax, mediastinal shift and hemorrhage are serious complications that require prompt surgical intervention.
11. Encourage the patient to breathe deeply and cough at frequent intervals.	11. Deep breathing and coughing assist in raising the intrapleural pressure and in clearing the bronchi, expanding the lung and preventing atelectasis.
12. Stabilize the drainage bottle by placing it in wooden blocks on the floor or in a special holder.	12. If any part of the apparatus is damaged, the closed system of drainage will be destroyed and the patient will be endangered by atmospheric pressure in the pleural space and the resultant collapse of lung. The drainage system must be kept air-tight to re-establish negative intrapleural pressure.
Caution visitors and personnel against handling equipment or displacing the drainage bottle.	

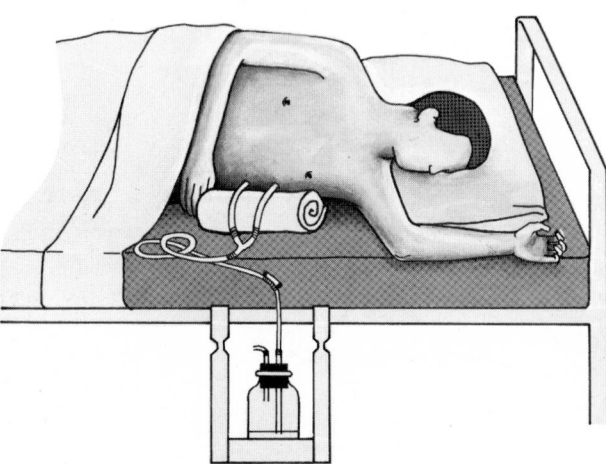

Figure 3-18. Placement of tubing while patient is in the lateral position. The nurse may readily observe the character of the drainage. A rolled towel is placed under the tubing to protect it from the weight of the patient's body. The arm and hand on the effected side should be put through range of motion exercises several times daily to avoid ankylosis of the shoulder and to assist in minimizing postoperative pain and discomfort.

Nursing Action	**Rationale/Amplification**
13. If the apparatus is damaged, clamp the bottle with a hemostat (close to the chest) immediately following expiration. Have 4 clamps (2 for each chest catheter) readily available (taped to the head of the bed) at all times.	13. Clamping the chest tube prevents disruption of the negative intrapleural pressure. However, if the patient shows symptoms of tension pneumothorax, the clamp may have to be released.
14. If the patient has to be transported to another area, place the drainage bottle below the chest level if he is lying on a stretcher and in his lap if he is in a wheelchair. Hemostats (clamps) should be attached to the patient's gown while he is transported.	14. The drainage apparatus must be kept at a level lower than the patient's chest to prevent backflow of fluid into the pleural space.
15. When assisting in removal of the tube a. Give the analgesic as ordered as this is a moderately painful procedure.	
b. Instruct the patient to exhale. The chest tube is withdrawn and a small gauze sponge is applied quickly and made airtight with snug-fitting adhesive.	b. During removal of the tube the chief precaution is to avoid the entrance of air into the pleural cavity.

Follow-up Phase

1. Rinse equipment and return to proper department (if not disposable).
2. Wash hands thoroughly before and after handling equipment.

CLINICAL CONDITIONS

Pulmonary Embolism

Pulmonary embolism refers to the obstruction of one or more pulmonary arteries by a thrombus (or thrombi) originating somewhere in the venous system or in the right side of the heart.

Predisposing Factors

1. Stasis of venous circulation especially in the blood vessels with injury to the endothelial lining which leads to intravascular clotting.
2. Most emboli originate in veins of the lower extremities or pelvic area.

Preventive Measures

1. Assess each patient with a high index of suspicion for pulmonary embolism.
2. Be aware of high-risk patients—trauma to pelvis (especially surgical), and lower extremities, obesity, varicose veins, pregnancy, congestive heart failure, myocardial infarction, malignant disease, postoperative patients.
3. Prevent stasis of blood in extremities due to dependent position of legs, prolonged sitting, immobility, constricting clothing.
   a. Instruct patient to wiggle toes, move feet, raise and lower legs every 15 minutes—to increase venous return.
   b. Apply fitted elastic stockings—to increase blood flow to deep leg veins.
   c. Elevate legs 15 to 20 degrees at periods—to minimize stasis.

    d. Avoid allowing legs and feet to dangle in a dependent position; have the patient place his feet on a chair when sitting on the edge of the bed (if bed is in high position).
4. Avoid hemoconcentration and immobilization of patients confined to bed.
5. Encourage higher levels of fluid intake during periods of immobility.
6. Avoid leaving catheters in veins (parenteral therapy, measurement of central venous pressure) for prolonged periods.
7. Use anticoagulant therapy for susceptible patients (myocardial infarction, pulmonary hypertension, etc.).
8. Assess for positive Homan's sign. (While patient is in supine position, lift leg and dorsiflex foot. Pain in the calf during this maneuver may indicate deep vein thrombosis.)

Clinical Manifestations

1. Underlying principles
    a. The size and location of the embolus determines the physiologic effect. Symptoms are therefore variable.
    b. The physiological effects develop from pulmonary artery obstruction.
    c. Small emboli tend to be multiple and recurrent.
2. Substernal pain with apprehension and a sense of impending doom; occurs when most of the pulmonary artery is obstructed.
3. Shortness of breath; weakness.
4. Pallor, cyanosis, tachyarrhythmias, clinical shock.
5. Engorgement of neck veins.
6. Right ventricular gallop rhythm.

Diagnostic Evaluation

1. Physical findings.
2. Chest roentgenogram.
3. Pulmonary angiogram (most effective).
4. Pulmonary scanning.
5. ECG (right ventricular strain pattern frequently seen).

Objectives of Treatment and Nursing Management

A. *To give anticoagulant therapy to prevent recurrence and extension of thromboembolism.*
1. Administer heparin (I.V. or I.M.) every 4 hours.
    Heparin has a rapid action, is easily reversible and apparently promotes resolution of the clot (see p. 233).
2. Adjust dosage as ordered to keep coagulation time or partial thromboplastin time within the therapeutic limit (about 3 times the normal baseline).
3. Assess patient for untoward bleeding.
4. Have protamine available until coagulation time is reduced during episodes of bleeding.
5. Use warfarin sodium (Coumadin) as anticoagulant after lung scan demonstrates improvement.
6. Adjust dose to provide a prothrombin time of 25% of normal.

NURSING ALERT: The prothrombin time is influenced by many drugs, especially aspirin.

B. *To restore cardiopulmonary physiology.*
  1. Provide respiratory assistance.
     a. Oxygen via face mask.
     b. Tracheal intubation if necessary (see p. 104).
  2. Monitor vital signs, ECG and arterial blood gases (p. 120).
  3. Give sedation as ordered; meperidine and morphine are usually avoided because of their hypotensive effects.
  4. Give digitalis and diuretics to support and assist heart function.
  5. Prepare patient for embolectomy (using cardiopulmonary by-pass technique) if hypotension, hypoxemia, etc. persist.

Teaching Emphasis
  1. See "Preventive Measures," page 155.
  2. Female patients who have experienced thromboembolism should be advised against taking oral contraceptives.

Pleurisy

Pleurisy (pleuritis) is inflammation of the pleura.
Fibrinous Pleurisy is deposition of a fibrinous exudate on the pleural surface.

Causes

May occur in the course of many pulmonary diseases:
  1. Pneumonia (bacterial, viral)
  2. Tuberculosis
  3. Pulmonary infarction, embolism
  4. Pulmonary abscess
  5. Upper respiratory tract infection
  6. Pulmonary neoplasm

Clinical Manifestations
  1. Chest pain—becomes severe, sharp and knife-like upon inspiration.
     a. Pain may become minimal or absent when breath is held.
     b. Pain may be localized or radiate to shoulder or abdomen.
  2. Intercostal tenderness.
  3. Pleural friction rub—grating or leathery sounds heard in both phases of respiration; heard low in the axilla or over the lung base posteriorly; may be heard only a day or so.
  4. Evidence of infection; fever, malaise, increased white cell count.

Diagnostic Evaluation
  1. Chest x-ray
  2. Sputum examination
  3. Examination from thoracentesis for smear and culture

Treatment and Nursing Management
Objective: To discover underlying condition.
  1. Treat the underlying primary disease (pneumonia, infarction, etc.). Inflammation usually resolves when the primary disease subsides.

2. Relieve the pain.
    a. Give prescribed analgesics.
    b. Splint the rib cage (Fig. 3-23) when the patient coughs.
    c. Apply heat or cold—to provide symptomatic relief.
    d. Instruct patient to lie on affected side occasionally—to splint chest wall.
    e. Assist with procaine intercostal block.
3. Watch for signs of development of pleural effusion (collection of fluid in pleural space)—shortness of breath, pain, local decreased excursion of chest wall.

The Pneumonias

Pneumonia is an inflammatory process of the lung air sacs commonly caused by infectious agents.*

Anatomical Classification

1. Pneumonitis—patchy or scattered pneumonia, often interstitial
2. Lobar Pneumonia—entire lobe of lung affected
3. Bronchopneumonia—disease process scattered throughout the lung

Mode of Transmission

Spread by droplets or by contact with infected patients or carriers.

Causes

1. Lowered resistance of host
2. Upper respiratory infection
3. Excessive intake of alcohol—alcohol suppresses body reflexes and white cell mobilization
4. Depression of central nervous system (drugs, head injury, etc.)
5. Cardiac failure
6. Debilitating illness
7. Superinfection in hospitalized patients
8. Exposure to intense cold, dampness
9. Any bronchial obstruction (chronic obstructive lung disease, cancer, asthma, etc.) associated with mucus formation
10. Bedridden immobile patients with shallow respiration (elderly, postoperative, etc.)

Preventive Measures

1. Natural resistance should be maintained (adequate nutrition, rest, exercise).
2. Upper respiratory infections, exposure to cold and excessive alcohol intake should be avoided.
3. Obliteration of cough reflex and aspiration of secretions should be avoided.
4. Highly susceptible persons should be vaccinated against influenza.
5. Adequate bronchial hygiene should be employed.
6. Patients should be turned every 2 hours and encouraged to breathe deeply, sigh and cough.

* See Table 3-4, page 162.

Unique Characteristics of Pneumonia

1. Pathogens producing pneumonia may be carried in nasopharynx of a healthy person.
2. Pathogens may invade tissues when the host's natural resistance is lowered.
3. Colds and upper respiratory tract infections lead to more serious illnesses by allowing bacterial invasion of lower respiratory tract.
4. Patients on high dosages of corticosteroids have a reduced resistance to infections.
5. Any condition interfering with normal drainage of the lung will predispose the person to pneumonia (i.e., cancer of the lung).
6. Postoperative patients may develop bronchopneumonia since anesthesia impairs respiratory defenses and decreases diaphragmatic movement.
7. Therapy of pneumonia depends upon laboratory identification of the agent causing the infection.
8. Recurring pneumonia often indicates underlying disease (cancer of the lung, multiple myeloma).

Objectives of Treatment and Nursing Management

A. *To identify the etiologic agent causing the pneumonia and determine the drug sensitivity.*
   1. Obtain freshly expectorated sputum for direct smear (gram stain) and culture.
      a. Be sure patient *coughs* up sputum, not saliva.
      b. Instruct patient to expectorate into sterile container for culture.
      c. Utilize percussion (p. 145) with or without IPPB treatment as directed; tenacious sputum may be liquefied by inhaling nebulized aerosol of water by mask.
   2. Collect blood for white blood count and bacterial culture.

B. *To treat the patient with prompt and effective antimicrobial chemotherapy.*
   1. Initiate therapy as soon as sputum for culture is obtained in acutely ill patients.
   2. Give parenteral antimicrobial therapy for severely ill patients.
      The dosage and route of administration depend upon the severity of the disease and the appearance of complications.
   3. Watch for continuing or recurring fever. Inadequate lung drainage or poor blood supply to involved lung may reduce amount of chemotherapeutic agent reaching invading organism.

C. *To clear the bronchi of increased secretions.*
   1. Humidify air to loosen secretions and improve ventilation.
   2. Encourage high level of fluid intake within limits of patient's cardiac reserve.
   3. Encourage the patient to cough. Avoid suppressing the cough reflex especially in patients sounding "bubbly."
   4. Control cough when coughing paroxysms cause serious hypoxia; give moderate doses of codeine.
   5. Avoid hypoxia in patients with existing heart disease (congestive heart failure, angina).

D. *To observe the patient carefully and continuously until clinical condition improves.*
   1. Remember that lethal complications may develop during the *early* period of antibiotic treatment.
   2. Assess for resistant fever or return of fever from:
      a. Drug allergy. Usually skin eruptions appear 7–10 days after the beginning of drug treatment.
      b. Drug resistance or slow response of a susceptible organism.

    c. Inadequate or inappropriate antimicrobial therapy.

    d. Superinfection.

    e. Sterile pleural effusion which subsides when fluid is removed by thoracentesis.

    f. Failure of pneumonia to resolve; raises suspicion of underlying carcinoma of bronchus.

    g. Pneumonia caused by unusual organisms (*Pneumocystis carinii*, etc.) or fungi or tuberculosis.

E. *To utilize supportive modalities of treatment.*

    1. Give oxygen when patient's condition indicates.

       a. Avoid high concentrations of oxygen in patients with chronic obstructive lung disease (bronchitis, emphysema). The use of high oxygen concentrations may worsen alveolar ventilation by removing patient's only remaining ventilatory drive.

       b. Monitoring the patient with arterial blood gas analysis will give precise guidance to the patient receiving oxygen therapy.

       c. Observe patient for cyanosis.

NURSING ALERT: Look for cyanosis of tongue which shows that a serious lack of arterial oxygen saturation exists.

---

       d. Assess patients with chronic ventilatory insufficiency (asthma, emphysema) for cyanosis and prepare for tracheostomy (p. 98) and mechanical ventilation (p. 137).

    2. Relieve the pleuritic pain.

       a. Avoid suppressing a productive cough.

       b. Avoid narcotics in patient with history of chronic obstructive lung disease.

       c. Administer moderate doses of codeine to relieve pleuritic pain.

       d. Assist with intercostal nerve block.

       e. Evaluate patient's sensorium before administering sedatives or tranquilizers to assess for signs and symptoms suggestive of pneumococcal meningitis.

NURSING ALERT: Restlessness, confusion, aggressiveness may well be due to cerebral hypoxia. In such instances sedatives are inappropriate.

---

    3. Maintain adequate hydration since fluid loss is high from fever, dehydration, dyspnea and diaphoresis.

    4. Encourage modified bedrest during febrile period.

    5. Treat abdominal distention due to air being swallowed during intervals of severe dyspnea.

       a. Give high concentrations of oxygen as oxygen is rapidly absorbed from intestines (except for patient with chronic obstructive lung disease).

       b. Use a rectal tube and give neostigmine methylsulfate (1:2000) to facilitate intestinal decompression.

       c. Pass nasogastric tube for acute gastric dilation (p. 387).

F. *To observe for complications.*

    1. Patients should respond to treatment within 24 hours. Observe for the following:

       a. Pleural effusion

       b. Sustained hypotension and shock, especially in gram negative bacterial disease, particularly in the elderly

    c. Meningitis

    d. Atelectasis (may occur at any stage of acute pneumonia)

    e. Toxic delirium *(This is considered a medical emergency.)*

    f. Lung abscess

    g. Congestive heart failure; cardiac arrhythmias

    h. Peripheral thrombophlebitis, with or without pulmonary emboli

  2. Employ special nursing surveillance for patients with the following conditions:

    a. Alcoholism or chronic obstructive lung disease; these persons as well as elderly patients may have little or no fever.

    b. Chronic bronchitis. It is difficult to detect subtle changes in condition as patient may have seriously compromised pulmonary function.

    c. Epilepsy; pneumonia may result from aspiration following a seizure.

    d. Delirium which may be caused by hypoxia, meningitis, delirium tremens of alcoholism

      (1) Prepare for lumbar puncture; meningitis may be lethal.

      (2) Assure adequate hydration and give mild sedation.

      (3) Give oxygen.

  3. Assess these patients for *unusual behavior,* alterations in mental status, stupor and congestive heart failure.

G. *To promote rehabilitation and convalescence.*

  1. Encourage chair rest after fever subsides; gradually increase activities.

  2. Encourage breathing exercises (p. 148) to clear lungs and promote full expansion and function after fever subsides.

  3. Instruct patient to report for follow-up x-rays as directed:

    a. Younger patients—films return to normal in 2–6 weeks.

    b. Patients over 60—films return to normal in 6 weeks or longer.

Chronic Bronchitis

Chronic bronchitis is a chronic productive cough associated with recurring infections of the lower respiratory tract often associated with reduced ability to ventilate the lungs.

Causes

  1. Infection—may follow pneumonia, acute bronchitis, etc.

  2. Chronic irritation—cigarette smoking, air pollution, dusts

  3. Hereditary factors

Altered Physiology

Infection, irritation, hypersensitivity → local hyperemia → hypertrophy and hyperplasia (abnormal increase in cells) of bronchi → increase in production of thick bronchial secretions → increase in goblet cells of epithelium → fibrosis and scarring of bronchioles → patchy atelectasis and swelling of bronchial walls of some alveolar units and hyperinflation of some alveolar units.

Clinical Manifestations

  Usually insidious, developing over a period of years.

  1. Recurrent bouts of coughing and expectoration

  2. Recurrent acute respiratory infections followed by persistent cough

TABLE 3-4. COMMONLY ENCOUNTERED PNEUMONIAS

Type	Organism Responsible	Manifestations
Pneumococcal pneumonia	*Diplococcus pneumoniae* (bacteria)	Sudden onset with shaking and chills Rapidly rising fever Cough with expectoration of purulent, rusty sputum Pleuritic pain aggravated by cough Grunting respirations with flaring of nares
Staphylococcal pneumonia	*Staphylococcus aureus* (bacteria)	Insidious development of cough with expectoration of yellow-blood-streaked mucus
Klebsiella pneumonia	*Klebsiella pneumoniae* (Friedländer's bacillus) (encapsulated gram negative aerobic bacillus)	Onset sudden with high fever, chills, pleuritic pain, hemoptysis Bloody gelatinous sputum present
Primary atypical pneumonia	Adenoviruses (Eaton Agent)	Onset usually insidious with low grade fever, *persistent hacking cough*, feeling of tightness in chest, generalized aching and prostration Sputum mucoid and blood-stained

3. Production of thick gelatinous sputum which is increased during superimposed infections
4. Wheezing and dyspnea as disease progresses

Clinical Features

1. Exacerbations of chronic bronchitis are most apt to occur during winter months—patients have bronchospasm due to inhalation of cold air.
2. A wide range of viral infections can produce acute episodes of bronchitis.
3. Secretions *must* be expelled or they produce chronic bronchial obstruction, air trapping, carbon dioxide retention, hypoxia and localized infection.
4. Progressive bronchitis will almost invariably result in obstructive bronchopulmonary disease (emphysema).

TABLE 3-4. COMMONLY ENCOUNTERED PNEUMONIAS (continued)

Clinical Features	Treatment	Complications
Herpes simplex lesions often present Usually involves one or more lobes	Penicillin G Tetracycline, erythromycin and cephalothin may be tried if patient is hypersensitive to penicillin	Shock Pulmonary edema Pulmonary effusion
Frequently seen in hospital setting Staphylococcal pneumonia is a necrotizing infection Treatment must be vigorous and prolonged due to disease's tendency to destroy the lungs Organism may develop rapid lung resistance Prolonged convalescence usual	Depends upon antibiotic sensitivity of organism Usually responds to chloramphenicol, erythromycin, oxacillin Rigid environmental control of air movement and laundry techniques required	Lung abscess Empyema
Tends to attack chronically ill, debilitated, alcoholic and elderly men Tissue necrosis occurs rapidly in lungs May be rapidly fulminating, progressing to fatal outcome High mortality rate	Intensive antimicrobial treatment (kanamycin, cephalothin, chloramphenicol, gentamycin)	Multiple lung abscesses with cyst formation Persistent cough with expectoration remains for prolonged period Empyema Pericarditis
Inflammatory infiltrate is primarily interstitial rather than alveolar.	Tetracycline	Pleural effusion Encephalitis

Diagnostic Evaluation

(See also p. 114.)

1. Chest roentgenogram—to exclude other diseases of the chest
2. Bronchoscopy—to rule out other causes of chronic cough
3. Bronchography studies
4. Lung function studies

Treatment and Nursing Management

Objectives: to maintain patency of peripheral bronchial tree.
to facilitate removal of bronchial exudates.

1. Control bronchial infection.
   a. Watch for changes in sputum pattern (nature, color, amount, thickness or decrease in) and changes in cough pattern.
   b. Treat recurrent bacterial infections with appropriate antibiotic therapy as directed by sensitivity studies.
2. Avoid bronchial irritation.
   a. Encourage patients to stop smoking as smoke inhalation causes an acute increase in airway resistance (bronchoconstriction) and smokers are more susceptible to respiratory infections.
   b. Look for other allergic factors by obtaining history, by doing skin tests when indicated, and observing factors that cause patient to cough.
   c. A change of occupation may be necessary.
3. Facilitate removal of bronchial exudates.
   a. Administer bronchodilator to relieve bronchospasm, reduce airway obstruction and thereby improve gas distribution and alveolar ventilation.
   b. Encourage high level of fluid intake to decrease sputum viscosity.
   c. Give IPPB treatment to facilitate removal of secretions and supply aerosolized medication to obstructed airways more effectively (see p. 134).
   d. Give adrenal corticosteroids to inhibit inflammatory responses when indicated— used when widespread bronchial infection and bronchial mucosal edema are present.
   e. See page 166 for other aspects of treatment which are similar to those of the patient with emphysema.
   f. See page 167 for patient teaching aspects (same as for emphysema).

Bronchiectasis

Bronchiectasis is dilatation of the bronchi resulting from pulmonary collapse and infection.

Causes

1. True cause of bronchiectasis unknown
2. Aspiration of foreign bodies, vomitus or material from upper respiratory tract
3. May follow sinusitis, pneumonia and repeated upper respiratory infections
4. Extrinsic pressure from tumors, dilated blood vessels, enlarged lymph nodes

Altered Physiology

Bronchial obstruction → infection → progressive fibrosis of involved areas → weakening of bronchial wall → stenosis of involved segments → stasis of infected secretions.

Clinical Manifestations

The patient experiences symptoms when he has superimposed infection.

1. Cough
2. Mucopurulent sputum
3. Hemoptysis
4. Recurrent pneumonia
5. Dyspnea (depending upon amount of lung tissue involved)

Diagnostic Evaluation

1. Chest roentgenogram (may reveal areas of atelectasis with widespread dilatation of bronchi)
2. Bronchogram to map the entire bronchial tree to determine the extent of bronchial dilation)
3. Bronchoscopy (usually shows purulent secretions from involved area)

Treatment and Nursing Management

1. Treat the patient during periods of acute infection.
   a. Employ judicious antibiotic therapy guided by sensitivity studies upon organisms cultured from sputum.
   b. Patients with repeated infections may be given small doses of antibiotics prophylactically during the winter months.
2. Empty the bronchi of their accumulated secretions.
   a. Use postural drainage to drain the bronchiectatic areas by gravity, thus reducing degree of infection and amount of secretions. (See p. 144.)
      (1) Postural drainage should be done 20 minutes twice daily or more frequently as clinical condition indicates.
      (2) Affected chest area may be percussed or "cupped" to assist in raising secretions. (See p. 145.)
   b. Encourage copious fluid intake.
   c. Utilize vaporizer to provide humidification and to keep secretions liquid.
   d. Eliminate smoking and dusts which are bronchial irritants that increase secretions.
   e. Give expectorants and bronchodilator drugs when indicated. (See treatment of patient with emphysema, p. 166.)
3. Employ surgical intervention when conservative treatment is inadequate.
   a. Segmental resection to spare as much healthy functioning lung parenchyma as possible. (See p. 175 for principles of nursing following chest surgery.)
   b. Evaluate for postoperative complications.
      (1) Pneumonia
      (2) Empyema
3. Patient teaching aspects (same as for patient with emphysema, p. 167).

Pulmonary Emphysema

Pulmonary Emphysema (chronic obstructive lung disease) is a complex and destructive lung disease characterized by distended alveoli due to chronic bronchial obstruction with subsequent loss of lung elasticity.

Altered Physiology

Chronic bronchial irritation and infection → edema → production of mucus → bronchospasm → constriction of bronchial lumen → loss of lung elasticity → bronchiolar collapse.

Causes

1. Cigarette smoking
2. Asthma and chronic bronchitis with repeated bronchial infections
3. Occupational hazards (dusts, etc.)
4. Genetic predisposition

Diagnostic Evaluation

1. Assessment of patient
2. Slowing of *forced expiration*
3. Chest roentgenogram
4. Pulmonary function studies

Clinical Manifestations

1. Dyspnea—slow in onset and steadily progressive.
2. Cough—aggravated by intercurrent respiratory infections.
3. Weakness, lethargy, anorexia, weight loss—due to hypoxia, increased respiratory muscular effort and respiratory acidosis.
4. Edema in patients with cor pulmonale (alteration of cardiac function due to impairment of lung function).

Complications

1. Respiratory acidosis
2. Congestive heart failure
3. Spontaneous pneumothorax
4. Overwhelming respiratory infections
5. Cardiac arrhythmias
6. Profound depression
7. Malnutrition

Objectives of Treatment and Nursing Management

A. *To maintain a patent airway—retained mucopurulent secretions perpetuate the problem.*
   1. *Eliminate all pulmonary irritants, particularly cigarette smoking.*
   2. Control bronchospasm—nearly all forms of pulmonary disease are accompanied by some degree of bronchospasm.
      a. Bronchospasm is detected by auscultation with a stethoscope.
      b. Administer prescribed bronchodilators which dilate airways by combating both bronchial mucosal edema and muscular spasm thus reducing airway obstruction.
         (1) Drugs may be administered orally, subcutaneously, intravenously, rectally or via nebulization (isoproterenol, racemic epinephrine, aminophylline).
         (2) Assess patient for cardiovascular side effects—tremor, tingling of extremities, tachycardia and excessive perspiration.
   3. Keep secretions liquefied.
      a. Encourage high level of fluid intake within the limits of the cardiac reserve.
      b. Give expectorants to alter bronchial secretions as directed.
   4. Give IPPB treatments to moisten secretions, increase alveolar ventilation and relieve respiratory insufficiency (see p. 134).
   5. Administer inhalations of nebulized water to humidify bronchial tree and liquefy sputum.
   6. Utilize positions of postural drainage as mucopurulent secretions produce and maintain airway obstruction (see p. 146).
   7. Prepare patient for bronchoscopic removal of secretions if he is unable to raise his sputum (see p. 118).
   8. Prepare patient for tracheostomy if indicated to permit more effective suctioning of secretions and to apply ventilatory assistance (see p. 98 and p. 137).
   9. *Give oxygen with extreme caution.*
      a. A patient with advanced emphysema has adapted to a high carbon dioxide level in his blood. With administration of a high concentration of oxygen, the patient's carbon dioxide is "washed out" thus eliminating his last stimulus to breathing.

> NURSING ALERT: Narcotics, sedatives and tranquilizers are often contraindicated. Watch for excessive somnolence due to hypercapnea or restlessness, aggressiveness or confusion due to hypoxemia.

    b. Monitor patient with arterial blood gas analysis (p. 120).

B. *To control infections in order to diminish inflammatory edema and allow bronchial mucosa to recover normal ciliary action.*
1. Obtain sputum for smear and culture.
2. Give prescribed antibiotics to control secondary bacterial infection in the bronchial tree thus clearing the airways.
3. Give adrenocortical steroids as prescribed; these drugs have an anti-inflammatory effect thus helping to relieve airway obstruction.

> NURSING ALERT: Watch for increased susceptibility to infections, gastrointestinal ulceration and bleeding tendencies.

C. *To maintain nutrition by liquid high protein feedings. Anorexia is a frustrating problem.*

D. *To educate the patient as follows:*
1. Accept the fact that therapy and medical supervision must be continued for a lifetime.
2. Become familiar with the nature of the disease and the *reasons* for the therapeutic regimen.
3. Study own life style and avoid energy wasting activities.
   a. Live within the limits that emphysema imposes.
   b. Adjust activities according to individual fatigue pattern.
   c. Breathe in a slow and relaxed manner during periods of physical activity.
4. Avoid exposure to respiratory irritants, i.e., fumes, dust, smoke, cold.
   a. Stop smoking!
   b. Stay out of extremely cold weather or keep a scarf over nose and mouth to warm inspired air.
5. Prevent and eliminate bronchial infections.
   a. Report any evidence of respiratory infection to the physician promptly, observe sputum and notify physician if there is any *change* in amount, character or color.
   b. Take prescribed antibiotic at the first sign of an infection.
6. Maintain general health in as optimal a condition as possible.
   a. Exercise to improve physical condition.
   b. Have rest periods before and after meals if eating produces dyspnea.
   c. Avoid overfatigue which is a factor in producing respiratory distress.
   d. Obtain immunization for influenza.
7. Reduce bronchial secretions.
   a. Maintain an adequate fluid intake—12 to 15 glasses daily.
   b. Use home humidifier.
   c. Follow postural drainage exercises as ordered.
   d. Take medications prescribed for cough and expectoration.
   e. Take bronchodilators as ordered.

8. Increase pulmonary ventilation:
     Use nebulization treatment consistently and faithfully.
     (1) Do the procedure immediately upon arising in the morning and before meals when indicated.
     (2) Inhale and exhale as evenly as possible during the treatment.
     (3) Try to cough *productively* after the treatment.
     (4) Observe oral hygiene after each treatment.
9. Do breathing exercises to strengthen muscles of expiration.
     a. Practice diaphragmatic breathing and pursed-lip breathing (see p. 148).
     b. Consciously use pursed-lip breathing during episodes of dyspnea.
     c. Maintain muscle tone of the body by regular exercise.

Lung Abscess

A *lung abscess* is a localized necrotic lesion in the lung characterized by cavity formation.

Etiology

1. Aspiration of infected material from upper respiratory tract.
     a. Blood after tonsillectomy
     b. Dental deposits
     c. Foreign body aspirated into lung
2. Bronchial obstruction (Usually a tumor causes obstruction to the bronchus with distal stasis and infection of secretions or there is necrosis within the tumor mass.)
3. Bacterial pneumonia
4. Tuberculosis
5. Vascular embolism
6. Chest trauma

Clinical Manifestations

1. The right lung is involved more frequently than the left—due to dependent position of its bronchus, the less acute angle which the right main bronchus forms within the trachea and its larger size.
2. In the initial stages, the cavity in the lung may or may not communicate with the bronchus.
3. Eventually the cavity becomes surrounded or encapsulated by a wall of fibrous tissue except at 1 or 2 points where the necrotic process extends until it reaches the lumen of some bronchus or pleural space and establishes a communication with the respiratory tract, the pleural cavity or both (bronchopleural fistula).

Symptoms

1. Cough
2. Fever and malaise—from segmental pneumonitis and atelectasis.
3. Headache, asthenia, weight loss
4. Pleuritic chest pain—from extension of suppurative pneumonitis to pleural surface.
5. Production of sputum—foul, yellow, green mucopurulent material which becomes profuse after abscess ruptures into bronchial tree.
6. Clubbing of fingers and toes—may signify underlying bronchogenic carcinoma.

Diagnostic Evaluation

1. History of patient.
2. X-ray of chest—for diagnosis and location of lesion.
3. Bronchogram—may be necessary to differentiate between lung abscess and bronchiectasis.
4. Direct bronchoscopic visualization—to exclude possibility of tumor or foreign body.
5. Leukocytosis in acute stage.
6. Sputum culture and sensitivity—to determine causative organism(s) and antibiotic sensitivity.
7. Dullness and bronchial breath sounds—may be heard over diseased segment.

Treatment and Nursing Management

Objectives: to establish edequate drainage.
to eradicate the infection.

1. Give appropriate antibiotic based upon sensitivity of organisms cultured—mixed infections are common and may require multiple antibiotics.
2. Carry out drainage procedures.
   a. Postural drainage—positions to be assumed depend upon the segmental localization of the abscess (see p. 146).
   b. Bronchoscopy may be necessary for removal of granulation tissue.
3. Measure and record the volume of sputum—to follow the course of healing.
4. Utilize supportive measures during the acute phase of illness.
   a. Give a high protein, high caloric diet—significant protein loss may occur when the patient is expectorating large quantities of sputum.
   b. Care for the patient having blood transfusions—anemia may be advanced in patient with infection.
5. Prepare for surgical intervention if indicated—usually done if patient shows little or no improvement in 4 to 6 weeks of medical treatment.
   a. Excision—frequently segmental resection or lobectomy is done as infiltrative pneumonitis surrounding the lung abscess pocket usually extends beyond the segmental confines of the lung.
   b. Incision and drainage—usually done for patients who cannot tolerate major thoracotomy (elderly patients, alcoholics, patients with low pulmonary functional reserve).
   c. See page 174 for caring for the patient having thoracic surgery.
6. Encourage the person to have patience—it may take 10 days to 4 months for the chest x-ray to be clear and the cavity to close.

Cancer of the Lung

Bronchogenic cancer refers to a malignant tumor of the lung arising within the wall or epithelial lining of the bronchus. The lung is also a common site of metastasis from cancer elsewhere in the body via venous circulation or lymphatic spread. Cancer of the pleura is uncommon.

Types

1. Squamous cell or epidermoid (most common)
2. Anaplastic
3. Adenocarcinoma

Predisposing Factors

1. Cigarette smoking—the amount, frequency and duration of smoking have positive relationship to cancer of the lung.
2. Industrial exposure to radioactive dusts, nickel, chromates, coal gas, arsenic and asbestos.

Preventive Measures

1. Maintain a high level index of suspicion on patients who are smokers—disease is insidious and exists before producing symptoms.
2. Encourage patients to abstain from cigarette smoking.
3. Recognize the presence of the tumor before symptoms appear.
   a. Continuous surveillance of smokers, especially those over 40.
   b. Chest roentgenograms at prescribed intervals.
4. Suspect cancer of the lung in patients who belong to a susceptible age group and have repeated unresolved respiratory infections.

Clinical Manifestations (usually occur late)

1. Cough—especially a new type or a changing cough
2. Hemoptysis
3. Thoracic discomfort; chest pain
4. Wheezing
5. Repeated infections of upper respiratory tract
6. General symptoms; weight loss, fatigue, anorexia.

Diagnostic Evaluation

1. Roentgenogram of chest—including fluoroscopy and tomography
2. Cytologic examination of sputum or saline washings from suspected bronchus
3. Bronchoscopy and biopsy (if possible)
4. Adrenal function tests preoperatively—under the stress of surgery the patient requires increased secretion of adrenocorticoids. (If the adrenal glands have been affected by metastatic cancer the patient may develop acute adrenal insufficiency.)

Treatment

1. Surgical removal of the lesion and regional lymph nodes
   a. Operation may be a segmental section, lobectomy or pneumonectomy depending on patient's clinical status and stage of disease.
   b. See page 174 for the nursing management of patient having thoracic surgery.
2. Treatment for inoperable cancer of the lung
   a. Radiotherapy—to decrease tumor size and relieve pressure on vital structures (see p. 882).
   b. Systemic chemotherapy—mechlorethamine hydrochloride (Mustargen)—for symptomatic control of metastatic disease (see p. 874).

Nursing Management

1. Prepare patient for surgical intervention if patient is a candidate for operation (see p. 174).
2. Support the patient receiving palliative treatment.
3. Treat underlying bronchitis or pulmonary infection.
   a. Bronchial drainage and removal of secretions

b. Bronchodilators and water vapor therapy

c. Antibiotics for infection

4. Give supplementary diet and encourage extra periods of rest.

5. Observe for central nervous system disturbances due to metastasis to brain, or a pain in the back, pelvis or extremities from bone metastasis.

6. See page 888 for nursing management of the patient with cancer.

7. See page 891 for the nursing management of the dying patient.

Chest Trauma*

Chest Trauma is an injury to the chest caused by any form of violence.

1. Chest injuries are potentially life-threatening because of disturbances to cardio-respiratory physiology.

2. Patients with chest trauma may have injuries to multiple organ systems.

Altered Physiology

1. In penetrating injuries, some air escapes into the pleural space. (Negative intra-pleural pressure is replaced by atmospheric pressure.)

2. A loss of negative pressure within the pleural cavity may cause collapse of the lung.

3. The change of pressure interferes with expansion of the uninvolved lung, and there is shifting back and forth of the collapsed lung and mediastinum.

4. This shifting interferes with filling of the right side of the heart, lessening cardiac output and causing cardiopulmonary collapse.

Emergency Management

The order of priority is determined by the clinical status of the patient.

Objective: to restore normal cardiorespiratory function as quickly as possible.

1. Assess condition of patient to determine his physiologic state.

2. Establish and maintain an open airway.

Aspirate secretions, vomitus and blood from nose and throat via:

(1) Tracheal aspiration if patient is unable to clear his tracheobronchial tree (see p. 105).

(2) Prepare for tracheostomy if necessary.

(a) Tracheostomy helps to obtain clear dry tracheobronchial tree, helps patient breathe with less effort, decreases amount of dead air space in the respiratory tree and reduces paradoxical motion.

(b) The use of a cuffed tracheostomy tube permits a closed system for air exchange when connected to a respirator.

3. Control hemorrhage.

4. Treat for shock. (Shock may be due to blood loss, impairment of cardiorespiratory function.)

a. Withdraw blood for cross-matching and other laboratory studies.

b. Using a large bore needle or cut-down, restore plasma volume to adequate levels—plasma, plasma expanders, electrolyte solution.

* See also page 911.

     c. Give infusion rapidly.

     d. Monitor repeated central venous pressure readings to prevent circulatory over-load (see p. 241).

  5. Close sucking wound of chest. *Make wound airtight* (see below).

Types of Chest Injuries

A. *Hemothorax*

Blood in the pleural cavity from injury to the intrathoracic organs or blood vessels of the chest wall.

  1. Blood in the pleural cavity produces a compression of the lung and can displace mediastinal structures.

  2. Patient may be asymptomatic or dyspneic, apprehensive or in shock.

  3. Treatment

     a. Continuous drainage of the pleural space with large bore intercostal tube.

        (1) 5th intercostal space is usually used but the level of tube insertion is usually determined by x-ray.

        (2) The thoracotomy catheter is sutured in position and connected to an under-water-seal drainage bottle (see p. 150).

     b. Give analgesics and assist patient to cough effectively (see p. 177).

B. *Pneumothorax*

Air in the pleural cavity occurring spontaneously from injury or disease. In patients with chest trauma it is usually the result of a laceration to the lung parenchyma, tracheo-bronchial tree or esophagus.

  1. Patient's clinical status depends upon the rate of air leakage and size of wound.

  2. A rapid flow of air into the pleural space will produce *tension pneumothorax* (air in the pleural cavity producing displacement of the mediastinum to the uninvolved side with resultant severe cardiorespiratory embarrassment).

  3. Treatment

     a. Small defects in lung will usually seal spontaneously.

     b. Chest-tube drainage (closed thoracotomy) of pleural space to evacuate air. (Chest tube connected to underwater-seal suction.)

     c. If tension pneumothorax is present, the pleural space is temporarily decompressed with a syringe attached to a 16–18 gauge needle inserted into the second inter-costal space (see p. 122).

C. *Sucking Wound of Chest*

Air passing through hole in the chest wall causing lungs to collapse and mediastinum to shift. There is an audible passage of air during inspiration and expiration.

  1. The negative intrapleural pressure is eliminated creating a disturbance in ventilation; this may cause rapid death by asphyxia.

  2. Treatment

     a. Close the chest wound immediately to restore adequate ventilation and res-piration.

     b. Instruct the patient to inhale and exhale forcefully against a closed glottis (Valsalva maneuver) as the pressure dressing is laid in place. (This maneuver helps to expand collapsed lung.)

     c. If necessary, prepare patient for surgical intervention or for catheter drainage of the pleural space (see p. 150). Thoracotomy tube is inserted after the emergency treatment above.

   d. If condition permits, place patient in semisitting position to permit greater ventilatory efficiency.

D. *Fracture of Ribs and Sternum* (most common chest injury)

  1. Manifestations
    a. Localized tenderness or crepitus (crackling) over fracture site.
    b. Chest pain referred to the fracture site.
    c. Painful, shallow respirations (due to splinting of involved chest).
  2. Pneumonitis is a complication of rib fracture if patient is **not** encouraged to deep breathe periodically.
  3. Intercostal nerve block of involved area is helpful in relieving pain.
  4. Analgesics (usually non-narcotic) to be given to assist patient to cough and deep breathe effectively.
  5. Strapping and tight binders are usually avoided as these limit respirations.

E. *Flail Chest*

Loss of stability of chest wall with subsequent respiratory impairment. This is usually the result of multiple rib fractures.

  1. Manifestations
    a. Pain, dyspnea, cyanosis
    b. Paradoxical (reverse of normal) movements of involved chest wall
  2. Objective of treatment: to stabilize the paradoxically moving chest.
    a. Tracheostomy and assisted ventilation instituted to correct cardiopulmonary derangement. (Respiratory assistance will control voluntary inspiration and expiration thus allowing fractured ribs to heal.)
    b. If necessary stabilize the flail segment of the chest by traction with weights and pulleys applied through wires or towel clips applied to broken portion of ribs (or by suction cups attached to skin).
    c. Utilize thoracotomy tube for associated hemothorax or pneumothorax.

F. *Wet Lung Syndrome*

Presence of fluid in the lungs (mucus, blood, serum)—as a result of severe chest injury and contusion of pulmonary tissue.

  1. Manifestations
    a. Constant loose cough, rattling, wheezing
    b. Rales present on auscultation
    c. Dyspnea, tachycardia and cyanosis
  2. Objective of treatment: to improve tracheobronchial drainage
    Encourage patient to cough.
    (1) Give manual support to the chest.
    (2) Give adequate analgesia to permit coughing.
    (3) Aspirate blood or air in pleural cavity. (See thoracentesis, p. 122.)
    (4) Assist with intercostal nerve block to relieve discomfort produced by coughing.
    (5) Give periodic IPPB to help clear tracheobronchial tree.
    (6) Administer bronchodilator drug if bronchospasm is present.
    (7) Prepare for tracheostomy with continuous ventilatory support if patient's respiratory efforts are exhausting him.

G. *Cardiac Tamponade*

Progressive collection of fluid or blood filling the pericardial space which interferes with diastolic filling of the ventricles.

1. Manifestations
   a. Faint heart sounds
   b. Narrowed pulse pressure
   c. Elevated venous pressure
   d. High central venous pressure; low arterial blood pressure
   e. Distended neck veins
   f. Dyspnea, cyanosis, shock

2. Treatment
   a. Pericardial aspiration (pericardiocentesis)—aspiration or drainage of the pericardium.
   b. Under local anesthesia the pericardial needle is inserted to the left of the xiphoid and fluid is removed. Repeated aspirations may be necessary.
   c. Open operation to control hemorrhage may be necessary if symptoms recur.

Thoracic Surgery

The Challenge: Meticulous attention must be given in the preoperative and postoperative care of patients undergoing thoracic surgery as these operations are wide in scope, obstructive pulmonary disease may be present and the margin of safety is apt to be narrow.

Preoperative Care

Objective: to ensure optimal patient condition for surgery.

A. *Determine the preoperative status of the patient, his physical assets and liabilities.*
   1. Assist the patient undergoing diagnostic studies.
      a. History and physical examination.
      b. Chest roentgenogram (see p. 116).
      c. Pulmonary function studies (p. 119)—to ascertain if patient will have sufficiently functioning lung tissue postoperatively.
      d. Special diagnostic studies as required (see p. 116).
      e. Base-line studies to ascertain any unsuspected abnormalities and to serve as a base-line reference during the postoperative period.
         (1) ECG—to disclose presence of arteriosclerotic heart disease or conduction defect.
         (2) Blood urea nitrogen—to obtain a "rough" measurement of renal function.
         (3) Blood sugar or glucose tolerance—to detect unrecognized diabetes.
         (4) Blood electrolytes, serum protein studies and blood volume determinations as indicated.
         (5) Arterial blood gas studies.
   2. Nursing assessment of the patient.
      a. What signs and symptoms are present?—cough, expectoration, hemoptysis, chest pain?
      b. What is his smoking history? How long and how much?
      c. What is the patient's cardiopulmonary tolerance while bathing, eating, walking, etc?
      d. What is the "physiologic age" of the patient?—general appearance, mental alertness, behavior, degree of nutrition?

    e. What is his breathing pattern?
    f. How much exertion is required to produce dyspnea?
    g. What are his personal preferences and dislikes?

B. *Improve alveolar ventilation*
1. Encourage the patient to stop smoking as this increases bronchial irritation.
2. Employ all measures to minimize pulmonary secretions.
    a. Measure sputum daily in patients with large volume of secretions to determine if volume of secretion is decreasing.
    b. Instruct the patient to cough against a closed glottis to increase intrapulmonary pressure.
    c. Humidify the air to loosen secretions.
    d. Administer bronchodilators for bronchospasm.
    e. Give antibiotics for infection.
    f. Give expectorants, enzymes and mucolytic agents as directed.
    g. Employ IPPB therapy to improve pulmonary ventilation (see p. 134).
    h. Carry out postural drainage positioning on patients with bronchiectasis, etc. (see p. 146).
    i. Teach diaphragmatic breathing preoperatively (see p. 148).
    j. Set up a schedule of breathing exercises that encourage the use of abdominal muscles (see p. 148).

C. *Evaluate cardiovascular and pulmonary status so that complications may be anticipated and prevented.*
1. Study the results of diagnostic tests to learn of existing deviations from normal.
2. Observe the patient and his reactions to various activities of daily living.
3. Give cardiac drugs to patients in congestive heart failure (see p. 276).
4. Correct anemia, dehydration and hypoproteinemia—intravenous infusions, tube feedings, blood transfusions as indicated.

D. *Prepare the patient for the surgical experience by offering reassurance, explanations and skillful preoperative nursing care.*
1. Orient the patient to events in the postoperative period.
    a. Cough and breathing routine.
    b. Presence of chest tube and drainage bottles.
    c. Oxygen therapy.
    d. Measures used to control discomfort.
2. Encourage expression of psychological and safety needs.

Postoperative Care

Objective: to restore normal cardiopulmonary function as quickly as possible.
1. Maintain an open airway.
2. Maintain constant nursing surveillance of the patient.
    a. Take blood pressure, pulse, respirations every 15 minutes as indicated, lengthening the time interval according to the patient's clinical status.
    b. Evaluate character of respirations and patient's color.
    c. Evaluate character of drainage from the chest-drainage bottles.
    d. Elevate the head of the bed to a 30- or 45-degree angle when the patient is oriented and his blood pressure is stabilized.

3. Aspirate all secretions with suctioning until patient is able to raise secretions effectively—endotracheal secretions are present in excessive amounts in post-thoracotomy patients due to trauma to the tracheobronchial tree during operation, diminished lung ventilation and cough reflex.

> NURSING ALERT: Look for changes in color and consistency of aspirated sputum. Colorless fluid sputum means improvement; thickening, opaque or colored sputum indicates dehydration or infection.

    a. Carry out tracheal aspiration on "wet" semicomatose patient to prevent atelectasis.
    b. Indications for tracheal aspiration are determined by chest auscultation.
    c. See page 105 for guidelines for tracheal aspiration.
    d. Sterile technique is mandatory.
4. Keep drainage bottles below the chest level unless they are clamped off.
5. Give oxygen in the immediate postoperative period to assure maximum oxygenation—respirations are still depressed and residual secretions in the peripheral respiratory passages may partially block gas exchange. Monitoring by means of arterial blood gas analysis may be necessary.
6. Avoid elevating the foot of the bed after thoracic surgery to prevent diaphragm from interfering with ventilation.

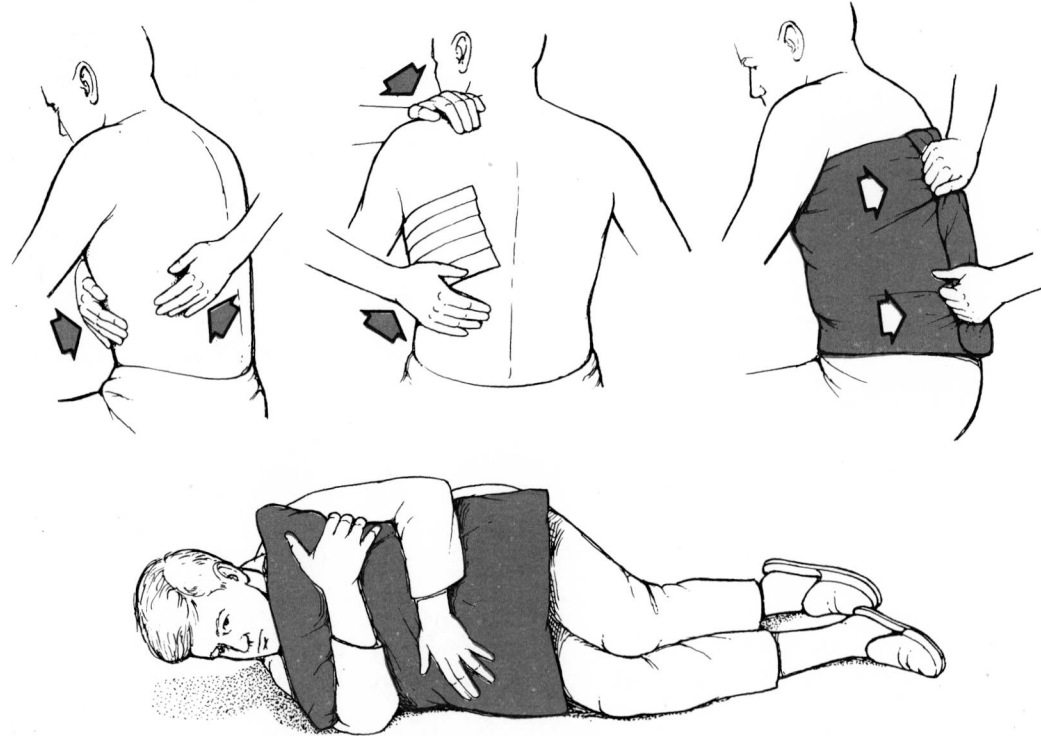

Figure 3-19. Promotion of an effective cough.

7. Give aerosol therapy to reduce viscosity of secretions.
8. Administer IPPB treatments in order to help expand the lung(s).
9. Listen to both sides of the chest with a stethoscope to determine if there are any changes in breath sounds.
   a. Are breath sounds normal indicating free flow of air in and out of lungs?
   b. Are breath sounds distant? Wheezing? Rales present?
10. Encourage and promote an effective cough routine (Fig. 3-19).
    a. Sit patient on side of bed with feet supported on a chair if his condition permits.
    b. Support the chest firmly over the operated side and against opposite chest to lessen incisional pain.
    c. Instruct the patient to cough against a closed glottis to increase intrapulmonary pressure.
    d. Assist the patient to cough at least every 1 or 2 hours during the first 24 hours and when necessary thereafter.
11. Maintain surveillance and careful management of the chest drainage system (except in patients with a pneumonectomy).* (See p. 150.)
12. Provide intelligent pain relief—pain limits chest excursions thereby decreasing ventilation.
    a. Severity of pain varies with type of incision and patient's reaction and ability to cope with pain.
    b. Narcotics and analgesics may assist patient to cough more effectively.
    c. Narcotics and analgesics may make some patients too somnolent to cough.
    d. Watch for signs of respiratory depression.
    e. Assist patient having an intercostal nerve block for pain control.
13. Record hourly urinary output—patient should excrete at least 30 ml. of urine hourly after surgery.
14. Administer blood and parenteral fluids at a slower rate after thoracic surgery—pulmonary edema due to transfusion overload is an ever present threat; following pneumonectomy the pulmonary vascular system has been greatly reduced.
15. Maintain care in positioning the postoperative thoracotomy patient.
    a. Position patient flat in bed at intervals unless this produces dyspnea.
    b. Position patient in a semi-Fowler's position—to permit residual air to rise to upper portion of pleural space and be removed via the upper chest catheter.
    c. Patients with limited respiratory reserve may not be able to turn on unoperated side—as this may limit ventilation of the operated side.
    d. A patient with a pneumonectomy is *not* turned on unoperated side—fluid in the pleural cavity will submerge the bronchial stump, and this will interfere with the drainage of secretions.
16. Anticipate and forestall complications.
    a. Hemorrhage
    b. Respiratory acidosis
    c. Pneumonitis; atelectasis
    d. Pulmonary edema
    e. Cardiac arrhythmias
    f. Renal failure
    g. Gastric distention—utilize nasogastric tube the first 24 hours.
17. Restore normal range of motion and function of shoulder and trunk.
    a. Encourage breathing exercises to mobilize thorax (see p. 148).
    b. Encourage skeletal exercises to promote abduction and mobilization of shoulder.

---

* A patient with a pneumonectomy does not have water-seal chest drainage as it is desirable that the pleural space fill with an effusion which eventually obliterates this space.

    c. Ambulate as soon as pulmonary and circulatory systems are compensated.

    d. Encourage progressive activities according to development of fatigue.

18. Patient Teaching Aspects;

    a. There will be some intercostal pain for a period of time which can be relieved by local heat and oral analgesia.

    b. Weakness and fatigability are common during first 3 weeks following a thoracotomy.

Tuberculosis

Microbiologic Review of Tuberculosis Bacillus (*Mycobacterium tuberculosis*)

1. Is a nonmobile aerobe which can be readily killed by heat, sunshine, drying, and ultraviolet light.
2. Reproduces slowly and may remain dormant for long periods of time.
3. Can be transmitted through the air in the residues of minute droplets of moisture projected when a person harboring the bacillus sneezes, coughs, laughs, etc.
4. As part of "droplet nuclei," is suspended in the air indefinitely and carried by air currents.
5. Can easily be inhaled via "droplet nuclei" and implanted on alveolar tissue because it is not filtered out by cilia.
6. Is also transmitted on larger particles, can be inhaled, but is filtered in the nasal and upper respiratory passages.
7. Can be adherent to fomites (substances other than food i.e., books, furniture, walls, floors, that may harbor and transmit infectious organisms but do not present an infection hazard).
8. When in the form of dried secretion, it is difficult to fragment; therefore, difficult to become airborne; those that do become airborne are unlikely to invade lung tissue.

Measures to Inhibit the Transmission of Droplet Nuclei

1. Place the tuberculosis patient on a *chemotherapeutic regimen.*

    a. Reduces the number of tubercle bacilli in the sputum.

    b. Lessens the amount of sputum produced.

    c. Reduces the frequency and force of coughing, thereby lessening the quantity of droplet nuclei.

2. Instruct the patient to *cover his nose and mouth* with disposable wipes *when sneezing, coughing or raising sputum;* provide him with a mask if he fails to do this properly.
3. *Provide effective ventilation* which will permit maximum diffusion of air particles.
4. If available, *use ultraviolet light* to kill tubercle bacilli.

    a. Recommended in areas likely to be occupied or frequented by individuals with undiagnosed or unsuspected tuberculosis or with diagnosed patients in the early phase of chemotherapy.

    b. Recommended in air-flow ducts during times of air recirculation.

5. *Initiate preventive chemotherapy* (chemoprophylaxis) for high-risk groups where tuberculosis is present.

    a. All recent converters (from negative to positive skin tests)

    b. Those not yet on chemotherapy

    c. Those under 20

    d. Those with concomitant diseases (diabetes, silicosis, etc.)

    e. Those on prolonged steroid therapy
    f. Patients with inactive tuberculosis who never received drug therapy or were given inadequate drug therapy.
  6. *Start a case-finding program.*
    a. Test all children.
      (1) Preschoolers
      (2) Those entering grade school
      (3) Those entering high school
    b. Prompt physical examinations for those
      (1) recently contacting a patient with early active tuberculosis
      (2) with questionable chest x-rays
      (3) with positive tuberculin skin test
      (4) known to have high incidence of tuberculosis
      (5) most likely to infect children, teachers, other school employees
    c. Educational program to encourage annual medical check-ups (including tuberculin tests).

Diagnostic Evaluation

  1. Tuberculin Skin Test (Mantoux)—the inoculation of tubercle bacillus extract into the skin on the inner aspect of the forearm.
    a. Purified protein derivative (PPD) or old tuberculin (OT) is injected intradermally.
    b. After 48 to 72 hours, the injection site is checked for inflammatory response:
        Induration measuring 5 mm. or more in diameter is considered positive.
  2. Heaf, Sterneedle, Tine and Mono-Vacc. are types of multiple-puncture tuberculin skin tests.
  3. Chest x-ray: 14″ × 17″ chest films have diagnostic value over microfilm.
  4. Sputum smear or culture
    a. Positive—presence of tubercle bacilli
    b. Negative—absence of tubercle bacilli

Contributing Conditions to the Development of Tuberculosis

  1. General physical debilitation
  2. Constant exposure to active tubercle bacilli
  3. Lowered resistance because of
    a. Pregnancy   d. Stress and emotional strain
    b. Presence of other diseases: diabetes, etc.   e. Recent gastrointestinal surgery
    c. Age: elderly and young including adolescents   f. Steroid therapy

Altered Physiology

  1. Tubercle bacilli infect the lung, forming a tubercle (lesion)
  2. The tubercle
    a. May heal leaving scar tissue.
    b. May continue as granuloma.
      (1) May heal.
      (2) May be reactivated.
    c. May eventually proceed to necrosis (death), liquefaction, sloughing and cavitation.
  3. The initial lesion may disseminate tubercle bacilli:
    a. By extension to adjacent tissues   c. Via lymphatic system
    b. Via bloodstream   d. Through the bronchi

Clinical Manifestations

1. Early manifestations are asymptomatic.
2. Later manifestations include fatigue, weight loss, anorexia, night sweating.
3. Afternoon temperature elevation, productive cough, blood-tinged sputum.

Clinical Classification

1. According to extent
   a. Minimal—one or more small lesions; no cavitation
   b. Moderately advanced—one or more lesions, slight to moderate density
      (1) Total dissemination—does not exceed volume of one lung
      (2) Total cavitation—does not exceed 4 cm.
   c. Far advanced—lesions or cavitation more extensive than in moderately advanced disease
2. According to disease activity
   a. Active.
   b. Quiescent, cavitary.
   c. Quiescent, noncavitary.
      (1) Negative bacteriologic findings at monthly intervals for 3 months.
      (2) Stable, slightly clearing or constricting lesions (x-ray) without visible cavitation.
   d. Inactive, cavitary.
   e. Inactive, noncavitary.
      (1) Negative bacteriologic findings at monthly intervals for 6 months.
      (2) Negative x-rays—stability and no evidence of cavitation.
   f. Activity undetermined.

Treatment and Nursing Management

1. Assess the patient.
   a. Collect information and evaluate health status.
      (1) Extent and activity of disease: clinical manifestations
      (2) Bacteriological status as determined by sputum cultures
      (3) Length of illness
      (4) Treatment regimen
      (5) Other health problems
      (6) History of tuberculosis in family
      (7) Plan for preventive therapy of family: skin testing, chest x-ray
2. Evaluate emotional reaction of the patient and his family.
   a. Patient's feelings about diagnosis and recommended treatment
   b. Family feelings about patient's diagnosis and treatment
   c. Psychosocial and cultural background of patient
3. Seek related significant data.
   a. Age, sex (psychosocial and biological aspects)
   b. Patient's parental family
   c. Patient's immediate family
   d. Occupation and income
   e. Recreational interests
   f. Education and hobbies
   g. Geographical background
   h. Socioeconomic background
   i. Patient's strengths and limitations

4. Initiate treatment:
    a. Two major emphases
        (1) Chemotherapy for the patient (see below)
        (2) Preventive chemotherapy for contacts
    b. Individualized care for the patient and his family
        (1) Stress importance of continuous, uninterrupted chemotherapy.
        (2) Recognize feelings of the patient and his reaction to his illness; assist him in accepting diagnosis and treatment.
        (3) Assist family in accepting the patient's diagnosis and treatment.
        (4) Instruct the patient and family according to their need.
5. Initiate respiratory isolation precautions of care in line with the bacteriologic nature of the tubercle organisms.
    a. Have patient wear a mask if he is unwilling or unable to cover his nose and mouth while in the communicable phase of the disease.
    b. Recognize that caps or gowns are unnecessary for the patient, hospital personnel or visitors because this disease is transmitted by "droplet nuclei" suspended in air currents. (Bacteria caught in or on clothing, etc., cannot be broken down and resuspended in the air in small enough particles for inhalation.)
    c. Dishes should be washed in hot, soapy water and rinsed in boiling water. (Electric dishwashers at home or hospital dishwashing procedures are sufficient.) Disposable dishes are preferred.
    d. Linens should be washed in hot, soapy water and dried in sunlight or dryers equipped with ultraviolet light.
    e. Burn food wastes or wrap in plastic bags for disposal with other garbage.
    f. Visitors need not be subjected to any restrictions.
    g. Segregate patient just prior to or early in chemotherapy phase; thereafter, he is given full hospital privileges like any other patient.
    h. The usual careful handwashing procedure for all nursing personnel is followed as when in contact with any other patient.
    i. Reading materials such as books, magazines, newspapers are handled with no restrictions on circulation to other patients.
    j. Primary tuberculosis (uncomplicated) in children is usually noninfectious because
        (1) Pulmonary lesions are minimal.
        (2) There is little or no cough.
        (3) Number of tubercle bacilli is low.
    k. Terminal housekeeping procedures are similar to that used for any hospitalized patient.

Chemotherapy and Chemoprophylaxis

A. *Major Features* (Clinical Effectiveness)

1. Is bacteriostatic.
2. Should be administered in combination with other antituberculosis drugs and without interruption to prevent development of resistant strains of tuberculosis organisms.
3. Is prescribed for at least 2 years.
4. Response noted by: (1) decrease in symptoms—cough, sputum, etc.; (2) improved chest x-rays and (3) negative sputum.
5. Has noninfectious nature.

TABLE 3-5. INITIAL OR PRIMARY TREATMENT DRUGS FOR TUBERCULOSIS

Medication	Isoniazid	Streptomycin
Abbreviation	INH	SM
Indications	Considered the drug of choice Used in combination with other anti-tuberculosis drugs in initial treatment regimens Used prophylactically for persons with tuberculin skin test reactions and for persons recently exposed to tuberculosis	Always used in combination with other chemotherapeutic agents to prevent the development of bacterial resistance
Contraindications	Epilepsy Suspicion of renal damage	Severe renal insufficiency
Administration	Oral	Intramuscular
Dosage	300 mg./day	1 gm. daily for no longer than 2 to 3 months, then 1 gm. twice a week; or 1 gm. twice a week from the onset
Absorption	Readily absorbed either orally or parenterally	Absorption is rapid and effective from intramuscular and subcutaneous sites
Distribution	Diffuses readily into all body fluids and cells	Little or no diffusion into the cerebral spinal fluid
Excretion	Mainly by the kidneys	By kidneys
Precautions	Give pyridoxine (Vit. B_6) to prevent or treat neurological manifestations	
Adverse reactions	Least toxic of primary drugs Toxic effects on peripheral and central nervous system: anesthesia, peripheral neuritis Convulsions, optic neuritis Metabolic acidosis, mental abnormalities, epigastric distress Hepatitis	Peripheral and central nervous system: labyrinth damage (ataxia), deafness, peripheral neuritis Blood dyscrasias Hypersensitivity reactions

B. *Susceptibility Studies* (to determine proper drug)
    1. Change if patient is hypersensitive.
    2. Change if patient fails to respond to therapy.

C. *Types of Antituberculosis Drugs*
    1. *Initial* (primary treatment drugs)—See Table 3-5.
       a. Isoniazid (INH)   c. Para-aminosalicylic acid (PAS)
       b. Streptomycin (SM)   d. Ethambutol (EMB)

TABLE 3-5 (continued)

Para-aminosalcylic Acid	Ethambutol
PAS	EMB
Used in auxiliary treatment of pulmonary and extrapulmonary tuberculosis	Used for initial treatment or retreatment of pulmonary tuberculosis Used in conjunction with other antituberculosis drugs
Hypersensitivity Demonstrated resistance of the tubercle bacillus to PAS	Hepatic abnormalities
Oral	Oral
8–12 gm. with or immediately after meals/daily	Initially 250 mg. twice a day. Increased by 125 mg. a day every 5 days until 1 gm. is being given daily
Readily absorbed from the gastrointestinal tract	Tends to be irregular
Appears in the pleural fluid but not in the cerebral spinal fluid	Rapidly and widely distributed; significant concentrations are present in the cerebral spinal fluid
More than 80% is excreted in the urine	Less than 1% is excreted in active form in the urine
	Give after meals to minimize gastric irritation Carry out blood and urine examinations and hepatic-function studies at regular intervals
Gastrointestinal tract irritation, anorexia, nausea, vomiting, diarrhea Reactions associated with hypersensitization, such as general malaise, joint pains, sore throat and skin eruptions Neurological manifestations Blood dyscrasias Hepatitis	Gastrointestinal irritation Hepatitis Difficulty in managing diabetes mellitus Allergic skin rashes Postural hypotension Mental depression Drowsiness Loss of visual acuity, difficulty in seeing the color green

2. *Secondary* (retreatment—used when tuberculosis bacilli are resistant to primary drugs)—See Table 3-6.

    a. Pyrazinamide (PZA)
    b. Ethionamide (ETHA)
    c. Cycloserine (CS)
    d. Kanamycin (KM)

    e. Viomycin (VM)
    f. Rifampin
    g. Capreomycin   } Research drugs
    h. Isoxyl

TABLE 3-6. RETREATMENT OR SECONDARY DRUGS FOR TUBERCULOSIS

Medication	Cycloserine	Kanamycin	Viomycin
Abbreviation	CS	KM	VM
Indications	Used in the treatment of pulmonary and extrapulmonary tuberculosis when the disease organisms are resistant to the primary drugs	Used in secondary treatment, often together with other tuberculostatic agents	Used in pulmonary and extrapulmonary tuberculosis Used only if patients are unable to tolerate streptomycin, para-aminosalicylic acid, or isoniazid or if the strain of *Mycobacterium tuberculosis* isolated from the lesions is resistant to these drugs.
Contraindications	Hypersensitivity Resistance of the disease organisms to the drug Renal insufficiency, epilepsy, psychiatric disorders In conjunction with other drugs	Renal insufficiency	Renal insufficiency
Administration	Oral	Intramuscular	Parenteral
Dosage	Daily dose: 0.5 gm.	Daily dose: 1 gm.	1 gm. every 12 hours every third day, alone or together with para-aminosalicylic acid
Absorption	Rapidly absorbed from the stomach and small intestine	If taken orally, it is poorly absorbed from the gastrointestinal tract	From the gastrointestinal tract it is limited
Distribution	Readily diffused throughout the body fluids and tissues	Diffuses significantly into the body fluids	Penetration into the central spinal fluid is poor
Excretion	By the kidneys	Mainly via kidneys	A large proportion of the drug is excreted in the urine
Precautions	Give pyridoxine (Vit. B_6) to prevent or control central nervous system toxicity	Pretreatment audiogram, BUN, and urinalysis, repeated frequently during treatment	Make audiometric determinations before initiation of therapy and at frequent intervals during treatment
Adverse reactions	Drowsiness, somnolence, dizziness, allergic dermatitis, hyperreflexia, mental confusion or convulsions, other mental symptoms	Toxicity to the 8th cranial nerve resulting in loss of hearing Vestibular dysfunction Renal irritation	Toxic manifestations involve the kidney, the labyrinth, and the electrolyte balance

D. *Follow-up Procedures with Chemotherapy*
  1. Determine whether patient is taking drug regularly.
  2. Make special evaluations:
     a. Bacteriological studies
     b. Chest x-rays
     c. Laboratory studies as required by individual patient
  3. Check for untoward side effects.
  4. Instruct patient regarding treatment and disease.
  5. Inform patient regarding other services.

E. *Clinical Management*
  1. Rarely requires isolation (noninfectious a few days after initiation of treatment).
  2. If hospitalization is required, it is usually for only a few weeks.
  3. Most patients return to work after a few weeks.

Basic Concepts in Tuberculosis Control

A. *Breeding Areas for Undiagnosed Tuberculosis*
  1. Institutions: mental hospitals, nursing homes, children's homes, penal institutions, etc.
  2. Large general hospitals
  3. Slum areas
  4. Migrant worker areas

B. *High-risk Groups*
  1. Persons in close contact with those having acute tuberculosis.
  2. Individuals reacting positively to tuberculin skin test.
     a. Those recently converted from negative to positive within the past year.
     b. Those having a reaction of 10 mm. or more induration.
     c. Those who are underweight.
     d. Those with questionable chest findings.
  3. Persons not reacting positively to tuberculin skin test but falling into one of the following categories:
     a. Those with low resistance to the disease or having some other debilitating disease, e.g., diabetes, silicosis.
     b. Those having had a gastrectomy.
     c. Those receiving steroid therapy.
     d. Those who are pregnant.
     e. The very young or very old.
     f. Those living in close-crowded conditions.

Tuberculosis Control Program

A. *Patient Priorities*
  1. Those diagnosed as having tuberculosis.
     a. Those who are newly diagnosed.
     b. All persons with positive sputum for tuberculous bacilli, especially where children are in close contact.
     c. Those with active, reactivated or quiescent tuberculosis.
  2. Those who are suspected of having tuberculosis but are undiagnosed.

3. Persons no longer receiving medical supervision.
    a. Have had tuberculosis.
    b. Have tuberculosis.
4. Patients who are on chemotherapy but take medications irregularly.
5. Persons who have stopped chemotherapy.
6. Former patients with inactive tuberculosis (not on chemotherapy).

B. *Who are the Contacts?*
    1. Newly diagnosed patients
    2. Persons in contact with someone who was not diagnosed as having tuberculosis until after he died.

C. *Who are the Reactors?* (exposure not known)
    1. Recent converters or those with reactions of 10 mm. or more.
    2. Those suspected because of questionable chest x-rays.
    3. Those who had contact with reactors.

Criteria for Evaluating a Tuberculosis Control Program*

CRITERIA	OBJECTIVE
1. Availability of services	1. To be available for all patients regardless of ability to pay and without residency requirements.
2. Treatment facilities	2. To utilize predominantly clinics and physician's offices. Utilize hospitals only when warranted.
3. Treatment success in initial phases	3. To reach 95% of all treated patients.
4. Duration of uninterrupted chemotherapy	4. To reach 100% completion by end of 12 months.
5. Status of sputum culture in patient's initial treatment	5. To reach 75% in 3 months. To reach 95% in 6 months.
6. Surgical treatment (resection)	6. Not to subject patients to surgery in initial treatment and rarely in retreatment.
7. Preventive therapy	7. To be initiated for every individual identified as a risk. (Criteria set up by Ad Hoc Committee on Evaluation, U. S. Public Health Service, Tuberculosis Branch.

° Adapted from: "Standards for Tuberculosis Treatment in the 1970's." A Statement by the Ad Hoc Committee on Quality Care for Tuberculosis, National Tuberculosis and Respiratory Disease Association, 1970.

BIBLIOGRAPHY

Conditions of the Nose and Throat

Books

Ballantyne, J., and Groves, J.: Scott-Brown's Diseases of the Ear, Nose and Throat, 3rd ed. Philadelphia, J. B. Lippincott, 1971.
Brunner, L. S., et al.: Textbook of Medical and Surgical Nursing, 2nd ed. Philadelphia, J. B. Lippincott, 1970, pp. 208–227.
Saunders, W. H., et al.: Nursing Care in Eye, Ear, Nose and Throat Disorders. St. Louis, C. V. Mosby, 1968.

Articles

Adler, S.: Speech after laryngectomy. Amer. J. Nurs., *69*:2138–2141, Oct. 1969.
Connor, G. H., et al.: Tracheostomy, when it is needed, how it is done, postoperative care. Amer. J. Nurs., 72:68–74, Jan. 1972.
Jacquette, G.: To reduce hazards of tracheal suctioning. Amer. J. Nurs., *71*:2362–2364, Dec. 1971.
Kearns, B.: Tracheostomy suctioning technique. Canad. Nurse, *66*:44–48, Feb. 1970.
Kirchner, J. A.: Cancer of the larynx. Hosp. Med., 8:65–78, Nov. 1972.
Pecora, D. V.: Transtracheal aspiration. Amer. Fam. Phys., *1*:99, March 1970.
Shelly, W. M., et al.: Cuffed tubes as a cause of tracheal stenosis. J. Thorac. Cardiovasc. Surg., 57:623, 1969.
Shim, C., et al.: Cardiac arrhythmias resulting from tracheal suctioning. Ann. Intern. Med., *71*:1149–1153, Dec. 1969.
Stivers, F. E., and Yarington, C. T.: Indications for tonsillectomy and adenoidectomy. Amer. Fam. Phys., *3*:72–77, March 1971.
Tardy, M. E., and Lederer, F. L.: Visual guide to the diagnosis of nasal lesions. Hosp. Med., *8*:8–33, Oct. 1972.
Thomas, A. N.: Management of tracheoesophageal fistula caused by cuffed tracheal tubes. Amer. J. Surg., *124*:181–189, Aug. 1972.
Ungvarski, P.: Mechanical stimulation of coughing. Amer. J. Nurs., *71*:2358–2361, Dec. 1971.
White, H. A.: Tracheostomy: care with a cuffed tube. Amer. J. Nurs., 72:75–77, Jan. 1972.

Conditions of the Chest

Books

Barach, A. L.: Treatment Manual for Patients with Pulmonary Emphysema. New York, Grune and Stratton, Inc., 1969.
Bates, D. V., et al.: Respiratory Function in Disease. Philadelphia, W. B. Saunders, 1971.
Belinkoff, S.: Introduction to Inhalation Therapy. Boston, Little, Brown and Co., 1969.
Brunner, L., et al.: Textbook of Medical-Surgical Nursing, 2nd ed. Philadelphia, J. B. Lippincott, 1970, pp. 228–301.
Dobkin, A. B. (ed.): Ventilators and Inhalation Therapy. Boston, Little, Brown and Co., 1972.
Egan, D. F.: Fundamentals of Inhalation Therapy. St. Louis, C. V. Mosby, 1969.
Fraser, R. G., and Paré, J. A. P.: Diagnosis of Diseases of the Chest. Philadelphia, W. B. Saunders, 1970.
Gibbon, J. H., et al.: Surgery of the Chest. Philadelphia, W. B. Saunders, 1969.
Hinshaw, H. C.: Diseases of the Chest. Philadelphia, W. B. Saunders, 1969.
Johnson, J., et al.: Surgery of the Chest. Chicago, Year Book Medical Publishers, Inc., 1970.
Kendig, E. L.: Pulmonary Disorders. Philadelphia, W. B. Saunders, 1972.

Lewis, E. P., and Browning, M. H.: Nursing in Respiratory Diseases. New York, The American Journal of Nursing Co., 1972.
Martin, J. D. (ed.): Trauma to the Thorax and Abdomen. Springfield, Charles C Thomas, 1969.
Montgomery, W. W.: Surgery of Upper Respiratory System. Philadelphia, Lea & Febiger, 1971.
Norris, W., and Campbell, D.: Anaesthetics, Resuscitation and Intensive Care. Baltimore, Williams and Wilkins, 1971.
Pace, W. R.: Pulmonary Physiology. Philadelphia, F. A. Davis, 1970.
Petty, T. L.: Intensive and Rehabilitative Respiratory Care. Philadelphia, Lea & Febiger, 1971.
Report of the Surgeon General: The Health Consequences of Smoking. Washington, D.C., U.S. Government Printing Office, 1972.
Rodman, T., and Sterling, F. H.: Pulmonary Emphysema and Related Lung Diseases. St. Louis, C. V. Mosby, 1969.
Secor, J.: Patient Care in Respiratory Problems. Philadelphia, W. B. Saunders, 1969.
Sweetwood, H.: Nursing in the Intensive Respiratory Care Unit. New York, Springer, 1971.
Young, J. A., and Crocker, D.: Principles and Practice of Inhalation Therapy. Chicago, Year Book Medical Publishers, Inc., 1970.

Articles

Barham, V. Z.: Changing the attitudes of hospital nurses—Tuberculosis Care 1971. Nurs. Outlook, 19:538–540, Aug. 1971.
Bocles, J. S., and Llamas, R.: Airway obstruction. Med. Clin. N. Amer. 55:445–455, March 1971.
Boush, S. F., et al.: Clinical physiologic and morphologic examination of the lung in patients with bronchogenic carcinoma and the relation of the findings to postoperative deaths. Amer. Rev. Resp. Dis., 101:685–695, May 1970.
"Chemoprophylaxis for the Prevention of Tuberculosis." A report of the Ad Hoc Committee on Chemoprophylaxis. Amer. Rev. Resp. Dis., 96:558, Sept. 1967.
Comroe, J. H. Jr., et al.: Screening tests of pulmonary function. New Eng. J. Med., 282:1249–1253, May 28, 1970.
Collart, M. E., et al.: Preventing postoperative atelectasis. Amer. J. Nurs., 71:1982–1987, Oct. 1971.
Crofton, J.: The chemotherapy of bacterial respiratory infections. Amer. Rev. Resp. Dis., 101:841–859, June 1970.
DeNardo, G. L., et al.: The ventilatory lung scan in the diagnosis of pulmonary embolism. New Eng. J. Med., 282:1334–1336, June 11, 1970.
Diagnostic Standards and Classification of Tuberculosis. New York, National Tuberculosis and Respiratory Disease Association, 1969.
Dines, D. E., and DeRemee, R. A.: Meaningful clues and physical signs in chest disease. Mod. Treat., 7:821–839, July 1970.
Dyer, E. D., et al.: Safe care of IPPB machines. Amer. J. Nurs., 71:2163–2166, Nov. 1971.
Epidemiology Program Center for Disease Control: Isolation Techniques for Use in Hospitals. PHS No. 2054, Washington, D.C., U.S. Government Printing Office, 1970.
Foley, M. F.: Pulmonary function testing. Amer. J. Nurs., 7:1134–1139, June 1971.
"Guidelines for the General Hospital in the Admission and Care of Tuberculosis Patients." By Ad Hoc Committee on the Treatment of Tuberculosis Patients in General Hospital, Amer. Rev. Resp. Dis., 99:631, April 1969.
"Intermittent Chemotherapy for Tuberculosis." A Statement by the Committee on Therapy. Amer. Thorac. Soc., Amer. Rev. Resp. Dis., 100:257–259, August 1969.
"Isolation Procedures for Tuberculosis Patients in General Hospitals." Tuberculosis-Respiratory Disease Association of New Jersey, 1971.
Kelly, H. B.: Patient population and treatment choices—Tuberculosis Care 1971. Nurs. Outlook, 19:541–542, Aug. 1971.
Lorin, M. I., and Denning, C. R.: Evaluation of postural drainage by measurement of sputum volume and consistency. Amer. J. Phys. Med., 50:215–219, Oct. 1971.

McCallum, H. P.: Emphysema: What is known and what remains obscure. Canad. Nurse, *68*: 27–33, Feb. 1972.

Moretz, W. H.: Pulmonary embolism. Hosp. Med., 7:128–144, March 1971.

Nett, L. M., and Petty, T. L.: Why emphysema patients are the way they are? Amer. J. Nurs., *70*:1251–1253, June 1970.

Olcott, C., et al.: Diagnosis and treatment of respiratory failure after civilian trauma. Amer. J. Surg., *122*:260–268, Aug. 1971.

Oslick, T.: Applied oxygen therapy. Amer. Fam. Phys. 5:113–121, May 1972.

Saklad, M.: Controlled ventilation. Mod. Treat., *6*:61–80, Jan. 1969.

Schwaber, J. R.: Evaluation of respiratory status in surgical patients. Surg. Clin. N. Amer., *50*: 637–644, June 1970.

Schwaid, M. C.: The impact of emphysema. Amer. J. Nurs., *70*:1247–1250, June 1970.

Scully, H. M.: A new look at pulmonary embolism. Surg. Clin. N. Amer., *50*:343–350, April 1970.

Shapiro, A. G., and Walker, C. G.: Respiratory intensive care. Med. Clin. N. Amer., *55*:1217–1231, Sept. 1971.

"Standards for Tuberculosis Treatment in the 1970's." A Statement by the Ad Hoc Committee on Quality Care for Tuberculosis, Amer. Rev. Resp. Dis., *102*:6, 1970.

Thomas, D. P.: The management of pulmonary embolic disease. Amer. J. Med. Sci., *259*:157–163, March 1970.

Ujiki, G. T., and Shields, T. W.: Newer trends in the diagnosis and treatment of bronchogenic carcinoma. Surg. Clin. N. Amer., *51*:183–193, Feb. 1971.

Ungvarski, P.: Mechanical stimulation of coughing. Amer. J. Nurs., *71*:2358–2361, Dec. 1971.

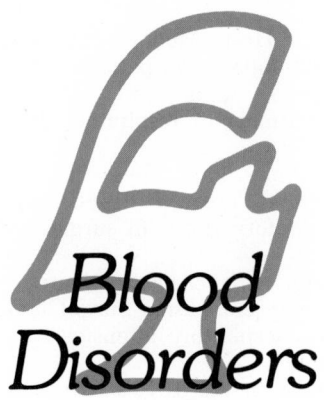

Blood Disorders

CELLULAR COMPONENTS OF NORMAL BLOOD

Erythrocytes (Red Blood Cells)

1. Comprise the vast majority of all blood cells; chiefly responsible for the color of blood.
2. Approximately 5 million erythrocytes in 1 cu. mm. of blood.
3. Normal red cell is a biconcave disk; red cell in normal blood has no nucleus.
4. Principal function is to transport oxygen—accomplished through the loose valence of an iron-containing pigment, hemoglobin, which accounts for 34% of mass of cells. Total normal concentration of hemoglobin—15 gm./100 ml. of blood.
5. Red blood cells are produced in red bone marrow which also provides most of the blood's leukocytes and all of its platelets.
   Red cells of normal adults found in short and flat bones—ribs, sternum, skull, vertebrae, bones of the hands and feet.
6. Bone marrow requires a number of nutrients, including iron, vitamin B_{12}, folic acid and pyridoxine for normal erythropoiesis (formation of red cells).
7. Normal life expectancy of a red cell is between 115 and 130 days—then eliminated by phagocytosis in the reticuloendothelial system, predominantly in spleen and liver.

Leukocytes (White Blood Cells)

1. Normally are present in a concentration of between 5000 and 10,000 cells in each cubic millimeter of blood (1 white cell for every 500–1000 red cells).
2. Leukocytes have a nucleus and are capable of active movement.
3. Major categories of leukocytes include the granulocytic series, lymphocytes, monocytes, and plasma cells.
4. Leukocytosis—white cell count over 10,000.
5. Leukopenia—white cell count below 5000.
6. *Granulocyte*—leukocytes produced in the marrow.
   a. Comprise 70% of all white cells.
   b. Called *granulocytes* because of the abundant granules contained in their cytoplasma, or *polymorphonuclear leukocytes* since their nuclei, when mature, are of a highly irregular, multilobed configuration.
7. *Lymphocytes*—a variety of leukocyte that arises in the thymus gland and lymph nodes; generally described as nongranular and including small and large varieties.
   a. Responsible for the immunologic competence of an individual.
   b. Comprise about 25% of the circulating white cells.
8. *Monocytes*—derived from components of the reticuloendothelial system (particularly spleen, liver and lymph nodes).
   a. Constitute a ready source of mobile phagocytes, congregating and performing their scavenging function at sites of inflammation and tissue necrosis.
   b. Account for about 5% of the white cell count.
9. *Plasmocytes*—formed in the lymph nodes and bone marrow.
   a. Are the main and probably sole source of the circulating immune globulins.
   b. Represent approximately 1% of the blood leukocytes.

Platelets (Thrombocytes)

1. Are the smallest and most fragile of the formed elements; are small particles (devoid of nuclei) that arise as a result of a fragmentation from giant cells called *mega-karyocytes* in the bone marrow.
2. Number approximately 250,000–500,000 platelets per cubic millimeter of blood.
3. Prime function to halt bleeding—accomplished by congregating and clumping at all sites of vascular injury and by plugging with their own substance the lumens of the bleeding vessel. As they disintegrate they release a constituent (platelet factor 3) which initiates clot formation in their immediate vicinity, thereby checking the flow of blood through the leakage of blood from the lacerated vessel.
4. Cause blood clots to shrink (retract), the effects of which is to draw together the margins of vascular defects, reduce their size and further stem the leakage.

COMMON PROBLEMS OF PATIENTS WITH BLOOD DISORDERS

The Problem	Nursing Management
Fatigue and weakness	Plan nursing care to conserve the patient's strength. Give frequent rest periods. Encourage ambulation activities as tolerated. Avoid disturbing activities and noise. Encourage optimal nutrition.
Hemorrhagic tendencies	Encourage patient to protect himself from injury. Keep the patient at rest during the bleeding episodes. Apply gentle pressure to the bleeding sites. Apply cold compresses to the bleeding sites when indicated. Avoid disturbing clots. Use topical hemostatic agents as directed. Use small gauge needles when administering medications by injection. Observe for symptoms of internal bleeding. Give a popsicle to the patient who is bleeding orally—induces vasoconstriction. Carry out serial hematocrit evaluations to determine if there is continued bleeding. Have a tracheostomy set available for the patient who is bleeding from the mouth or throat; observe for signs of asphyxiation. Transfuse the patient with appropriate agents.
Ulcerative lesions of the tongue, gums or mucous membranes	Avoid irritating foods and beverages. Give frequent oral hygiene with mild, cool mouthwash solutions. Use cotton-tipped applicators or soft-bristled toothbrush. Keep the lips lubricated. Give mouth care both before and after meals.

The Problem	Nursing Management
Dyspnea	Elevate the head of the bed. Use pillows to support the patient in the orthopneic position. Administer oxygen when indicated. Prevent unnecessary exertion. Avoid gas-forming foods.
Bone and joint pains	Relieve pressure of bedding by using a cradle. Administer either hot or cold compresses as directed. Provide for joint immobilization when ordered.
Fever	Administer cool sponges. Give antipyretic drugs as ordered. Encourage liberal fluid intake unless contraindicated. Maintain a cool environmental temperature.
Pruritus or skin eruptions	Keep the patient's fingernails short. Use soap sparingly. Apply emollient lotions in skin care.
Anxiety of patient and his family	Explain the nature, the discomforts and the limitations of activity associated with the diagnostic procedures and treatments. Encourage the patient to verbalize his *feelings*. Offer the patient the service of listening. Display an empathetic and accepting attitude. Promote the patient's relaxation and comfort. Remember the patient's individual preferences. Promote the sense of independence and self-care within the patient's limitations. Encourage the family to participate in the patient's care (as desired). Create a comfortable atmosphere for the family to visit with the patient.

BLOOD AND BONE MARROW SPECIMENS

Blood may be obtained by (1) skin puncture (finger puncture) or (2) venipuncture.

A *skin puncture* is performed when only a small amount of blood is needed (for red and white blood cell counts, hemoglobin and hematocrit determinations, reticulocyte counts, blood films for differential smear).

A *venipuncture* is a puncture of a vein to obtain blood; used when larger amounts of blood are needed.

GUIDELINES: *Obtaining Blood by Skin Puncture*

Equipment

Disposable lancet	Slides
Pipette and tubing	Alcohol sponges and dry sterile sponges

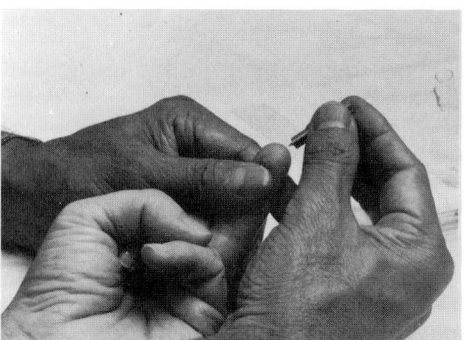

Figure 4-1. To obtain blood sample, hold finger so that fingertip becomes red. The lancet has a flange (or guard) to prevent it from being inserted too deeply.

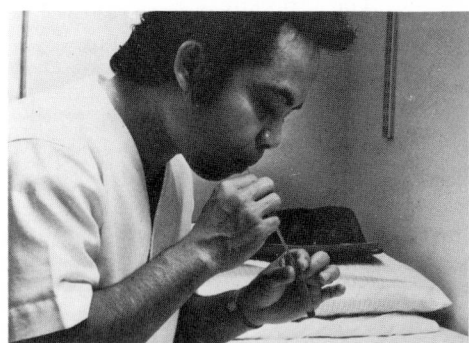

Figure 4-4. The blood is dispensed into Drabkins solution for hemoglobin determination.

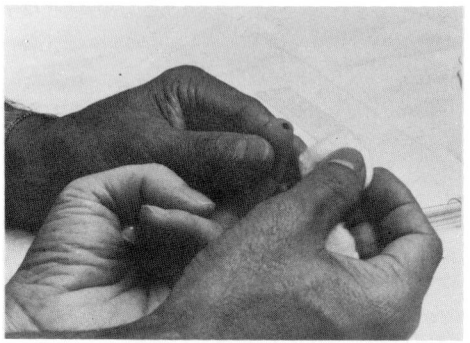

Figure 4-2. The first drop of blood is wiped away with dry cotton so that the ensuing blood will form a round drop.

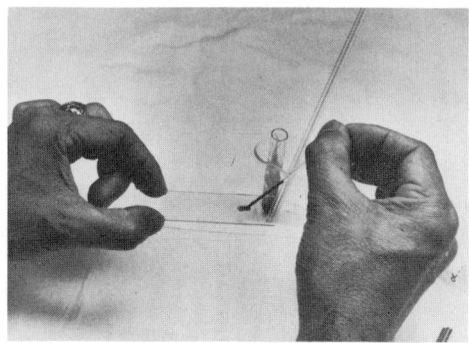

Figure 4-5. A drop of blood is placed on the slide.

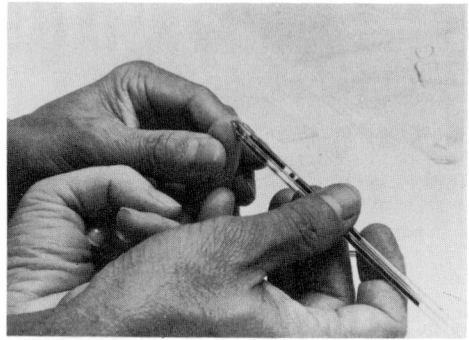

Figure 4-3. The blood is drawn up into capillary tube. The nurse is bracing the finger of his right hand on the side of the patient's finger to stabilize the patient's finger and keep the tip of the capillary tube in the drop of blood.

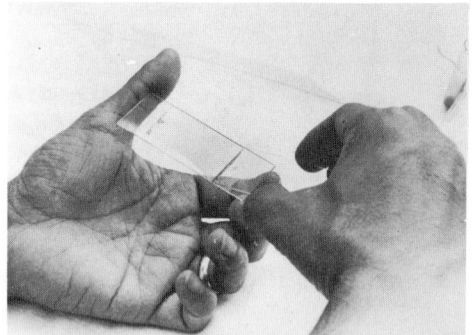

Figure 4-6. The blood is smeared over the slide.

Procedure

Nursing Action	***Rationale/Amplification***

Performance Phase

1. Cleanse site (preferably ball of finger) with alcohol and dry with sterile gauze square.

2. Create stasis by pressing on the distal joint of the finger to produce redness at the end of the finger.
3. Use a sterile disposable lancet (Fig. 4–1).

4. Prick the skin sharply and quickly with the lancet.
5. Release pressure on the finger. Wipe off the first drop of blood (Fig. 4–2).

6. Allow the blood to flow freely with an adequate puncture.
7. Obtain the blood sample (Fig. 4–3).
   a. Fill the pipette (Fig. 4–4).
   b. Make blood slides according to the study ordered (Fig. 4–5 and 4–6).
8. Apply pressure over the wound with a dry gauze sponge until bleeding stops.

1. If skin is wet with alcohol the blood will hemolyze; also it will not collect into a compact drop but will run down the patient's finger.

3. This avoids the possibility of the transference of the hepatitis virus.
4. Pricking the skin sharply and quickly minimizes pain and produces a free-flowing sample.
5. Epithelial or endothelial cells may be found in the first drop of blood and render the count inaccurate.
6. Pressing out the blood dilutes it with tissue fluid.

GUIDELINES: *Obtaining Blood by the Syringe Method*

Veins Used

Median basilic vein in antecubital area
Wrist

Dorsum (back) of hand
Top of foot

Equipment

70% alcohol and tincture of iodine
Dry sterile sponges

5 and 10 ml. syringe
20 gauge needle(s)

Procedure

Nursing Action	***Rationale/Amplification***

Performance Phase

1. Reassure patient. Explain that relatively little blood will be taken.

2. Instruct the patient to extend his arm; the arm should be held straight at the elbow.
3. Apply the tourniquet directly above the elbow with just sufficient pressure to prevent venous return.
4. Inspect the area to visualize the vein. Palpate the vein.
5. Cleanse the skin with iodine and alcohol. Dry.

1. The patient is reassured when the nurse displays self-assurance and competence in relating to people and when performing technical skills.

3. A tourniquet increases venous pressure and makes the vein more prominent and easier to enter.
4. Select a vein that is visible, palpable and well-fixed to surrounding tissue.
5. Cleansing the skin reduces pathogens.

Nursing Action	**Rationale/Amplification**
6. Fix chosen vein with the thumb and draw the skin taut immediately below the site before inserting needle.	6. The vein may roll beneath the skin when the needle approaches its outer surface (especially in elderly and extremely thin patients).
7. Insert the needle, bevel up, at a 30-degree angle so that it enters the skin first and then the vein.	7. When the needle point enters the lumen of the vein, blood will enter the tip of the syringe.
8. Release the tourniquet.	
9. Obtain blood sample by *gently* pulling back on the plunger.	9. Use minimal suction to prevent hemolysis of blood and collapse of the vein.
10. Withdraw the needle slowly.	10. Slow withdrawal of the needle is less painful.
11. Apply gauze over the puncture site firmly for 2–4 minutes.	11. Firm pressure over the puncture site prevents leakage of blood into surrounding tissues with subsequent hematoma development. Merely flexing the arm may not prevent a hematoma as the vein can slip to the side of the area where pressure is applied.
12. Make the blood smear from the needle as desired.	
13. Remove the needle from the hub of the syringe. Gently eject the blood sample into a test tube containing an anticoagulant.	13. Slowly transfer the blood into the test tube *without* forming bubbles.
14. Place stopper on the test tube.	
15. Invert the tube gently several times to mix blood with anticoagulant.	
16. Label specimens correctly and send to laboratory immediately.	16. Specimens should go to the lab with a minimum of delay for optimum reliability.

GUIDELINES: *Bone Marrow Aspiration and Biopsy*

Bone marrow aspiration or biopsy is done so that specimens of bone marrow can be obtained for establishing a diagnosis.

Purposes

1. To diagnose hematologic disease—enables the precursors of cells in peripheral blood to be examined and their relative numbers determined.
2. To follow the course of disease and the patient's response to treatment.
3. To diagnose diseases other than pure hematologic disorders such as primary and metastatic tumors, infectious diseases, certain granulomas and parasitic infestations.
4. To isolate bacteria and other pathogenic agents by culture or animal inoculation.

Complications

1. Osteomyelitis (rare)
2. Bleeding and hematoma in patients with bleeding disorders
3. Puncture of vital organs if biopsy is too deep

Contraindications

Hemophilia and related hemorrhagic disorders

Equipment

Bone marrow aspiration tray
  Marrow aspiration needles with stylets
  Sterile towels
  25 and 22 gauge needles
  Two 20-ml. syringes
  Three 5-ml. syringes
  Local anesthetic (1% procaine or xylocaine)

Sterile gloves
Skin antiseptic
Laboratory equipment:
  Coverslips
  Microscopic slides
  Test tubes (plain and heparinized)
Scalpel blade and handle

Procedure

Nursing Action	Rationale/Amplification

Preparatory Phase

1. Explain the procedure to the patient.

    1. An explanation helps the patient to cope with anticipated stress.

2. Give medication—meperidine (Demerol)—if ordered; usually not necessary.

    2. Demerol may be used as an analgesic and sedative for apprehension.

3. Place the patient in supine position.

4. Shave area. The following sites may be used:
  a. Sternum
  b. Iliac crest—(anterior and posterior spines)
  c. Spinous processes of vertebrae (T10 through L4)

    4. The marrow of the sternum and the marrow of the iliac crest are used commonly for obtaining aspirations.

STERNAL ASPIRATION

Performance Phase (by physician)

1. The skin is prepared and the site infiltrated with procaine or xylocaine.

2. The site selected is usually the midsternal line at the level of the 2nd interspace.

    2. The sternum is thinner and marrow more plentiful between the sternal interspaces.

3. The marrow needle with stylet in place is inserted through the cortex of the bone with a slight twisting motion. The physician usually feels a "give" in the marrow needle when the marrow cavity has been penetrated.

    3. A sternal puncture is considered more dangerous than other sites because of its proximity to vital structures in the mediastinum.

4. The stylet is removed and a syringe attached to the hub of the needle. The plunger is withdrawn slowly until marrow appears in the syringe (0.2–0.5 ml. of fluid is aspirated).

    4. The marrow will appear as whitish granular particles through the bloody aspirate.

5. Warn the patient that he will feel pain.

    5. The pain is caused by suction of the syringe and lasts only a few seconds.

6. The syringe is removed and the marrow expressed onto a slide or watch glass.

    6. If repeated aspirations result in no marrow it indicates that the sternal marrow is not suitable for aspiration.

7. The needle is removed.

    7. If the patient has thrombocytopenia, pressure should be applied 5 to 10 minutes.

8. Pressure is applied over the puncture site until bleeding (if any) ceases.

ILIAC CREST ASPIRATION/BIOPSY

Performance Phase (by physician)

ANTERIOR APPROACH

1. Position the patient prone or on his side.
2. The needle is passed into the cavity of the ilium 2 cm. behind and 2 cm. below the anterior superior iliac spine and perpendicular to the flat surface of the bone.
3. A small hammer may be used to tap the needle gently in place, but this is rarely necessary.

    2. Pain is an indicator that the needle is within the marrow cavity.

    3. The bone of the iliac crest is harder than that of the sternum.

POSTERIOR APPROACH

1. Position the patient on his side.
2. The needle is passed along an anesthetized tract that runs behind the prominence of the posterior iliac spine and at right angles with the anterior abdominal wall.
3. Instruct the patient to lie on his affected side after the procedure.

    3. Lying on the affected side promotes hemostasis.

Follow-up Phase

1. Give mild analgesic if needed.
2. Assess patient for discomfort, continued bleeding and untoward symptoms.

TRANSFUSION THERAPY

Blood

1. Whole blood is used for acute hemorrhage and hypovolemic shock (actual or potential).
2. Fresh blood (i.e., blood stored less than 24 hours) is indicated for:
   a. Patients requiring multiple transfusions
   b. All exchange transfusions
   c. Postoperative transfusions following extracorporeal circulation with stored blood
   d. Patients with certain specific hemorrhagic disorders who are bleeding actively or who are anemic as the result of recent bleeding (i.e., hemophilia A, factor V deficiency complicating severe liver disease or coumarin therapy, severe thrombocytopenia)
   e. See page 199 for technique of administration

Blood Components

A. *Packed Red Cells*—erythrocytes from a unit of blood with most of plasma removed; contains a minimum of plasma colloids and imposes less risk of circulatory overload.
   1. Packed red cells provide erythrocytes in a minimal volume of fluid; oxygen-carrying capacity is treated directly.
   2. Used for:
      a. Patients with severe anemia who have relatively normal blood volume
      b. Patients with risk of heart failure
      c. Transfusion of infants

3. Packed cells are administered through a large bore needle at a flow rate slower than whole blood.

B. *Platelet Transfusions*—given to patients with dangerous degrees of thrombocytopenia (decrease of platelets in circulating blood) to control or prevent bleeding.
   1. Viable platelets may be supplied in form of:
      a. Fresh blood—replaces red cells and platelets.
      b. Platelet-rich plasma (PRP)—contains 80–90% of original platelets.
      c. Platelet concentrates (PC)—retains nearly all original platelets in a viable state but the volume is reduced.
         Eliminates risk of circulatory overloading.
   2. The quantity of platelets needed to elevate the recipient's platelet count from a hemorrhagic to a safe level (e.g., from 5000–50,000/cu. mm.) represents the harvest from at least 4–6 units of donor blood.

C. *Whole Plasma*—fluid portion of the blood in which corpuscles are suspended.
   1. Clinical Usefulness
      a. Treatment of clotting defects—all of the plasma factors can be supplied rapidly without overexpanding the patient's blood volume.
      b. Correction of hypovolemia due to selective loss of plasma—mainly in burned patients.
      c. Correction of hypovolemia in acute blood loss when whole blood is not immediately available.
   2. Plasma that has been separated from stored blood (or has been stored in the liquid state after separation) contains the stable clotting factors VII, IX, X and XI.
   3. As a plasma expander for hypovolemia or as an exogenous source of plasma albumin for hypoalbuminemia, whole plasma has largely been replaced by pure preparations of serum albumin and other plasma fractions that are comprised largely of albumin.
   4. *Freshly Frozen Plasma*—plasma which has been separated immediately from freshly donated blood and then promptly frozen.
      Factor V (one of the accelerators of prothrombin conversion) and factor VIII (the antihemophilic factor) are retained by this process.
   5. *Factor VIII Concentrates* (There are 13 named and numbered clotting factors.)
      a. Antihemophilic cryoprecipitate—effective in treatment of hemophilia
      b. Glycine precipitate
   6. *Human Serum Albumin and other Albumin Preparations*
      Clinical usefulness
      (1) To expand blood volume in patients in hypovolemic shock.
      (2) To elevate the circulating albumin in patients with hypoalbuminemia.
   7. *Human Fibrinogen*
      Used for congenital and acquired hypofibrinogenemia complicated by active bleeding.

GUIDELINES: *Administering Blood Transfusions*

Blood Transfusion is the introduction of blood into the body circulation.

Purposes
1. To restore circulating blood volume.
2. To replace clotting factors.
3. To improve oxygen-carrying capacity.

Equipment

Blood administration set (disposable)   Blood as ordered
Needles, No. 18–19 gauge   Alcohol and iodine sponges/tourniquet
Normal saline infusion

Procedure

Nursing Action	Rationale/Amplification
Preparatory Phase	
1. Make sure that the blood has been typed and cross matched.	1. Typing is done to establish the blood group (A, B, AB or O) and Rh factor; a cross match is done to establish the compatibility between the patient's blood and the donor's.
2. Give the blood within 20 minutes after taking it from the blood bank.	2. Storage at 1–6° C. should be maintained until just before administration. Rapid deterioration of the red blood cells can occur with uncooled blood.
3. Inspect the blood for gas bubbles and any abnormal color or cloudiness.	3. Gas bubbles may indicate bacterial growth; abnormal color or clouding may warn of hemolysis.
Performance Phase	
1. *Check the labels identifying the donor and recipient blood (number and type) and confirm the identity of the patient who is to receive it:* Call the patient by his full name, check his identification wrist band, check his chart to make sure of his number and type.	1. Meticulous attention to detail is essential to avoid giving the wrong blood to the wrong patient which may cause a fatal reaction.
2. Take the patient's T.P.R. (temperature, pulse, respiration)	2. Base-line temperature, pulse and respiration measurements are used for later comparisons.
3. Prepare the saline solution.	
4. Select a suitable vein (see p. 53). Cleanse skin thoroughly (alcohol and iodine). Allow to dry.	4. Skin cleansing is done to remove skin bacteria and sebum.
5. Perform the venipuncture (see p. 51).	
6. Allow 50 ml. of saline to run into the patient's vein.	6. Normal saline is used to flush the tubing before blood is started.
7. Allow the blood to run through the blood transfusion set.	7. A filter is located between the container and the flow indicator to screen out particles that can embolize. Precipitation of platelets, leukocytes and fibrin may clog the administration set.
8. Hang the unit of blood about a meter (3–4 feet) above the level of the patient's heart.	8. The rate of flow is determined by the height at which the bottle is suspended and the size of the needle.
9. Discontinue the saline infusion and start the blood.	
10. DO NOT GIVE MEDICATIONS IN THE BLOOD. DO NOT GIVE 5% DEXTROSE IN WATER IN BLOOD.	10. Dextrose does not contain electrolytes and can cause hemolysis and clotting in the I.V. tubing.

(see p. 53); (see p. 51)

Nursing Action	**Rationale/Amplification**
11. Adjust the rate of blood flow to 20 drops per minute during the first 15 minutes of the transfusion. *Stay with the patient for at least 15 minutes after the start of the transfusion.* Then adjust the rate to 4 ml. (42 drops) ° per minute if the patient's condition permits. At this rate approximately 500 ml. of blood will be transfused in 2 hours.	11. Symptoms of an untoward reaction are usually manifested during the infusion of the initial 50 to 100 ml. of blood. If the transfusion is stopped early, acute renal necrosis and death rarely occur.
12. Give the blood at a slower rate if the patient is elderly or has heart disease.	12. Too rapid administration of blood may overload a precarious circulatory system and induce congestive heart failure and pulmonary edema.
13. Monitor central venous pressure through a separate infusion line for patients with circulatory overload problems.	
14. Watch the patient carefully. Monitor the vital signs hourly or more frequently as indicated.	14. A change in the condition of the patient may signal the development of a transfusion complication.
15. Change the administration set (tubing, filter) if another unit of blood is to be given.	15. The filter may become clogged after a unit of blood has been given.

Complications

NURSING ALERT: Transfusion therapy (whether of whole blood or blood components) entails a number of calculated risks. Some of these potential complications cannot be prevented with absolute certainty. There is a significant incidence of morbidity and mortality associated with administration of a blood transfusion.

Circulatory Overloading

Due to administration of excessive volume or at a rate faster than the heart can accept.

Assess for rise in venous pressure, distended neck veins, dyspnea, cough, rales heard in base of lungs.

NURSING INTERVENTION

1. Prevent by using packed cells, proper spacing of transfusions and give at rate within circulatory reserve of patient.
2. Monitor C.V.P. of patients with heart disease.
3. Stop transfusion immediately.
4. Place patient upright with his feet in a dependent position.
5. Prepare to digitalize the patient as directed.

Transmission of Disease

The virus of hepatitis and malaria parasites may be transmitted from donor to recipient via infected blood.

1. Screen donors carefully.
2. Reject donors with history of hepatitis or jaundice or if the laboratory test is positive for Australia Antigen.
3. Only albumin, gamma globulin, frozen red cells and plasma protein fractions are considered hepatitis free.

Pyrogenic Reactions (Febrile Reaction)

Usually due to presence of leuko-agglutinins or platelet agglutinins in patient or to antigens in transfused blood.

1. Stop transfusion.
2. Substitute new container of blood.

° Using the Baxter Blood Administration Set—calibrated at 10 drops/ml.

Symptoms: (may occur after transfusion is discontinued):
   a. Sudden chilling and fever
   b. Headache
   c. Nausea and vomiting

3. Take temperature ½ hour after chill and as indicated thereafter.
4. Give aspirin to reduce fever.

Bacterial Contamination
Due to transfusion of bacteria or their toxins in the blood.

Symptoms:
   a. High fever (over 38.4° C./101° F.)
   b. Intense flushing
   c. Severe headache or substernal pain
   d. Vomiting; diarrhea
   e. Hypotension; shock-like state

1. Before transfusion, inspect blood for gas bubbles and change in color.
2. Stop transfusion.
3. Obtain cultures of donor's blood—(and recipient's blood)—send remainder of blood to the lab.
4. Treat septicemia as directed—antibiotics, intravenous fluids, fresh transfusion, vasopressors.

Allergic Reactions
Blood of allergic patient may contain antibodies capable of reacting with allergens in the donor's blood.

Symptoms:
   a. Flushing
   b. Itching and rash
   c. Urticaria (hives)
   d. Asthmatic wheezing
   e. Laryngeal edema

1. Screen and reject all donors with known allergies.
2. Give prophylactic antihistamine or steroids *before* blood is started to patients known to have severe allergic attacks.
3. Prepare epinephrine if respiratory distress is severe.

Hemolytic Reaction or Incompatibility
   (most severe)
Hemolysis occurs when incompatible red cells are injected into the patient's circulating blood. It may cause oliguric renal failure and death.

Clinical Manifestations:
   a. Chilliness
   b. Feeling of head fullness
   c. Oppressive feeling in chest
   d. Sharp pain in lumbar area
   e. Distention of neck veins
   f. Tachycardia
   g. Tachypnea
   h. Fall in blood pressure and vascular depression

1. Positively identify patient and blood before transfusion is started.
2. Stay with patient during the first 15 minutes that he is receiving transfusion—if transfusion is stopped early, fatal untoward reaction may be halted.
3. Administer blood at 20 drops/minute during this period.
4. Stop transfusion.
5. Recross match immediately—patient may need further transfusions.
6. Monitor blood pressure.
7. Insert indwelling catheter; monitor hourly urinary output.
8. Send sample of patient's blood and urine to lab for presence of hemoglobin—indicative of intravascular hemolysis.
9. Treat hypovolemia—transfusion of compatible blood, plasma, plasma volume expanders.

10. Treat acute renal failure—due to hemoglobin deposition in nephron.
    a. Give mannitol as directed to initiate diuresis—renal toxicity is affected by rate of urinary excretion and pH.
    b. Give bicarbonate—to alkalinize urine and to help prevent precipitation of hemoglobin within renal tubule.

Hyperkalemia (potassium excess)

Symptoms:

  a. Nausea, colic, diarrhea
  b. Muscular weakness
  c. Paresthesia of hands, foot, tongue, face
  d. Flaccid paralysis
  e. Apprehension
  f. Slowed pulse rate
  g. Cardiac arrest

1. Avoid using old blood—stored blood causes potassium levels to increase.

Hypocalcemia (calcium deficit)

Calcium deficit can occur with administration of large volume of citrated blood.

Clinical Manifestations:

  a. Tingling of fingers and in circumoral region
  b. Muscular cramps
  c. Hyperactive reflexes
  d. Convulsions
  e. Carpopedal spasms of hands
  f. Laryngeal spasms

1. Clamp the tubing and notify the physician.

Air Embolism (may occur if blood is transfused under pressure)

1. Clamp tubing.
2. Position patient on his left side in a slight Trendelenburg position—to divert air from pulmonary tract.

ANEMIA

The term *anemia* implies an abnormally low number of circulating red cells or a decreased concentration of hemoglobin in the blood.

Altered Physiology

1. The appearance of anemia reflects (1) marrow failure, (2) excessive red cell loss or (3) both.
2. Marrow failure may occur as a result of a nutritional deficiency, toxic exposure or tumor invasion, or from unknown causes.
3. Red cells may be lost through hemorrhage or hyperhemolysis (increased destruction).
   a. This problem may be rooted in some red-cell defect that is incompatible with normal red-cell survival or is explainable on the basis of some factor extrinsic to the red cell that promotes red-cell destruction.

    b. Red-cell lysis occurs mainly within the phagocytic cells of the reticuloendothelial system, notably within the liver and spleen.

    c. As a by-product of this process, bilirubin, formed from hemoglobin within the phagocyte, enters the bloodstream, and an increase in hemolysis is promptly reflected by an increase in total plasma bilirubin.

        (1) Normal concentration of total plasma bilirubin—1.0 mg./100 ml. or less.

        (2) Levels above 1.5 mg./100 ml. produce visible jaundice of sclerae.

Clinical Manifestations

1. Pallor
2. Susceptibility to fatigue
3. Increased cardiac output
4. Predisposition to angina pectoris or congestive heart failure
5. Disturbed mental cerebration; dizziness

Severity of Symptoms Dependent Upon

1. The speed with which the anemia has developed
2. Its prior duration, i.e., how chronic it is
3. The metabolic requirements of the particular patient
4. Any other disorders currently afflicting the patient
5. Special complications or concomitant features of the condition producing the anemia

Iron Deficiency Anemia

Iron deficiency anemias are conditions in which the total body iron content is decreased below a normal level.

Etiology

Iron deficiency develops when the body's need for iron exceeds the supply.

1. Excessive bleeding from menorrhagia or from bleeding in gastrointestinal tract, etc.
2. Impaired gastrointestinal absorption of iron—small bowel disease, postgastrectomy.
3. Inadequate dietary sources of iron
4. Increased iron requirements—during pregnancy, periods of rapid growth, menstruation (average of 20 mg. of iron lost per menstrual cycle).

Dietary Implications

1. Average person ingests 10–15 mg. of iron daily in food iron and inorganic iron salts; less than 10% of all iron ingested (including food and iron supplements) is absorbed.
2. Approximately 6 mg. of iron is ingested per 1000 calories.
3. The average diet usually will maintain normal iron balance unless there is abnormal drain of iron (bleeding, pregnancy).
4. Food sources of iron
    a. Meat, fish, poultry and eggs
    b. Green leafy vegetables, potatoes, dried fruits, enriched bread and cereal products, whole grains, dried beans
5. Ascorbic acid has been shown to enhance iron absorption.

Clinical Manifestations

Reduction in hemoglobin concentration decreases the capacity of the blood to transport and deliver oxygen to the tissues.

1. Fatigue
2. Headache, dizziness, tinnitus
3. Palpitations and dyspnea
4. Paresthesias
5. Pallor of mucous membranes

Treatment

1. Recognize and correct the underlying cause.
   Assist in the search for the site of chronic blood loss.
2. Correct the hemoglobin and tissue iron deficiency with the administration of the prescribed iron preparation.
3. Encourage the selection of a well-balanced diet.

A. *Oral Iron Therapy*

1. Choice of iron depends on (1) patient tolerance, (2) gastrointestinal absorption, (3) dosage according to estimate of hemoglobin deficiency.
2. Oral Iron Preparations
   a. Ferrous sulfates (Feosol, Fer-In-Sol, Ironate, Irosul)
   b. Ferrous gluconate (Fergon, Nionate)
   c. Ferrous fumarate (Ircon, Tolferain, Firon, Fumiron)
   d. Preparations of iron with other compounds
   e. Molybdenized iron (Mol-Iron, Mol-Iron Chronosules)
3. Nursing Emphasis
   a. Iron preparations are absorbed at all levels of the gastrointestinal tract below the stomach; maximal absorption occurs in the duodenum.
   b. Give iron with or immediately after meals to minimize gastric irritation.
   c. Educate patient to anticipate a certain amount of dyspepsia from time to time.
   d. Iron salts alter the color of the stools; tell the patient to expect color changes (dark green to black).
   e. Ferrous sulfate is apt to deposit on the teeth and the gums; advise patient to use frequent oral hygiene measures.
   f. The dosage of iron may be gradually increased over a few days.
   g. If gastrointestinal side effects are troublesome the dosage may have to be cut in half.
   h. Iron administration should be continued several months after hemoglobin levels return to normal—to ensure replenishment of the iron stores.
   i. Emphasize that the patient should take his iron faithfully.

B. *Parenteral Iron Therapy*

1. Parenteral iron therapy is given (1) when the patient is unable to tolerate iron preparations orally, (2) when the patient has severe gastrointestinal disorders or (3) when a rapid response is required.

NURSING ALERT: Extravasation of medication results in painful local induration. Systemic reactions (flushing, nausea, vomiting, myalgia and fever) may occur.

---

2. Parenteral Iron Preparations
   a. Dextriferron (Astrafer)

        b. Iron dextran (Imferon)
        c. Iron sorbitol complex (Jectofer)—may cause patient's urine to turn black on standing.
    3. Technique of Parenteral Iron Administration
        a. Discard needle that is used to draw medication into syringe; use a fresh needle for injection.
        b. Draw 0.5 ml. of air into syringe before injecting medication.
        c. Use a needle 5 cm. (2 inches) long—medication is injected deep into muscle.
        d. Retract the skin over the muscle *laterally* before inserting needle.
        e. Inject the medication and 0.5 ml. of air following the medication—to prevent leakage along injection tract when needle is withdrawn.

Pernicious Anemia

Pernicious anemia is a megaloblastic anemia due to vitamin B_{12} deficiency caused by lack of the intrinsic factor in the gastric juice.

Altered Physiology

    1. Pernicious anemia is produced by a defect in the gastric secretory function, the gastric juice being devoid of a material (intrinsic factor) that is necessary for the absorption of vitamin B_{12} (extrinsic factor) from the lower portion of the ileum, the only site where vitamin B_{12} can be absorbed.
    2. Vitamin B_{12} is the extrinsic factor necessary for the maturation of red blood cells.
    3. The basic defect in pernicious anemia appears to involve the synthesis of a nucleoprotein (DNA) required for nuclear division.

Clinical Manifestations

    1. Symptoms due to anemia
        a. Pallor
        b. Dyspnea or orthopnea
        c. Angina pectoris
        d. Edema of legs
    2. Symptoms due to physiologic changes in gastrointestinal tract
        a. Sore mouth with smooth red "beefy" tongue
        b. Loss of appetite
        c. Indigestion and epigastric discomfort
        d. Recurring diarrhea or constipation
        e. Weight loss
    3. Symptoms due to neurologic changes (occurs in high percentage of untreated patients)
        a. Tingling and numbness or burning pain (paresthesias) involving hands and feet
        b. Loss of position sense, leading to disturbances of gait
        c. Disturbances of bladder and bowel function
        d. Irritability
        e. Depression
        f. Paranoia and delirium

Diagnostic Evaluation

1. Blood smear—reveals marked variation in size and shape of cells and a variable number of unusually large cells containing abundant hemoglobin.
2. Gastric analysis—the gastric juice lacks free hydrochloric acid.
3. Schilling test (administration of radioactive vitamin B_{12} by mouth and subsequent measurement of its excretion in the urine).
   Shows that there is lack of ability to absorb vitamin B_{12} normally.
4. Bone marrow aspiration—reveals megaloblastic marrow.
5. Gastroscopy—gastric mucosa appears thin and gray.
6. Low serum B_{12} analysis.

Treatment

Objectives: to support the patient during the acute phase of his illness.
to give enough antianemic factor (vitamin B_{12}) to produce a remission.
to help the patient accept that he must be on vitamin B_{12} maintenance for his lifetime.

A. *Treatment During Acute Stage*
1. Give cyanocobalamin (vitamin B_{12}) 100 μg. intramuscularly 3 times weekly until the blood values return to normal.
   a. Reticulocytes begin to increase on 4th day after therapy is started; normal hemoglobin values are obtained in approximately 6 weeks.
   b. Patient begins to improve in general well-being and mental status in a few days.
   c. *Recent* neurological changes will usually be reversed.
2. Give transfusion of packed cells very slowly (if ordered).
   a. Transfusions are only given to patients whose anemia is life-threatening (symptoms of hypoxia to heart or brain).
   b. Place the patient in a sitting position in bed.
      Too rapid administration of transfusion to patient with pernicious anemia may produce acute pulmonary or cerebral edema.
3. Support the patient with neurological involvement (see p. 765 for management of patient with neurogenic bladder).

B. *Maintenance Therapy*
1. Impress upon the patient that vitamin B_{12} must be continued for his lifetime.
   a. Maintenance dose schedule—100 μg. monthly.
   b. Teach patient and family or have a visiting nurse give the maintenance therapy.
   c. Untreated pernicious anemia is fatal.
2. Instruct the patient to report for follow-up examinations every 6 months for hematocrit and physical examination.
      Patients with pernicious anemia have a higher incidence of gastric cancer; therefore periodic stool examinations for occult blood should be made.
3. Following total gastrectomy, patient should receive maintenance dose of vitamin B_{12} (100 μg. I.M.) as often as indicated—removal of gastric fundus deprives the patient of all intrinsic factor; may take as long as 10 years for clinical symptoms to appear due to small amount of daily vitamin B_{12} required and the large body stores available for use.

Aplastic Anemia

Aplastic anemia is a condition of bone marrow failure which results in markedly reduced production of all blood cells (erythrocytes, leukocytes and platelets [pancytopenia]).

Causes

1. Congenital (Fanconi's anemia)—congenitally constituted defect in the bone marrow.
2. Idiopathic—approximately 50% of aplastic anemia cases are of unknown etiology.
3. Ionizing radiation—therapeutic, industrial or laboratory accidents.
4. Chemical compounds—benzol (dry-cleaning agents)—may induce permanent bone marrow damage.
5. Drugs—antibiotics (chloramphenicol), analgesics, anticonvulsants, hypoglycemia agents, diuretics, antihistamines, insecticides, others.

Clinical Manifestations

1. Anemia, pallor, weakness—resulting from depression of hemoglobin and rapidity of blood change.
2. Infections with high fever—resulting from granulocytopenia.
3. Purpura and bleeding from gums, nose, gastrointestinal tract, urinary tract—resulting from thrombocytopenia.

Diagnostic Evaluation

1. Peripheral blood smear
   a. Red cell count may be below 1 million/cu. mm.
   b. White blood count may be less than 2000/cu. mm.
   c. Platelet count may be less than 30,000/cu. mm.
   d. This pancytopenia reflects failure of the marrow to produce and deliver the formed elements in the blood.
2. Bone marrow aspiration—bone marrow is hypoplastic or aplastic; reduction of its cellular elements with an almost complete absence of hemopoietic activity.

Clinical Course

1. Bone marrow failure cannot usually be reversed by any known agent.
2. The patient's clinical course may range from a few weeks to 4 years or longer.
3. Approximately half of the patients with aplastic anemia die of the disease, usually from *hemorrhage, infection* and *complications of chronic anemia.*

Treatment

Objectives: to bring the patient to remission.
      to prolong his survival time with supportive therapy.

1. Attempt to identify and remove the underlying toxic agent(s).
   a. Question patient regarding all agents (chemicals, drugs) to which he has been exposed.
   b. Instruct patient to eliminate exposure to toxins and discontinue all unnecessary medications.
2. Support the patient who has bone marrow failure.
   a. Give packed red cells carefully—to maintain hemoglobin level compatible with patient's activities and to relieve symptoms of dyspnea, palpitation and weakness.

b. Give transfusion of whole blood for hemorrhagic emergencies.

c. Give platelet transfusions—to arrest bleeding in patient hemorrhaging from thrombocytopenia.

d. Keep patient receiving multiple transfusions over a period of time under careful nursing surveillance—transfusion complications usually develop with these patients (see p. 201).

   (1) Assess for chills, fever, shock.

   (2) Patients receiving many transfusions may develop *hemosiderosis* (excess iron stores in the tissues).

3. Give corticosteroids—to help bring a remission; may also modify bleeding tendencies of patients with thrombocytopenia.

4. Give agents to attempt to stimulate marrow function and bring about a remission.

   a. Androgens

      (1) Fluoxymesterone (Halotestin)

      (2) Oxymetholone (Adroyd, Anadrol)

      (3) Testosterone enanthate (Delatestryl)

   b. Cobaltous chloride

5. Watch for evidences of infection—patients with aplastic anemia are susceptible to infections due to low leukocyte count and prolonged treatment with corticosteroids.

   a. Utilize reverse isolation techniques on patient with pronounced leukopenia.

   b. Treat infections with antibiotics.

      (1) Long-term antibiotic therapy may cause enteritis and diarrhea from changes in intestinal flora.

      (2) Generalized moniliasis may also occur in weakened patients taking antibiotics for prolonged periods.

6. Prepare patient for splenectomy (see p. 229) if indicated—the spleen destroys large numbers of white cells and platelets; splenectomy may cause slight elevation of hemoglobin levels and decrease the transfusion requirements.

POLYCYTHEMIA VERA

Polycythemia vera (erythremia) is a disease of unknown cause characterized by an increase of red blood cells. There may be an increased production of myeloid leukocytes and even of platelets.

Secondary polycythemia commonly accompanies cardiac and pulmonary diseases.

Altered Physiology

1. Altered physiology due to increased blood viscosity and hypermetabolism

2. Increased supply of precursor cells (to the erythroid, meloid and megakaryocytic line)

3. Striking increase in total blood volume; gradually increasing blood viscosity

4. Engorgement of all organs with blood

5. Hyperplasia of all bone marrow elements

6. Enlargement of spleen

Clinical Course

1. Insidious and gradual onset—probably measured in years.

2. Clinical course of long duration—10 to 20 years.

3. More frequent in males; most common during middle and later years of life.
4. Peptic ulcers are common in these patients; cerebral, gastrointestinal and nasal hemorrhages may occur at any time during the course of the disease.

Clinical Manifestations

This is a multiple organ system disease.
1. Weakness and fatigue
2. Headache, dizziness, impaired mental ability, visual disturbances
3. Pruritus
4. Plethoric appearance
5. Reddish-purple hue of the face, lips, hands, feet and buccal cavity; aggravated by cold
6. Peripheral vascular complaints
7. Paresthesia
8. Splenomegaly producing abdominal discomfort
9. Elevated systolic blood pressure
10. Hepatomegaly (late in course of disease)

Diagnostic Evaluation

1. Elevated red cell mass (8–10 million/cu. mm.)
2. Elevated white blood cells (10,000–50,000) and platelets (300,000–600,000/cu. mm.)
3. Elevated leukocyte alkaline phosphatase test
4. Increased cellular activity of bone marrow

Treatment

Objective: to reduce the red cell mass (e.g., normalize the hematocrit)
1. Assist with phlebotomy (venesection) to correct blood viscosity and circulating abnormalities.
   a. 500 ml. of blood removed every 2 to 3 days until hematocrit reaches desired level (less than 50%).
   b. Repeated phlebotomies may be performed to lower hemoglobin and hematocrit and red cell mass to normal ranges; usually done for younger patients early in course of disease.
2. Give chemotherapy for myelosuppression (suppress bone marrow function).
   a. Chlorambucil (Leukeran) is drug of choice.
   b. ^{32}P (radiophosphorus) I.V. or oral—reduces myelopoiesis
      With radiophosphorus the incidence of terminal leukemia is thought to be increased.
   c. Busulfan (Myleran)
   d. Melphalan (Aleran)
   e. Cytosine arabinoside
   f. Cyclophosphamide (Cytoxan)
   g. See page 881 for nursing support of patient receiving chemotherapy.
3. Prepare the patient for radiation to the bone marrow—to reduce the tremendous proliferation of red cells, white cells and platelets (alternative to chemotherapy).
   Spleen may be irradiated to relieve pressure symptoms of enlarged spleen.

4. Evaluate and treat for complications—the clinical course of polycythemia is determined by the development of complications.
    a. Thrombotic complications—due to hypervolemia and hyperactivity of the hematopoietic tissues.
        Includes deep vein thrombophlebitis, myocardial and cerebral infarction and thrombotic occlusion of the splenic hepatic, portal and mesenteric veins.
    b. Hemorrhage—bleeding occurs spontaneously from engorgement of capillary beds.
    c. Peptic ulcers—from increased gastric secretion.
    d. Gout—from overproduction of uric acid (exact mechanism unknown).
    e. Congestive failure—from increased blood volume and hypertension.
    f. Patients with polycythemia vera frequently progress into myeloid leukemia and myelosclerosis.

AGRANULOCYTOSIS

Agranulocytosis (agranulocytopenia) is a depression of the granulocytic (mainly neutrophilic) leukocyte formation with an extreme decrease in the number of white cells in the blood (leukopenia).

Etiology
1. Hypersensitivity to certain drugs—may suppress bone marrow activity and decrease production of white blood cells.
    a. Aminopyrine (frequent and serious offender)
    b. Anticonvulsants
    c. Phenothiazines
    d. Tranquilizers
    e. Antithyroid drugs
    f. Sulfonamides and their derivatives
    g. Certain antibiotics (chloramphenicol)
    h. Agents that regularly depress leukopoiesis (alkylating agents, antimetabolites)
2. Viral diseases
3. Overwhelming bacterial infections
4. Neoplastic disease of the bone marrow

Clinical Course
Spontaneous restoration of marrow function (except in patients with neoplastic disease); often occurs in 1 to 3 weeks if death from infection can be averted.

Clinical Manifestations
1. Chills, fever, extreme weakness
2. Sore throat, ulcerations of mucosa of mouth and pharynx (agranulocytic angina); throat becomes increasingly sore and eventually gangrenous
3. Regional adenopathy
4. Extreme prostration

Diagnostic Evaluation

Blood—shows leukopenia (500–2000/cu. mm.) with reduction in polymorphonuclear
    cells
Bone marrow—appears hypoplastic

Treatment

Objectives: to eliminate the factor responsible for the bone marrow suppression.
                to prevent and treat infection until the bone marrow has returned to normal.
1. Take the patient off the offending drug—recovery can take place in less than a week.
   Warn the patient to avoid re-exposure to offending drug.
2. Prevent and treat infection.

NURSING ALERT: Granulocytes are the first barrier to infection. In patients with agranulocytosis, infection develops rapidly and may soon become overwhelming.

---

    a. Place the patient on reverse isolation precautions—to reduce exposure to infection.
    b. Obtain blood samples and throat culture for bacterial culture and antibiotic
       sensitivity testing.
    c. Give antibiotic on basis of culture and sensitivity test.
3. Utilize measures to support the patient and increase comfort.
    a. Use nursing and therapeutic measures to relieve throat pain.
       (1) Hot saline throat irrigations—to clear the throat of necrotic detritus and
           exudate
       (2) Ice collar—to relieve pain
       (3) Antipyretic drug and fever sponge—to reduce fever
       (4) Analgesic (codeine, meperidine)—for pain
       (5) Anesthetic lozenges—to relieve pharyngeal pain.
    b. Encourage patient to remain on bedrest.
    c. Give high vitamin, high caloric, semisolid or liquid diet.

Complications

1. Sepsis
2. Bronchial pneumonia
3. Hemorrhagic necrosis of mucous membrane lesions

LEUKEMIA

The *leukemias* are neoplastic disorders of the blood-forming tissues (spleen, lymphatic system and bone marrow). They are characterized by widespread proliferation within the bone marrow and other blood-forming tissues of immature precursors of one of the types of leukocytes. The leukemic process drastically reduces the production of the principal constituents of normal blood, resulting in anemia and increased susceptibility to infection and hemorrhage.

Classification

Classified according to the white cell affected.
1. Lymphocytic—affects lymphocytes
2. Myelocytic (granulocytic or myelogenous leukemia)—affects the granulocytes
3. Acute or chronic

Predisposing Factors

1. Etiology unknown
2. Exposure to radiation
3. Chemical agents—benzene
4. Infectious agents—viruses (currently being investigated)
5. Genetic abnormalities—increased risk of leukemia in patients with Down's syndrome (see p. 1362).

Acute Leukemia

Clinical Manifestations

Produced by proliferation and infiltration of bone marrow and other organs by immature white blood cells of the lymphocytic or granulocytic group.

1. Easy fatigability and general malaise, pallor—from anemia caused by depressed erythropoiesis, hemorrhage and hemolysis.
2. Persistent fever of unknown cause.
3. Enlarged lymph nodes and spleen; abdominal discomfort—from local tissue invasion.
4. Bone pain, arthralgia—from expanding marrow in bone and gout of hyperuricemia.
5. Bleeding of gums, epistaxis or petechiae, prolonged bleeding following a surgical procedure—from thrombocytopenia (lowered platelet count).
6. Tachycardia, weight loss, dyspnea on exertion, intolerance to heat—from increased metabolism.
7. Leukemia infiltration of the skin.
8. Cerebral hemorrhage, cranial nerve paralysis, increased intracranial pressure—from neurological complications.
9. Pain—from infarction; particularly the spleen.

Diagnostic Evaluation

1. Blood evaluation—total peripheral white count varies widely (10,000–100,000/ cu. ml.).
2. Bone marrow biopsy—characteristically large percentage of bone marrow's nucleated cells are immature leukocyte forms called "blasts."
3. Lymph node biopsy.
4. Chest x-ray—to detect mediastinal node and lung involvement.
5. Skeletal x-ray—to detect skeletal lesions.

Treatment

Objective: to provide the patient with as long and as normal a life as possible.

A. *Chemotherapy*
1. The drugs are classified on the basis of their effects on cell chemistry (see pp. 874–878 for complete list of drugs used in cancer chemotherapy).
2. Objective of Chemotherapy
   To induce remission (disappearance of all abnormal cell forms in the bone marrow and peripheral blood).

B. *Underlying Principles of Chemotherapy*
1. Chemotherapy destroys abnormal leukemic cells, causes bone marrow suppression and depresses the patient's immunological defense mechanism.

2. Drugs are usually given in combination at high dose levels to produce greater leukemic cell damage.
3. Drugs used in leukemia are limited in usefulness by *toxicity* and *decreased effectiveness.*
4. To achieve remission, doses of the drugs must be increased to nearly intolerable levels of toxicity.
5. The nursing management of the patient with acute leukemia includes constant assessment of the patient for effects of drug toxicity.

C. *Some Drugs Used in Acute Leukemia*
   1. Antimetabolites—compete with the natural metabolite thus blocking the pathway for the synthesis of DNA or another cellular constituent thereby blocking cell growth.
      Amethopterin (Methotrexate)
      6-mercaptopurine
      Arabinosyl cytosine (Ara-C)—inhibits DNA synthesis
   2. Alkylating agents—cell poisons; may exert their anti-cancer effects by a direct chemical interaction with the DNA of the cell.
      Cyclophosphamide (Endoxan, Cytoxan)
   3. Antibiotics—inhibits synthesis of cell proteins.
      Daunomycin
   4. Plant alkaloids.
      Vincristine (Oncovin)—blocks the process of cell division
   5. Hormones—suppress the growth of lymphocytes.
      Adrenal cortical steroid (prednisone)
   6. Other drugs:
      L-asparaginase—an enzyme which breaks down asparagine, an amino acid frequently required by leukemic cells for cell growth.

Nursing Management

A. *Constant Nursing Surveillance of Patient Receiving Chemotherapy.*
   1. Obtain base-line information before chemotherapy is started.
      a. Know the patient's "normal, T.P.R. and B.P."
      b. Follow the W.B.C., differential count, hemoglobin measurements, platelet counts—to be aware of the drug's effect on the body.
      c. Weigh the patient once or twice weekly.
      d. Assist with bone marrow aspirations as directed (see p. 193).
   2. *Watch for toxic manifestations during chemotherapy.*
      a. Monitor intravenous infusion of drugs—may cause local irritation in the veins; patient may complain of burning sensations during infusions of methotrexate and prednisone.
         (1) Adjust infusion flow to a slower rate.
         (2) Change position of extremity to prevent muscular cramping.
         (3) Patient may complain of nausea, vomiting and burning sensation along the gastrointestinal tract during or immediately after drug infusion.
      b. Watch for mouth ulcers—frequently occur when patient is taking methotrexate.
         Offer medicated mouth rinses frequently to relieve oral discomfort.
      c. Expect the patient to experience loss of hair during antitumor therapy—alopecia occurs in 40–65% of patients receiving vincristine.
         Encourage the patient to experiment with wigs, hair pieces, head scarfs.

  d. Assess patient for footdrop, weakening hand grasp, ptosis of eye lids—vincristine may cause neuropathy.

  e. Assess for constipation and abdominal pain—vincristine may produce adynamic ileus.

  f. Watch for personality changes, fluid retention, hypertension and gastric ulcers—occurs with prednisone therapy.

  g. Watch for other drug side effects—diarrhea, maculopapular rash, stomatitis, phlebitis, bone marrow depression, evidences of cardiac toxicity (tachycardia, arrhythmias, tachypnea, dyspnea).

  h. Take serial ECG readings as prescribed—cardiac toxicity is associated with certain antitumor drugs.

B. *Supportive Measures for Patient with Leukemia or Lymphoma*

 1. Underlying Consideration: Failure to improve is usually due to complications—infection and hemorrhage.

 2. *Objective:* To control complications so that chemotherapeutic agents can demonstrate their effectiveness.

 3. To eliminate the morbidity and mortality resulting from hemorrhage.

  a. Major cause of hemorrhage is thrombocytopenia (decrease in platelets).

  b. Risk of hemorrhage is high at platelet levels below 10,000 (normal; 250,000–500,000 platelets/cu.mm.).

  c. Prepare the patient for a transfusion of compatible platelets.
    Platelet transfusion may need to be repeated 2–3 times weekly—average platelet half-life is 3–5 days.

 4. To prevent and treat infection—the major morbidity and mortality associated with leukemia; bone marrow invasion of the leukemic cell line prevents normal production and maturation of granulocytes.

  a. Monitor the concentration of circulating granulocytes.
    Concentrations below 1000 cu. mm.—serious danger of infection.

  b. Recognize infection promptly.
    Monitor temperature at regular intervals—fever is major symptom for recognizing infection.

  c. Give appropriate antibiotic—obtain blood cultures and identification of infecting organism.

  d. Be aware that certain gram negative organisms and fungi are major causes of morbidity and mortality in patients undergoing chemotherapy.

 5. To prevent infectious complications by control of environmental contamination.

  a. Laminar air-flow room—a unidirectional air-flow "barrier" that establishes an air environment in which the infection-prone patient is free from contact with exogenous microorganisms (see Fig. 17-2).

  b. Life-island unit—patient is placed inside plastic tent which provides a positive barrier between the patient and outside environment. (Currently being replaced by laminar air-flow rooms.)

  c. Utilize all appropriate measures to reduce environmental contamination when special units are not available (reverse isolation).

C. *Other Measures*

 1. Assist the patient to accept and participate in his therapeutic regimen.

  a. Give expert physical care and support—encourages the patient to endure much discomfort associated with treatment.

    b. Help the patient to mobilize his defenses to cope with his physiologic and emotional distress.
2. Control the pain and discomfort.
    a. Use milder analgesics when possible; change to a stronger narcotic as the patient's condition requires.
    b. Give tranquilizers as directed to enhance the effects of narcotics.
    c. Give antiemetic medication ½ hour before meals—to help assuage the patient's nausea; sedatives may also be helpful.
3. Maintain oral intake between 3–4 liters daily—to prevent precipitation of uric acid crystals in the urine; overproduction of uric acid is due to the tremendous proliferation of blood cells and the destruction of these cells by antileukemic agents.
4. Control fever—employ fever sponges, increased fluid intake, antipyretic drugs.
5. Give frequent and special mouth care—to remove dried blood, combat odor and soothe oral ulcerations.
    a. Alternate solutions of mouth wash, dilute hydrogen peroxide solution and glycerine and lemon solutions.
    b. Use cotton applicators instead of a toothbrush when there is oral bleeding.
    c. Cleanse and lubricate the lips and nostrils—to prevent drying and cracking.
    d. Offer a soft diet if indicated—to reduce mechanical irritation to the gums.
6. Demonstrate continuing concern for the welfare of the patient. (See p. 192 for a review of other salient principles of nursing care.)

Chronic Lymphocytic Leukemia

Chronic lymphocytic leukemia is a type of leukemia characterized by lymphoid hyperplasia and infiltration involving any part of the body in which there is lymphoid tissue.

Clinical Features
1. Occurs most frequently between age 45 and 60.
2. Insidious onset; symptoms closely resemble those of chronic myelogenous type (p. 217).

Clinical Manifestations
1. Gradual appearance of generalized lymph node enlargement.
2. Anemia, fever, cachexia and hemorrhagic features.
3. Possible leukemic infiltrations in retinae of eyes and in skin. (Skin may become pruritic and bronzed.)
4. Ascitic and pleuritic fluid infiltrations.

Treatment
Objective: to achieve a remission of symptoms.

A. *Asymptomatic patient with chronic lymphocytic leukemia*
1. May not require treatment for a period of years.
2. Support the patient with optimum nutrition, rest, exercise, recreation and mental activity.

B. *Symptomatic patient* (with massive adenopathy, severe anemia, thrombocytopenia, skin involvement, recurring infections)
    1. For anemia—from blood loss, replacement of bone marrow by leukemia cells:
        a. X-ray therapy for local disease
        b. Corticosteroids (prednisone)—to control hemolytic element
        c. Chemotherapy (especially chlorambucil [Leukeran])—for generalized disease
        d. Transfusions
            (1) Whole blood for hemorrhage
            (2) Packed red blood cells—when hemolysis or bone marrow failure exists.
    2. For adenopathy
        Supervoltage x-ray therapy for localized nodes, masses or splenomegaly
    3. For hemorrhage—may occur when severe thrombocytopenia and purpura are present or when bleeding, secondary to peptic ulcer, occurs as a complication of corticosteroid therapy.
        Transfusions to replace blood loss.
C. *Chemotherapy*—Brings symptomatic relief; decreases size of lymph nodes and spleen
    1. Chlorambucil (Leukeran)
    2. Triethylenemelamine (TEM)
    3. Cyclophosphamide (Cytoxan)
    4. Corticosteroids (prednisone)

Nursing Management

See page 881 for nursing support of patient receiving chemotherapy and page 214 for other aspects of management of a patient with leukemia.

Chronic Granulocytic Leukemia

Chronic granulocytic (myelocytic, myelogenous) leukemia is a condition characterized by white cell counts ranging from 100,000–1,000,000/cu.mm.; a high percentage of these leukocytes are immature cells. The condition is associated with great enlargement of the spleen and liver but little swelling of the lymph glands.

Clinical Features

1. Appears most often between age 35 and 45.
2. Gradual insidious onset.

Clinical Manifestations

1. Pallor, palpitations—from anemia.
2. Dragging sensation or enlargement of left side of abdomen—from splenic enlargement.
3. Weakness, loss of weight, cachexia—from increased metabolic rate from progress of disease.
4. Tenderness and pain in long bones (particularly tibia, ribs, sternum)—due to invasion by the abnormal marrow.

Treatment

Objective: to achieve a remission of symptoms.
1. Irradiation methods
    a. Whole body irradiation by an external source, preferably supervoltage; e.g., Cobalt-60 (^{60}Co).
    b. Internal irradiation with radioactive phosphorus (^{32}P).
    c. Extracorporeal irradiation of blood.
    d. Local irradiation to spleen, liver or area of local infiltration.
2. Chemotherapy
    a. Busulfan (Myleran)—drug of choice
    b. Melphalan (Alkeran)
    c. Cyclophosphamide (Cytoxan)

Nursing Management

See page 881 for nursing support of patient receiving chemotherapy, and page 214 for other aspects of management of a patient with leukemia.

MALIGNANT LYMPHOMAS

The *lymphomas* are a group of neoplastic diseases of the lymphoid and reticuloendothelial systems characterized by enlargement of the lymph glands and spleen. The major lymphomas are Hodgkin's disease, lymphosarcoma and reticulum cell sarcoma.

Altered Physiology

1. Lymphomas generally originate in lymph nodes and grow and spread to other lymph tissues.
2. Organs and tissues of the lymphoid and reticuloendothelial system (spleen, liver, GI tract, bone marrow, lungs and skin) may also become primary sites of malignant lymphomas.
3. Two principal cell types in lymphatic tissue
    a. Lymphocytes
    b. Reticulum cells (histocytes)
        (1) Each of these may undergo neoplastic transformation leading to the cell production of a malignant lymphoma.
        (2) The variety of lymphoma produced is determined by the type and maturity of the particular cell that is involved.

Hodgkin's Disease

Hodgkin's disease is a malignant disease of unknown etiology that originates in the lymphoid system and involves predominantly the lymph nodes. It may occur in nearly any lymphoid mass of tissues: spleen, bone marrow, alimentary tract.

Altered Physiology

1. The malignant cell of Hodgkin's disease is the "Reed-Sternberg" cell which is a gigantic atypical tumor cell, morphologically unique and of uncertain lineage (probably a reticulum cell).

2. The different histopathologic types of Hodgkin's disease are associated with varying prognoses.
3. Hodgkin's disease shows a highly predictable pattern of spread usually via the lymphatic channels from one chain of lymph nodes to another, often to the spleen and ultimately to extra lymphatic sites.

Clinical Manifestations

1. Painless enlargement of lymph nodes on one side of neck
2. Generalized pruritus (itching), sweating, weight loss
3. Progressive anemia
4. Slight to high fever
5. Enlargement of lymph nodes in other regions of the body.
6. Enlargement of mediastinal and retroperitoneal lymph nodes produces pressure symptoms
   a. Dyspnea from pressure against the trachea
   b. Dysphagia from pressure against the esophagus
   c. Laryngeal paralysis due to pressure against the recurrent laryngeal nerve
   d. Brachial, lumbar or sacral neuralgias due to pressure on the nerve
   e. Edema of the extremities due to pressure on the veins
   f. Enlargement of spleen and liver
7. Effusions into the pleura or peritoneum
8. Obstructive jaundice

Diagnostic Evaluation

1. Biopsy of lymph node(s) to identify characteristic histologic features
2. Complete blood count
3. Chest x-ray
4. Roentgenographic skeletal survey
5. Strontium-85 bone scan
6. Bone marrow biopsy
7. Liver function tests and scan
8. Inferior caval venography
9. Lymphangiogram
   a. Reveals size of lymph nodes
   b. Detects abdominal lymph node enlargements which may not be seen or felt by ordinary means
10. Laparotomy with splenectomy, open liver biopsy, biopsy of para-aortic lymph nodes: these procedures are important in determining prognosis and treatment.

Staging of Hodgkin's Disease

Stage I: Disease limited to a single node or 2 contiguous anatomic regions.

Stage II: Disease involves more than 2 regions or 2 noncontiguous regions but is confined to one side of the diaphragm only.

Stage III: Disease is present both above and below the diaphragm but does not extend beyond lymph node chains, spleen or the oronasopharyngeal tonsils.

Stage IV: Disease has extended to the bone marrow, lung parenchyma, pleura, skin, gastrointestinal tract, liver or other extra lymphoid tissues.

Treatment

A. *Concepts*
   1. Irradiation is treatment of choice for early stages; given with gamma rays from a cobalt-60 unit or with high energy x-rays from a linear accelerator. *The most important factor in treatment is the radiation dose administered.*
   2. Hodgkin's disease may be permanently eradicated from any site that has received 4000 to 4500 rads within the space of 4 weeks. Megavoltage radiation techniques permit the delivery of such a dose to one or more entire lymph node chain.
   3. Areas of the body in which the lymph node chains are located can tolerate doses of this magnitude without serious damage (as can the area of the spleen and the oronasopharynx); vital structures such as the lungs, liver, and kidneys are protected by lead shields.

B. *Treatment for Advanced Hodgkin's Disease*
   Objectives: to produce tumor regression and remission.
   to relieve pressure on a vital organ (brain, kidney, bronchi).
   1. Radiation alone may be used as a palliative measure, or a combination of radiotherapy and chemotherapy may be used.
   2. Chemotherapy is used since Hodgkin's disease is considered a drug-responsive tumor:
      a. Drugs are given in combination (2 to 4 drugs) each attacking the tumor-cell population at a different point in the metabolic pathway.
      b. Dosage depends on patient's status and his response to treatment.
      c. Toxicity of these drugs often overlap, especially bone marrow suppression.
   3. Types of drugs
      a. Alkylating agents
         (1) Nitrogen mustard; gives a more rapid response to toxic patient.
         (2) Cyclophosphamide (Cytoxan) can be given orally; relatively low in toxicity and has a platelet-sparing effect.
      b. Vinca alkaloids; vinblastine (Velban) or vincristine (Oncovin)
         Assess for bone marrow toxicity, leukopenia, transient gastrointestinal disturbances.
      c. Methylhydrazine derivatives (procarbazine)—useful to patients who are no longer responsive to other agents.
      d. Corticosteroids (prednisone)
      e. Other agents: L-Asparaginase

Nursing Management
   1. Support patient having toxic effects from chemotherapy (see p. 881).
      a. A sedative administered in the evening after drug administration may help control acute symptoms.
      b. Encourage the patient that the therapy will end in "a period of time"—serves as an incentive for the patient to continue with therapy.
   2. Give laxatives and stool softeners to control constipation that accompanies chemotherapy.
   3. Anticipate that patients on chemotherapy will develop leukopenia, thrombocytopenia and anemia (see p. 881).
   4. Prepare patient for surgical excision of localized lymph nodes if indicated (may be followed by radiation therapy).
      Surgery may also be used to alleviate complications caused by pressure or obstruction due to tumor masses.

Lymphosarcoma

Lymphosarcoma is a malignant growth of lymphocytes in lymphoid tissue characterized by progressive generalized lymphadenopathy, splenomegaly and involvement of one or more nonlymphoid organ systems. Marrow damage, manifested by anemia and thrombocytopenia, and immune dysfunction, with heightened susceptibility to bacterial and mycotic infections are also especially pronounced in patients with lymphosarcoma.

Clinical Manifestations

1. Painless generalized lymphadenopathy—usually in neck, nasopharynx, oropharynx and tonsillar areas, gastrointestinal tract, mediastinum, abdomen
2. Fatigue—attributable primarily to anemia from impaired erythropoiesis and hemolysis.
3. Malaise, anorexia, weight loss
4. Fever and sweating
5. Abdominal distention—due to enlargement of spleen

Diagnostic Evaluation

1. Biopsy of lymph node(s)—reveals destruction of node architecture and replacement by abnormal cells
2. Chest x-ray—to detect hilar adenopathy
3. Bone marrow aspiration and biopsy—may reveal hypercellular marrow with lymphocytes
4. Serum-protein immunoelectrophoresis—may reveal an increase or decrease of one or more of the immunoglobulins
5. Lymphangiogram
6. Laparotomy

Treatment and Nursing Management

Objective: to induce a remission
1. Staging of the disease (similar to Hodgkin's disease, see p. 218) is done to determine extent of disease and is a determinant of prognosis for survival.
2. Prepare the patient for irradiation—done for localized disease or symptomatic tumor masses.
3. Give chemotherapy as directed—used for systemic disease (multiple lymph-node bearing sites and organ involvement).
   a. The following drugs are usually used in combination to bring about a remission.
      (1) Cyclophosphamide (Cytoxan)
      (2) Vincristine (Oncovin)—patient will usually develop alopecia and symptoms of neurotoxicity
      (3) Prednisone
   b. See page 881 for discussion of nursing support of patient receiving chemotherapy.
4. Prepare the patient for splenectomy if indicated (p. 229); corrects hypersplenism, removes symptomatic abdominal masses, may decrease transfusion requirements and increase tolerance to irradiation and chemotherapy.
5. Be on constant vigil for complications.
   a. *Infection*—by bacteria, viruses (usually herpes type), fungi; due to deficiencies of cellular immunity.
   b. *Anemia*—from bone marrow invasion, hemorrhage, chemotherapy, hypersplenism, failure of bone marrow, hemolysis.

  c. *Spinal cord compression*—from lymphomatous infiltration.
  d. *Hyperuricemia*
 6. See also discussion on the care of patients with Hodgkin's disease (p. 220).

Multiple Myeloma

Multiple myeloma (plasma cell myeloma; plasmocytoma) is a malignant disease of plasma cells that infiltrates bone and soft tissues. The cause is unknown.

Altered Physiology

1. This tumor has its origin and principal location in the bone marrow, with involvement of the lymph nodes, liver, spleen and kidneys occurring as a later development and less prominent feature.
2. There is widespread proliferation of immature plasma cells in the marrow cavity throughout the skeleton.
3. Bones most commonly affected are those which are the site of active hemopoietic marrow—spine, skull, ribs, sternum, pelvis, upper ends of humerus.
4. The malignant plasma cells usually produce abnormal amounts of an immunoglobulin or parts of an immunoglobin protein (Bence Jones protein) that can usually be detected in serum or urine by immunoelectrophoresis.
5. There is a constant threat of hypercalcemia, hypercalciuria, and hyperuricemia due to skeletal destruction.

Clinical Manifestations

1. Constant severe bone pain, especially on movement
 a. Backpain—the most characteristic symptom
 b. Skeletal lesions—producing swelling, tenderness, pain, *pathological fractures*
2. Anemia—due to replacement of marrow with neoplastic plasma cells
 May be associated with thrombocytopenia and granulopenia—causes increased susceptibility to infection and abnormal bleeding.
3. Marked weight loss
4. Symptoms of renal failure—due to precipitation of the immunoglobulin in the tubules.
5. Bleeding tendency—due to the immunoglobulin interfering with the clotting mechanism.

Diagnostic Evaluation

1. Bone marrow biopsy—shows evidence of increased numbers of abnormal plasma cells in the marrow (neoplastic cells comprise 30–95% of entire bone marrow population; normal is 5%)
2. Bence Jones protein in urine (see above)
3. Elevated total protein in blood—due to presence of elevated immunoglobulin (gamma globulin)
4. Elevated blood calcium level
5. Skeletal x-ray—numerous areas of localized bone destruction may be visible; one-fourth of patients show diffuse demineralization of the skeleton (osteoporosis)
6. Elevated erythrocyte sedimentation rate

7. Immunoelectrophoresis (serum and concentrated urine)—gives positive indication of multiple myeloma

Treatment and Nursing Management

Objectives: to decrease tumor mass.

to control pain.

A. *Decrease the tumor mass and relieve bone pain.*
  1. Give the appropriate chemotherapy (the foundation of treatment).
     Drugs may be given as single agents or in combination.
     (1) Phenylalanine mustard—melphalan (Alkeran)
     (2) Cyclosphosphamide (Cytoxan)
     (3) Steroid hormone (prednisone)—may stimulate bone marrow regeneration, decrease hypercalcemia and give a sense of well-being; used as an adjunct in chemotherapy.
     (4) Androgens—occasionally produce an increase in red cell volume
     (5) Fluorides—to reduce bone pain and promote recalcification of bone.
  2. See page 881 for supportive care of patient receiving chemotherapy.
B. *Give attentive and supportive care*
  1. Keep the patient ambulatory unless lesion in spine produces danger of cord compression—bone pain and fracture immobilization of the patient lead to infection and osteoporosis.
     a. Avoid immobilization.
     b. *Watch for pathological fractures*
        (1) Avoid excessive lifting and straining.
        (2) Use analgesics, supportive splints and back brace for pathology of spine.
        (3) Local irradiation may be employed to achieve mobilization.
        (4) Calcium and fluorides may be given to reduce bone pain and promote recalcification.
  2. Evaluate for spinal cord compression—from extradural plasmacytomas
     a. Radiation therapy—to prevent paraplegia
     b. Laminectomy for decompression—for cord compression or vertebral fracture
  3. Watch for recurrent infections—patient has impaired capacity for antibody production.
     a. Assess for symptoms of bacterial pneumonia.
     b. Give gamma globulin as indicated.
  4. Assess the patient for signs and symptoms of renal insufficiency—from precipitation of Bence Jones protein in renal tubules or from pyelonephritis, hypercalcemia, amyloidosis (hypercalcemia may result from bony destruction and immobilization).
     a. Encourage liberal fluid intake—to prevent protein precipitation and to minimize hypercalcemia.
     b. Avoid dehydration which can precipitate acute renal failure

---

NURSING ALERT: Patients with multiple myeloma should not be put on fasting regimens for x-rays, lab tests, etc.

---

   c. Maintain fluid and electrolyte balance.
   d. Treat urinary infections promptly (see p. 480).
   e. Give prednisone as ordered—may be used in management of hypercalcemia.

5. Treat concomitant anemia—occurs in most patients.
   a. Give blood transfusions for patients with severe anemia.
   b. Administer chemotherapy, steroid hormones, androgens—may improve anemia.
6. Be aware of the complications.
   a. *Infection*—from decrease in normal circulating antibodies due to proliferation of abnormal plasma cells which produce ineffective globulins; extensive bone marrow involvement causes leukopenia; chemotherapy and radiotherapy also cause marrow depression; steroid hormones increase susceptibility to infection.
   b. *Neurologic complications*
      (1) Paraplegia—from collapse of supporting structures or from cord compression of plasma cell tumors
   c. *Bone complications*—pathologic fractures
   d. *Hematologic complications*—anemia and pancytopenia
   e. *Renal complications*
      (1) Renal failure—from plugging of renal tubules by proteinaceous casts
      (2) Renal stones from hypercalcemia—due to bone destruction and increased bone resorption
      (3) Infiltration of kidney from plasma cells, etc.

Mycosis Fungoides

Mycosis fungoides is a cutaneous lymphoma that may progress to involve the lymph nodes and other internal organs. The late stage of the disease closely resembles Hodgkin's disease.

Clinical Manifestations

1. Generalized severe itching—may last for several years.
2. Erythematous, urticarial, eczematous or psoriasis-like lesions—there are exacerbations and remissions of these eruptions.
3. Ulcerating and necrotic tumors of the skin—lesions become indurated and more fungoidal until they are mushroom-like growths (scarlet or purplish in color), varying in size from 1–15 cm.; the body may be covered with these lesions.
4. Patient usually dies from systemic lymphoma.

Diagnostic Evaluation

Biopsy of skin lesion—gives distinctive diagnostic pattern of mycosis fungoides.

Treatment and Nursing Management

Objective: to bring about a remission
1. Radiation is applied by electron beam—gives very little skin penetration and permits total body irradiation without visceral damage; used primarily when there is no evidence of systemic involvement.
2. Chemotherapy—to arrest the disease.
   a. Nitrogen mustard—administered parenterally and topically
   b. Azaribine (Triazure)—antimetabolic agent
   c. Corticosteroids—given topically and systemically.
3. Support the patient who has painful ulcerative lesions.
   a. Place bed cradle over patient when he is unable to tolerate the weight of the bed clothing on his skin lesions.

b. Apply bacteriostatic ointment (as prescribed) to lesions as a prophylaxis against infection and to promote comfort by excluding air from open nerve endings.

c. Administer analgesics for pain.

d. See page 220 for discussion of the nursing management of patients with Hodgkin's disease.

BLEEDING DISORDERS

Vascular Purpuras

The term, *purpura*, refers to extravasation (escape) of blood into the skin and mucous membranes. Purpuras may occur spontaneously as an isolated phenomenon or as an accompaniment of obvious disease.

Related Conditions

1. *Petechiae*—small pinpoint hemorrhages under the skin
2. *Ecchymoses*—escape of blood into tissues producing a large bruise.
3. Petechiae and ecchymoses may occur as the result of vascular rupture, permitting the leakage of blood into the subcutaneous tissue of the mucous membranes.
4. *Symptomatic or secondary purpura*—certain types of bloodstream infections (e.g., meningococcemia and infectious endocarditis) exhibit this phenomenon due to damage to the vascular walls by the infectious agent.
5. Severe arterial hypertension—may cause the patient to bruise easily.
6. *Anaphylactoid purpura*—generally regarded as an allergic disorder in which there are various skin lesions (purpuric and otherwise) and episodes of arthritis, abdominal pain, hematuria, gastrointestinal hemorrhages and fever.
   a. Attacks last several weeks and recur for years.
   b. Steroid therapy is often effective.
7. *Familial hemorrhagic telangiectasia*—a hereditary disorder manifested by an abnormal tendency to bleed and bruise.
   a. Precise nature of defect is obscure.
   b. Condition does not respond to any proved method of treatment.
8. *Toxic purpura*—a condition observed after exposure to certain drugs and poisons.
9. *Vitamin C deficiency.*
10. *Diabetes mellitus*—causes increased vascular fragility.
11. *Aging*
12. *Polyarteritis*

Thrombocytopenic Purpura

Thrombocytopenic purpura refers to purpura (extravasation of blood into skin) which is accompanied by reduction in the number of circulating platelets. It is a hemorrhagic disorder due to platelet deficiency and characterized by purpuric bleeding.

Causes

1. Idiopathic thrombocytopenic purpura
2. Decreased formation of platelets from chemical, vegetable, animal or physical agents or from infections or as part of the picture of various blood disorders

3. Excessively rapid destruction of platelets—immune mechanism, systemic lupus erythematosis
4. Sequestration of platelets in the spleen (hypersplenism of cirrhosis, leukemia lymphoma

Clinical Manifestations

1. May appear abruptly or slowly; disorder may wax and wane.
2. Bleeding—mild to severe (thrombocytopenia not usually accompanied by bleeding unless the platelet count falls below 50,000/cu.mm.).
   a. Skin lesions—small red hemorrhages; do not blanche on pressure.
   b. Purpuric lesions may occur in vital organ (brain).
   c. Bleeding may occur from nose, mouth, uterus.

Laboratory Manifestations

1. Low platelet count (below 50,000/cu.mm.)
2. Prolongation of bleeding time (8–60 minutes or more; normal 30 seconds to 6 minutes)
3. Positive tourniquet test—intracutaneous oozing of bleeding when capillary pressure is increased by tourniquet

Treatment and Nursing Management

Objectives: to search for possible causes of bleeding
to treat patient during spontaneous bleeding episodes

1. Give adrenal corticosteroids (prednisone)—may produce improvement by reducing bleeding (by affecting blood vessels, resulting in decreased capillary fragility, or by elevating the level of circulating platelets) (probably by suppressing immunologic or other factors producing decreased platelets).
2. Support the patient receiving transfusions.
   a. Transfusions of fresh whole blood (blood collected within 4 hours)—fresh blood is a source of platelets as well as plasma-clotting factors.
      Given to enhance hemostasis during bleeding episodes, to restore circulating blood volume and to correct anemia.
   b. Transfusions of platelets (in form of fresh whole blood, platelet-rich plasma, platelet concentrates).
      Used in treating patients with thrombocytopenia secondary to bone marrow suppression caused by drugs (chemotherapy).
3. Prepare the patient for a splenectomy (see p. 229).
   Splenectomy may bring about an improvement (in 85% of patients) by elevating platelet levels, by removing major site of platelet sequestration or by removing from production site a factor that inhibits platelet production.
4. Give immunosuppressive therapy—used for patients who do not respond to corticosteroids or splenectomy.
   Azathioprine (Imuran) has been used with some success.
5. Utilize other measures to help the patient.
   a. Avoid unnecessary trauma (I.M. injections, etc.).
   b. Keep patient on bedrest during periods of active bleeding.
   c. Administer iron salts (ferrous sulfate, p. 205) for iron deficiency anemia from chronic blood loss.

    d. Suppress menstrual flow (by oral progestational-estrogenic agents) if patient has recurrent menometrorrhagia.

    e. Avoid aspirin—interferes with the hemostatic function of platelets.

CLOTTING DEFECTS

Hemophilia

Hemophilia is a hereditary coagulation disorder (see p. 1167).

Acquired Defects in Coagulation

Acquired defects in coagulation may be associated with many conditions including:

Vitamin K deficiency
Administration of coumarin-indanedione anticoagulant drugs
Heparin therapy
Diseases of the liver
Disseminated intravascular clotting
Uremia
Transfusion-induced clotting factor deficiency

Vitamin K Deficiency

A. *General Considerations*

    1. Vitamin K is obtained partly from diet and partly from bacterial action in the intestinal tract.

        a. Foods high in vitamin K—leafy vegetables (spinach, cauliflower, cabbage, kale, dandelion greens).

        b. Vitamin K is not absorbed in the absence of bile salts.

B. *Causes*

    1. Interference with flow of bile salts into gastrointestinal tract—obstructive jaundice, biliary fistula

    2. Impaired intestinal absorption (sprue, steatorrhea, gastrocolic fistula, regional enteritis)

    3. Extensive surgical resection of small bowel

    4. Dietary deprivation

    5. Therapy with broad spectrum antibiotics

C. *Clinical Manifestations*

    1. Ecchymoses

    2. Epistaxis

    3. Gingival bleeding

    4. Hematuria

    5. Hematemesis and melena

    6. Menorrhagia

    7. Operative and postoperative bleeding

D. *Treatment*

    Administer vitamin K via oral or parenteral routes—bleeding will cease in 3–4 hours, clotting activity rises and by 24–48 hours the prothrombin time will be within normal limits.

        a. Phytonadione (Mephyton, AquaMEPHYTON)

        b. Menadione sodium bisulfate (Hykinone)

        c. Menadiol sodium diphosphate (Synkayvite; Synkamin)

Bleeding Due to Ingestion of Coumarin-Indanedione Anticoagulant Drugs

A. *Causes*

Bleeding may develop from long-term use of coumarin or indanedione anticoagulant drugs that are used in the treatment of thromboembolic disorders.

> NURSING ALERT: Laboratory determinations of the anticoagulant status should be carried out on patients taking anticoagulant drugs who have had a change in physical condition or have had other drugs suddenly introduced or withdrawn. The anticoagulant dosage must be appropriately adjusted in these circumstances.

B. *Clinical Manifestations*
1. Bleeding in G.I. tract or central nervous system
2. Ecchymoses
3. Hematomas
4. Epistaxis
5. Hematuria
6. Vaginal bleeding

C. *Treatment*
1. Administer vitamin K (phytonadione, [Mephyton]) orally, subcutaneously or intramuscularly.
2. Nursing precautions—pain, swelling and tenderness occasionally occur at site of subcutaneous or intramuscular injection.
3. Nursing priorities for administration of phytonadione:
   a. Dilute with 0.9% sodium chloride solution, 5% dextrose solution or 5% dextrose and sodium chloride.
   b. Give infusion immediately after admixture with diluent.
   c. Give at slow rate (not to exceed 5 mg. per minute)—rapid administration produces flushing, peculiar taste sensations, vertigo, tachycardia, hypotension, dyspnea, and profuse sweating.

Heparin Therapy as a Cause of Bleeding

Heparin therapy is given for thromboembolic disorders (see p. 228).

A. *Causes*
1. Overdosage of heparin
2. Trauma
3. Ulceration
4. Surgery

B. *Complications*
1. Cerebral hemorrhage
2. Hemoptysis
3. Bleeding from pre-existing gastrointestinal lesions and from sites of surgery or trauma

C. *Treatment*
1. Stop heparin therapy immediately
2. Give protamine sulfate as directed.

Deficiency of Prothrombin Conversion Accelerators

1. Hemorrhagic disorders have occurred as a result of deficiency states involving both factors responsible for accelerating the conversion of prothrombin to thrombin; i.e., the stable factor or serum prothrombin conversion accelerator (SPCA) and the labile factor.

2. The net result of such a deficiency is equivalent to that caused by a lack of prothrombin.
3. Treatment consists of administration of fresh whole blood or plasma.

Hypofibrinogenemia

A deficiency in fibrinogen, the precursor of fibrin (the substance of the clot) may be an inherited trait or may be due to eclampsia or prolonged surgical procedures accompanied by massive hemorrhages that deplete the available supply of this factor in the circulating blood.

1. The result is a hemorrhagic diathesis with uncontrollable bleeding from all sites where there is blood vessel damage.
2. Treatment:
   Injections of purified fibrinogen fractionated from human plasma.

SPLENECTOMY

Splenectomy is removal of the spleen. It is useful in severe forms of autoimmune diseases (thrombocytopenia purpura, acquired hemolytic anemia).

Indications for Splenectomy

1. Rupture of the spleen—most common indication
   a. History of injury
   b. Persistent abdominal pain
   c. Abdominal rigidity, rebound tenderness, shock
2. Tumor of the spleen
3. For hematologic disorders
   a. Idiopathic thrombocytopenic purpura
   b. Splenomegaly of undetermined cause
   c. Chronic splenomegaly
   d. Acquired hemolytic anemia

Nursing Management

A. *Preoperative Care*

1. Administer whole blood if rupture of the spleen has occurred.
   Give fresh blood for patients with disorders of coagulation.
2. Prepare to give increased dosages of steroids preoperatively if patient is receiving steroids.
3. Assist patient who is having a gastric tube inserted preoperatively (see p. 383)—to keep the stomach deflated during the operative procedure.

B. *Postoperative Care*

1. See page 49 for general aspects of nursing management following abdominal surgery.
2. Watch for the developments of *complications.*

NURSING ALERT: There is a high rate of complications following splenectomy related to the indications for the procedure and co-existing disease.

---

a. Thrombosis—thrombosis often follows a few days after splenectomy; platelet count of 3 to 5 times normal values may occur; this postoperative physiological thrombocytosis may be conducive to thromboembolic complications.
   (1) Abdominal discomfort and fever may be caused by thrombi lodging in branches of portal system.
b. Atelectasis of left lower lobe with pneumonia—operations on left upper quadrant predispose to limited diaphragmatic movement.
c. Subdiaphragmatic abscess—assess for persisting fever.
d. There is a higher rate of septicemia in children following splenectomy (up to a year or longer).

BIBLIOGRAPHY

Books

Brinkhous, K. M. (ed.): Hemophilia and New Hemorrhagic States. Chapel Hill, University of North Carolina Press, 1970.
Britton, C. J. C.: Disorders of the Blood. New York, Grune and Stratton, Inc., 1969.
Brunner, L., et al.: Textbook of Medical-Surgical Nursing, 2nd ed. Philadelphia, J. B. Lippincott, 1970, pp. 302-325.
Frankel, S., et al.: Gradwohl's Clinical Laboratory Methods. St. Louis, C. V. Mosby, 1970.
Izak, G., and Lewis, S. M.: Modern Concepts in Hematology. New York, Academic Press, 1972.
Laufman, H., and Erichson, R. B.: Hematologic Problems in Surgery. Philadelphia, W. B. Saunders, 1970.
Nursing Dept of the Clinical Center, National Institutes of Health: Nursing Care of Patients in the Laminar Air Flow Room. Washington, D.C., U.S. Government Printing Office, 1971.
Ratnoff, O. D.: Treatment of Hemorrhagic Disorders. New York, Harper and Row, 1968.

Articles

Bergeron, J.: A patient's plea: Tell me, I need to know. Amer. J. Nurs., 71:1572–1573, August 1971.
Devita, V. T., et al.: Combination chemotherapy in the treatment of advanced Hodgkin's disease. Ann. Intern. Med., 73:881–895, Nov. 1970.
Henry, J. B.: Iron-deficiency anemia. Postgrad. Med., 51:163–166, June 1972.
Hugos, R.: Living with leukemia. Amer. J. Nurs., 72:2185–2188, Dec. 1972.
Hyatt, D. F., et al.: Splenectomy for lymphosarcoma. Surg. Gynecol. Obstet., 131:928–932, Nov. 1970.
Lee, B. J.: The management of plasma cell neoplasms. Med. Clin. N. Amer., 55:703–719, May 1971.
Lessin, L. S., and Rosse, W. F.: Diagnosis, mechanisms and treatment of hemolytic anemias. Mod. Treat., 8:321–350, May 1971.
McArthur, J. R., et al.: Melphalan and myeloma. Ann. Intern. Med., 72:665–670, May 1970.
McDonald, C. J., and Calabresi, P.: Azaribine for mycosis fungoides. Arch. Derm., 103:158–167, Feb. 1971.
Rosenbaum, D. L.: The diagnosis and management of Hodgkin's disease: current concepts. CA, 20:287–297, Sept.-Oct. 1970.
Skarin, A. T., et al.: Lymphosarcoma of the spleen. Arch. Intern. Med., 127:259–265, Feb. 1971.
Wilson, P.: Iron-deficiency anemia. Amer. J. Nurs., 72:502–504, March 1972.

5

Conditions of the Cardiovascular System

1. Heart Disorders

MANIFESTATIONS OF HEART DISEASE

The patient's symptoms of heart disease depend on:
1. Nature of cardiopathy
2. Resultant physiological disturbances in circulation

Dyspnea

Dyspnea is undue breathlessness; an awareness of discomfort associated with breathing.

A. *General Features*
   1. Cardiac dyspnea is due to increased effort in breathing from a reduction of lung capacity as a result of pulmonary venous congestion.
   2. Dyspnea due to heart disease is usually rapid and shallow.
   3. The threshold (tolerance) for dyspnea varies with the individual.
B. *Types of Dyspnea*
   1. *Exertional dyspnea*—breathlessness upon moderate exertion which is relieved by rest; seen in congestive heart failure, chronic pulmonary disease.
   2. *Orthopnea*—shortness of breath when lying down which is relieved by promptly sitting upright.
      a. Usually due to stasis of blood in lungs, indicating left ventricular failure, mitral disease.
      b. May be from cardiac insufficiency or pulmonary insufficiency.
   3. *Paroxysmal nocturnal dyspnea*—sudden dyspnea at night while lying down, due to left ventricular insufficiency, pulmonary edema, mitral stenosis.
   4. *Cheyne-Stokes respiration*—periodic breathing characterized by gradual increase in depth of respiration followed by a decrease in respiration resulting in apnea; periods of hypernea alternating with periods of apnea.
      a. Cheyne-Stokes respiration is usually considered a serious sign.
      b. Associated with left ventricular failure, cerebral vascular disease.
C. *Nursing Assessment of Dyspnea*
   1. What precipitates or relieves the dyspnea?
   2. What position does the patient assume?
   3. What is the skin color? Pallor? Cyanosis?

Chest Pain

A. *Cardiac Causes of Chest Pain*
   1. Usually from ischemia due to stimulation of afferent nerve endings in the myocardium by metabolites resulting from oxygen deficiency in heart muscle—due to coronary artery disease (angina pectoris, p. 259; myocardial infarction, p. 261).
   2. Excruciating pain—due to acute dissecting aneurysms of the aorta.
   3. Sharp precordial pain (over heart area) aggravated by deep breathing—indicates acute pericarditis.
   4. Anxiety is a common cause of chest pain.
B. *Nursing Assessment of Patient with Chest Pain*
   1. How intense is the pain—dull, sharp, boring, crushing, tearing?
   2. Where is pain located? Does it radiate?
   3. What is the time and mode of onset?
   4. How long does the episode last?
   5. What factors precipitate pain (breathing, coughing, swallowing, rapid walking)?
   6. What factors alleviate pain (rest, change in position)?

Edema

Edema is an abnormal accumulation of serous fluid in the connective tissues.

A. *General Features*
   1. Cardiac causes of edema—congestive heart failure
   2. Other causes of edema—sodium retention, liver disease, hypoproteinemia, venous or lymphatic obstruction

B. *Types*
   1. Ascites—excessive fluid in peritoneal cavity
   2. Hydrothorax—excessive fluid in the pleural cavity
   3. Anasarca—gross generalized edema
C. *Nursing Implications*
   1. In heart conditions the location of edema is influenced by gravity. Fluid collects in the lower parts of the body (dependent edema).
      a. Evaluate for edema of ankles and feet in the ambulatory patient.
      b. Evaluate for edema of sacral area and posterior thighs in patients confined to bed.
   2. Avoid undue pressure on edematous areas. Edematous patients are prone to develop decubitus ulcers.

Palpitation

Palpitation is a rapid, forceful or irregular heart beat felt by the patient.

A. *General Features*
   1. The patient complains of pounding, jumping, stopping sensations in his chest.
   2. May be associated with heart disease—enlargement of heart, disturbances of rhythm.
   3. Other causes—anxiety, fever, anemia, thyroid disturbances.
B. *Nursing Implications*
   1. Take ECG during episodes of palpitation—to help establish the diagnosis.
   2. Count radial, carotid and apical pulses. (See nursing the patient with an arrhythmia, p. 254.)

Hemoptysis

Hemoptysis is coughing up of blood.
   1. Small quantities of dark clotted blood—indicates mitral stenosis.
   2. Admixture of blood and pus—indicates pulmonary suppuration.
   3. Pink, frothy sputum—indicates acute pulmonary edema.
   4. Blood-streaked sputum—indicates acute pulmonary congestion.
   5. Frank hemoptysis—due to lung pathology (see p. 112).

Fatigue

   1. Fatigue in the presence of heart disease is produced by low cardiac output.
   2. Fatigue related to effort—indicates advanced heart disease, congestive heart failure, mitral stenosis.

Syncope and Fainting

   1. May be caused by anoxemia or reduced cardiac output with resulting inadequate circulation.
   2. Also seen in arrhythmias, atrioventricular block, carotid-sinus sensitivity.

Cyanosis

Cyanosis is a bluish discoloration of the skin and mucous membranes.

A. *Types of Cyanosis*
   1. Central cyanosis—low oxygen saturation of arterial blood.
   2. Peripheral cyanosis—reduction of oxyhemoglobin in capillaries from slow circulation —results from reduced cardiac output due to mitral stenosis, pulmonary stenosis, heart failure.

B. *Cardiac Causes of Cyanosis*
1. Congenital heart disease—due to contamination of arterial stream by venous blood.
2. Congestive heart failure and pulmonary edema—due to circulatory hypoxia from circulatory failure.

C. *Nursing Appraisal of Cyanosis*
1. Look at lobes of ears, fingernail beds, mouth under the tongue, mucous membranes, malar eminences.
2. Give oxygen when indicated.

Abdominal Pain or Discomfort

1. Epigastric (upper abdominal) pain—due to myocardial infarction, distention of liver capsule from congestive heart failure.
2. Severe abdominal pain—may be due to dissecting abdominal aorta, rupture of aortic aneurysm.

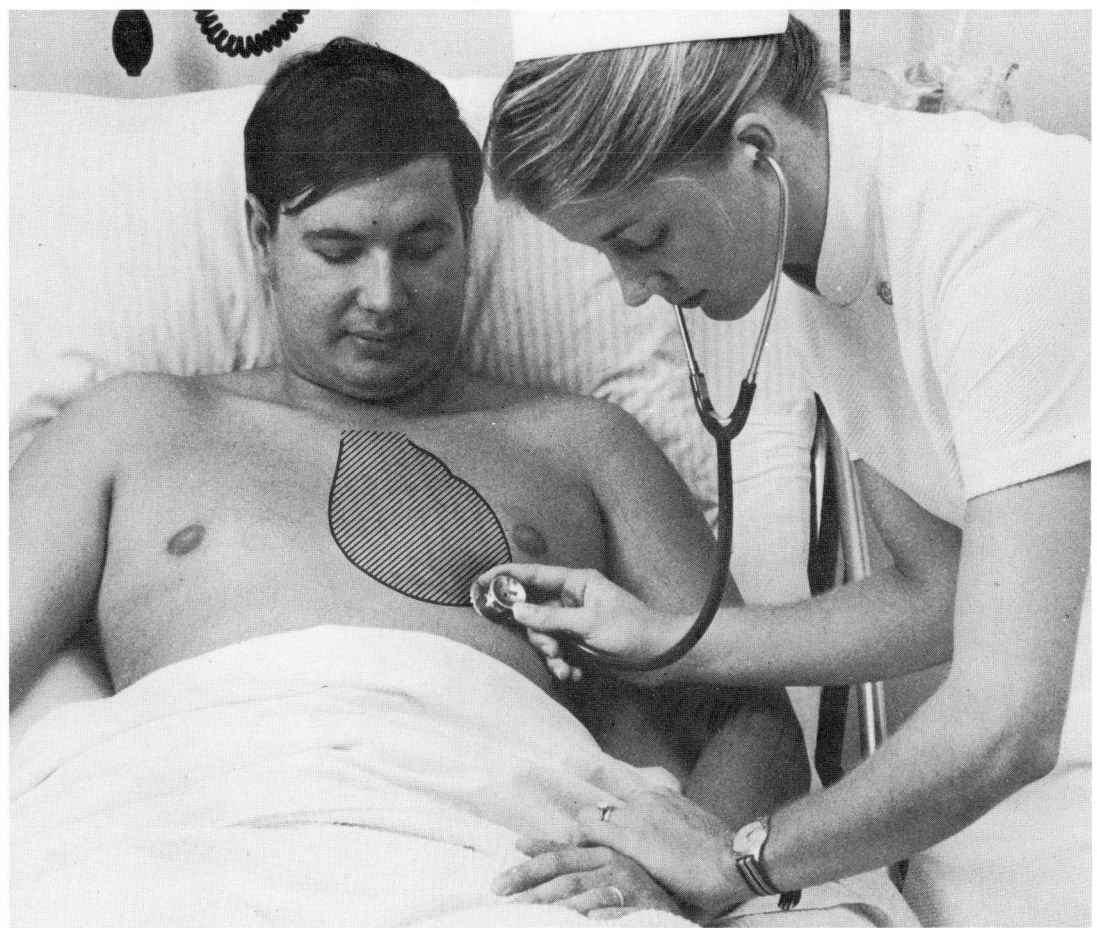

Figure 5-1. Heart auscultation.

3. Intermittent abdominal pain (related to food intake)—indicates circulatory insufficiency of mesenteric arteries.

Other Manifestations of Heart Disease

1. Distention of neck veins—pressure on liver may produce distention of neck veins (hepatojugular reflux), congestive heart failure, pericardial compression due to effusion or constrictive pericarditis.
2. Digital clubbing (clubbing of fingers)—due to cyanotic congenital heart disease, bacterial endocarditis.
3. Jaundice—congestive heart failure associated with severe liver congestion.

DIAGNOSTIC EVALUATION FOR HEART DISEASE

Heart Auscultation

1. Heart auscultation requires knowledge, experience and a "listening ear" tuned in to hear each event of the cardiac cycle.
2. Heart auscultation should be systematic, and the stethoscope should "inch" from one area to another.
3. Listen for rate and regularity of rhythm.
   a. Determine if an irregularity is related to respiratory movements.
   b. Evaluate the sequence in which an irregularity occurs.
4. During auscultation, the examiner assesses the venous pulse, feels the pulsation of the right carotid artery and the radial artery, feels precordial movement and listens to the heart (Fig. 5-1).
5. The reader is referred to a book on physical examination for a complete discussion of heart examination and auscultation.

Cardiographic Studies

1. *Electrocardiogram*—a graphic record of electric potential generated by electrical activity of the heart.
   a. ECG is obtained by placing leads on various body parts (Fig. 5-2) and recording the electrical impulse as a tracing on a strip of paper or on the screen of an oscilloscope.
   b. ECG interpreted rather than "read." Note patient's age, blood pressure and medications (especially digitalis).
   c. Clinical usefulness—evaluation of conditions that interfere with normal electrophysical function—disturbances of rhythm, disorders of cardiac muscles, enlargement of chambers of heart, electrolyte disturbances. (For a more detailed account of electrocardiograms see pp. 289-295.)
2. *Ballistocardiogram*—a graphic recording of the movement of the body generated with each heart beat—provides information on strength and coordination of cardiac contraction.
3. *Phonocardiogram*—a graphic recording of heart sounds. (An electrocardiogram may be recorded simultaneously.)
   a. Identifies and differentiates various sounds.
   b. Affords permanent record for future comparison.

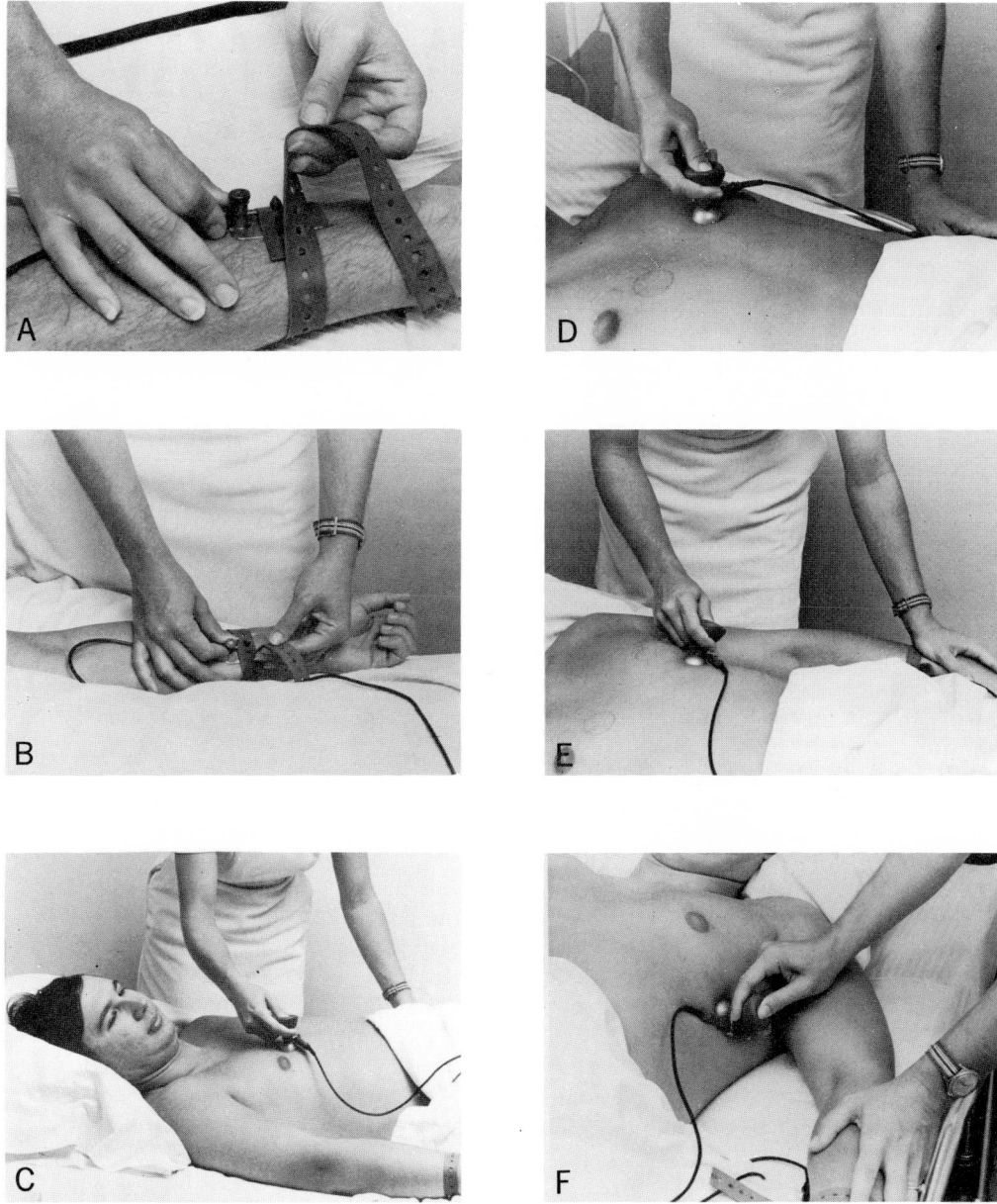

Figure 5-2. Technique of applying an ECG limb lead.

    (A) It should be attached securely but not snugly.
    (B) Apply the limb lead to the left arm.
    (C) V1 chest lead.
    (D) V2 chest lead.   (V3 chest lead is placed slightly to left of V2.)
    (E) V4 chest lead.
    (F) V5 chest lead.   (V6 chest lead would be slightly lower in the midaxillary line.)

4. *Echocardiography* (ultrasound cardiography)—a record of high frequency sound vibrations which have been sent into the heart through the chest wall.
5. *Vectorcardiography*—a method of recording the magnitude and direction of the electrical action of the heart in the form of a vector loop—obtained by simultaneous recording of the 3 standard limb leads, employing a cathode-ray oscilloscope.

Roentgenologic Studies

1. *Chest x-ray*—determines heart size, contour and position.
2. *Planigraphy* (body section radiography)—identifies cardiac contour which may be obscured by regular x-ray; identifies and localizes intracardiac and vascular calcification.
3. *Fluoroscopy*—assesses unusual cardiac contours, cardiac and vascular pulsations.
4. *Cinefluorography*—fluoroscopic image is photographed on motion picture film.
5. *Angiocardiography*—injection of contrast media into the vascular system to outline the heart and blood vessels accompanied by serial roentgenograms; valuable in study of aortic or mitral valve insufficiency by observing dye refluxing through incompetent aorta.

    Selective angiocardiography—injection of contrast media through a catheter directly into one of the heart chambers or greater vessels and recording the angiocardiogram by means of a rapid film changer or motion picture camera.
6. *Thoracic aortography*—a study of the aortic arch and its great vessels by means of contrast media and rapid serial roentgenography.
    a. Approach may be intravenous, translumbar or retrograde femoral.
    b. Nursing Implications
        (1) Keep the patient in a fasting state prior to the x-ray examination. The colon should be cleansed with castor oil and enemas.
        (2) Limit patient's activities for approximately 12 hours after procedure.
        (3) Patient may complain of mild headache or discomfort in groin, depending on route of administration.
7. *Coronary arteriography*—a radiopaque catheter is introduced into the right brachial artery (via open arteriotomy), passed into the ascending aorta and manipulated into appropriate coronary artery under fluoroscopic control.
    a. Used as an evaluation tool before coronary artery surgery or myocardial revascularization.
    b. Used to study suspected congenital anomalies of the coronary arteries.
8. *Cardiac catheterization*—introduction of radiopaque catheter into vein (usually left antecubital) under fluoroscopic guidance into right atrium, right ventricle and pulmonary artery.
    Left heart catheterization (transseptal)—a catheter is passed into the right atrium; a hollow needle is passed up through the catheter and is used to puncture the septum separating the right and left atria. A second catheter is then passed through the needle into the left side of the heart.
    a. Clinical Usefulness
        (1) Measures oxygen concentration and pressure in the various heart chambers.
        (2) Provides blood samples for analysis.
        (3) Measures cardiac output.
        (4) May be used adjunctively with intracardiac electrocardiography or phono-cardiography.
        (5) Calculates the flow of blood in cardiac shunts.

    b. Complications of Heart Catheterization and Implications for Nursing Assessment
       (1) Arrhythmias, syncope, vasospasm may develop.
       (2) Myocardium may be damaged during selective angiography.
       (3) Thrombophlebitis of vein used for catheterization may result.
       (4) Great vessels of heart may be perforated.
    c. Nursing Concern Preceding Heart Catheterization
       (1) Know which approach is to be used in order to anticipate possible complications.
       (2) Withhold food and fluid 6 hours before procedure—to ensure a basal metabolic rate and prevent vomiting and aspiration.
       (3) Ascertain history of previous allergies.
       (4) Be sure that patient has received premedication as directed.
    d. Nursing Concerns During and Following Heart Catheterization
       (1) During the procedure the patient is monitored electrocardiographically and viewed with the oscilloscope. Appropriate resuscitative equipment should be readily available.
       (2) After the procedure, record the blood pressure and pulse every 15 minutes (or more often as the patient's condition indicates) until vital signs are stable.
       (3) Check peripheral pulses, extremity temperature and color—to determine signs of arterial insufficiency.
       (4) Check dressings for tightness, bleeding and underlying hematoma.

Circulation Time

Circulation time measures the velocity of blood flow and helps distinguish between cardiac and pulmonary edema.

    1. Arm to tongue—rapid injection (I.V.) of sodium dehydrocholate (Decholin sodium) in a peripheral vein. The time when the injection is given to the time when the patient complains of a bitter taste is measured with a stop watch.
    2. Arm to lung—intravenous injection of either ether or paraldehyde. The end point is reached when the odor of the drug is smelled on the patient's breath or when the patient begins to cough.
      a. Normal arm to tongue time—9–16 seconds
      b. Normal arm to lung time—4–6 seconds

Blood Studies*

    1. *Antistreptolysin titer*—measurement of blood antibodies against streptococcus; shows whether a patient has had a recent infection.
    2. *Sedimentation rate*—speed of sedimentation of red cells of blood that is expressed in millimeters per hour. The test is elevated when an inflammatory process is present; also used as a test for rheumatic fever.
    3. *C-reactive protein (CRP)*—a blood test that is a sensitive indicator of inflammation of infectious or noninfectious origin.
    4. *Blood culture*—test to detect presence of bacteria in circulating blood. Clinical usefulness in cardiology—indicates bacterial endocarditis.
    5. *Blood electrolytes* (potassium, sodium, calcium)—to determine patients with heart failure or renal disease (especially if treated with digitalis or diuretics).

---

* Normal range of values depends on laboratory methods used.

6. *Blood enzymes*—measurement of enzymes may help diagnose the specific site of injury.

Rationale of blood enzyme studies—heart muscle is rich in enzymes which release different biochemical reactions. The serum activity of these enzymes may be changed by myocardial infarction; serum activity of enzyme may *increase* as result of damage to skeletal muscle, liver, brain, kidney, and other organs.

a. Serum glutamic oxaloacetic transaminase (SGOT)—range, 8–40
b. Serum glutamic pyruvic transaminase (SGPT)—range, 8–38
c. Serum lactic dehydrogenase (SLD)—range, 120–270
d. Creatine phosphokinase (CPK)—measures more specifically the presence of heart muscle cell damage—male 0–20 I.U./L.—female 0–14 I.U./L.

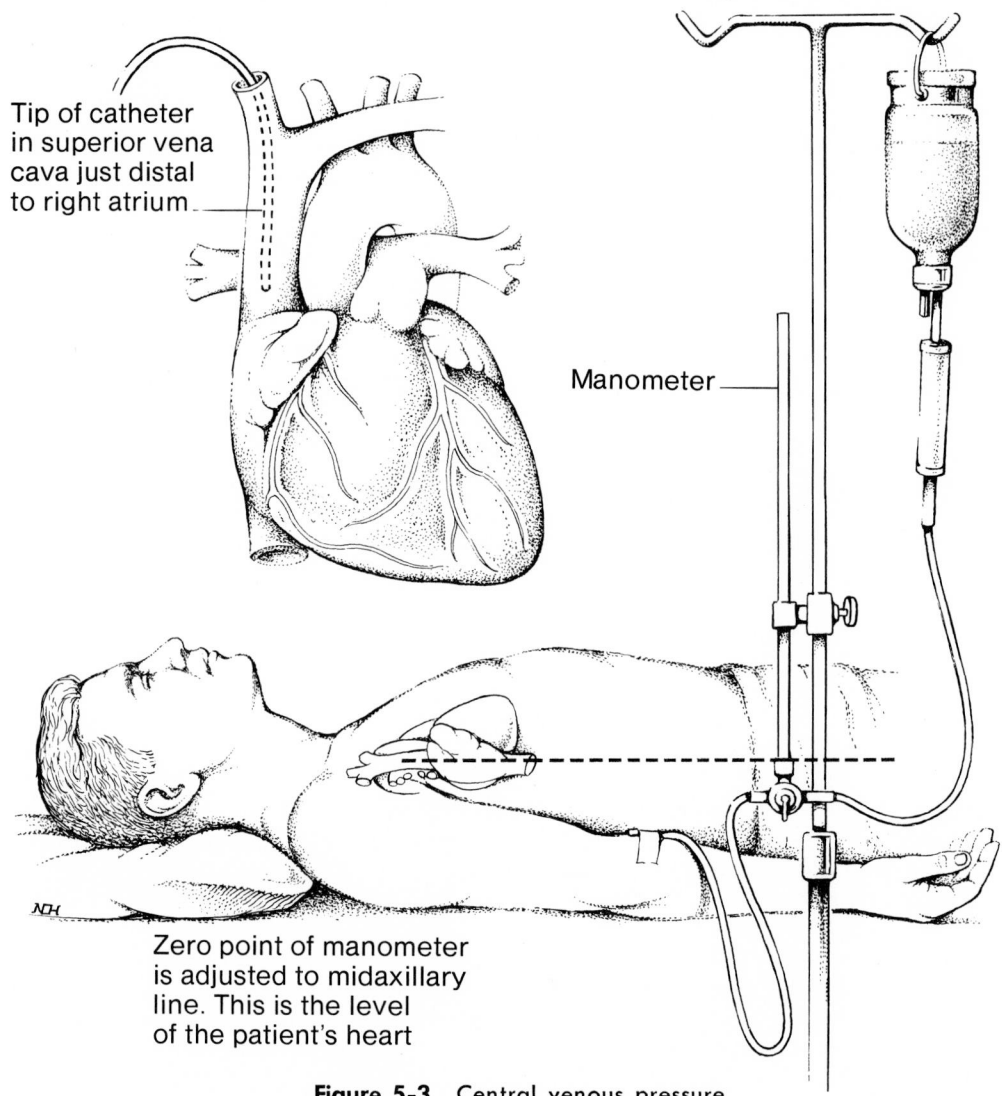

Tip of catheter in superior vena cava just distal to right atrium

Manometer

Zero point of manometer is adjusted to midaxillary line. This is the level of the patient's heart

Figure 5-3. Central venous pressure.

GUIDELINES: *Measuring Central Venous Pressure*

Central venous pressure is a measurement that indicates the competency of the right heart to accept and expel the blood returned. It provides an index of right atrial filling pressure. Vascular pressure is measured by the height of a column of water or mercury (Fig. 5-3).

Purposes

1. To indicate right ventricular function.
2. To reflect relationship between blood volume and cardiac competence.
3. To indicate status of patient in shock or response to treatment.
4. To serve as a guide in early recognition of congestive heart failure.
5. To give direct access to active circulation to serve as a route for infusions and medications.
6. To permit withdrawal of blood for blood samples and phlebotomy.
7. To offer route for insertion of intracardiac pacing electrode.

Vein Sites for Catheter Placement

Basilic   Cephalic
Brachial   External and internal jugular

Equipment

Venous pressure tray   Infusion solution and infusion set
Cutdown tray   Intravenous pole

Procedure

Nursing Action	Rationale/Amplification
Preparatory Phase	
1. Place patient in a supine position.	1. It is preferable to obtain serial C.V.P. measurements with patient in the same position. If the patient has had extensive chest surgery or is suffering from respiratory distress his bed may be elevated and subsequent readings taken in this same bed position.
2. Assemble and hang infusion set and tubing on infusion pole.	
3. Attach the external end of the catheter to the water manometer.	
4. Attach manometer to a 3-way stopcock on I.V. pole with adhesive so that the zero point on the manometer is at a level with the patient's heart (at the patient's midaxillary line) (Fig. 5-3).	
5. Mark the midaxillary line on the patient.	5. To ensure a constant base line.
6. Fill the catheter-manometer system with saline solution up to the 10-cm. mark on the manometer.	6. The I.V. tubing is filled by releasing the clamp between the fluid container and the stopcock handle.
Performance Phase	
1. The catheter is usually threaded through the arm vein (basilic vein at antecubital fossa) or a neck vein into the superior vena cava just before it enters the right atrium of the heart.	1. Catheter position may be confirmed by portable chest x-ray.

Nursing Action	Rationale/Amplification
2. When the catheter enters the thorax an inspiratory fall and expiratory rise in venous pressure is observed.	2. Fluid level fluctuates with respiration and rises sharply with coughing.
3. The patient is usually monitored on the ECG while the catheter is being inserted.	3. When the tip of the catheter contacts the wall of the right atrium or right ventricle, it may produce aberrant impulses and disturb the cardiac rhythm.
4. The infusion (drip) rate is adjusted to allow the solution to flow into the patient's vein at rate of flow prescribed.	4. An infusion may cause a significant increase in venous pressure if more than 20 ml./minute is administered.

5. Take the venous pressure readings as directed:
  a. Place the patient flat in bed.
  b. Turn stopcock to allow infusion solution in manometer to flow into patient's veins. Hold the zero point of the manometer level at the right atrium by holding the zero point at the marked midaxillary line.
  c. Observe the drop in level of solution in manometer. Record in centimeters the level at which the solution stabilizes. If pressure readings are made from antecubital vein, place patient's arm at level of his heart and abduct the arm to avoid any compression of veins in the axilla.
  d. Turn the stopcock again to allow solution in I.V. bottle to flow into patient's veins.
	b. When the stopcock is turned to connect the manometer to the intravenous catheter, fluid in the column falls until it balances the central venous pressure in the superior vena cava.
	c. The fluid level indicates the central venous pressure measured in centimeters of water.

6. The normal venous pressure is 3–10 cm. of water (2–8 mm. Hg).	6. The normal value of venous pressure varies from patient to patient.
7. C.V.P. may be monitored continuously or intermittently. The course of serial C.V.P. values is more important than a single measurement.	7. Central venous pressure is a continuously changing and dynamic measurement.
8. Assess the patient's clinical condition frequently.	8. Central venous pressure is interpreted by considering the patient's entire clinical picture: hourly urine output, heart rate, blood pressure, blood volume and cardiac output measurements. It reflects the combination of adequate cardiac pumping action, blood volume and vascular tone.
9. Flush the catheter at intervals with dilute solutions of heparin.	9. Flushing the catheter prevents obstruction by blood clots.

10. Observe the patient for complications:
  Sepsis
  Embolization or clot at catheter tip
  Hemothorax, hydrothorax, pneumothorax
  Injuries to peripheral nerves and arteries
  Arrhythmias
  Perfusion of myocardium
  Intravenous infusion overload	

Follow-up Phase

1. Clean and dispose equipment in proper place.

SPECIAL NURSING MEASURES

GUIDELINES: Assisting the Patient Undergoing Pericardiocentesis (Pericardial Aspiration)

Pericardiocentesis is the puncturing of the pericardium in order to aspirate pericardial effusion, thereby relieving cardiac tamponade.

Cardiac tamponade is compression of the heart by blood, effusion or a foreign body in the pericardial sac thereby restricting normal heart action.

Signs and Symptoms of Cardiac Tamponade

1. Rising venous pressure (20 cm. or more)
2. Falling arterial blood pressure
3. Narrowing pulse pressure (difference between systolic and diastolic pressures)
4. Small quiet heart (evidenced by fluoroscopy and chest auscultation)
5. Paradoxical pulse—lessening of pulse amplitude during inspiration and prompt reappearance of pulse with expiration
6. Apprehension
7. Dyspnea
8. Pallor or cyanosis
9. Characteristic posture—sitting upright and leaning forward

Purpose

To remove fluid from the pericardial sac caused by:
Pericarditis
Effusion from malignant neoplasm or lymphoma
Trauma to heart and chest
Acute rheumatic fever

Equipment

Pericardiocentesis tray
Intracath set
Skin antiseptic
1–2% procaine
Sterile gloves

ECG for monitoring purposes
Sterile ground wire—to be connected between pericardial needle and V-lead of ECG (optional)
Apparatus for artificial respiration
Defibrillation equipment

Sites for Pericardiocentesis (Fig. 5–4)

1. Subxiphoid—needle inserted in the angle between left costal margin and xiphoid
2. Near cardiac apex, 2 cm. inside left border of cardial dullness
3. To the left of the 5th or 6th interspace at the sternal margin
4. Right side of 4th intercostal space just inside border of dullness

Procedure (Fig. 5–4)

Nursing Action	Rationale/Amplification
Preparatory Phase	
1. Premedicate patient with barbiturate, morphine or meperidine and atropine as prescribed.	1. Premedication helps reduce apprehension.
2. Place the patient in a comfortable position with the head of the bed or treatment table raised to a 60-degree angle.	2. The position makes it easier to insert needle into pericardial sac.

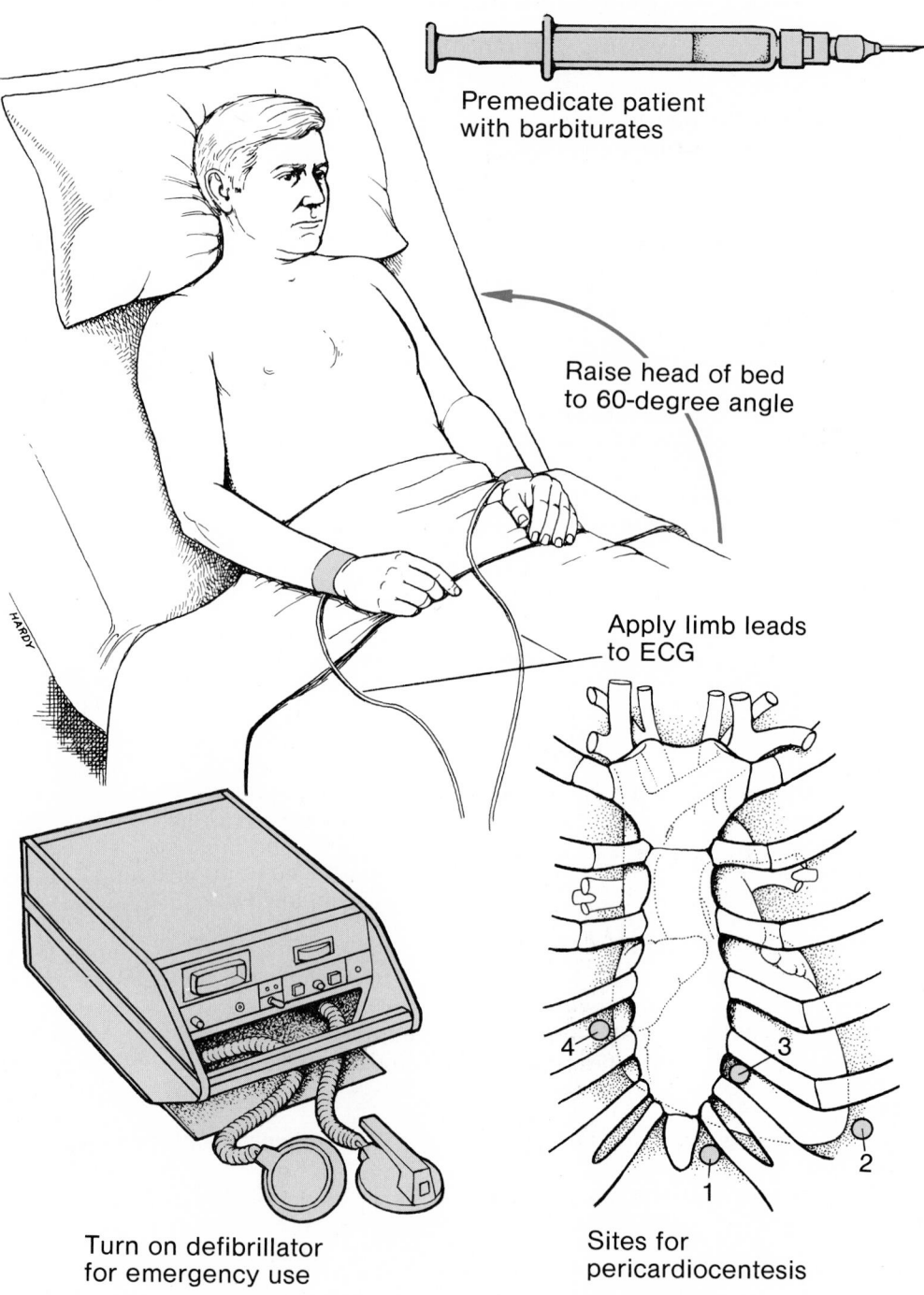

Premedicate patient
with barbiturates

Raise head of bed
to 60-degree angle

Apply limb leads
to ECG

Turn on defibrillator
for emergency use

Sites for
pericardiocentesis

Figure 5-4. Preparing patient for pericardiocentesis.

Nursing Action	**Rationale/Amplification**

3. Apply the limb leads of the ECG to the patient. Turn on the defibrillator for emergency use.
3. In case procedure has severe adverse effect.

4. Open the tray, using aseptic technique.

Performance Phase (by physician)

1. The site is prepared with skin antiseptic and the area draped with sterile towels and injected with procaine solution.

2. The pericardial aspiration needle is attached to a 20-ml. syringe by a 3-way stopcock. The V-lead (precordial lead wire) of the ECG is attached to the hub of the aspirating needle by a sterile wire and alligator clips or clamp.
2. The ECG is turned on for constant monitoring purposes.

3. The needle is advanced slowly until fluid is obtained.
3. Fluid is generally aspirated at a depth of 3–4 cm.

4. When fluid is obtained a hemostat is clamped on the needle at the chest wall.
4. This prevents movement of the needle and further penetration while fluid is being removed.

5. Monitor the patient's ECG, blood pressure and venous pressure constantly.
5. A marked elevation of the ST segment or P wave indicates that the myocardium has been entered producing a localized current of injury. If this happens the needle is withdrawn a few millimeters. This method is used when repeated drainage is necessary.

6. If a large amount of fluid is present a polyethylene catheter may be inserted through a needle (an intracath) and left in the pericardial sac and attached to a drainage bottle.

7. Watch for presence of bloody fluid. If blood accumulates rapidly, an immediate thoracotomy and cardiorrhaphy (suturing of heart muscle) is indicated.
7. Pericardial fluid may be due to trauma. Pericardial blood does not clot while blood obtained from inadvertent puncture of one of the heart chambers *does* clot.

Follow-up Phase

1. Place patient in intensive care unit or cardiac care unit.
1. Following pericardiocentesis careful monitoring of blood pressure and venous pressure will be necessary to indicate possible recurrence of tamponade. A repeated aspiration is then necessary.

2. Watch for decline of venous pressure and rising systolic blood pressure after procedure.
2. In the presence of these signs the patient is probably experiencing cardiac tamponade.

3. Auscultate the area over the heart.
3. Listen for decrease in intensity of heart sounds indicating recurring cardiac tamponade.

4. Prepare for surgical intervention (thoracotomy, see p. 174) if:
   a. Pericardial fluid repeatedly accumulates or
   b. The aspiration is unsuccessful or
   c. Complications develop

5. Assess for complications:
   Inadvertent puncture of heart chamber
   Arrhythmias
   Puncture of lung, stomach or liver
   Laceration of coronary artery or myocardium

GUIDELINES: *Cardiopulmonary Resuscitation for Cardiac Arrest*

Cardiac arrest is the sudden and unexpected cessation of the heart and effective circulation.

A. *Causes*
1. Ventricular fibrillation
2. Cardiac asystole
3. Cardiovascular collapse
4. Acute myocardial infarction
5. Anaphylactic reaction
6. Acute airway obstruction
7. Surgery
8. Accidents (electrocution, drowning, inhalation of toxic gases)

B. *Signs and Symptoms*
1. Immediate loss of consciousness
2. Absence of pulses
3. Absence of audible heart sounds
4. Convulsions (may or may not present)
5. Dilation of pupils of eyes (begins in 45 seconds)

Purpose

To *promptly* establish effective circulation and ventilation.

Equipment

Arrest board   Defibrillator
Oral airway   Emergency cardiac drugs
Rebreathing bag

Procedure

Nursing Action	*Rationale/Amplification*
Performance Phase	
1. Note the time as soon as cardiac arrest is determined. a. Use bedside call system; telephone to summon help. b. Start elapsed time clock if available.	NURSING ALERT: Lack of effective circulation to the central nervous system of more than 4 to 6 minutes may result in irreversible changes.
2. Administer 1 or 2 sharp blows over lower sternum.	2. Cardiac standstill may sometimes be terminated by a sharp blow, particularly if asystole is mechanism of arrest.
START ARTIFICIAL VENTILATION	
1. Clear airway of foreign material.	
2. Hyperextend (tilt back) head and pull jaw forward.	2. This tends to lift the tongue off the back wall of the pharynx and open the airway.
3. Insert oropharyngeal tube if available.	
4. *Ventilate the patient.* Inflate the patient's lungs by forcing a full breath through a mouth-to-mouth airtight seal.	4. With each attempted inflation, the patient's chest should rise to a visible degree. Absence of chest expansion indicates airway obstruction. Keep the jaw pulled forward during ventilation to relieve obstruction.
5. Provide 12 breaths per minute. (Utilize bag and mask if someone is available to operate.)	

Nursing Action	**Rationale/Amplification**
Start External Cardiac Massage	External cardiac compression is necessary to circulate blood that has been oxygenated by artificial ventilation.

Nursing Action

START EXTERNAL CARDIAC MASSAGE

1. Place patient on firm surface.

2. Place the heel of one hand on the lower half of the sternum and place the opposite hand on top of the first hand.
3. Using the rescuer's weight, quickly and forcefully depress the lower sternum 3.7–5 cm. (1½–2 inches).
   Then suddenly release the sternal pressure.

4. Use 60–80 compressions/minute.

5. Deliver 1 deep breath for each 5 cardiac compressions, without interruption of compression rhythm.
6. Palpate for carotid pulse and look at size of response of pupils.

UTILIZE APPROPRIATE DRUG THERAPY

1. Prepare epinephrine (0.5–1 mg.) which may be given every 5 minutes until normal sinus rhythm and adequate cardiac output return.

2. Prepare I.V. sodium bicarbonate (44 mEq.) to be given every 5–10 minutes. (Dosage determined by blood pH data.)

3. Utilize ECG monitoring to determine type of cardiopulmonary arrest.

4. Defibrillate the heart with a 200–400 watt seconds direct current shock across the heart if ventricular fibrillation has occurred. (Use lidocaine hydrochloride if defibrillation is unsuccessful or if fibrillation recurs.)

Rationale/Amplification

External cardiac compression is necessary to circulate blood that has been oxygenated by artificial ventilation.

1. A firm surface supports the spine and allows the heart to be compressed between it and the sternum.

3. Each compression forces blood from the heart into the arterial system.

   Rapid sternal release facilitates filling of the right heart from the great veins and the left heart from the pulmonary veins.

5. If only 1 person is available alternate 30 seconds of external massage with 5 seconds of ventilation.
6. The presence of a palpable carotid pulse and constriction of the pupils are evidence of effective circulation of oxygenated blood.

1. Epinephrine is a cardiotonic and vasopressor drug. It is administered intravenously (if an I.V. route is already available) or directly into the heart via a long needle. After drug is injected into the heart, the heart must be externally massaged in order to deliver the drug to the coronary circulation.
2. Marked metabolic acidosis occurs at the time of cardiac arrest and persists during cardiopulmonary resuscitation since perfusion of body tissues is far below normal.
3. If asystole or profound cardiovascular collapse is found, continue mouth-to-mouth ventilation and external massage. Additional epinephrine, sodium bicarbonate and calcium chloride or lactate are usually given.
4. Continue to use cardiotonic, vasopressor and antacid drugs if external cardiopulmonary resuscitation is prolonged since artificial circulation causes severe acidosis.

Postresuscitative Care

Maintain adequate peripheral blood pressure.

1. Give norepinephrine (or other vasoconstrictors) following resuscitation of the arrested heart if hypotension remains.
   a. Give infusion of 5% dextrose in water or 5% dextrose in normal saline.

      b. Check blood pressure every 2 minutes after drug is given until desired blood pressure is obtained.

      c. Stay with patient while he is receiving norepinephrine.

  2. Watch ECG tracings for evidence of improvement or deterioration.

  3. Keep careful intake and output record.

      a. Use mannitol for postresuscitation oliguria or anuria.

      b. Observe for evidences of dehydration.

      c. Carry out serial nonprotein nitrogen determinations if there is evidence of renal damage.

  4. Watch for postresuscitative convulsions (may arise from cerebral anoxic complications).

      a. Control seizures with intravenous administration of sodium amobarbital (Amytal) during the acute phase.

      b. Give daily maintenance dose of diphenylhydantoin (Dilantin) if necessary.

  5. Observe for respiratory depression.

      a. Patient may require prolonged mechanical artificial ventilation in the postresuscitative period—prevents cerebral congestion and edema, combats metabolic acidosis and lessens the work of breathing.

      b. Utilize tracheal suctioning in the immediate postresuscitation period—to prevent complications resulting from aspirated or retained secretions.

GUIDELINES: *Direct Current Countershock Procedure for Ventricular Fibrillation*

Countershock is the use of electrical discharge to patient's chest wall to terminate ventricular fibrillation.

A *defibrillator* is an instrument that delivers an electric shock to the heart to convert ventricular fibrillation to normal sinus rhythm. (Defibrillators are also used to convert other abnormal cardiac rhythms.)

Purpose

To terminate ventricular fibrillation

Equipment

Defibrillator with paddles
Conduction jelly (electrode jelly)
Resuscitative equipment

Procedure

Nursing Action	Rationale/Amplification
Performance Phase	
1. Expose the patient's anterior chest.	1. This procedure should be carried out immediately after ventricular fibrillation is detected to minimize cerebral and circulatory deterioration.
2. Turn on the electric power and charge the cardioversion circuit to 400-joule setting.	2. The machine's dial should always be left in this position. The shock is measured in *joules* (sometimes called watt-seconds).

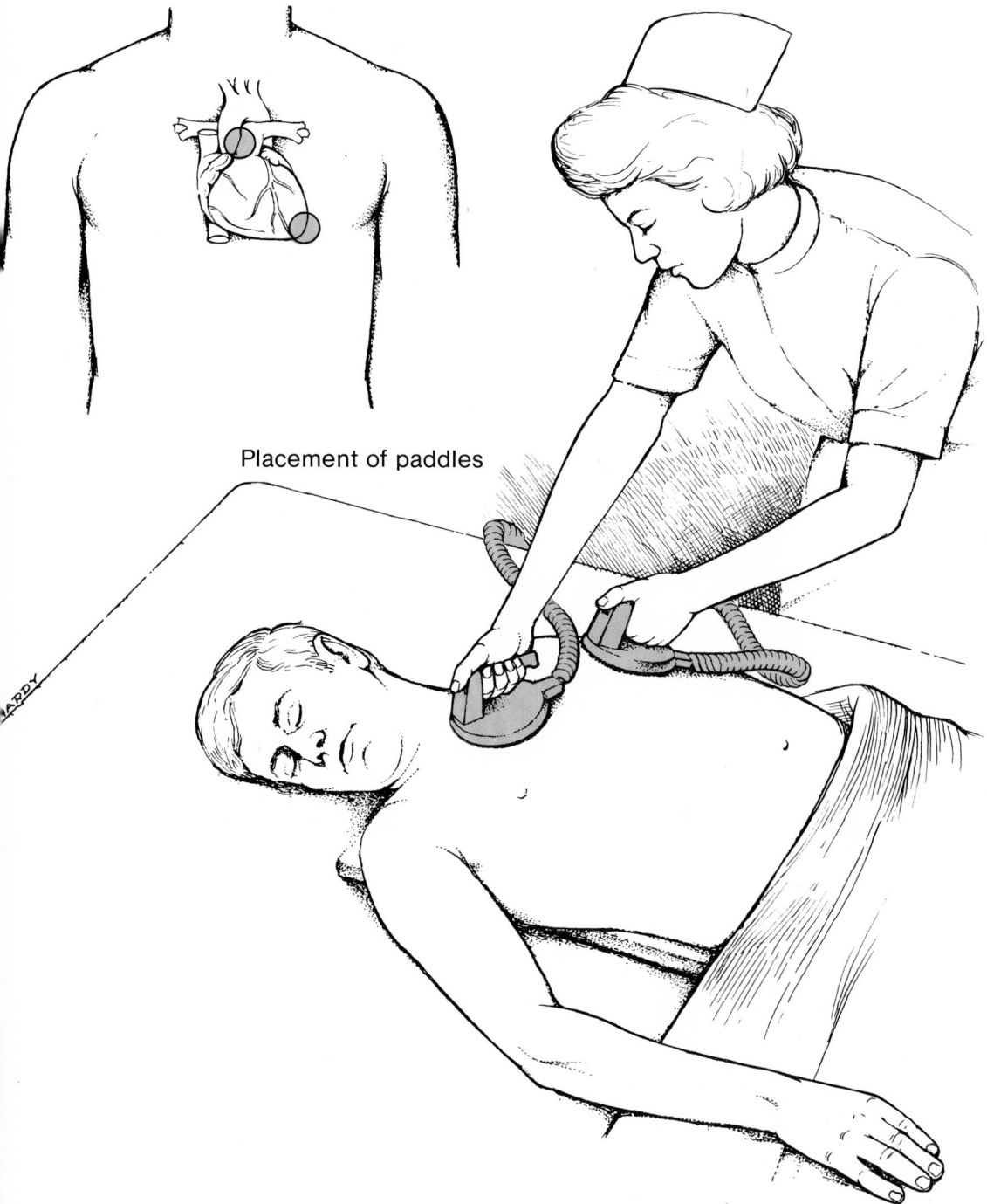

Placement of paddles

Figure 5-5. Closed-chest defibrillation.

Nursing Action	**Rationale/Amplification**
3. If the machine has a synchronization circuit for reversion of tachyarrhythmias, make sure that it is not activated.	3. If this is not done the apparatus fruitlessly seeks a nonexistent QRS complex before firing the electrical discharge, regardless of how often the manual discharge button is pressed.
4. Apply electrode paste to the paddle electrodes if they are not routinely kept in tubs of paste at all times.	4. The electrode paste helps provide better contact and prevents skin burns.
5. Place the paddle electrodes on the chest along the longitudinal axis of the heart; i.e., with one paddle centered over the right 2nd intercostal space parasternally and the other centered over the presumed location of the cardiac apex (Fig. 5-5).	5. If anteroposterior paddles are used, the anterior paddle is held with pressure on the midsternum while the patient lies on the posterior paddle which is placed in the intrascapular region.
6. GIVE THE COMMAND TO STAND CLEAR OF PATIENT AND THE BED.	6. If a person touches the bed, he may act as a ground for the current and receive a shock.
7. Administer the electrical shock by pressing the discharge button.	7. Remove paddles from the patient immediately after the shock is administered.
8. Re-examine the monitored electrocardiogram to determine if further shocks are necessary, either immediately or after appropriate drug therapy.	

GUIDELINES: *Application of Rotating Tourniquets*

Rotating tourniquets refers to a technique whereby tourniquets are systematically rotated on the extremities to remove a volume of blood from the central circulation in order to decrease venous return.

Purpose

To pool the blood temporarily in the extremities in order to reduce venous return to the heart.

Underlying Principles

1. Three of the 4 extremities are compressed while 1 extremity is usually free at all times.
2. No single extremity should be compressed continuously for more than 45 minutes.
3. Tourniquets may have to be rotated at 5-minute intervals on the elderly to prevent gangrene and other complications.
4. These principles are important so that the risks of phlebothrombosis and fatal pulmonary embolism are reduced.

Equipment

Equipment for extremity compression
   4 sphygmomanometer cuffs or
   4 tourniquets, 61 cm. (2 feet) long with outside diameter 0.8–3.8 cm. (5/16 to 1-1/2 inches) or
   Equipment designed to inflate and deflate blood pressure cuffs automatically (Danzer apparatus)
Small towels
Watch—to note time interval
Work sheet

Procedure

Nursing Action	Rationale/Amplification
Performance Phase (Fig. 5-6)	
1. Explain to the patient (if his condition permits) the purpose of the compression and that the skin of the extremities may become discolored.	1. To relieve anxiety.
2. Take the blood pressure.	2. Initial blood pressure reading serves as a base line for future comparison.
3. Apply the 4 blood pressure cuffs (or Danzer apparatus if available) to extremities and inflate 3 to a pressure less than the systolic blood pressure; or	3. Venous flow must be occluded but arterial flow must not be impeded.

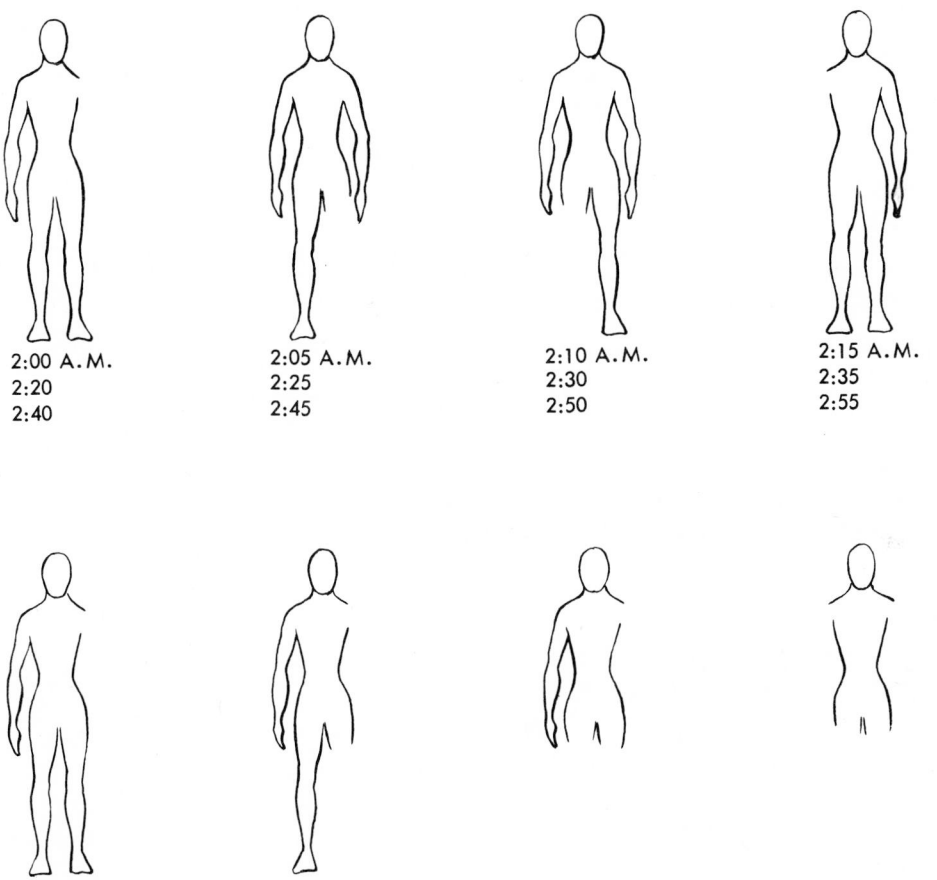

2:00 A.M.
2:20
2:40

2:05 A.M.
2:25
2:45

2:10 A.M.
2:30
2:50

2:15 A.M.
2:35
2:55

3:00 A.M.

3:05 A.M.

3:10 A.M.

3:15 A.M.

Figure 5-6. Rotating tourniquet technique. This illustration shows the timing of compression and the rotation sequence and release of tourniquets. This was prescribed for 1 hour starting at 2 A.M. Anatomy shown in figures indicates extent of circulation.

Nursing Action	**Rationale/Amplification**
4. Apply tourniquets as high as possible on 3 extremities. Place tourniquets over gown or small towel in a definite rotation pattern.	4. Tourniquet should be placed in such a way that the arterial pulse can be palpated. One extremity should be free of a tourniquet during each time interval.
5. Release 1 tourniquet every 15 minutes. Then apply a tourniquet to the previously free extremity.	5. The venous outflow in any 1 extremity will be occluded for 45 minutes and unoccluded for 15 minutes.
6. Rotate tourniquets in a definite clockwise pattern.	
7. Monitor blood pressure every few minutes after tourniquets have been applied.	7. Application of tourniquets may precipitate hypotension in some patients.
8. Measure urinary output at frequent intervals. (Usually an indwelling catheter is used.)	8. Watch for sudden reduction in plasma volume with hypotension and oliguria after administration of rapid-acting diuretics (ethacrynic acid, furosemide).
9. Remove 1 tourniquet at a time according to the specified time interval (usually 15 minutes) at the completion of the rotation.	9. Releasing the tourniquets 1 at a time prevents a sudden increase in circulatory blood volume thus preventing circulatory overload.

Follow-up Phase
1. Record starting time of procedure, rotation intervals, clinical response, medications given and the time tourniquets were discontinued.

CARDIAC ARRHYTHMIAS

Arrhythmia is a clinical disorder of the heart beat; it may include a disturbance of rate, rhythm (sequence) or both. Arrhythmias are derangements of heart function and not of heart structure.

Etiology

1. Arrhythmias due to organic heart disease
   a. Inflammatory heart disease
   b. Degenerative heart disease (atherosclerosis)
   c. Congenital heart disease
   d. Hypertensive heart disease
2. Arrhythmias due to disturbances of other organ systems
   a. Diseases of central nervous system—from sympathetic and vagal stimulation
   b. Pulmonary disease
   c. Endocrine disorders (hyper- and hypothyroidism, hypoglycemia, diabetic ketoacidosis)
   d. Gastrointestinal disorders (fluid and electrolyte imbalance)
   e. Renal disorders (renal failure)
3. Arrhythmias from other causes
   a. Drugs (digitalis intoxication, quinidine, procaine amide)
   b. Infection
   c. Disturbances of electrolyte balance
   d. Anemia
   e. Following cardiac surgery

Classification of Arrhythmias Based on Disturbed Physiology

1. Disturbance of impulse formation—heart beat activated for one or more beats by a pacemaker other than the SA node.
2. Disturbances of conduction—due to delayed transmission in impulse or failure of some impulses to be conducted or to a block at the affected site.
3. Combined disorders—combination of abnormally rapid impulse formation and decreased ability to conduct the impulses.

Common Disturbances of Rhythm*

1. *Premature contractions (beats) of the heart (extrasystoles)*—those arising outside the normal sinus pacemaker.
2. *Sinus tachycardia*—heart rate over 100 beats per minute.
3. *Sinus bradycardia*—unduly slow heart action; below 60 beats per minute.
4. *Paroxysmal atrial tachycardia*—a period of rapid heart beats which begins and ends suddenly.
5. *Atrial flutter*—rapid heart beat almost always caused by organic heart disease. ECG is usually necessary to differentiate atrial flutter from other disorders of the heart beat.
6. *Atrial fibrillation*—disorganized and uncoordinated twitching of atrial musculature at ventricular rates of 160 to 200 beats per minute.
7. *Paroxysmal ventricular tachycardia*—a series of successive ventricular premature beats which usually occur in presence of severe myocardial damage.
8. *Ventricular fibrillation*—complete disorganization of the heart beat; if not immediately treated ventricular fibrillation produces cardiac arrest.

Nursing Alert: Suspect ventricular fibrillation when palpable pulse and audible heart sounds suddenly disappear and the blood pressure is unobtainable.

Ventricular fibrillation must be treated within 4 minutes.

1. Carry out closed chest resuscitation (p. 246).
2. Maintain respiration and oxygenation.
3. Do external defibrillation of the heart.
4. Give appropriate drugs and fluid therapy (see p. 247).

---

9. *Heart block*—impairment of the conduction of the electrical impulses of the heart between the atria and ventricles producing a partial or complete heart block.
10. *Complete heart block*—a permanent or episodic condition in which the pacing impulses from the SA node are blocked with the result that the ventricles beat independently of the atria. Complete heart block is a major indication for pacing.
11. *Stokes-Adams syndrome*—a deficiency of cerebral blood flow due to a slowing of heart rate or ineffective ventricular contraction and output during tachyarrhythmias.
    a. Signs and symptoms
       (1) Transient faintness—blackouts, fainting
       (2) Dizziness
       (3) Sudden syncope, convulsions and cerebral seizures
       (4) Cardiac arrest and shock

* See pages 296–315 for more detailed discussion.

b. Treatment
   (1) Give isoproterenol via intravenous infusion for acute attack.
   (2) Utilize temporary pacing of the heart (transvenous pacing).
   (3) Prepare patient for implantation of permanent cardiac pacemaker (see p. 257).

Clinical Manifestations

(Depends on ventricular rate, condition of heart and patient's psychological reaction.)

1. Symptoms and signs of rapid arrhythmias
   a. Palpitation
   b. Dizziness and fainting
   c. Throbbing in head and neck
   d. Shortness of breath
   e. Precordial discomfort and pain
   f. Anxiety
2. Symptoms and signs of slow heart action (bradyarrhythmia)
   a. Shortness of breath
   b. Fatigue on exertion
   c. Dizziness and fainting—may indicate syncopal attacks, leading to convulsive seizures

Clinical Effects

1. Some arrhythmias are relatively harmless while others are harbingers of cardiac arrest.
2. Cardiac arrhythmias can reduce cardiac output, lower the blood pressure and decrease blood perfusion of the brain, heart, kidneys, gastrointestinal tract, muscles and skin.
3. Cardiac arrhythmias often produce attacks of transient cerebral ischemia with complete stroke.
4. Arrhythmias can precipitate congestive heart failure or angina pectoris in certain patients.
5. Bradyarrhythmias (rate below 50) predispose to electrical instability of the heart.
6. A marked degree of disability may accompany an arrhythmia.

Treatment

1. Depends on:
   a. Type of arrhythmia
   b. Underlying cause
   c. Associated clinical condition
   d. Presence of hypotension or shock-like state
2. Methods available
   See Table 5-1, p. 255.

Nursing Assessment

1. How does the patient describe his symptoms?
2. What is the duration and frequency of the arrhythmia?
3. Evaluate the patient's general appearance: pallor, cyanosis, sweating—may indicate peripheral arteriolar constriction.
4. Observe carotid pulsation: Rapid and vigorous? Irregular with varying amplitude?
5. Listen to the heart beat with a stethoscope.
   a. Listen for rate, presence of irregularity, increase in intensity of first heart sound.
      (1) 30 beats or lower—complete AV block, partial AV block or sinus bradycardia.
      (2) 40–60 beats per minute—varying degrees of AV block, atrial tachycardia with block, etc.

TABLE 5-1. METHODS AVAILABLE IN TREATING CARDIAC ARRHYTHMIAS

A. Drugs	D. Electrical devices
B. Respiratory maneuvers	E. Surgical procedures
C. Mechanical maneuvers	F. Various combinations of these methods

I. *To Increase Cardiac Automaticity*
   A. Sympathomimetic amines (e.g., isoproterenol, epinephrine)
   B. Parasympathetic blocking agents (e.g., atropine, methantheline)
   C. Alkalinizing solutions (e.g., sodium bicarbonate, molar sodium lactate)

II. *To Decrease Cardiac Automaticity*
   A. *Vagal Stimulation:* Often efficacious in supraventricular tachycardia (atrial or junctional)
      1. Drugs (e.g., digitalis, neostigmine)
      2. Mechanical means (carotid sinus or ocular pressure)
         a. Use of emetics (ipecac, apomorphine)   *c.* Blowing in balloon or bag
         b. Finger in throat   *d.* Right atrial stimulation
   B. *Drugs that Slow Tachyarrhythmias and Tend to Abolish Premature Beats (Atrial and/or Ventricular):*
      1. Quinidine   6. Beta blocking agents (propranolol and alprenolol)
      2. Procaine amide   7. Diphenylhydantoin
      3. Potassium   8. Antazoline
      4. Lidocaine   9. Digitalis (occasionally)
      5. Bretylium

III. *Vasopressor Drugs*
   A. Norepinephrine   C. Methoxamine
   B. Metaraminol

IV. *Electrolytes*
   A. Restore alteration in pH to normal   C. Magnesium
   B. Potassium   D. Calcium

V. *Other Drugs*
   A. Antihistamines
   B. Antithyroid drugs (e.g., propylthiouracil, ^{131}I)
   C. Corticoids (e.g., hydrocortisone, DCA)
   D. Sedatives and tranquilizers (e.g., barbiturates, meprobamate, chlordiazepoxide, diazepam)

VI. *Respiratory Maneuvers*
   A. Valsalva maneuver
   B. Breath-holding maneuver

VII. *Mechanical Maneuvers*
   A. Carotid sinus pressure
   B. Thumping on precordium
   C. Cardiopulmonary resuscitation (closed chest; rarely, open chest)

VIII. *Electrical Devices*
   A. Pacemaker   B. Defibrillator
      1. Internal   C. Electric countershock
      2. External   D. Carotid sinus stimulator

IX. *Surgical Procedures*
   A. Thoracotomy with manual cardiac systole
   B. Sympathectomy
   C. Surgical interruption of accessory pathway in refractory PAT (paroxysmal atrial tachycardia) associated with W–P–W (Wolff–Parkinson–White Syndrome)

(From Bellet, S.: Clinical Disorders of the Heart Beat. Philadelphia, Lea & Febiger, 1971.)

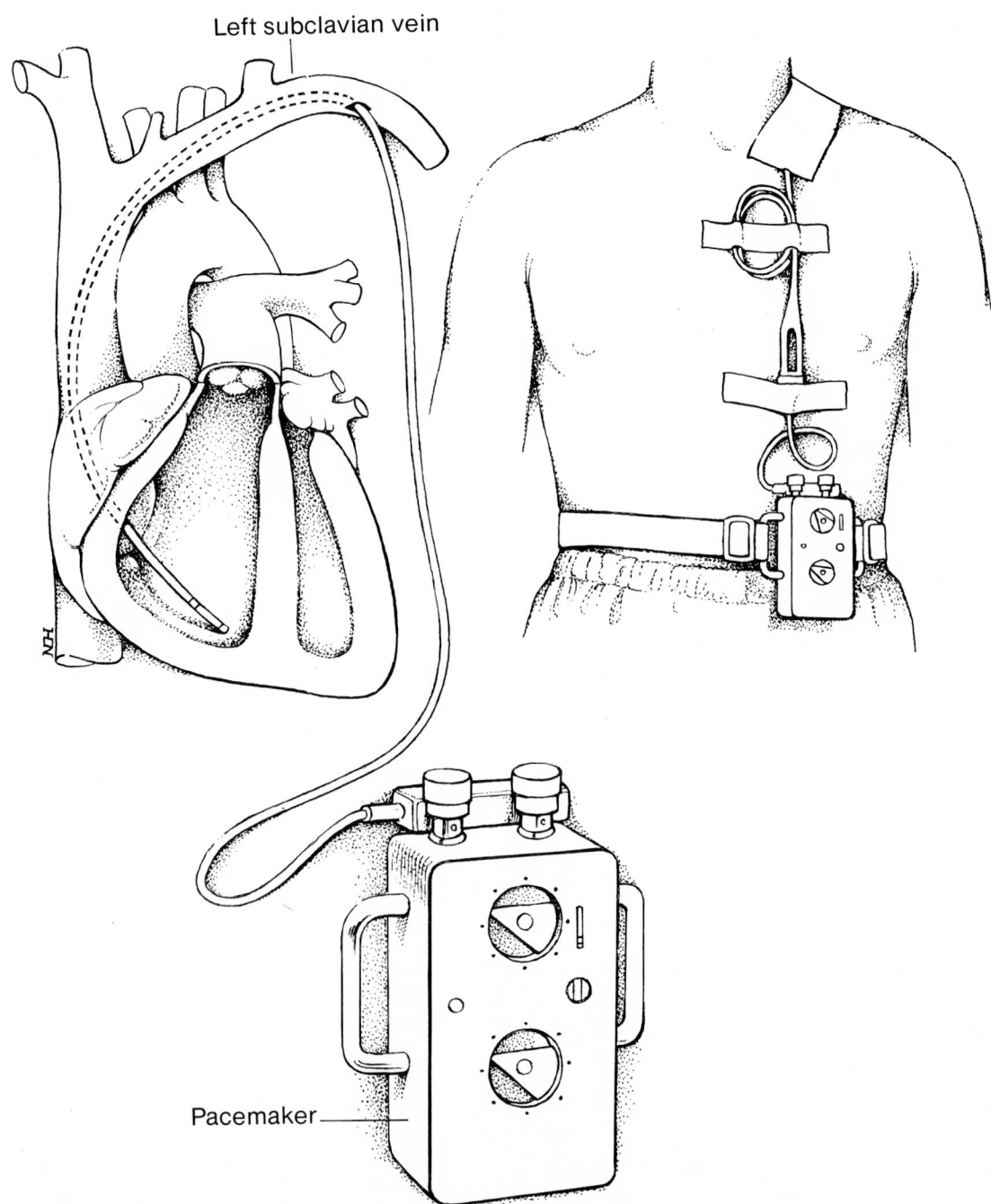

Figure 5-7. Cardiac pacemaker.

(3) 60–110 beats per minute—sinus arrhythmia, premature beats, AV heart block, atrial fibrillation, atrial flutter.

(4) 140–180 beats per minute—atrial tachycardia, atrial flutter, junctional or ventricular tachycardia.

   b. If possible have an electrocardiogram taken during an episode of arrhythmia.

   c. Take the blood pressure and pulse.

6. Evaluate for:

   a. Mental confusion with arrhythmia—indicates cerebral ischemia

   b. Presence of signs and symptoms of congestive heart failure—may indicate arrhythmia causing serious effect

   c. Chest pains with arrhythmia—due to myocardial ischemia.

Cardiac Pacing

A *pacemaker* is an electronic device that provides repetitive electrical stimuli to the heart muscle for the control of heart rate. It initiates and maintains the heart rate when the natural pacemakers of the heart are unable to do so (Fig. 5-7).

Component Parts of a Pacemaker

1. Generator—contains the power, including a battery

2. One or more electrodes which are in contact with area to be paced

3. Cable wire (used occasionally to connect generator and electrodes)

Underlying Principles

1. Artificial pacemakers vary in design and usage according to the type and severity of the condition requiring treatment.

2. A temporary pacemaker may be strapped to the patient's waistline or attached to his arm via an elastic compression bandage.

3. A permanent pacemaker is implanted within the body or may consist of both implanted and external units.

4. The stimuli from the pacemaker travel through wire electrodes that approach the heart through a vein leading to the vena cavae and right atrium or by direct penetration of the chest wall or via a subcutaneous tunnel from implanted units.

Clinical Indications

1. Heart block (especially those complicated by Stokes-Adams syndrome)

2. Tachyarrhythmias

3. Arrhythmias following acute myocardial infarction

4. Following open heart surgery

Types of Pacemakers

1. *Demand (standby; synchronous)*—this unit discharges if the patient's conduction is not complete; it senses the rate or amplitude of the QRS complex. A demand pacer allows the patient to function on his own and emits a stimulating impulse only when the patient does not trigger his own.

2. *Asynchronous*

   a. *Fixed rate*—this unit stimulates the ventricle at a preset constant rate that is independent of the patient's rhythm. However, it can compete with the patient's own rhythm.

   b. *Variable rate*—this unit has a control that permits the physician to vary the fixed rate of stimulation.

Approaches to Pacemaker Implantation

1. *Transthoracic*—placement of 2 electrodes on the chest in order to allow electric stimulation to the heart to promote systolic contraction.
2. *Direct pacing*—the electrode is placed in contact with the heart. Direct pacing may be *epicardial* or *endocardial*.
   a. *Epicardial implantation*—implantation of the electrode system directly on the outside of the left ventricle with the electrodes just penetrating the myocardium. This is done via a thoracotomy. The generator is placed subcutaneously in a skin pocket above or below the waistline.
   b. *Endocardial implantation*—insertion of a thin, pacing electrode near the apex of the right ventricle via the neck vein. Endocardial pacing may be *temporary* or *permanent*.
      (1) *Temporary (transvenous) pacing*—is usually an emergency procedure performed when medications (isoproterenol and epinephrine) are ineffective. Temporary pacing may be done for hours, days or weeks and is usually continued until a permanent pacemaker is installed.
         (a) Improves cardiac output and coronary, cerebral and renal blood flow.
         (b) Controls ventricular tachycardia and fibrillation.
         (c) Allows complete control of heart rate during surgery.
         (d) Permits observation of effects of pacing on heart function so that optimum pacing rate for the patient can be selected before permanent pacemaker is implanted.
      (2) *Permanent Pacing*—a permanent pacemaker battery unit is implanted in a pocket under the skin and connected to the heart by:
         (a) Myocardial electrodes.
         (b) An electrode catheter which is inserted through a vein and positioned near the apex of the right ventricle (most common). The peripheral end of the electrode is connected to the generator which is implanted underneath the skin of the right or left pectoral region.

Complications

1. Battery failure (failure of electronic components) (See p. 259.)
2. Breakage or dislocation of electrodes
3. Infection at site of pacemaker or electrode implantation
4. Perforation of right ventricle by catheter tip
5. Blood clot formation at electrode tips
6. Increased pacing threshold causing cessation of pacing rate
7. Interference with pacer stimuli from:
   a. Electrocautery and electrocoagulating equipment
   b. Diathermy equipment
   c. Microwave ovens

Nursing Management

1. The patient is monitored by ECG following implantation of the pacemaker—high risk if electrode is displaced soon after insertion.
   a. See nursing management after chest surgery, page 174, if patient has implantation via thoracotomy.

b. Know what type of pacer the patient has and what rate it has been set to fire. This information should be recorded on the chart and Kardex.
c. The patient with a temporary or line-operated pacemaker must be placed in an electronically safe environment. Only a qualified electrician can ascertain such a condition. The nurse must have special training in electrical hazards.
2. Inspect the site under the pressure dressings for hematoma.
3. Keep the intravenous infusion running—to combat dehydration and to have a readily accessible vein in the event an arrhythmia occurs.
4. Give analgesic drugs to relieve pain.
5. Carry out a comprehensive teaching and rehabilitation program.
   a. Teach the patient to check his own pulse daily. Report immediately any deviation (5 beats below or 5 beats above the preset level) from normal.
   b. Advise patient to report signs and symptoms of dizziness, fainting, palpitation, chest pain—indicative of pacemaker failure.
   c. Encourage patient to have regular periodic examination including ECG, chest x-ray and other tests to monitor function and integrity of electronic equipment.
   d. See that the patient has a copy of his ECG tracing (according to agency policy) —for future comparison so that rate changes and decreases in amplitude may be noted.
   e. Inform the patient to expect to have a battery change within 18 to 24 months.
   f. Watch for interference with pacemaker stimuli by extraneous electrical signals from electrical motors and appliances, microwave ovens, diathermy machines, etc.
   g. Advise patient to avoid working with faulty electrical equipment and poorly grounded equipment.
   h. Advise patient to wear loose fitting clothing around the area of pacemaker implantation.
   i. Patient should wear identification (bracelet) that lists pacemaker type, rate, physician's name and the hospital where the pacemaker was inserted.

ATHEROSCLEROTIC HEART DISEASE

Angina Pectoris

Angina pectoris is a clinical syndrome characterized by paroxysms of pain or oppression in the anterior chest produced as a result of insufficient coronary blood flow and myocardial hypoxia.

Altered Physiology

Atherosclerosis of major vessels → diminution of coronary blood flow → increased cardiac work → increased myocardial oxygen need → anginal pain.

Etiology

1. Usually due to atherosclerotic heart disease—is almost invariably associated with a significant obstruction of a major coronary artery.
2. May be from severe aortic stenosis or insufficiency, aortitis, hyperthyroidism, anemia, tachycardia.

Clinical Manifestations

Pain—(probably caused by metabolic changes produced by ischemia).
1. *Location*—behind middle or upper third of sternum (retrosternal) felt deep in chest. Patient may make a fist over site of pain.
2. *Radiation*—usually radiates to neck, jaw, shoulders and upper extremities.
    a. Frequently may be localized.
    b. Patient often experiences a tightness, choking or strangling sensation.
3. *Character*—constricting, oppressive, strangling, vice-like, insistent quality.
    a. May be mild to severe.
    b. May produce numbness or weakness in arms, wrist, hands.
    c. Accompanied by severe apprehension and feeling of impending death.
4. *Duration*—attack usually lasts less than 3 minutes.
    Attacks occurring when patient is at rest—persist 5–15 minutes.

NURSING ALERT: Suspect an impending myocardial infarction if anginal pain lasts more than one-half hour.

---

5. *Factors Precipitating Pain*
    a. Exertion
    b. Exposure to cold
    c. Eating a heavy meal
    d. Emotion and excitement

Treatment and Nursing Management

Objectives: to reduce the discrepancy between myocardial oxygen demands and the available supply of oxygen.
    to relieve pain.

A. *Drug Therapy*
    1. Nitroglycerin (glyceryl trinitrate sublingual tablets, 0.15–0.60 mg.)
        a. Decreases coronary vascular resistance and increases coronary blood flow.
        b. Should be used before pain develops if possible.
        c. Pain relief begins in ½–3 minutes. Prompt response to nitroglycerin usually distinguishes cardiac from noncardiac pain.
        d. Dosage may be repeated in a few minutes for a total of 3 tablets if relief not obtained.
        e. Patient may complain of fullness or pounding in head.
        f. Should be used prophylactically to avoid pain known to occur with certain activities (sexual intercourse, stair climbing, exposure to cold).
        g. Record should be kept of number of tablets taken—to evaluate any change in anginal pattern.
        h. Precautions against nitroglycerin becoming inactivated should be taken.
            (1) Inactivated by heat, moisture, air, light, time.
            (2) Should be kept in dark bottle, with main supply refrigerated.
            (3) Should not be carried close to body or in a metal pill box.
            (4) Supply should be renewed every 6 months.
    2. Amyl-Nitrate (0.3-ml. ampules)
        a. Ampules crushed and vapor inhaled.
        b. Drug acts in 10 seconds.
        c. Should be given when patient is lying down—causes peripheral arterial vasodilation and a fall in blood pressure.

3. *Drugs to lessen frequency of anginal attacks*
   a. Long-acting nitrites
      (1) Erythrityl tetranitrate (Cardilate) 10–30 mg.
      (2) Pentaerythrityl tetranitrate (Peritrate) 10 mg., 3 times daily
      (3) Isosorbide dinitrate (Isordil) 5–30 mg., 3–4 times daily (a long-acting sublingual vasodilator)
   b. Beta-adrenergic blocking agent
      Propranolol hydrochloride (Inderal)—slows heart rate and decreases myocardial contractility thereby conserving myocardial oxygen supply.
      Given daily in divided doses. (Dosage variable ranging according to patient's cardiac status.)

B. *Patient Education*
   1. Avoid activities known to cause anginal pain—sudden exertion, walking against the wind and after meals, exposure to cold, life stresses.
   2. Stop physical activity when pain occurs—relief should be afforded in a few minutes.
   3. Control the pain.
      a. Take nitroglycerin sublingually (under tongue) for feelings of chest oppression or constriction—*use before pain develops.*
         (1) Repeat dosage in a few minutes for total of 3 tablets if relief not obtained.
         (2) Note the time it takes for nitroglycerin to relieve pain.
         (3) Use nitroglycerin prophylactically to avoid pain known to occur with certain activities (sexual intercourse, stair climbing, exposure to cold).
         (4) Make certain that nitroglycerin is not inactivated.
            (a) Nitroglycerin inactivated by heat, moisture, air, light, time.
            (b) Keep in dark bottle; main supply should be refrigerated.
            (c) Renew supply every 6 months.
            (d) Do not carry nitroglycerin close to the body or in metal pill boxes.
         (5) Keep a record of number of tablets taken—to evaluate any change in anginal pattern.
      b. Take other medication as directed by physician.
   4. Stop smoking—smoking produces tachycardia and raises the blood pressure thus increasing work load of the heart.
   5. Reduce weight (if necessary)—to reduce cardiac work.
   6. Engage in a regular graded program of exercise—keep exercise below pain threshold.
   7. Change attitudes and living habits to adapt to life stresses.

Myocardial Infarction

Myocardial infarction is a process by which myocardial tissue is destroyed in regions of the heart that are deprived of their blood supply after closure of the coronary artery or one of its branches, either by a thrombus or by obstruction of the vessel lumen by atherosclerosis.[*]

Causes

1. Atherosclerotic heart disease
2. Hypertension
3. Diabetes

[*] See page 340, arteriosclerosis and atherosclerosis.

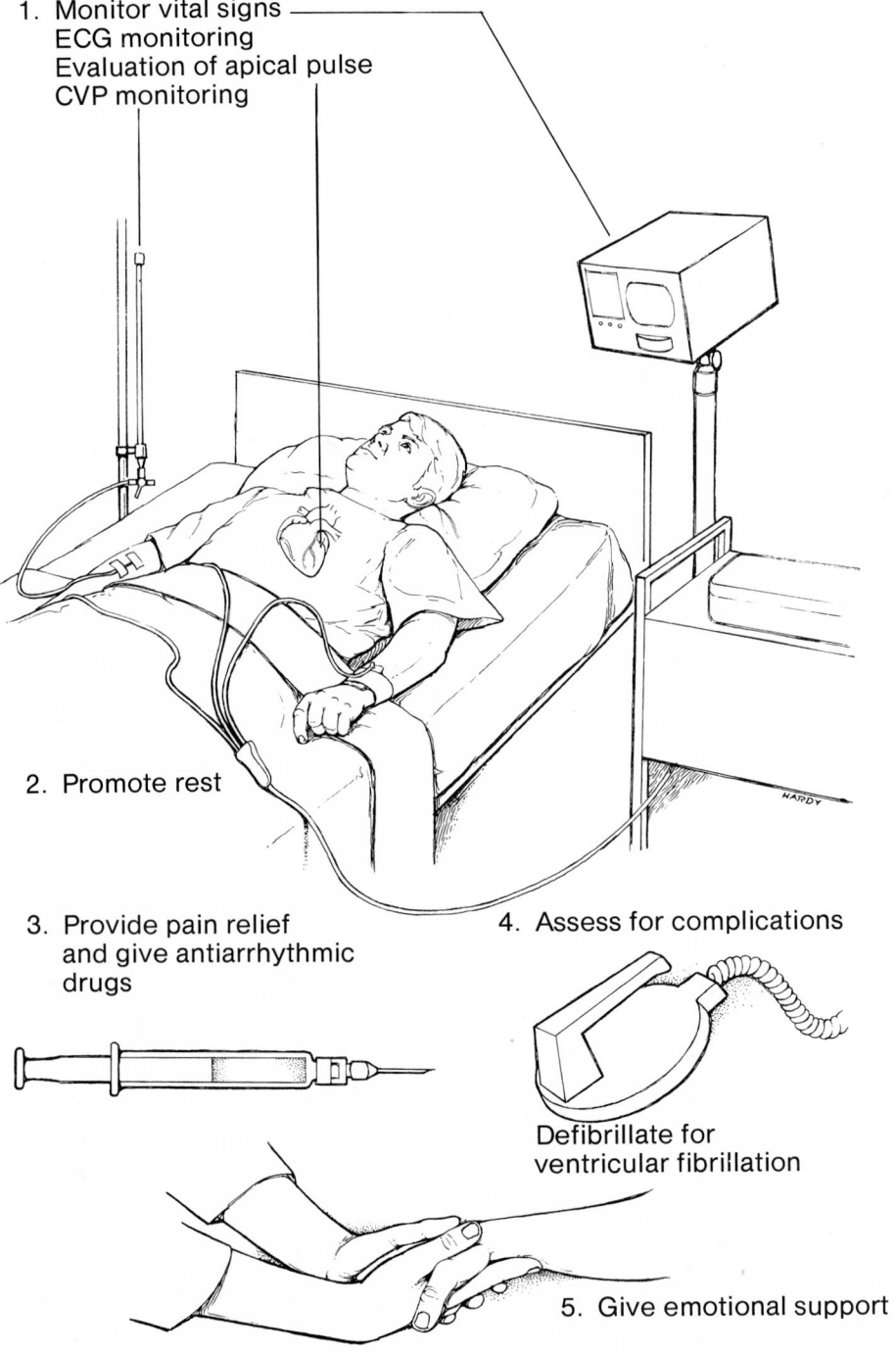

1. Monitor vital signs
   ECG monitoring
   Evaluation of apical pulse
   CVP monitoring

2. Promote rest

3. Provide pain relief
   and give antiarrhythmic
   drugs

4. Assess for complications

Defibrillate for
ventricular fibrillation

5. Give emotional support

Figure 5-8. Myocardial infarction.

Clinical Manifestations

1. Chest pain—steady, constrictive pain not relieved by rest or nitrites; pain may radiate widely
2. Profuse perspiration, moist clammy skin with pallor
3. Drop in blood pressure
4. Dyspnea, weakness and fainting
5. Nausea and vomiting
6. Tachycardia or bradycardia

NURSING ALERT: Many patients do not have symptoms; these are the "silent coronaries." Nevertheless there is still resultant damage to the myocardium.

Objectives of Treatment and Nursing Management (Fig. 5-8)

A. *To provide constant nursing surveillance during the critical phase of the illness.*
   1. Measure and record vital signs—to determine the presence of impending complications, especially arrhythmia and shock.
      a. Assess both radial and apical pulse rates—tachycardia, bradycardia and pulse deficits indicate impending arrhythmias.
      b. Count respirations—tachypnea indicates congestive failure, pulmonary embolism.
      c. Evaluate blood pressure—low arterial blood pressure is an indicator of shock which is a dangerous complication in acute myocardial infarction.
      d. Attach ECG monitoring electrodes—a myocardial infarction produces distinctive ECG changes (pathological Q waves or loss of R-wave potential).
      e. Monitor the central venous pressure of an acutely ill patient (see p. 241)—central venous pressure reflects the state of the intravascular blood volume and the competence of the right ventricle. It indicates impending shock and assesses the patient's response to therapy.
   2. Relieve the patient's pain and anxiety—anxiety increases the heart rate, raises the blood pressure and causes the adrenal glands to release epinephrine which may produce an arrhythmia.
      a. Give analgesic medication within prescribed limits.
      b. Monitor the blood pressure, pulse and respiratory rate before administering narcotics—narcotics depress arterial pressure and may contribute to the development of shock.
      c. Give humidified oxygen inhalations—to supply oxygen to hypoxic heart muscle.
      d. Offer intelligent reassurance and endeavor to assist the patient to establish a positive attitude toward his illness.

B. *To be alert for developing complications.*
   1. Know the signs of deficient peripheral blood flow which causes cardiogenic shock.
      a. Reduced blood pressure
      b. Reduction of urinary output (30 ml./hour or less)
      c. Cool moist skin; may be peripheral cyanosis—from systemic vasoconstriction caused by reduction in cardiac output
      d. Restlessness, apathy, lessening of responsiveness—inadequate cerebral perfusion
      e. Metabolic acidosis (low arterial pH, low pCO_2 and elevated blood lactate concentration—poor tissue perfusion and tissue hypoxia)
   2. Be alert for arrhythmias, thromboembolism, congestive heart failure.

C. *To increase the blood flow to the vital organs if the patient is in cardiogenic shock.*
   1. Give plasma volume expanders intravenously (Dextran) if central venous pressure is not elevated and if the patient's condition indicates.
   2. Give vasoconstrictor drugs (norepinephrine; metaraminol)—to raise aortic pressure if patient is hypotensive.
      a. Drugs given in 500 ml. of 5% dextrose.
      b. Adjust rate of flow according to patient's blood pressure response—usually enough to raise systolic pressure to 100 mm. Hg.
   3. Give vasodilator drugs if peripheral blood flow is reduced and arterial blood pressure is not low—to promote increased blood flow by decreasing vasoconstriction.
      a. Give isoproterenol when prescribed.
      b. Monitor arterial pressure to prevent severe hypotension.
   4. Give antiarrhythmia agents—serious arrhythmias may follow myocardial infarction.
      a. Give I.V. lidocaine—avoid cardiac depressant effect of large doses.
      b. Prepare patient for transvenous pacing if his condition indicates. (See p. 258.)

D. *To make critical observations about the patient's physiological status and his response to therapy.*
   1. Watch the ECG monitor—this provides the constant information needed for optimal arrhythmia prevention and treatment.
   2. Monitor the urine output hourly—rate of urine formation reflects status of patient.
      a. Measure urine osmolarity—an indicator of changing fluid status.
         (1) Urine osmolarity levels exceeding 700 mOsm—marked concentration; reveals fluid deprivation.
         (2) Urine osmolarity levels at 275–350 mOsm—isomolar urine; indicates neither concentration nor dilution of urine.
         (3) Urine osmolarity levels less than 200 mOsm—excretion of excess water; usually a desirable renal response.
      b. Give furosemide as ordered intravenously—to maintain urinary output over 30 ml. hourly.
   3. Palpate the radial, carotid and femoral pulses—to note their *quality* especially if auscultatory blood pressure readings are difficult to obtain.
   4. Evaluate for restlessness and anxiety—may be prodromal signs of shock.
   5. Be alert for waxing and waning ischemic chest pain.
   6. Assist with the measurement of arterial blood gases—to determine arterial oxygen saturation.
   7. Watch for signs of dyspnea, cough, rhonchi or rales—premonitory signs of congestive heart failure.

E. *To provide nursing support through the patient's convalescence.*
   1. Avoid sudden physical effort.
   2. Assist patient to bedside commode.
   3. Give diet as tolerated—depending on patient's circulatory status.
      a. Restrict sodium.
      b. Avoid iced drinks—ingestion of cold fluids may trigger an arrhythmia.
   4. Assist the patient to make the modifications in his life style consistent with long-term rehabilitation goals.
      a. Avoid physiologic and psychogenic stresses.
      b. Encourage active motion of all joints as condition permits—especially put shoulder girdle muscles through range of motion to prevent anterior chest wall pain.

c. Plan a program of daily graded exercise—to stimulate the development of collateral circulation.

5. Prepare patient for myocardial revascularization procedure if he is a candidate.
   a. Coronary artery by-pass procedures are used for patients with coronary occlusive disease and angina pectoris that is refractory to treatment.
      (1) Direct anastomosis of reversed segments of saphenous vein between the ascending aorta and the patent segments of one or more of the 3 major arteries.
      (2) Anastomosis of the internal mammary artery directly into the coronary arterial bed.
   b. See page 284 for care of the patient having heart surgery.

ENDOCARDIAL DISEASE

Endocarditis is an exudative and proliferative inflammatory alteration of the endocardium (inner lining of the heart).

Infectious endocarditis (bacterial endocarditis) is an infection of the valves and inner lining of the heart caused by direct invasion of bacteria leading to deformity of the valve leaflets.

Etiology

1. Bacteria—streptococcus (majority caused by *Streptococcus viridans*), enterococci (10%), pneumococcus, staphylococcus
2. Other organisms—fungi and Rickettsia

Characteristics

1. Infectious endocarditis usually develops on a cardiac valve already injured by other disease (rheumatic fever and congenital defects) or on abnormally vascularized valves.
2. Rheumatic fever precedes infectious endocarditis in the majority of cases.
3. May follow cardiac surgery—especially when prosthetic devices (valves) are used.

Altered Physiology

1. Characterized by bacteria lodging on endocardium of valves (usually mitral and aortic). The bacteria multiply—fibrin and platelet thrombi are deposited, forming vegetations (verrucae). The vegetations on the affected endocardial surface may embolize to various organs and tissues.
2. Embolization may occur to spleen, kidney, central nervous system and lungs. Observe patient for petechiae of skin and mucous membranes.

Clinical Manifestations

Nonspecific; develop from destruction of heart valves, from embolization of fragments of vegetations and from toxicity of the infection.

1. Fever
   a. Intermittent, irregular, mild
   b. May be absent in patients receiving antibiotics or corticosteroids, the elderly or patient with congestive heart failure or uremia
2. Chills, diaphoresis
3. Anorexia, weight loss

    4. Petechiae—located in mucous membranes of mouth
    5. Anemia
    6. Heart murmur (apical, systolic)

Diagnostic Evaluation

    1. Blood culture—serial blood cultures are drawn to document the presence of continuous bacteremia and to determine etiologic agent.
    2. Sensitivity studies—to determine the antibiotic for treatment.
    3. Determination of serum bactericidal level of antibiotic—patient's serum containing the administered antibiotic is titered against the causative organism; helps determine the optimum dosage of antibiotic.

Treatment and Nursing Management

    1. Treat with bactericidal (capable of destroying bacteria) antibiotic.
       a. Penicillin G (drug of choice)—20 million to 40 million units I.V. daily.
       b. Methicillin, oxacillin, ampicillin or streptomycin—given when patient cannot tolerate penicillin because of hypersensitivity reactions.
       c. Intravenous route usually used for long-term administration of parenteral antibiotics.
       d. Adequate dosages are necessary—to kill every organism in every vegetation.
       e. Patient usually hospitalized 4 to 8 weeks—cure of infectious endocarditis depends on adequate dosages of antibiotic.
       f. Blood culture taken periodically—to monitor efficiency of therapy.
    2. Take temperature at regular intervals—course of fever is evaluated to determine effectiveness of treatment.
    3. Give supportive care for possible complications.
       a. Persistence of fever from:
          (1) Inadequate antibiotic therapy
          (2) Drug sensitivities (especially to penicillin)
          (3) Superimposed infection on valves
          (4) Thrombophlebitis
       b. Embolism to other organ systems
          (1) Peripheral arterial emboli—hemiplegia or aphasia
          (2) Infarction of bowel, kidney, spleen
          (3) Acute arterial insufficiency to an extremity
       c. Congestive heart failure
       d. Renal involvement
    4. Educate the patient as to the necessity of follow-up visits to doctor or clinic—valve deformities caused by bacterial infection, healing and scarring are sequelae of infectious endocarditis.

Preventive Measures

    1. Give antibiotic prophylactically in susceptible patients (those with rheumatic or congenital heart disease) undergoing surgical procedures that cause transient bacteremia.
       a. Dental manipulations   d. Instrumentation of genitourinary tract
       b. Oral surgery   e. Surgery of lower intestinal tract
       c. Bronchoscopy   f. Childbirth
    2. Procaine penicillin (or erythromycin for penicillin-sensitive patient) is the drug of choice.

RHEUMATIC HEART DISEASE

Rheumatic heart disease is damage done to the heart, particularly the valves, by one or more attacks of rheumatic fever. There is valvular deformity with associated compensatory changes in the size of the heart chambers and the thickness of their walls.

Role of Streptococcal Infection

Rheumatic fever is a disease which is a sequelae of Group A streptococcal respiratory infection. Rheumatic fever is probably a sensitivity reaction precipitated by streptococci.

A. *Symptoms of Hemolytic Streptococcal Infection*
   1. Sudden onset of sore throat; throat reddened with exudate
   2. Swollen tender lymph nodes at angle of jaw
   3. Headache and fever

Nursing Alert: Some cases of streptococcal throat infection are relatively asymptomatic.

B. *Diagnostic Evaluation*
   Throat culture—to determine presence of streptococcal organisms
C. *Treatment of Streptococcal Infection*
   1. Penicillin G for 10 days—to eradicate streptococci
   2. Erythromycin for patients sensitive to penicillin

Clinical Manifestations of Rheumatic Fever

   1. Fever, rapid pulse
   2. Perspiration
   3. Polyarthritis
   4. Carditis
   5. Chorea (irregular, jerky, involuntary and unpredictable muscular movements)
   6. Subcutaneous nodules
   7. Erythema

Laboratory Evaluation

   1. Sedimentation rate—increases during acute phase of infection
   2. C-reactive protein—reveals rheumatic activity
   3. Antistreptolysin titer—an increase indicates infection

Treatment and Nursing Management

   1. Limit physical activity during the acute phase—patient should rest in bed as long as signs of active carditis are present.
   2. Eradicate hemolytic streptococcus—utilize penicillin therapy
      a. Procaine penicillin, 600,000 units, 1–2 times daily for 10 days.
      b. *Or* Benzathine penicillin, 900,000–1,200,000 units, single dose.
   3. Give salicylates or corticosteroids to suppress rheumatic activity by controlling toxic manifestations, lessening constitutional symptoms and improving well-being of patient.
      a. Salicylates
         (1) Give after meals—to reduce gastric irritation.
         (2) Give vitamins K and C—to prevent hemorrhage if large doses of salicylates are continued for long period.

(3) Assess for toxic signs of salicylates—nausea and vomiting, gastric distress, tinnitus, headache.
  b. Corticosteroid therapy—given for very ill patients with carditis
    (1) Steroids are started with large doses and decreased according to patient's clinical response.
    (2) Steroids must be withdrawn gradually—to prevent reappearance of signs and symptoms of acute rheumatic fever.
    (3) Sodium is restricted—retention of sodium and fluids and loss of potassium are apt to occur with steroid therapy.
4. Give liquid high carbohydrate diet during acute febrile period; diet is liberalized after fever subsides.
5. Instruct the patient that he will need continuous penicillin prophylactic therapy—to prevent streptococcal infections and the possibility of recurrent attacks of rheumatic fever.

Complications

1. Valvular deformities of the heart
2. Pericarditis or bacterial endocarditis
3. Congestive heart failure

MYOCARDITIS

Myocarditis is an inflammatory process involving the myocardium.

Etiology

Follows infection:
  Bacterial—beta hemolytic streptococcus
  Viral—Coxsackie group, influenza, viral pneumonia, mumps, infectious mononucleosis
  Mycotic—actinomycosis, blastomycosis, moniliasis
  Parasitic—trichinosis
  Protozoal—trypanosomiasis (Chagas' disease), malaria
  Spirochetal—syphilis

Clinical Manifestations

A. *Symptoms*
  1. Depend on type of infection, degree of myocardial damage, capacity of myocardium to recover and host resistance.
  2. Fatigue and dyspnea
  3. Palpitations
  4. Occasional precordial discomfort
B. *Clinical Findings*
  1. Cardiac enlargement
  2. Cardiac murmur—abnormal heart sound; sounds like fluid passing an obstruction
  3. Pericardial friction rub
  4. Gallop rhythm—a tripling or quadrupling of heart sounds resembling the galloping of a horse, heard upon auscultation

5. Pulsus alternans—a pulse in which there is regular alternation of weak and strong beats
6. Fever with tachycardia
7. Evidence of development of congestive heart failure

Treatment and Nursing Management

1. Give specific therapy for underlying disease. (Example: antibiotic for hemolytic streptococci)
2. Restrict physical activity—to reduce work load of heart.
   a. Prolonged bedrest may be required—until there is reduction in heart size and improvement of function.
   b. Assess for clinical evidence that disease is subsiding—evaluate pulse, heart sounds, temperature, etc.
3. Treat the symptoms of congestive heart failure (see p. 275).
   a. Restrict activity—to reduce systemic oxygen requirements.
   b. Give digitalis—augments myocardial contractility and slows heart rate.

> NURSING ALERT: Patients with myocarditis are sensitive to digitalis—assess for toxic symptoms (see p. 277).

   (1) Evaluate patient's pulse and apical rate for signs of tachycardia and gallop rhythm—indicates that congestive heart failure is recurring.
   (2) Evaluate for evidences of arrhythmia—*patients with myocarditis are prone to develop arrhythmias.*
      (a) See page 255 for management of arrhythmias.
      (b) Place patient in unit with continuous cardiac monitoring if evidences of an arrhythmia develop.
      (c) Have equipment for resuscitation, cardiac defibrillation and cardiac pacing available in event of life-threatening arrhythmia.
4. Watch for evidences of embolic phenomena—emboli from venous thrombosis and mural thrombi occur frequently.

PERICARDITIS

Pericarditis is an inflammation of the pericardium, the membranous sac enveloping the heart. *Pericardial effusion* is an outpouring of fluid into the pericardial cavity. *Constrictive pericarditis* is a condition in which there is a chronic inflammatory thickening of the pericardium compressing the heart so that it is unable to expand to normal size during diastole. The signs and symptoms are those of heart failure.

Etiology

1. Nonspecific:
   Usually occurs secondarily or as a complication of some other disease—uremia, metastatic tumors, etc.
2. Infection
   a. Bacteria—staphylococcus, meningococcus, streptococcus, pneumococcus, gonococcus (commonly follows rheumatic fever and pneumonia)

    b. Virus
    c. Fungus
    d. Tuberculosis
 3. Disorders of connective tissues and allergies—lupus erythematosus, periarteritis nodosa
 4. Myocardial infarction
 5. Neoplastic processes; following irradiation of mediastinal tumors
 6. Trauma

Clinical Manifestations

 1. Pain in anterior chest—may vary from mild to sharp and severe; located in precordial area—may be relieved by leaning forward
 2. Dyspnea—from compression of heart and surrounding thoracic structures
 3. Fever, sweating, chills—due to inflammation of pericardium
 4. Arrhythmias
 5. Pericardial friction rub—scratchy, grating or creaking sound
    Nursing implication: Listen with the diaphragm of stethoscope held tightly against the thorax.

Diagnostic Evaluation

Diagnostic roentgenogram—shows increase in heart size, bulging of lower part of cardiac silhouette. Pericardial fluid may cause roentgenographic changes.

NURSING ALERT: Normal pericardial sac contains less than 50 ml. of fluid; pericardial fluid may accumulate slowly to 100–150 ml. without noticeable symptoms. However, a rapidly developing effusion can cause decreased cardiac output and venous return producing *cardiac tamponade.* (See p. 243.)

Treatment and Nursing Management

 1. Utilize *anticipatory nursing.* Be alert to the possibility of cardiac tamponade. Intervention with pericardiocentesis (pericardial aspiration) is indicated immediately. (See p. 243.)
 2. Encourage the patient to remain on bedrest while he is having chest pain, fever and friction rub.
 3. Give medications as indicated.
    a. Meperidine or morphine—for pain relief during acute phase.
    b. Salicylates—to relieve pain and hasten reabsorption of fluid in patients with rheumatic pericarditis.
    c. Corticosteroids—to control symptoms, to hasten resolution of inflammatory process in the pericardium and to prevent recurring pericardial effusion.
    d. Isoniazid and streptomycin—for specific treatment of tuberculosis (producing pericarditis).
 4. Assist patient to increase his activity gradually—if pain, fever or friction rub appears, bedrest should be resumed.

ACQUIRED VALVULAR DISEASE OF THE HEART

Causes

1. Rheumatic fever
2. Congenital aortic stenosis
3. Traumatic lesions of aortic valve
4. Syphilis

Altered Physiology

1. Inflammatory process → thickening and retraction of valve cusps → fusion and shortening of chordae tendineae → inadequate closure of valve.
2. Mitral valve most commonly involved (85%) followed by aortic, tricuspid and pulmonary valves.
3. Patients with valvular disease usually develop congestive heart failure.

Diagnostic Evaluation

1. Chest x-ray—to determine size and shape of heart
2. Fluoroscopy—to detect intracardiac calcification
3. Cardiac catheterization
   a. To observe and record intracardiac pressure and oxygen saturation of blood in each heart chamber
   b. To receive information regarding presence of shunts
   c. To calculate cardiac output
4. ECG—to detect atrial and ventricular hypertrophy, myocardial infarction and to diagnose disturbances of rhythm
5. Angiography—used as part of diagnostic cardiac catheterization

Aortic Stenosis

Aortic stenosis is a narrowing of the orifice between the left ventricle and the aorta. The obstruction to the aortic outflow places a pressure load on the left ventricle resulting in hypertrophy and failure. It is often the result of rheumatic fever or arteriosclerosis.

Clinical Manifestations

1. Exertional dyspnea and fatigue
2. Slow pulse
3. Blood pressure variable; lower in severe cases
4. Loud rough systolic murmur over aortic area
5. Syncope
6. Angina pectoris
7. Symptoms of congestive heart failure

Treatment

1. Management of angina pectoris and congestive heart failure as outlined on pages 259 and 274.
2. Surgical intervention (See p. 284 for care of patient undergoing heart surgery.)
   a. Valvotomy (done mainly in children)
   b. Replacement of valves by prosthetic valves of synthetic material or homograft aortic valves

Aortic Insufficiency

Aortic insufficiency (regurgitation) is caused by inflammatory lesions that deform the flaps so that they fail to completely seal the aortic orifice during diastole. It usually follows endocarditis of the rheumatic type or bacterial type but occasionally is due to syphilis or congenital abnormality.

Clinical Manifestations

(Patient usually asymptomatic for long period)
1. Dyspnea—paroxysmal nocturnal dyspnea
2. Symptoms of congestive heart failure
3. Systolic murmurs at base and apex
4. Wide pulse pressure
5. Water-hammer pulse—large, strong pulse related to an increased rate of left ventricular pressure or to a large left ventricular stroke volume with decreased peripheral resistance.

Treatment

Surgical intervention—replacement of damaged valve with ball valve prosthesis.

Mitral Stenosis

Mitral stenosis is progressive thickening and contracture of valve cusps with narrowing of orifice and progressive obstruction to flow. It is almost always rheumatic in origin.

Clinical Manifestations

1. Dyspnea
2. Pulmonary congestion or hemoptysis, cough, orthopnea
3. Angina pectoris
4. Systemic embolism
5. Arrhythmias
6. Characteristic murmur—diastolic rumble on opening snap with an increased first sound

Treatment

1. Medical treatment
   a. Prevent rheumatic recurrences with antibiotic therapy.
   b. Treat the developing congestive failure—digitalis, sodium restriction, limitation of activity (p. 274).
   c. Control atrial fibrillation.
2. Surgical intervention
   a. Closed technique—mitral commissurotomy (valvotomy)—to rupture the fused commissures of the mitral valve.
   b. Open technique—replacement of mitral valve with prosthetic valve.

Mitral Insufficiency

Mitral insufficiency (regurgitation) is incompetence and distortion of the mitral valve. Valvular movement is more restricted than in mitral stenosis and valvular calcification is usually more extensive. It is almost always rheumatic in origin.

Treatment

Surgical intervention—replacement with prosthesis; either ball valve or disc type. This procedure is done when there is extensive calcification and destruction of the chordae tendineae.

Tricuspid Stenosis

Tricuspid stenosis is restriction of the tricuspid valve orifice from commissural fusion and fibrosis usually following rheumatic fever. (May be congenital.) It is commonly associated with diseases of the mitral valve.

Clinical Manifestations

1. Systemic venous hypertension
2. Symptoms of right-sided heart failure—edema, bloating
3. Diastolic murmur

Treatment

Patient may have mitral and aortic disease which must be corrected.
Valvuloplasty

Tricuspid Insufficiency

Tricuspid insufficiency results from fibrosis and contraction of the valve leaflets.

Clinical Manifestations

Right-sided heart failure
Edema, dyspnea, atrial fibrillation

Treatment

1. Surgical treatment of associated mitral valve disease
2. Tricuspid valvuloplasty

Pulmonary Valve Lesions

(See pediatric text, p. 1172.)

Treatment and Nursing Management of Valvular Diseases of the Heart

Treatment

1. Conventional medical treatment is employed until the patient shows progressive signs of heart decompensation and his life expectancy appears limited.
   a. Control of arrhythmias
   b. Treatment of congestive heart failure (See p. 277).
   c. Prevention of rheumatic occurrences by means of antibiotic therapy

2. Surgical intervention for valvular disease
   a. Replacement of diseased valve with prosthetic device.
      (1) Caged-ball or disc prostheses
      (2) Mitral valve replacement
      (3) Aortic valve replacement
   b. Reconstructive procedures
   c. Aortic valve homografts

Nursing Management

A. *Preoperative Care*
   1. Stop digitalis and diuretics at least 2 days before surgery—to avoid digitoxic arrhythmias precipitated by cardiopulmonary bypass.
   2. Administer vitamin K preoperatively—to return prothrombin time to normal.
   3. Obtain serum electrolytes, blood urea nitrogen, hemogram, ECG, chest x-rays—for base-line studies and for future comparisons.
   4. Give antibiotics (penicillin or penicillin substitute) if directed—thought to decrease incidence of postoperative endocarditis.
   5. See page 285 for other preoperative considerations.

B. *Postoperative Care*
   1. See page 286 for postoperative care of patient undergoing cardiac surgery.
   2. Begin anticoagulant therapy 5–7 days following insertion of valve prosthesis; this is continued indefinitely.
   3. Listen to the apical heart beat—expect to hear a delayed opening "click" following insertion of valve prosthesis.
      a. Evaluate for development of cardiac murmurs.
      b. Reassure the patient that the sound from his prosthesis is a normal one after this type of surgery.
   4. Antibiotics are given for approximately 1 month following valve replacement.
   5. Cardiac glycosides are usually given 3–6 months after valve replacement—to improve cardiac function and control arrhythmias.

CONGESTIVE HEART FAILURE

Heart failure is failure of the heart to pump an adequate amount of blood necessary for venous return and for the metabolic requirements of the body.

Congestive heart failure is the occurrence of circulatory congestion from decreased myocardial contractility resulting in inadequacy of cardiac output to maintain the blood flow to body organs and tissues.

Causes

1. Secondary to myocardial disease—myocardial infarction, myocarditis
2. Tachyarrhythmias, bradyarrhythmias
3. Pulmonary embolism
4. Hemorrhage and anemia
5. Anesthesia and surgery
6. Transfusions or infusions, corticosteroids, estrogens
7. Thyrotoxicosis

8. Pregnancy
9. Infections
10. Physical and emotional stress
11. Hypertension
12. Excessive sodium intake

Clinical Manifestations

(Patient usually has combination of symptoms; any system may be involved.)

A. *Left-sided Heart Failure*
1. Congestion occurs mainly in the lungs.
2. Fatigability—from insomnia, nocturia, dyspnea, cough, low cardiac output, catabolic effect of chronic failure
3. Dyspnea on exertion—paroxysmal nocturnal dyspnea (due to reabsorption of dependent edema that has developed during the day)—orthopnea
4. Cough—may be dry, unproductive; often occurring at night
5. Insomnia—often due to Cheyne-Stokes respiration
6. Hemoptysis
7. Restlessness (common in elderly)
8. Rales—usually present with pulmonary congestion; not a reliable sign of heart disease

B. *Right-sided Heart Failure*
1. Usually occurs relatively late
2. Unexplained weight gain
3. Upper abdominal pain—due to liver congestion when venous pressure increases
4. Nocturia—diuresis occurs at night with rest and improved cardiac output
5. Excessive sweating—from increased adrenergic activity
6. Weakness
7. Anorexia and nausea—from edema of the bowel
8. Pitting edema—becomes obvious only after retention of at least 4.5 kg. (10 pounds) of fluid

Complications

1. Intractable heart failure—patient becomes progressively refractory to therapy (not yielding to treatment)
2. Pulmonary infarction
3. Myocardial failure
4. Digitalis toxicity—from overdosage, decreased renal function and potassium depletion
5. Cardiac arrhythmias
6. Pneumonia

Diagnostic Evaluation

1. Cardiovascular findings
   a. Cardiomegaly (hypertrophy of the heart)—detected by physical examination and x-ray
   b. Ventricular or atrial gallop—heard on auscultation, ECG
   c. Rapid heart rate

      d. Development of pulsus alternans—detected by palpation or by use of blood pressure cuff
      e. Distended neck veins
      f. Hepatomegaly (enlargement of the liver)
  2. ECG
  3. X-ray—to evaluate heart size; show lung fields (for pleural effusion)
  4. Pulmonary function studies—may show depressed ventilatory function
  5. Liver function studies—altered from hepatic congestion

Medications

A. *Cardiac Glycosides* (Digitalis)
    1. *Drug Selection and Dosage*

CARDIAC GLYCOSIDES

| Cardiac Glycoside | Digitalizing Dose* | | Maintenance Dose* |
	Oral	Parenteral	Oral
Digitalis (whole leaf)	1000–1500 mg.	———	100 mg.
Digitoxin	1.2–1.5 mg.	1.2 mg.	0.1 mg.
Digoxin	1.5–3 mg.	0.75–1 mg.	0.25–0.75 mg.
Lanatoside C (Cedilanid)	6 mg.	———	1 mg.
Deslanoside (Cedilanid D)	———	1.2–1.8 mg. (6–8 ml.)	———
Acetyldigitoxin	1.6–2.4 mg.	1.8 mg.	0.1–0.2 mg.
Gitalin (Gitaligin)	4–6 mg.	———	0.5 mg.
Ouabain	———	0.25–0.5 mg.	———

* Review package insert before administering medication as dosage, sizes of tablets and ampules may change.

    2. *Underlying Principles*
      a. Increases force and efficiency of cardiac contractions
        (1) Increases cardiac output by enhancing force of contraction of ventricle.
        (2) Slows heart rate reflexly via the vagus.
        (3) Decreases right atrial pressure.
        (4) Decreases venous pressure.
        (5) Promotes diuresis—increasing circulation gives less time for sodium reabsorption—increases excretion of sodium and water.
      b. Slows the conduction of impulses through the AV node—prolongs refraction period of the node.
        (1) Prolongs PR interval.
        (2) Reduces ventricular rate.

3. *Clinical Uses*
   a. Congestive heart failure
   b. Atrial fibrillation
   c. Atrial flutter
   d. Supraventricular paroxysmal tachycardia
   e. Before cardiac surgery
4. *Nursing Considerations and Actions*

> NURSING ALERT: The incidence of digitalis toxicity is high because of the narrow margin between the therapeutic and toxic doses. Toxic effects do not always appear in a predictable manner.

   a. Watch for toxic effects—*arrhythmias* (most important toxic effect), *anorexia,* nausea, vomiting, bradycardia, headache and malaise.
   b. Assess clinical response of patient as to relief of symptoms (lessening dyspnea, orthopnea, rales, hepatomegaly, peripheral edema).
   c. Elderly patients tolerate digitalis therapy poorly—due to impaired renal function.
   d. Sensitivity to digitalis is increased in acute myocardial infarction.
   e. Potassium is given to overcome arrhythmias produced by digitalis toxicity.
   f. Assess for symptoms of electrolyte depletion—lassitude, apathy, mental confusion, anorexia, decreasing urinary output, azotemia—in patients taking digitalis.
   g. The following factor(s) may increase toxicity or decrease therapeutic usefulness:
      (1) Inadequate digitalis dose
      (2) Concurrent kidney disease
      (3) Level of potassium ions
      (4) Physiologic and emotional stresses
      (5) Diuretic therapy
      (6) Diarrhea
      (7) Loss of appetite

B. *Diuretics*—agents which increase the rate of urine flow.
   1. *Action of Diuretics*
      a. Dependent upon functionally active kidneys.
      b. Most diuretics interfere with reabsorption of electrolytes by kidney, promoting water loss secondarily.
   2. *Dosages*
      a. Determined by patient's daily weight, clinical signs and symptoms.
      b. Usually given in divided doses except for furosemide.
   3. Most commonly used diuretics
      See Table 5-2.

Treatment and Nursing Management

Objective: to reduce the cardiac load by:
      a. lessening the tissue demands for blood
      b. eliminating factors that stimulate the heart action.

A. *Rest*

Place the patient at rest—to reduce the work of the heart, increase the cardiac reserve, diminish blood pressure, decrease work of respiratory muscles and slow the heart rate.
   1. Ascertain the amount of activity that can be done without producing discomfort.
      a. Provide bedrest in semirecumbent position or in armchair in air conditioned room —this position reduces venous return to the heart and lungs, alleviates pulmonary congestion and reduces pressure on the diaphragm by the liver.
      b. Assess the patient's response to rest—are his symptoms alleviated?

TABLE 5-2. FREQUENTLY USED DIURETICS

Diuretic Agent	Actions and Uses	Nursing Considerations
Thiazides Chlorothiazide (Diuril) Hydrochlorothiazide (HydroDiuril, Esidrix, Oretic) Flumethiazide (Ademol) Benzthiazide (ExNa) Hydroflumethiazide (Saluron) Bendroflumethiazide (Naturetin)	Most widely used diuretics. Used in treatment of edema and congestive heart failure, retention of sodium due to steroid therapy. Act in the proximal tubules to inhibit sodium, chloride and water reabsorption.	Watch for side effects from electrolyte imbalance — hypokalemia (weakness). May cause mild gastrointestinal symptoms: nausea, vomiting, diarrhea. Assess patient for dizziness, paresthesias. Give supplementary potassium (potassium chloride syrup 3 times daily). NURSING ALERT: Give potassium chloride syrup well diluted; concentrated solutions may produce lesions of the intestines. Thiazides may precipitate an attack of gout or accentuate hyperglycemia in the diabetic.
Potassium-sparing Diuretics Spironolactone (Aldactone)	Inhibits action of aldosterone in distal tubule and reduces reabsorption of sodium and chloride. Gives gradual diuretic effect. Used in treatment of cirrhosis and edema when other diuretics are toxic or ineffective.	Spironolactone is usually given in combination with a thiazide diuretic. Watch for side effects—skin rash, gynecomastia.
Triamterene (Dyrenium)	Appears to interfere with the exchange of sodium, potassium and hydrogen in the distal tubule. Usually used as an adjunct to thiazide therapy.	Triamterene may cause elevation in blood urea. Watch for nausea, vomiting, mild diarrhea, weakness, headache, skin rash.
Sulfonamide Derivatives Chlorthalidone (Hygroton) Quinethazone (Hydromox)	Less potent than thiazides. Has a relatively prolonged diuretic action; 2–3 days.	Chlorthalidone can cause hypokalemia and hypochloremic alkalosis. Chlorthalidone therapy may precipitate an acute attack of gout.
Mercurial Diuretics Meralluride sodium with theophylline (Mercuhydrin) Mercaptomerin sodium (Thiomerin) Mercurophylline (Mercuxanthin)	Mercurial diuretics have been largely replaced by thiazides. Act on proximal tubules to produce sodium diuresis with limited depletion of potassium. Reserved for patients with severe dyspnea or massive edema who require profuse diuresis or those who do not respond to thiazides.	Mercurials are given intramuscularly. Watch for symptoms of chloride depletion—weakness, apathy, somnolence, disorientation, delirium.

TABLE 5-2. FREQUENTLY USED DIURETICS (continued)

Diuretic Agent	Actions and Uses	Nursing Considerations
Potent Diuretics Furosemide (Lasix)	Usually reserved for patients who do not respond to thiazide diuretics. Blocks the reabsorption of sodium and water in proximal renal tubule and interferes with reabsorption of sodium in ascending limb of loop of Henle and in the most proximal portion of the distal tubule.	Acts almost immediately when given by I.V. May produce *profound diuresis.* Watch for nausea, vomiting, diarrhea, skin rash, pruritus, blurring of vision, postural hypotension.
Ethacrynic Acid (Edecrin)	Blocks the reabsorption of sodium within ascending limb of loop of Henle.	Ethacrynic acid causes rapid electrolyte and fluid loss resulting in excessive dehydration, hypokalemia and hypotension. Watch for nausea, vomiting, diarrhea, *deafness,* metabolic acidosis, precipitation of gout. Maximum activity is reached in 2 hours; diuresis persists 6–8 hours.

2. Provide for rest and sleep—patients with congestive heart failure have a tendency to be restless at night from cerebral hypoxia with superimposed nitrogen retention.
   a. Give oxygen during acute stage—to diminish work of breathing and increase the comfort of the patient.
   b. Give appropriate sedation—to relieve insomnia and restlessness.
      (1) Give small doses of morphine (per order) for extreme dyspnea.
      (2) Give chloral hydrate (0.5–1 gm.) as needed for sleep.
   c. Raise head of bed 20–25 cm. (8–10 inches) on blocks.
   d. Keep a night light on in the room.
3. Increase the patient's activities gradually.
   a. Alter or modify patient's activities—to keep within the limits of his cardiac reserve.
   b. Observe the pulse response to increased activities.
4. Observe for the complications of bedrest—phlebothrombosis and pulmonary embolism.
   a. Encourage patient to do deep breathing and leg exercises—improves muscle tone, aids in venous return to the heart.
   b. Use bedside commode—to avoid straining at the stool which may precipitate a pulmonary embolism.
   c. Utilize sedatives carefully—to prevent respiratory depression, immobility of patient and delayed detoxification of drugs due to hepatic congestion.
5. Provide for psychological rest—emotional stress may produce changes in pulse rate, stroke volume, cardiac output, peripheral resistance, salt and water metabolism.
   a. Offer careful explanations and answers to patient's questions.
   b. Give intelligent and reasonable reassurance.

B. *Drug Therapy*

DIGITALIS

Administer digitalis (see p. 276)—to increase the force of myocardial contraction and produce a stronger systolic contraction of the heart and slow the heart rate, resulting in increased cardiac output, decreased venous pressure and blood volume and diuresis, thereby relieving edema.

1. *Principles underlying digitalis therapy*
   a. The initial saturating dose is given to digitalize the patient—this is done until the first toxic symptoms appear.
   b. The patient is then given a daily dose just adequate to replace the drug that is destroyed or excreted (minimal effective dose)—to maintain digitalis effect without toxicity.
2. Take apical pulse rate before administering digitalis.
3. Withhold digitalis if patient develops anorexia, cardiac arrhythmias, (bradycardia, premature ventricular contractions, bigeminy, atrial fibrillation, etc.)
4. Give *written instructions* to the elderly patient (and his family) concerning digitalis administration.
5. Make sure the patient has a check-off system that will show whether or not he has taken his medication.
6. Assess the patient for symptoms of digitalis intoxication.
   a. *Anorexia,* nausea, vomiting (early symptoms)
   b. Alterations in heart rate and rhythm (arrhythmias)
   c. Headache, fatigue, malaise, drowsiness
   d. Blurred vision

DIURETIC

1. Give prescribed diuretic—to promote excretion of sodium and water through the kidneys (see Table 5-2).
2. Give diuretic early in the morning.
3. Keep input and output record as directed—patient may lose large volume of fluid after a single dose of diuretic.
4. Weigh patient daily—to determine if edema is being controlled.
5. Assess for weakness, malaise, muscle cramps—diuretic therapy may produce hypovolemia and electrolyte depletion, namely hypokalemia.

C. *Diet*

1. Give the prescribed low sodium diet (Table 5-3)—to rid the body of extracellular fluid retention.
2. Teach the patient the importance of adhering to the low sodium diet.
   a. Sodium is present in all foods in varying amounts
   b. Moderate sodium restriction—about 3 gm. of sodium daily
   c. Severe sodium restriction—about 0.5–1 gm. of sodium daily
3. Make the diet as palatable as possible.
   a. Use flavorings, spices, herbs and lemon juice.
   b. Avoid salt substitutes in the presence of renal disease.
4. Offer small frequent feedings—to avoid excessive gastric filling and abdominal distention with subsequent elevation of diaphragm that causes decrease in lung capacity.
5. Teach the patient to rinse the mouth well after using tooth cleansers and mouthwashes—some of these contain large amounts of sodium.
6. Teach the patient that sodium is present in alkalizers, cough remedies, laxatives, pain relievers, etc.
7. Give the patient written dietary instructions.

TABLE 5-3. SODIUM-RESTRICTED DIET*
(500 mg.; 1800 calories)†

Category	Allowed	To be Avoided
Dairy Products		
Milk	2 glasses	Salt or monosodium glutamate
Cheese	¼ cup unsalted cottage cheese 1 ounce low sodium dietetic cheese	Ice cream Sherbet
Fat		Malted milk
	Unsalted butter or margarine	Milk shakes
	Unsalted cooking fat or oil	Chocolate milk
	Unsalted French dressing	Condensed milk
	Unsalted mayonnaise	
	Unsalted nuts	Regular butter or margarine
	Heavy or light cream	Commercial salad dressing
		Bacon or bacon fat
Eggs	1 egg daily	Olives
		Salted nuts
		Party spreads and dips
Meats, Fish, Fowl	Fresh, frozen or dietetic canned meat or poultry; beef, lamb, pork, veal, fresh tongue, liver, chicken, duck, turkey, rabbit Fresh or dietetic canned (not frozen) fish	Brains or kidneys Canned, salted or smoked meat (Bacon, bologna, corn or chipped beef, frankfurters, ham, meats koshered by salting, luncheon meats, salt pork, sausage, smoked tongue) Frozen fish fillets, canned, salted or smoked fish, canned tuna or salmon Shellfish—clams, crabs, lobsters, oysters, scallops, shrimp, etc.
Vegetables	Fresh, frozen or canned dietary vegetables except those listed	Canned vegetables or vegetable juices unless they are low sodium dietetic Frozen vegetables if processed with salt Artichokes, beet greens, beets, carrots, celery, chard, dandelion greens, whole hominy, kale, mustard greens, sauerkraut, spinach, white turnips
Fruits	Any fruit or fruit juice (if sugar has not been added)	Fruits canned or frozen in sugar (because of the extra calories)

* From Sodium-restricted Diet, 500 mg. American Heart Association.

† For a 250-mg. sodium diet, use low sodium milk (either low sodium whole milk or low sodium powdered milk) instead of regular milk.

For 1000-mg. sodium diet, follow 500-mg. sodium diet, plus 1 of the following for the additional 500 mg. of sodium.

¼ teaspoon salt (scant)	Average serving of cooked cereal, rice, spaghetti, noodles, hominy, etc. seasoned with salt
¾ teaspoon monosodium glutamate	1 cup drained sauerkraut
½ bouillon cube	1 average frankfurter
1 cup tomato juice	1½ ounces ham

TABLE 5-3. SODIUM-RESTRICTED DIET
(500 mg.; 1800 calories)† (continued)

Category	Allowed	To be Avoided
Breads, Cereals, Cereal Products	Low sodium bread, rolls, crackers Dry cereals (puffed rice, puffed wheat, shredded wheat) Plain unsalted matza Unsalted melba toast Macaroni or noodles Spaghetti, rice, barley Unsalted popcorn Flour	Regular breads, crackers Commercial mixes Cooked cereals containing a sodium compound Dry cereals other than those listed or those having more than 6 mg. of sodium in 100 gm. of cereal Self-rising cornmeal or self-rising flour Potato chips Pretzels Salted popcorn
Miscellaneous	Coffee, tea, coffee substitutes, lemons, limes, plain unflavored gelatin, vinegar, cream of tartar, potassium bicarbonate, sodium-free baking powder, yeast	Instant cocoa mixes, other beverage mixes, including fruit-flavored powders, fountain beverages, including malted milk, soft drinks (both regular and low calorie), any kind of commercial bouillon (cubes, powders or liquids), sodium cyclamate and sodium saccharin, commercial candies, commercial gelatin desserts, regular baking powder, baking soda (sodium bicarbonate), rennet tablets, molasses, pudding mixes

Patient Teaching

Teach the patient measures to prevent recurrence of congestive heart failure.
1. Take the digitalis *exactly* as prescribed.
2. Stay on the sodium-restricted diet.
3. Set up a regularly scheduled program of rest.
4. Treat all infections promptly.
5. Adhere to the program of diuretic therapy.

ACUTE PULMONARY EDEMA

Acute pulmonary edema is a dramatic event characterized by sudden and rapid transudation of fluid from the pulmonary capillaries into the alveoli, usually following acute left ventricular failure.

> NURSING ALERT: Acute pulmonary edema is a true medical emergency as it is a life-threatening syndrome.

Causes

1. Acute left ventricular failure
2. Congestive heart failure
3. Circulatory overload—intravenous infusions, blood transfusions
4. Central nervous system injuries
5. Mitral valve disease
6. Infection and fever

Clinical Manifestations

1. Coughing and restlessness during sleep (premonitory symptoms)
2. Extreme dyspnea and orthopnea—patient usually uses accessory muscles of respiration
3. Cough with varying amounts of white or pink-tinged frothy sputum
4. Extreme anxiety and panic
5. Noisy breathing—inspiratory and expiratory wheezing and bubbling sounds
6. Cyanosis with profuse perspiration
7. Rapid pulse

Treatment and Nursing Management*

Objective: to reduce transudation of fluid into alveoli by:

   a. reducing right atrial inflow of systemic venous blood
   b. increasing left ventricular output

1. Take steps to reduce the right atrial inflow of systemic venous blood (retard venous return).
   a. Place patient in upright orthopneic position, head and shoulders up, feet and legs down—to favor pooling of blood in dependent portions of body.
   b. Give morphine (10–15 mg.) every 2–4 hours—to allay the acute anxiety and decrease respiratory effort, thereby allowing better oxygen exchange and inducing sleep.
      (1) Morphine is *not* given if pulmonary edema is caused by cerebral vascular accident or occurs in the presence of chronic pulmonary disease or cardiogenic shock.
      (2) Watch for excessive respiratory depression.
      (3) Have morphine antagonist available—(naloxone hydrochloride, [Narcan]).
   c. Give oxygen in high concentration (100%)—to relieve hypoxia and dyspnea and to decrease pulmonary capillary permeability.
      (1) Oxygen must be given with high enough pressure to provide blood oxygenation and to overcome the pressure barrier of the edema fluid.
      (2) Oxygen may be given by slight IPPB (if shock is not present), by mask or by oropharyngeal catheter.
   d. Give injections of diuretics (ethacrynic acid, furosemide) I.V.—to reduce blood volume and pulmonary congestion by producing a prompt diuresis.
      (1) Insert an indwelling catheter.
      (2) Profuse diuresis may result 15 minutes after administration.
      (3) Watch for falling blood pressure, increasing heart rate and decreasing urinary output—indicates that the total circulation is not tolerating diuresis.
      (4) Watch for signs of urinary obstruction in patients with prostatic hypertrophy.
   e. Utilize rotating tourniquets (see p. 250)—to produce venous stasis in extremities thus reducing venous return to the heart.
      (1) Apply tourniquets to extremities.
      (2) Rotate tourniquets every 15 minutes.
      (3) Do not use tourniquets when patient is in shock.

* Many of these steps of management are carried out simultaneously or in as rapid a sequence as possible.

f. Utilize phlebotomy (rapid withdrawal of blood from a peripheral vein)—to decrease venous return and produce a corresponding decline in right ventricular output. Phlebotomy is usually done if attack is precipitated by overadministration of blood or infusion fluids.

Save the blood as it may be needed in treatment of shock if there has been extensive infarction.

g. Stay with the patient and show a confident attitude—presence of another person is therapeutic as the acute anxiety of the patient tends to intensify the severity of his condition. (Arterial vasoconstriction diminishes as anxiety is relieved.)

2. Increase left ventricular output.
   a. Give a rapid-acting digitalis preparation intravenously (ouabain, lanatoside C)—improves strength of cardiac contraction and cardiac stroke output.

Exercise extreme care in giving digitalis to previously digitalized patient.

   b. Administer aminophylline—to decrease bronchospasm and increase cardiac output.
      (1) Give aminophylline very slowly intravenously—syncope and sudden death may follow too rapid administration.
      (2) Watch for falling blood pressure—may be a dangerous complication.

NURSING ALERT: Use extreme care in transfusing or infusing elderly or cardiac patients.

3. Educate the patient as follows in order to prevent recurrences of pulmonary edema
   a. Restrict sodium.
   b. Take diuretics and digitalis exactly as directed.
   c. Sleep with head elevated (on 10-inch blocks).
   d. Avoid excessive and sudden physical exertion.
   e. Weigh daily—to determine need for additional diuresis.
   f. Treat all infections promptly with antibiotics.

HEART SURGERY

Cardiac Conditions Requiring Surgery

(Surgical procedures have been established for the following conditions:)*

A. *Congenital Disease of the Heart and Great Vessels*

Patent ductus arteriosus†
Coarctation of aorta†
Atrial septal defect (secundum)
Atrial septal defect (primum)
Ventricular septal defect
Endocardial cushion defect
Tetralogy of Fallot
Valvar pulmonic stenosis
Valvar aortic stenosis
Subvalvar aortic stenosis
Transposition of great vessels
Tricuspid atresia
Truncus arteriosus
Aortic septal defect
Aortic vascular ring†
Mitral stenosis
Mitral insufficiency
Congenital origin of left coronary artery from pulmonary artery
Coronary arteriovenous fistula

* Adapted from Report of Inter-society Commission for Heart Disease Resources. Circulation, 44:228, Sept. 1971. By permission of the American Heart Association.
† Ordinarily, cardiopulmonary bypass is not required.

B. *Acquired Disease of the Heart and Great Vessels*

Mitral stenosis	Direct myocardial trauma
Mitral regurgitation	Traumatic rupture of aorta
Aortic stenosis	Saccular thoracic aneurysm
Aortic regurgitation	Fusiform thoracic aneurysm
Constrictive pericarditis*	Dissecting aortic aneurysm
Heart block*	Aorto-coronary sinus fistula
Coronary artery occlusive disease	Tricuspid stenosis
Ventricular aneurysm	Aneurysm sinus of Valsalva
Acute ventricular septal defect	Massive pulmonary embolism

Preoperative Nursing Management

1. Bring the patient to the peak of his physical and psychological capabilities.
2. Support the patient undergoing diagnostic studies to determine the type and severity of specific lesions. (Also serves as a base line for postoperative evaluation.)
   a. Cardiac catheterization   d. Electrocardiogram
   b. Angiography   e. Chest roentgenogram
   c. Pulmonary function
3. Assess hematological (blood) status.
   a. Complete blood count
   b. Antibody screen
   c. Preoperative coagulation survey (coagulation time, plasma prothrombin time, serum prothrombin time, platelet count)—extracorporeal circulation will affect certain coagulation factors.
      (1) Patients with congestive failure may have decreased prothrombin time—from hepatic congestion.
      (2) Patients with cyanotic heart disease may have increased amounts of platelets and fibrinogen.
4. Evaluate patient's emotional tenor and try to reduce his anxieties—patients undergoing heart surgery are more anxious and fearful than other surgical patients.
   a. Encourage the patient to express what he feels and thinks.
   b. Help the patient to mobilize his defenses and cope with his fears.
   c. Clarify the information previously given him by the cardiovascular surgeon.
   d. Anticipate and answer the patient's questions.
      (1) Ask the patient what he *wants* to know.
      (2) Establish a relationship of trust.
   e. Reinforce and accelerate education of patient as day of operation approaches.
   f. Expect some patients to have psychological and psychiatric problems from prolonged illness.
5. Teach effective deep breathing and cough routine.
6. Know the preoperative conditions which predispose to postoperative respiratory complications.
   a. Pulmonary hypertension   d. Pulmonary sepsis
   b. Pulmonary congestion or edema   e. Elderly or debilitated patient
   c. Pre-existing lung disease
7. Encourage the patient to stop smoking—smoking increases incidence of postoperative respiratory complications.

---

* Ordinarily, cardiopulmonary bypass not required.

8. Assess the patient's reactions to medications—these patients are usually on multiple drugs.
   a. Digitalis
      (1) Patient may be receiving large doses to improve myocardial contractility.
      (2) Drug may be stopped several days before surgery—to avoid digitoxic arrhythmias from cardiopulmonary bypass.
   b. Diuretics
      (1) Assess patient for potassium depletion and volume depletion (weakness, postural hypotension)—all diuretics produce potassium loss, and severe diuresis may cause a decrease in blood volume.
      (2) Give potassium supplement if patient is on prolonged diuretic therapy—to replete body stores.
      (3) Determine if patient has taken corticosteroids or reserpine within a year prior to surgery.
      (4) Question if patient has any drug sensitivities—especially to antibiotics, opiates and sedatives.
      (5) Have the patient keep a written record of his weight several weeks before surgery.
9. Keep the patient as active as possible preoperatively.
10. Notify the blood bank of anticipated needs—open heart surgery may require 15–20 units of fresh whole heparinized blood.

Postoperative Nursing Management

1. Evaluate the patient closely and continuously to prevent complications.
2. Employ physiologic monitoring* during immediate postoperative period. Patient is usually in intensive unit 48–72 hours.
   a. Intra-arterial pressure—to determine cardiovascular status. Residual vasoconstriction following extracorporeal circulation makes blood pressure auscultation unreliable. Blood pressure is the most important physiological parameter to follow.
   b. Central venous pressure (see p. 241)—indicates blood volume and cardiac performance.
   c. Weight and intake and output—to determine patient's fluid requirements.
   d. Urine output (urinary output recorded every ½–1 hour)—an index of adequacy of cardiac output and peripheral perfusion.
   e. Serial hematocrit, serum electrolytes (sodium, potassium, carbon dioxide and chloride), BUN—metabolic acidosis and electrolyte imbalance can occur after use of pump oxygenator.
   f. ECG monitoring—cardiac arrhythmias frequently occur after heart surgery; low cardiac output is dangerous.
   g. Daily chest x-ray—to evaluate presence of hemothorax, pleural effusion, atelectasis, state of lung expansion, presence or absence of pulmonary vascular congestion.
3. Assure adequate oxygenation in the early postoperative period. Respiratory insufficiency is common following open heart surgery.
   a. Employ assisted or controlled ventilation (endotracheal or nasotracheal tube)—

* Monitoring equipment is valuable only when it is understood and used correctly. The clinical assessment of the patient by the nurse is indispensable to patient care.

adequacy of assisted ventilation is assessed by patient's clinical status and by direct measurement of tidal volume and blood gases.

b. Remove tracheobronchial secretions carefully (see p. 115)—prolonged aspiration leads to hypoxia and possible cardiac arrest.

c. Promote coughing, deep breathing and turning.

d. Monitor arterial blood gases.

e. Ventilate with supplemental oxygen.

f. Prepare for tracheostomy if assisted ventilation must be prolonged.

g. Administer digitalis and diuretics—trauma of operation may produce mild ventricular failure.

h. Restrict fluids (per order) for first few postoperative days—danger of pulmonary congestion from excessive fluid intake.

4. Assess for cardiac failure (low cardiac output syndrome). Following cardiovascular surgery the cardiac output may decrease. Low cardiac output causes deficient blood perfusion to different organs.

  a. Inspect patient for:

    (1) Cool, slightly cyanotic skin

    (2) Constricted or collapsed veins on back of hand

    (3) Restlessness or lethargy

    (4) Reduced arterial blood pressure

    (5) Diminished urinary output (less than 30 ml. of urine/hour)

  b. Treatment of cardiac failure

    (1) Give infusions to elevate central venous pressure.

    (2) Correct acidosis with infusion of sodium bicarbonate (50–200 mEq.).

    (3) Give cardiac inotropic drugs (norepinephrine, metaraminol) carefully.

    (4) Administer oxygen by mask or use artificial ventilation if respiratory insufficiency continues.

5. Assess for bleeding syndromes and hemorrhage. Blood clotting mechanisms are usually transitory following cardiopulmonary bypass; however, a significant platelet deficiency is usually present.

  a. Evaluate for presence of *cardiac tamponade* (see p. 243)—may occur in association with persistent excessive bleeding and malfunction of chest tube drainage.

  b. Give aminocaproic acid (Amicar) following bypass—to neutralize fibrinolytic activity.

  c. Watch for steady and continuous drainage of blood (100 ml. or more/hour for 3 hours).

    (1) Measure total amount and *rate* of drainage.

    (2) Transfuse patient with appropriate amounts of blood when indicated.

    (3) Some blood loss is to be expected after cardiac surgery.

  d. Watch oscillation (fluctuation) of chest tube (see p. 150). Freely fluctuating tube indicates that clotted blood is not collecting in thorax and that the tube is patent. Abrupt cessation of chest drainage suggests obstruction of chest tube.

6. Evaluate for sudden life-threatening arrhythmias—from hypoxia or hypercapnia, myocardial infarction, metabolic acidosis, hypokalemia, restlessness and pain. Patients with advanced myocardial disease or potassium depletion are more apt to develop arrhythmias but any arrhythmia may arise following cardiac surgery.

  a. Monitor patient constantly on ECG oscilloscope 2–3 days following surgery.

  b. Watch for ventricular extrasystoles—may be prodromal sign of bigeminy, ventricular tachycardia or ventricular fibrillation.

    c. Keep patient on controlled postoperative ventilation and monitor arterial blood gases—to prevent respiratory acidosis and arterial hypoxemia.

    d. Sedate patient adequately—to help patient tolerate endotracheal tube and cope with ventilatory sensations and to reduce his fear.

    e. Prevent metabolic acidosis by administering sodium bicarbonate or THAM.

    f. Maintain serum potassium between 4.5–5.0 mEq. per liter.

    g. Give coronary vasodilators as directed.

7. Evaluate for central nervous system complications. Advanced age, low arterial pressure during perfusion and prolonged bypass produce central nervous system damage after open heart surgery.

    a. Watch for convulsions from focal injury to central nervous system.

       (1) Prepare for tracheostomy—to facilitate removal of secretions and assist ventilation if patient has frequent convulsions.

       (2) Control convulsions with prescribed dosage of diphenylhydantoin (Dilantin).

    b. Watch for altered state of consciousness, stupor or coma.

    c. Control fever associated with central nervous system injuries with hypothermia mattress.

    d. Evaluate for symptoms of postperfusion psychosis—may result from disturbances in cerebral circulation.

       (1) Give appropriate sedation.

       (2) Watch patient carefully to avoid bodily injury. (Pad side rails.)

       (3) Reassure the patient's family that psychiatric disorders following heart surgery are usually transient.

8. Watch for signs of renal failure. Renal injury may be caused by deficient perfusion, hemolysis or transfusion incompatibility.

    a. See page 472 for management of patient with renal failure.

    b. Employ peritoneal dialysis (see p. 476) for severe renal insufficiency. (Renal insufficiency may produce serious cardiac arrhythmias.)

9. Watch for febrile complications. Fever almost always follows extracorporeal circulation.

    a. Control higher degrees of fever by use of a hypothermia mattress.

    b. Evaluate for atelectasis or pleural effusion if fever persists.

    c. Watch for "pericardiotomy syndrome"—may occur in any patient who has had pericardium opened; cause is not known.

       (1) Symptoms and signs—prolonged fever, pericardial friction rub, pericardial and pleural effusions.

       (2) Treatment—prednisone; 50–60 mg. daily (used diagnostically and therapeutically).

    d. Evaluate for urinary tract infection—a cause of postoperative fever.

    e. Bear in mind the possibility of bacterial endocarditis if fever persists (see p. 265).

10. Assess for psychological problems—stress of severe cardiac disease, cardiac surgery and postoperative intensive care may produce psychologic aberrations of varying severity.

    a. Watch for paranoid delusions, visual and auditory hallucinations, depression and agitation associated with disorientation—these reactions may last 3–5 days.

    b. Give mild sedation as required.

    c. Have nurse in constant attendance.

    d. If possible, remove patient from intensive unit to his own room.

    e. Offer reassurance, kindness and attention to patient's needs.

f. Have a system of communication (slate, paper and pencil) for patient who cannot speak with endotracheal tube in position.
11. Help the patient accept the responsibility of continuing follow-up care by instructing him as follows:
    a. Report for frequent postoperative examinations to assess progress.
    b. Inform the patient of the necessity of receiving antibiotics at times of predictable risk of endocarditis—dental work, oral and genitourinary surgery.
    c. Encourage graded exercise within limits of cardiac capability. Exercise has physical and psychological benefits.
       (1) Most patients are fairly inactive 1 month after returning home and resume normal activity in 3 months.
       (2) Patients with valve replacements may require 3–4 months to convalesce.

2. Essentials of Basic Electrocardiography

THE ECG AND HEART PHYSIOLOGY

The Electrocardiogram (ECG)

1. Is nothing more than a recording of the heart's electrical impulse.
2. The heart is stimulated to contract and thus pump blood to the body organs because of the electrical pulsation which begins at the top of the heart and travels inferiorly.
3. To record the impulse, electrodes do not have to be placed directly on the heart, but can be placed on the extremities where heart's activity can be sensed (Fig. 5-9).

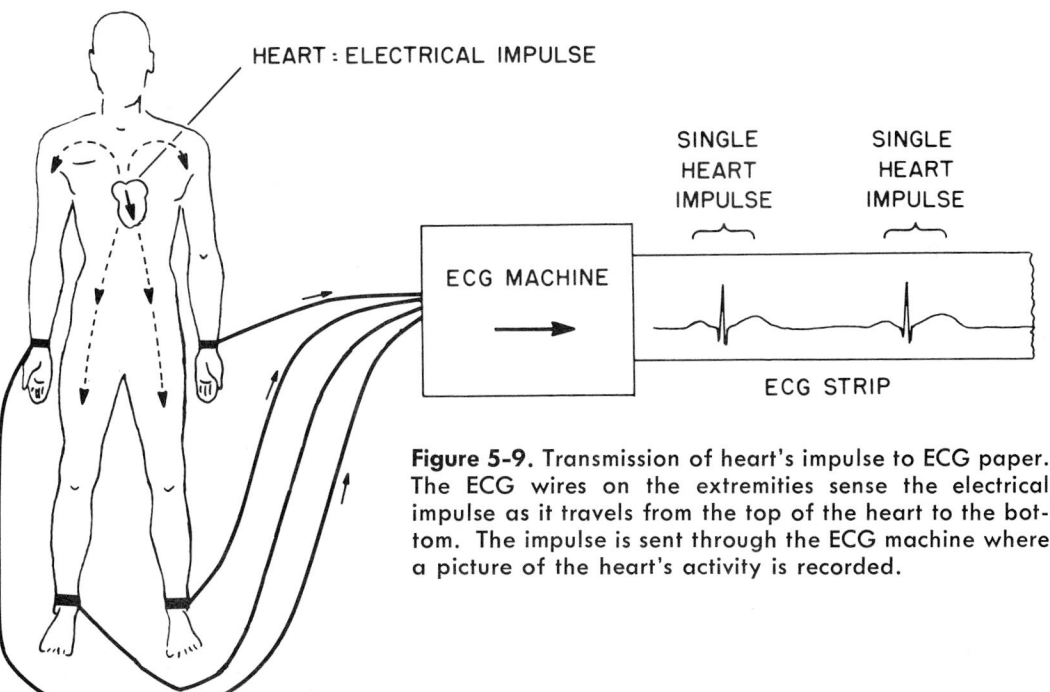

Figure 5-9. Transmission of heart's impulse to ECG paper. The ECG wires on the extremities sense the electrical impulse as it travels from the top of the heart to the bottom. The impulse is sent through the ECG machine where a picture of the heart's activity is recorded.

Clinical Use of ECG

An electrocardiogram can be helpful in diagnosing the following:
1. Myocardial infarction and arteriosclerotic heart disease
2. Cardiac arrhythmias
3. Cardiac enlargement
4. Electrolyte abnormalities (especially potassium and calcium)
5. Pericarditis (inflammation of the pericardial sac which surrounds the heart)
6. Pericardial effusion (fluid in the pericardial sac which can restrict the heart's pumping ability)

Heart Anatomy and Physiology (Fig. 5-10)

1. The normal electrical impulse of the heart, which inscribes the ECG and causes the heart to contract, begins in the SA node (sinoatrial node, sinus node or normal physiological pacemaker).
2. The SA node occupies the superior aspect of the right atrium.
3. The impulse, after beginning in the SA node, travels across the atria, causing them to contract and pump blood into the ventricles.
4. The impulse then hits the AV node (atrioventricular node) which lies between the atria and ventricles.
5. The impulse is somewhat delayed in the AV node and then travels down the ventricles, causing them to contract and thus pump blood to the body organs.
6. Both the SA and AV nodes have 2 main nerve systems connected to them which control the rate at which the heart beats.
   a. Sympathetic nerves—cause the heart rate to increase.
   b. Parasympathetic nerves (vagus nerve)—slow the heart rate.

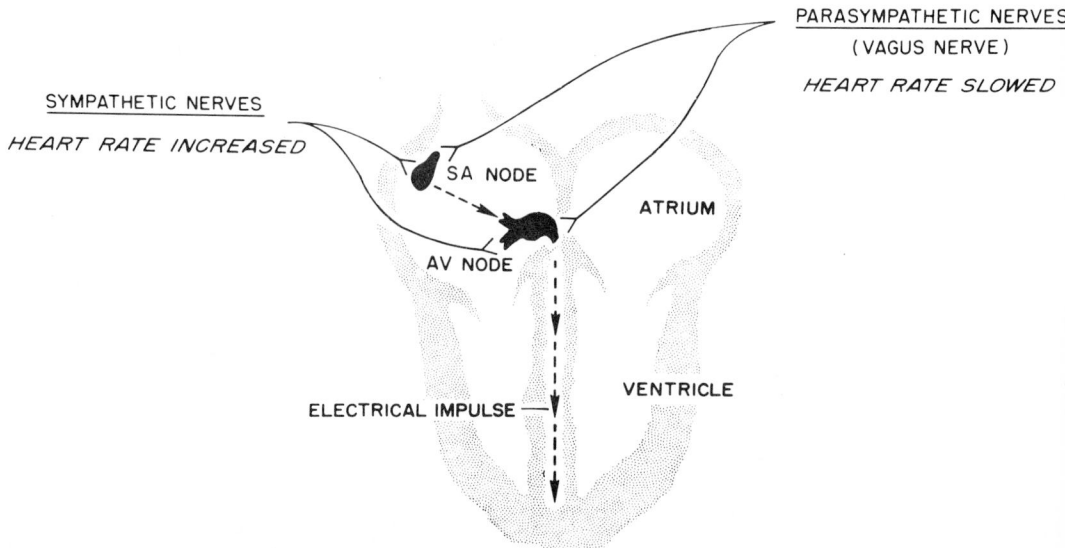

Figure 5-10. Heart Physiology. Pictured is the pathway of the normal electrical impulse which inscribes the ECG and causes the heart to contract and pump blood. Also shown are the nerves which regulate the heart rate.

Normal ECG

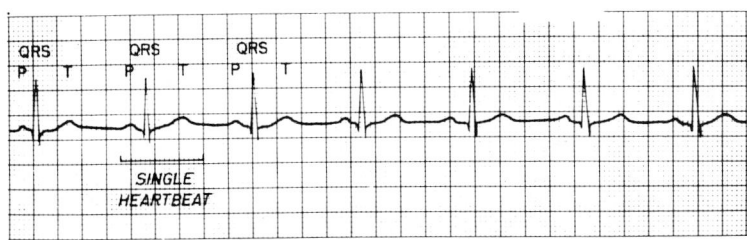

Figure 5-11. A normal ECG.

1. Figure 5-11 represents a normal ECG.
2. Each heart beat manifests as 3 major deflections.
   a. P wave
   b. QRS complex
   c. T wave
3. The QRS complex is composed of 3 parts:
   a. Q wave—the first downward deflection
   b. R wave—the first upward deflection
   c. S wave—the first downward deflection after the R wave
4. Beats come at regular intervals (normal sinus rhythm), indicating the impulse is originating properly from the sinus node.

ECG Waves Related to Heart Anatomy (Fig. 5-12)

1. *The P wave*—begins in the SA node and can be thought of as representing the cardiac electrical impulse traveling through the *atria*.
2. *QRS complex*—represents the impulse going through the *ventricles*. It begins in the AV node which lies atop the ventricular chambers.
3. *T wave*—does not represent an impulse going through any specific chamber but is a pure electrical phenomenon and signifies recovery of the electrical forces (*repolarization*).

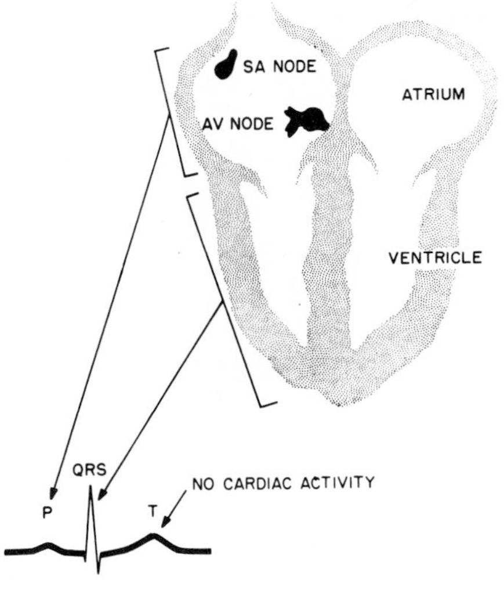

Figure 5-12. ECG waves related to heart anatomy. The electrical impulse is shown traveling through the chambers of the heart and thus inscribing the normal ECG of 1 heart beat. The P wave represents atrial activity and the QRS complex is derived from ventricular stimulation.

ECG Paper (Fig. 5-13)

1. Vertical lines—measure the *magnitude* of the electrical impulse.
2. Horizontal inscriptions—represent the *time* it takes for an impulse to travel over cardiac tissue.
3. In vertical axis—each small block is 1 mm.
   1 darker large block is 5 mm.
4. In horizontal axis—1 small block represents .04 second
   1 darker large block represents .20 second

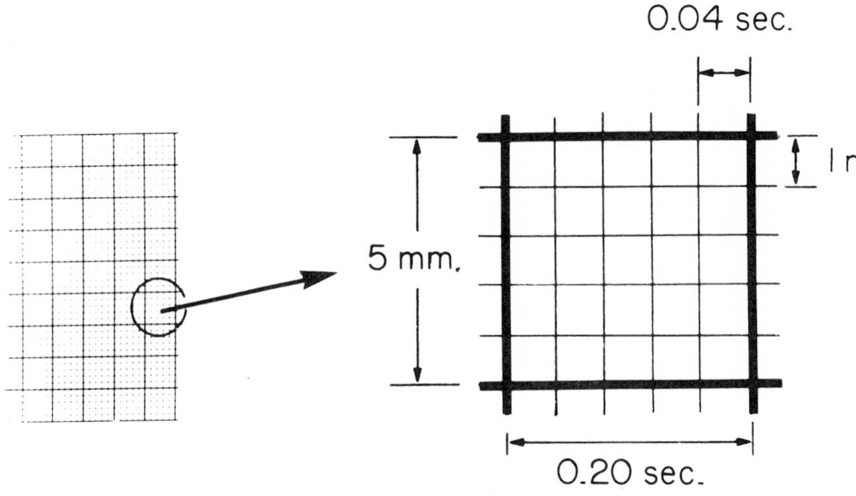

0.04 sec.

1 mm.

5 mm.

0.20 sec.

Figure 5-13. Meaning of blocks on ECG paper. All one really needs to remember is that 1 small block is 1 mm. tall and .04 second wide.

Determination of Cardiac Rate on ECG Paper

1. Cardiac rate can be obtained by dividing the number of heavily lined large blocks between each QRS complex into 300.
2. The number 300 is used because 300 large blocks represent 1 minute on the ECG paper.
   Examples: If there are 3 large blocks between each QRS complex, the rate would be 100 beats per minute (300 divided by 3 = 100). (See Fig. 5-14.)
   If there are 2½ blocks between each QRS complex, the rate would be 120 beats per minute.

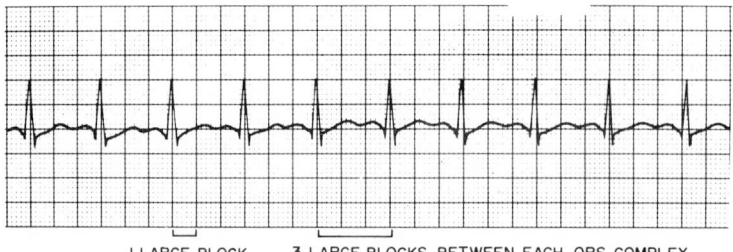

1 LARGE BLOCK   3 LARGE BLOCKS BETWEEN EACH QRS COMPLEX

Figure 5-14. Determination of rate. There are 3 large blocks between each QRS complex. By dividing 300 by 3, the rate is 100 beats per minute.

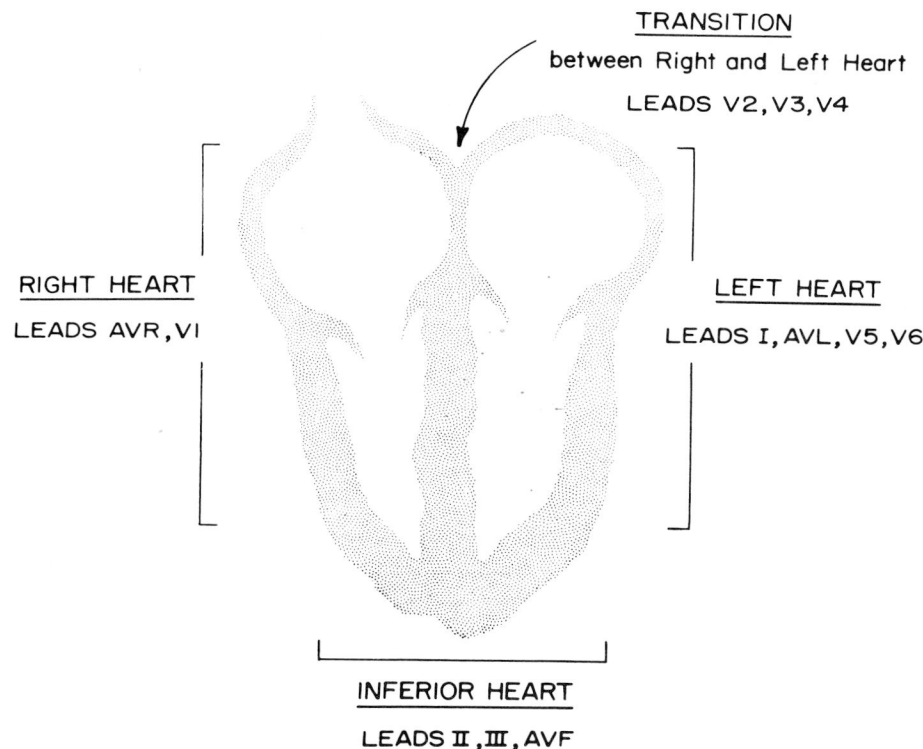

Figure 5-15. ECG leads related to heart anatomy.

ECG Leads

1. Standard ECG machines have a dial which turns to 1 to 12 leads (I, II, III, AVR, AVL, AVF, V1, V2, V3, V4, V5, V6).
2. Each leads sees and records the heart's electrical impulse from a different anatomical position relative to the heart's surface.
3. Letter designations can be confusing; thus position of each lead must be memorized.
4. The area of the heart represented by each lead is shown in Figure 5-15.
5. Location of leads helps to localize cardiac pathology.

Significance of Each ECG Wave and Interval

A. *P Wave* (Fig. 5-16a)
   1. P wave represents the atrial contraction.
   2. Enlargement of the P-wave deflection indicates enlargement of the atrium as might occur in mitral stenosis. (The atrium enlarges in mitral stenosis because the mitral opening between the atrium and ventricle is small, causing blood to back up, which in turn forces the atrial wall to expand.)
   3. P wave is considered enlarged if it is over 3 mm. tall (3 small blocks) or .12 second wide (3 small blocks).

B. *PR Interval* (Fig. 5-16b)
   1. Starts at the beginning of the P wave and extends to the onset of the Q wave.
   2. At normal rates, the PR interval should not exceed .20 second (5 small blocks).

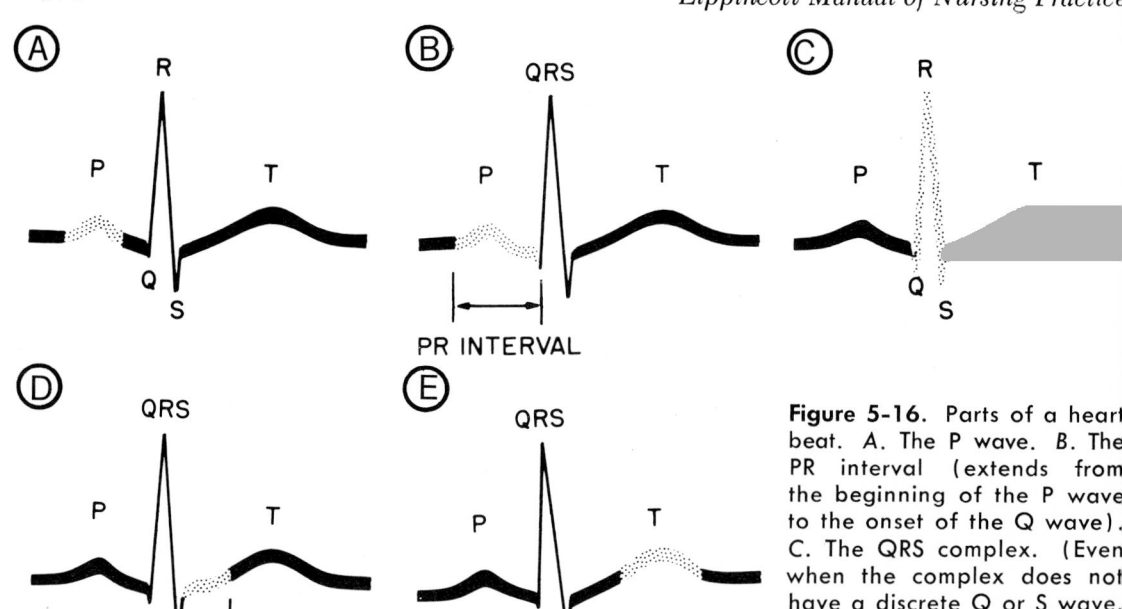

Figure 5-16. Parts of a heart beat. *A.* The P wave. *B.* The PR interval (extends from the beginning of the P wave to the onset of the Q wave). *C.* The QRS complex. (Even when the complex does not have a discrete Q or S wave, it is still referred to as the QRS complex to denote a ventricular impulse and to provide simplicity and uniformity.) *D.* The ST segment begins at the termination of the S wave and ends at the beginning of the T wave. *E.* The T wave.

3. This interval increases in length in arteriosclerotic heart disease and in rheumatic fever.
4. The PR interval is prolonged because the heart tissue covered by the PR interval (namely the atrium and AV node area) is scarred or inflamed and the impulse is forced to travel at a slower rate.

C. *The QRS Complex* (Fig. 5-16c)
1. Q wave (first downward stroke)—when it becomes large it is indicative of an old myocardial infarction.
2. The R wave (first upward deflection)
   a. Becomes increased in amplitude when the ventricle enlarges as occurs in most types of heart diseases. (Overwork of a specific part of the heart causes enlargement.)
   b. May become small when the heart is compressed by fluid as in a pericardial effusion.

D. *The ST Segment* (Fig. 5-16d)
1. Begins at the end of the S wave (the first downward deflection after the R wave) and terminates at the beginning of the T wave.
2. Is elevated above the base line on the ECG strip in an acute myocardial infarction or in pericarditis.
3. Becomes depressed when the heart muscle is getting a decreased supply of oxygen or when a patient is taking digitalis.

4. Becomes long in hypocalcemia. (Hypocalcemia occurs most commonly in chronic renal disease because the scarred kidneys cannot excrete phosphate. Since phosphate and calcium maintain a reciprocal balance in the body fluid, the elevated phosphate causes a depression in the calcium level.)
5. Becomes shorter in hypercalcemia, which is most commonly seen in metastatic carcinoma because the tumor erodes the bones and spills calcium into the serum.

E. *The T Wave* (Fig. 5-16e)
1. Represents no cardiac activity, but reflects the electrical recovery of the ventricular contraction. (An electrical impulse is the flow of electrons; the T wave is inscribed when these electrons migrate back to their resting position after traversing the heart muscle to make it contract.)
2. Is flat when the heart is not receiving enough oxygen (arteriosclerotic heart disease).
3. May be inverted in a myocardial infarction.
4. May be made tall by an elevated serum potassium.
5. Should not be over 10 mm. (10 small blocks) high in the precordial leads (those that are placed on the chest) and should not be over 5 mm. in the remaining leads.

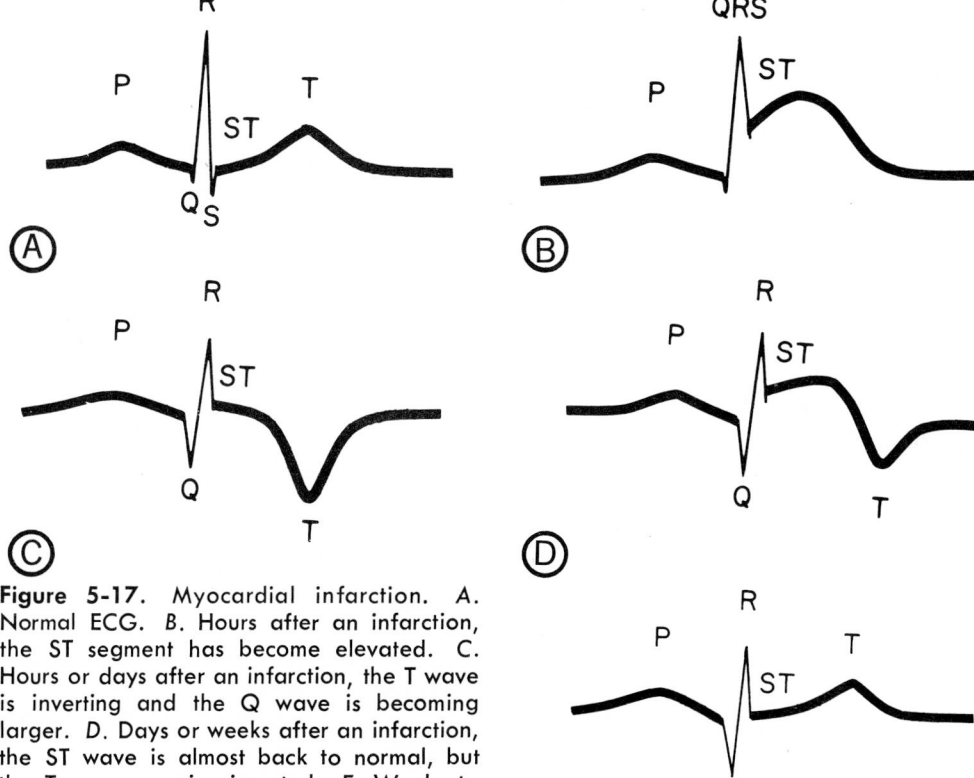

Figure 5-17. Myocardial infarction. A. Normal ECG. B. Hours after an infarction, the ST segment has become elevated. C. Hours or days after an infarction, the T wave is inverting and the Q wave is becoming larger. D. Days or weeks after an infarction, the ST wave is almost back to normal, but the T wave remains inverted. E. Weeks to months after an infarction, the T wave has become upright again and the only residual of a myocardial infarction may be an abnormally large Q wave.

ECG INTERPRETATION OF MYOCARDIAL INFARCTION

ECG Interpretation (Fig. 5-17)

NOTE: Approximately 15% of patients suffering a myocardial infarction have *no changes* on the initial tracing. Therefore, if a person has symptoms compatible with a heart attack and has a normal ECG, he should nevertheless be admitted to the hospital for observation and further electrocardiograms.

1. Elevation of ST segment is first finding.
2. T wave inversion follows.
3. Then a large Q wave appears.
    a. As infarct heals, Q wave may remain as the only stigmata of an old coronary occlusion. (In AVR a large Q wave is normal.)
    b. Q wave can be considered abnormal if it is over .04 second wide (1 small block is .04 second) or if it is greater in depth than ⅓ the height of the QRS complex (Fig. 5-18).

ECG INTERPRETATION OF CARDIAC ARRHYTHMIAS

NOTE: The lower the ectopic focus resides in the heart, the more lethal the arrhythmia becomes.

Sinus Tachycardia

Sinus tachycardia can be defined as a cardiac rate of over 100 beats per minute. All the complexes are normal, but their rate is excessive.

Altered Physiology

The impulse begins normally in the SA node but comes at a faster rate secondary to increased sympathetic nerve stimuli.

Causes

1. Exercise
2. Anxiety
3. Fever
4. Shock

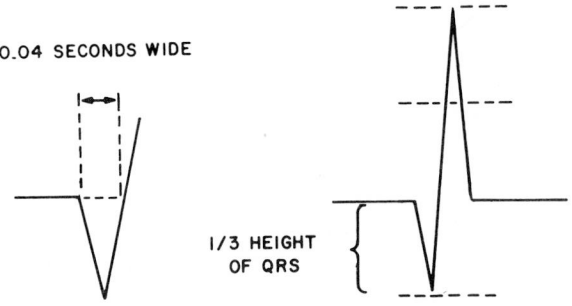

0.04 SECONDS WIDE

1/3 HEIGHT OF QRS

Figure 5-18. Abnormal Q wave. A Q wave is considered abnormal when it is over .04 second (1 small block on the ECG paper) or over one-third the height of the QRS complex. This usually indicates an old myocardial infarction.

Mechanism of Sinus Tachycardia

Normal Pathway

Sinus Tachycardia Pathway

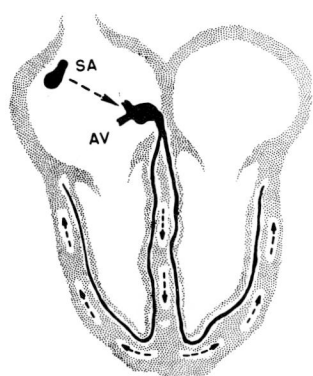 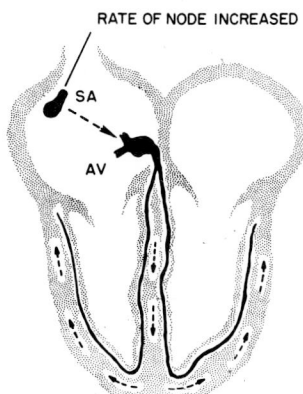

The pathway of sinus tachycardia is the same as a normal sinus rhythm, but the number of impulses per minute is greater in sinus tachycardia.

ECG of Sinus Tachycardia

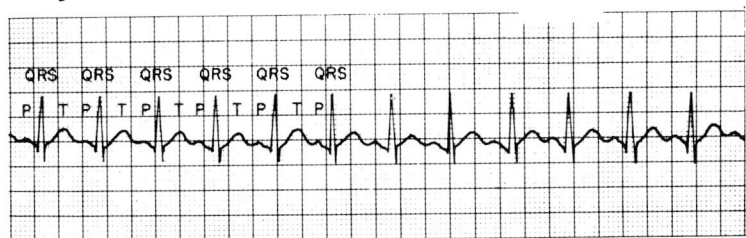

The P wave, the QRS complex and the T wave are all normal. The only abnormality is a rate of over 100.

Treatment

Since sinus tachycardia is usually a compensatory rhythm, treatment is directed at the primary causes which usually are not cardiac.

Sinus Bradycardia

Sinus bradycardia is defined as a heart rate below 60. All the complexes are normal.

Etiology

1. Seen *normally* in well-trained athletes.
2. May be secondary to certain drugs such as digitalis or morphine.
3. Also seen in myocardial infarction at which point it could be detrimental to the patient who is already in a compromised cardiac state.

Complications

Slow rate and low cardiac output can cause:
    Fainting (Stokes-Adams syndrome) or
    Congestive heart failure (Heart cannot pump all the fluid presented to it, result-
    ing in stasis or "congestion" of the blood in the lungs and other body tissues.)

Mechanism of Sinus Bradycardia

Normal Pathway   Sinus Bradycardia Pathway

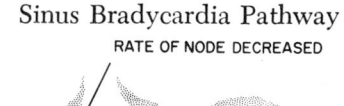

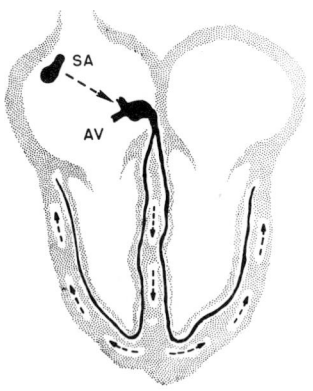
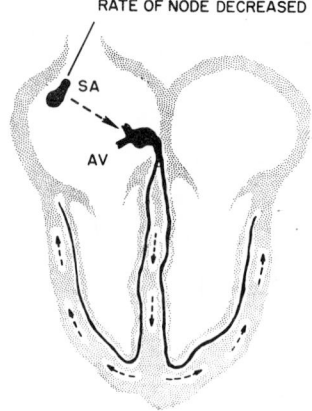

The pathway of sinus bradycardia is identical to that of normal sinus rhythm, but the
rate is slower.

ECG of Sinus Bradycardia

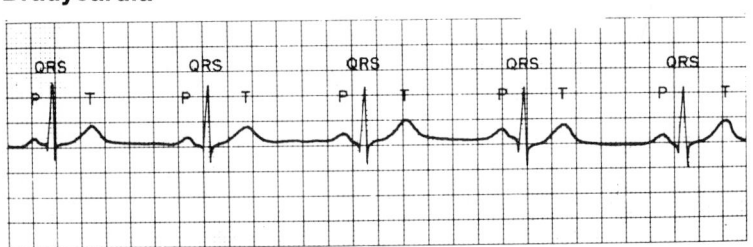

The only abnormality is a rate below 60 beats per minute.

Treatment

1. Rarely has to be treated.
2. If congestive failure or fainting occurs, treatment should be initiated immediately to
   increase the heart rate.
   a. Give 0.5–1 mg. of atropine by I.V. push (inhibits the vagal or the "slowing" nerve
      and therefore makes the heart go faster).
   b. If patient becomes resistant to atropine, the rate can be increased by adding 1 mg.
      of isoproterenol (Isuprel) to 250 ml. of 5% glucose in water and initially running
      the solution at about 10 drops per minute. (Stimulates the sympathetic or "fast"
      nerve of the heart.) (Atropine can be prepared more quickly and is less toxic
      to the heart than Isuprel.)

    c. The heart rate can be increased or decreased by adjusting the rate of fluid administered.

    d. An electrical pacemaker may be necessary in refractory cases or when the fluid load becomes excessive.

Sinus Arrhythmia

Sinus arrhythmia is normally found in children and young adults and is characterized by a heart rhythm that is normal in every way except for irregularity.

Etiology

1. On inspiration the heart rate increases and on expiration the heart rate decreases.
2. Inspiration tends to inhibit the vagus nerve (slows the heart) and causes an acceleration of the cardiac rate.

Mechanism of Sinus Arrhythmia

Normal Pathway

Sinus Arrhythmia Pathway

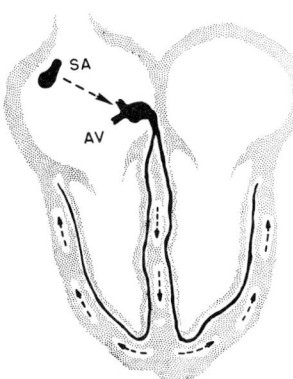
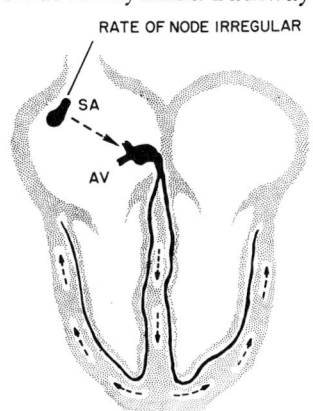

The pathway of sinus arrhythmia is the same as the normal sinus rhythm; the only differential point is the regularity of the impulses.

ECG of Sinus Arrhythmia

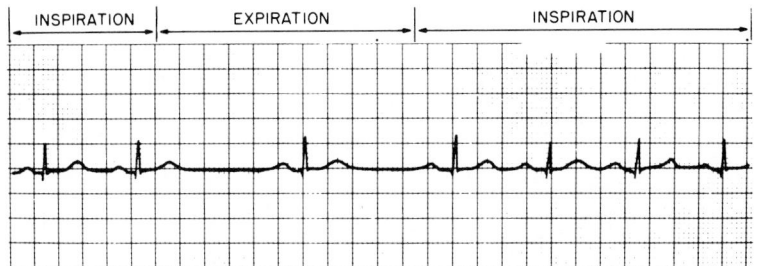

All the complexes are normal; only the rate is irregular—varying with respiration. The rate increases with inspiration and decreases with expiration.

Treatment

Since sinus arrhythmia is usually normal no treatment is necessary.

Premature Atrial Contractions (PAC's)

PAC's constitute a very common rhythm disturbance and are seen in both normal and abnormal hearts. They rarely cause symptoms and are felt to be of little consequence except when they occur frequently, at which time they may tend to deteriorate into other more serious arrhythmias.

Altered Physiology

1. Beats occur *early* in cycle and begin in the atrium, but *outside* the sinus node where normal impulses originate.
2. Since the atrial pathway is abnormal, the P wave is distorted.
3. Since ventricular activation is undisturbed, the QRS is normal.

Mechanism of a PAC

Normal Pathway   PAC Pathway

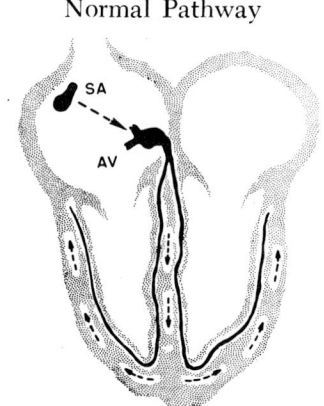
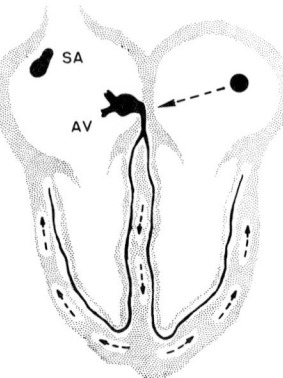

The PAC begins in the atrium outside the SA node.

ECG of a PAC

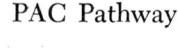
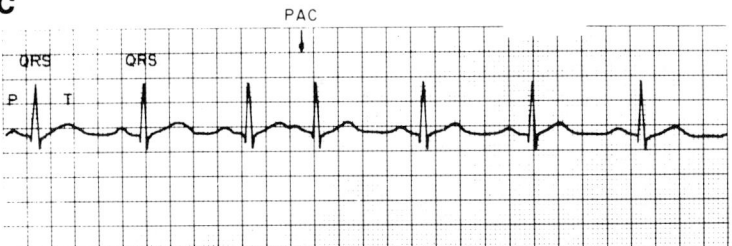

1. PAC comes early in the cycle.
2. P wave is abnormally shaped.
3. QRS complex is normal.

Treatment

1. Most of the time PAC's do not need to be treated.
2. Quinidine, which is a good suppressant of atrial ectopic beats, may be used when the patient requires therapy.

Paroxysmal Atrial Tachycardia (PAT)

PAT is a common arrhythmia seen in young adults and is usually found in normal hearts. There is a rapid heart rate which ranges from 140–250 beats per minute with an average of about 180 beats per minute.

Clinical Manifestations

Patient will complain of a pounding or fluttering in the chest associated with shortness of breath and fainting—due to rapid heart rate.

Altered Physiology

1. Begins in an ectopic focus of the atrium outside the sinus node.
2. Its pathway over the heart is similar to that of a PAC. Thus PAT may be considered as a rapid succession of PAC's.
3. The P wave (atrial wave) is distorted because the pathway over the atrium is abnormal. (Most of the time the rate is so fast, that the P wave is not seen since it is buried in the previous complex.)
4. The QRS complex (ventricular wave) is normal because the route of the cardiac impulse after penetrating the AV node is undisturbed.

Mechanism of PAT

Normal Pathway

PAT Pathway

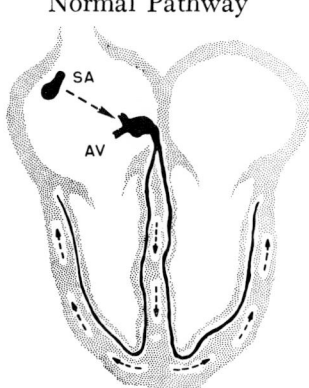 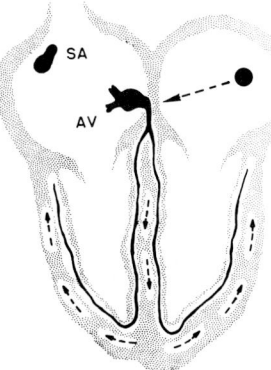

An impulse traveling along the abnormal PAT pathway (right) produces an abnormal P wave and a normally shaped QRS complex (ventricular wave). Notice that the focus of the PAT is the same as a PAC.

ECG of PAT

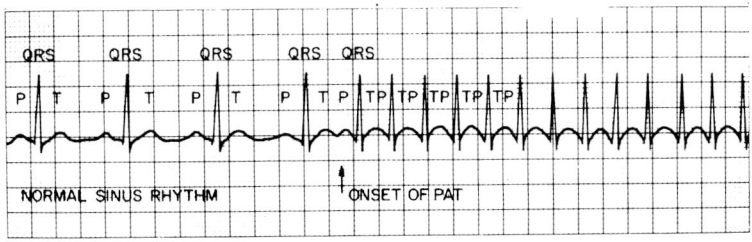

1. The rate is very rapid over 140 per minute (higher than in sinus tachycardia).
2. P waves cannot be seen since they are superimposed within the T wave of the preceding beat. If the P waves were seen they would be abnormal in configuration.
3. The QRS complex is normal.

Treatment

1. Since cardiac arrest can occur with any mode of treatment for PAT, an ECG machine should remain attached to the patient, an I.V. started and appropriate resuscitation equipment, including a defibrillator, should be at hand.
2. If the patient is relatively asymptomatic and stable, giving a simple sedative and waiting 5–10 minutes may result in spontaneous conversion of PAT.
3. Start by stimulating the right carotid sinus (an area of dense nerve supply) of the carotid artery for several seconds or gagging the patient with a tongue depressor in an effort to terminate the arrhythmia. These maneuvers work by stimulating the vagus nerve which puts a "break" on the heart.
4. If the above procedure is not effective and if the blood pressure is low (many patients with PAT have a systolic pressure about 90 mm.Hg), a slow drip of metaraminol (Aramine), I.V., can be started.
    a. Add 100 mg. of Aramine to 500 ml. of 5% glucose in water and run the I.V. initially at 10 drops per minute.
    b. Gradually increase the rate of the infusion until the PAT terminates, at which time the I.V. should be stopped (usually a matter of seconds). (See Fig. 5-19.)
    c. Do not raise the systolic blood pressure above 180. This drug increases the blood pressure, which, in turn, stimulates the vagus nerve to inhibit the ectopic focus of the atrium.
    d. If the patient is already hypertensive (rare), Aramine should not be used.
    e. Some authorities do not use a vasopressor such as Aramine because of the occasional report of a cerebral vascular accident, but this complication has usually occurred when the drug is used in bolus form. Instead of Aramine, they prefer a fast-acting digitalis preparation which works in part by stimulating the vagal nerve.
5. In an unusual case, in which the preceding steps are ineffective or contraindicated, 1–3 mg. of propranolol (Inderal)—a sympathetic nerve blocker—may be given by I.V. at a rate of no greater than 1 mg./minute.
6. In the extreme case when the patient is in congestive heart failure, D.C. synchronized electrical shock (cardioversion) should be instituted instead of giving Inderal.

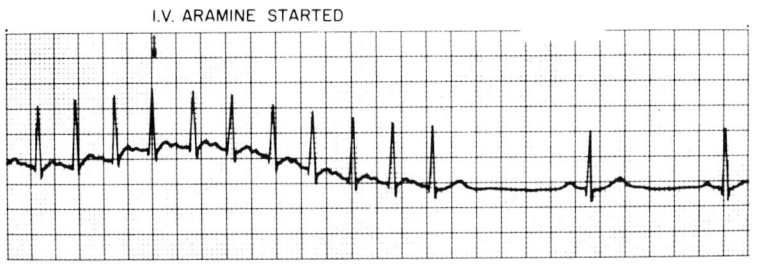

Figure 5-19. Termination of PAT. The ECG illustrates PAT being terminated with a slow I.V. infusion of Aramine.

a. Initial shock—can be 50–100 watt-seconds (joules).
b. Electrical shock stops the heart and allows it to begin again normally at the SA node.

Atrial Flutter

Atrial flutter is a rapid, regular "fluttering" of the atrium.

Altered Physiology

1. P waves take on a "sawtooth" appearance because they are coming from a focus other than the sinus node and are coming at a very rapid rate.
2. As in PAC or PAT, the impulse comes from *one* ectopic focus in the atrium but the *atrial* rate (not pulse or ventricular rate) is between 250 and 350 per minute for PAT.
   The following over-simplified arbitrary rule may be used to distinguish the atrial arrhythmias from each other:
   Atrial rate in sinus tachycardia goes up to 140/minute.
   Atrial rate in PAT is between 140–250/minute.
   Atrial rate in atrial flutter is between 250–350/minute.
3. Atrial flutter occurs usually in a pathological heart (usually arteriosclerotic or rheumatic), as contrasted to PAT which many times is associated with a normal heart.
4. Since the abnormality is above the AV node, the QRS complex (ventricular wave) is normal in configuration.
5. Since the P waves are coming so rapidly, the AV node cannot accept and conduct each one; therefore, there is some degree of "blockage" at the AV node.
   Example: If the atrial rate is 300, the ventricular rate (which is the same as the pulse rate) might be 150, since the AV node is not able to conduct every atrial impulse because of the excessive rapidity. In this instance, the "block" is said to be 2:1 since there are 2 atrial impulses per 1 ventricular response.
6. The 2:1 block is the most common block in atrial flutter.
7. Most cases of PAT do not exhibit a block since P waves are not occurring as fast as in a flutter. Thus all the impulses are transmitted by the AV node to the ventricles.

Mechanism of Atrial Flutter

Normal Pathway

Atrial Flutter Pathway

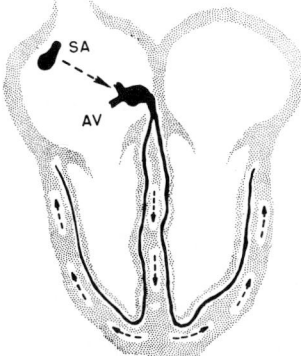
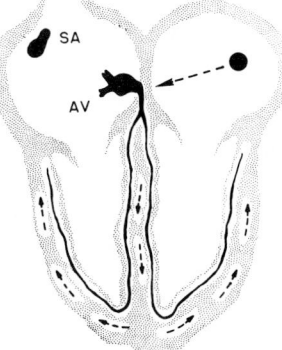

The pathways for atrial flutter are the same as for PAC and PAT, but in atrial flutter the ectopic impulse fires at a faster rate.

ECG of Atrial Flutter

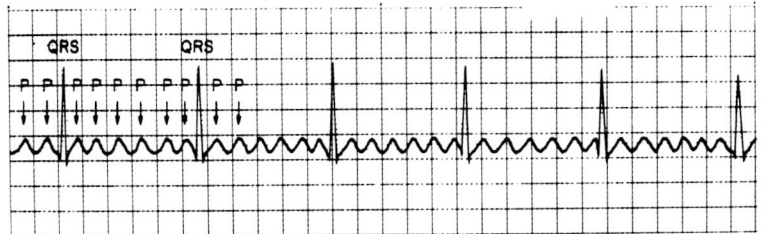

1. The arrows indicate the P waves that are coming from the fast ectopic focus in the atrium.
2. Notice that not every P wave stimulates a QRS complex (ventricular wave).
3. Since the abnormality present in the heart is above the AV node, the QRS complexes that appear are normal in configuration.

Treatment

1. Classic initial treatment is digitalis which partially blocks the AV node and allows fewer P waves to pass through the ventricles and thus slows the pulse rate.
2. The fast pulse rate must be slowed down (ventricular rate) because the heart is not given enough time to fill itself with blood when it is contracting rapidly, which causes the blood to back up in the body tissues leading to congestive failure.
3. Cardioversion
    a. Tried when the patient is not tolerating the arrhythmia well.
    b. Atrial flutter responds well to cardioversion at a relatively low wattage (50–100 watts/second).

NURSING ALERT: When a patient is taking digitalis, cardioversion can be dangerous since a lethal arrhythmia may be precipitated.

Atrial Fibrillation

Atrial fibrillation is an atrial arrhythmia occurring at an extremely rapid and uncoordinated rate. The atria produce impulses so rapidly that the ventricles are not capable of responding to every atrial beat; therefore, only a small percentage of atrial stimuli excite the ventricles. Since the atrial rate is irregular, the ventricular rate (pulse rate) will also be irregular.

Etiology

Usually seen in patients with arteriosclerotic or rheumatic heart disease.

Altered Physiology

1. Arteriosclerosis leads to scarring of the atrium and thus disruption of the normal course of the P wave (atrial wave).
2. P waves are replaced by irregular rapid waves each of which is different in configuration from the other.
3. P waves (often called fibrillatory waves) assume different shapes because they are coming from different foci in the atrium. (In atrial flutter the P waves are very regular and uniform since they come from one focus.)

4. Because P waves are coming at variable intervals, the QRS complexes assume an irregular rhythm and thus the patient's pulse is irregular. (The configuration of the QRS is normal since the conduction tissue beyond the AV node has not been critically involved with the arteriosclerotic process as yet.)
5. Because P waves are coming so fast, all of them do not pass on to the ventricles because of normal refraction of the AV node. Thus the atrial rate is usually much faster than the ventricular rate.
6. Occasionally, the ventricular rate is very fast because the AV node is blocking relatively fewer beats than normal. If this is the case, atrial activity may not be seen because the QRS complexes are so close together since their rate is so rapid, thus making it difficult to define the arrhythmia.

NOTE: General rule: If *normal* QRS complexes are present at a very rapid rate so that atrial activity cannot be seen and the rhythm is *irregular,* the probable diagnosis is atrial fibrillation.

Mechanism of Atrial Fibrillation

Normal Pathway   Atrial Fibrillation Pathway

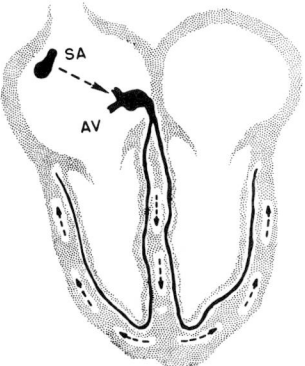 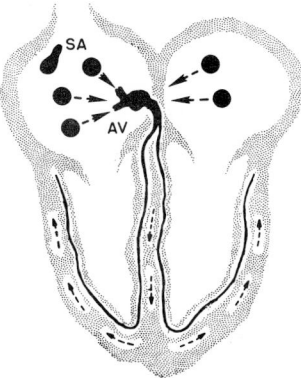

1. In atrial fibrillation many ectopic foci are present in the atrium (right).
2. Since each small atrial wave comes from a different focus and travels a different route, the shape of each atrial wave (P wave) is different.

ECG of Atrial Fibrillation

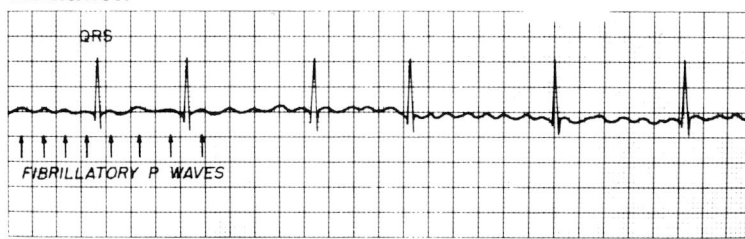

1. Note the small, irregular fibrillating P waves (arrow).
2. As with atrial flutter, only an occasional P wave travels through the AV node to form a QRS complex, but since these complexes come at irregular intervals in atrial fibrillation, the ventricular rate is irregular.
3. Each P wave is different in shape because it is coming from a different focus in the atrium.

Treatment

1. Depends on patient's clinical condition, cardiac rate and drug status.
2. For average patient who is not critical and not on digitalis, the following treatment is common:
   a. 0.5 mg. of I.V. digoxin, given over a 5-minute period under ECG control.
   b. After 2 hours, an additional 0.25–0.5 mg. is given, depending on the ECG and the patient's condition. (Total I.V. dose before oral maintenance therapy is 0.75–1.5 mg.)
3. If atrial fibrillation is an immediate life-threatening emergency (rare):
   a. Cardioversion may be started with 100 watt-seconds.
   b. As with atrial flutter, cardioversion becomes somewhat of a risk when the patient is taking digitalis.
   c. In contrast to atrial flutter, atrial fibrillation is more difficult to correct to normal sinus rhythm with electric countershock.

AV Block

AV block means that the AV node is diseased and has difficulty conducting the atrial waves (P waves) into the ventricles.

Causes

1. Arteriosclerosis
2. Myocardial infarction

Types of AV Block

1st degree
2nd degree
3rd degree

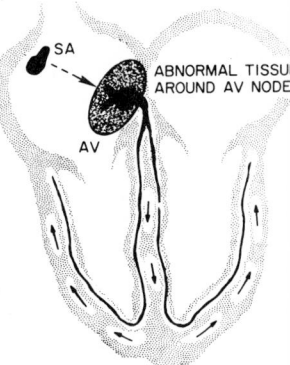

Mechanism of AV Blocks

1. Abnormal tissue around and in the AV node causes physiological blockage of the atrial impulse into the ventricles.
2. In 1st degree block—the impulses are merely slowed.
3. In 2nd degree block—only a portion of the atrial impulses penetrate to the ventricles.
4. In 3rd degree block—no atrial impulse enters the ventricles so that the atria and ventricles are beating independently.

NORMAL AV
CONDUCTION

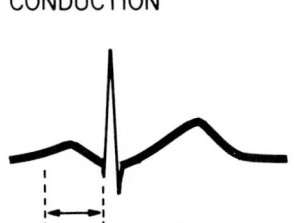

PR = 0.16 sec.

FIRST DEGREE
AV BLOCK

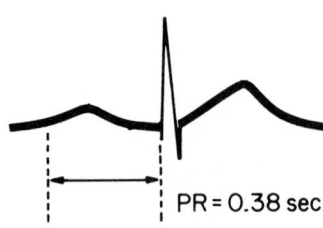

PR = 0.38 sec.

Figure 5-20. 1st degree AV block. Since the tissue around the AV node is abnormal, the impulse takes longer to traverse this area which leads to a prolonged PR interval.

1st Degree AV Block (Fig. 5-20)

1. The PR interval is prolonged. (The PR interval represents the impulse going through the atrium and the area of the AV node.) It should not exceed 0.20 second (5 small blocks on ECG paper when 1 block equals .04 second).
2. Since the atrial and AV nodal tissues are diseased, the electrical impulse takes a longer time to traverse its pathway as reflected by the increased length in the PR interval.
3. All P waves penetrate the ventricles to form QRS complexes (in contrast to 2nd and 3rd degree block).

2nd Degree AV Block

1. Some P waves do not pass through the ventricles, but others do.
2. A ratio of 2:1, 3:1, 4:1 or any such combination appears on ECG. (Figure 5-21 represents a 2:1 ratio.)
3. 2nd degree block is distinguished from 3rd degree block by the fact that some P waves conduct QRS complexes and others do not.

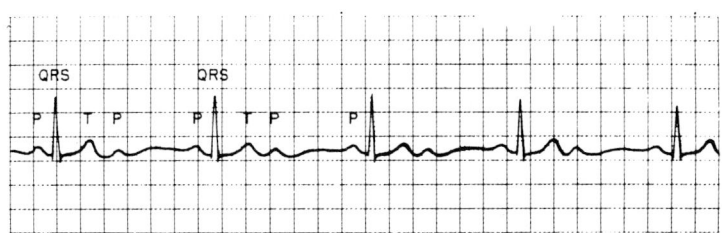

Figure 5-21. 2nd degree AV block. Some P waves pass through to the ventricles but others do not.

3rd Degree AV Block

1. Also called a complete AV block.
2. *No* P waves penetrate the AV node to the ventricles; therefore, the P waves and QRS complexes are beating *independently*.
3. P waves are seen before the QRS complexes, but the PR interval varies and there is no constant relationship of the P waves to the QRS complexes (Fig. 5-22).
4. The pulse rate is usually slow since the ventricles are beating at their own inherent rhythm which is about 35 beats per minute.

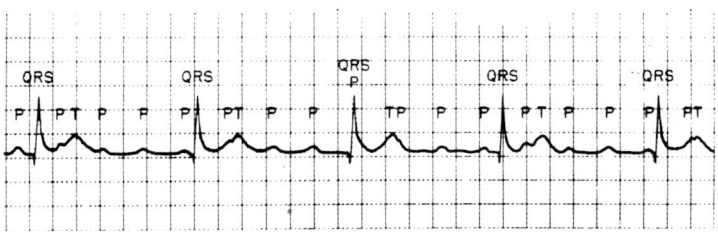

Figure 5-22. 3rd degree AV block. The P waves and QRS complexes are beating independently of each other.

Treatment of AV Blocks

1. 1st degree block
   No treatment is needed.
2. 2nd degree block
   a. When certain types of 2nd degree heart block occur in a myocardial infarction many cardiologists insert a pacemaker which is activated when the cardiac rate falls to unacceptable levels.
   b. To increase rate while awaiting a pacemaker, atropine, 0.5–1.0 mg. may be given I.V.
   c. If the rate cannot be maintained with atropine, 1 mg. of isoproterenol (Isuprel) added to 250 ml. of 5% glucose in water may be infused by the "piggyback" technique to stimulate the heart to function at an acceptable rate.
3. 3rd degree heart block
   a. In myocardial infarction, 3rd degree block is frequently treated with a pacemaker
   b. While awaiting insertion of the pacemaker, patient may be maintained on atropine or isoproterenol (Isuprel) as in 2nd degree block.

The Artificial Pacemaker

A. *Normally Functioning Pacemaker* (Fig. 5-23)
   1. The ECG of a patient with a normal functioning artificial pacemaker shows a *vertical line* just at the beginning of the QRS complex. This represents the electrical stimulus of the artificial pacemaker.

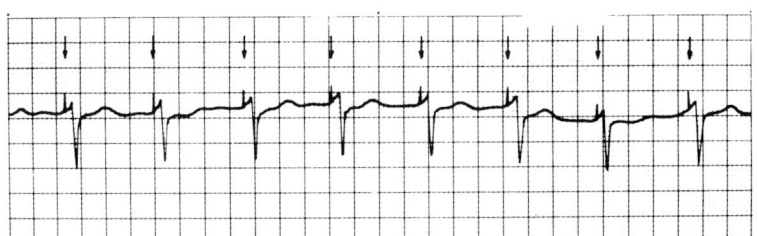

Figure 5-23. Normal pacemaker function. In this ECG each QRS complex is preceded by a small vertical line (arrows) which represents the electrical stimulus of the artificial pacemaker.

B. *Poorly Functioning Pacemakers*
   1. Due to lack of contact between pacing catheter and heart wall.
      a. May occur when patient performs a sudden movement.
      b. Appears on ECG when the small vertical pacemaker stimulus is *not* followed by a QRS complex (Fig. 5-24).
   2. Due to malfunctioning:
      a. Examples: wires break or disconnect from pacemaker.
         battery fails to function.
      b. Noted on ECG by the absence of vertical pacer lines (Fig. 5-25).

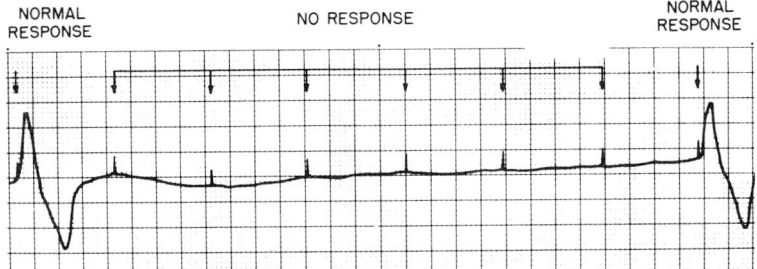

Figure 5-24. Poor pacemaker contact. Notice that the first and last pacemaker stimuli are followed by ventricular complexes and that the other pacemaker deflections failed to produce a cardiac impulse because of the lack of pacemaker contact with the heart wall.

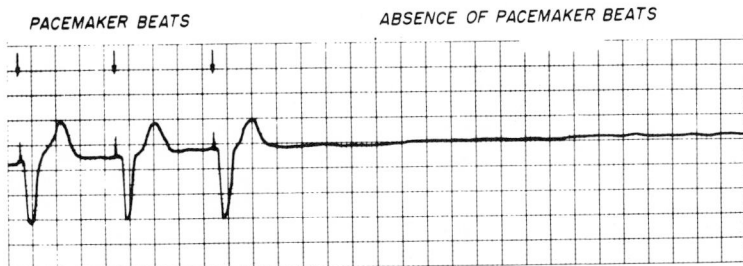

Figure 5-25. Malfunctioning pacemaker. Notice the eventual absence of pacemaker stimuli which in this case resulted in cardiac standstill. This patient had a faulty pacemaker.

Premature Ventricular Contractions (PVC's)

Premature ventricular contractions represent one of the most easily recognized rhythm disturbances seen on an ECG. They occur in all forms of heart disease and are seen in the majority of patients with myocardial infarction. They occur frequently in normal hearts and can be secondary to smoking, coffee or alcohol. While not usually symptomatic, PVC's, when frequent, may cause palpitations.

Altered Physiology

1. Contractions come early in the cycle and originate in the ventricle *below* the AV node.
2. QRS configurations are wide and bizarre, since a PVC does not begin normally and therefore does not follow the true conduction path in the ventricle.

Mechanism of a PVC

Normal Pathway   PVC Pathway

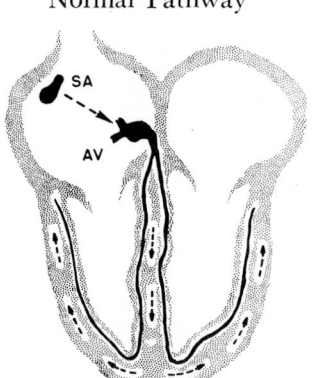
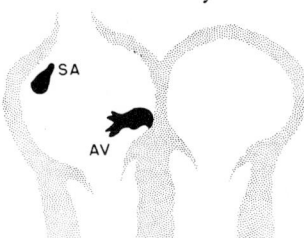

Since a PVC begins in the ventricle outside the AV node a bizarre ventricular QRS complex will be inscribed.

ECG of PVC's

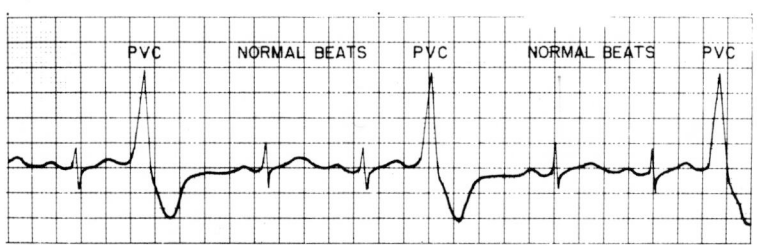

PVC's come early in the cycle and are wider than the normal beat.

Dangers of PVC's

PVC's are especially dangerous when they:
1. Occur more frequently than 1 in 10 beats
2. Occur in groups of 2 or 3
3. Are landing near the T wave
4. Take on multiple configurations, since this indicates that the PVC's are coming from different foci which in turn means that the ventricle is more irritable.

Treatment

If a patient has an infarct, PVC's are vigorously treated since they *can precipitate ventricular fibrillation by hitting a T wave.*
1. Lidocaine (Xylocaine) can be given—PVC's are usually seen with a cardiac rate of over 60 per minute; lidocaine (a cardiac muscle suppressant) is drug of choice because PVC's are most likely coming from an irritable focus such as an infarct.
   a. Dosage: 75–100 mg. I.V., as a bolus over a 2-minute period.
   b. Repeat in 2–3 minutes.
   c. If effective, a continuous I.V. drip of lidocaine should be started with a delivery of 1–3 mg. per minute.

(1) Addition of a 50-ml. bottle of 2% lidocaine to 1000 ml. of 5% glucose in water, will give 1 ml. of fluid a concentration of 1 mg. of lidocaine.

(2) Most I.V. sets are calibrated to deliver 1 ml. in 10 drops of fluid.

(3) If above concentration results in too much fluid for the patient, the amount of lidocaine should be increased in the I.V. solution.

2. If heart rate is *slow* secondary to a myocardial infarction involving the heart's normal physiological pacemaker (SA node), PVC's may occur as a compensatory mechanism to maintain a reasonable rate so as to provide some type of cardiac contraction to pump blood to the body tissues. (A PVC does not pump as much blood as a normal impulse from the SA node, but it does provide some circulation.)

  a. Xylocaine would be contraindicated since it would decrease circulation by extinguishing the PVC's which are pumping needed blood.

  b. Atropine is treatment of choice in this case (a slow rate resulting in PVC's).

    (1) Increases the sinus node rate which in turn would terminate the inefficient ectopic beats by replacing them with normal impulses.

    (2) Dosage: 0.5–1.0 mg., I.V.

Ventricular Tachycardia

Ventricular tachycardia is one of the dreaded complications of a myocardial infarction and can be considered as multiple (3 or more) consecutive premature ventricular contractions occurring from an ectopic focus below the AV node in the ventricles, causing the complexes to be wide and bizarre in configuration.

Dangers of Ventricular Tachycardia

1. Leads to a reduced cardiac output (the ventricles are not being stimulated normally from the AV node, but from a focus farther down in the ventricle wall which leads to an incomplete and inefficient contraction of the heart muscle).
2. Is a precursor to ventricular fibrillation where there is no cardiac output.

Mechanism of Ventricular Tachycardia

Normal Pathway   Ventricular Tachycardia Pathways

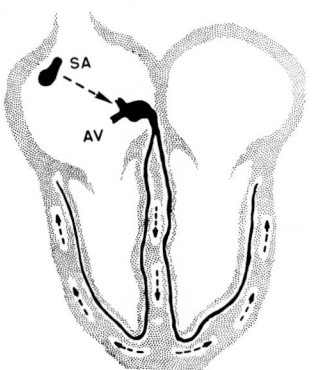 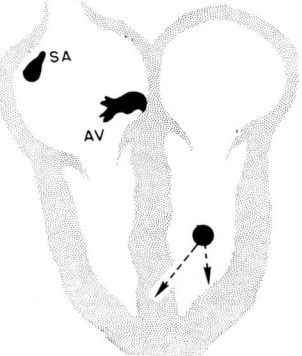

1. Pathway is the same as for PVC since ventricular tachycardia can be considered as a series of PVC's.
2. Like the PVC's, the complexes of ventricular tachycardia show a bizarre configuration.

ECG of Ventricular Tachycardia

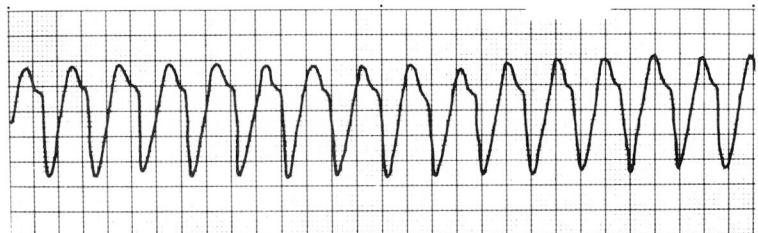

1. Since this arrhythmia begins below the AV node, the atria are beating independently
2. In 20% of patients where the ventricular rate is not too fast and where the ventricular complexes are not too wide, P waves can be seen, which are independent of the QRS complexes.
3. The rate is fast and the QRS are wide. A width equivalent to 0.12 second (3 small blocks) or more is considered abnormal for a QRS complex.

Treatment

1. If patient is tolerating the arrhythmia fairly well:
   a. Give lidocaine (Xylocaine)
      (1) 75–100 mg. I.V. as a bolus over a 2-minute period.
      (2) Repeat in 2 or 3 minutes.
      (3) If effective a continuous I.V. drip of lidocaine should be started with the delivery of 1–3 mg. per minute.
      (4) If a 50-ml. bottle of 2% lidocaine is added to 1000 ml. of 5% glucose in water, 1 ml. will contain 1 mg. of lidocaine.
         Most I.V. sets are calibrated to deliver 1 ml. in 10 drops of fluid. If concentration results in too much fluid for the patient, the amount of lidocaine should be increased in the I.V. solution.

> NURSING ALERT: Because the heart muscle is weakened, the cardiac patient should not receive excessive fluid since this may precipitate congestive failure.

2. Cardioversion
   a. Used when lidocaine does not work or if patient is not tolerating the arrhythmia well.
   b. Start with about 200 watt-seconds.

   Cardioversion is a *timed* electric shock delivered by a machine which is set so that its electrical output does not hit a T wave which is considered the vulnerable period on the cardiac cycle. If an electrical shock such as that from an external source or from an electrical impulse within the heart itself (such as a PVC) hits the T wave ventricular fibrillation may ensue. If not terminated, ventricular fibrillation results in death.

Ventricular Fibrillation

Ventricular fibrillation is a lethal condition seen most commonly in the setting of a myocardial infarction. The patient will die within minutes if the arrhythmia is not terminated.

Altered Physiology

1. The heart is being stimulated simultaneously from numerous ectopic foci throughout the ventricles; therefore, there is no effective contraction of the cardiac musculature and thus no pulse.
2. Characterized by totally irregular appearance on ECG.

Mechanism of Ventricular Fibrillation

Normal Pathway   Ventricular Fibrillation Pathway

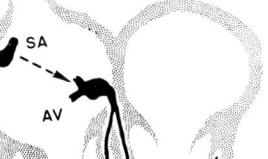
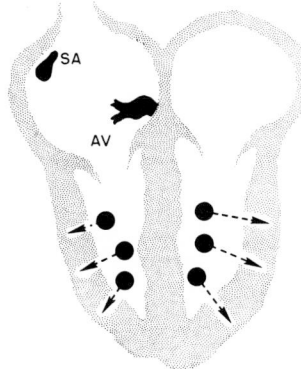

In ventricular fibrillation there are multiple ectopic foci in the ventricle which prohibits an effective heart beat.

ECG of Ventricular Fibrillation

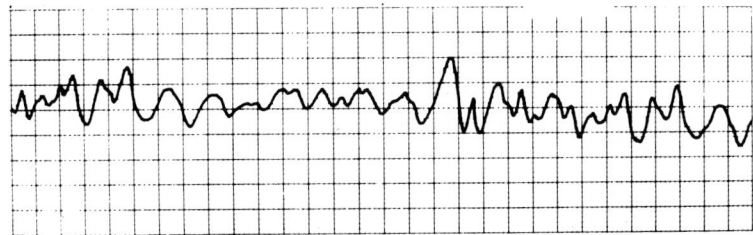

The complexes are completely distorted and irregular.

NOTE: It is extremely important to be sure that the chaotic undulations on the ECG do not represent artifact since movement by the patient or the monitor wires can give the same appearance. If the patient is alert or has a pulse, the rhythm is *not* ventricular fibrillation.

Treatment

Electrical defibrillation at 400 watt-seconds, the highest energy capability of the machines now available. (In children, start with 200 watt–seconds.)

1. If successful, the defibrillation shock stops the erratic uncoordinated electrical activity of the ventricle. After a moment the heart resumes its normal innate rhythm from the SA node.

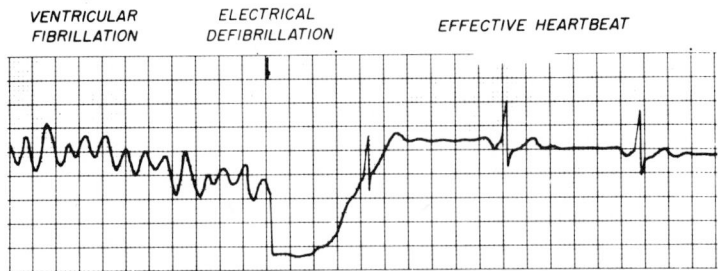

2. Differs from cardioversion in that no timing is necessary with the defibrillation shock since there are no T waves in ventricular fibrillation.
3. Paddle Placement (Fig. 5-26)
   a. The center of 1 paddle is applied just to the right of the upper sternum in the 2nd interspace.
   b. The rim of the other paddle is placed just below the left nipple.
   c. Paddles should be well lubricated and be in firm contact with the skin.
4. See pages 248-250.

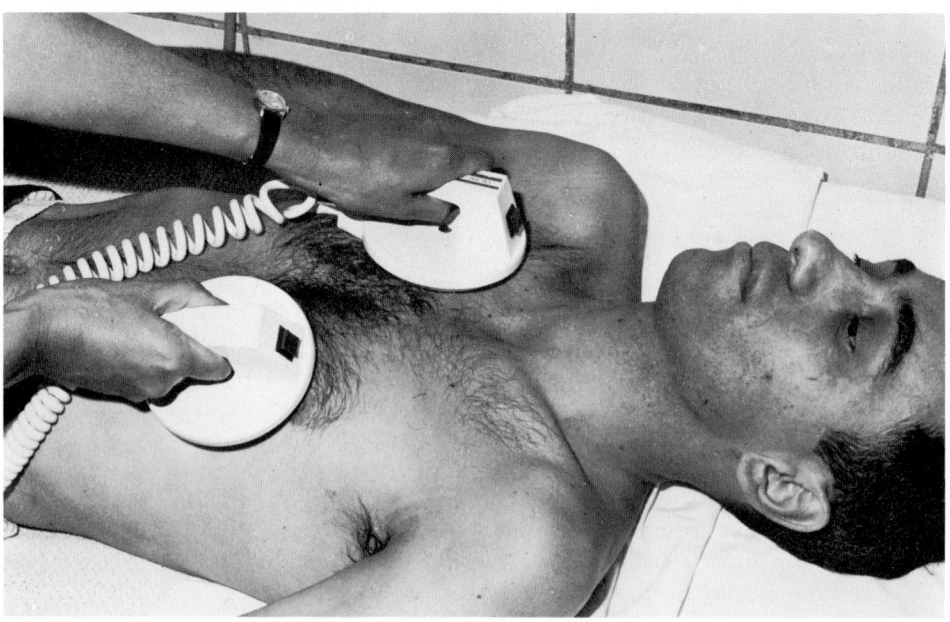

Figure 5-26. Paddle placement in ventricular defibrillation.

SUMMARY: EMERGENCY DIAGNOSIS AND TREATMENT OF ARRHYTHMIAS

Type of Arrhythmia	Appearance of ECG	Treatment	Pathway
Normal rhythm		None.	
Sinus tachycardia		Treat cause.	
Sinus bradycardia		Atropine, Isuprel, or pace-maker when condition is pathological.	
Sinus arrhythmia		None.	
PAC's		Usually none. Quinidine may be used.	
PAT		Carotid sinus pressure or metaraminol (Aramine).	
Atrial flutter		Digitalis if rate is above 100. Cardioversion is very effective.	
Atrial fibrillation		Digitalis if rate is above 100, and if fibrillation is not caused by too much digitalis. Cardioversion may be effective.	
AV Blocks 2nd degree		Atropine, Isuprel, or pace-maker.	
3rd degree		Atropine, Isuprel, or pace-maker.	
PVC's		No treatment if benign. Lidocaine (Xylocaine) in most patients. Atropine if basic rhythm is slow.	
Ventricular tachycardia		Cardioversion or lidocaine.	
Ventricular fibrillation		Electrical defibrillation.	

3. *Vascular Disorders*

Vascular disorders refer to conditions of the blood vessels.

Peripheral vascular disease (PVD) refers to disease of the blood vessels that supply the extremities: veins, arteries and lymphatics.

PATHOPHYSIOLOGIC MANIFESTATIONS OF VASCULAR DISORDERS

Nature of the Disorder

1. Long-term. This is often discouraging to the patient: treatment may be painful and tedious; healing is slow.
2. Appears minor, but hospitalization or disability may last for months before healing takes place.
     Patient may have financial concerns and may worry about loss of job, separation from family and community responsibilities.
3. Elderly are especially prone to peripheral vascular disease.
4. This condition is often compounded with other medical problems, such as diabetes.
5. Recurrence of the condition is frequent with concomitant incapacitation.

Thrombus and Embolus Formation

1. *Thrombus*—a blood clot which partially or completely occludes a blood vessel.
    a. Thrombosed vessel—an occluded vessel
    b. Thrombosis—the condition of having a thrombosed vessel
2. Spontaneous clotting of the blood will not occur unless there is damage to the intimal surface of the vessel wall.
    a. Injury by trauma
    b. Inflammation
    c. Degenerative changes due to arteriosclerosis
3. Injured intima—causes platelets to collect, fibrin to form, and thrombus to develop.
4. *Embolus*—a fragment of a thrombus or a thrombus that has broken away from the point of formation.
    a. Embolism—the process of an embolus moving through a blood vessel and arriving at a narrowing of the vessels thereby occluding it
    b. Air embolism—a bubble of air in the bloodstream
    c. Fat embolism—a plug of fat in the bloodstream

Ischemia

Ischemia is a lack of blood supply to meet tissue needs. This can develop as a result of:

1. Gradual occlusion of the lumen of the artery by fatty deposits (atherosclerosis).
2. More rapid development of ischemia due to a blood clot (thrombus) occurring at the atherosclerotic site.
3. Rapid occlusion of an artery when a free-flowing clot (embolus) lodges at a bifurcation or narrowing of the vessel.

Coldness

1. Due to deficient blood supply to a part even though the environment is warm.
2. One extremity may be compared to another to note the difference.
3. The patient notices that the part feels uncomfortably cold.

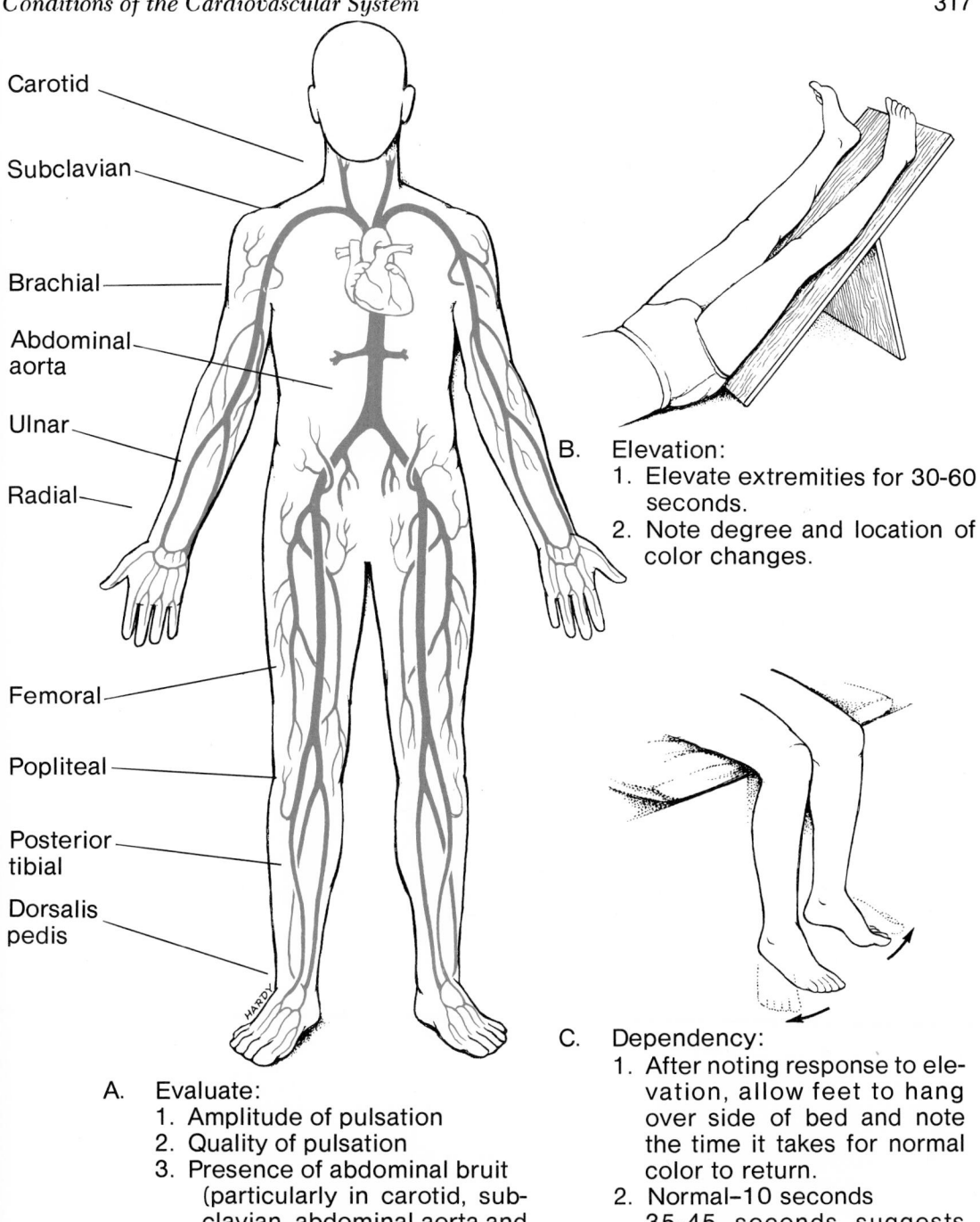

Carotid

Subclavian

Brachial

Abdominal aorta

Ulnar

Radial

Femoral

Popliteal

Posterior tibial

Dorsalis pedis

B. Elevation:
  1. Elevate extremities for 30-60 seconds.
  2. Note degree and location of color changes.

C. Dependency:
  1. After noting response to elevation, allow feet to hang over side of bed and note the time it takes for normal color to return.
  2. Normal—10 seconds 35-45 seconds suggests marked impairment.
  3. Dependent rubor may develop if ischemia is severe.

A. Evaluate:
  1. Amplitude of pulsation
  2. Quality of pulsation
  3. Presence of abdominal bruit (particularly in carotid, subclavian, abdominal aorta and femoral arteries)
  4. Color and temperature of skin
  5. Postural changes (See B and C)

Figure 5-27. Salient points in evaluating peripheral arterial insufficiency.

Pallor (Paleness)

1. Normally the pink hue of the skin is due to adequate superficial circulation.
2. Diminished blood supply produces a paleness or lack of color.
3. Blanching occurs when the part is elevated above the level of the heart.

Rubor (Redness)

1. Instead of a normal rosy-pink, the part may be reddish-blue. This is due to injury of superficial blood vessels causing them to remain dilated.
2. Circulation is impaired.
3. Anoxia or coldness may be the cause of rubor.

Cyanosis (Blueness)

1. Less than normal oxygen is in the blood.
2. Blood supply is deficient but not to the point of causing blanching.

Pain

1. Due to inadequate blood supply.
2. This is common but varies with the condition.
   a. May be constant and severe, i.e., ulceration.
   b. May be burning with a feeling of heaviness, i.e., varicosities.
3. When it occurs only after a certain amount of exercise, it is called *intermittent claudication.* (This disappears after rest, but returns with exercise.)
4. When it occurs at rest (rest pain), it may be due to an embolus or other severe circulatory impairment such as an ulcer or gangrene.

Tests to Determine Vascular Conditions (Fig. 5-27)

A. *Oscillometry*
  1. Degree of arterial occlusion may be measured by an oscillometer which measures pulse volume. One extremity may be compared to the other.
  2. An inflatable cuff is wrapped around the extremity, and the *oscillometric index* is determined by inflating the cuff and reading the dial.
  3. Normal readings (points of pressure at which circulation ceases)
     a. Lower extremity

Midthigh	4–16 mm./Hg
Upper third of leg	3–12 "
Above ankle	1–18 "
Foot	0.2–1.0 "

     b. Upper extremity

Upper arm	4–16 mm./Hg
Elbow	3–12 "
Wrist	1–10 "
Hand	0.2– 2 "

B. *Angiography*—an x-ray visualization of the vascular tree after the injection of a radiopaque dye (renografin).
  1. Inform the patient that he may experience an intense burning sensation in the area where the solution is injected. This will last for only a few seconds.
  2. Note any evidence of allergic reaction to the dye; this may occur as soon as the dye is injected or it may be delayed and occur when the patient reaches his room.

a. Perspiring, dyspnea, nausea, vomiting
b. Rapid heart rate, numbness of extremities
c. Treatment
(1) Notify physician.
(2) Have adrenalin available for injection, as well as antihistamine drugs and oxygen.
3. Postangiography care
a. Encourage patient to remain in bed for 24 hours.
b. Observe injection site.
(1) Signs of inflammation or local thrombosis—redness, swelling
Therapy—Notify physician.
(2) Evidence of bleeding
Therapy
(a) Apply pressure dressing.
(b) Notify physician.
c. Check for arterial occlusion.
(1) Note extremity pulses including quality.
(2) Observe color (pallor or cyanosis).
(3) Ask patient about sensation of feeling (pain, numbness).

C. *Exercise Tolerance*—the measurement of the amount of exercise the involved part can tolerate before pain is experienced.

D. *Skin Temperature Studies*

Objective determination of skin temperature suggesting the degree of arteriospasm; e.g., noting differences between 2 extremities when individual is placed in a new environment: coolness of 1 extremity.

E. *Intermittent Claudication Determination*
1. At rest, blood supply is adequate.
2. Following exercise, such as walking, running or climbing stairs, a severe cramping pain develops in those muscle areas not receiving an adequate blood supply.
3. Upon resting, pain is relieved; metabolites are carried away and normal blood ratio to tissue demand is restored.
4. Measurement
a. Have patient walk up steps, counting the number before pain occurs.
b. Use a foot-pedal device which lifts a weight when pressed.
(1) Normally, fatigue occurs in 5–10 minutes.
(2) The person with arterial occlusion complains of pain in less than a minute.

F. *Lumbar Sympathetic Block*
1. Used to evaluate peripheral circulation in the legs.
2. Procedure
a. Local anesthetic is injected into retroperitoneal space, blocking sympathetic ganglionic cord and affecting legs.
b. Sympathetic nerves control tension of muscles in blood vessels; a block causes vasodilation of vessels.
c. Arteriosclerotic vessels are not capable of dilating.

G. *Plethysmography*—electronic measurement of pulse volume in peripheral vessels
1. Determines state and patency of arterial system.
2. Provides a method of monitoring changes in the peripheral vascular system.
3. The small "strip" of graphic record may be compared with later measurements.

GENERAL MANAGEMENT OF PATIENTS WITH VASCULAR DISORDERS

Therapeutic Modalities in Increasing Blood Supply to Tissues

Postural Therapy

Objective: to permit intermittent filling and emptying of capillaries, veins and arteries.

Observation: Arterial blood supply to a section or part of the body can be increased by positioning it lower than the heart (gravity-assist).

A. *Walking*—a simple but very effective exercise.
   1. A level surface is preferred.
   2. Encourage patient to set realistic goals; each week these goals may be extended in keeping with his tolerance.
   3. Use assistive devices as necessary—walker, cane, etc.
   4. Evaluate patient's ability to climb stairs.

B. *Jogging*—a means of stimulating collateral blood flow not only to legs but also to the myocardium.
   May be practiced as long as it is comfortable and pleasurable.

C. *Buerger's exercises*—prescribed according to condition of extremities and the condition of the patient.
   1. Elevate extremity for a minute.
   2. Place extremities in a dependent position until cyanosis or rubor becomes maximal.
   3. Lie with extremities horizontal for a minute.
   4. See Buerger-Allen exercises below.

D. *Oscillating bed*—provides postural exercises using a passive method.
   1. Aids indirectly in prevention of pressure areas—decubitus ulcers.
   2. Prescribed according to patient needs.
   3. Explain to the patient that the bed will assist in his circulatory difficulty.
      a. Explain how the bed is turned on, regulated and stopped.
      b. Inform him as to whether he can stop for meals, treatments, rest periods, etc.
   4. Proceed gradually with motion of the bed to eliminate the possibility of headache, dizziness or nausea.
   5. Follow prescribed cycle for the individual patient.
      Cycle: Degree of angle and the length of time to be elevated
             Degree of angle and the length of time to be lowered
   6. Prevent the patient from slipping downward by providing a padded footboard.

E. *Buerger-Allen exercises*—exercises by which gravity alternately fills and empties the blood vessels.
   1. Procedure
      a. Begin with patient lying flat in bed. Elevate legs to above level of heart—2 minutes or until blanching takes place.
      b. Allow legs to be dependent; exercise feet—3 minutes or until legs are pink.
      c. Instruct patient to lie flat—5 minutes.
      d. Repeat a, b and c 5 times; do entire set 3 times a day.
   2. Tolerance and proper pacing
      a. Advise patient to rest when he feels pain.

  b. Avoid chilly environment since it causes vasoconstriction which in turn causes pain when patient exercises.

  c. Maintain stability particularly if postural hypotension is a problem.

 3. Comfort

  a. Improvise equipment in order to achieve comfortable support for the patient in the leg-elevated position.

  b. Well-padded straight-back chair can be placed on the bed so that the back of the chair supports the leg—top of chair is toward the top of the thigh.

  c. Overbed table may be used with a pillow.

Thermotherapy

> NURSING ALERT: When heat is applied externally to an extremity—circulation is increased. When applied to diseased tissues—tissue may be damaged, destroyed or become necrotic. When applied to diseased tissues—sensations are impaired; may result in damaging burn and necrosis.

A. *Dry Heat*

 1. Warm Water Bottles

  a. Check temperature of water before filling bottle—not to exceed 48.8°C. (120°F.).

  b. Apply cover to bottle so that it does not come in direct contact with skin.

 2. Heat Cradle (thermostatically controlled or regulated with electric bulbs).

  a. Pad metal edges of cradle to prevent injury to extremities.

  b. Control temperature so that it will not exceed 32.2°C. (90°F.).

  c. Ensure that bulbs are not likely to be touched by extremity (usually legs and feet).

  d. Higher temperatures would stimulate metabolism (not desired).

  e. Reduce temperature if patient complains of pain in extremity.

 3. Ultrasound (acoustic vibration with frequencies beyond human ear perception).

  a. Useful in small areas where deeper penetration of heat is desired and where circulation needs to be stimulated.

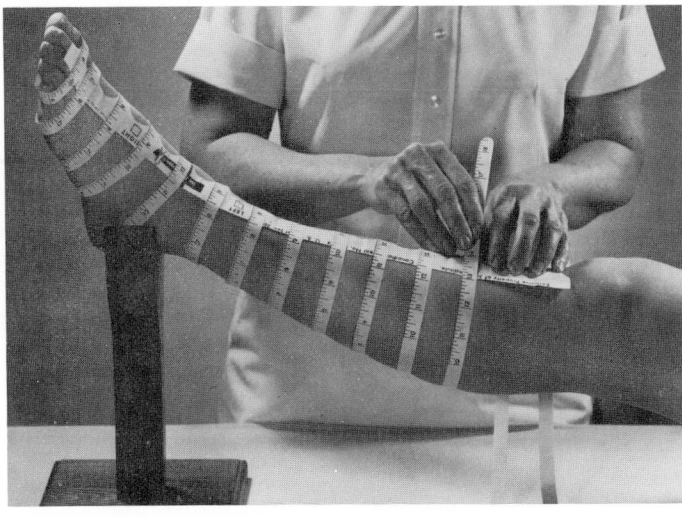

Figure 5-28. By using a special measuring tape, exact measurements of the extremity can be obtained. Measurements are taken while the patient is lying down with the extremity slightly elevated. The foot is in a normal relaxed position. The horizontal spine of the measuring tape is placed anteriorly; key cross straps are fastened and then each succeeding strap is fastened. All straps are calibrated in centimeters. When properly and completely fastened, this measuring device can be cut according to directions and sent to the manufacturer for made-to-order support. (Courtesy Jobst.)

        b. Application time is under 10 minutes.

        c. Avoid areas where metal sutures may be present.

    4. Paraffin Bath (see p. 805).

B. *Moist Heat*

    1. Hydrotherapy

        a. Sitz baths—used for perineal therapy (see p. 424, rectal surgery).

        b. Basin—for hands or feet with prescribed temperatures and for prescribed times.

    2. Whirlpool bath.

        a. In addition to moist heat, the effect of agitated water provides hydromassage.

        b. May be used for 1 or 2 extremities, or the whole body.

    3. Warm compresses.

        a. Applied directly to the skin.

        b. When hot, apply over toweling.

Pressure Gradient Therapy (Compression Devices and Garments)

A. *Cuffs, Sleeves or Boots*

    1. Circulator—electrically produced air pressure which alternately inflates and deflates a boot in which the extremity is encased.

        Rhythm of occlusion and release as well as pressure can be regulated, such as gradual pressure build-up for 45 seconds, alternating with 15-second release phase.

    2. Pressor sleeve or boot—a plastic tube filled with air

        a. Can be maintained at low pressure for several hours.

        b. Can be regulated to function intermittently. (Useful in lymphedema of arm following mastectomy, see p. 563).

Put on supports early in the morning, before swelling occurs.

Always begin with supports "inside-out"... as they are when you receive them.

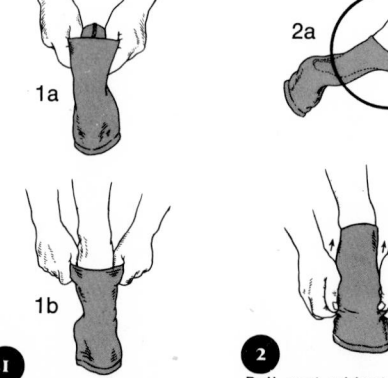

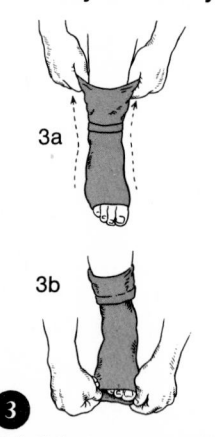

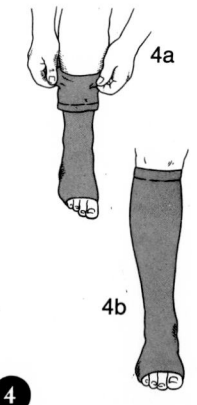

1   Sit with feet in easy reach. Support must be "inside out," with its foot inverted back to heel. Seam faces down (sketch 1a). Grasp each side firmly and pull onto foot (sketch 1b).

2   Pull past midpoint of heel (sketch 2a), so support will not slip back. Then, reach just beyond toes and grasp fabric between fingers and start pulling over foot. Pull from sides ... never by seams.

3   Pull all the way up past ankle (sketch 3a). Seat heel in place. Pull foot portion of support out toward tips of toes (sketch 3b) to set fabric evenly on foot. Allow to settle back normally.

4   Using short (2 inches at a time) snappy pulls (sketch 4a) pull support up to point it was measured to end (sketch 4b). Smooth evenly down leg. **Never allow top to roll or turn down.**

Figure 5-29. Method of applying supporting hose. (Courtesy Jobst.)

B. *Elastic Garments*

  1. Support to an extremity can be tailor-made: A unique measuring tape was devised by Jobst* so that exacting "fabric" pressures are produced with their custom-made venous pressure gradient supports (Fig. 5-28).
  2. Method of applying supporting hose is demonstrated in Figure 5-29.

Anticoagulant Therapy

Normal Physiology

Normal mechanisms responsible for hemostasis (blood coagulation).

A. *Vascular Factors*

Increased fragility—tendency to break up on slight provocation (subnormal resistance) due to quality or quantity of intercellular "cement."

B. *Extravascular Factors*

These include thromboplastin ingredients that operate less effectively than normal due to:

  a. Inadequacy of platelets
  b. Deficiency in some activating component

C. *Platelets*

  1. Form clumps mechanically at the margin of a damaged blood vessel—they plug the hole.
  2. Release vasoconstricting substances.
    a. 5-hydroxytryptamine
    b. Adrenalin
  3. Contribute to formation of fibrin by:
    a. Accelerating manufacture of thromboplastic substances
    b. Acting as a thromboplastin
    c. Hastening the conversion of prothrombin to thrombin
    d. Accelerating the changing of fibrinogen to fibrin
  4. Assist in contracting the clot, thereby extending process of coagulation.
      Upon contraction, clot squeezes out excess thrombin which invades adjacent blood to cause more fibrin formation.

D. *Plasmatic Factors*

Fibrinogen—largest of plasma proteins

  a. Negatively charged terminal groups (glutamic acid) are split off by proteolytic enzyme, thrombin.
  b. Without these negative charges, fibrinogen molecules come together and fuse (polymerization), forming fibrin (a network of interwoven strands).
  c Fibrin is further stabilized by cross linkage.

Composite Physiologic Action of Anticoagulants

  1. Extrinsic prothromboplastin (tissue)
  2. Intrinsic ingredients (blood)—plus:
  3. Plasma Factors (V, VII, and X)—acting in presence of:
  4. Ionized calcium—assist in converting:

* The Jobst Institute, Toledo, Ohio 43601.

5. Prothrombin to thrombin
6. Thrombin and fibrinogen form fibrin

Clinical Indications

(Authorities disagree as to the justification of long-term use of anticoagulants in various disease entities.)

1. *Venous thrombosis* because of the dangers of thrombophlebitis and phlebothrombosis and the danger of emboli.
2. *Pulmonary embolism,* prophylactically if it is known a patient is suspect; also indicated during recovery phase to prevent further clot formation.
3. *Patient susceptible to embolism*—rheumatic heart disease, atrial fibrillation, preoperative surgical patients undergoing vascular surgery, and patients who have undergone vascular surgery including mitral or aortic valve replacement.
4. *Coronary occlusion with myocardial infarction.*
5. *Cerebral vascular accident caused by emboli or cerebral thrombi*—to reduce sludging of blood: useful in prevention and treatment of strokes.

Contraindications

1. May cause spontaneous bleeding, therefore not used when there is evidence of weakened blood vessel walls.
2. Individuals with peptic ulcer and chronic ulcerative diseases are considered poor risks.
3. Should not be given following neurosurgery because of danger of hemorrhage in brain or spinal cord.
4. Liver disease rules out anticoagulants because of interference with plasma protein clotting factors.
5. Liver and kidney insufficiency diseases preclude their use because of difficulty in metabolizing and eliminating anticoagulants, resulting in toxicity and difficulty responding to antidotal medication.
6. Poor follow-up by patients; unless the patient cooperates by reporting for blood tests, etc., he should not be on anticoagulants.

Types of Anticoagulants

	Generic Name	Proprietary Name
Heparin sodium	Heparin	Panheprin
		Lipo-Hepin
Oral		Liquaemin
Coumarin derivatives	Bishydroxycoumarin	Dicumarol
	Warfarin sodium	Coumadin
		Panwarfin
		Athrombin
	Acenocoumarol	Sintrom
	Phenprocoumon	Liquamar
Indanedione derivatives	Anisindione	Miradon
	Diphenadione	Dipaxin
	Phenindione	Danilone
		Eridione
		Hedulin

Heparin Sodium

A. *Pharmacologic Action*
   1. Affects coagulation time by its effect on the clotting mechanism.
   2. Inactivates thromboplastin, which in turn interferes with changing of prothrombin to thrombin.
   3. Inactivates any thrombin which manages to form.
   4. Decreases the adhesiveness of platelets.
   5. Promotes resolution of a newly formed clot.
   6. Does not dissolve the fibrin of a well-established clot.

B. *Advantages*
   1. Chief advantage is its rapid action which makes it the medication of choice in emergency situations and for short-term therapy.
   2. When administered by vein, it acts within seconds and is predictable and controllable (action time intramuscularly or subcutaneously is 30 minutes).
   3. Its effect can be readily neutralized by injecting protamine sulfate or other heparin antagonists intravenously.
   4. It has little cumulative effect and dissipates quickly (within 4 hours).

C. *Disadvantages*
   1. Chief disadvantage is that it must be given parenterally; it is unsuitable for long-term maintenance therapy.
   2. For continued effectiveness, heparin must be given frequently intravenously or by infusion which obviously requires hospitalization of patients.
   3. Heparin is expensive—8 times as expensive as oral anticoagulants.

D. *Side Effects and Contraindications*
   1. Bleeding from mucous membranes may occur; therefore, heparin should not be given to those patients listed under Contraindications (p. 324), to those who have lost large areas of skin, or those with clotting-factor deficiencies.
   2. Allergic reactions may be apparent in those sensitive to substances of animal origin —redness, itchy skin, urticarial wheals.

E. *Antidotes*
   1. Protamine sulfate—this should be available on the department where the patient is receiving heparin anticoagulant therapy.
   2. Blood transfusion.

Coumarin and Indanedione

A. *Most Commonly Used and Administered by Mouth*
   1. Bishydroxycoumarin (Dicumarol)
   2. Warfarin sodium (Coumadin)

B. *Pharmacologic Action*
   1. Acts on reducing blood coagulability by its effect on prothrombin activity.
   2. Prevents vitamin K from participating in the liver's "synthesizing of proteins" process in the clotting action.
   3. Failure of Factor VII is the primary deficiency leading to prolonged clotting time.
   4. Has no effect on clotting factors already in circulation—hence, the delayed action of these drugs is noted later and can be measured by prothrombin time tests.

C. *Prothrombin Time Testing*
1. Normal prothrombin time—11 to 13 seconds.
2. By lengthening the prothrombin time to about 24–30 seconds, coagulability of blood is lowered to lessen thrombosis and yet prevent spontaneous bleeding from developing. This would be the *desired therapeutic range*.

D. *Prothrombin Activity*
Prothrombin range may also be reported in percent of normal—the activity of the plasma prothrombin
1. Desired therapeutic range is 20–30% of normal.
2. Probability of hemorrhage exists when activity is less than 10% of normal. In other words, when prothrombin activity lessens, hypoprothrombinemia increases.

E. *Advantages*
1. Is convenient since it is given by mouth.
2. Unnecessary to keep the patient in the hospital.

F. *Disadvantages*
1. Effects are unpredictable; dosage varies from one person to another and even from one time to another in the same patient.
2. Because the prothrombin level must be tested frequently, laboratory facilities must be available. (This often is a problem.)
3. There is a cumulative effect:
    Dicumarol has a slow onset (2–3 days) and extended cumulative effect (up to 9 days after last dose).
    Coumadin onset occurs within 18–24 hours; cumulative effect lasts up to 7 days.
    Phenindione onset is within 10–12 hours; effects disappear after 24–48 hours; however, there are side effects with which to reckon.

G. *Antidotes to Coumarin Anticoagulants*
1. Administer vitamin K—phytonadione (aquaMEPHYTON) be vein, or Mephyton tablets by mouth.
    Brings prothrombin levels back to safe levels within 4–12 hours.
2. Provide fresh whole blood if immediate antidote action is required, e.g., physical injury, or other urgent emergency.

Nursing Management
1. Since heparin is given along with longer lasting hypoprothrombinemic agents, for the first few days of treatment, each day's medication orders should be checked *after* reports of daily prothrombin time tests are known.
2. Have on hand the antidotes of anticoagulants being used:
    Heparin—protamine sulfate
    Coumarin—vitamin K (phytonadione, Mephyton)
3. Note that the relatively long duration of action of oral anticoagulants makes it easier to maintain low prothrombin levels for long periods.
4. Observe carefully for any possible signs of bleeding and report immediately so that anticoagulant dosage may be reviewed and altered if necessary:

    a. Urine—note evidence of hematuria.

    b. Stool—check for tarry color.

    c. Emesis basin following tooth brushing—note any pink or bloody return.

5. Later, when anticoagulant medication is stabilized, patient must be reminded to keep prothrombin test appointments as scheduled—once a week or however often they are required.

6. Inform patient of precautions to take and observations to make while on anticoagulant therapy after he leaves the hospital.

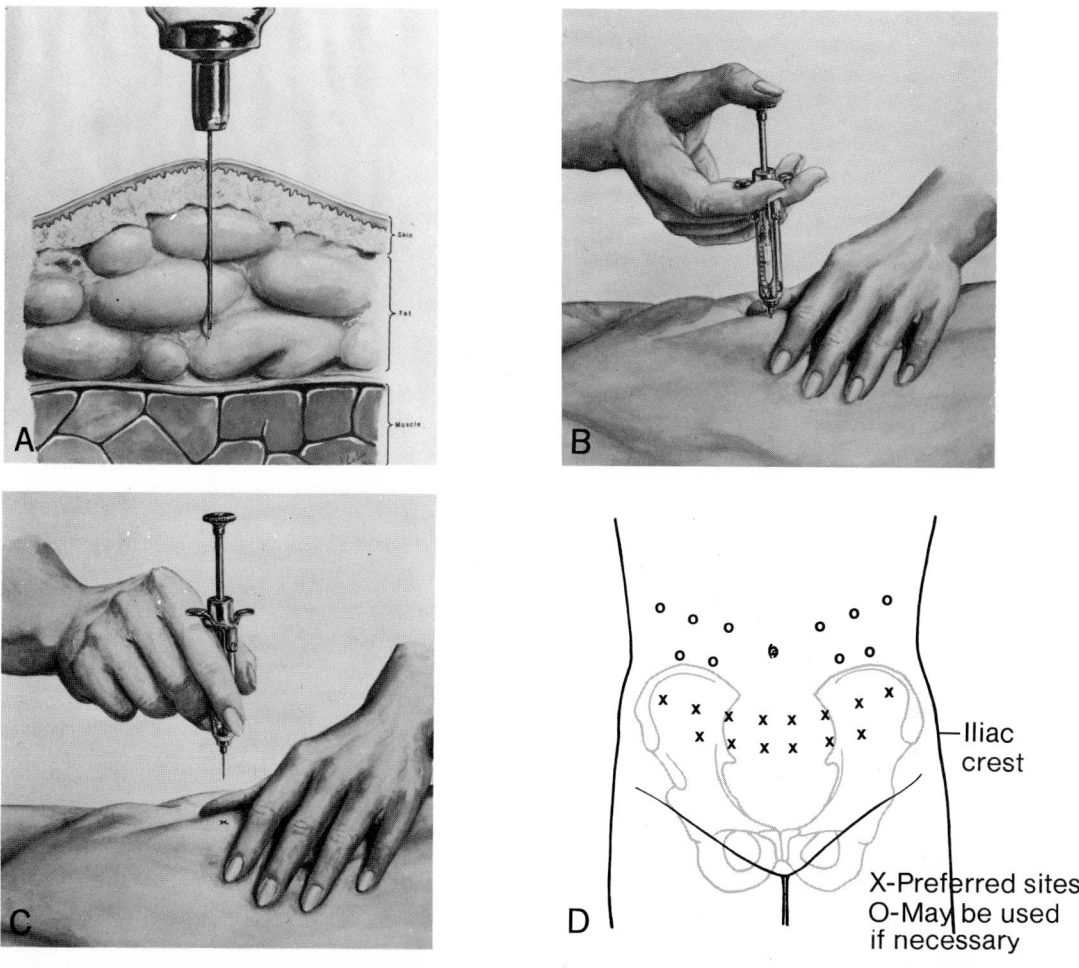

Figure 5-30. Subcutaneous injection indicating technique and sites for heparin therapy. *A.* When prolonged therapy is indicated, heparin is most conveniently given subcutaneously into the fatty tissue which is a distinct layer beneath the skin. *B.* Gently accumulate a well-defined roll of skin without pinching. *C.* Insert the needle directly through the skin at a right angle (see *A*). *D.* Since the site of injection of heparin must be changed each time heparin is administered, a suggested division of the abdomen into suitable areas is indicated. Do not inject into a bruised area or within 5 cm. (2 inches) of the umbilicus or any scar. (Courtesy, Wyeth Laboratories, Philadelphia, Pa.)

Observe for signs of developing toxicity.
    (1) Skin discoloration or bruises on arms or legs
    (2) Undue oozing from small skin abrasions
    (3) Frequent nosebleeds
    (4) Blood in urine

NOTE: Patients on phenindione produce orange or broth-colored urine: when acidified, this coloration disappears. With true hematuria, acid does not affect color.

    (5) Red or tarry stools
    (6) Severe or long-lasting headaches or stomach pain
    (7) Excessive menstrual flow
    (8) Any bleeding
 7. If prolonged diarrhea occurs, anticoagulant requirements increase.
 8. Drug interactions
    a. If infection exists and antibiotics are required, anticoagulant therapy requirements increase.
    b. Recognize that aspirin and salicylates interfere with the same clotting mechanisms that coumarin-type medications act on; hence avoid these drugs unless specifically approved by the physician.
    c. Advise patient to avoid drinking alcoholic beverages to excess since this may affect absorption of vitamin K or anticoagulant from the intestines.
    d. Note that multivitamin supplements may contain vitamin K—patients on these will require a higher dose of anticoagulant.
    e. Report use of mineral oil since it can cause vitamin K deficiency because it interferes with absorption of fat-soluble vitamins.
    f. Note that barbiturates increase metabolism of coumarin medications which means an increased dose of anticoagulants is in order.

GUIDELINES: *Subcutaneous Injection of Heparin*

Purpose

When prolonged therapy is indicated, heparin may be given subcutaneously directly into fatty tissues (Fig. 5-30).

Equipment

1- or 2-ml. syringe
Fine sharp needle, No. 25, 1.6 cm. (⅝ inch) long
Skin antiseptic

Considerations

 1. Most convenient sites are along lower abdominal fat pad to avoid pain and hematoma formation.
 2. Areas such as the thigh muscles should be avoided because of the possibility that drug will diffuse along fascia layers, leading to retroperitoneal bleeding.

Procedure

Nursing Action	Rationale/Amplification
Performance Phase	
1. Sponge the area gently with alcohol. Do not rub!	1. Rubbing or pinching skin might initiate damage to the tissue; heparin would aggravate the problem.
2. Accumulate a well-defined roll of skin—without pinching.	
3. Holding the shaft of the syringe in dart fashion (Fig. 5-30*B*) insert needle directly through the skin at a right angle into the subcutaneous fatty layer.	
4. Move right hand in position to direct plunger.	
a. Do not move needle tip once it is inserted.	a. Hemorrhage or tissue damage could be initiated.
b. Do not pull back on plunger for testing.	
5. Firmly push plunger down as far as it will go. (Fig. 5-30*C*)	5. This ensures administration of total dose of heparin.
6. When injection has been made, withdraw needle gently at the same angle that it entered, releasing skin roll as you withdraw.	6. To minimize tissue damage.
7. Press an alcohol sponge to the site for a few seconds.	7. To minimize ooze or bleeding.
Follow-up Care	
1. *Do not rub the area. Instruct patient not to rub area.*	1. Rubbing would enhance the likelihood of tissue damage.
2. *Site of Injection*	

    a. Change site of injection each time heparin is administered.
    b. Figure 5-30*D* shows a suggested division of abdomen into suitable areas.
    c. A chart can be marked with time, date and measured dosage so that rotation of sites can be assured.

Nursing Management of the Patient with a Peripheral Vascular Problem

Nursing Objectives

A. *To encourage patient to avoid those practices which cause vasoconstriction in the vessels of the extremities.*
    1. Impress the patient with the dangers of smoking, especially inhaling.
    2. Promote an atmosphere that is devoid of emotional tension; restrict those visitors who appear to upset the patient.
    3. Maintain a warm and properly humidified environment.
    4. Prevent the wearing of constricting garments, such as girdles, garters, belts.
    5. Utilize analgesic and tranquilizing medications as required to keep the patient comfortable.

B. *To encourage the following measures and activities to increase the blood flow to the patient's extremities.*
    Instruct the patient as follows:
    1. Wear warm clothing before going out into cool air; protect hands and feet with lamb's wool lining in gloves and boots.

2. Take a warm bath to offset chilling; replace vigorous rubbing of the skin after a bath with gentle patting.
3. Avoid excessive heat to extremities such as using a hot water bottle, electric pads, etc. since this increases metabolism which in turn demands more oxygenated blood.
4. Sleep with the head of the bed elevated about 20.3 cm. (8 inches); wear bedsocks to keep feet warm if necessary.
5. Walking is the best form of exercise; otherwise, active or passive exercises to the extremities are recommended.
6. Take prescribed vasodilating medications even though they may not appear to help; at times they maintain the status quo and keep the problem from worsening.
7. Administer antilipemic drugs to retard progress of concomitant sclerotic disease by reducing serum lipids.
8. Use antihypertensive drugs with caution—may decrease renal circulation or cause cerebral hypoxia.

C. *To recognize the signs and symptoms indicative of circulatory disturbances affecting peripheral tissues.*
   1. Pain in the extremity—(Note whether this occurs at rest, with limited activity, or with more pronounced exercise.)
   2. Color changes of the skin or nails—pallor, pink, rubor, cyanotic
   3. Impaired or peculiar growth of nails
   4. Evidence of scleroderma—shiny taut skin
   5. Discrepancy in size of one extremity when compared to contralateral (or opposite) extremity
   6. Enlarged or abnormal pulsations of veins
   7. Temperature variations: abnormally cold or abnormally warm
   8. Indications of ulcerations, necrosis or gangrene

D. *To keep metabolic demands on the body at a minimum.*
   Instruct the patient as follows:
   1. Take precautions to prevent injury and infection particularly of the extremities.
   2. Practice daily hygienic cleanliness and care of the feet: proper trimming of nails, avoiding strong medications, utilizing lamb's wool for pressure areas, wearing proper size shoes and hosiery.
   3. Avoid exposure to cold or excessive heat.
   4. Recognize the limitations of exercising; set up a reasonable rest plan.
   5. Remain in bed if there is evidence of necrosis, ulceration or gangrene.

Foot Care in the Patient with a Vascular Disorder

Patient Instruction

1. Keep the feet clean to prevent irritation and infection.
   a. Wash daily with a bland soap and warm water.
   b. Dry thoroughly, paying particular attention to the areas between the toes; pat rather than rub dry.
   c. Apply lanolin or petrolatum to prevent drying and cracking of skin.
   d. Wear clean hose daily: woolen socks for winter, cotton for summer.

2. Avoid injury, excess pressure or other irritants to the feet.
   a. Shoes
      (1) Wear properly fitting shoes with a comfortable heel.
      (2) Check inside of shoe to avoid wearing shoes with protruding seams, torn lining, piercing nails or faulty lumps.
      (3) Wear shoes when out of bed; avoid going barefoot.
      (4) Break in new shoes gradually; alternate with an older pair.
      (5) Leather shoes are preferred to rubber because the latter interferes with proper circulation.
      (6) Allow wet or damp shoes to dry slowly on shoe trees to prevent misshaping.
   b. Hose
      (1) Wear proper length and size; hose too short compress toes; hose too long wrinkle and exert pressure on skin.
      (2) Avoid seams, holes or lumpy darned areas.
      (3) Use bedsocks rather than hot water bottle or heating pad if feet are cold in bed.
      (4) Use woolen or cotton hose; they absorb moisture; nylon is not as absorbent.
      (5) Avoid constricting garments: foundation garments, garters and even support hose unless they are specifically prescribed.
   c. Pedicure
      (1) Trim toenails straight across after soaking the feet in warm water.
      (2) Place wisps of cotton under corner of great toenail if there is a tendency toward ingrown toenails.
      (3) Have a podiatrist cut corns and calluses; do not use corn pads or strong medications.
   d. Heat and Cold
      (1) Keep feet warm; avoid exposure to cold for long periods of time.
      (2) Use heating devices only on advice of physician; excess heat can be as damaging as insufficient warmth.
      (3) Rely on warm socks, fleece-lined boots or mitts, light-weight blankets, etc., rather than heating extremities near a fire, oven or radiator.
   e. General Measures
      (1) Avoid areas where injury to feet is likely, e.g., crowded subways, construction areas, sports show, etc.
      (2) Prevent sunburn in the summer and avoid wading in very cold water.
3. Prevent pressure on feet; rest and exercise in moderation.
   a. Place a pillow under covers at end of bed to provide a footrest and prevent weight of top bedding from exerting pressure on toes.
   b. Avoid remaining in one position for long periods of time.
   c. Do not cross legs when sitting because of pressure on nerves and blood vessels.
   d. Elevate feet on a chair or footstool with proper support of leg; do this about 15 minutes every 2 hours.
4. If damage or injury occurs to any part of foot or leg report to physician.
   a. Redness, swelling, irritation, blistering
   b. Itching, burning—athlete's foot
   c. Bruises, cuts, unusual appearance of skin.

PHLEBOTHROMBOSIS

Phlebothrombosis is the formation of thrombi in a vein.

Etiology

1. May occur as a postoperative complication.
2. Occasionally associated with abdominal cancers, particularly those involving the head and tail of the pancreas.

Clinical Manifestations

1. Minimal local and constitutional symptoms or signs
2. Calf pain that is aggravated when foot is dorsiflexed with the leg in extension (Fig. 5-31)
3. Slight swelling around ankle; obvious prominence of leg veins in affected leg

> NURSING ALERT: Do not massage the leg; this may dislodge blood clot and cause pulmonary embolism.

Preventive Measures

1. Encourage early ambulation in surgical patients—exercises for the bedridden patient to prevent venous stasis.

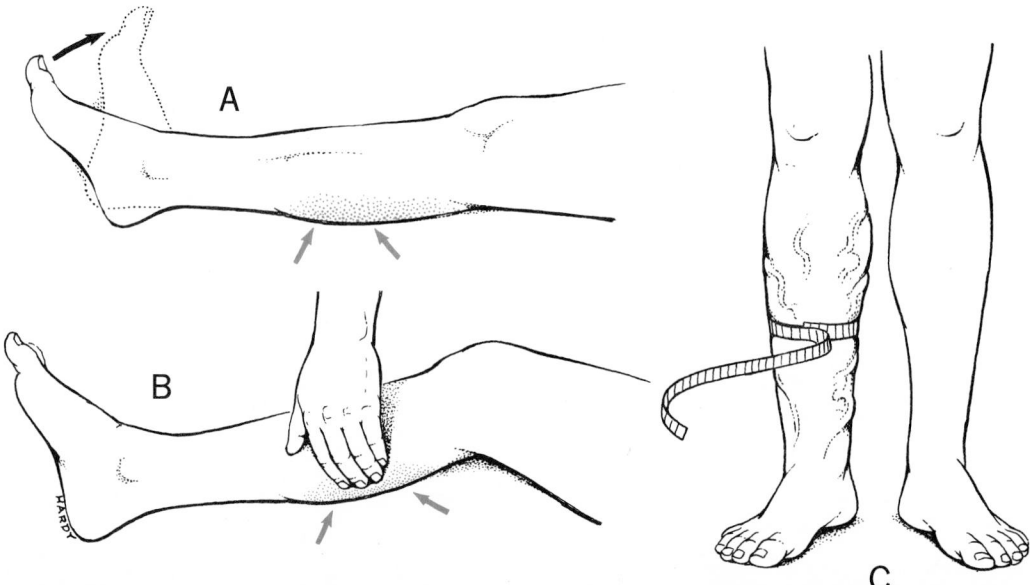

Figure 5-31. Assessment of Signs and Symptoms of Phlebothrombosis. A. With the leg in extension, the patient complains of pain in the calf on dorsiflexion (Homan's sign); note arrow indicating pain site. B. Gentle compression reveals tenderness of the calf muscles (note arrow). C. The affected leg may swell; veins are more prominent and may be palpated easily.

2. Suggest deep breathing exercises that produce increased negative pressure in the thorax which in turn assists in emptying large veins.
3. Recommend properly applied elastic stockings for the bedridden patient—to increase deep venous blood circulation. (Remove twice daily and check for skin changes or calf tenderness.)

Treatment

1. Administer anticoagulation therapy (see p. 323).
2. Maintain adequate hydration of patient to increase circulatory volume.
3. Keep patient in bed; do not massage or actively exercise the legs.
4. Elevate foot end of bed 20.3 cm. (8 inches) to prevent stasis and to promote systemic circulation.
5. Apply local heat for symptomatic relief.
6. After 1 or 2 days, if all local signs have disappeared, ambulate patient.

Complications

1. Pulmonary embolus—can result in sudden death (see p. 155)
2. Pulmonary hypertension—leading to cor pulmonale
3. Phlebothrombosis—may lead to thrombophlebitis or ileofemoral phlebothrombosis

PHLEBITIS OR THROMBOPHLEBITIS

Phlebitis is an inflammation of the walls of a vein.

Thrombophlebitis is a condition in which a clot forms in a vein secondary to phlebitis or due to partial obstruction of the vein.

Etiology

1. Injury (bruise) to a vein
2. Extension of an infection of tissues surrounding the vessel
3. Varicose veins as a complication
4. Continuous pressure of a tumor or aneurysm
5. Pregnancy when the women must be in bed for a prolonged time
6. Unusual activity in a person who has been sedentary

NURSING ALERT: In thrombophlebitis, the clot or portion of it may be dislodged and swept into the pulmonary circulation as an embolus.

Clinical Manifestations

1. Earliest signs—assumption of "frog-leg" position (leg externally rotated, knee flexed)
2. Stiffness or soreness in the calf and edema
3. Pain in upper posterior calf on dorsiflexion of the foot (Homan's sign)
4. Muscle ache—may be falsely assumed to result from wearing flat bedroom slippers postoperatively.

Signs of Obstruction due to Occluding Thrombus

1. Swelling, particularly in loose connective tissue of popliteal space, ankle or supra pubic area
2. Vasospasm—following subsidence of vasospasm, there may be mild to deep cyanosis
3. Increasing warmth of the leg or area

Preventive Measures

1. Initiate early ambulation as soon as possible in postoperative patient.
2. Avoid placing the extremities in one position for a period of time.

Treatment

Objective: to achieve early resolution of thrombi and prevention of sequelae.

1. Avoid massaging or rubbing calf because of the danger of breaking up the clot which can then circulate as an embolus.
2. Check with physician as to proper position of the extremity since there may be differences of opinion.
   a. Some recommend elevation—reduces venous congestion and edema
   b. Others do not recommend elevation—prevents possibility of releasing emboli
3. Apply heat in the form of hot wet dressings or a heat cradle to promote circulation and comfort.
4. Place the patient on anticoagulant therapy (see p. 323).

Patient Instruction

1. Wear elastic stockings all day.
2. Avoid standing for more than one-half hour—thereafter elevate extremity for 15 minutes.
3. Elevate leg when sitting or sleeping.
4. Exercise extremity for 5 minutes out of every hour.
5. Take precautions against injury.

Postphlebitic Syndrome

Postphlebitic syndrome is a form of chronic venous stasis and may be initiated as a residual effect of phlebitis.

Etiology

1. Smaller vessels have dilated because main channel for returning blood from the leg to the heart was blocked by a thrombus.
2. Valves of diseased veins can no longer prevent backflow, thereby leading to→ chronic venous stasis→swelling and edema→superficial varicose veins.
3. Lower leg becomes discolored due to venous stasis and pigmentation ulceration (postphlebitis).

Altered Physiology

1. Pressure in veins at ankle is much greater than normal—leading to transudation of fluid from intravascular to interstitial space.
2. Stasis, intractable induration, chronic edema, discoloration, pain, venous congestion ulceration, recurrent thrombosis→cellulitis.

Treatment

1. Best treatment is prevention of those actions which precipitate the condition.
2. After this syndrome has developed, only palliative and symptomatic treatment is possible because the damage is irreparable.
3. Patient should:
   a. Wear elastic stockings to prevent edema.
   b. Avoid sitting or standing for long periods of time.
   c. Elevate legs on a chair 5 minutes every 2 hours.
   d. Elevate legs above level of head by lying down (2–3 times daily).
   e. Raise foot of bed 15–20 cm. (6–8 inches) at night to allow venous drainage by gravity.
   f. Apply bland oily lotions to prevent scaling and dryness of skin.
   g. Avoid constricting bandages.
   h. Prevent injury, bruising, scratching or other trauma to skin of leg and foot.

VARICOSE VEINS

Primary varicose veins—bilateral dilation and elongation of saphenous veins; deeper veins are normal.

Incidence

This is a common venous disorder of the lower extremity; 10% of the population is affected.

Etiology

1. Dilation of the vein prevents the valve cusps from meeting; this results in increased back-up pressure to be passed into the next lower segment of the vein. The combination of vein dilation and valve incompetence produces the varicosity (Fig. 5-32).
2. Varicosities may occur elsewhere in the body such as the esophageal and hemorrhoidal veins.
3. Predisposing factors
   a. Hereditary weakness of vein wall
   b. Long-standing distension of veins brought about by pregnancy, obesity or prolonged standing
   c. Old age in which tissue elasticity is lost

Clinical Manifestations

1. Disfigurement due to large, discolored, tortuous leg veins
2. Easy leg fatigue, cramps in leg, heavy feeling, increased pain during menstruation, nocturnal muscle cramps

Complications

1. Leg edema, pain from superficial thrombosis
2. Skin infection and breakdown, producing ulcers
3. Hemorrhage due to the weakening of the vein wall and pressure upon it

Diagnostic Evaluation

A. *Trendelenburg Test*—for valvular competence
1. Have the patient lie down; elevate leg 65 degrees to allow veins to empty.
2. Apply tourniquet high on upper thigh to constrict superficial veins (not deep veins)
3. Instruct patient to stand with tourniquet in place.

a. Veins fill slowly from below in 20–30 seconds. Rate of filling not accelerated when tourniquet is removed.	a. Considered normal
b. Veins fill rapidly from below. Lower-leg "blown out" may be evident. Rate of filling not accelerated when tourniquet is removed.	b. Incompetence of communicating veins of lower leg

4. Remove tourniquet

a. Rapid flow of blood down saphenous vein from above.	a. Incompetence of valves of saphenofemoral and superficial veins
b. If in addition to 3b, there is rapid flow of blood downward	b. Incompetence of saphenofemoral veins, valves, superficial veins and valves of communicating veins

B. *Venography*—injection of radiopaque substance into deep veins, followed by observation of blood flow and valve action via x-ray.
1. If dorsal vein of foot is used, dye seems to seep into superficial veins.
2. If dye injection is done directly into medial malleolus to the marrow cavity, regional or general anesthesia is required (because of pain).

Treatment and Nursing Management

A. *Medical Treatment* (nonoperative)
   Patient is instructed to:
1. Avoid activities that cause venous stasis by obstructing venous flow.
   a. Wearing tight garters, tight girdle
   b. Sitting or standing for prolonged periods of time
   c. Crossing the legs at knees for prolonged periods while sitting (reduces circulation by 15%)
2. Control excess weight gain.
3. Wear firm elastic support as prescribed, from toe to thigh when in upright position. Put elastic stockings on in bed before getting up.
4. Elevate foot of bed 15–20 cm. (6–8 inches) for night sleeping.
5. Avoid injury of legs.

B. *Surgical Treatment*
1. Indications
   a. Progressively advancing varicosities
   b. Stasis ulceration
   c. Cosmetic needs
2. Surgery—high ligation at saphenofemoral junction and stripping of saphenous vein from there to ankle. Any remaining dilated veins may be sclerosed with injection of sodium morrhuate (or similar sclerosing agent).

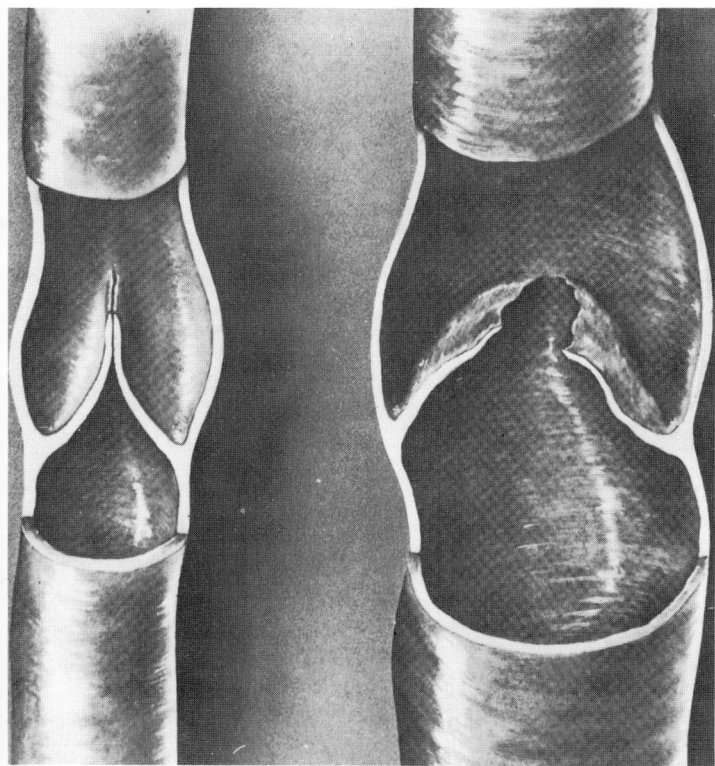

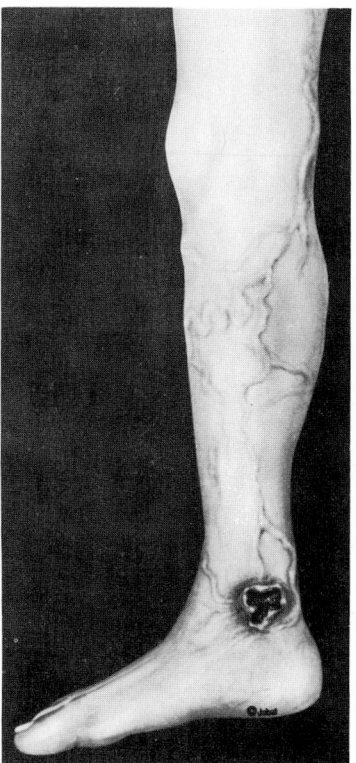

Figure 5-32. Valve incompetence develops as dilatation of a vessel prevents effective approximation of the valve cusps. (Courtesy, Jobst.)

Figure 5-33. Diagram showing leg ulcer resulting from concomitant postphlebitis and varicose veins. (Courtesy, Jobst.)

3. Postoperative nursing care and support
   a. The legs are encased in pressure bandages from the toes to the groin for at least a week; thereafter for a month. Elastic stockings are also worn.
   b. Administer analgesics as required and encourage the patient to walk; support him if necessary.
   c. Observe circulation to detect constriction or hemorrhage.
   d. Note that complaints of patchy numbness can be expected but should disappear in less than a year.
   e. Prevent venous stasis and instruct patient how to avoid this problem.
   f. Recognize that varicosities may recur; therefore conservative measures, learned preoperatively, should be continued.

LEG ULCERS

Incidence
1. Occurrence is increasing with greater numbers being found in the older age group.
2. Postphlebitic syndrome and varicose veins account for most leg ulcers (Fig. 5-33).
3. Burns, sickle-cell anemia and neurogenic disorders account for the remaining ulcers of the leg.

Diagnostic Evaluation

Phlebography
1. A radiopaque dye is injected into a foot or ankle vein and forced into the deep system.
2. Films are taken before and after exercises.
3. Normal results show intact deep venous circulation and good valves.
4. Exercise clears dye from the deep veins after the test is completed.

Objectives of Treatment and Nursing Management

A. *To promote rest and reduce the inflammation.*
   1. Elevate the leg and maintain bedrest.
   2. Initiate proper cleansing routine.
      a. Handle leg very gently.
      b. Use mild soap, warm water and cotton balls.
   3. Remove devitalized tissue.
      a. Flush out necrotic materials with hydrogen peroxide.
      b. Apply enzymatic ointments such as fibrinolysin and desoxyribonuclease, combined-Bovine (Elase) and proteolytic enzymes with neomycin (Biozyme).

B. *To stimulate healing by reducing the infection and providing physiological and nutritional support.*
   1. Administer antibiotic therapy based on culture and sensitivity studies.
   2. Participate in physiotherapy and maintain a regular exercise program.
   3. Control excess weight and provide proper vitamin and protein dietary supplements.
   4. Apply gold leaf (done in some clinics) directly over ulcer site to stimulate formation of granulation tissue.

C. *To stimulate and maintain healthy tissue in the surrounding skin near the ulcer.*
   1. Use sterile saline compresses if area is inflamed or oozing.
   2. Apply compression bandages to the leg (Unna's boot or zinc oxide paste bandage). (See below.)

D. *To employ more radical procedures if the ulcer does not heal during ambulatory conservative treatment.*
   Radically excise the ulcer and cover the remaining tissue with skin grafts.

E. *To encourage the patient who is likely to get discouraged during prolonged treatment.*
   1. Stress the importance of following explicitly the recommendations of the physician-nurse team.
   2. Explain the hazards of trying other remedies on his own at home.
   3. Indicate that the treatment may be long but that patience is an important aspect.
   4. Maintain healthy tissue when the ulcer is healed by continuing with the safeguards as practiced before, because breakdown of healthy tissue unfortunately is frequent.

GUIDELINES: *Applying an Unna's Paste Boot*

Unna's paste boot is a treatment for varicose ulcers consisting of a paste dressing made of gelatin, zinc oxide and glycerin, which is applied to the leg and then covered with an elastic bandage. A commercially prepared gauze bandage impregnated with the zinc oxide, glycerin and gelatin is available.

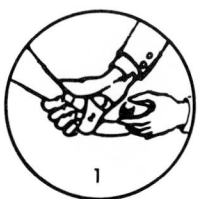 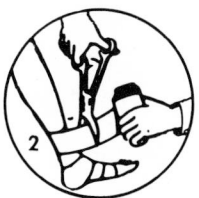 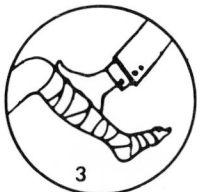 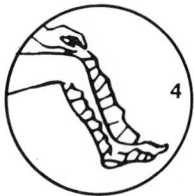

1. Apply right from can. Hold knee in slight flexion. Pad instep and ankle with cotton wad. Start at inner ankle. Make overlapping turns. Figure of eight turn around ankle joint. Use firm equal compression up to the knee.

2. If a turn does not fit snugly, nip edges with scissors or cut bandage off and start a new turn.

3. Mold cast during application with free hand until cast appears even and smooth. Make a cut 2″ long below knee to avoid constriction. Cover cast with loosely woven gauze bandage.

4. Patient can be fully ambulatory. Boot is usually changed once a week. Remove by cutting with scissors.

Figure 5-34. Application of gelatin compression boot. (Manufactured by Graham-Field surgical Co., Inc., New Hyde Park, N.Y.)

Purpose

To treat hard-to-heal ulcers and edema.

Equipment

375 ml. of hot water   400 ml. of glycerin
200 gm. of gelatin   100 gm. of zinc oxide (pulverized)

Procedure

Preparatory Phase

1. Dissolve gelatin in hot water.
2. Mix glycerin and zinc oxide until smooth and add to the dissolved gelatin.
3. Cook for 30 minutes in a double boiler.
4. Allow to become lukewarm before application. (If it is too cool, it will harden.)

Nursing Action	Rationale/Amplification
Performance Phase (Fig. 5-34)	
1. Cleanse, dry and elevate leg for 1 hour prior to applying paste.	1. Reduces venous pool of blood which is an objective of therapy.
2. Apply a sterile dressing over the ulcer; bandage leg with a layer of 5–7.5 cm. (2- or 3-inch) gauze bandage. a. Avoid wrinkling. b. Provide uniform snugness.	2. Provides optimum clean environment to stimulate healing and comfort.
3. Use a 76 cm. (30-inch) brush to paint the leg from the metatarsals to the knee.	3. Introduce paste thoroughly into the bandage.
4. Alternate a layer of bandage and more paste until about 3 or 4 layers of each are applied or until desired thickness is obtained.	4. Gives the leg rigidity.
5. Have patient remain for a half hour.	5. To permit boot to dry and to check circulation.
6. If toes are warm, if color is good and if no edema occurs, discharge patient.	

Follow-up Phase

1. Change boot every 3 or 4 days.
2. As edema subsides and ulcer heals, a change once every week or 10 days is sufficient.

ARTERIAL EMBOLISM

Causes

1. Arterial emboli originate from thrombi in the heart chambers following coronary occlusion due to atrial fibrillation or myocardial infarction.
2. Arteriosclerosis may cause roughening or ulceration of atheromatous plaques.

Clinical Manifestations

1. Acute pain—severe
2. Loss of function—motor and sensory
   a. Paralysis of part   ⎫ Due to embolic block of artery
   b. Anesthesia of part   ⎬ Due to associated vasomotor reflex
   c. Pallor and coldness   ⎭

Treatment and Nursing Management

1. Heparin should be administered intravenously to reduce tendency of emboli to form or expand—useful in smaller arteries.
2. Surgical intervention (embolectomy) is essential when an embolus blocks a large artery, such as the iliac.
3. Postoperative nursing management
   a. Encourage activity in the leg to prevent stasis—obtain specific recommendations from surgeon as to type and duration of exercises.
   b. Administer anticoagulants with full cognizance of what to watch for.
      (1) Inspect for bleeding anywhere including surgical wound; this may be indicative of overdose of heparin.
      (2) Monitor vital signs.
      (3) Recognize cardiovascular history of this patient; hence be able to assess cardiac and circulatory manifestations.

ARTERIOSCLEROSIS AND ATHEROSCLEROSIS

Arteriosclerosis is an arterial disease manifested by a loss of elasticity and a hardening of the middle layer of the vessel wall.

Atherosclerosis is a type of arteriosclerosis, manifested by the formation and collection of deposits containing cholesterol, fatty acids and other substances along the inner wall (intima) of an artery.

Significance

1. Arteriosclerosis is the chief cause of death in the U.S.
2. One of the major clinical manifestations of arteriosclerosis is coronary heart disease
3. Studies indicate that arteriosclerotic heart disease is preventable if attention is paid to "risk" factors.

Etiology

(A combination of many factors)
1. Predisposition of arteriosclerosis is thought by many authorities to be inheritable.
2. Other etiologic factors include metabolic disturbances, arterial hypertension.

3. Commonly associated with diabetes mellitus, chronic nephritis, hypertension (arterial).
4. Risk Factors
   a. Age—death rate in white males between 25–34 is 10 per 100,000
      death rate in white males between 55–64 is 1000 per 100,000
   b. Sex—death rate in ages 35–44 in white males is 6 times greater than in females.
   c. Emotional tension
   d. Elevated serum lipids
   e. Hypertension
   f. Cigarette smoking
   g. Obesity
   h. Impaired glucose tolerance (diabetes mellitus)
   i. Physical inactivity—hence substantial collateral circulation is not established
   j. Gout—uric acid levels of 6.9 mg./100 ml. and above
   k. Hardness of drinking water; some authorities report that the softer the water, the higher the mortality from cardiovascular conditions.

Altered Physiology

1. Arteriosclerosis → narrowing of arterial vessels → malnutrition of tissue cells → ischemic necrosis → fibrosis → sclerosis.
2. Sclerosis → degeneration of major organs due to lack of blood supply (nutrition): brain, myocardium, kidney.
3. Calcium deposits in the media of arterial vessel cause loss of elasticity.
4. Atheromas (plaque-like deposits) of cholesterol, fatty acids and often calcium form on intima of arterial vessels (atherosclerosis).
5. Dislodging of plaque may occur or a thrombus may be formed near the plaque; subsequent embolus may cause arterial occlusion and infarction in distant body sites.
6. Arteriosclerosis tends to be localized rather than generalized.
7. After menopause, women are no longer protected by estrogen.

General Patient Assessment

1. Arteriosclerosis is a generalized vascular disease; however, it varies from patient to patient in that it may affect one area more than another.
2. Often it limits itself to a segment of the vascular tree.
3. Five areas which are the most dangerous and cause disturbing symptoms are:
   a. Brain—cerebroarteriosclerosis   d. Kidneys
   b. Heart—coronary artery disease   e. Extremities
   c. Gastrointestinal tract
4. Prognosis depends upon the greatest area of weakness.

Treatment

1. Since arteriosclerosis and atherosclerosis affect many different parts of the body, treatment is described where the major condition occurs. For example: angina pectoris and myocardial infarction are brought about by athersclerosis of coronary arteries; treatment is discussed under the disease entity.
2. Attention is directed to reducing risk factors such as avoiding tension, reducing excess weight, giving up cigarette smoking, controlling diabetes, and adjusting diet to reduce cholesterol intake (Table 5-4).

TABLE 5-4. LOW CHOLESTEROL DIET
(High in Polyunsaturated Fatty Acids)

Category	Allowed	To be Avoided
Dairy Products		
Milk	Skim milk	Whole milk, cream, cocoa
Cheese	Fat-low or uncreamed cottage cheese	Other
Fat	Corn oil, cottonseed oil, soybean oil, safflower oil	Butter, margarine, coconut oil, olive oil, lard
Eggs	None	Eggs in any form
Meats, Fish, Fowl	Beef—lean, eye, tenderloin Lamb—leg Veal Poultry Fish (excluding shell fish)	Organ meats, pork, ham, cold cuts, frankfurters, goose, duck, fatty meats, bacon, sausage, canned meats, shellfish
Soups and Broths	Fat free broths, bouillon consomme	Creamed soups
Vegetables	All—recommended 1 yellow and 1 green daily	Omit only those which may cause discomfort
Fruits	Any fruit or juice	None
Breads, Cereals, Macaroni Products	Breads permissible made of recommended oils Cereals—all Whole grain recommended	Biscuits, muffins, pancakes, doughnuts, sweet rolls, pastry Cereals—none
Desserts	Fruits, gelatin, sherbet, puddings made with skim milk or fruit juice Angel cake	Whip cream desserts, pies, cake, cookies (unless made with allowed fat or oil) Puddings, custard, ice cream (unless made with skim or nonfat milk)
Beverages	Carbonated beverages, tea, coffee	
Condiments and Miscellaneous	Candy — gumdrops, hard candy, mint patties, honey, jam, jellies Seasonings, herbs, relishes	Candy made with chocolate, buttercream or coconut Potato chips French fried potatoes Sauces, gravies

ARTERIOSCLEROSIS OBLITERANS

Arteriosclerosis obliterans is a condition in which the vascular system of the leg becomes blocked.

Incidence

Men affected more than women.

Clinical Manifestations

Symptoms appear gradually
1. Coldness of extremity
2. Color change—pallor
3. Decrease in size of leg
4. Intermittent claudication (see p. 319)
5. Tingling, numbness of toes
6. Later pain, even when leg is at rest
   Occurs at night requiring patient to get out of bed to walk to relieve pain
7. Cramp-like excruciating pain in calf muscles
8. Ulcers of toes and feet develop

Treatment and Nursing Management

Objectives: to preserve the extremity.
to relieve the intermittent claudication.

See page 329, General Management of the Patient with a Peripheral Vascular Problem.

THROMBOANGIITIS OBLITERANS
(Buerger's Disease)

Thromboangiitis obliterans is a disease characterized by inflammation in the arteries, veins and nerves usually of the lower extremities. It is associated with venous and arterial thrombosis and frequently leads to gangrene.

Etiology

1. Primarily affects males between the ages of 20 and 45.
2. Incidence has decreased in the last several years.

Altered Physiology

1. Structural changes in the walls of the arteries and veins produce a roughening of the intima; a thrombosis then results.
2. Arterial involvement predominates over venous involvement.
3. Coronary, abdominal visceral, and cerebral vessels may be involved in the late stages of the disease.

Clinical Manifestations

1. Onset may be gradual or sudden.
2. Coldness, numbness, tingling or burning sensation in extremities.
3. Intermittent claudication—cramps in the legs after exercise but relieved with rest.
4. Painful red lumps appear under the skin, heal and migrate to nearby areas as phlebitis shifts.
5. More persistent pain is noted in the pregangrenous stage; this becomes more severe when ulcers are present or gangrene has begun.
6. Symptoms are aggravated by smoking, chilling and emotional disturbances.
7. Dependent position of extremity—rubor
   Elevated above heart level—pallor } Indicative of arterial insufficiency
8. Coldness of extremity is common.
9. Arterial pulses are diminished or absent as the disease advances.

Objectives of Treatment and Nursing Management

A. *To improve circulation of the extremities and maintain cleanliness to prevent the spread of the disease.*

Instruct patient as follows:

1. Wash feet with a bland soap and warm water.
2. Pat the washed areas dry with a soft towel; powder unbroken skin.
3. Massage the extremities gently with a bland lubricating oil.
4. Wear clean fresh socks or stockings each day.
5. Initiate Buerger-Allen exercises (see p. 320) if intermittent claudication is in evidence.

B. *To urge a therapeutic health regime in blocking the spread of the disease.*

Instruct patient as follows:

1. Avoid smoking in any form because of its vasoconstricting effect.
2. Obtain rest so as to minimize the demands on the circulatory system.
3. Maintain adequate hydration to assist in avoiding stasis in the affected vessels.

C. *To protect the extremities from trauma and infection.*

Instruct patient as follows:

1. Wear properly fitting shoes and hosiery.
2. Protect the feet from chilling and exposure to cold.
3. Avoid overheating leg by injudicious use of hot water bottles or heating pads.
4. Never use circular garters, constricting bands or garments which would impair circulation.
5. Seek medical attention for evidence of tissue disturbance, e.g., color changes, blister development, abrasion, infection, changes in sensation such as tingling, numbness or pain.

D. *To perform a temporary sympathetic block in selected patients.*

1. Inject lumbar sympathetic ganglia and cord with procaine.
2. Abolish vasoconstricting influence of the sympathetic nervous system.
3. Evaluate effects of the temporary block; if definitely favorable, a lumbar sympathectomy may be done for more permanent effect.

E. *To initiate more drastic attempts to curb the spread of the disease.*

1. Recognize that amputation of a part, such as toes, may be necessary if necrosis develops.
2. Be prepared to repeat the process if gangrene develops in other toes or foot.

DISEASES OF THE AORTA

Aortitis

Aortitis is inflammation of the arch of the aorta.

Types of Aortitis

A. *Arteriosclerotic Aortitis*

1. Accompanies the generalized disease of arteriosclerosis.
2. Appears after the age of 60.
3. Causes pain, dilatation (aneurysm), aortic valve insufficiency.
4. Degeneration and sclerosis of entire surface of intima occur.

B. *Luetic Aortitis*

1. Appears before age of 50.
2. Begins at root of aorta and spreads in patch-like areas over normal intima.
3. Symptoms are variable—may be severe or mild.
   a. Sensations of substernal oppression or weight (vise-like pains)
   b. Sudden attacks of dyspnea may be agonizing and last 5–15 minutes.
      Accompanied by tachycardia, deep cyanosis, profuse perspiration.
   c. Symptoms lead to aortic insufficiency.

Diagnostic Evaluation

Aortic insufficiency without associated mitral lesion, paroxysmal dyspnea, anginal attacks or aneurysm suggest luetic aortitis.

Treatment and Prognosis

1. Antiluetic therapy for luetic aortitis (see p. 841)
2. Damage cannot be repaired completely.
3. If untreated, over two-thirds of patients die within 1 year.

Aortic Aneurysm

Aneurysm is a distention of a vessel

Types of Aneurysms

1. Mycotic aneurysm—very small distended vessel due to infection
2. Saccular aneurysm—somewhat larger distention of a vessel projecting from one side
3. Fusiform aneurysm—distention of the whole artery

Etiology

1. Local infection, pyogenic or luetic
2. Congenital weakness of vessels
3. Arteriosclerosis
4. Most aneurysms are found in the thorax—most of these affect the aortic arch

Clinical Manifestations

A. *Subjective Symptoms*

1. At first no symptoms; later symptoms are similar to congestive heart failure or to a pulsating tumor mass in the chest.
2. Pain and pressure symptoms
   a. Constant, boring pain because of pressure, or
   b. Intermittent and neuralgic pain because of infringement on nerves
3. Dyspnea causing pressure against trachea
4. Cough, often paroxysmal and brassy in sound
5. Hoarseness, voice weakness or complete aphonia resulting from pressure against recurrent laryngeal nerve
6. Dysphagia due to impingement on esophagus
7. With luetic aortic aneurysm there may be anginal and paroxysmal dyspnea due to concomitant luetic aortitis

B. *Objective Signs*
1. Edema of chest wall
2. Dilated superficial veins on chest
3. Cyanosis because of vein compression of chest vessels
4. Ipsilateral dilatation of pupils due to pressure against cervical sympathetic chain
5. Pulse difference in 2 wrists if aneurysm interferes with circulation in left subclavian artery
6. Abnormal pulsation may be apparent on chest wall—due to erosion of aneurysm through rib cage

Diagnostic Evaluation
1. Fluoroscopy will reveal pulsating tumor.
2. Angioaortogram allows visualization of vessels and aneurysm.

Treatment and Nursing Management
1. If untreated, the prognosis is poor
2. Abdominal aortic aneurysm
   a. Surgery to excise area affected.
   b. Replacement of excised segment by a bypass graft.
3. Dissecting aneurysm of aorta
   a. This is a type of aneurysm in which there is a tear in the intima of a blood vessel; as a result of pressure, blood splits the wall and may produce a large hematoma or may continue to rip the wall.
   b. Symptoms resemble coronary occlusion; diagnosis is confirmed by aortography
   c. Prognosis is poor but surgical removal of involved aneurysm and replacement of segment with a graft may be effective.
4. Peripheral vessel aneurysms
   a. May involve renal artery, subclavian artery, popliteal artery (knee).
   b. These produce a pulsating mass and interference with peripheral circulation distal to it.
   c. Replacement grafts are used to repair these aneurysms.

RAYNAUD'S DISEASE

Raynaud's disease is a peripheral vascular disorder of the hands (occasionally the feet, less often the nose, ears, chin) in which there is paroxysmal contraction of the arteries.

NOTE: *Raynaud's phenomenon* is a symptom not only of Raynaud's disease but also of other conditions:
1. Intermittent changes in color of the skin of fingers, toes, and less commonly the nose and ears:
2. Pallor phase—arteries and arterioles completely occluded
3. Cyanotic phase—spasm causes partial occlusion of affected vessels
4. Rubor phase—a period of hyperemia

Etiology
The disease occurs most exclusively in females between the ages of 20 and 40.

Causes

1. Cause is unknown; however, there appears to be a hereditary predisposition.
2. It appears to be related to emotional stress and exposure to cold.

Altered Physiology

1. There is an abnormality of the peripheral sympathetic nervous system—sympathetic overactivity leading to toxic contraction of arterioles.
2. Intermittent vasospasm may completely interfere with the arterial blood flow to the fingers or toes leading to ischemia, pallor, coldness, prickling feeling, pain and numbness.
3. Responding, the capillaries become dilated because of an increase in metabolites; color changes from pallor to cyanosis.
4. Following the spasm, circulation is re-established; color changes from cyanotic to rubor to normal pink.
5. With repeated vasospasms, the artery wall thickens and thrombosis may develop, leading to occlusion, cyanosis, coldness, numbness, atrophy, gangrene.

Clinical Manifestations

1. Gradual onset: pallor of 1 or 2 fingers or toes when exposed to cold—then all digits may become involved.
2. Upon relaxation of vasospasm, tissue temperature change may move rapidly from cold to warm.
3. Nerve sensations may be apparent: tingling, numbness, dull ache.
4. Skin may appear white, smooth, taut, shiny; nail deformity may eventually occur.
5. Continued bouts of vasospasm may gradually progress to ulceration and gangrene.

Treatment

Objective: to relieve and prevent vasospasm.

1. Relief from emotionally stressful experiences may be in order since emotional stress appears to contribute to vasospasm.
2. Exposure to cold which causes vasoconstriction should be avoided.
3. Patient should eliminate smoking which has a tendency to constrict the peripheral vascular system.
4. Vasodilators are administered. Doses are gradually increased until therapeutic effect is noted or adverse effects which suggest stopping increments.

Medication	Adverse Effects
1. Phenoxybenzamine Hydrochloride (Dibenzyline)	Headache, tachycardia, nasal congestion, orthostatic hypotension.
2. Cyclandelate (Cyclospasmol)	Headache, nausea, heavier than usual perspiration, vertigo, flushing, tingling.
3. Azapetine Phosphate (Ilidar)	Fever, general weakness, vertigo, gastrointestinal upset, drowsiness, orthostatic hypotension, nasal congestion.
4. Tolazoline Hydrochloride (Priscoline)	Gastrointestinal upset, orthostatic hypotension, chilliness, tachycardia, palpitations.

5. Regional sympathectomy may be considered if condition worsens and does not respond to above measures; such surgery would remove vasoconstricting impulses.
   a. In most patients, this appears to have only transient benefit; a few patients have had significant improvement.
   b. If Raynaud's phenomenon is secondary to other underlying diseases, results of sympathectomy are poor.
6. Amputation may be necessary if gangrene affects digits (rare).

Patient Teaching

1. Think through the possible causative factors which provoke a spasm; these should be avoided.
2. Utilize insulating clothing when it is necessary to go out into the cold: wool gloves and socks, fleece-lined boots and footwear, etc.
3. Avoid exposing hands to cold objects such as reaching into the freezer, handling a cold, ice-filled glass, etc.
4. Give up smoking; consider moving to a warmer climate, if possible.

HYPERTENSION

Hypertension is an abnormal condition of the small vessels of the arterial system in which the systolic or diastolic blood pressure is elevated.

Normal Physiology

1. *Normal blood pressure* (normotension) is the pressure of the blood within the systemic arterial system. It ranges from 100/60 to 140/90.
2. *Systolic pressure* represents the greatest pressure of the blood against the wall of the vessel following ventricular contraction.
3. *Diastolic pressure* represents the least pressure of the blood against the wall of the vessel following closure of the aortic valve.
4. *Pulse pressure* represents the difference between the systolic and diastolic readings— the range of pressure in the arteries.
5. The *mean arterial pressure* is the average pressure attempting to push blood through the circulatory system.
   This can be determined electronically or mathematically as well as by using an intra-arterial catheter and mercury manometer.
   Mathematical determination. (Slightly less than average of systolic and diastolic)
   Mean arterial pressure = ⅓ systolic pressure + ⅔ diastolic pressure
      Example: for a blood pressure of 130/85
      Mean arterial pressure is 100 mm. Hg
      Kidney function requires a minimum of 70 mm. Hg (mean arterial pressure)
6. *Basal blood pressure* is the lowest blood pressure taken in supine position after several days of hospitalization without treatment.
   Basal sitting pressure and basal standing pressure are often taken for later comparison.

Factors Affecting Pressure of Blood

Blood volume, peripheral resistance, blood viscosity, cardiac output.
1. Blood pressure = cardiac output × total peripheral resistance
   a. Pressure varies with exercise, emotional reaction, sleep, digestion, time of day.
   b. Such functions as renal, adrenal, vascular and neurogenic functions affect blood pressure.
2. Higher blood pressure = increased cardiac output × greater total peripheral resistance (circulatory overload).
3. Lower blood pressure = lessened cardiac output × lesser total peripheral resistance.
4. Increased diastolic pressure due to peripheral resistance indicates decreased size or diameter of arterioles: These are affected by sympathetic stimulation, hereditary factors, more vasopressor hormones in the blood.
5. Increased systolic pressure indicates increased cardiac output and systolic hypertension which is always secondary.

Incidence

1. It is estimated that between 5 and 15% of the population in the U.S. is hypertensive.
2. Onset of hypertension occurs in the early 30's. Because hypertension is asymptomatic, it is usually untreated for at least 20 years.
3. Hypertension is more common but better tolerated in women than in men.
4. Hypertensive women tend to be obese; hypertensive men do not appear to differ from other men in stature.
5. There is a higher incidence in the black race.

Etiology and the Significance of Blood Pressure Elevation

1. Cause is unknown; however, there are several hypotheses:
   a. Hyperactivity of sympathetic vasoconstricting nerves
   b. Presence of blood component which contains a vasoconstrictor that acts upon smooth muscle, thereby making it sensitized to constrictor substances
   c. Increased cardiac output followed by arteriole constriction
   d. Familial tendency
2. Individual tolerance of increased blood pressure varies; however, there is direct correlation between increase in blood pressure and the rate at which atherosclerosis and arteriosclerosis develop.
3. Onset of hypertension occurs in the early 30's; because it is asymptomatic, it is usually untreated for at least 20 years.
4. Rising blood pressure adversely affects the brain, the heart and the kidneys.
   a. Heart—myocardial infarction, congestive heart failure
   b. Kidney—nephrosclerosis, kidney failure
   c. Brain—headache, encephalopathy, cerebral hemorrhage, cerebrovascular accident
   d. Eye—papilledema, swelling of optic disc
5. Emotional stress exacerbates the problem.
6. Obesity and diabetes mellitus are associated with hypertension.

Diagnostic Evaluation

1. Diastolic blood pressure greater than 95 mm. Hg
2. Ruling out of other factors: emotional upset, arteriosclerosis, etc.
3. Urine catecholamine determination (24-hour specimen to determine epinephrine and norepinephrine values)
4. Ophthalmoscopy to detect vascular changes in the capillaries
5. Surgically correctable causes
   a. Coarctation of aorta
   b. Renal disease
   c. Adrenal tumors
6. Review history
   Use of oral contraceptives
7. Assess damage—ascertain effect on kidneys, heart and blood vessels

Classification of Hypertension

A. *Primary or Essential Hypertension* (approximately 90% of patients with hypertension)
   1. With a diastolic pressure of 90 mm. Hg or higher and an absence of other causes of hypertension, the condition is said to be primary hypertension.
   2. Genetic factors contribute to this condition; patterns of the patient indicate his being hyperactive to internal and external stimuli.
   3. Benign—the presence of hypertension for years without manifesting any symptoms.
   4. Malignant—a sudden and severe acceleration in arterial pressure producing many symptoms and vascular damage.

B. *Secondary Hypertension*
   1. Occurs in approximately 5–10% of patients with hypertension.
   2. More common in men and in black race.
   3. Apparently follows other pathology.
      a. *Renal pathology* which may lead to hypertension
         (1) Congenital anomalies, pyelonephritis, renal artery obstruction, acute and chronic glomerulonephritis
         (2) Reduced blood flow to kidney (such as atherosclerotic plaque)—release of *renin*
            (a) Renin reacts with serum protein in liver (alpha-2-globulin)—angiotensin I; this plus an enzyme—angiotensin II—leads to increased blood pressure.
            (b) Symptoms: proteinuria, polyuria, elevated blood pressure.
            (c) Therapy—endarterectomy, bypass graft, nephrectomy; blood pressure is reduced following correction of initial problem.
      b. *Coarctation of Aorta* (stenosis of aorta)
         (1) Blood flow to upper extremities is greater than flow to lower extremities—hypertension of upper part of body.
         (2) Correction—removal of stenosed section of vessel; anastomosis or graft to eliminate area.
      c. *Endocrine Disturbance*—causing elevated blood pressure may be due to pheochromocytoma
         (1) Pheochromocytoma—causes a release of epinephrine to norepinephrine and a rise in blood pressure
         (2) Adrenal cortex tumors lead to an increase in aldosterone secretion and an elevated blood pressure

(3) Cushing's syndrome leads to an increase in adrenocortical steroids and hypertension.
d. *Retinal Changes*
   (1) Optic disc—blurring of disc margins and contour changes
   (2) Papilledema—choked disc
   (3) Arterial diameter lessened
e. *Arteriosclerosis*—renal pathology

Phases of Hypertension and Therapeutic Approach

A. *Prehypertensive Phase*
1. Characteristics
   a. Blood pressure elevation—no vascular change
   b. Systole below 200 mm. Hg
      Diastole below 100 mm. Hg
   c. Headache, giddiness, insomnia, forgetfulness, irritability, epistaxis
   d. Pressure elevation may be the only sign for 10 or 15 years before other symptoms appear.
2. Therapy
   Relief of symptoms only

B. *Benign or Early Phase*
1. Characteristics
   a. Systole below 200 mm. Hg
   b. Diastole above 90 mm. Hg
   c. Headache, giddiness, insomnia, forgetfulness, irritability, epistaxis, blurring of vision, shortness of breath, anginal pain.
2. Therapy
   a. Periodic check-up; treat as an outpatient.
   b. If under age 40, antihypertensive drugs such as methyldopa, hydralazine, guanethidine are considered. (See p. 353.)
   c. Initiate treatment in high-risk patients: young, black race, males, patients with family history of hypertension.

C. *Moderately Severe Phase*
1. Characteristics
   a. Systole above 200 mm. Hg
   b. Diastole above 100 mm. Hg—no evidence of vascular damage
2. Therapy
   a. Rauwolfia, thiazide
   b. Reduce weight, salt restriction
   c. Prophylaxis against cerebral hemorrhage
3. Characteristics—with onset of arteriosclerosis, hypertension increases and diastolic blood pressure is persistently elevated:
   Therapy:
   (1) If exceeding 130 mm. Hg (diastole), hospital rest is recommended.
   (2) Immediate treatment if the following are present:
       (a) Convulsive movements   (c) Severe occipital headache
       (b) Abnormal neurologic signs   (d) Pulmonary edema
   (3) Watch blood pressure; reduce gradually and avoid wide pressure variations— note that bringing pressure down to the usual normal may not be tolerated.
   (4) Measure and record urinary output.

D. *Malignant Phase*
1. Blood pressure may elevate very rapidly with serious damage to vital organs.
   a. Hypertensive encephalopathy or cerebrovascular accident
        Progressive headache—stupor—convulsions
   b. Eye effect—visual impairment, hemorrhage, papilledema, exudates
   c. Kidney effect
      (1) Blood flow decreased, vasoconstriction   (4) Specific gravity down
      (2) B.U.N. more than 100 mg./100 mm.   (5) Proteinuria
      (3) Plasma renin activity
   d. Epigastric pain
   e. Left ventricular failure
   f. Morning headache, nausea and vomiting
2. Therapy
   a. Hospitalization—up to 6 weeks or until blood pressure is well controlled (average diastolic pressure below 100 mm. Hg—in sitting position)
   b. Reduce pressure with ganglionic blocking agents combined with chlorothiazide

Treatment

Objectives: to delay the progress and control the disease.
            to recommend supportive psychotherapy in some form if it will lessen vasocon striction.

A. *General Considerations*
1. Diagnostic Assessment of the Patient.
   a. Blood pressure is determined with patient in resting, sitting and supine position
   b. Electrocardiogram is taken to establish a base line
   c. Chest x-rays are taken to determine cardiac size
   d. Urinalysis and B.U.N., specific gravity, and protein studies are ordered to indicate status of kidney function
   e. Optic fundus is examined—to note edema, spasm, hemorrhage
   f. Neurologic tests are run to detect cerebral damage
2. Type of Therapy.
   a. Therapy is prescribed on an individual basis, depending upon blood pressure, the extent of vascular damage, and whether hypertension is primary or secondary
   b. Assess vital signs and evaluate function of the vital organs.
   c. Inform the patient of the significance of avoiding excess fat and salt in the diet
   d. Initiate a program of weight reduction if obesity is a problem.
   e. Help the patient to understand the importance of giving up smoking.
   f. Instruct patient that he must learn to rest, eat light meals, refrain from running up stairs, etc.
   g. Emphasize the importance of gaining a relaxed attitude toward living.
   h. Select medications with regard to creating complementary combinations, mini mizing side effects and meeting the individual patient's needs.
3. Onset of Complications
   a. Pathology
      (1) Elevate diastolic pressure→strain on arterial wall→thickening and calcifica cation of arterial media (sclerosis)→narrowed blood vessel lumen.
      (2) Sclerosis of vessels→increased wall permeability→deposits placed on intima and media of vessels→cerebral, myocardial, or renal ischemia.

b. Cerebrovascular affectations
   Changes are determined by the type of onset of symptoms
   (1) *Rapid*
       (a.) Cerebral hemorrhage→headache, increase in cerebrospinal pressure→ papilledema→retinal hemorrhages→hemiplegia→coma
       (b.) Cerebral thrombosis→tingling sensations→numbness, limb paresis→ aphasia
       (c.) Subarachnoid hemorrhage→stiffness of neck→pupil dilatation on side of hemorrhage→blood cells in cerebrospinal fluid→unconsciousness
   (2) Neurological changes with recovery in a few hours→cerebrovascular spasms
   (3) *Slow*
       Gradual vascular insufficiency

TABLE 5-5. ANTIHYPERTENSIVE DRUGS

Drug	Action	Clinical Effect	Side Effects and Pertinent Points
Rauwolfia Alkaloids			
Rauwolfia (Raudixin) Reserpine (Serpasil) Deserpidine (Harmonyl) Syrosingopine (Singoserp)	Blocks epinephrine and norepinephrine at intraneuronal level. Decreases peripheral resistance. Readily absorbed from gastrointestinal tract; metabolic products are excreted in urine	Antihypertensive effect is mild and slow in onset. Relieves patient's reaction to emotional stress	Cumulative effects are noted with rauwolfia. (Observe for these even over a long period of time.) Nasal stuffiness — fluid retention. Increased appetite—weight gain. Increased gastrointestinal motility. Diarrhea. Bradycardia. Drowsiness and dizziness. Excessive sedation—depression. Peptic ulceration
Diuretics			
Saluretics (sodium-excreting diuretics) potentiates action of hypotensive drugs. Benzothiazides	Antihypertensive action thought to be due to decreased circulating blood volume and decreased cardiac output. As treatment continues, blood volume and cardiac output return to original level, but dropped blood pressure continues and systemic peripheral resistance decreases.	Sodium is reduced, thereby removing some extracellular fluids → decreased volume of circulating fluids → lessened cardiac output → lowered arterial blood pressure	Potassium depletion may occur depending upon dosage and duration of benzothiazides. Use these drugs cautiously on patients with kidney problems. Hypercalcemia may be a problem. Photosensitivity or skin irritation may be noted.

TABLE 5-5. ANTIHYPERTENSIVE DRUGS (continued)

Drug	Action	Clinical Effect	Side Effects and Pertinent Points
Aldosterone antagonists Spironolactone (Aldactone)	Produces natriuresis (loss of sodium)	Decreases potassium excretion and causes some potassium retention	Epigastric distress, drug rash Breast tenderness or gynecomastia Drowsiness NURSING ALERT: Aldactone should not be given to patients with renal impairment because of the danger of hypercalcemic acidosis.
Decarboxylase Inhibitors Alpha Methyldopa (Aldomet)	Initiates norepinephrine —fails to carry vasoconstrictor alert to blood vessels	Decreased peripheral vascular resistance → decreased blood pressure Used in presence of chronic renal insufficiency	Postural hypotension Watch for kidney toxicity and hepatitis Drowsiness—disappears after a period of time Dry mouth Depression—feeling of unreality Grippe-like pains

Veratrum Alkaloids
Hydralazine (Apresoline)
	Interferes with sensory receptors in the myocardium
	Acts directly on vascular (arteriolar) smooth muscle to decrease peripheral resistance.
		Increases cardiac output
		Increases pulse rate
		Increases renal blood flow
		More pronounced effect on diastolic than systolic blood pressure
		Chief Use: Patients with hypertension complicated by renal insufficiency — (since it does not affect renal function and does not depend on kidney for inactivation)
		Expected clinical signs with dosage higher than 50 mg. daily
		Headache, palpitation, flushing, dyspnea on exertion
			Headache, dizziness (disappears in 7–10 days if drug is continued)
			Tachycardia
			Palpitation, precordial pain
			Anorexia
			Nausea, vomiting
			Diarrhea
			Varying degrees of:
			  Nasal congestion
			  Conjunctivitis
			  Febrile reaction

TABLE 5-5. ANTIHYPERTENSIVE DRUGS (continued)

Drug	Action	Clinical Effect	Side Effects and Pertinent Points
Sympatholytic Agents			
Guanethidine (Ismelin)	Prevents release of nor-epinephrine at sympathetic myoneural junction ("clinical sympathectomy")	Bradycardia Decreases cardiac output and renal blood flow Decreases central venous pressure Orthostatic hypotension *Chief Use:* For moderate or severe hypertension which cannot be controlled satisfactorily with other antihypertensive drugs. Effective with nonazotemic patients.	Orthostatic and exercise hypotension (Caution patient not to stand up rapidly, to sit or lie down if dizziness occurs and lessen dose.) Diarrhea (may be explosive)—may lead to fecal incontinence—control with atropine or other parasympatholytic drug (propantheline) Dry mouth, nasal stuffiness Muscle tremor, weakness Impotence

B. *Pharmacotherapy*

Nursing Considerations

1. Be familiar with the action and side effects of antihypertensive drugs (Table 5-5).
2. Recognize the potent and distressing side effects of these drugs on some patients—individuals react differently.
3. Note the importance of relaying the observations of patient reactions to a medication so that the physician may adjust dosage or type of drug.
4. Instruct patient going home regarding nature of his medications: dosage, frequency, expected effects and untoward signs.
5. Hypotensive drugs are used singly or in combination; they can lower pressure to a desired level.
6. Side effects, unfortunately, often accompany drug administration.
7. Diuretics are effective drugs in treating patients with hypertension; usually thiazides are used first and when no longer effective, a change is made to mercurials.
8. Ganglionic blocking agents are no longer used to any extent.

C. *Parenteral Treatment*

Objective: to reduce diastolic pressure to 110 mm. Hg, then initiate oral therapy.

1. Used in hypertensive emergencies.
   a. Diastolic blood pressure over 150 mm. Hg
   b. Pulmonary edema, cerebral hemorrhage, encephalopathy in combination with diastolic pressure over 120 or 130.
2. Patient must be hospitalized and monitored constantly.
   a. Record blood pressure frequently.
      Some drugs such as trimethaphan and pentolinium require blood pressure to be taken every 5 minutes.

TABLE 5-6. DRUGS FOR PARENTERAL TREATMENT OF HYPERTENSION

Drug	Action	Side Effects and Pertinent Points
1. Trimethaphan camsylate (Arfonad)	Has immediate antihypertensive effect—its effect disappears when infusion is discontinued.	Extremely dangerous medication requiring physician monitoring constantly.
2. Diazoxide (Hyperstat)	Orally—mildly antihypertensive Intravenously—strongly antihypertensive Causes lowering of blood pressure by direct arterial dilatation with an increase in cardiac output and renal blood flow.	Salt is restricted to prevent salt and water retention.
3. Hydralazine (Apresoline)	Effective in treating hypertensive patients with acute glomerulonephritis. Onset of action in 10–20 minutes. Maximum response—1 hour. Persists—12 hours.	Monitor blood pressure every 15 minutes.
4. Methyldopa (Aldomet)	Effective in lowering blood pressure in 4–6 hours and extends 10–16 hours after injection.	Sedation sometimes occurs as a result of this medication but usually wears off in a few days when a maintenance dose is established. Watch for kidney toxicity.
5. Pentolinium (Ansolysen)	Administered intramuscularly, usually into deltoid muscles. Acts within 3 minutes with maximal effects occurring in 15 minutes.	Apply tourniquet above injection site if severe hypotension results. Place patient in sitting position or with head elevated.

      b. Evaluate changes in cerebral status.
      c. Measure urine output accurately.
      d. Be prepared to administer vasopressors if severe hypotension develops.
   3. Medication.
      See Table 5-6, above.

D. *Surgery* (Sympathectomy)
Sympathectomy is not being done as much as heretofore—it is not curative.

Objective: to lower blood pressure effectively without producing severe postural hypotension.
   1. *Indications*
      a. Blood pressure not lowered by medical therapy.
      b. There is severe kidney involvement.
      c. Indications of cerebral dysfunction.
   2. *Surgery*
      10th thoracic ganglion is resected on through the 1st or 2nd lumbar ganglion.

3. *Postoperative Results*
   a. Orthostatic hypotension may result when the patient assumes standing position abruptly.
   b. Blood pressure drops because there is a pooling of blood in the dependent vessels.
4. *Nursing Management Postoperatively*
   a. Recognize that the patient has an increased sensitivity to change in the body position.
   b. Note that the patient may feel faint in moving to the standing position.
   c. Initiate gradually the activity of walking.
   d. Provide a binder or corset that compresses blood vessels thereby avoiding a sudden drop in blood pressure on patient's rising.
   e. Apply elastic bandages or elastic stockings if the patient is going to sit—to decrease pooling of the blood in the legs.
   f. Expect lack of perspiration in areas deprived of sympathetic innervation; conversely, expect excessive perspiration in remaining areas.
   g. Provide the patient with extra covering to prevent undue loss of body heat or fluids.

Nursing Management

1. Recognize the varying effect of certain factors on symptoms of a patient with primary hypertension.
   a. Age, sex, occupation, race, environment, emotional response of the individual, etc.
   b. Understanding of his problem and his rapport with physician, nurse, etc.
   c. Ability to adapt and adjust his activities in line with the prescribed therapeutic regimen.
2. Enlist the patient's cooperation in redirecting his life-style in keeping with the guidelines of therapy.
   a. Present an instructional pattern to fit individual requirements.
   b. Reassure patient when encouragement is needed; the modifications required must appear meaningful to him.
3. Present a coordinated and complementary plan of guidance.
   a. Be aware of the dietary plan developed for this particular patient.
   b. Be available when the physician visits the patient so that his approach and instructions to the patient are known.
   c. Solicit the assistance of the patient's wife or husband and inform them regarding the total treatment plan.
   d. Inform the patient of the meaning of the various diagnostic and therapeutic activities to minimize his anxieties and solicit his cooperation.
4. Measure the blood pressure of the patient under the same conditions each day.
   a. Place patient in the desired position, sitting, standing, etc., according to the preferences of the physician.
   b. Mark the blood pressure reading to indicate patient's position and the arm used: L (lying), St. (standing), R.A. (right arm), L.A. (left arm)—Example: L.A. 152/78/68 St.
   c. Note that muffling may occur at pressures 7–10 mm. Hg higher than direct intra-arterial diastolic pressures. Record 2 readings for the diastolic pressure if required: (130/95/99). The middle figure indicates sign change or occurrence of muffling and final disappearance.

5. Observe patient for signs of cerebral nervous system complications.
   a. Note signs of confusion, irritability, lethargy, disorientation.
   b. Listen for complaints of headache, difficulty with vision; be alert for evidence of nausea or vomiting.
   c. Be prepared to offer protection to the patient if he exhibits convulsions—padded bed sides, nonrestrictive garments, anticonvulsive medications.
6. Prevent those reactions or activities which will increase arterial pressure.
   a. Avoid situations which might engender feelings of anxiety, anger or annoyance in the patient. Psychological stress has a direct effect on physiological function.
   b. Prevent alterations in the ordinary functions of eating, sleeping or elimination which might lead to discomfort or annoyance: Physiological disturbance may increase stress reaction.
   c. Provide rest period and maintain a pleasant comfortable environment.
      (1) Advise patient to rest for a short time before and after eating.
      (2) Remind him to rest during the waking hours for a full hour.
   d. Serve food in small quantities more frequently than in 3 heavier meals.
      (1) Cardiac output increases with food intake.
      (2) Blood pressure is elevated with large intake of fluids.
      (3) Sodium intake may be restricted depending upon severity of hypertension.
7. Practice supportive psychotherapy by observing the patient's reaction, appearance and personality as he relates to the professional staff, visitors, ancillary personnel, etc.
   a. Permit his expression of feelings; promote positive reactions; analyze negative reactions in an attempt to avoid their recurrence.
   b. Note side-reactions which can be easily missed; investigate these.
      (1) Failure to make "eye-to-eye" contact in conversation
      (2) Suggestion of uneasiness, nervousness, restlessness
      (3) Side remarks or "under-the-breath" comments
8. Develop a plan of instruction which will be practiced when the patient goes home.
   a. Instruct him regarding proper method of taking his blood pressure at home and at work if his physician so desires. (Some authorities recommend this practice.) Inform him of the readings which should be reported to the physician.
   b. Plan his medication schedule so that the many medications are given at proper and convenient times; set up a daily check list for him to record taking the medication.
   c. Determine recommended dietary plans, e.g., extent of salt restriction, exchange foods, etc.
9. Assist the patient in coping with the side effects of the therapeutic medications.
   a. Recognize that the drugs used to control effectively the elevated blood pressure will very likely produce side effects.
   b. Warn the patient of the possibility of hypotension occurring following the intake of certain drugs.
      (1) Instruct him to get up slowly to offset the feeling of dizziness.
      (2) Encourage him to lie down immediately if he feels faint.
   c. Alert patient to expect such effects as nasal congestion, asthenia (loss of strength), anorexia (loss of appetite), orthostatic hypotension (dizziness on changing position).
   d. Inform the patient that the goal of treatment is to control the patient's blood pressure, reduce the possibility of complications and utilize the minimum number of drugs with least dosage necessary to do the task.

10. Educate the patient to be aware of toxic manifestations and report them so that adjustments can be made in his individual pharmacotherapy.
    a. Note that dosages are individualized; therefore, they may need to be adjusted since it often is impossible to predict reactions.
    b. Remember that certain conditions produce vasodilatation—a hot bath, hot weather, febrile illness, consumption of alcohol.
    c. Be aware that blood pressure is increased when circulating blood volume is reduced—dehydration, diarrhea, hemorrhage.
    d. Suspect the presence of edema as a reportable symptom particularly when guanethidine and ganglioplegic agents are taken; these medications are less effective in the presence of edema.

THE LYMPHATIC SYSTEM

The *lymphatic system* is a network of vessels and lymph that are interrelated with the circulatory system. It removes tissue fluid from intercellular spaces and protects the body from bacterial invasion. Lymph nodes are located along the course of the lymphatic vessels and filter lymph before it is returned to the bloodstream.

Significance of Lymphangiography

Radiologic visualization of the lymphatic system is possible when a dye is injected into the lymphatic vessels of the hands or feet.

Means of detecting lymph-node involvement by metastatic carcinoma, lymphoma or other inaccessible sites (except by surgery) such as the pelvis, retroperitoneum, deep axilla.

Lymphangitis

Lymphangitis is an acute inflammation of lymphatic channels.

Etiology

Arises most commonly from a focus of infection in an extremity.

Clinical Manifestations

1. Displays characteristic red streaks that extend up an arm or leg from an infection—not localized—septicemia.
2. Produces general symptoms: high fever, chills.
   Produces local symptoms: local pain, tenderness, swelling along involved lymphatics.
   Produces local lymph node symptoms: enlarged, red, tender (acute lymphadenitis).
   Produces an abscess: necrotic, pus-producing (suppurative lymphadenitis).

Treatment and Nursing Management

1. Administer chemotherapeutic agents since causative organisms usually are streptococci and staphylococci.
2. Treat affected part by rest, elevation and the application of hot, moist dressings.
3. Incise and drain if necrosis and abscess formation takes place.

Acute Cervical Adenitis

Acute cervical adenitis is an acute infection of the lymphatic glands of the neck. It is usually secondary to an infection of the mouth, pharynx or scalp.

Etiology

1. Usually cervical adenitis is secondary to an infection of the mouth, pharynx or scalp.
2. Occurs more frequently in children.
   a. Inspect teeth, tonsils, etc., since they are often foci of infection.
   b. Examine scalp for evidence of pediculosis.

Clinical Manifestations

1. Swelling on one side of neck: markedly tender and edematous.
2. Systemic signs indicative of an infection: temperature elevation, malaise, increased pulse, etc.
3. Process continues to abscess formation and spontaneous rupture if not incised.

Treatment

1. Determine the source of infection and treat it.
2. Administer antibiotics.
3. Apply warm moist compresses to localize infection.
4. Incise and drain; continue with moist warm compresses until drainage ceases and infection is cleared.

Lymphedema

Lymphedema is an obstruction to the lymph flow in an extremity which produces a swelling of the tissues particularly in the dependent position.

Clinical Manifestations

Obstruction may be in lymph nodes as well as the lymphatic vessels
   a. Observed in arm following radical mastectomy (see p. 563).
   b. Noted in lower extremity associated with varicose veins or chronic phlebitis.

Treatment and Nursing Management

1. Apply elastic bandages or stocking.
2. Keep patient at rest with affected part elevated, each joint higher than the preceding one.
3. Administer diuretics to control excess fluid.
4. Give antibiotics as prescribed.

BIBLIOGRAPHY

Heart Disorders

Books

Andreoli, K. G., et al.: Comprehensive Cardiac Care. St. Louis, C. V. Mosby, 1971.
Armington, Sister Catherine, and Creighton, H.: Nursing of People with Cardiovascular Problems. Boston, Little, Brown and Co., 1971.

Bellet, S.: Clinical Disorders of the Heart Beat. Philadelphia, Lea and Febiger, 1971.
Brunner, L., et al.: Textbook of Medical-Surgical Nursing, 2nd ed. Philadelphia, J. B. Lippincott, 1970, pp. 359–427.
Burch, G. G.: A Primer of Cardiology. Philadelphia, Lea and Febiger, 1971.
Chung, E. K.: Principles of Cardiac Arrhythmias. Baltimore, Williams and Wilkins, 1971.
Conn, H. L., Jr., and Horwitz, O.: Cardiac and Vascular Diseases. Philadelphia, Lea and Febiger, 1971.
Duffy, M., et al. (eds.): Current Concepts in Clinical Nursing. St. Louis, C. V. Mosby, 1971, pp. 291–315.
Friedberg, C. K. (ed.): Physical Diagnosis in Cardiovascular Disease. New York, Grune and Stratton, 1969.
Furman, S., and Escher, D.: Principles and Techniques of Cardiac Pacing. New York, Harper and Row, 1970.
Hurst, J. W., and Logue, R. B. (eds.): The Heart. New York, McGraw-Hill, 1970.
Julian, O. C.: Cardiovascular Surgery. Chicago, Year Book Medical Company, 1970.
Kernicki, J., et al.: Cardiovascular Nursing. New York, G. P. Putnam's Sons, 1970.
Lewis, E. P. (ed.): Nursing in Cardiovascular Diseases. New York, American Journal of Nursing Co., 1971.
Neville, W. E.: Care of the Surgical Cardiopulmonary Patient. Chicago, Year Book Medical Publishers, Inc., 1971.
Norman, J. C. (ed.): Cardiac Surgery. New York, Appleton-Century-Crofts, 1972.
Pitorak, E., et al.: Nurse's Guide to Cardiac Surgery and Nursing Care. New York, McGraw-Hill, 1969.
Riehl, C. L.: Coronary Nursing Care. New York, Appleton-Century-Crofts, 1971.
Rodman, T., et al.: The Physiologic and Pharmacologic Basis of Coronary Care Nursing. St. Louis, C. V. Mosby, 1971.
Russek, H. I., and Zohman, B. L.: Coronary Heart Disease. Philadelphia, J. B. Lippincott, 1971.
Sanderson, R. G.: The Cardiac Patient. Philadelphia, W. B. Saunders, 1972.
Sharp, L., and Rabin, B.: Nursing in the Coronary Care Unit. Philadelphia, J. B. Lippincott, 1970.
Stephenson, H. E.: Cardiac Arrest and Resuscitation. St. Louis, C. V. Mosby, 1969.
Stock, J. P. P.: Diagnosis and Treatment of Cardiac Arrhythmias. New York, Appleton-Century-Crofts, 1970.
Whipple, G. H.: Acute Coronary Care. Boston, Little, Brown and Co., 1972.
Zohman, L. R., and Tobis, J. S.: Cardiac Rehabilitation. New York, Grune and Stratton, 1970.

Articles

Bain, B.: Pacemakers and the people who need them. Amer. J. Nurs., 71:1582–1585, Aug. 1971.
Barstow, R. E.: Nursing care of patients with pacemakers. Cardio-Vasc. Nurs., 8:7–10, March-April 1972.
Barry, E. M., et al.: Hospital program for cardiac rehabilitation. Amer. J. Nurs., 72:2174–2177, Dec. 1972.
Boyek, J.: What heart patients want to know—and what to tell them. Nursing '72, 2:38–42, May 1972.
Brener, E. R.: Surgery for coronary artery disease. Amer. J. Nurs., 72:469–473, March 1972.
Carnes, G. D.: Understanding the cardiac patient's behavior. Amer. J. Nurs., 7:1187–1188, June 1971.
Davis, M. Z.: Socioemotional component of coronary care. Amer. J. Nurs., 72:705–709, April 1972.
Escher, D. J. W.: Medical aspects of artificial pacing of the heart. Cardio-Vasc. Nurs., 8:1–5, Jan.-Feb. 1972.
Fowler, N. O. (ed.): Treatment of cardiac arrhythmias. Mod. Treat., 7:13–227, Jan. 1970.
Gazes, P. C.: Adams-Stokes syndrome: indications for permanent pacemakers. Postgrad. Med., 50:199–203, Oct. 1971.

Germanin, C. P.: Exercise makes the heart grow stronger. Amer. J. Nurs., *72*:2169–2173, Dec. 1972.

Hochberg, H. M.: Effects of electrical current on heart rhythm. Amer. J. Nurs., *71*:1390–1394, July 1971.

Husni, E. A., et al.: Elastic compression of the lower limbs: merits and hazards. Amer. Heart J., *82*:132–133, July 1971.

Jarvis, D.: Open heart surgery. Patients' perceptions of care. Amer. J. Nurs., *70*:2591–2593, Dec. 1970.

Kos, B., et al.: Teaching patients about pacemakers. Amer. J. Nurs., *71*:523–527, March 1971.

Kouchoukos, N. T., and Kirklin, J. W.: Coronary bypass operations for ischemia heart diseases. Mod. Conc. Cardiovasc. Disease, *41*:47–51, Oct. 1972.

Lamberton, M. M.: Cardiac catheterization: anticipatory nursing care. Amer. J. Nurs., *71*:1718–1721, Sept. 1971.

Lawson, M.: Progressive coronary care. Heart and Lung, *1*:240–253, March-April 1972.

Lehmann, Sister J.: Auscultation of heart sounds. Amer. J. Nurs., *72*:1242–1246, July 1972.

Littmann, D.: Stethoscopes and auscultation. Amer. J. Nurs., *72*:1238–1241, July 1972.

Nelson, C. L., and Esselstyn, C. B.: Cardiac and renal surgery. Surg. Clin. N. Amer., *51*:1009–1242, Oct. 1971.

Mayer, J.: Low-sodium diets. Postgrad. Med., *49*:193–195, June 1971.

Ochsner, J. L.: Surgery for myocardial revascularization. Postgrad. Med., *49*:127–129, April 1971.

Pinneo, R. (ed.): Symposium on concepts in cardiac nursing. Nurs. Clin. N. Amer., *7*:411–585, Sept. 1972.

Scannell, J. G., et al.: Optimal resources for cardiac surgery. Circulation, *44*:221–236, Sept. 1971.

Walters, M. B., et al.: Complications with central venous catheters. JAMA, *220*:1455–1457, June 12, 1972.

Williams, T. W., et al.: Management of bacterial endocarditis—1970. Amer. J. Card., *26*:186–191, Aug. 1970.

Vascular Conditions

Books

American Heart Association: Recommendations for Human Blood Pressure Determination by Sphgmomanometer, 1967.

Brunner, L. A., et al.: Textbook of Medical and Surgical Nursing, 2nd ed. Philadelphia, J. B. Lippincott, 1970, pp. 326–358.

Conn, H. L., and Horwitz, E.: Cardiac and Vascular Disorders. Philadelphia, Lea & Febiger, 1971.

Fairbairn, J. F., et al.: Peripheral Vascular Diseases, 4th ed. Philadelphia, W. B. Saunders, 1972.

Hume, M., Sevitt, S., and Thomas, D. P.: Venous Thrombosis and Pulmonary Embolism. Cambridge, Harvard University Press, 1970.

Review of Modern Medicine: Hypertension and the Cardiovascular System. Minneapolis, Minnesota, Modern Medicine Publications, 1972.

Szelagyi, D. E.: Surgery of the Peripheral Arteries—Principles of Preoperative, Intraoperative, and Postoperative Management. *In* Kinney, et al. (eds.): Manual of Preoperative and Postoperative Care, 2nd ed. Philadelphia, W. B. Saunders, 1971.

Wilkins, R. W., Hollander, W., and Chobanian, A. V.: Evaluation of Hypertensive Patients. Ciba: Clinical Symposia, Vol. 24, No. 2, 1972.

Articles

Boyle, E.: Biological patterns in hypertension by race, sex, body weight, and skin color. JAMA, *213*:1637–1643, Sept. 7, 1970.

Caldwell, J. R., et al.: The dropout problem in antihypertensive treatment. J. Chr. Dis., *22*:579–592, Feb. 1970.

Cox, M., and Wear, R. F.: Campbell's soup program to prevent atherosclerosis. Amer. J. Nurs., 72:253–259, Feb. 1972.

Dodd, H.: Varicose veins and venous disorders of the lower limb. Nurs. Mirror, Part I *135*:42–47, Nov. 17, 1972; Part II *135*:46–51, Nov. 24, 1972.

Fries, E. D.: Medical treatment of chronic hypertension. Mod. Conc. Cardiovas. Dis., *40*:17–22, April 1971.

Gifford, R. W.: Raynaud's disease. Hosp. Med., *6*:37–53, March 1970.

Gross, H., Hasson, J., and Solomon, S.: Anticoagulant therapy: a critique. Amer. Fam. Phys., *3*:87–91, June 1971.

Hunter, J. A.: Surgery of venous and thromboembolic disease. Surg. Clin. N. Amer., *51*:99–110, Feb. 1971.

Husni, E. A.: The postphlebitic limb. Hosp. Med., *7*:73–91, Oct. 1971.

Husni, E. A., et al.: Elastic support of the lower limbs in hospital patients. JAMA, *214*:1456–1462, Nov. 23, 1970.

Jackson, B. S.: Chronic peripheral arterial disease. Amer. J. Nurs., 72:928–934, May 1972.

Kaufman, H.: Deep vein thrombophlebitis. Arch. Surg., 99:489–493, Oct. 1969.

Lord, J. W., Jr.: Varicose veins: a surgeon's view. Hosp. Med., 5:61–77, July 1969.

Postgraduate Medicine: Hypertension and Renal Disease. Postgrad. Med., *52*: No. 3, Sept. 1972.

Roos, D. B.: Plethysmography. Surg. Clin. N. Amer., *49*:1333–1342, Dec. 1969.

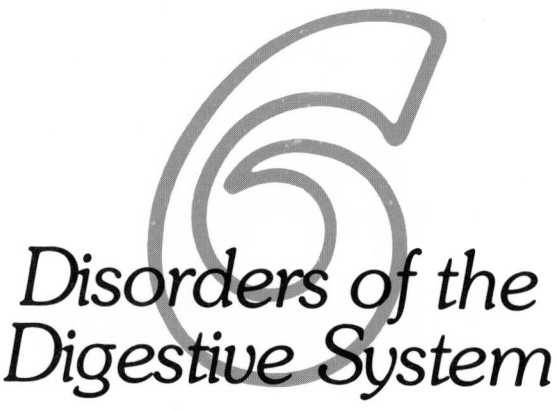

Disorders of the Digestive System

1. Conditions of the Mouth, Neck and Esophagus

SPECIFIC MOUTH LESIONS

Cancer of the Lip

Predisposing Factors

1. Chronic irritation, i.e., from a warm pipe stem or prolonged exposure to wind and sun.
2. Tendency for leukoplakia to progress to epidermoid lip cancer.

Clinical Manifestations

1. Occurs most frequently on lower lip, in men, as a chronic ulcer.
2. Painless indurated ulcer with raised edges.

Treatment

Objective: to remove malignancy with best cosmetic result
1. Small lesions are excised liberally.
2. V-excision is the simplest form of treatment for cancer of the lip. The lip is reconstructed by approximating the layers of the mucous membrane, subcutaneous tissues and the skin.
3. More extensive resection involves excising half of the lip or the entire lip.
4. If lesion involves more than one-third of lip, best treatment may be radiotherapy.
5. If lymph nodes involved, a radical neck dissection is indicated (see p. 370).

Nursing Management

A. *For V-excision*
1. Observe appearance of lip for uncontrolled bleeding forming a hematoma. If untreated,
   a. Undue pressure on mucous membrane results in sloughing.
   b. Cosmetic results are poor.
2. Avoid trauma to incision when the patient eats.
   a. Keep a small dressing over lip.
   b. Feed patient liquids and blenderized foods through straw or nasal tube.
3. Observe for possible secondary infection.

B. *For More Extensive Resection* (excision of half or entire lip)
1. Preoperative nursing management
   Provide meticulous oral hygiene (particularly in presence of infected teeth, gingivitis and a generally poor mouth condition)—to avert infection in the incision line, thereby interfering with proper healing.
2. Postoperative nursing management
   a. Observe incision to detect signs of inflammation or infection.
   b. Aspirate oral secretions frequently to keep mouth clean and to avoid crusting of secretions around sutures.
   c. Note any swelling around incision which might indicate onset of infection or slow bleeding.
   d. Prevent the patient from exerting undue strain on operated lip when eating, talking, smiling, laughing or using other facial expressions.
   e. Feed patient preferably via a nasogastric tube to prevent strain on suture line.
   f. Offer sips of water, crushed ice, or tea to keep oral mucous membrane moist and free of drying secretions.
   g. Liberalize light liquid nourishment by mouth about the 5th day.
   h. Permit soft or semi-solid foods after 10 days.

Cancer of the Tongue

Anterior Tongue

A. *Manifestations*
1. A small ulcer (or thickening) on the anterior undersurface of lateral aspects of tongue that has not healed in 3 weeks
2. Pain or soreness of tongue on eating hot or highly seasoned foods
3. Limitation of motion of tongue

4. With spread of growth to neighboring structures
   a. Excessive salivation, blood-tinged sputum
   b. Slurred speech, trismus (contraction of mastication muscles)
   c. Pain on swallowing liquids
5. If untreated
   a. Inability to swallow
   b. Earache, face-ache and toothache
   c. Inability to eat or sleep
   d. Cervical lymph node metastasis
   e. Hemorrhage
   f. General debilitation

B. *Objectives of Treatment*
   To remove the malignancy and salvage as much of the tongue as possible.
   1. When limited to one side of tongue, hemiglossectomy may be done.
   2. With more spread, a glossectomy is usually done.
   3. With metastasis, surgical dissection may be combined with radiation.

C. *Postoperative Medical and Nursing Management*
   See below, Cancer of the Mouth

Posterior Tongue

A. *Manifestations*
   Symptoms are less obvious
   1. Slight dysphagia, sore throat
   2. Salivation
   3. Blood-tinged sputum

B. *Treatment*
   Poor prognosis
   1. It is a difficult site for effective radiation
   2. Total glossectomy is very mutilating

C. *Postoperative Medical and Nursing Management*
   See page 368, Cancer of the Mouth, and page 888, Advanced Cancer Nursing Care

Cancer of the Mouth

Incidence

1. Cancer of the mouth accounts for 3% of all cancer deaths in this country
2. Males afflicted 3½ times more than females.
3. Lesions of lips and tongue account for half of mouth cancer.

Clinical Manifestations

A. For precancerous mouth lesions—leukoplakia buccalis, keratosis labialis
   1. Pearly patches—1 or 2 small thin, often crinkled areas on mucous membranes of the tongue, mouth, or both, due to
      a. Keratinization of mucosa
      b. Sclerosis of underlying tissue
   2. Later, most of tongue and mouth may become covered
      a. Creamy white, thick, fissured mucous membrane
      b. Sometimes desquamates, leaving a beefy-red base

B. For cancerous lesions
   1. White patchy area, sore spot or ulcer on lips, gums or mouth which fails to heal
   2. Swelling, numbness or loss of feeling in the part

Preventive Measures

Eliminate causes of chronic irritation.
   1. Proper dental care—remove or repair jagged, carious and infected teeth.
   2. Reduce or eliminate smoking and chewing tobacco—also pipe smoking if it irritates the lip.
   3. Restrict or eliminate ingestion of highly spiced foods.
   4. If syphilis is suspected, seek treatment (see p. 840).

Diagnostic Evaluation

   1. Roentgenogram of head and neck to determine involvement.
   2. Cytologic examination of sputum.
   3. Biopsy of suspected tissue.

Treatment

   1. Surgical removal of lesion and perhaps regional lymph nodes. Operation may be glossectomy, radical neck dissection, depending on patient's clinical status and stage of disease (see p. 370).
   2. For inoperable cancer (see p. 888).
       a. Radiotherapy to decrease cancer size
       b. Systemic chemotherapy to slow tumor growth

Nursing Management

A. *Preoperative Care*
   1. Provide optimum mouth care.
       a. Proper care of teeth because they are essential to mastication.
           (1) Regular dental care
           (2) Good nutrition
       b. Mouth cleanliness to reduce incidence of infectious disease such as mumps, surgical parotitis.
           (1) Brush teeth frequently.
           (2) Use oxygen-releasing and antimicrobial mouth-rinsing solutions.
           (3) If patient is a mouth-breather, use swabs of mineral oil with lemon juice.
           (4) Apply lanolin to dry and cracking lips.
           (5) Remove dentures and clean frequently.
       c. Adequate fluid intake, particularly in debilitated patients who are prone to mouth infections.
       d. Stimulation of flow of saliva.
           (1) Offer chewing gum.
           (2) Encourage patient to suck lemon sour balls, a fresh lemon or orange slices.
           (3) Administer antibiotics as prescribed to assist in control of infection.
   2. Promote optimum physical condition and psychological adjustment.
       a. Maintain a good nutritional level.
       b. Assess patient's reaction to his condition.

(1) Correct any misinformation.

(2) Evaluate his apprehension and offer emotional support.

(3) Determine physician's objectives for patient's rehabilitation.

3. Care for mouth lesions and control mouth odors.
   a. Feeding problems
      (1) Use straws, teaspoon, feeders, etc.
      (2) Provide food that is soft, liquid and nonirritating—not too hot or cold or highly seasoned.
      (3) Serve small, frequent meals attractively.
   b. Excessive salivation and mouth odors
      (1) Insert gauze wick in corner of mouth; place basin conveniently to catch drippings.
      (2) Use small rubber catheter and suction.
      (3) Encourage use of mouthwashes, particularly oxidizing agents: potassium permanganate, 1:10,000; hydrogen peroxide half strength.
      (4) Use power spray.
4. Provide regular preoperative care (see p. 42).

B. *Postoperative Care*
1. Maintain a patent airway.
   a. Place patient in prone position, supine position with head turned to side, or laterally—position should facilitate drainage.
   b. Suction as required; precautions necessary to avoid injury to suture line and sensitive tissues.
2. Keep mouth clean for comfort and to assist in healing process.
   a. Mouth irrigations, using normal saline, diluted hydrogen peroxide, sodium bicarbonate, or alkaline mouthwashes.
   b. Gentle lavaging, using a catheter between cheek and teeth to loosen mucus.
   c. Power spray to clean inaccessible spaces.
   d. A vaporizer will provide moisture to traumatized tissue and discourage crusting.
3. Encourage speech rehabilitation and social adjustment.
   a. Supply pad and pencil or "magic slate" so that patient can express his needs and thoughts.
   b. Allow him to have his meals in privacy if he desires.
   c. Encourage his family and friends to visit so that he is aware others care for him.
   d. Assist him in caring for his personal appearance.
   e. Observe closely for indications of his needs which may be communicated in other ways.
   f. Refer him to a speech pathologist or therapist if the services of this specialist are indicated.
   g. Be consistent with emotional support.
4. Provide an environment conducive to the patient's recovery.
   a. Maintain proper humidification and aeration of room.
   b. Prevent odors by removing soiled dressings; use effective and pleasant deodorizers.
   c. Inform patient that his general throat discomfort is due to endotracheal anesthesia and will improve in a few days.
5. Prepare patient for convalescence and extended care at home.
   a. Provide detailed instructions to the patient or a member of his family.

b. If suctioning is required, instruct as to method, type of equipment and where it can be obtained.

c. Emphasize adequate nutrition—proper consistency, proper seasoning and right temperature. Suggest commercial baby foods or the use of a blender if available.

d. Repeat the details of good mouth care and cleanliness of dressings.

e. Review signs of obstruction, hemorrhage, infection and depression and what to do about them if they are evident.

RADICAL NECK DISSECTION FOR MALIGNANCY

Objective: to remove all lymph-node-bearing tissue on the involved side of the neck.

Scope of Surgery—Removal of all tissue under the skin from the ramus of the jaw down to the clavicle; from midline back to the angle of the jaw. This includes: sternocleidomastoid muscle, other smaller muscles, jugular vein in the neck.

Concomitant Surgery—Tracheostomy (see p. 98)

Nursing Management

A. *Preoperative Care*

Preoperative care including diagnostic evaluation—see specific related condition, such as Cancer of Mouth, p. 367, Cancer of the Esophagus, p. 372, etc.

B. *Postoperative Care*

Postoperative nursing objectives are based on the following patient concerns.

1. His ability to breathe normally
   a. Place him in Fowler's position.
   b. Observe for signs of respiratory embarrassment, such as dyspnea, cyanosis, edema.
   c. Evaluate vital signs which may suggest hemorrhage or infection onset.
   d. Note condition of dressings to detect early signs of hemorrhage.

2. His ability to swallow
   a. Observe for throat irritation: edema, clearing of throat.
   b. Note how he accepts liquids: refusal may mean difficulty in swallowing which in turn may be indicative of superior laryngeal nerve damage.
   c. Encourage coughing to remove secretions.
   d. Allow patient to assume sitting position to bring up secretions (the nurse should support his neck with her hands).
   e. Suction secretions if patient is unable to bring them up himself.

3. His wound healing
   a. Reinforce pressure dressings from time to time to assist in obliterating dead spaces and providing immobilization.
   b. Observe dressings for evidence of hemorrhage and constriction which may affect respiration.
   c. If suction drainage (Hemovac) is used, approximately 80–120 ml. of serosanguineous secretions are drawn off during the first postoperative day; this diminishes with each day.
   d. Apply aeroplast or other antiseptic plastic sprays to protect the wound.

4. His ability to communicate
   a. Inform the patient that temporary hoarseness can be expected with extensive neck surgery and tracheostomy.
   b. Encourage him to write messages for first few days.
5. His appearance
   a. Respect his desire for privacy during treatments, dressing change, and feedings.
   b. Inform his visitors of his appearance before they see him so that their expressions do not cause him to be upset.
   c. Provide frequent aeration of the room and utilize deodorants to prevent unpleasant odors.
   d. Observe for lower facial paralysis since this may indicate facial nerve injury.
   e. Watch for shoulder dysfunction which may follow resection of spinal accessory nerves.
      (1) Utilize postoperative muscle exercises and muscle re-education.
      (2) Work with the patient to obtain good functional range of motion.
6. His prognosis
   a. Encourage the patient to verbalize his concerns and feelings.
   b. Consult the physician to determine the nature and extent of explanation and prognosis he has given to the patient.
   c. Encourage the patient to seek confirmation of his personal philosophy and religious beliefs if this would provide answers for him.
   d. Accentuate the positive.
   e. Encourage the patient to participate in his plan of care.

Hemorrhage as a Major Complication Following Mouth Surgery and Radical Neck Dissection

Principal Causes of Sudden Hemorrhage Following Surgery

1. Loose ligature around a large vessel
2. Sudden distention of tied off blood vessel followed by rupture
3. Slipping of ligature that may occur in violent coughing spasm
4. Rupture of a vessel due to trauma incident during surgery
5. Rupture of a vessel weakened by erosion, tumor or slough
6. Sloughing associated with secondary infection.

Treatment

A. *Immediate Treatment for Sudden Hemorrhage*
   1. Pressure over the common carotid and internal jugular vessels in the neck may be life saving.
   2. Have someone notify surgeon immediately.
   3. Treat patient for shock.

B. *Definitive Treatment*
   1. Surgical intervention to repair vessel defect
   2. Correct fluid and blood loss with proper replacement
   3. Initiate postoperative monitoring program until vital signs remain consistently normal for this patient.

CONDITIONS OF THE ESOPHAGUS

Cancer of the Esophagus

Incidence

1. Benign tumors and sarcomas of esophagus are rare.
2. About 80% of cancers of the esophagus involve men.
3. Middle third of esophagus is most involved.
4. Carcinoma of esophagus is responsible for 2% of all cancer deaths in the United States.
    a. Usually this is a geriatric patient who also has pulmonary and cardiovascular disorders.
    b. Proximity of lesion to vital body structures, e.g., heart and lungs; lymph-node-spread is easy and rapid.
    c. Before significant symptoms occur, the tumor has already invaded surrounding structures.

Causes

1. Chronic trauma—frequent use of alcohol, tobacco, spicy foods, hot Oriental tea.
2. Poor mouth hygiene.

Clinical Manifestations

1. Intermittent and increasing difficulty in swallowing. At first only solid foods give trouble then as growth progresses and obstruction becomes more complete, even liquids have trouble passing into stomach.
2. Regurgitation of food and saliva occurs.
3. Hemorrhage may take place.
4. Progressive loss of weight and strength due to starvation.
5. Later symptoms: substernal pain, hiccough, respiratory difficulty, foul breath.

Diagnostic Evaluation

1. Roentgenogram and esophagoscopy
2. Bronchoscopy—usually performed with lesions in the upper two-thirds of the esophagus in order to determine tracheal involvement and whether the lesion can be removed
3. Cytologic and tissue biopsy

Treatment

1. Surgery is the only hope of cure.
2. Lesions of middle and lower esophagus are excised.
    a. Portion of esophagus containing tumor is removed.
    b. Continuity of gastrointestinal tract is reformed by bringing the stomach into the chest and implanting proximal end of esophagus into it.
    c. Chest drainage of pleural cavity is carried out (see p. 150).
3. Lesions in middle and upper third, particularly, are often not suitable for excision.
    a. Some clinics report success with implanting jejunum or a plastic tube to bridge the involved area.

  b. Radiation therapy is used either before or after surgery depending upon surgeon's preference.
  c. If growth is inoperable, a gastrostomy (see p. 395) may be performed as a palliative procedure to permit administration of food and fluids.

Nursing Management

Principles are similar to those given for Radical Neck Dissection (p. 370) and Thoracic Surgery (p. 174).

Esophageal Trauma

Esophageal trauma is injury to the esophagus caused by external or internal insult.
  1. Externally—stab or bullet wounds, crush injuries, etc.
  2. Internally—swallowed foreign bodies, i.e., metal objects, fishbones, dental appurtenances, poison (e.g., lye burn).

Treatment and Nursing Management

Objectives: to institute emergency life-saving treatment.
  to restore continuity of esophagus.
  to facilitate healing and prevent infection and constriction.

  1. Assess condition of patient to determine his physiologic needs.
  2. Maintain open airway. Often, difficulty in respiration is due to edema of throat or a collection of mucus in pharynx.
  3. Control hemorrhage if present.
  4. Treat for pain and shock. (Shock may be due to hemorrhage, impairment of cardio-respiratory function.)
  5. Provide high fluid intake; may require parenteral therapy.
  6. For external wound:
     a. Initiate emergency first-aid wound care and prepare for surgery (see p. 42).
     b. Maintain feeding through a nasogastric tube.
  7. For internal chemical damage, give specific antidote.
     a. A gastrostomy may be performed, either as a temporary or a permanent means of feeding the patient (see p. 395).
     b. Resulting strictures may be relieved by dilating the narrow esophagus with bougies.
     c. Reconstructive surgery may be necessary to create a new passageway for food between pharynx and stomach.
  8. For swallowed foreign bodies.
     a. When foreign body is made of metal, such as bobby and safety pins, needles, jacks, nails, etc., it is not considered safe to allow object to make its way through gastrointestinal tract.
     b. Usually these can be removed with the aid of an esophagoscope.
     c. A skilled operator is required; magnets can be used on end of retrieving instrument passed through esophagoscope.

Achalasia (Cardiospasm)

Cardiospasm or *achalasia* refers to a benign stenosis of the lower end of the esophagus often with a marked dilatation of the upper esophagus. It is a neuromuscular disorder due to absent or defective nerves (myenteric plexus) going to the involuntary muscles in the esophagus.

Clinical Manifestations

1. Loss of peristaltic activity
2. Failure of esophageal sphincter to relax (cardiospasm) as food approaches this area during the swallowing process
3. Difficulty in swallowing, substernal pressure, fullness and regurgitation
4. Weight loss followed by marked emaciation

Diagnostic Evaluation

1. Roentgenogram including barium swallow
2. Patient's history and dietary maladjustment

Treatment

1. Medical or Minor Surgical
   Dilating agents such as French bougies or mercury-weighted dilators.
2. Major Surgical
   a. Esophagomyotomy—a division of muscular fibers enclosing the narrowed esophagus permitting mucosa to pouch out through the divided area in muscle layers.
   b. Cardiomyotomy—when above operation is extended to include cardiac end of stomach.

Nursing Management

Incisional approach determines nature of postoperative care, thus, an incision through chest implies nursing care similar to a thoracotomy (see p. 174).

Esophageal Diverticulum

An *esophageal diverticulum* is an outpouching of the wall usually in the cervical posterior side.

Types

1. Zenker's—upper end of esophagus
2. Traction—near Tracheal bifurcation
3. Epiphrenic—lower third of esophagus

Clinical Manifestations

1. Difficulty in swallowing, fullness in neck, a feeling that food stops before it reaches the stomach.
2. Belching, gurgling or coughing brought about by diverticulum becoming filled with food or liquid. This is regurgitated and may irritate the trachea.
3. Foul odor to breath caused by decomposing of food in pouch (diverticulum).

Diagnostic Evaluation

1. Roentgenograms using barium
2. Esophagoscopy contraindicated because of danger of perforation of diverticulum leading to mediastinitis.

Treatment

1. Evaluate nutritional state to determine dietary needs.
   With swallowing difficulty, diet is limited to those foods that pass more easily.
   (1) Blenderized meals
   (2) Vitamin supplements
2. Surgical intervention, usually using a vertical incision; however, some surgeons prefer a transverse cervical incision.
   a. Caution taken to avoid injury to common carotid artery and internal jugular vein.
   b. Sac is dissected free and then excised flush with esophageal wall.
   c. If transthoracic approach is used, nursing management is similar to that described for chest operations (see p. 174).
   d. Nasogastric tube inserted.

Nursing Management

1. Institute nasogastric feedings utilizing fluids.
   a. Irrigate tube carefully with water following each feeding.
   b. Record kind and amount.
2. Observe wound for evidence of leakage from esophagus—may lead to fistula formation.
3. If patient is tolerating liquid diet well, consider offering a bland diet.

Esophageal Varices

See pages 439–442.

2. *Gastrointestinal Conditions*

MAJOR MANIFESTATIONS OF GASTROINTESTINAL DISTURBANCE

Anorexia, Nausea, Vomiting

Normal Physiology

A. *Appetite*—a desire for food, or an agreeable attitude toward ingesting food, often specific kinds of food.
   1. The frontal and parietal areas of the brain are known to be associated with appetite.
   2. Desire for food is associated with increased rates of gastric hydrochloric acid secretion, with gastric hyperemia and hypermotility.
B. *Hunger*—a strong sensation or urge to eat following a period of fasting.
   1. Hunger is temporarily associated with rhythmic contractions of the stomach.
   2. The precise mechanisms by which hunger is produced is unknown; it is related to a low blood-sugar level.
C. *Satiety*—a condition following consumption of sufficient food to meet present requirements.

Anorexia

Lack of appetite for food; lack of interest in all food.
1. Associated with a disinterest in consumption of even those foods which ordinarily one has great interest in and liking for.
2. Associated with decreased secretion of gastric hydrochloric acid.
3. Possible causes
   a. Unpleasant or upsetting experiences
   b. Apprehension, fear and anxiety
   c. Excitement, both pleasurable and desirable

Nausea

A most unpleasant sensation usually associated with a distinct revulsion toward the ingestion of food; it may or may not precede vomiting.
1. Very often, anorexia leads to nausea and vomiting. However, either of these states may occur without the others.
2. Associated with decreased motor activity of the stomach, pallor of gastric mucosa and contraction of proximal duodenum.
3. Frequently associated with evidence of diffuse autonomic discharge: profuse watery salivation, sudden drenching perspiration, tachycardia.
4. Difficult to describe by many patients:
   a. Vague unpleasantness in epigastrium
   b. Distressing feelings in the throat
   c. Vague unpleasantness spread diffusely in abdomen (must be distinguished from mild visceral abdominal pain)

Vomiting

Sudden forceful expulsion of stomach contents through the mouth.
1. Vomiting center is located in the medulla.
2. May or may not be preceded by nausea and retching.
3. Exaggerated and often extreme vasomotor activities may immediately precede and accompany the vomiting act; watery salivation, sweating, pulse rate change, vasoconstriction and pallor.
4. Tachycardia prior to vomiting becomes bradycardia during process.
5. Incited by neuromuscular "reverse peristalsis" or mechanical obstruction.

Nursing Management

1. Observe the preliminary symptoms.
   a. Patient is often lightheaded, weak and dizzy.
   b. Irregularity of respiration before and during vomiting.
   c. Blood pressure may fall before and then fluctuate during vomiting.
2. Observe character and quantity of expectorated material
   a. Yellowish or greenish color—may contain bile
   b. Fecal—may indicate intestinal contents or intestinal obstruction
   c. Bright red blood—may indicate hemorrhage from gastric ulcer
   d. Coffee-ground—may indicate digested blood from peptic ulcer bleeding or small intestinal hemorrhage
   e. Undigested food—may indicate gastric tumor or ulcer obstruction

    f. Odorless

    g. Sour smelling

    h. Liquid

    i. Containing mucus or pus.

3. Be aware of progression of events when there is a diminution of intake and output—weight loss, dehydration, fluid and electrolyte imbalance:
   a. Skin becomes dry and loses turgor
   b. Poor mouth hygiene leading to halitosis
4. Recognize progression of events which might lead to shock, tachycardia, hypotension, urine oliguria.

Disturbances Associated with Anorexia, Nausea and Vomiting

A. *Psychic and Neurological Factors*
1. Life situations that evoke subjective manifestations of fear, frustration, depression and anxiety may be associated with these symptoms.
2. *Anorexia* is commonly a manifestation of a depressed state which can lead to a profound impairment of food intake and possibly anorexia nervosa.
3. *Nausea and Vomiting*
   a. Occurring on a psychic basis
      (1) Frequently occurs during or shortly after meals
      (2) Often unaccompanied by nausea and retching
      (3) Frequently does not empty stomach
      (4) After vomiting, patient may desire to continue to eat
      (5) No recurrence of vomiting occurs.
   b. Reflecting oxygen deprivation in association with:
      (1) Severe anemia
      (2) Excessive blood loss
      (3) Diminished cardiac output
      (4) Increased intracranial pressure
      (5) Vascular shock
      (6) Reduction in environmental oxygen
   c. Projectile type associated with increasing intracranial pressure
      (1) Commonly not preceded by nausea.
      (2) May indicate meningitis, internal hydrocephalus, space-occupying lesion, cerebellar lesions.
   d. Accompanying migraine headache
      (1) Hypoxemia affecting the vomiting center
      (2) Vascular changes
      (3) Associated visual disturbances
   e. Caused by unusual stimulation of labyrinth of the ear.

B. *Drugs and Toxic Agents*
1. Pathophysiologic Effect
   a. Medullary chemoreceptor zone may be stimulated.
   b. Direct effect on gastrointestinal organs brought about by mercury.
   c. Stimulation of hypothalamus nuclei brought about by alcohol, apomorphine, emetine, histamine, epinephrine.
2. Mucosal damage of upper gastrointestinal tract caused by mercury, ammonium chloride, copper sulfate, aminophylline, sodium salicylate

C. *Intra-abdominal Disorders*
   1. Mechanical obstruction in gastrointestinal tract (see p. 407)
   2. Intra-abdominal inflammatory disorders
D. *Nausea and Vomiting of Pregnancy* (see p. 951)
E. *Other Factors*
   1. Febrile illness
   2. Uremia (see p. 475)
   3. Motion sickness
   4. Meniere's disease (see p. 715)

Nursing Management

   1. Observe and assess status of patient when he experiences anorexia, nausea, and vomiting. Note the effect of these symptoms on the patient generally:
      a. Food and fluid intake
      b. Balance between intake and output
      c. Effect on body weight, indicating malnutrition
      d. Character and amount of vomitus
      e. Effect on patient's activity—malaise or apathy
      f. Changes in patient's skin color and turgor and in mucous membranes
      g. Note other fluid losses—perspiration, feces, urine fluid and electrolyte balance which may result in dehydration
   2. Improve psychological desire for food in order to overcome anoxemia, nausea and vomiting.
      a. Determine patient's eating habits, cultural preferences, etc.
      b. Include patient's family in soliciting information.
      c. Encourage adequate rest before, during and after his meal; allay anxiety.
      d. Prepare patient for his meals by being certain he has had good oral hygiene, is comfortable and has clean bedding and clothing.
      e. Promote physical comfort of patient so that he may enjoy his food and not be distracted by discomfort during or after his meal.
      f. Protect his environment from noise, foul odors, confusion, too many visitors, etc.
      g. Serve food in attractive appearance and appropriate quantity.
      h. Be sure that food is served at proper temperature.
   3. If patient is nauseated but does not vomit:
      a. Reduce environmental stimuli

Visual	other "sick" patients
	soiled dressings
Olfactory	drainage bottle
(Sensory)	colostomy cauterization
	bed pan
Auditory	noise

      b. Encourage rest and deep breathing.
      c. Cater to patient's preferences in food.
      d. Limit size of servings.
      e. Remove meal tray as soon as he is finished.
      f. If he does vomit, carefully observe vomitus and remove promptly; clean area and patient if necessary and offer mouthwash.

4. Provide opportunity for patient to express his feelings.
   a. Keep channels of communication open.
   b. Provide time to allow patient to talk.
5. Correlate administration of medication with needs of the patient.
   a. If patient has pain, administer analgesics.
   b. If patient is tired and exhausted, sedatives may be ordered.
   c. If patient appears tense and worried, tranquilizers may be indicated.

Constipation and Diarrhea

Constipation

Constipation is a deficiency in output of waste through the intestinal tract.
Obstipation is absence of intestinal output (no stool).
1. Gross deviation in pattern of intestinal elimination is indicative of a disturbance in homeostasis.
2. Constipation is usually caused by altered routine in dietary and activity patterns, by drugs such as morphine and codeine, by mechanical obstruction or surgery, or by psychological factors resulting from restricted use of toilet facilities.
3. Manifestations of constipation include changes in color, consistency and ease of expulsion—darker, harder and difficult or painful to pass.

Diarrhea

Diarrhea is loose and watery stools.
1. When related to infection, stools are loose, watery and frequent.
2. Color changes are produced by presence of abnormal constituents.
   a. "Tarry"—may indicate digested blood which may originate in upper G.I. tract.
   b. Bloody—may indicate hemorrhage which may originate in rectal or anal region.
   c. Dark green—may indicate excessive bile.
   d. Other—indicates dietary excesses or effect of medications.

NURSING ALERT: Alteration in bowel habits, such as constipation, then diarrhea, then constipation, followed by diarrhea may mean partial obstruction.

Nursing Management

A. *Constipation and Diarrhea*
1. Disturbances in elimination produce psychological discomfort; conversely, psychological deviation can produce elimination disturbances.
2. Assist patient in overcoming correctable problems by:
   a. Affording privacy
   b. Helping patient approach as near-normal position during evacuation as possible
   c. Providing comfort measures such as warmed bedpan
   d. Providing sufficient time and a schedule as close to the patient's own as possible.

B. *Constipation*
1. Correct dietary habits to include adequate fluids, fresh fruits, roughage.
2. Suggest a small glass of prune juice or lemon juice in warm water each morning.

3. Encourage a regular time for evacuation each day.
4. Suggest a bulk-forming laxative such as Metamucil that does not irritate the bowel. One heaping teaspoonful in a glass of water, once or twice daily, followed by a second glass of water.

C. *Diarrhea*
1. Have required facilities readily available.
2. Pay particular attention to proper hand and body hygiene since diarrhea may be infectious.
3. Use talcum powder or emollients to prevent skin excoriation.
4. Provide dry and clean bed linen and clothing.
5. Administer fluids and anti-diarrheal medications as prescribed.

DIAGNOSTIC STUDIES FOR GASTROINTESTINAL CONDITIONS

Radiography

Roentgenography of the Gastrointestinal Tract (G.I. Series)

1. The entire gastrointestinal tract can be delineated by x-rays following the introduction of barium sulfate as the contrast medium.
2. Barium is a tasteless, odorless, completely insoluble powder:
    a. It can be ingested in an aqueous suspension for upper gastrointestinal tract study (upper G.I. series).
    b. It can be instilled rectally for visualization of the colon (barium enema).
3. The fasting patient is required to swallow barium under direct fluoroscopic examination.
    a. Esophagus
       (1) Patency and calibre noted—may indicate anatomical and functional derangement.
       (2) Abnormally enlarged right atrium noted—impinges on esophagus.
       (3) Esophageal varices noted—indicates liver cirrhosis.
    b. Stomach
       (1) Motility and thickness of gastric wall noted.
       (2) Spasms, ulcerations, malignant infiltrates and anatomic abnormalities noted.
       (3) Pressure from outside of stomach detected.
       (4) Patency of pyloric valve observed.
    c. Small Intestine
       Barium swallow or a continuous infusion of a thin barium sulfate suspension via duodenal tube may be done to visualize jejunum and ileum.
4. During fluoroscopic examination, roentgenograms are taken for permanent records.

Nursing Management and Patient Instruction
1. The patient is to receive nothing by mouth after midnight prior to the test.
2. During this interim, the patient is to receive no purgative, however mild, and no other medication unless specifically ordered.
3. The patient remains in a fasting state until the last roentgenogram is taken.

Roentgenography of the Colon: Barium Enema

The fasting patient receives a rectal instillation of a barium sulfate suspension which is viewed in the fluoroscope and then filmed. If adequately prepared fluoroscope will reveal:

a. Colon—contour of entire colon is visible.
b. Cecum and appendix—contour and motility observed.

Nursing Management and Patient Instruction

1. Explain to the patient:
   a. What the x-ray procedure involves
   b. That proper preparation provides a more accurate view of the tract
   c. That it is important to retain the barium so that all surfaces of the tract are coated with opaque solution.
2. Empty the intestinal tract by giving laxatives, enemas, or rectal suppositories as prescribed before the examination.

NURSING ALERT: Use nursing judgment regarding the administration of cathartics or enemata in the presence of acute abdominal pain or obstruction.

---

3. Restrict food and fluids for the examination.
4. Administer an oil-retention enema or laxative such as magnesium citrate following the barium enema to completely evacuate the barium.
5. Permit patient to eat following the examination since he has been fasting and is undoubtedly hungry.

Examination of Gastrointestinal Contents

Stool Specimen

1. The stool is examined for its amount, consistency and color; a screening test for melena is also done. Normal color varies from light to dark brown depending on urobilin content. Special tests may be for fecal urobilinogen, fat, nitrogen, parasites, food residue, and other substances.
2. Various foods and medications affect stool color:

Meat protein—dark brown	Calomel—green
Spinach—green	Bismuth, Iron, Charcoal—black
Beets—red	Barium—milky white
Cocoa—dark red or brown	Upper G.I. bleeding—tarry black
Senna or santonin—yellowish	Lower G.I. bleeding—bright red bloody

   Considerable quantities hemoglobin—occult blood (not visible to naked eye)
3. Characteristic clinical entities: (stool)
   a. Bulky, greasy, foamy, foul in odor, gray in color with silvery sheen—steatorrhea
   b. Light gray "clay-colored" (due to absence of urobilin "acholic")—biliary obstruction
   c. Mucus or pus visible—chronic ulcerative colitis
   d. Small, dry, rocky-hard masses—constipation, obstipation, fecal obstruction

Nursing Management
 1. Use a tongue blade to place a small amount of stool in a disposable waxed container.
 2. Save a sample of any fecal material if it is unusual in appearance—worms, blood or blood-streaked, unusual color, much mucus.
 3. Send specimen to be examined for parasites to the laboratory immediately so that the parasites may be observed under microscope while viable, fresh and warm.
 4. Tests for melena: Usually based on benzidine, guaiac, or orthotolidin reaction.

Stomach Contents (Gastric Analysis via Nasogastric Tube)

 1. Stomach contents are evacuated to determine secretory activity of the gastric mucosa, presence or retention of gastric contents in patients suspected of having pyloric or intestinal obstruction.
 2. A 12-hour overnight gastric analysis may be done to test volume excreted as well as concentration of acid. (Zollinger-Ellison syndrome.)

Nursing Management
 1. Withhold food and fluids for 6 to 8 hours before the test is to be done.
 2. Pass the nasogastric tube (see Guidelines, p. 383); the patient may sit in a back-supporting chair in preference to being in bed.
 3. Verify that the tube is in the stomach by testing aspirated secretions with litmus paper (blue litmus turns pink in the presence of acid).
 4. Secure tube to nose and encourage the patient to relax.
 5. Collect a fasting specimen; then administer histamine phosphate 0.2 mg. subcutaneously—stimulates gastric secretions.
 6. Be alert for the patient who is sensitive to histamine; have epinephrine available to treat shock, should it occur.
 7. Collect 3 more specimens at 10- to 20-minute intervals.
 8. Label specimens and send to the laboratory.
 9. Withdraw nasogastric tube and make patient comfortable:
    a. Suggest mouth care
    b. Offer breakfast.

Tubeless Gastric Analysis

 1. Whereas analysis of gastric contents via the nasogastric tube provides the means for quantitative analysis, the tubeless analysis merely enables the determination of acidity or its absence.
 2. May be done to detect gastric achlorhydria.

Nursing Management
 1. Instruct the patient to fast for several hours.
 2. Administer a gastric stimulant such as caffeine or histamine phosphate.
 3. One hour later, administer 2 gm. of a cation resin containing 90 mg. of azure A (Azuresin or Diagnex Blue) with 240 ml. of water.
 4. Resin in the stomach will react with free hydrochloric acid (if this is present) to produce a substance which will be absorbed from the small intestine and excreted by the kidneys.
 5. Test results: If dye is detectable in the urine in 2 hours, the patient has free hydrochloric acid in the stomach.

GUIDELINES. *Nasogastric Intubation*

Purposes

1. To remove fluid and gas from the gastrointestinal tract (decompression).
2. To determine the amount of pressure and motor activity in the gastrointestinal tract (diagnostic studies).
3. To treat patients with mechanical obstruction and bleeding within the upper gastrointestinal tract.
4. To administer medications and feeding (gavage) directly into the gastrointestinal tract.
5. To obtain a specimen of gastric contents for laboratory studies.

Equipment

Nasogastric tube—usually Levin (rubber or plastic, 12 to 18 F.)—preferably disposable (Plastic tubes are less irritating than rubber.)
Water-soluble lubricant
Clamp for tubing
Towel and emesis basin
Glass of water and straw

Procedure

Preparatory Phase

1. Explain procedure to patient and tell him how mouth breathing and swallowing can help in passing the tube.
2. Have patient in a sitting or high Fowler's position with neck hyperextended; place a towel across his chest.
3. Determine with the patient what sign he might use, such as raising his index finger, to indicate "wait a few moments" because of gagging or discomfort.
4. Remove dentures if tube is to be passed through mouth.
5. For rubber tubing, place in ice chilled water to firm tubing.
6. For plastic tubing it may be firm enough; if too stiff, dip in warm water.
7. Mark distance tube is to be passed by measuring as indicated in Figure 6-1. This will ensure the passage of the tubing into the stomach.

Nursing Action	**Rationale/Amplification**
Performance Phase	
1. Lubricate tube for about 15–20 cm. (6 to 8 inches) with water-soluble jelly.	1. Lubrication reduces friction between mucous membrane and tube.
2. Lift head before inserting tube into nostril and gently pass it into the posterior nasopharynx aiming downward and backward.	2. Passage of tube is facilitated by following the natural contours of the body.
3. When tube reaches the pharynx, the patient may gag; allow him to rest for a few moments.	3. Gag reflex is triggered by the presence of the tube.
4. Have patient hold his head in a normal position; offer him several sips of water sucked through a straw. Advance tube as he swallows.	4. Normal head position makes swallowing easier. Swallowing facilitates passage of tube.
5. Continue to advance tube gently each time patient swallows.	

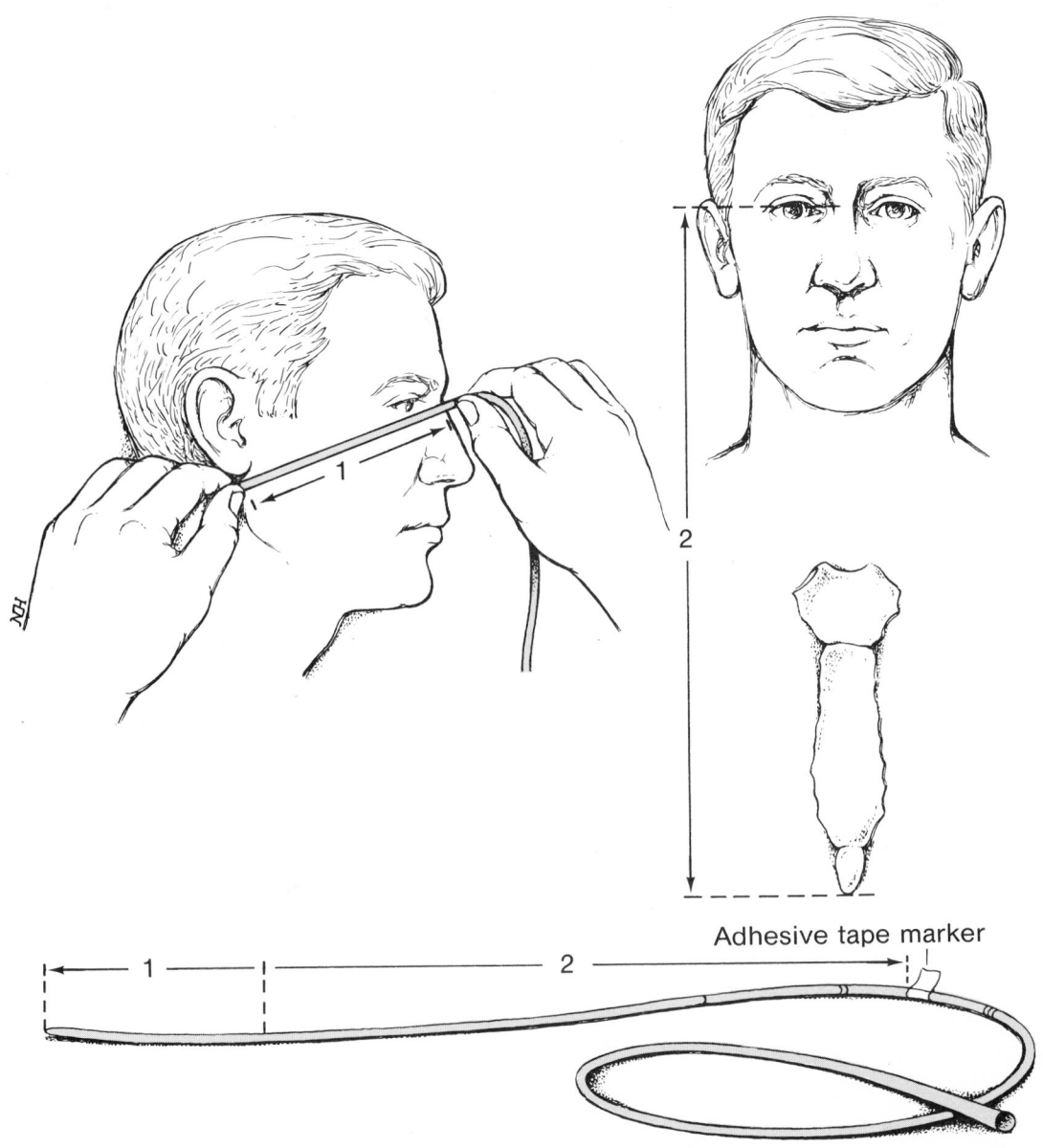

Figure 6-1. To measure the distance a Levin tube is to be passed in a patient (to insure that it enters the stomach): (1) Measure the distance on the tube from the patient's tragus (ear lobe) to bridge of nose, plus (2) the distance from the bridge of the nose to the bottom of the xyphoid process. Mark this distance with a piece of adhesive tape. Note that the Levin tube usually has circular marks on the tubing—when it is in the patient's stomach, it is between the 2nd and 3rd circular markings.

Nursing Action	Rationale / Amplification
6. If obstruction appears to prevent tube from passing, do *not* use force. Rotating tube gently may help. If unsuccessful, remove tube and try other nostril.	6. Avoid discomfort and trauma to patient.
7. If there are signs of distress such as gasping, coughing or cyanosis, immediately remove tube.	
8. To check whether the Levin tube is in the stomach:	
a. Aspirate contents of stomach with a 20-ml. syringe.	a. Aspirated stomach contents would indicate that the tube is in the stomach.
b. Place end of tube in a glass of water.	b. Paroxysms of coughing would indicate the tube is in the trachea.
c. Place a stethoscope over epigastrium; inject 5 ml. of air into Levin tube.	c. Air can be detected entering stomach rather than the bronchus.
9. Adjust tubing after these tests to proper position in the stomach.	

Follow-up Phase

1. Anchor tube with hypoallergenic tape.	
a. Prevent patient's vision from being disturbed.	
b. Prevent tubing from rubbing against nasal mucosa.	b. To make the patient as comfortable as possible.
2. Anchor the tubing to the patient's gown.	2. To permit mobility of patient.
3. Clamp the tube until the purpose for inserting the tube is about to take place.	

NURSING ALERT: All enteric tubes must be irrigated at regular intervals with small volumes of saline to ensure patency.

---

4. Administer oral hygiene frequently. Cleanse tubing at nostril. Utilize a decongestant spray.	4. To promote patient comfort.

Before Removing Nasogastric Tubing

1. Be certain that gastric drainage is not excessive in volume nor from the small bowel.
2. Ensure, by auscultation, that audible peristalsis is present.
3. Determine whether the patient is passing flatus so that abdomen is not distended.

NURSING ALERT: Recognize the potential for complications when intubation is prolonged—nasal erosion, sinusitis, esophagitis, gastric ulceration, and pulmonary infection.

GASTRIC CONDITIONS AND TREATMENT

Peptic Ulcer

A *peptic ulcer* is an excavation found in the mucosal wall of the stomach, in the pylorus, or in the duodenum due to the erosion of a circumscribed area of its mucous membrane.

Predisposing Factors

1. Emotional stress.
2. Eating hurried and irregular meals.
3. Excessive smoking or drinking of coffee or alcohol.
4. Seasonal occurrence.
5. Drugs (salicylates, reserpine, phenylbutazone, steroids, aminophylline, etc.) are irritating to the mucous lining of the stomach and pylorus.
6. Genetic susceptibility.

Incidence

1. Duodenal ulcer is found most frequently in the 25–40 age group and in males 4 times more than females.
2. Gastric ulcer occurs most frequently in the 40–55 age group and in males 2½ times more often than females.
3. Five to 15% of population in U.S.A. have ulcers; only one half the cases are recognized.
4. Duodenal ulcers occur 10 times more frequently than gastric ulcers.
5. No significant racial or national difference.
6. Duodenal ulcer occurs more frequently in patients with type O blood.

Altered Physiology

1. Overstimulation of secretory mechanisms.
2. Failure of the mechanisms inhibiting secretion.
3. Failure of mechanisms for neutralizing hydrochloric acid.
4. Failure of epithelium to regenerate rapidly.
5. Failure of epithelium to secrete an adequate quantity of mucus.
6. Poor epithelial blood supply.

Preventive Measures

Points of Emphasis in Posthospital Patient Education

1. Establish regular eating habits.
2. Avoid foods that are difficult to digest or irritating—fried foods, highly seasoned foods, alcohol, and coffee.
3. Follow a regular exercise and rest program.
4. By-pass stress situations inasmuch as they stimulate gastric secretion and motility.
5. Avoid irritating drugs, such as aspirin, steroids, etc. If it is necessary to take these medications, ingest milk and crackers between meals and at bedtime for buffering action.
6. Be aware of high-risk tendency due to familial history of peptic ulcer.
7. Eliminate smoking because smoking increases the secretion of acid by the stomach.

Clinical Manifestations

A. *Underlying Principles*
1. More apt to be in the duodenum than in the stomach (ratio of 10 to 1).
2. Occurs only in the areas of the gastrointestinal tract that are exposed to hydrochloric acid and pepsin (Fig. 6-2).

B. *Pain*
   1. Gnawing sensation (sharply localized in midepigastrium or in the back) or dull, burning sensation (heartburn).
   2. Recurs from 1 to 3 hours after meals.
   3. Is relieved promptly by food or alkalies.

C. *Vomiting*
   1. May or may not be preceded by nausea.
   2. Usually follows a bout of pain.
   3. Pain is relieved when this occurs.

D. *Eructation*
   1. Due to increased air swallowing.

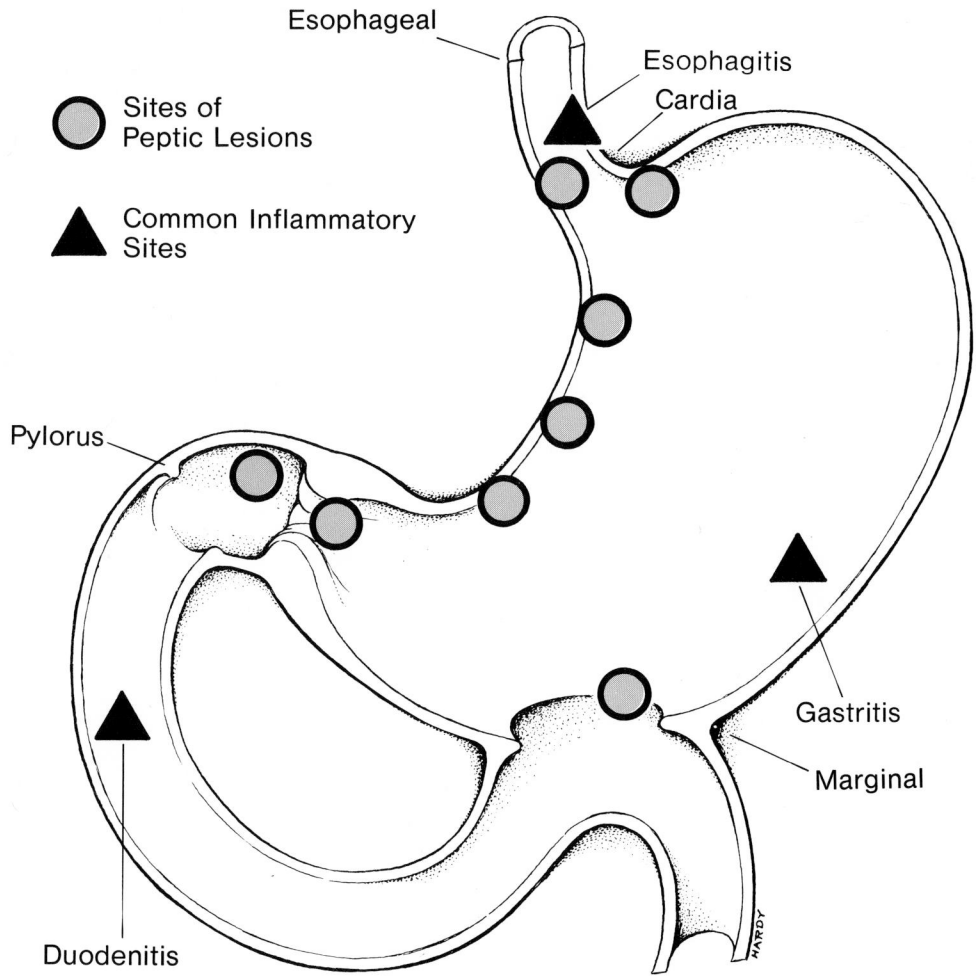

Figure 6-2. "Peptic" lesions may occur in the esophagus, stomach or duodenum. Note peptic ulcer sites and common inflammatory sites (esophagitis, gastritis, and duodenitis).

Diagnostic Evaluation

A. *Observation, History and Nursing Assessment*
   1. Where is the pain? Does it radiate? How long does it last?
   2. Is pain relieved by food or alkalies?
   3. Is there a history of tension, problem-situations, anxiety?
   4. Was there ingestion of known drug-irritants?
   5. Does patient smoke and/or consume alcohol?
   6. Are his symptoms accentuated in the spring or fall?

B. *Upper G.I. Series* (see p. 380)

C. *Associated Diseases*
   Associated occasionally with: hyperparathyroidism, polycythemia vera, chronic liver disease, chronic respiratory disease, uremia.

Objectives of Treatment and Nursing Management

A. *To promote an atmosphere conducive to physical and mental rest*
   1. Encourage bedrest to reduce physical activity and to separate patient from his usual environment.
   2. Offer sedatives or tranquilizers to lessen the response to stimuli and to promote relaxation and sleep.
   3. Provide frequent feedings, antacids and other medications given on time.
   4. Inform visitors to avoid upsetting conversation.

B. *To relieve pain and discomfort, and to promote healing through the control of gastric acidity by using antacids and antisecretory medications.*
   1. Administer antacid medications to neutralize hydrochloric acid and relieve pain.
   2. Administer anticholinergic drugs to suppress gastric secretions and to delay gastric emptying.
   3. Encourage hydration to minimize side-effects of anticholinergic medications.

C. *To reduce motor and secretory activities of the stomach by means of a therapeutic diet.*
   1. Serve bland protein foods to buffer gastric acidity.
   2. Include fat foods to stimulate the production of enterogastrone which decreases gastric secretion and motility.
   3. Give small servings to reduce the work of the gastrointestinal tract.
   4. Provide frequent feedings to neutralize gastric secretions and dilute stomach contents.
   5. Avoid caffeinated beverages.
   6. Avoid spicy foods and fried foods.
   7. Include iron and ascorbic acid to facilitate tissue repair.
   8. Discourage smoking because it increases the secretion of stomach acid.

D. *To assist the patient in understanding how chronic his problem is and the very real part he has in controlling it.*
   1. Emphasize the need to avoid anxiety-producing situations.
   2. Alert him to the irritating nature of certain drugs to the gastric mucosa.
   3. Review the reasons for smaller meals and midmeal snacks.
   4. Suggest the elimination of smoking; suggest switching from coffee and cola to decaffeinated beverages.

5. Recommend skim milk and less fattening foods not only to keep weight under control but also to prevent atherosclerosis and coronary artery disease.
6. Remind patient to consult his physician if he develops an infection such as an upper respiratory infection.

Complications

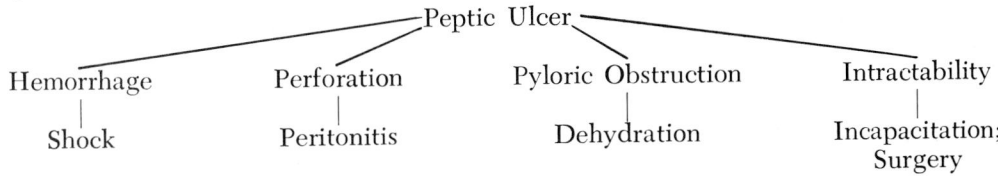

Hemorrhage	Perforation	Pyloric Obstruction	Intractability
Shock	Peritonitis	Dehydration	Incapacitation; Surgery

A. *Hemorrhage*
   1. Accounts for 40% mortality.
   2. Manifestations
      a. Giddiness, faintness, out of breath with slight exertion.
      b. Tachycardia, sweating and coldness of extremities.
      c. Slight hemorrhage producing black, tarry stool (test for occult blood).
      d. Large amount of bleeding and vomiting.
   3. Medical and Nursing Intervention
      a. Encourage bedrest and take vital signs frequently.
      b. Give meperidine (Demerol) for restlessness or pain; but, be on alert for shock.
      c. Employ nasogastric suction to empty stomach of clots and gauge rate of bleeding.
      d. Give whole blood and/or plasma to keep circulating blood volume at a safe level, usually a unit of blood every 8 hours for 48 hours.
      e. Note color, consistency and volume of stools and vomitus.
      f. Provide treatment if patient goes into oligemic shock (see p. 76).

B. *Perforation*
   1. Clinical Manifestations
      a. Severe upper abdominal pain, persisting and increasing in intensity.
      b. Vomiting.
      c. Pain may be referred to shoulders (phrenic nerve irritation).
      d. Abdomen—extremely tender, board-like rigidity.
      e. X-ray of abdomen; 50–75% free air visible.
      f. Shock.
   2. Surgical Intervention
      Immediate—to close perforation, plication of ulcers is performed (see Postoperative Care, p. 393).

C. *Pyloric Obstruction*
   1. Etiology
      Area around pyloric sphincter becomes scarred and stenosed from spasm, edema or scar tissue formed when ulcer alternately heals and breaks down. Inflammation, muscle spasm or edema may cause a temporary obstruction.
   2. Major Manifestations
      Nausea and vomiting, constipation and weight loss.

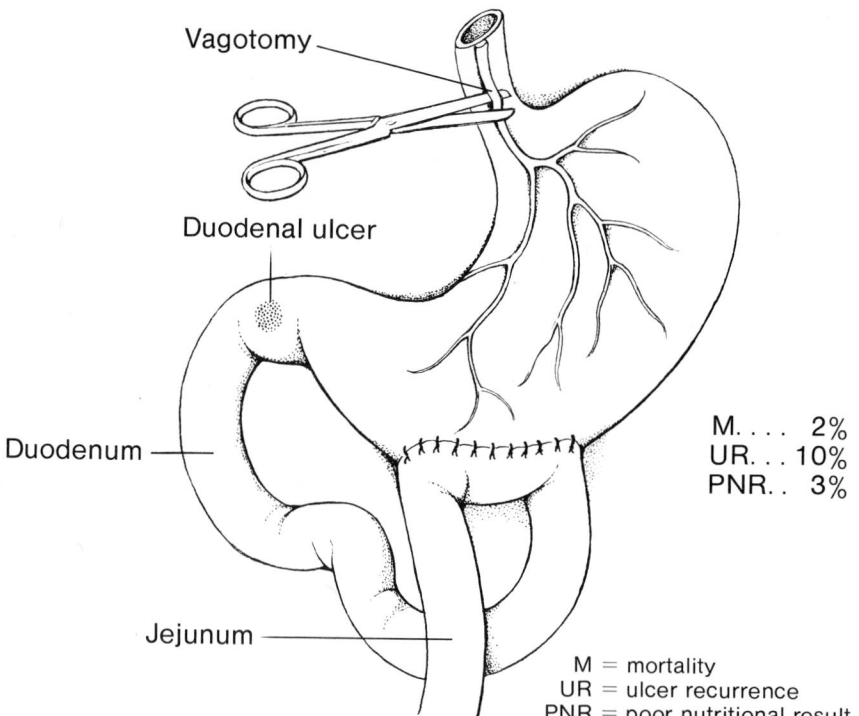

M. . . . 2%
UR. . . 10%
PNR. . 3%

M = mortality
UR = ulcer recurrence
PNR = poor nutritional result

Figure 6-3. Gastrojejunostomy and vagotomy.

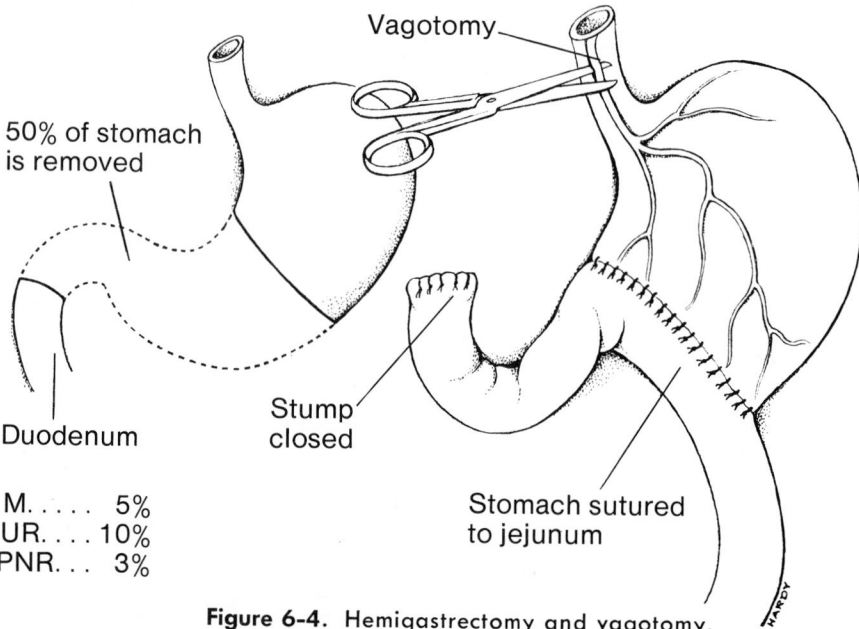

M. 5%
UR. . . . 10%
PNR. . . 3%

Figure 6-4. Hemigastrectomy and vagotomy.

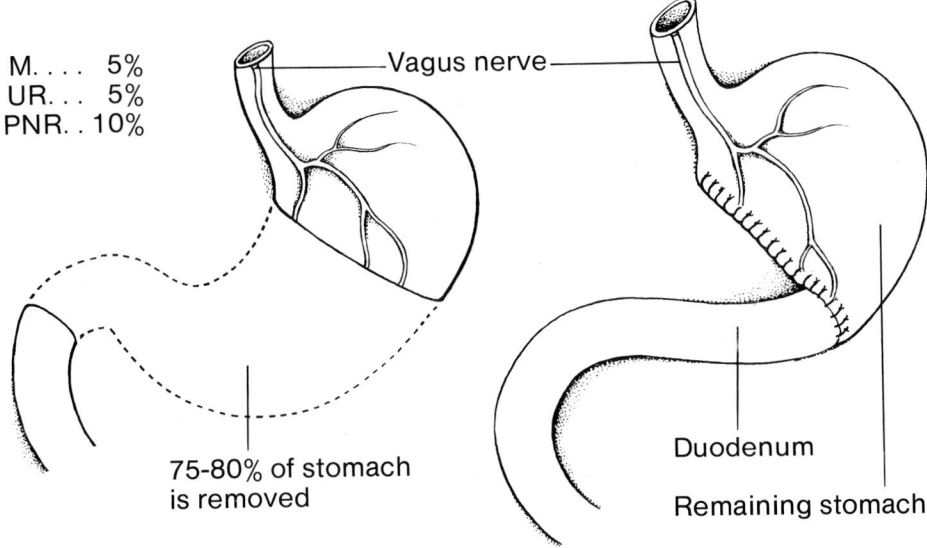

M. . . . 5%
UR. . . 5%
PNR. . 10%

Vagus nerve

75-80% of stomach
is removed

Duodenum

Remaining stomach

Figure 6-5. Subtotal gastrectomy.

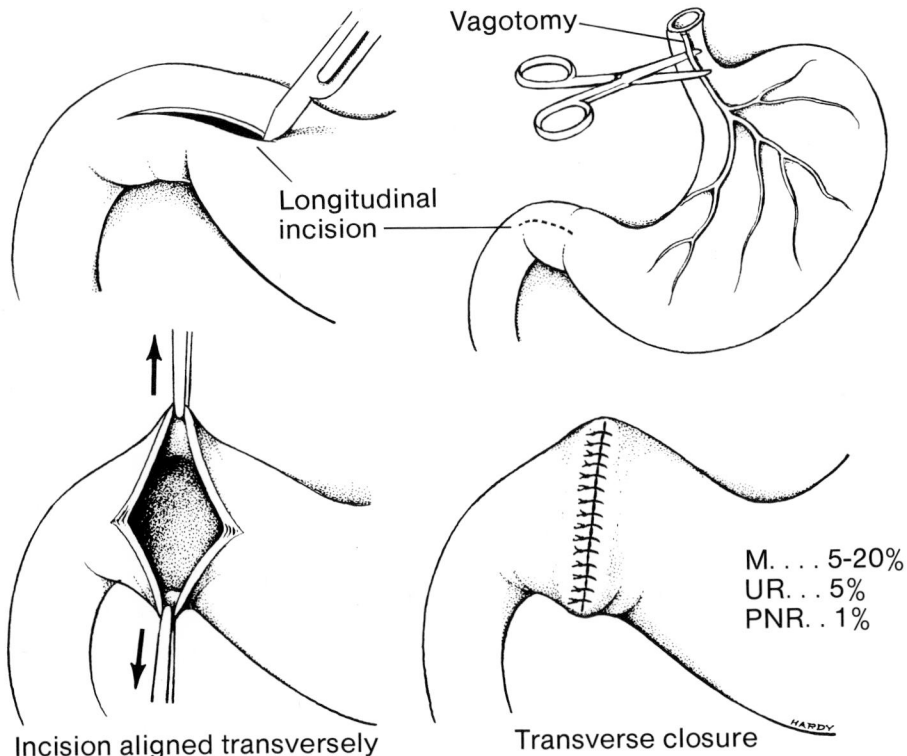

Vagotomy

Longitudinal
incision

Incision aligned transversely

Transverse closure

M. . . . 5-20%
UR. . . 5%
PNR. . 1%

Figure 6-6. Vagotomy and pyloroplasty.

3. Medical and Nursing Intervention
    a. Gastric decompression and intravenous fluids.
    b. Surgery may follow if clinical course is prolonged.
D. *Intractability*—the failure of medical management to accomplish healing of the ulcer usually calloused posterior ulcer penetrating into pancreas.
    1. Manifestations
        Pain continues without adequate relief from milk or antacid.
    2. Surgical Intervention
        a. Vagotomy and gastrojejunostomy—to abolish cephalic phase of secretion.
        b. Vagotomy and hemigastrectomy—to abolish cephalic and gastric phase of secretion.
        c. Gastric resection—to abolish acid-secreting parietal cells.

Surgical Treatment

Surgery is required in only about 15–20% of ulcer patients; operation is individualized based on patient's age, ability to withstand procedure, preoperative nutritional status and particular indication.

Objectives:

1. To relieve complications
    a. Perforation (described p. 389)
    b. Hemorrhage (described p. 389)
    c. Pyloric obstruction (described p. 389)
    d. Intractability (described above)
2. To treat the tendency to ulcer formation

Types of Gastric Operations

A comparison of these may be made for the following:

M—mortality rate; UR—ulcer recurrence; PNR—poor nutritional result.

A. *Gastrojejunostomy and Vagotomy* (Fig. 6-3)

The jejunum is sutured to the stomach to provide a 2nd outlet of gastric contents. Severed vagus nerve reduces secretions and movements of the stomach (90% good results).

B. *Hemigastrectomy and Vagotomy* (Fig. 6-4)

The resected portion includes the first part of the duodenum, the pylorus and at least one-half of the stomach. The stump of the duodenum is closed by suture and the side of the jejunum is anastomosed to the end of the stomach.

C. *Subtotal Gastrectomy* (Fig. 6-5)

The resected portion includes the first part of the duodenum, the pylorus and from two-thirds to three-quarters of the stomach. The duodenum is anastomosed to the remaining portion of the stomach.

D. *Vagotomy and Pyloroplasty* (Fig. 6-6)

A longitudinal incision is made in the pylorus and it is closed transversely to permit the muscle to relax and to establish an enlarged outlet.

Nursing Management

See page 393, for managing the patient undergoing a gastric resection.

Gastric Cancer

ancer of the stomach accounts for about 20,000 annual deaths in the United States—usually ersons of middle age. (See p. 872, Cancer Mortality by Site.) There has been a decrease i incidence in U.S.A. over the last 2 decades for unknown reasons.

Clinical Manifestations

. *Early Manifestations*
1. Progressive loss of appetite
2. Noticeable change in, or appearance of, gastrointestinal symptoms—gastric fullness, dyspepsia of more than 4 weeks duration
3. Blood in the stools
4. Vomiting which may indicate pyloric obstruction or cardiac-orifice obstruction
5. Occasionally, vomiting that has a coffee-ground appearance due to slow leaks of blood from ulceration produced by the cancer.

. *Later Manifestations*
1. Pain is a late symptom often induced by eating and relieved by vomiting.
2. Weight loss, loss of strength, anemia, metastasis, hemorrhage, obstruction.

Diagnostic Evaluation

1. Patient's history—weight loss and loss of strength over several months.
2. Cytologic examination of gastric juice which may show cancer cells.
3. Palpable mass near pylorus.
4. Suspicion of metastasis by palpable lymph nodes—surface of liver, skin at umbilicus, supraclavicular nodes, etc.
5. Roentgenology, fluoroscopy and gastroscopy.

Treatment

1. The only successful treatment of gastric cancer is surgical removal.
2. If tumor is localized to stomach and can be removed, chances are good that the patient can be cured.
3. If tumor has spread beyond the area that can be excised surgically, cure cannot be accomplished.

    Palliative surgery may be performed such as total gastrectomy, subtotal gastrectomy, entero-anastomosis to maintain continuity of the gastrointestinal tract.

Gastric Resection

Gastric resection is the surgical removal of part of the stomach.

Objectives of Treatment and Nursing Management

A. *To promote comfort and wound healing by relieving the patient of pain and discomfort*
1. Frequently turn the patient and encourage deep breathing to prevent vascular and pulmonary complications.
2. Institute nasogastric suction to remove fluids and gas in the stomach.

3. Provide conscientious mouth care to prevent mouth dryness.
4. Administer parenteral antibiotics to prevent infection.
5. See that patient has nothing by mouth until ordered (to promote gastric woun healing).

B. *To meet nutritional needs of the patient*
1. Give intravenous fluids to prevent shock and to provide adequate fluid an electrolytes.
2. Give fluids by mouth when audible bowel signs are present.
3. Increase fluids according to patient's tolerance.
4. Offer a bland diet with vitamin supplements when patient's condition permits.
5. Give protein-vitamin supplements to foster wound repair and tissue building.
6. Avoid foods that may trigger "dumping syndrome."

C. *To anticipate complications in order to prevent them*
1. Shock and Hemorrhage
   a. Evaluate status of blood pressure, pulse and respiration.
   b. Observe patient for evidence of apathy, apprehension, air hunger, pallor o clammy skin.
   c. Check the dressings and drainage bottle frequently for evidence of bleeding.
   d. Administer fluid and blood as ordered.
2. Cardiopulmonary Complications
   a. Encourage the patient to cough and take deep breaths to produce ventilatory exchange and enhance circulation.
   b. Assist the patient to turn and move, thereby mobilizing secretions.
   c. Promote ambulation as ordered to increase respiratory exchange.
3. Thrombosis and Embolism
   a. Initiate a plan of self-care activities to promote circulation.
   b. Encourage early ambulation to stimulate circulation.
   c. Prevent venous stasis by use of elastic stockings if indicated.
   d. Check for tight dressings or binder that may restrict circulation.
   e. See also page 316.
4. "Dumping Syndrome"
   Instruct the patient as follows:
   a. Eat small frequent meals rather than large meals.
   b. Avoid meals high in sugars and salt.
   c. Reduce fluids with meals but take them between meals.
   d. Take anticholinergic medication before meals (if ordered) to lessen gastrointes- tinal activity.
   e. Relax when eating; eat slowly and regularly.
   f. Take a rest after meals.
5. Adjustment to Self-care and Return to the Community
   a. Emphasize the importance of avoiding stress situations.
   b. Review nutritional requirements and regime with patient.
   c. Stress the importance of vitamin B_{12} supplements.
   d. Encourage follow-up visits with the physician.
   e. Recommend annual blood studies and medical check-ups for any evidence of pernicious anemia or other problems.

Gastrostomy

A gastrostomy is an opening into the stomach performed for the *purpose* of administering ood and fluids when a complete obstruction of the esophagus exists. The obstruction may e due to scar-tissue contracture such as may result from a lye burn or a carcinomatous rowth. A gastrostomy may also be done occasionally in the unconscious or debilitated atient.

Preoperative Patient Care

1. Explain the nature of the problem to the patient and the recommended treatment; use simple line drawings for clarification.
2. Achieve adequate fluid, electrolyte and nutritional balance by administering the required foods and fluids.
3. Immediate preoperative care is similar to that described on page 42.

Surgery

1. Frequently performed under local anesthesia.
2. The anterior gastric wall is incised through a left rectus incision.
3. A tube is inserted and held in place with several purse-string sutures. The tube may be a rubber tube or a Foley catheter inflated with 5 to 8 ml. of water or air and pulled taut to the abdominal wall (Fig. 6-7).
4. The skin is closed close to the tube to prevent leakage.
5. The tube is clamped at all times except for feedings.

GUIDELINES: Assisting the Patient with Gastrostomy Feedings

Purpose

To provide a means of alimentation when the oral route is inaccessible.

Types of Feedings

1. Powdered feedings that are easily liquified are commercially available.
2. Food blender is very useful in preparing a normal diet; psychologically it is more acceptable, since fiber and residue content are retained and good bowel function is promoted.
3. Prepare a tray containing a funnel, tubing and adaptor plus water at room temperature.
4. Pour feeding into a graduated container; warm to 37.8°C. (100°F.) in a basin of water.

Procedure

Preparatory Phase

1. Begin feeding the patient when peristalsis has returned.
2. Place patient in high Fowler's position unless contraindicated.
3. Place a half-sheet or bath towel over upper half of patient; fold top bedding down to cover the patient from the waist downward. This permits a space for gastrostomy tube exposure.

GASTROSTOMY FEEDING

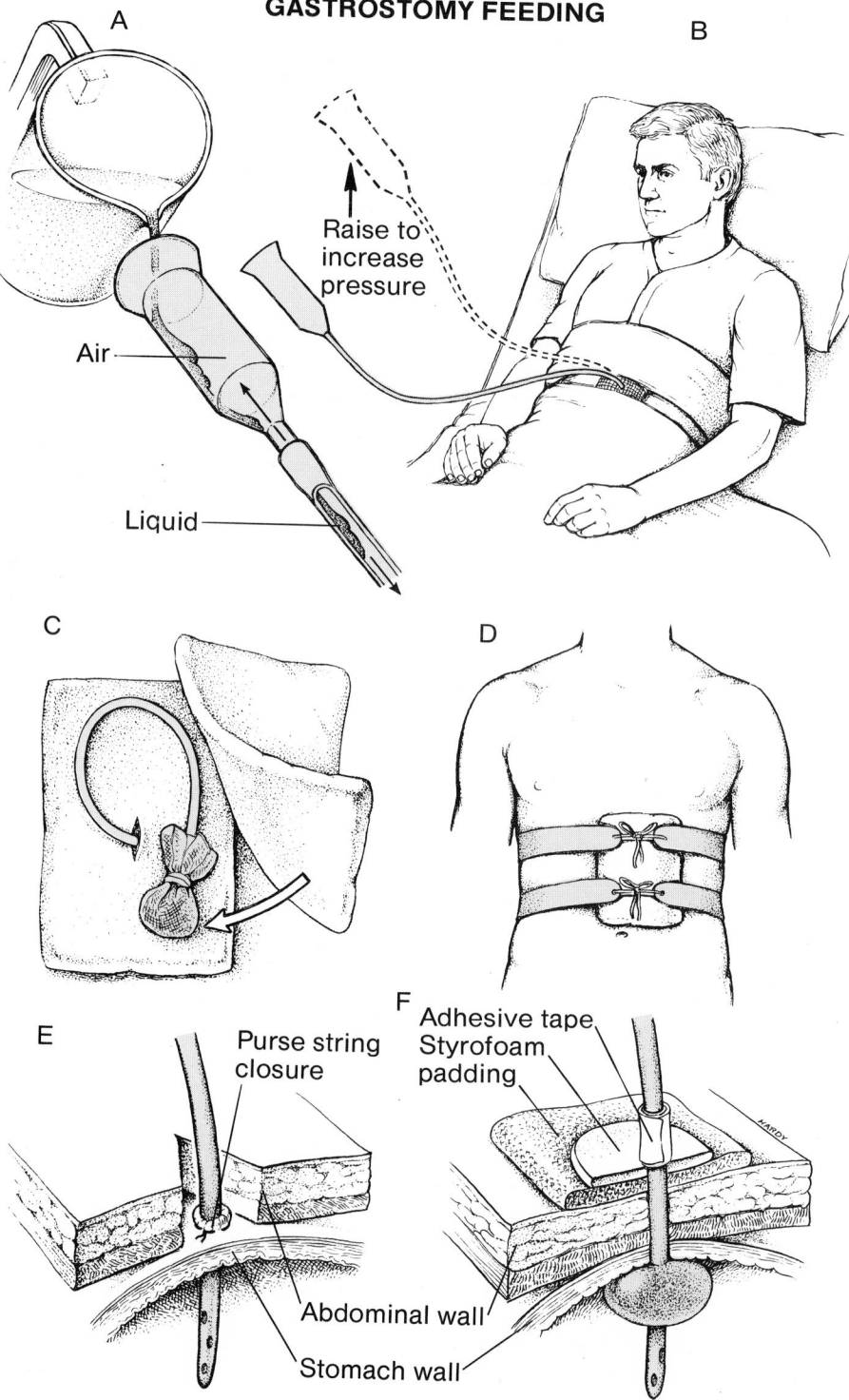

A

Air

Liquid

Raise to increase pressure

B

C

D

E

Purse string closure

Abdominal wall

Stomach wall

F

Adhesive tape
Styrofoam padding

Nursing Action (Fig. 6-7)	**Rationale / Amplification**

erformance Phase

Connect funnel to tubing and connecting tube.

Uncover opening of gastrostomy (or jejunostomy) tube and insert connecting tube.

Pour feeding into tilted funnel, unclamp tubing and allow fluid to flow into the stomach by gravity.

Regulate flow by raising or lowering receptacle.

2. Provides a receptacle for feeding that will lead into gastrostomy tube.

3. Tilting the funnel allows air bubbles to escape; when tubing is unclamped, air bubbles will not enter stomach.

4. Raising increases pressure; lowering decreases pressure.

NURSING ALERT: Force should not be used nor should feeding be given directly from the refrigerator; such action would cause abdominal discomfort to the patient.

NURSING ALERT: If there appears to be an obstruction, stop feeding and report the problem.

. After each feeding, the tube should be irrigated with water (room temperature) and clamped.

. Apply a small dressing over the tube opening, using a rubber band to keep it in place (Fig. 6-7).

. Twist a thin strip of adhesive around tube and attach firmly to abdomen, or coil the tubing on a dressing.

. Cover tubing with a dressing and apply a firm abdominal binder to hold in place.

5. A water flush will prevent the tube from clogging and will assist in keeping it clean.

6. This will keep the tube opening clean for the next feeding.

7. Prevents the tubing from being accidentally pulled out of the stomach.

8. Provides maximum mobility for the patient.

Patient Education

1. Since the tube should be changed every 2 or 3 days, the patient may be taught how to do it. (The tube should be clean but not necessarily sterile.)

2. The patient should learn how to feed himself. (He can learn what foods may be taken.)

Figure 6-7. A. By tilting the receiving receptacle, feeding can be poured to allow air bubbles to escape. B. Liquid feeding is poured and permitted to flow into the stomach by gravity. Raising the funnel can increase pressure; lowering it can decrease pressure. At the end of the feeding, flush tubing with water. C. Following the feeding, disconnect catheter and cover the outlet with a sterile gauze square; fasten with a rubber band. Coil tubing on dressing. D. Cover tubing with a dressing or abdominal pad; close using Montgomery straps. E. A gastrostomy tube may be a rubber perforated tube; the stomach may be pulled upward and fastened with sutures to prevent leakage. F. Another method is to use a Foley catheter as the gastrostomy tube. It is inflated with 5 ml. of water or air and pulled snugly against upper gastric wall. This tube is anchored in place with tape which rests on a cushion of styrofoam or padding. The nurse recognizes the extra precaution required in handling this latter type of gastrostomy.

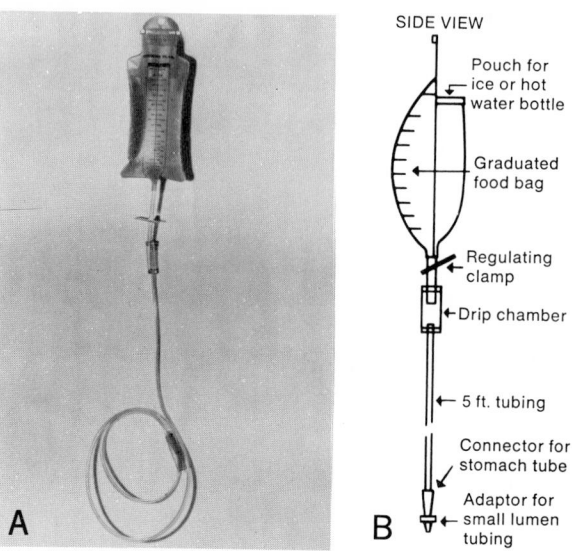

SIDE VIEW

Pouch for ice or hot water bottle

Graduated food bag

Regulating clamp

Drip chamber

5 ft. tubing

Connector for stomach tube

Adaptor for small lumen tubing

A   B

Figure 6-8. Kangaroo tube-feeding s keeps food solutions warm or cold long as desired. A. 1000-ml. feedir bag is of clear plastic and shows bo volume issued and consumed. Cle polyvinyl drip chamber permits visu check on flow rate. Feeding chamb may be filled and sealed by dietitic thus eliminating need for intermedia containers. This is a sterile disposab product. (Courtesy Chesebrough-Pond Inc.)

3. Skin requires special care
   a. It can be irritated by action of gastric juices that leak out.
   b. Daily dressing of wound averts skin maceration.
   c. Bland ointment, such as zinc oxide or petrolatum, can be applied to area aroun the tube.
4. After several weeks, the tube may be removed and inserted only for feedings.

GUIDELINES: *Gastric Gavage, Using the Kangaroo Tube Feeding Set*

Purpose

1. To keep the feeding at the proper temperature.
2. To administer the feeding slowly to the patient.
3. To regulate rate at which feeding is flowing.

Equipment

Kangaroo tube feeding set* (Fig. 6-8).
Small hot water bag or ice cubes, whichever is desired.
Prescribed feeding.

Procedure

(See p. 383 for Insertion of Nasogastric tube)
(See p. 395 for Surgical Insertion of Gastrostomy tube)

* Chesebrough-Pond's Inc.

Nursing Action	**Rationale/Amplification**
Hang feeding bag on I.V. pole with clamp on tubing closed.	1. To prepare for reception of liquid feeding.
Pour feeding into bag; fasten top of bag.	2. Directions are on bag.
Place small hot water bag or ice cubes in pouch.	3. To control temperature of feeding as prescribed.
Clear air from tubing by allowing solution to run through to emesis basin; connect tubing to gastrostomy tube.	4. To prevent air bubbles from entering stomach thereby causing discomfort.

ollow-up Phase

Care for patient's gastrostomy tubing as described on pages 396-397.
Rinse bag with water and hang to dry. With proper care, the bag may be re-used several times for the patient.
Check on the patient's comfort; record the nature of the feeding and the amount given.

INTESTINAL CONDITIONS AND TREATMENT

Medical and Nursing Management of the Patient Undergoing Major Intestinal Surgery

reoperative Objectives

. *To insure that the general physical condition of the patient is the best possible.*

1. Administer parenteral therapy to correct fluid and electrolyte imbalance.
2. Correct nutritional deficiencies: protein supplements, between meal feedings.
3. Provide blood replacement to overcome losses sustained by bleeding, infection and neoplasm.
4. Assist with diagnostic studies as they relate to the evaluation of the cardiopulmonary, hepatorenal bodily functions.
5. Give the patient psychological support as he encounters the stresses of accepting the diagnosis, surgery, and possibly a colostomy.
6. Insert an indwelling catheter immediately prior to going to the operating room.
7. Oversee general personal cleanliness to minimize skin and wound infection postoperatively.

B. *To reduce bacteria in the intestinal tract to prevent postoperative infection.*

1. Administer antibiotic agents to suppress aerobic colon microflora.
   Combinations of kanamycin or neomycin with tetracycline, erythromycin or lincomycin.
2. Reduce content of colon.
   a. Give low residue diet and, when required, change to liquid diet.
   b. Offer laxatives as prescribed.
   c. Administer enemas or colonic irrigations.
3. Decompress gastrointestinal tract by means of indwelling gastrointestinal tube to control distention and vomiting.
   Miller-Abbott or Cantor tube.

Postoperative Objectives

A. *To meet nutritional needs by administering fluids, electrolytes and nutrients.*
1. Utilize intravenous catheter if intravenous therapy is to continue several days. Observe tissue for infiltration of fluid.
2. Maintain meticulous mouth hygiene while patient is on parenteral therapy.

B. *To promote proper functioning of nasogastric decompression and patient comfort.*
1. Observe and record quality and quantity of aspirated material.
2. Lubricate nostrils with water-soluble lubricant.
3. Humidify room to prevent dryness of mucous membranes.
4. Turn patient frequently to minimize discomfort.
5. Remove tube (when required) upon re-establishment of peristalsis (determined by auscultation, passage of flatus rectally).

C. *To alleviate psychosocial concerns of patient.*
1. Encourage patient to express concerns and questions. (See Colostomy and Ileostomy Management if these are pertinent, pp. 414 and 412.)
2. Administer analgesics according to needs.
3. Promote restfulness with appropriate nursing measures prior to giving sedation o hypnotics.

D. *To prevent complications by recognizing early signs.*
1. Evaluate vital signs and recognize patterns of development that may suggest hemor rhage, infection, shock, obstruction, etc.
2. Stress preventive measures, such as turning frequently, maintaining fluid balance encouraging coughing, emphasizing cleanliness.

E. *To prepare a plan for convalescence and follow-up care.*
1. Encourage ambulation and self-care activities.
2. Stimulate appetite by promoting those measures that will make patient want to eat what he should eat.
3. Help patient set goals toward which he can progress.
4. Emphasize the importance of follow-up visits to evaluate healing process, genera physical and psychological adjustment.

Ulcerative Colitis

Ulcerative colitis is an ulcerative and inflammatory disease of the colon and rectum.

Etiology and Incidence
1. Unknown (idiopathic); however, there are several unproven possibilities:
    a. Emotional response alters blood supply to colon mucosa which eventually causes ulceration.
    b. Unidentifiable organisms cause pathology.
    c. A combination of causative factors: infection, stress, allergy, autoimmunity.
2. Most common in young adulthood and middle life; almost equal between sexes (slightly more in females); more prevalent among Jews; highest among 3rd and 4th decades, familial incidence.

Clinical Manifestations

1. Multiple ulcerations, diffuse inflammation and desquamation of the colonic epithelium.
2. Self-perpetuating destructive infection of the mucosal lining of the large intestine.
3. Weight loss, fever, dehydration, anorexia, nausea and vomiting, anemia, cachexia.
4. The disease begins in the rectum and sigmoid and spreads upward, eventually involving the entire colon.
5. It is a serious disease accompanied by systemic complications and high mortality rate.

Diagnostic Evaluation

1. Stool examination to rule out dysentery.
2. Sigmoidoscopy, proctoscopy.
3. Barium enema x-ray.
   NOTE: If disease is in acute stage, cathartic may be contraindicated because it may cause exacerbation and lead to toxic megacolon.
4. Careful clinical assessment to rule out diverticulitis, cancer, etc.

Complications

1. Skin ulcers
2. Arthritis
3. Malnutrition
4. Anemia
5. Abscess formation
6. Stricture
7. Erythema nodosum
8. Amyloidosis
9. Malignancy

Objectives of Treatment and Nursing Management

A. *To combat infection and toxic state.*
   1. Administer nonabsorbable sulfa drugs, penicillin or streptomycin as prescribed.
   2. Give ACTH and adrenal steroid hormones as ordered (when other measures are unsuccessful) to combat inflammatory reaction, promote a feeling of well-being and decrease patient's toxic symptoms.
   3. For severe proctitis, nightly rectal instillations of prednisolone acetate (30 mg.) dissolved in 50 ml. of tap water, may produce a remission of symptoms.

B. *To promote rest and relaxation of intestinal tract.*
   1. Give sedatives and tranquilizers not only for general rest but also to allow peristalsis to slow down and afford rest to infected bowel.
   2. Be aware of the possibility of pressure sores in this patient because of malnourishment and enforced inactivity, especially if he is very thin.
   3. Administer tincture belladonna or atropine as prescribed to lessen gastric motility; kaolin and pectin may also be ordered to coat and soothe mucosa.
   4. Relieve painful rectal spasms (produced by frequent diarrheal stools) with anodyne suppositories.
   5. Give antispasmodics, if ordered, with caution since they may be instrumental in producing toxic megacolon.
   6. Report any evidence of sudden abdominal distention since it may precipitate toxic megacolon.

C. *To meet nutritional and fluid needs of the body.*
   1. If patient is acutely ill, maintain on parenteral replacement of vitamins, fluids and electrolytes.

TABLE 6-1. DIETS VARYING IN RESIDUE*

Very Low Residue

Foods	Allowed	Omitted
Dairy Products		
Milk	If allowed: milk, buttermilk, yoghurt, cream (Boiled or evaporated milk may be tolerated better than pasteurized)	Usually milk and milk drinks
Cheese	Cottage cheese only, if tolerated	Other cheeses
Fat	Butter, margarine	Salad dressing, fried foods
Eggs	Cooked, poached, scrambled in double boiler	
Meats, Fish, Fowl	Ground, tender meat; Minced chicken and fish Broiled or baked chicken, lamb, veal, white fish	Luncheon meats, frankfurters, pork and pork products, smoked or salted meats, sausage
Soups and Broths	Broth only	Any other
Vegetables	Unseasoned vegetable juices in limited amounts	Any other
Fruits	Fruit juices, preferably citrus in limited amounts if allowed	Any other
Breads, Cereals, Macaroni Products	Refined, enriched bread and cereals only; macaroni, spaghetti, noodles, white crackers	Bread or crackers containing whole grain flour or bran; quick breads, whole grain cereals
Desserts	Ices, ice cream, junket, cereal puddings, custard, gelatin, plain cake, and cookies	Any other No fruits and nuts
Beverages	Tea, postum; coffee as permitted; milk and milk beverages only if tolerated	Usually milk and milk drinks
Condiments and Miscellaneous	Salt in small quantities; sugar	Spices, salted foods, pickles, nuts, olives, relishes, fried foods

* 1. The omission of roughage will prevent irritation of the inflamed colon (e.g., ulcerative colitis).
  2. The high protein, high caloric diet will help to restore better nutritional status in this patient who is usually debilitated.
  3. Vitamin and iron supplements are recommended.

2. Provide a well-balanced, bland, low residue, high protein diet to correct malnutrition (Table 6-1).
3. Determine which foods agree with this patient and which do not. Modify diet plan accordingly.
4. Bolster with supplemental vitamin therapy including vitamin K.
5. Avoid cold fluids inasmuch as they increase gastric motility.
6. Administer proper electrolytes which have been lost in diarrheal bouts.

TABLE 6-1. DIETS VARYING IN RESIDUE (continued)

Low Residue

Foods	Allowed	Avoid
Dairy Products		
Milk	If allowed: milk, buttermilk, yoghurt, cream	Usually milk and milk beverages
Cheese	Cottage cheese, cheddar	Strongly flavored cheese
Fat	Butter, margarine	
Eggs	Cooked, poached, scrambled in double boiler	Fried
Meat, Fish, Fowl	Tender chicken, white fish, sweetbreads; ground beef and lamb	Corned beef, frankfurters, luncheon meat, pork, sausage, tough meat
Soup and Broths	Broth Strained cream soups	Any other
Vegetables	Vegetable juice; vegetable puree; cooked asparagus tips, carrots; potatoes (boiled, mashed, creamed, scalloped, baked)	Strong vegetables: broccoli, brussel sprouts, cabbage, cauliflower, onion, cucumber, pepper, corn
Fruits	Fruit juice; fruit puree, ripe bananas; cooked peeled apples, apricots, peaches, pears, plums	Raw fruits, stewed and canned berries, pineapple, canned fruits with skins
Bread, Cereals, Macaroni Products	Refined, enriched bread and cereals only; macaroni, spaghetti, noodles, white crackers	Fresh bread, whole grain breads, graham crackers, pretzels, bran and sweet rolls
Desserts	Ices, ice cream, junket, cereal puddings, custard, gelatin, plain cake and cookies; all without fruits and nuts	None with fruits, nuts, or spices, gingerbread, cakes, pies, pastries
Beverages	Tea, coffee; carbonated beverages	Alcoholic beverages, milk, unless physician allows
Condiments	Salt and sugar only	Mustard, spices, catsup, chili sauce

7. Administer blood transfusions and iron to correct existing anemia.
8. Carefully note fluid intake and output and character of bowel movements.

D. To cope with and correct psychological disturbances.

1. Offer psychological support.
2. Educate the patient to accept and learn to live with this chronic disease. This is done on a long-range basis.
3. Recognize that psychotherapy during the acute phases of this illness may do more harm than good.
4. Indicate by actions and expressions that you, the nurse, are responsible for and care for him. Good nurse-patient relationship enables him to satisfy his dependency needs.

5. Solicit the assistance of the family in helping to understand the patient; visa versa assist the family in understanding the patient.
6. Following surgery, when patient has an ileostomy, it is helpful if he is visited b someone who has had a similar operation and made a good adjustment.

E. *To prevent complications.*
   1. Observe for signs of colonic perforation and hemorrhage.
   2. Assess carefully the behavior of the patient and all his complaints.

Surgical Treatment and Nursing Management

A. *Indications and Contemplated surgery.*
   1. Approximately 20% of patients in the United States require surgical intervention.
   2. Recommended when no improvement occurs through conservative means: evidence by continued deterioration, such as profuse bleeding, perforation, stricture formatio and indications of malignancy developing.
   3. Total colectomy and permanent ileostomy recommended.

B. *Preoperative Physical and Psychological Preparation*
   1. Institute an intensive program of fluid, blood and protein replacement.
   2. Administer chemotherapy and antibiotics to reduce intestinal organisms.
   3. Recognize psychological needs of this patient:
      a. Fear, anxiety, and discouragement accompany diarrhea.
      b. Hypersensitivity may be evident.
      c. Let him know his complaints are understood.
   4. Encourage patient to talk; listen to what he says is bothering him.
   5. Answer his questions relative to the permanent ileostomy he is about to have.

C. *Postoperative Care Including Ileostomy Management*
   (See Management of Patient having Major Intestinal Surgery, p. 399.)
   (See Conditions: Caring for a Patient with an Ileostomy, p. 412.)

Diverticulosis and Diverticulitis

Diverticulum is a pouch or saccular dilatation leading out from a tube or main cavity (Fig. 6-9) *Diverticulitis* is an inflammation of diverticula.
Diverticulosis is the condition when an individual has multiple diverticula.

Predisposing Factors

   1. May be congenital.
   2. Weakening and degeneration of muscular wall of the intestine causing herniation o the lining mucous membrane.
   3. Mechanical pressure, such as constant pulling from outside intestinal wall or pressure from within.
   4. Chronic overdistention of large bowel.

Incidence

   1. Diverticula of large bowel occurs in 5–10% of adults—of these, ⅓ may experience diverticulitis.
   2. Usually occurs in individuals over 40 years of age.

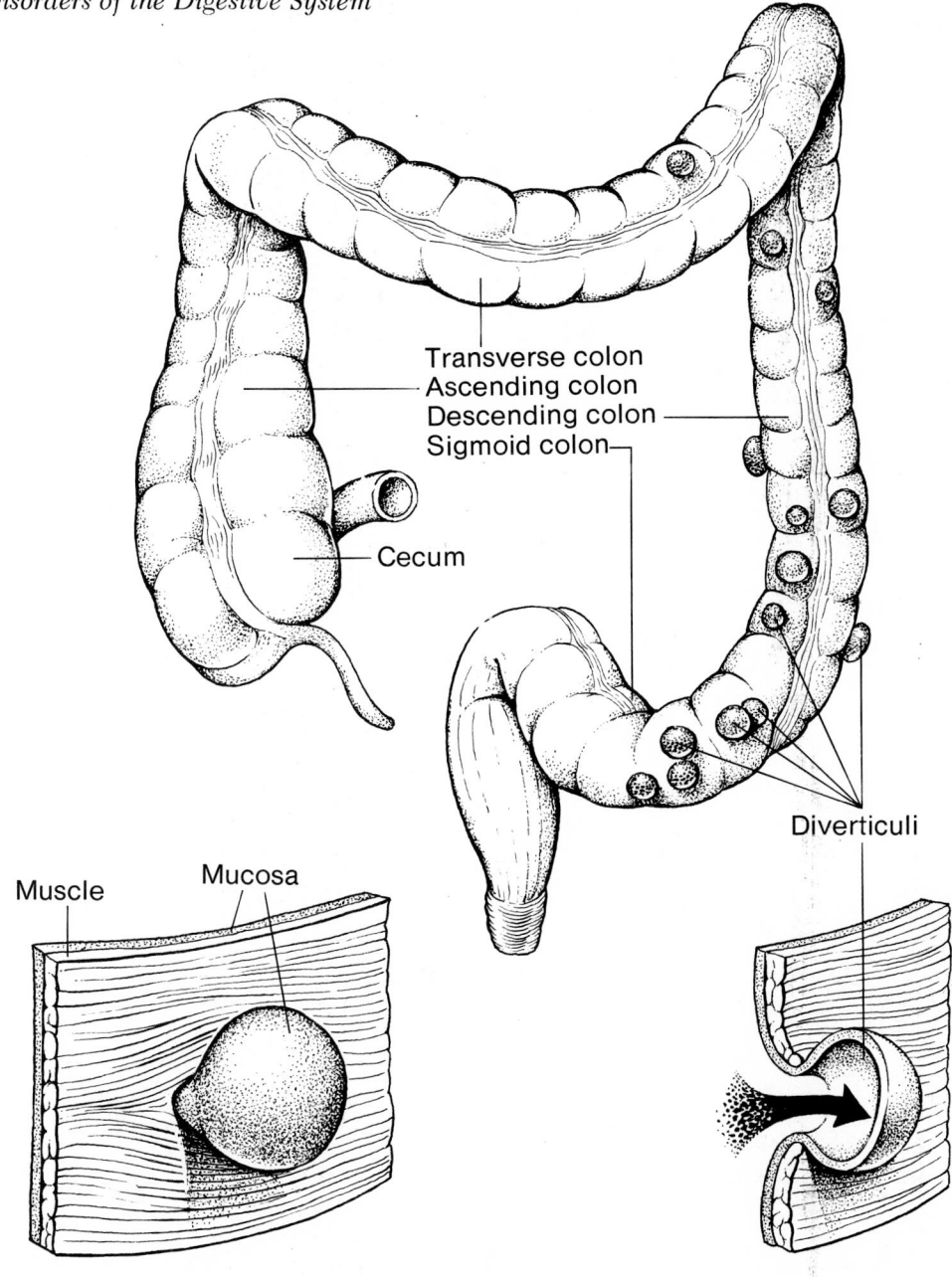

Transverse colon
Ascending colon
Descending colon
Sigmoid colon

Cecum

Diverticuli

Muscle   Mucosa

A diverticulum is formed by the herniation of the intestinal mucosa through the weakened muscular wall

Fecal matter accumulates within the diverticulum

Figure 6-9. Diverticula are most common in the sigmoid colon; they diminish in number and size as the colon approaches the cecum. Diverticula are rarely found in the rectum.

Clinical Manifestations

A. *General Clinical Signs*
   1. May occur in acute attacks or persist as a long drawn out smoldering infection.
   2. Tends to spread to surrounding bowel wall, causing irritability and spasticity of colon.
   3. When infections are severe, perforation of colon can occur, leading to peritonitis.
   4. When infection is less acute but slowly progressive, extensive scarring and abscess formation involving bowel wall may occur, with the possibility of lower bowel obstruction.

B. *Specific Clinical Signs*
   1. Moderately severe acute diverticulitis
      a. Crampy pain in lower left quadrant of abdomen.
      b. Flatulence, slight nausea, low-grade fever.
   2. Milder form of diverticulitis
      a. Bouts of soreness, mild lower abdominal cramps.
      b. Bowel irregularity, constipation and diarrhea.
   3. Hemorrhage occurs in 10–20% of patients.
      a. Not persistent but may be massive.
      b. May be rectal bleeding only (not massive).
   4. Fever and leukocytosis

Diagnostic Evaluation

   1. Fluoroscopy and x-ray with barium enema.
   2. Sigmoidoscopy may be helpful.

Treatment

A. *During acute episode*
   1. Maintain fluid and nutritional requirements with intravenous therapy; give nothing by mouth.
   2. Maintain antibiotic therapy to reduce infection.

B. *Dietary*
   1. Elimination of roughage from diet will prevent irritation of the inflamed colon.
   2. Sample of a very low residue diet:
      Breakfast: Cream of wheat, light cream, postum, sugar
      Midmorning: Cookie with warm milk or malted milk
      Lunch: Vegetable juice, creamed chicken (sm. pieces) on toast, milk
      Midafternoon: Custard (not cold)
      Dinner: Broth, cream cheese and jelly sandwich, gelatin
      Evening: Cookie with warm milk or malted milk
   3. Foods considered as roughage and to be avoided:
      a. Meat fibers (but not tender meats), clams, oysters
      b. Sweet potatoes, whole grain rice, whole wheat bread.
      c. Carrots, corn, beets

      d. Spinach, lettuce, cabbage, celery
      e. Olives, garlic, pickles, nuts
  4. High protein and high caloric diet to restore a better nutritional status.
  5. Vitamin and iron supplements to supplement dietary requirements.

C. *Surgical*
  1. If there is little response to medical treatment or if complications occur such as hemorrhage, obstruction, or perforation, surgery is necessary.
  2. Preparation for surgery:
      a. Low residue diet or nothing by mouth.
      b. Antimicrobials, systemic and intestinal surface-acting, to reduce bowel bacterial flora, diminish bulk of stool and soften fecal mass for easier movement.
      c. Cleansing enemas may be ordered.
  3. Resection of segment of intestine involved with diverticula, reuniting (anastomosing) two ends to maintain continuity.
  4. Temporary colostomy is sometimes performed to divert fecal stream (see p. 414).

D. *Community Nursing and Patient Education*
  Objective: to prevent recurrence
  1. Maintain a low residue diet.
  2. Establish regular bowel habits to promote regular and complete evacuation.
  3. Continue under periodic medical supervision and follow-up.

Intestinal Obstruction

Intestinal obstruction is an interruption in the normal flow of intestinal contents along the intestinal tract.

Types of Obstruction

  1. Mechanical—a physical block to passage of intestinal contents without disturbing blood supply of bowel.
      a. *Location*
      Extrinsic, e.g., adhesions, hernia
      Intrinsic, e.g., hematoma, tumor
      Luminal, e.g., foreign body, fecal impaction, polyp
      b. *Clinical Pattern*   *Incidence*

Clinical Pattern	Incidence
High small-bowel (jejunal) }	80%
Low small-bowel (ileal) }	
Colonic	20%

  2. Paralytic (neurogenic; adynamic) ileus
      Peristalsis is ineffective (diminished motor activity perhaps due to toxic or traumatic disturbance of autonomic nervous system); no physical obstruction and no interrupted blood supply.
  3. Obstruction by strangulation
      Blood supply compromised leading to gangrene of bowel.

Causes

1. Mechanical (extramural)
   a. Adhesions—postoperative
   b. Hernia
   c. Carcinomatosis
   d. Volvulus (loop of intestine twisted)
2. Mechanical (intramural)
   a. Carcinoma
   b. Hematoma
   c. Intussusception (telescoping of intestine)
   d. Stricture or stenosis (scarring)
3. Paralytic
   a. Back injuries, fractures
   b. Postoperative kidney surgery
   c. Peritonitis
   d. Wound dehiscence (breakdown)

NOTE:
1. In postoperative patients, 90% of mechanical obstructions are due to adhesions.
2. In unoperative patients, hernia is the most common cause of obstruction.

Altered Physiology

1. Disturbed physiology as a result of mechanical small intestine obstruction results in increased peristalsis, distention by fluid and gas, and increased bacterial growth.
2. Extracellular fluid (interstitial and plasma) volume contracts thereby leading to shock.

Diagnostic Evaluation

1. Obstruction may be partial or complete.
2. Seriousness depends upon area of bowel affected, extent of blockage and degree of interrupted blood supply.
3. Small bowel obstruction is serious because of persistent vomiting and acute electrolyte imbalance.
   a. Alkalosis (loss of hydrogen ion)
   b. Severe dehydration and acidosis (water and sodium loss from small intestine).
4. Partial obstruction which has developed slowly produces mild symptoms.
5. Colonic obstruction even if complete is less serious if blood supply is not interrupted.
6. "Closed-loop" obstruction is a condition where the intestinal segment is occluded at both ends, preventing either the downward passage or the regurgitation of intestinal contents.

Clinical Manifestations

1. Simple mechanical—high small bowel
   Colic (cramps) mid to upper abdomen, some distention, early bilious vomiting, increased bowel sounds, minimal diffuse tenderness.
2. Simple mechanical—low small bowel
   Significant colic (cramps) midabdominal, considerable distention, some vomiting—later feculent, increased bowel sounds and "rush" sounds, minimal diffuse tenderness.
3. Simple mechanical—colon
   Cramps (mid-to-lower abdomen), later distention appears, then vomiting may be present (feculent), bowel sounds usually increased, minimal diffuse tenderness, fever, peritoneal irritation, increased white blood cell count, toxicity, shock.

4. Strangulation

   Symptoms are initially those of mechanical obstruction but later rapid progression: Pain is severe, continuous, localized; moderate distention, persistent vomiting, usually decreased bowel sounds, marked localized tenderness.

5. Paralytic ileus

   Gaseous distention is prominent, abdomen is tense, pain is dull and diffuse, obstipation (intractable constipation) rarely complete since small amounts of flatus may be passed, peristalsis is usually depressed and bowel sounds are infrequent, vomiting occurs only after eating.

NOTE: Due to loss of water, sodium and chlorides, signs of dehydration become evident: intense thirst, drowsiness, general malaise, aching; tongue becomes parched, face appears pinched, abdomen becomes distended. Shock may result (pulse increasingly rapid and weak, temperature and blood pressure lowered, skin pale, cold, clammy) ending in death.

Treatment and Nursing Management

A. *Initial Nursing Assessment and Care*

1. Describe accurately the nature and location of the patient's pain, the presence of distention, absence of flatus or defecation; the overview of symptoms is important in differentiating intestinal obstruction from other more benign conditions.
2. Measure, record and chart vital signs including blood pressure every 4 hours.
3. Measure and record accurately all intake and output.
4. Save any stool that may be passed; this is to be tested for occult blood.
5. Anticipate physician's request for urinalysis, hemoglobin determination and blood cell counts.
6. Recognize the patient's concern and initiate measures to secure his cooperation and confidence in the staff.
7. Undertake measures to prepare the patient for surgery since most problems of mechanical obstruction require surgical correction.

B. *Medical and Surgical Management*

1. Relieve distention by introducing long gastrointestinal tube; this can be passed more effectively with the patient lying on his right side; begin to suction to remove gas and fluid.
2. Correct fluid imbalance by initiating
   a. $Na+$, $K+$, plasma substitutes
   b. Ringer's lactate to correct interstitial fluid deficit
   c. Dextrose/water to correct intracellular fluid deficit.
3. Administer antibiotics (neomycin and kanamycin) and possibly a broad spectrum agent to lessen the possibility of infection, particularly peritonitis.
4. Recognize that giving an enema may distort an x-ray picture by introducing gas into the tract distal to the obstruction. An enema may make a partial obstruction worse, hence is contraindicated.
5. Prevent strangulation by carefully assessing status of patient; if pain increases in intensity, localizes or becomes continuous it may herald strangulation.

6. Detect early signs of peritonitis, such as rigidity and tenderness in an effort to mini-mize this complication.
7. Relieve obstruction by releasing, removing or repairing the cause of the obstruction; this is done surgically in most instances. Complete small bowel obstruction and colon obstruction requires an operation for relief. When tube suction therapy does not help after 12 hours, surgery is indicated.
   a. *Resection* of obstructing lesion and end-to-end anastomosis is done when no evi-dence of peritonitis and only minimal edema exist; this requires a proximal colos-tomy to decompress new anastomosis.
   b. Resection of all necrotic intestine is necessary.
   c. A tube *enterostomy* may be done by introducing a catheter into distended bowel; the other end of catheter is brought out through the abdominal wall via a separate incision.
   d. A *loop colostomy* is done when relief is sought by drawing a proximal loop or segment of colon up to the skin surface and opening it as a colostomy; the distal portion of colon is treated later.

C. *Postoperative Care*
   1. To meet fluid and nutritional needs, administer large amounts of fluids, keep accurate intake and output records.
   2. For an enterostomy, connect tube to drainage bottle at side of bed; expect consider-able amount of fecal drainage during the first 12–15 hours (500–1000 ml.).
      a. Observe frequently the patency of drainage equipment.
      b. If there is difficulty with drainage, it may be necessary to inject 15 ml. of warm saline into the enterostomy tube every 2–4 hours with approval of physician.
      c. Protect skin around enterostomy tube with triamcinolone acetonide (Kenalog) spray followed by a light dusting of nystatin powder (Mycostatin).
   3. Follow additional postoperative care described on page 399, Major Intestinal Surgery.

Cancer of the Colon

Incidence
1. Cancer of the colon and rectum will account for over 79,000 deaths—the second highest overall death rate in the U.S. for any site.
2. Males and females affected equally.
3. Two-thirds occur in patients over 50.
4. Five-year survival is 40–50% (best of visceral cancers).

Etiology
1. Familial polyposis (numerous pedunculated growths arising from mucosa and extending into lumen of intestine).
2. Chronic ulcerative colitis—definite risk of colon cancer.
3. Diverticulosis and cancer may be found together—no definite evidence that diverti-cula is significant in the development of cancer.

Clinical Manifestations

1. Distribution of cancer in the colon is usually as follows:

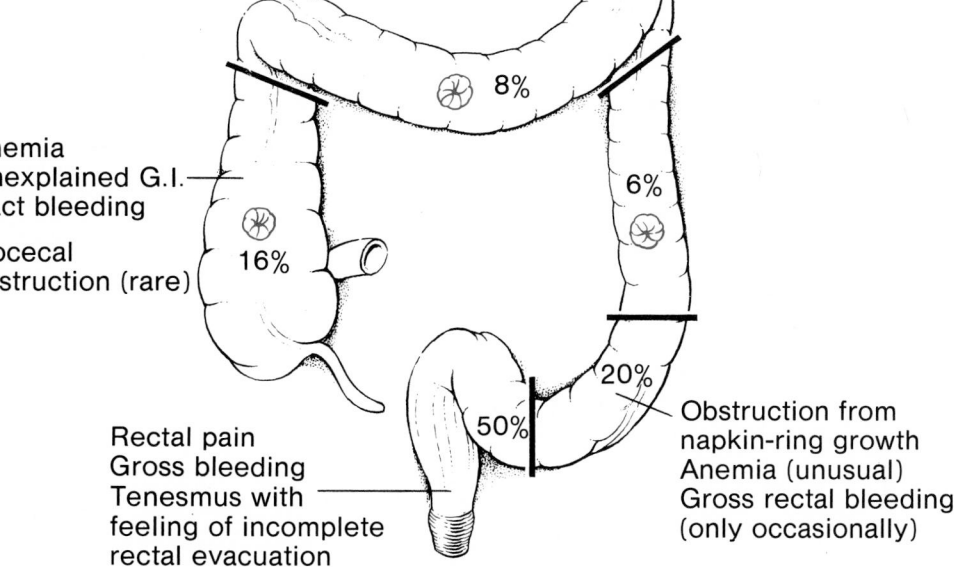

Anemia
Unexplained G.I.
tract bleeding

Iliocecal
obstruction (rare)

16%

8%

6%

20%

50%

Rectal pain
Gross bleeding
Tenesmus with
feeling of incomplete
rectal evacuation

Obstruction from
napkin-ring growth
Anemia (unusual)
Gross rectal bleeding
(only occasionally)

Figure 6-10. Distribution of cancer in the colon.

2. Most common symptoms:
   a. Blood in stools—causing anemia, obstruction and perforation.
   b. Partial obstruction—causing constipation alternating with diarrhea, lower abdominal pains (crampy), distention.
   c. Additional signs—progressive weakness, anorexia, weight loss, shortness of breath, anginal pain, anemia.

Diagnostic Evaluation

1. Digital rectal examination—half of all colon and rectal cancers are found this way.
2. Sigmoidoscopy—⅔ of all colon and rectal cancer can be seen and biopsied.
3. Stool examination for blood.
4. Blood-hemoglobin determination for anemia.
5. Barium enema—especially significant in unexplained abdominal mass.
6. Napkin-ring-type outline clearly indicates obstruction and possible tumor.
7. Silicone foam enema—expelled silicone cast may show indentations suggestive of cancer of polyps.
8. Cystoscopy may be significant in detecting spread of malignancy.

Treatment

A. *Diagnosis Confirmed by*
   1. Removing rectosigmoid polyps through sigmoidoscope for histologic study.
   2. Removing polyps above rectosigmoid by laparotomy (if other symptoms are present) to verify diagnosis.

B. *Surgical Therapeutic Plan*
   1. Recommend total colectomy for patient with familial history of polyposis even before cancer confirmed.
   2. Most common operative procedures:
      a. Wide segmental resection of colon and mesentery with anastomosis, or
      b. Abdominoperineal resection with colostomy
      c. Even more extensive surgery involving removal of other organs if cancer has spread—such as to the bladder, uterus, small intestine, groin, etc.
      d. If cancer is extensive and it may not be in the patient's best interest to do radical surgery, palliative treatment by radiation may be done using radon seed implantation (combined surgery and preoperative radiation therapy is being studied in several clinics).

Nursing Management

A. *Preoperative Care*
   1. Meet nutritional needs of patient by serving a high caloric, low residue diet for several days prior to surgery if condition permits.
   2. Reduce bacterial count of colon by administering antibiotics as prescribed: phthalyl-sulfathiazole (Sulfathalidine), kanamycin.
   3. Observe and record fluid losses such as may be sustained by vomiting and diarrhea.
   4. Chart and report any complaints of abdominal pain with a description of nature and location.
   5. Assist with and maintain nasogastric suction to minimize postoperative distention.
   6. Elicit any concerns or questions patient may have regarding postoperative dependency, etc.
   7. Prepare patient immediately preoperatively by adequate shaving of area. (See page 399 for Care of Patient Having Major Intestinal Surgery.)

B. *Postoperative Care*
   See page 400.

GUIDELINES: *Changing an Ileostomy Appliance*

Purposes

   1. To prevent leakage (bag is usually changed every 2–4 days).
   2. To permit examination of skin around stoma.
   3. To assist in controlling odor.

Time

   1. Early in morning before breakfast or 2–4 hours after a meal when the bowel is least active.

2. Immediately if patient is complaining of burning or itching underneath the disk or has pain around the stoma.

Equipment

Duplicate ileostomy appliance with belt.
Solvent—medicine dropper
Karaya powder, karaya ring (self-adhering appliance)
Gauze dressings
Emesis basin

Procedure

Nursing Action	Rationale/Amplification
Preparatory Phase	
1. Have patient assume a relaxed position.	1. Encourage patient participation and understanding so that eventually he will be able to change appliance himself.
2. Explain details of this activity to patient.	
3. Expose ileostomy area; remove ileostomy belt.	
4. Position lamp; wash hands.	
Performance Phase	
1. Apply solvent (using medicine dropper) around edge of disk; gradually peel disk from skin.	1. Alternating solvent application with careful lifting of disk prevents skin damage.
2. Moisten skin with solvent, using a saturated cotton ball.	2. This prevents debris accumulation which could cause skin irritation.
3. Wash skin with warm water and soap using a soft washcloth.	3. Patient could take a shower or bath at this time. If stoma is discharging, cover with a dressing and plastic such as Saran Wrap; seal with Micropore tape.
4. Spray dry skin thoroughly with triamcinolone acetonide (Kenalog) spray or dust with nystatin (Mycostatin) powder.	4. Corticosteroid spray or antibiotic powder protects skin.
5. Moisten a karaya gum washer, wait until it is tacky and then apply over the stoma.	5. Gum karaya protects the skin while permitting healing underneath.
6. Apply adhesive disk on the faceplate of the pouch against washer; press firmly for a few minutes until adherence is assured.	6. Seal-tight adherence results only when both parts are tacky before being pressed together.
7. Check the pouch bottom for closure; use rubber band or clip provided.	7. Proper closure controls leakage.
Follow-up Phase	
1. Dispose waste materials.	
2. Clean ileostomy bag by washing in soap and water.	2. Preserve life of appliance and control odor.
3. Soak in deodorant solution; or rinse in solution of 60 ml. (2 oz.) distilled vinegar to 1 liter water.	3. Deodorizing agents should be effective but not destructive to rubber.

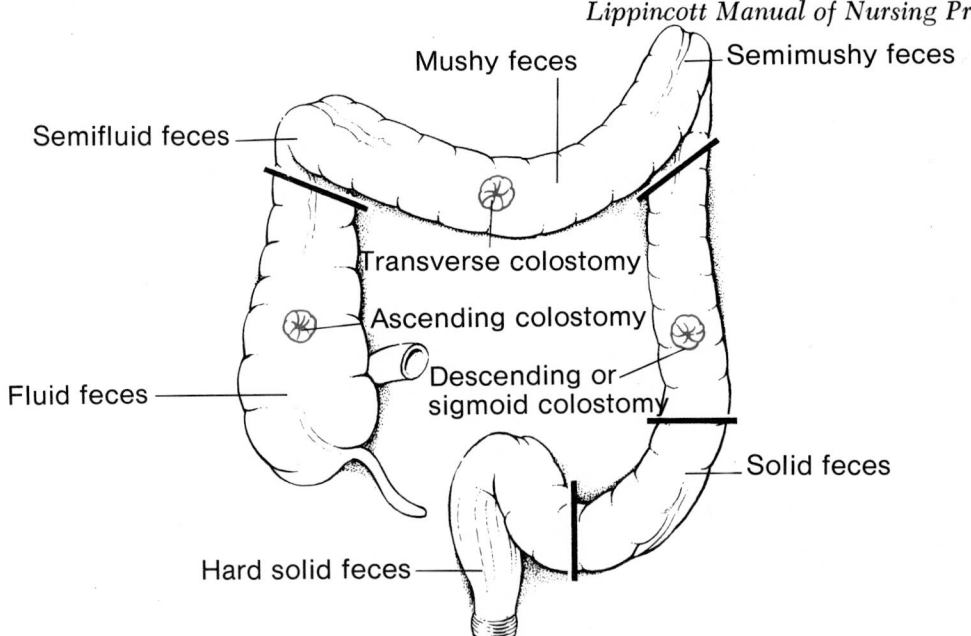

Figure 6-11. A diagrammatic representation of the placement of permanent colostomies and the nature of the discharge at these sites.

GUIDELINES: *Irrigating a Colostomy*

A *colostomy* is a temporary or permanent opening of the colon through the abdominal wall (an
abdominal anus). Placement of colostomy will influence the nature of the discharge (Fig. 6-11).
The *stoma* is that part of the colon that is brought above the abdominal wall in a colostomy.

Purposes

1. To empty the colon of its contents: fecal, gas, mucus.
2. To cleanse the lower intestinal tract.
3. To establish a regular pattern of evacuation so that normal life activities may be
   pursued.
4. To prevent intestinal obstruction.
5. To prevent skin excoriation due to irritating fecal contents.

Equipment

1. Reservoir for irrigating fluids: enema bag, irrigating can, large bulb syringe
2. Irrigating fluid: tap water or warm saline—4 ml. of salt to 500 ml. of water (1 t. salt
   to 1 pt. water); total solution—1000–2000 ml. at 40.5°C. (105°F.)
3. Tubing, connecting tubes, and clamp: rubber or plastic tubing; preferable clamp—
   one that can be opened with one hand.
4. Irrigating tip: soft rubber catheter—No. 22 or No. 24 with or without wide-cone
   irrigating tip.
5. Irrigating bag or sheath: self-adhesive (adhering) or held in place with a belt. (A
   plastic or rubber sheet can be used as a trough in place of bag or sheath.)
6. Newspaper or plastic bag: to collect soiled dressings and disposable bag.
7. Petrolatum and toilet tissues.

Procedure

Preparatory Phase

1. Select a suitable time, preferably after a meal, so that this hour fits into patient's posthospital pattern of activity.
2. Hang irrigating reservoir with solution 45–50 cm. (18–20 inches) above stoma.
3. Have patient sit in front of toilet commode.
4. Remove soiled dressings and place in bag.

Nursing Action	Rationale/Amplification
Irrigation	
1. Apply irrigating vessel or sheath (if available) to stoma.	1. Unnecessary; however, if available, it helps to control odor and splashing.
2. Attach tubing to bag and irrigating tip; allow some of solution to flow through catheter.	2. By releasing air bubbles in the set-up, air is not introduced into the colon to cause crampy pain.
3. Insert catheter gently about 10–15 cm. (4–6 inches); move it in and out a number of times while solution slowly flows.	3. This cleanses and clears terminal end of colon up to 15 cm. (4 inches). Solution flowing slowly helps to relax bowel and facilitates passage of tube.

> NURSING ALERT: Finger dilatation of any stoma is not advised (it may be done by the physician on rare occasion). Dilatation may cause tearing of mucosa and skin leading to infection, fibrosis and stricture formation.

Nursing Action	Rationale/Amplification
4. Allow fluid to enter colon; if cramping occurs, clamp off tubing and allow patient to rest before progressing.	4. Painful cramps are usually caused by too rapid flow or too much solution.
5. Remove catheter when the patient has taken as much solution as possible—about 5–10 minutes.	
6. Allow fecal material to flow (through sheath) into toilet; most of fecal material will be expelled in 15–20 minutes.	6. Gravity and peristaltic action will promote expulsion in about 20 minutes; however, it may require longer time.
7. If available, apply sealable type bag to permit his moving about.	
8. If fluid is not evacuated, siphon off.	
Follow-up	
1. Cleanse area with mild soap and water; pat dry.	1. Cleanliness and dryness will provide patient with hours of comfort.
2. Replace colostomy dressing or pouch; karaya powder or karaya ring may be used.	
3. Clean equipment with soap and water; dry before being stored in well-ventilated area.	3. This will control odor and prolong life of equipment.

GUIDELINES: *Bulb Syringe Method* of Irrigating a Colostomy*

Purposes

1. By using smaller quantities of solution, fecal return is stimulated rather than flushed out with larger quantities of fluid.
2. Fluid is prevented from being trapped in the colon.

* Adapted from Postel, A. H.: Training the Patient in the Bulb Syringe Method of Colostomy Irrigation. New York, Department of Surgery in collaboration with The Institute of Physical Medicine and Rehabilitation, New York University Medical Center, 1965.

Equipment

240-ml. (8-oz.) soft rubber bulb syringe with flexible plastic or rubber tip
1-liter (32-oz.) pitcher for water
Plastic ring—7.5-cm. (3-inch) diameter
Disposable plastic drainage sheath—45-cm. (18-inch) long and plastic ring
Petrolatum

Procedure

Nursing Action	*Rationale / Amplification*

Preparatory Phase

1. Collect equipment and fill pitcher with water; place within reach of patient.

2. Have patient sit on toilet.

   2. This approach lends itself to a more normal evacuation position.

3. Pull one end of drainage sheath through plastic ring (a) and carefully fold edge over ring (b).

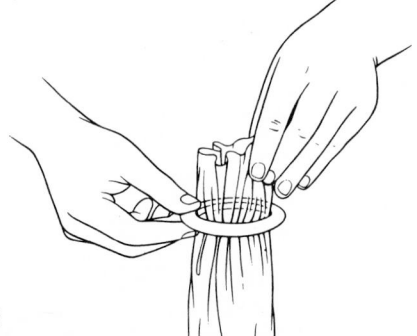

a

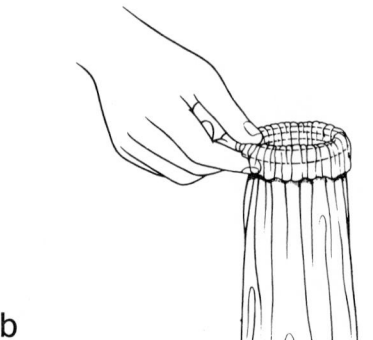

b

4. Place plastic-covered ring over stoma and secure ring to the body using patient's elastic colostomy belt (c). Place opposite end of sheath between patient's legs so that outflow is directed into toilet (d).

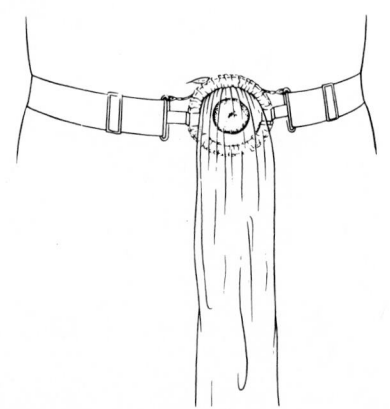

c

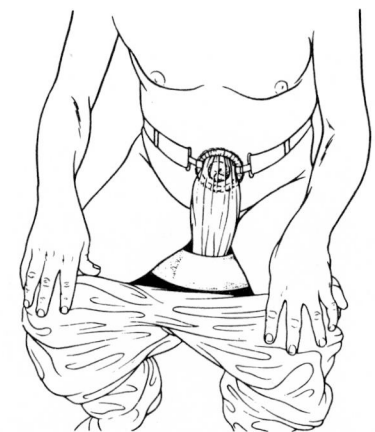

d

5. Pierce hole in sheath to permit insertion of tip of syringe.

   5. By placing hole above the stomal opening, fluid leakage is avoided.

Nursing Action | **Rationale/Amplification**

Irrigation

1. Fill bulb syringe with tepid water; expel all air.

   1. Air introduced into colon may cause distention and cramp-like pain. It may also prevent a good fecal return. Purpose is to stimulate peristalsis.

2. Lubricate tip and insert about 7.5–12.5 cm. (3–5 inches) into stoma.

3. Use both hands to apply continuous pressure on bulb to permit a steady flow of water (a & b).

   3. Even pressure is more relaxing and likely to aid peristalsis.

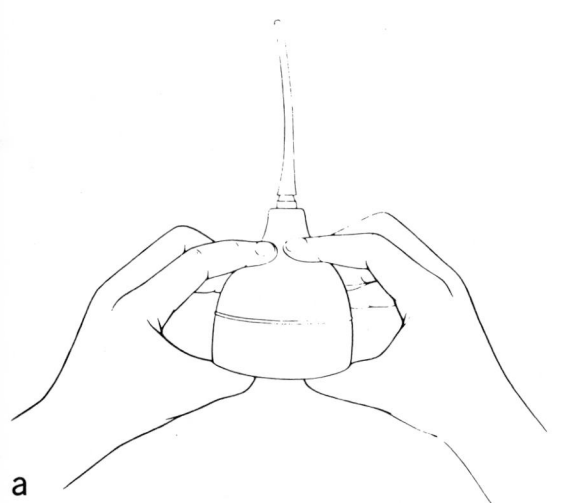

a

Nurse uses thumbs to compress bulb.

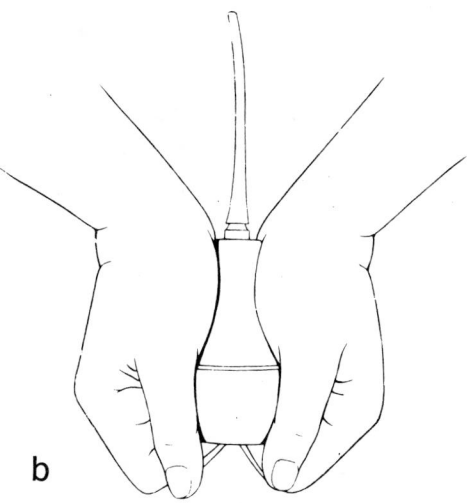

b

Patient uses fingers to compress bulb.

4. When syringe is empty, continue to maintain pressure on bulb as syringe is withdrawn from stoma.

   4. Pressure must be maintained on bulb as it is withdrawn so that aspiration of feces or fluid into syringe is prevented.

5. Repeat steps 1 through 4, not more than 2 more times (3 bulbfuls altogether).

   5. To use more than 720 ml. (24 oz.) may cause retention of fluid.

6. Instruct patient to massage lower abdomen and area around stoma; also he may take deep breaths. Usually 15–20 minutes are required to complete the irrigation.

   6. To facilitate an adequate return.

7. Skin and stoma care are the same as follow-up procedure (p. 415). The patient may find he needs to wear the bag for a very short time, or it may not even be necessary.

   7. A small dressing (4″ x 4″) applied to stoma is usually all that is required. During the day, a girdle or shorts may keep dressing in place. At night, tape may be necessary.

Appendicitis

Acute appendicitis is an inflammation of the appendix due to an infection. It is usually always a surgical problem.

Incidence

1. Occurs most frequently in young adults but may occur in any age group.
2. Incidence of appendicitis in U.S. has been decreasing during the past decade.

Clinical Manifestations

1. Begins with a progressively severe generalized or upper abdominal pain.
2. Within a few hours, the acute tenderness becomes localized in the right lower quadrant (McBurney's point).
3. Anorexia, slight or moderate temperature elevation, and perhaps nausea and vomiting occur.

Diagnostic Evaluation

1. Physical examination noting especially location and localization of pain, rebound tenderness, etc.
2. Blood studies with particular attention to white count; urinalysis.
   A white blood count reveals a moderate leukocytosis.
3. Careful history to rule out other possibilities.

Treatment and Nursing Management

A. *Palliative Preoperative Care*
1. Place patient in comfortable position to relieve abdominal pain and tension—usually Fowler's position.
2. See that patient takes nothing by mouth—to decrease peristalsis. Note time and nature of last meal.
3. Place ice bag to right lower quadrant—NEVER HEAT because of the possibility of causing a rupture of appendix and peritonitis.
4. Do not administer cathartics—for the same reason as preceding precaution concerning heat.
5. Frequently evaluate vital signs—to assess progression of infection.
6. When diagnosis of acute appendicitis is made, administer chemotherapy and/or antibiotics.

NOTE: If there is evidence that perforation has occurred recently and a generalized peritonitis has developed, conservative treatment is instituted (see p. 419).

B. *Operative*
1. If diagnosis of acute appendicitis is established, a simple appendectomy is performed.
2. Because patient will obtain relief from pain, he usually accepts surgery very willingly which affords a smooth recovery.
3. Anesthetic may be general or spinal.
4. Incision may be McBurney, muscle-splitting or gridiron, or right rectus.

C. *Postoperative Care* (see also p. 49)
1. Without drainage
   a. Following recovery from anesthetic, Fowler's position is maintained, morphine is given every 3 or 4 hours, and fluids and food are given as tolerated.
   b. Enema given 3rd postoperative day.
   c. Stitches removed between 5th and 7th day (usually in physician's office).
2. With drainage
   Treat same as for peritonitis (see p. 419).

Meckel's Diverticulum

Meckel's diverticulum is a congenital abnormality of the ileum consisting of a blind pouch resembling the appendix.

Incidence

(A disease of "two's")
1. Such a diverticulum observed in about 2% of the population.
2. More common in men than women; 2–1.
3. Usually opens into ileum about 2 feet proximal to ileocecal valve.
4. Two complications: Inflammation and bleeding.

Significance

1. Not infrequently the mucosal lining is composed of misplaced ectopic linings such as gastric or pancreatic and this tends to ulcerate and bleed (hemorrhage).
2. It may become inflamed leading to intestinal obstruction, perforation and peritonitis.

Clinical Manifestations

1. Abdominal pain which is umbilical in location.
2. Possibly passage of blood in stools—not bright red or tarry but rather dark crimson.

Treatment

Similar to that for an appendectomy (p. 418).

Peritonitis

Peritonitis is an inflammation of the peritoneal cavity.

Etiology

Bacterial infections: point of origin may be gastrointestinal disease or infection from the ovaries, uterus or extraperitoneal organs (i.e., inflammation of the kidney).

Clinical Manifestations

(Dependent upon location and extension of inflammation.)
1. Diffuse type of abdominal pain—tends to become constant, localized and more intense.
2. Abdomen becomes extremely tender, muscles become rigid; rebound tenderness and ileus may be present.
3. Usually nausea and vomiting—peristalsis diminishes.
4. Elevation of temperature and pulse as well as leukocyte count.

Objectives of Treatment and Nursing Management

A. *To remove cause of the infection*
1. If localized:
   a. If acutely inflamed appendix—an appendectomy is called for.
   b. If ruptured duodenal ulcer—ulcer closed or plicated.
2. If not localized, patient is acutely ill.

B. *To combat infection and promote patient comfort.*
   1. Give nothing by mouth—to reduce peristalsis; ensure meticulous oral hygiene.
   2. Provide fluids by vein to establish adequate fluid level and to promote adequate urinary output so that toxins are eliminated.
   3. Record accurately intake and output including the measurement of vomitus.
   4. Administer antibiotics as prescribed.
   5. Observe and describe symptoms accurately: pain and tenderness have a tendency to shift and must be reported precisely.
   6. Reassure the patient and establish his confidence because he usually realizes the seriousness of his condition.

C. *To promote recovery and reduce the possibility of complications.*
   1. Following recovery from anesthetic, place patient in Fowler's position to facilitate drainage.
   2. Administer fluids by vein since nothing is given by mouth initially.
   3. Prevent nausea and vomiting by use of nasogastric suction; institute proper nursing measures for nasal and oral comfort.
   4. Reduce parenteral fluids and increase oral food and fluids when
      a. Temperature and pulse rate come down.
      b. Abdomen becomes soft.
      c. Peristaltic sounds return (determined by abdominal auscultation).
      d. Flatus is passed and patient has bowel movements.
   5. Be alert for possibility of complications: Report immediately
      a. Wound evisceration—"It feels as if something just gave way."
      b. Abscess formation—an area of abdomen is tender or painful.

Abdominal Hernia

A *hernia* is a protrusion of viscus through the wall of the cavity in which it is normally contained. It is often called a "rupture."

Incidence

   1. Occurs 3 times more frequently in men than women; may occur at any age.
   2. Results from congenital or acquired weakness of the abdominal wall.
   3. Tends to increase in size and occurrence with increase in intra-abdominal pressure brought about by coughing, straining or pressure from a nearby tumor.

Classification

A. *According to Area*
   1. Inguinal
      a. In male—due to weakness in abdominal wall where spermatic cord emerges; enters inguinal canal and then scrotum.
      b. In female—due to weakness in abdominal wall where round ligament is located; enters inguinal canal and then labia.
         (1) Direct inguinal   (2) Indirect inguinal
             Medial-to-deep epigastric artery   Lateral-to-deep epigastric artery
             Majority are acquired   Majority are congenital
   2. Femoral
      a. Occurs most often in women.
      b. Located below Poupart's ligament (below groin).

3. Umbilical
   a. Results from failure of umbilical orifice to close.
   b. Occurs most often in obese women and children.
4. Ventral or incisional
   a. Due to weakness in abdominal wall.
   b. May occur following impaired healing of incision because of drainage, infection, etc.

B. *According to Severity*
1. Reducible—the protruding mass can be replaced in abdomen.
2. Irreducible—the protruding mass cannot be moved back into abdomen.
3. Incarcerated—an irreducible hernia in which the intestinal flow is completely obstructed.
4. Strangulated—an irreducible hernia in which the blood and intestinal flow are completely obstructed.
   Symptoms—pain, vomiting, swelling of hernial sac, fever, lower abdominal signs of peritoneal irritation.

Treatment

A. *Mechanical* (reducible hernia only)
   A *truss* is an appliance having a pad that is held snugly in the hernial orifice.
1. Does not cure a hernia—it prevents abdominal contents from entering hernial sac.
2. May be used in treatment of hernia in adults when, because of disease or age, it is inadvisable to perform surgery.

B. *Surgical*
   Recommended to correct the hernia before a strangulation occurs which then becomes an emergency situation.
1. Hernial sac is dissected free.
2. Contents of sac are replaced in abdominal cavity.
3. Neck of sac is ligated.
4. Muscle and fascial layers are sewed together firmly to prevent a recurrence. If this is not possible, synthetic mesh may be sutured over area.

Nursing Management

A. *Preoperative*
1. If hernia is strangulated, emergency conditions prevail. (See p. 407, *Intestinal Obstruction.*)
2. If surgery is elective, patient is usually in good physical condition.
3. Shave suprapubic region and anterior surface of upper thigh.
4. Observe for upper respiratory infection—if present, surgery will be postponed because coughing or sneezing postoperatively may break the sutures.

B. *Postoperative*
1. Ambulate patient in a day or two.
2. Take following measures for scrotal edema or swelling.
   a. Bedrest
   b. Ice pack, scrotal suspensory for support
3. Observe for urinary retention.

C. *Patient Instruction*
1. Athletics and extremes of exertion are not permitted for 6 to 8 weeks.

ANORECTAL CONDITIONS AND TREATMENTS

Ischiorectal Abscess

An *ischiorectal abscess* is a localized infection in the fatty tissue near the rectum.

Treatment

Incision and drainage

Fistula in Ano

A *fistula in ano* is an abnormal opening from the skin near the anus winding tortuously into the anal canal; because it is an infectious area, pus leaks outward.

Treatment

1. Surgical identification of path of fistula.
2. Cutting fistula open followed by insertion of packing.

Fissure in Ano

A *fissure in ano* is a longitudinal ulcer (a crack which does not heal) in the anal canal, associated frequently with constipation and excruciating pain on defecation.

Treatment

1. Dilatation of anal sphincter
2. Excision of fissure

Hemorrhoids

Hemorrhoids are varicose veins of the anal canal; *external* hemorrhoids appear outside the external sphincter whereas *internal* hemorrhoids appear above the internal sphincter. When blood within the hemorrhoids becomes clotted and infected, the hemorrhoids are referred to as *thrombosed*.

Predisposing Factors

1. Pregnancy
2. Chronic constipation
3. Hereditary factors

Clinical Manifestations

1. Itching
2. Constipation
3. Bleeding during stool
4. Pain (more noted in external hemorrhoids)

Diagnostic Evaluation

Anoscope or proctoscope visualization for internal hemorrhoids.

Treatment

1. Medical
   a. Medication and foods to keep stools soft
   b. Application of witch hazel compresses
   c. Frequent sitz baths
2. Surgical
   a. Dilatation of rectal sphincter
   b. Ligation and excision of hemorrhoid
   c. Insertion of drainage tube to permit escape of flatus and blood; or application of Gelfoam or Oxycel gauze to control bleeding.

Pilonidal Cyst

A *pilonidal cyst* is a cyst located in the intergluteal cleft on the posterior surface of the lower sacrum; hair frequently protrudes from sinus openings giving the cyst its name—pilonidal (a nest of hair).

Clinical Manifestations

1. Rarely produces symptoms until early adult life when infection produces drainage followed by the development of an abscess.
2. Trauma may be a factor in cyst development.

Treatment

1. Antibiotics are administered.
2. When abscess develops, incision and drainage is indicated.
3. Radical dissection indicated when abscesses recur or secondary sinus infection develops.
4. Healing takes place by granulation since defect may be too large to heal with suturing.

Nursing Objectives and Management in Caring for Patients with Rectal Problems

Preoperative Care

A. *To recognize the psychosocial concerns of the patient with a rectal problem.*
   1. Be an understanding and concerned listener when this patient relates problems of a personal nature.
   2. Insure and respect his privacy when attending to personal hygiene, examinations and treatments.
   3. Do not minimize complaints of discomfort.

B. *To assess nature of the rectal problems in order to assist physician in approaching an accurate diagnosis.*
   1. Observe the stool for evidence of bleeding. Is stool mixed or coated with blood?
   2. Determine presence of pain during and after evacuation. Is there associated abdominal pain? How long does it last?
   3. Describe the problem in the patient's words when recording.
   4. Note presence of a discharge. Is it purulent, bloody?

Postoperative Care

A. *To promote comfort of patient and healing of wound.*
1. Be gentle in changing dressings, shaving, irrigating or administering perineal care
2. Use petrolatum gauze in protecting edges of wounds (ex. following incision and drainage of ischiorectal abscess, excision of pilonidal sinus) to prevent crusting and the dressings from sticking to wound.
3. Provide sitz baths when recommended; adjust temperature of solution and provide a comfortable position for the patient.
4. Apply ointments (dibucaine-containing) and analgesic sprays to promote desensitization of area.
5. Keep the perineal area clean to minimize or eliminate infection; presence of *B. col* demands meticulous cleanliness to prevent infection and promote healing.
6. Change patient's position from side to side to prevent added discomfort of pressure areas; use air ring properly inflated—not too full.
7. Prevent constipation by proper attention to diet needs of patient; give mineral oil or mild cathartic only as prescribed.
8. Encourage voluntary voiding to avoid catheterization; this may be facilitated by getting patient out of bed.
9. Observe vital signs and dressings for evidence of hemorrhage, particularly following hemorrhoidectomy.

B. *To prepare patient for posthospital convalescence.*
1. Instruct patient regarding perianal hygiene to minimize the possibility of infection; avoid rubbing area with toilet tissue.
2. Apply wet dressings (equal parts of witch hazel and water) to relieve edema.
3. Advise patient regarding dietary effect on stool formation.
4. Avoid cathartics so that stool is formed rather than soft or liquid.
5. Recommend hot sitz baths or hot compresses to relieve painful sphincter spasm.

3. Conditions of the Hepatic and Biliary System

MANIFESTATIONS OF DISORDERS OF THE LIVER

Jaundice (Icterus)

The condition of the body when all tissues including the sclerae and skin assume a yellow or greenish-yellow tinge due to an increased concentration of bilirubin in the blood. (See p. 429 for types of jaundice.)
1. Normal bilirubin concentration in blood is 0.1–1.0 mg./100 ml. of blood.
2. Over 3.0 mg./100 ml. of blood, jaundice can be detected.

Abnormal Bleeding Tendencies of G.I. Tract and Nutritional Deficiencies

1. Because of blood coagulation defects, gastrointestinal hemorrhage may occur as well as bleeding gums, blood in urine, rectal bleeding, tarry stool.
2. Minor skin trauma may produce ecchymosis (black and blue marks).
3. Following all types of intramuscular and intravenous injections, it is necessary to apply pressure for longer than usual and to observe for hematoma.

4. Inability of malfunctioning liver cells to metabolize certain vitamins.
   Deficiencies:
   a. Thiamine   Vitamin A deficiency, beriberi, polyneuritis, Wernicke-Korsakoff psychosis.
   b. Riboflavin   Skin and mucous membrane lesions.
   c. Vitamin K.   Hypoprothrombinemia, spontaneous bleeding and ecchymosis.
   d. Vitamin C   Hemorrhagic lesions of scurvy.
   e. Folic acid   Macrocytic anemia.
5. Hence, the extreme importance of supplementing the diet of the patient with chronic liver disease with vitamins A, B complex, C and K.

Excessive Water Retention, Edema and Ascites

1. Tissue edema and intra-abdominal fluid are manifestations of intense sodium and water retention combined with potassium excretion.
2. Protein deficiency and disturbed kidney function are also instrumental in fluid retention.

Impairment of Central and Peripheral Nervous System

1. Pyridoxine deficiency can result in nervous irritability and in convulsive seizures in children.
2. Thiamine deficiency may lead to polyneuritis and Wernicke-Korsakoff psychosis.
3. Hypersensitivity results from infectious agents, anoxia and presence of certain drugs and toxins.

DIAGNOSTIC EVALUATION OF LIVER DISEASE

GUIDELINES: *Assisting with Liver Biopsy*

Liver biopsy is the sampling of liver tissue by needle aspiration.

Purpose

To establish a diagnosis of liver disease by histologic study of liver tissue.

Equipment

Sterile aspiration syringe and biopsy needle (Silverman)
Local anesthetic
Skin antiseptics, sterile fenestrated towel, gloves
Glass slides, specimen bottles and/or test tubes

Procedure

Preparatory Phase
1. Verify that the patient has had prothrombin tests and blood typing by checking the chart.
2. Determine availability of compatible blood inasmuch as these patients often have clotting defects.
3. Determine and record patient's pulse, respiration, arterial pressure and prothrombin time immediately before the biopsy in order to have a base line of comparison with the postbiopsy condition of the patient.
4. Explain the steps of this procedure to the patient to reduce his concerns and gain his cooperation.

Nursing Action	Rationale/Amplification

Performance Phase

1. Place patient flat in bed with arm under head and face turned left.
2. Expose the upper abdomen in readiness for skin disinfection and local anesthetic injection.
3. Determine biopsy site—usually between 6th and 7th intercostal space.
4. Instruct the patient to inhale and exhale deeply 3 or 4 times, then to exhale and hold his breath.
5. The physician introduces biopsy needle via intercostal or subcostal route into the liver, aspirates tissue and withdraws.
6. As soon as needle is withdrawn, inform patient to resume normal breathing.

2. For optimum exposure and comfort of patien the right hypochondriac region is treated as surgical area to minimize danger of infection

4. Holding one's breath immobilizes the ches wall and diaphragm; this helps to prevent the needle from penetrating the diaphragm and also minimizes the possibility of injuring the liver.

6. Actual insertion and withdrawal of needle takes about 10 seconds.

Follow-up Phase

1. Following biopsy, assist the patient to turn on his right side, place a pillow under his lower rib cage and advise him to remain quiet for several hours.
2. Determine and record the patient's pulse and respiratory rates and his blood pressure at frequent intervals until they stabilize.
3. Recognize that an inceasing pulse and falling blood pressure may be indicative of hemorrhage; note any indication of pain.

1. Compressing the liver against the chest wal near the biopsy site, reduces the possibility o bleeding.

2. The nurse needs to be aware of the possible complications of liver biopsy; hemorrhage and bile peritonitis. Anticipatory nursing include early recognition of symptoms.

LIVER DIAGNOSTIC STUDIES

Test and Purpose	Normal	Clinical and Nursing Significance
Bile Formation and Secretion		
1. *Serum bilirubin (van den Bergh)* Measures bilirubin in the blood; this determines the ability of the liver to conjugate and excrete bilirubin. Bilirubin is a product of the breakdown of hemoglobin.		
Direct (conjugated)—water soluble	0.05–1.4 mg./100 ml.	Abnormal in biliary and liver disease causing jaundice clinically.
Indirect (free or unconjugated)—insoluble in water	0.4–0.8 mg./100 ml.	
Total serum bilirubin	0.0–0.9 mg./100 ml.	
2. *Urine bilirubin* Not normally found in urine, but if serum bilirubin is elevated, some may spill into urine.	None	Mahogany-colored urine; when specimen is shaken, yellow tint to foam can be observed. If pyridium is being taken, there will be a false positive bilirubin reaction (Mark lab. slip if this medication is being taken.)

LIVER DIAGNOSTIC STUDIES *(continued)*

Test and Purpose	Normal	Clinical and Nursing Significance
3. *Urobilinogen* Formed in small intestine by action of bacteria on bilirubin.	Urine urobilinogen 0–1.16 mg./24 hr. Fecal urobilinogen 40–280 mg./24 hr.	Urine specimen is collected over 2-hr. period; place in dark brown container and send to lab. immediately to prevent disintegration. If patient is receiving antibiotics, mark lab. slip to this effect since production of urobilinogen can be falsely reduced.

Protein Studies

Test and Purpose	Normal	Clinical and Nursing Significance
1. *Albumin and globulin measurement* Is of greater significance than total protein measurement. Albumin—produced in liver Globulin—produced in lymphatics, spleen, and bone marrow Total serum protein	3.5–5.5 gm./100 ml. 1.5–3.0 gm./100 ml. 7.0–8.0 mg./100 ml.	As one increases, the other decreases, hence Albumin ↓ cirrhosis chronic hepatitis edema, ascites Globulin ↑ cirrhosis liver disease chronic obstructive jaundice viral hepatitis
2. *Prothrombin test* Prothrombin is manufactured in the liver; its rate is influenced by the supply of vitamin K.	100% return to normal	Prothrombin time may be prolonged in liver disease; in severe liver cell damage, prothrombin time will not return to normal with vitamin K.
3. *Serum flocculation* Measures liver parenchymal cell function. Cephalin flocculation—to determine if increase in gamma globulin when decrease in albumin Thymol turbidity—reaction of gamma globulin and lipids	0–14 units 0–5 units	Positive reaction indicates parenchymal cell damage—cirrhosis, hepatitis. Elevated in cirrhosis, hepatitis. NOTE: May be elevated in arthritis, rheumatic fever.

Carbohydrate Metabolism

Test and Purpose	Normal	Clinical and Nursing Significance
1. *Galactose tolerance* To determine glycogenic function of liver (Normally liver converts galactose to glycogen, and large amounts will be absorbed, not excreted.) Blood determination: Administer intravenous galactose 1 ml./50% sol./kg. body weight. Draw blood at half-hour intervals every 2 hours.	Galactose removed from blood in 1 hr. and 15 min.	Abnormalities: If after 75 min., large amounts of galactose are found in the blood, indication is liver disease, cirrhosis, acute hepatitis.

LIVER DIAGNOSTIC STUDIES (continued)

Test and Purpose	Normal	Clinical and Nursing Significance

2. *Glucose tolerance*
Procedure
Collect fasting blood and urine specimens as base samples.
Administer oral glucose (Glucola—a carbonated cola preparation)
Draw blood samples: at 30-, 60-, 120-, 180-min. intervals.
Collect urine samples: at 30-, 60-, 120-, 180-min. intervals.
This test may be done using intravenous glucose.
  For those unable to tolerate oral glucose:
  If gastrointestinal absorption is impaired.
	Glucose level should return to normal in 1–2 hours.	Administer glucose and see to it that specimens are collected on time.
		Prolonged high glucose levels—indicate impaired glucose utilization by body tissues.
		
		Similar to intravenous galactose tolerance test.

Fat Metabolism 1. *Cholesterol and phospholipids* It is possible to measure lipid metabolism by determining cholesterol and phospholipid levels.	Ester: 150–250 mg./100 ml. 60% of total	Serum lipid level lower in parenchymal liver disease. Serum lipid level increased in biliary obstruction.
Liver Detoxification 1. *Bromsulphalein excretion (BSP test)* Liver serves to excrete dyes from body via bile. The dye is nontoxic, given intravenously and removed from the blood by the liver cells, stored, conjugated and excreted. Draw blood from opposite arm 30 min. and 1 hour after injection.	 After 1 hour, less than 5% of dye should be retained.	Administer dye according to body weight: 2 mg./kg. body weight. Observe patient closely for: urticaria, nausea, vomiting, dizziness, allergic reaction. Have available epinephrine in case of anaphylactic reaction. Recognize that local reaction at injection site may occur; instruct patient not to bend arm after injection, and apply gentle pressure to prevent extension of irritation. If local reaction: Apply hot pack for comfort and to hasten absorption. NOTE: Since Telepaque interferes with liver uptake of this substance, notify laboratory if patient has taken Telepaque recently. *Abnormalities:* Increased retention occurs in cirrhosis, infectious hepatitis, advanced carcinoma.

LIVER DIAGNOSTIC STUDIES (*continued*)

Test and Purpose	Normal	Clinical and Nursing Significance
2. *Serum alkaline phosphatase* Since bile disposes this enzyme, any obstruction in bile passages will cause an elevation.	Varies with method: 2–5 Bodansky units.	*Abnormalities:* Elevated in obstructive jaundice, liver metastasis. Also elevated in osteoblastic diseases, Paget's disease, and hyperparathyroidism.
Enzyme Production 1. SGOT—serum glutamic oxaloacetic transaminase 2. SGPT—serum glutamic pyruvic transaminase 3. LDH—lactic dehydrogenase All 3 are useful in measuring extent of liver damage.	10– 40 units 5–35 units 165–400 units	Since an elevation in these indicates organ damage, encourage patient to limit his activity. Rest will provide more oxygen for cells and alleviate further cell damage. NOTE: Opiates may also cause a rise in SGOT and SGPT.

JAUNDICE

Hemolytic Jaundice

Hemolytic jaundice is attributable to abnormally high concentration of bilirubin in blood exceeding the capacity of normal liver cells to excrete it.

1. Encountered in patients with hemolytic transfusion reactions, hereditary spherocystosis, autoimmune hemolytic anemia, erythroblastosis fetalis, and other hemolytic disorders.
2. Bilirubin in the blood is "free" and unconjugated.
3. In feces and urine, urobilinogen is increased; urine is free of bilirubin.
4. Prolonged jaundice leads to formation of "pigment stones" in gallbladder. Extremely severe jaundice (free bilirubin elevated: 20–25 mg./100 ml.) causes brain-stem damage.

Hepatocellular Jaundice

Hepatocellular jaundice is due to an inability of diseased liver cells to clear the normal amount of bilirubin from the blood.

A. *Predisposing Conditions*
1. Infection—infectious hepatitis, homologous serum hepatitis, yellow fever virus.
2. Drug or chemical toxicity—carbon tetrachloride, chloroform, phosphorus, arsenicals, ethanol.

B. *Types of Hepatocellular Jaundice*
1. Cirrhosis of the liver; usually attributed to excessive alcohol ingestion (see p. 434).
2. Viral-caused liver cell necrosis.

C. *Clinical Manifestations*
1. Mildly or severely ill patient.
2. Lack of appetite, nausea, loss of vigor and strength, weight loss.
3. Elevated SGOT (serum glutamic oxaloacetic transaminase) and SGPT (serum glutamic pyruvic transaminase)—2 enzymes that are liberated with cellular necrosis and rise in bloodstream.
4. Rise in BSP (bromsulphalein), bilirubin alkaline phosphatase, urobilinogen in urine
5. Abnormal serum proteins in prolonged illness; prothrombin time increased.
6. Headache and chills possible in infectious condition.

Obstructive Jaundice

Causative Factors
1. Extrahepatic obstruction—caused by blockage of bile duct by gallstone, tumor, inflammatory process or an enlarged gland pressing on the duct.
2. Intrahepatic obstruction—caused by pressure on the channels due to inflammation and swelling of liver substance or inflammatory exudate from ducts themselves.
   a. Certain drugs may cause this. e.g., "cholestatic" agents: phenothiazine derivatives (Thorazine), perphenazine (Trilafon), sulfonamides, tolbutamide (Orinase) and other antidiabetic drugs, thiouracil, a p-aminobenzoic acid (PABA).
   b. Symptoms—due to damming back of bile, it is reabsorbed by blood
      Skin jaundice, scleral yellow
      Deep orange-colored urine
      White or clay-colored stools
      Itchy skin and dyspepsia
   c. Laboratory signs
      SGOT and SGPT do not rise
      Bilirubin and alkaline phosphatase do rise.

Objectives of Nursing Management

A. *To control pruritus and make the patient more comfortable.*
1. Use starch or baking soda baths, soothing lotions, such as calamine.
2. Administer antihistamines, cholestyramine (Cuemid; Questran), tranquilizers and sedatives if ordered; use these with caution to avoid further damage.
3. Assist patient in reducing the strong tendency to scratch his skin:
   a. Resort to activities which can divert his attention.
   b. Keep nails trimmed and clean.
   c. Avoid excessive top bedding.
   d. Give soothing massages particularly at night in preparing patient for sleep since this is an especially likely time to scratch.
   e. Provide clean white gloves to use at night if he scratches subconsciously.

B. *To support the patient psychologically.*
1. Instruct staff to avoid remarks or facial expressions which the patient can interpret as referring to his unusual appearance.
2. Notify visitors in a like manner to avoid embarrassing the patient.
3. Encourage patient to talk about his problems and listen to his expressions of concern.
4. Use discretion by not placing patient's bed in a position where he can look at himself in the dresser mirror.

HEPATITIS

Hepatitis is an inflammation of the liver.

Significance
1. From a public health point of view one is concerned with ease of disease transmission and morbidity.
2. From a socioeconomic point of view one is concerned with prolonged loss of time from school and employment.

Preventive Measures
1. Stress importance of proper public and home sanitation.
2. Recognize merits of conscientious surveillance in the proper and safe preparation and dispensation of food.
3. Promote effective health supervision in schools, dormitories and camps.
4. Initiate and support health education programs.

Types of Hepatitis
1. Type A hepatitis (infectious hepatitis, IH virus)
   Also called epidemic hepatitis, catarrhal jaundice
2. Type B hepatitis (serum hepatitis, SH virus)
   Also called homologous serum jaundice.

Diagnostic Evaluation
1. By radioimmunoassay test, the presence of Australian antigen, (HB Ag) is detected in individuals who have infectious or serum hepatitis.
2. By the (HB Ag) test, detection of hepatitis is possible before the patient becomes clinically ill.
3. SGPT levels.

Type A Hepatitis

Epidemiology
1. Causative agent—filtrable virus
2. Mode of transmission
   a. Fecal-oral route; respiratory possible
   b. Blood transfusion, blood serum or blood plasma from a carrier or infected person
   c. Contaminated equipment: syringe and needles
   d. Contaminated food, milk, or shellfish, polluted water
3. Incubation—2–7 weeks; average 4 weeks
4. Occurrence
   a. Worldwide—sporadic or epidemic
   b. Fall and winter months
   c. Usually in children and young adults

Clinical Manifestations
1. Pre-icteric
   a. Headache, fever, anorexia, nausea, vomiting, abdominal tenderness, pain palpable over liver
   b. Respiratory manifestations

2. Icteric phase
    a. Urine—dark.
    b. Liver—enlarged, jaundice noted.
    c. Nausea, vague epigastric distress, heartburn, flatulence.

Treatment and Nursing Management

1. Isolate patient to minimize contacts.
2. Assist with laboratory diagnostic studies such as transaminase and serum bilirubin.
3. Provide tissues and paper bags for nasal and throat secretions; incinerate.
4. Handle bedpan carefully; clean thoroughly and restrict its use to the same patient Continue this pattern for at least 3 weeks.
5. Ascertain nature of sewage disposal; if questionable, after diagnosis is verified, utilize chemical disinfection before disposal.
6. Instruct and supervise patient to ensure meticulous personal hygiene habits.
7. Use disposable syringes and needles when such are required; label clearly all labora tory specimens as coming from a patient with hepatitis.
8. Provide diet that is nutritious and appealing to the patient; small, frequent feeding may be in order:
    a. Offer a large breakfast inasmuch as anorexia worsens later in the day.
    b. Restrict use of alcohol.
    c. Advise patient to avoid eating raw or insufficiently cooked shellfish.
9. Admonish patient not to give blood as a donor in the future.
10. Give gamma globulin to close contacts of the patient, particularly members of hi family.
11. Impress on the patient the importance of careful follow-up visits including laboratory and physical examinations until laboratory results have returned to normal levels.
12. Correct any unsanitary condition in patient's area of contact.

Type B Hepatitis

Epidemiology

1. Causative agent
    a. Filtrable virus
    b. Australia antigen (1963—Blumberg)
2. Mode of transmission
    a. Parenteral route
        Blood transfusion from an infected person
        Contaminated needles, syringes
    b. Skin puncture—medical or dental instruments
3. Incubation—2–5 months (average 2½–3 months)
4. Occurrence
    a. Worldwide
    b. Recipients of blood and blood products

Diagnostic Evaluation

1. Counterelectrophoresis (CEP)
2. "Sandwich" counterelectrophoresis (SCEP)

Clinical Manifestations

1. Usually more insidious than infectious hepatitis with similar symptoms
2. Enlarged liver, splenomegaly
3. Brown urine (possible)

Treatment and Nursing Management

1. Encourage bedrest until the symptoms have subsided; restrict activities until the liver is no longer enlarged and the serum bilirubin is normal.
2. Obtain serum bilirubin and transaminase twice weekly to determine disease status.
3. Supplement the diet with vitamins, particularly vitamin B Complex, protein and carbohydrates.
4. Administer alkalies to counteract gastric acidity.
5. Give soporofics for rest and relaxation.
6. Recognize that recovery is slow and prolonged; increase activities as tolerated.

HEPATIC COMA

Causes

1. Incomplete metabolizing of protein fragments by the diseased liver—manifestation of profound liver failure.
2. Biochemical abnormalities responsible are not known; however, the accumulation of significant amounts of nitrogenous substances, particularly ammonia, in the blood are believed to be highly suspect.

Precipitating Factors

1. Progressive hepatocellular disease not associated with any acute irritation of the liver.
2. Increased sources of ammonia in the blood; azotemia, high protein diet, gastrointestinal bleeding, following administration of ammonium chloride, thiazides.
3. Infections, paracentesis, acute alcoholism, hypotension, shock, general anesthesia, minor surgery, hypokalemia, alkalosis, administration of sedatives, or narcotics.
4. Portacaval shunts, especially if protein is not restricted postoperatively in the diet.

Clinical Manifestations

1. Minor mental aberrations—patient slightly confused, has faraway look in his eyes and drowsing tendency in daytime, becomes untidy and confused and displays inappropriate behavior.
2. Motor disturbance—coarse or "flapping" tremor especially of hands, hyper-reflexia.
3. Progression to gross disturbances of consciousness.
4. Complete disorientation to time and place; eventual coma.

Altered Physiology

A. *Problems*

1. Disruption of enzymatic function.
2. Failure of liver cells to detoxify the ammonia (by converting to urea).
3. Aggravation comes from accumulation of ammonia in blood.

B. *Sources of Ammonia.* It comes from bloodstream as a result of
   1. Its absorption from *gastrointestinal tract* (largest source)
      Enzymatic and bacterial digestion of protein; increases blood ammonia
      a. Increases, as a result of
         (1) Gastrointestinal bleeding
         (2) High protein diet
         (3) Ingestion of ammonium salts (diuretic: ammonium chloride)
         (4) Bacterial growth in small bowel (infection)
         (5) Uremia
      b. Decreases
         (1) Elimination of protein from diet.
         (2) Intestinal antibiotics—neomycin, kanamycin, chlortetracycline.
   2. Its production by metabolizing *kidney* tissue (deamination of various amino acids)
      a. Increases with
         (1) Diuretics (steroids, chlorothiazide)
         (2) Restriction of dietary sodium (hyponatremia)
         (3) Potassium depletion (hypokalemia)
   3. Its liberation from contacting *muscle* cells
      a. Increases during exercise.

Treatment

   1. Begin early to control coma and eliminate precipitating causes.
   2. Arrest gastrointestinal bleeding.
      a. If upper gastrointestinal bleeding, constant gastric aspiration may be required.
      b. If bleeding has ceased, administer a cathartic or enema.
   3. Cancel orders for an ammonium product.
   4. Greatly reduce dietary protein—if patient begins to improve, gradually increase protein intake.
   5. Administer antibiotics to reduce intestinal flora of organisms: neomycin, tetracycline or other broad spectrum antibiotics.
   6. Correct electrolyte abnormalities, especially hypokalemia.

Nursing Management

   1. Observe patient's neurologic status such as his ability to perform simple arithmetic calculations and his handwriting (keep a daily record and note differences).
   2. Weigh him daily and keep an intake and output record.
   3. Be alert for any signs of infection including infections of upper respiratory tract.
   4. If hepatic coma is anticipated, reduce the patient's protein intake and administer antibiotics as prescribed for control of enteric infection.
   5. Administer sedatives and analgesics sparingly.
   6. See page 728 for nursing the unconscious patient.

HEPATIC CIRRHOSIS

Cirrhosis means scarring.

Classification of Hepatic Cirrhosis

   1. Laennec's portal cirrhosis
      a. Scar tissue surrounds portal area.
      b. Most commonly due to chronic alcoholism.

2. Postnecrotic
    a. Broad bands of scar tissue.
    b. Due to previous acute viral hepatitis.
3. Biliary
    a. Scarring around bile ducts and lobes of liver.
    b. Results from chronic biliary infection and obstruction.
    c. Much more rare than Laennec's and postnecrotic.

Etiology and Clinical Manifestations

1. Cirrhosis of the liver is characterized by repeated occurrences of death of the liver cells, replacement with scar tissue and regeneration of liver cells.
2. Malnutrition is the chief cause, very often coupled with a history of alcoholism. Protein deficiency rather than alcohol toxicity is thought to be the chief antagonist.
3. Onset is insidious—it may be developing and progressing over many years.
4. Twice as many men as women are affected; age group predominately is from 40–60 years.

Altered Physiology

1. Early in disease—gastrointestinal disturbances, fever and liver enlargement due to cells being loaded with fat; as tissue is replaced, scars contract and become smaller, the surface becomes rough and hobnail.
2. Later—chronic failure of liver function and obstruction of portal circulation.
    a. Congestion of spleen, pancreas, gastrointestinal tract.
        (1) Chronic dyspepsia, change in bowel habits—diarrhea, constipation
        (2) Gradual weight loss, spider telangiectasis (dilated superficial arterioles)
        (3) Ascites, diuresis
        (4) Obstruction of portal circulation, causing portal hypertension, esophageal varices, internal hemorrhoids
    b. Chronic failure of liver function
        (1) Plasma albumin is reduced which leads to edema
        (2) Deficiencies of vitamins A, C, and K because of inadequate formation, utilization and storage of these vitamins, causing avitaminosis
        (3) Chronic gastritis and poor gastrointestinal function leading to anemia
        (4) Increasing weakness, leading to depression, wasting, delirium, coma, and, eventually death.

Treatment

1. Prevent further damage to the liver.
2. Offer supportive care of the patient; bedrest is recommended when fever, infection, deteriorating liver function occur.
3. Maintain adequate nutritional levels—moderately high protein, high caloric diet:
    a. Provide protein within ability of liver to handle it.
    b. Restrict alcohol.
4. Restrict salt intake when fluid retention occurs.
5. Protect patient from infections and toxic agents.
6. Administer bile salts if jaundiced, to assist in absorption of vitamin A and synthesis of vitamin K.

7. Provide vitamins A, B complex, D, and K to compensate for liver's inability to store them.
8. Give folic acid to correct folic acid deficiency anemia.
9. Control or reduce pruritus in patients with liver disease and retention of bile salts—administer cholestyramine (Cuemid).

Nursing Management

1. Instruct and prepare patient for the very many laboratory and x-ray studies needed.
   a. Diagnostic evaluation and nursing implications (see p. 425).
   b. Liver studies and nursing significance (see p. 426).
2. Evaluate nutritional status and needs.
   a. Offer small frequent meals rather than 3 large meals.
   b. Consider patient preferences in food.
   c. If patient is severely anorexic or nauseated and eating poorly, tube feeding may be necessary; include milk and starch hydrolysate (Dextri-maltose).
   d. Supplement diet with protein—powdered Sustagen and Protanal (low sodium).
   e. Give pancreatin (if diarrhea and steatorrhea) to permit better tolerance of diet.
3. Adjust nutritional offerings if the patient has ascites or edema.
   a. Restrict sodium intake to 200–500 mg. daily.
   b. Maintain normal protein, caloric and vitamin intake.
   c. Avoid table salt, salty foods, salted margarine and butter as well as all ordinary frozen and canned foods.
   d. Use "salt" substitutes to enhance flavor such as lemon juice, oregano, thyme; commercial salt substitute should be cleared by physician.
   e. Encourage use of powdered low-sodium milk and milk products.
   f. If water accumulation is not controlled on above regimen, resort to the following:
      (1) Limit sodium allowance to 200 mg. daily.
      (2) Restrict fluids if serum sodium is low.
      (3) Administer oral diuretics (Hydrodiuril); perhaps injections of a mercurial diuretic (Mercuhydrin) may be necessary.
   g. Abdominal paracentesis is avoided as long as possible (if necessary, see Procedure, p. 437).
4. Assist the patient in overcoming anorexia, weight loss and fatigue.
   a. Encourage him to eat all meals and supplementary feedings by serving them with eye-catching appeal, in small servings, and in small frequent meals.
   b. Recognize the effect of esthetic factors—control odors, disturbing conversations, unpleasant situations.
   c. Eliminate alcohol but encourage high protein and high caloric intake.
   d. Give supplementary vitamins (A, B complex, C and K).
   e. Conserve patient's energy so that total food intake is not expended to replace energy requirements.
5. Observe skin and control pruritus.
   a. Provide good skin care; bathe without soap; apply soothing lotions.
   b. Keep patient's fingernails short to prevent him from scratching his skin.
   c. Administer cholestyramine (Cuemid) as prescribed for pruritus with fruit juices or applesauce; be alert for side effects of nausea, diarrhea or constipation.

6. Be cognizant of signs of hematemesis and melena.
   a. Assess for anxiety, weakness, restlessness, epigastric fullness as possibly heralding hemorrhage.
   b. Take and record vital signs frequently.
   c. Administer vitamin C as prescribed.
   d. Observe each stool for color, consistency and amount.
   e. Record nature, amount and time of vomiting.
   f. Offer refreshing mouthwash after meticulous mouth care.
   g. Note patient's reaction frequently as he receives a blood transfusion.
7. Anticipate manifestations of hemorrhage such as ecchymosis, petechiae, epistaxis and nose bleeds; initiate preventive measures.
   a. Maintain a safe environment to prevent injury.
   b. Avoid trauma such as forceful nose blowing, use of hard toothbrush, large gauge needles for injection.
   c. Apply pressure to small bleeding sites; record their nature and location.
   d. Encourage intake of foods high in vitamin C.
8. Recognize signs of increasing stupor, notify physician and initiate nursing measures as follows:
   a. Be alert for evidences of mental changes, lethargy, hallucinations.
   b. Avoid giving patient narcotics and barbiturates.
   c. Restrict dietary protein; offer small high caloric feedings frequently.
   d. Protect patient by keeping him in bed; pad side-rails.
   e. Arouse patient at intervals.
   f. Limit visitors.
   g. Provide constant nursing surveillance and emphasize sensitivity to patient's changes and needs.
9. Instruct patient regarding precautions and regimen to follow upon his discharge from the hospital.
   a. Stress the necessity of giving up alcohol completely; this may require the skillful assistance of a trusted friend, religious adviser, psychiatrist, or Alcoholic Anonymous.
   b. Provide written dietary instructions, emphasizing the restriction of sodium.
   c. Emphasize the significance of rest, a sensible way of life and an adequate well-balanced diet.
   d. Involve the person closest to him (usually spouse) because recovery often is not easy and slipbacks are common; a close trusted helper can help patient over the rough spots.

GUIDELINES: *Assisting With Abdominal Paracentesis*

Paracentesis (abdominal) is the withdrawal of fluid from the abdominal cavity.

Purposes

1. To remove accumulated fluid from the abdominal cavity to relieve pressure on
   a. Diaphragm, which impairs breathing
   b. Bladder, which causes frequency.
2. As an alternate procedure to using diuretics (for releasing accumulated fluid) when such therapy might precipitate hepatic coma.
3. For diagnostic purposes.

Danger and Complications

1. In chronic liver disease, paracentesis may precipitate hepatic coma.
2. Shock and hypovolemia can occur if fluid from general circulation shifts to abdomen to replace withdrawn fluid; this can be minimized if paracentesis fluid is not completely withdrawn or if lost fluid is replaced in kind by parenteral administration of human albumin (salt poor).

Equipment

Sterile paracentesis tray and gloves
Procaine hydrochloride 1%
Drape or cotton blankets
Scultetus binder

Pail
Skin preparation tray with antiseptic
Specimen bottles and laboratory forms.

Procedure

Nursing Action	*Rationale/Amplification*
Preparatory Phase	
1. Have patient void before treatment is begun.	1. This will lessen the danger of accidentally piercing the bladder with the trocar.
2. Position patient in Fowler's position with back, arms and feet supported (sitting on the side of the bed is frequently used position).	2. Patient is more comfortable and a steady position can be maintained.
3. Drape patient with sheet exposing abdomen.	3. Minimizes exposure of patient and keeps him warm.
Performance Phase	
1. Assist physician in preparing skin with antiseptic solution.	1. This is considered a minor surgical procedure requiring aseptic precautions.
2. Open sterile tray and package of sterile gloves; provide anesthetic solution.	
3. Position bucket and be prepared to place end of rubber tubing into bucket.	
4. Assess pulse and respiratory status frequently during procedure; watch for pallor, cyanosis or syncope (dizziness).	4. Preliminary indications of shock must be watched for. Keep emergency stimulants available.
5. Physician administers local anesthesia and introduces trocar with obturator through small incision into peritoneum.	
6. After obturator is withdrawn, rubber tubing is attached to trocar sheath.	6. Fluid flows out by gravity.
7. Apply dressing when trocar is withdrawn.	7. Elasticized adhesive patch is effective, serving as water-proof-adhering dressing.
Follow-up Phase	
1. Assist patient to be comfortable after treatment.	
2. Record amount and kind of fluid removed, number of specimens sent to laboratory, patient's condition through the treatment.	
3. Check blood pressure and vital signs every half hour for 2 hours, every hour for 4 hours, and every 4 hours for 24 hours.	3. Close observation will detect poor circulatory adjustment and possible development of shock.
4. Usually a dressing is sufficient; however, if the trocar wound appears large, the physician may close the incision with sutures.	

BLEEDING ESOPHAGEAL VARICES

Esophageal varices are dilated tortuous veins found in the submucosa of the lower esophagus; they may extend up in the esophagus and down into the stomach.

Causes

1. Nearly always due to portal hypertension which may result from obstruction of the portal venous circulation and cirrhosis of the liver.
2. Abnormalities of the circulation in splenic vein or superior vena cava.

Altered Physiology and Symptoms

1. Increasing portal vein obstruction—venous blood returning to right atrium from intestinal tract and spleen seeks new pathways, thus imposing strain on esophageal veins.
2. Usually no symptoms are produced by dilated veins unless mucosa becomes ulcerated.
3. Hematemesis and melena plus a history of alcoholism tend to point toward esophageal varices; bleeding may also result from gastritis or duodenal ulcer.
4. The strain of coughing or vomiting may cause esophageal rupture, hemorrhage and death.
5. Irritation of vessels by poorly chewed foods may cause esophagitis, esophageal rupture, hemorrhage and death.

Diagnostic Evaluation

1. Liver function tests include bromsulphalein retention, serum transaminase, bilirubin, serum proteins, alkaline phosphatase.
2. Esophagoscopy may confirm the diagnosis since the varices can be seen; however, many physicians are reluctant to insert an endoscope because of the danger of initiating hemorrhage or rupturing the esophagus.
3. Portal vein pressure above 250 mm. of water is abnormal; this can be measured in the operating room by introducing a needle into spleen.
4. Splenoportography using diodrast can be effective when studied as a series of x-ray plates or done as a segmental roentgenogram; extensive collateral circulation of esophageal vessels may be indicative of varices.

Treatment and Nursing Management

1. Initiate measures to overcome blood loss.
   a. Replace blood with fresh whole blood.
      (1) Ammonia content is lower than in stored blood.
      (2) Coagulation effect is greater particularly if the patient has severe liver disease.
   b. Administer vitamin K intramuscularly or intravenously.
2. Recognize the importance of controlling hemorrhage.
   a. Purpose
      (1) To lessen transfusion requirements.
      (2) To reduce large amounts of blood in gastrointestinal tract.
      (3) To avoid hepatic coma.
   b. Methods
      (1) Administer Vasopressin—to reduce portal pressure and to initiate hemostasis.
      (2) Ice-water lavage of stomach (gastric hypothermia) may temporarily control bleeding.

(3) Esophageal tamponade—pressure is exerted on the cardiac portion of the stomach and against the bleeding varices by a double balloon tamponade (Sengstaken-Blakemore tube) (See below).
(4) Treat bleeding by resorting to sedation and complete rest of the esophagus (parenteral feedings); avoid straining and vomiting and continue gastric suction.
(5) Initiate vitamin-K therapy; multiple blood transfusions.

GUIDELINES: *Using the Sengstaken-Blakemore Tube to Control Esophageal Bleeding*

Purposes

1. To exert pressure on the cardiac portion of the stomach and against bleeding varices by a double balloon tamponade.
2. To reduce transfusion requirements.
3. To prevent blood accumulation in the gastrointestinal tract which could precipitate hepatic coma.

Equipment

Sengstaken-Blakemore tube	Towel and emesis basin
Basin with cracked ice	Glass of water and straw
Clamp for tubing	Flashlight

Procedure

Preparatory Phase

1. Provide nursing support by reassuring patient that this procedure will help to control his bleeding.
2. Explain procedure to patient and tell him how breathing through the mouth and swallowing can help in passing the tube.
3. Elevate head of bed slightly unless patient is in shock.

Nursing Action	Rationale/Amplification
Performance Phase	
1. Check balloon by trial inflation to detect leaks.	1. This is best done under water because it is easier to see escaping air bubbles.
2. Chill the tube, then lubricate it before physician passes it via mouth or nose (preferable).	2. Chilling will make the tube more firm and lubrication will lessen friction.
3. After the tube has entered the stomach, the stomach balloon is inflated and pulled back gently to exert force against cardia, then the esophageal bag is inflated. These are tied with double ties to prevent leakage. (See Fig. 6-12)	3. The triple-lumen tube provides 2 channels to inflate each compression bag, one in stomach and one in esophagus. Balloons are inflated using a manometer to measure pressure to 25 or 30 mm.Hg; position of balloons is verified by fluoroscope.
4. Traction is placed on the tubing where it enters the nose of the patient.	4. This keeps balloons in position and assists in exerting proper pressure.
5. Gastric suction may be attached to the 3rd outlet of the catheter.	5. By using suction and irrigating the tubing hourly, it is possible to tell how well the bleeding is controlled by the appearance of the drainage.
6. Some physicians circulate ice water through the stomach balloon to assist in controlling hemorrhage.	6. Constriction of blood vessels by pressure and lower temperature can control bleeding.

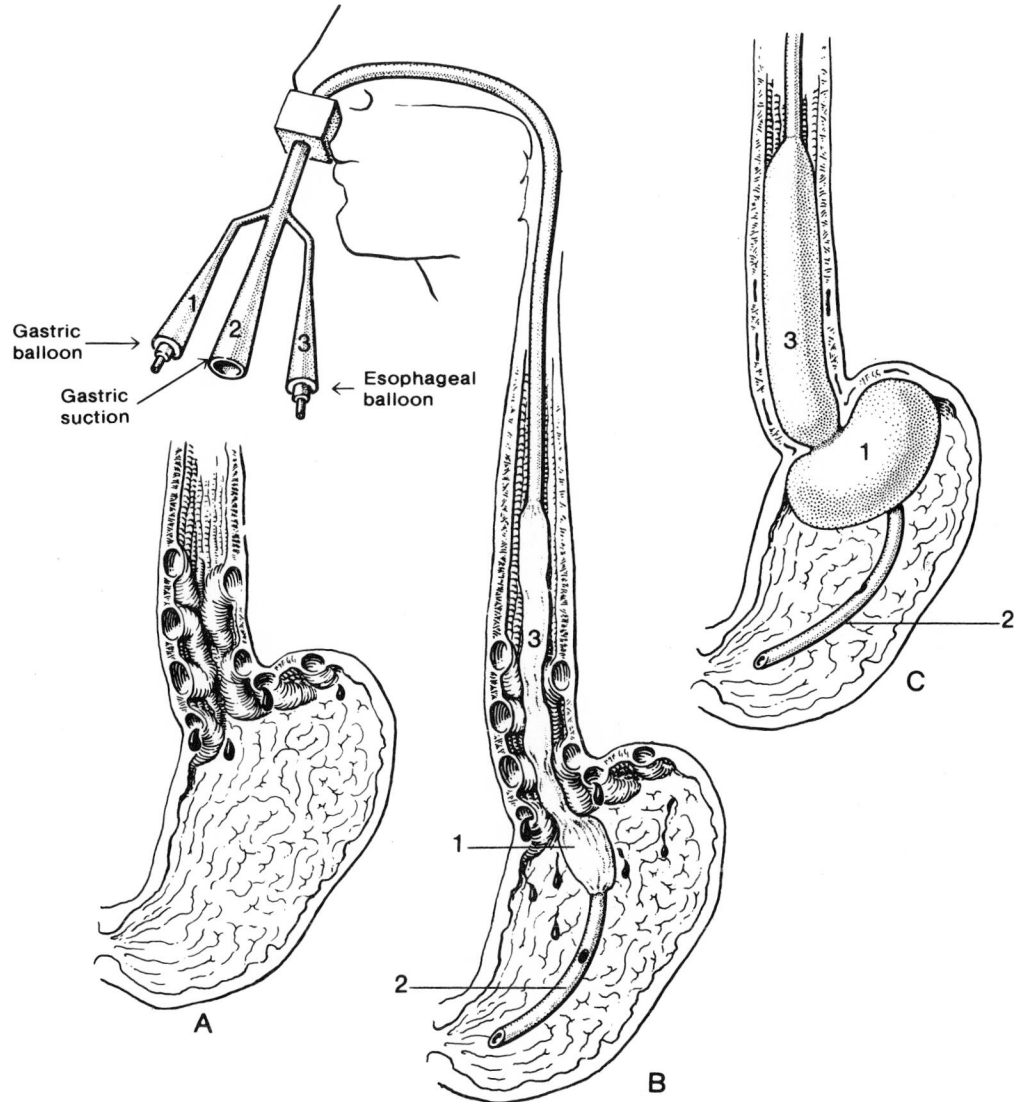

Figure 6-12. Diagram showing esophageal varices and their treatment by a compressing balloon tube (Sengstaken-Blakemore). *A.* Dilated veins of the lower esophagus. *B.* The tube is in place in the stomach and the lower esophagus but is not inflated. *C.* Inflation of the tube and the compression of the veins which can be obtained by inflation of the balloon. (From Brunner, et al.: *Textbook of Medical and Surgical Nursing,* 1st ed. Philadelphia, J. B. Lippincott.)

Nursing Action	Rationale/Amplification
7. Deflate tube at 8- or 12-hour intervals for 5 minutes.	7. To prevent erosion and necrosis of esophagus or stomach.
8. Pressure on tubes and traction are released in 2–4 days.	8. If bleeding is controlled, the tubing is removed in 24 hours.

Nursing Responsibilities

1. Maintain constant vigilance while balloons are inflated in the patient.
2. Keep balloon pressures at required level to control bleeding. (Hemostats are utilized as clamps.)
3. Observe and record vital signs frequently—bleeding, shock, etc.
4. Be alert for chest pain—may indicate injury or rupture of esophagus.
5. Irrigate suction tube as ordered; observe and record nature and color of aspirated material.
6. Keep head of bed elevated to avoid gastric regurgitation and to diminish nausea and a sense of gagging.
7. Maintain nutritional and electrolyte levels parenterally or by feedings through the tube.
8. Provide tissue-wipes for the patient to expectorate saliva inasmuch as he cannot swallow when the esophageal balloon is inflated.
9. Note nature of breathing: if counterweight pulls the tube into oropharynx, the patient may be asphyxiated.

NURSING ALERT: Keep a pair of scissors taped to the head of the bed. In the event of *acute respiratory distress*, use the scissors to cut across tubing (to deflate both balloons) and remove tubing.

DISEASES OF THE BILIARY (GALLBLADDER) SYSTEM

Incidence

1. About 500,000 persons a year in the U.S. are hospitalized for gallbladder disease; ⅔ of these are treated surgically.
2. Women acquire the disease more frequently than men; 4 to 1.
3. Patients are usually past 40, multiparous and overweight.

   NOTE: Preventive emphasis is on losing weight and avoiding fatty foods.

Types of Gallbladder Disease

(Chole—gallbladder)
Cholecystitis—inflammation of the gallbladder
Cholelithiasis—stones in the gallbladder
Choledocholithiasis—stones in the common duct.

Diagnostic Evaluation

A. *Cholecystography*—is used to visualize the shape and position of the gallbladder

NOTE: This test is only effective if the liver cells are functioning properly and are capable of excreting the radiopaque dye into the bile.

1. *Purpose*
   a. To detect gallstones.
   b. To estimate ability of gallbladder to fill, concentrate its contents, contract and empty in a normal manner.

2. *Method*
   a. Because gallstones are rarely radiopaque, it is necessary to fill the gallbladder with a radiopaque dye which permits stones to show up as shadows.
   b. Iodide-containing dye is excreted into bile by the liver and concentrated in the gallbladder.
      (1) By mouth
         (a) Contrast media may be given by mouth: (Ex.: Telepaque, Priodax, Oragrafin, Teridax, Monophen).
         (b) Iodide preparation is usually given in oral doses of 2–3 gm. approximately 10–12 hours before x-ray.
      (2) Intravenously
         (a) Intravenous cholecystography involves giving an iodide (e.g., Cholografin) about 10 minutes before x-ray.
         (b) Nothing by mouth from the time of iodide administration to time of x-ray to prevent contraction of gallbladder and expulsion of contrast medium.

3. *Patient Preparation*
   a. At least 1 hour after the evening meal, the patient takes the prescribed tablets or capsules of iodide preparation by mouth.
   b. These tablets are taken one at a time at 3- to 5-minute intervals with at least 8 oz. of water.
   c. From this time to bedtime, nothing is taken by mouth except water; from midnight on, water is also excluded. (If nausea or vomiting occurs, notify physician; test may be postponed.)
   d. No laxatives are given during this time; however, a saline enema is given on the morning of the x-ray.
   e. Breakfast is withheld and patient goes to x-ray.
   f. Right upper abdominal quadrant is x-rayed.
   g. The patient is fed a fatty meal containing cream, butter or eggs to test contractility of the gallbladder.
   h. X-ray examination is repeated at intervals until gallbladder has expelled dye and becomes invisible (Graham-Cole).

B. *Cholangiography*—(dye is injected directly into biliary tree)
   1. Advantages
      a. Visualization is accomplished regardless of the state of liver function.
      b. All components of the biliary tree can be observed: hepatic ducts within liver, common hepatic duct, cystic duct, gallbladder.
   2. Clinical Usefulness
      a. In differentiating hepatocellular jaundice from jaundice due to biliary obstruction.
      b. In locating stones within bile ducts.
      c. In detecting and diagnosing cancer of the biliary system.
      d. In investigating gastrointestinal symptoms of patients who had cholecystectomy.
   3. Patient Preparation
      a. The patient is dehydrated by restricting his fluid intake.
      b. Enema is given early in morning of test.
      c. A sedative is given at least 1 hour before the x-ray.

d. Dye (Ex. Urokon Sodium) is injected either intravenously (results not as conclusive), or directly into the common duct.
   (1) Operatively; this can be done during surgery.
   (2) Postoperatively; by injecting dye into the common duct drain.
e. Following the x-ray, regardless of method of dye injection, as much as possible of the dye and bile are aspirated to prevent leakage into the peritoneal cavity thus avoiding a possible bile peritonitis.

Types of Gallbladder Surgery

1. *Cholecystostomy*—opening of gallbladder to remove stones, bile or pus; a tube is then sutured into the gallbladder for drainage.
   NOTE: When patient returns to the Recovery Unit, this drainage tube is connected to a drainage bottle.
2. *Cholecystectomy*—removal of the gallbladder after ligation of the cystic duct and artery; done in most situations of acute or chronic cholecystitis. A drain (penrose type) may be inserted in the gallbladder bed to permit drainage into dressings.
3. *Choledochostomy*—an opening into the common duct for the purpose of removing obstructing stones; a drainage tube is inserted into the duct which needs to be connected to a drainage bottle. Usually a cholecystectomy is done at this time because the gallbladder often contains stones also.

Preoperative Nursing Management

1. Diagnostic evaluation
   a. Gallbladder x-rays (see p. 442)
   b. Chest roentgenogram
   c. Examination of urine and stool
   d. Blood studies including liver function tests (see p. 426)
2. It may be necessary to administer vitamin K and blood transfusions to elevate a low prothrombin.
3. Proper nutritional levels may require supplements of protein hydrolysate to aid in wound healing and to prevent liver damage.
4. Adequate instruction regarding immediate postoperative requirements such as turning and deep breathing to prevent hypostatic pneumonia, a common postoperative complication.

Postoperative Nursing Objectives and Management

1. To prevent respiratory complications which are common in obese patients and in those having upper abdominal incisions.
   a. Encourage the patient to take 10 deep breaths hourly and to turn frequently.
   b. Administer analgesics as ordered to permit patient to take deep breaths comfortably (may be painful otherwise).
   c. Place patient in low Fowler's position to facilitate lung expansion.
   d. Activate and ambulate as early as permissible; apply a scultetus binder if it will make the patient more comfortable.
   e. Since he may still have a drainage bottle, place it in his pocket or fasten so that it is at desired level.

2. To promote drainage from T-tube or cholecystostomy tube until normal flow of bile is established.
    a. Place patient in low-Fowler's position and later semi-Fowler's position as tolerated to facilitate drainage.
    b. Connect drainage tube to drainage bottle at side of bed; observe for kinking, twisting and blockage of tubes.
    c. Check postoperative orders regarding positioning of drainage bottle; often the bottle or tubing is elevated so that bile drains through the apparatus only if pressure develops in the system. This is done purposely to prevent total bile loss and to promote normal bile flow through the common bile duct.
    d. Allow enough tubing leeway to permit the patient to be turned without dislodging tubes.
    e. Observe, describe and record amount and character of drainage frequently.
    f. After 5 or 6 days of drainage, the T-tube may be clamped 1 hour before and after each meal to allow bile to flow into duodenum to aid in digestion. (Done with physician's permission.)
    g. T-tube drain may be removed from 1 to 2 weeks. Cholecystostomy tube is removed from 6 weeks to 6 months. Drainage tube from gallbladder bed may be removed in 5 to 6 days.
3. To maintain fluid and nutritional needs of the postoperative biliary patient.
    a. Intravenous fluids are usually initiated; fluids by mouth are given in 24 hours.
    b. Insert nasogastric tube to relieve distention and promote normal peristalsis.
    c. An enema is usually given after 72 hours after which the patient is offered a soft, low fat diet.
    d. If necessary to feed the patient his own bile (in chronic biliary drainage) it may be best not to tell the patient what the liquid is other than it is to stimulate his appetite; bile may be chilled, strained and diluted with grape or other fruit juice.
    e. Provide diets which are low in fats and high in carbohydrate and proteins (fatty foods are usually avoided because they cause nausea).
    f. It may be necessary to continue to give vitamin K.
4. To observe color changes in skin, sclerae and stool which will indicate whether bile pigment is disappearing from blood and draining again into the duodenum.
    a. Note color and consistency of all stools; chart an accurate description.
    b. Send specimens of urine and stool to the laboratory at frequent intervals for examination of bile pigments.
    c. Observe skin and sclerae for yellowish color which would indicate bile-flow obstruction.
5. To protect skin around incision site due to bile seepage.
    a. Change the outer dressings frequently to provide for absorption of drainage; Montgomery straps may facilitate dressing changes.
    b. Apply skin pastes of zinc oxide or petrolatum to prevent the bile drainage from attacking and digesting the skin.
6. To stress elements in posthospital care which will assist patient in his convalescence.
    a. Encourage his continuing a nutritious diet while avoiding fats (Table 6-2).
        (1) The amount and type of fat in the diet appears to be related to lipid levels in the blood.
        (2) The diet may be modified in the treatment of atherosclerosis as to the total amount and the kind of fat (saturated vs polyunsaturated fat).
        (3) Total fat may be reduced in diseases of the gallbladder.
    b. Emphasize importance of follow-up visits to his physician.

TABLE 6-2. FAT CONTROLLED DIET

Category	Allowed	Avoid
Daily products		
Milk	Skim milk	Whole milk and cream.
Cheese	Cottage cheese	Other cheeses
Eggs	One egg 4 times a week	Fried eggs
Meats, fish, fowl	Lean meat, fish or fowl	Fried meats, fish or fowl, ham, pork, sausage
Soups and broths	Any made of the foods allowed	
Vegetables	Any except those to avoid	Any which cause distress: broccoli, brussels sprouts, cabbage, cucumbers, onions, cauliflower, green pepper, radishes, sauerkraut, turnips, dried beans and peas.
Fruits	Any fruit or juice except those excluded	Apples, melon, avocado
Breads, cereals, macaroni products	Whole grain breads Whole grain cereals	None
Desserts	Fruits Gelatin desserts Puddings Angel cake Fruit whips Sherberts	Desserts made from whole milk, eggs and cream Pastries, ice cream, chocolate
Beverages	Carbonated beverages Tea, coffee, fruit juices	Only milk beverages
Condiments and miscellaneous	All	None

4. Conditions of the Pancreas*

ACUTE PANCREATITIS

Acute pancreatitis is an inflammation of the pancreas brought about by the digestion of this organ by enzymes, particularly trypsin, an enzyme it produces.

Etiology

1. Unknown.
2. Associated with blockage of ampulla of Vater by gallstones causing activation of pancreatic enzymes.
3. Associated with spasm and edema of ampulla of Vater following duodenitis.
4. May occur as a complication of mumps or bacterial disease.
5. Associated with excessive intake of alcohol.

* For discussion of diabetes mellitus see pages 638-661.

Clinical Manifestations

A. *Acute Interstitial Pancreatitis*
1. Pancreatic edema and escape of enzyme into nearby tissues and peritoneal cavity.
2. Fat necrosis of omentum caused by pancreatic lipase.
3. Increase in peritoneal fluid.
4. Abdominal and back pain.
5. Nausea, vomiting.
6. Tenderness across upper abdomen.
7. Elevated blood lipase and amylase.

B. *Acute Hemorrhagic Pancreatitis*
1. A more advanced form of acute interstitial pancreatitis.
2. Enzymatic digestion of gland more widespread.
3. Tissue becomes necrotic—blood escapes into pancreas and retroperitoneally.
4. Severe abdominal and back pain.
5. Symptoms similar to acute interstitial pancreatitis only more severe.
6. Blood lipase and amylase elevated.

Treatment and Nursing Management

1. Relieve discomfort and pain to control restlessness which increases body metabolism causing stimulation of enzyme secretions.
   a. Give meperidine (Demerol); this is preferred because it depresses the central nervous system. (Opiates on the other hand may produce spasm of biliary-pancreatic ducts.)
   b. Encourage patient to assume position of comfort. Turn frequently to prevent pulmonary-vascular complications.
2. Decrease pancreatic secretions by reducing stimulation.
   a. Give nothing by mouth to eliminate chief stimulus to enzyme secretion.
   b. Offer anticholinergic medications as ordered to assist in reducing pancreatic secretions by suppressing vagal mechanisms.
   c. Initiate nasogastric suction to remove hydrochloric acid from stomach thus preventing release of secretin; adynamic ileus is also prevented.
      (1) Record color and nature of gastric secretions.
      (2) Measure secretions at periodic intervals.
   d. Maintain the comfort of the intubated patient.
      (1) Assist patient in cleansing and refreshing mouth care.
      (2) Apply lubricant to external nares to prevent irritation of mucous membrane and skin.
      (3) Alternate side-positioning to prevent esophageal and gastric irritation by tube.
      (4) Provide cool mist vapor therapy to increase humidity and control drying of mucous membrane.
3. Provide medications to correct deficiencies and prevent complications.
   a. Give parenteral fluids: electrolytes, blood and plasma to meet body's nutritional needs, replace losses and combat shock. Keep accurate intake and output record.
   b. Administer antibiotics to ward off secondary infection or abscess formation.
   c. If marked hyperglycemia occurs, give insulin in small doses (crystalline insulin at 6-hour intervals) rather than long-acting insulin.
4. Support cardiopulmonary system in acute hemorrhagic pancreatitis.
   a. Provide blood, plasma, dextran to maintain blood volume.
   b. Maintain surveillance of vital signs—initiate IPPB therapy when required.

   c. Keep the body metabolism of the patient low.
      (1) Administer oxygen therapy if breathing is labored.
      (2) Keep patient in bed to control overexertion.
      (3) Turn on air-conditioning to keep body heat under control.
5. Manage recovery phase and offer guidelines to the patient to prevent future attacks of pancreatitis.
   a. By the 5th or 6th day, offer the following:
      (1) Small amounts of clear-fat liquids
      (2) Anticholinergics parenterally or orally
      (3) Nonabsorbable antacids hourly
   b. Instruct the patient as follows:
      (1) Gradually resume normal diet.
      (2) Avoid alcohol and excessive use of coffee since they increase pancreatic secretion.
      (3) Avoid spicy foods and heavy meals because they are gastric stimulants.
      (4) Maintain a calm, even temperament; avoid emotional upsets.
   c. Urge follow-up visits with physician. (Biliary tract studies and surveillance may uncover the cause of the pancreatitis.)

CHRONIC PANCREATITIS

Chronic pancreatitis is a chronic fibrosis of the pancreas with obstruction of its ducts and destruction of its secreting cells.

Incidence
1. Men between 45 and 60.
2. Follows repeated attacks of acute interstitial pancreatitis.
3. May be a history of prolonged use of alcohol.

Clinical Manifestations
1. Recurrence of severe upper abdominal and back pain (morphine often does not relieve pain), vomiting, low grade fever.
2. Protein and fat digestion is disturbed because of deficient pancreatic juice.
3. Steatorrhea, stools which are frequent, frothy and foul-smelling with high fat content because of faulty fat digestion.
4. Later, calcium stones form in the duct as calcification develops; with obstruction; jaundice is noted.

Diagnostic Evaluation
1. Serum amylase and lipase to determine whether elevated.
2. Stool examination to measure fecal fat and trypsin content.
3. Arteriography and x-ray may show fibrous tissue and calcification.

Treatment and Nursing Management
1. A bland low fat diet is offered to the patient in 6 feedings daily.
2. Rich, stimulating foods which would stimulate pancreatic action are to be avoided.
3. Antacids and anticholinergic medication are given to reduce acid which would stimulate the release of secretin and enhance pancreatic activity.

4. Pancreatic insufficiency is controlled by giving medication containing amylase, lipase and trypsin—Pancreatin, Cotazym, Viokase.
   Administer with antacids, if not enteric coated, at mealtime.
5. Bile salts may be given to prevent further loss of fat, to facilitate digestion and absorption of vitamins A, D, E, K.
6. Since these patients often develop diabetes, the nurse should be alert for symptoms such as polydipsia, polyuria, weakness, polyphagia or weight loss and report these to physician.
7. The use of alcohol to relieve pain should be discouraged since this will aggravate the pancreatitis.
8. Surgical aspects are similar to biliary tract surgery (see p. 444).
9. Nature of surgery is determined by identifying the cause
   a. With gallbladder disease—biliary tract surgery to explore common bile duct, choledocholithotomy (removing stones in duct) and cholecystectomy (removing gallbladder).
   b. Sphincterotomy—dividing sphincter of Oddi to improve drainage of common bile duct.

PANCREATIC CYSTS

Pancreatic cysts are collections of fluid walled off by fibrous tissue in the pancreas, usually resulting from local necrosis at the time of acute pancreatitis.

Clinical Manifestations

1. Cysts may attain considerable size.
2. Because they occur in posterior peritoneum, they may exert pressure against stomach or colon.

Treatment

1. Symptoms of secondary infection may require surgery for drainage.
2. Drainage may be established into gastrointestinal tract or through skin surface.

Nursing Management

1. Recognize the irritating qualities of the pancreatic enzyme; meticulous skin care is required.
2. Maintain adequate drainage, avoiding tube dislodgment.

PANCREATIC TUMORS

Cancer may arise in the head, body or tail of pancreas; insulin-secreting pancreatic islet cells may or may not be involved.

Clinical Manifestations

1. Obstruction of the flow of bile produces jaundice, clay-colored stools and dark urine.
2. Disease usually occurs in older thin men; chronic alcoholism may be a contributing cause.

3. Weight loss, severe and constant pain, nausea and vomiting are common symptoms with diarrhea and steatorrhea.
4. Differentiation must be made from jaundice due to biliary obstruction due to a stone in the common duct.

Treatment

A. *Reasons for Surgery*
    1. Impacted gallstone is removed if present.
    2. Tumor is removed if it has not invaded important surrounding structures.
B. *Nature of Surgery*
    1. Whipple Resection—removal of head of pancreas, adjacent stomach, distal portion of common duct.
    2. If Whipple cannot be done, jaundice may be relieved by diverting bile from gallbladder into jejunum (cholecystojejunostomy).

Nursing Management

1. Because of the patient's poor nutritional state, it is a challenge to maintain adequate caloric levels. A bland, low fat diet is recommended plus whatever he can tolerate without overeating.
2. Medium-chain triglycerides are better tolerated causing less fat excretion.
3. Alcohol to be avoided.
4. Anticholinergics used.
5. See management of the patient undergoing major gastrointestinal surgery (p. 399) and biliary surgery (p. 444).

BIBLIOGRAPHY

Conditions of the Mouth, Neck and Esophagus

Books

Brunner, L. S., et al.: Textbook of Medical and Surgical Nursing, 2nd ed. Philadelphia, J. B. Lippincott, 1970, pp. 428–447.

Articles

Alexander, R. E.: Hospitalized dental patients: The nurse's role. RN, 32:52–55, April 1969.
Burdette, W. G.: Esophageal carcinoma. Amer. Fam. Phys., 5:88–96, May 1972.
Byrd, D. L., et al.: Open and closed reductions for fractures of facial bones. AORN J., 15:53–58, Feb. 1972.
Cady, B.: Carcinoma of the oral cavity. Surg. Clin. N. Amer., 51:537–551, June 1971.
Myers, E. N.: Rehabilitation after radical surgery of the tongue. AORN J., 11:55–59, Feb. 1970.
———: The toluidine blue test, in lesions of the oral cavity. CA-A J. Clin., 20:135–139, May-June 1970.
Oral Manifestations of Systemic Disorders. (Special Issue), Postgrad. Med., Jan. 1971.
Tarsitano, J. J., et al.: Nursing care after oral surgery. Amer. J. Nurs., 69:1493–1496, July 1969.
Trodahl, J. N., et al.: White lesions of the mouth. Hosp. Med. 7:6–25, Nov. 1971.

Gastrointestinal Conditions

Books

Brunner, L. S., et al.: Textbook of Medical and Surgical Nursing, 2nd ed. Philadelphia, J. B. Lippincott, 1970, pp. 448–503.
Colostomy, Ileostomy, and Ureterostomy Care: A Guide of Practical Information for Nurses. American Cancer Society, Cuyahoga Unit, Ohio, 1970.
Given, B. A., and Simmons, S. J.: Nursing Care of the Patient with Gastrointestinal Disorders. St. Louis, C. V. Mosby, 1971.
Spiro, H. M.: Clinical Gastroenterology. New York, Macmillan, 1970.
Turnbull, R. B.: The care of intestinal stomas. *In* Kinney, J. M. (ed.): Manual of Preoperative and Postoperative Care. Philadelphia, W. B. Saunders, 1971, pp. 391–410.
Welch, C. E.: The colon and rectum. *In* Kinney, J. M. (ed.): Manual of Preoperative and Postoperative Care. Philadelphia, W. B. Saunders, 1971, pp. 411–424.

Articles

Belinsky, I., Shinya, H., and Wolff, W. I.: Colonofiberoscopy: technique in colon examination. Amer. J. Nurs., 73:306–308, Feb. 1973.
Berland, T.: Peptic ulcer—the quiet epidemic. Pub. Affairs Committee, Pamphlet No. 472, Dec. 1971.
Buchan, D. J.: Mind-body relationships in gastrointestinal disease. Canad. Nurse, 67:35–37, March 1971.
DeLuca, J. C.: The ulcerative colitis personality. Nurs. Clin. N. Amer., 5:23–34, March 1970.
Edwards, D. A. W.: Changing ideas about hiatal hernia. Postgrad. Med., 52:161–165, Oct. 1972.
Engel, S.: Gastrostomy. Surg. Clin. N. Amer., 49:1289–1295, Dec. 1969.
Flynn, W. E.: Managing the emotional aspects of peptic ulcer and ulcerative colitis. Postgrad. Med., 47:119–122, May 1970.
Gibbs, G. E., and White, M.: Stomal care. Amer. J. Nurs., 72: 268–271, Feb. 1972.
Gutowski, F.: Ostomy procedure: nursing care before and after. Amer. J. Nurs., 72:262–267, Feb. 1972.
Helping your ostomy patient to cope. Nurs. Update, 3: (No. 10), Oct. 1972.
Hoerr, S. O., and Hertzer, N. R.: Current concepts of diagnosis and management of cancer of the stomach. Hosp. Med., 8:58–74, May 1972.
Jackson, B.: Ulcerative colitis from an etiological perspective. Amer. J. Nurs., 73:258–261, Feb. 1973.
Jacobson, M. J.: Hiatal hernia—changing concepts of treatment. Amer. Fam. Phys., 3:106–112, May 1971.
Kegney, F.: Psychosomatic gastrointestinal disturbances: A multifactor interactional concept. Postgrad. Med., 47:109–113, May 1970.
Kirsner, J. B.: The challenging ulcerative colitis. Postgrad. Med., 49:109–112, March 1971.
Kratzer, G. L.: Modern management of hemorrhoids. Amer. Fam. Phys., 6:82–88, Sept. 1972.
Mowchenko, G.: Care of patients with gastrointestinal diseases that have a psychological component. Canad. Nurse, 67:38–40, March 1971.
Nichols, R. L., and Condon, R. E.: Antibiotic preparation of the colon: failure of commonly used regimens. Surg. Clin. N. Amer., 51:223–231, Feb. 1971.
Roy, R., Sauer, W., et al.: Experience with ileostomies. Amer. J. Surg., 70:77–86, Jan. 1970.
Sill, A. R.: Bulb-syringe technique for colonic stomal irrigation. Amer. J. Nurs., 70:536–537, March 1970.
Symposium on acid-peptic disease. Surg. Clin. N. Amer., 51: (No. 4), Aug. 1971.
Tarsitano, J. J., et al.: Nursing care after oral surgery. Amer. J. Nurs., 69:1493–1496, July 1969.
Williams, L. F. Jr.: The acute abdomen. Amer. J. Nurs., 71:299–303, Feb. 1971.

Conditions of the Hepatic and Biliary System

Books

Brunner, L. S., et al.: Textbook of Medical and Surgical Nursing, 2nd ed. Philadelphia, J. B. Lippincott, 1970, pp. 504–531.

Puestow, C. B.: Surgery of the Biliary Tract, Pancreas and Spleen, 4th ed. Chicago, Year Book Medical Publishers, Inc., 1970.

Schiff, L. (ed.): Diseases of the Liver. Philadelphia, J. B. Lippincott, 1969.

Sherlock, S.: Diseases of the Liver and Biliary System, 4th ed. Philadelphia, F. A. Davis, 1968.

Articles

Blumberg, B. S.: Australia antigen—what it means to the hospital clinician. Res. Staff Phys., *18*:66–84, Sept. 1972.

Danzinger, R., et al.: Dissolution of cholesterol gallstones by chenodeoxycholic acid. New Eng. J. Med., *286*:1–7, Jan. 6, 1972.

Monroe, L. S.: Cholangitis. Hosp. Med., *5*:111–122, Oct. 1969.

Simmons, S., and Given, B.: Acute pancreatitis. Amer. J. Nurs., *71*:934–939, May 1971.

Small, D. M.: Gallstones: diagnosis and treatment. Postgrad. Med., *51*:187–193, Jan. 1972.

Stefanini, P., et al.: Surgical treatment of chronic pancreatitis. Amer. J. Surg., *124*:28–30, July 1972.

Ward R., et al.: Hepatitis B antigen in saliva and mouth washings. Lancet, *2*:726–727, Oct. 7, 1972.

Conditions of the Pancreas

Books

Brunner, L. S., et al.: Textbook of Medical and Surgical Nursing, 2nd ed. Philadelphia, J. B. Lippincott, 1970, pp. 534–539.

Friesen, S. R.: The Endocrine Pancreas. *In* Kinney, J. M. (ed.): Manual of Preoperative and Postoperative Care. Philadelphia, W. B. Saunders, 1971, pp. 518–528.

Articles

Bowden, L.: Cancer of the pancreas. CA-A J. Clin., *22*:275–283, Sept.-Oct. 1972.

Simmons, S., and Given, B.: Acute pancreatitis. Amer. J. Nurs., *71*:934–939, May 1971.

7

Conditions of the Kidney, Urinary Tract and Reproductive System

453

1. *Renal and Genitourinary Conditions*

MANIFESTATIONS OF DISORDERS
OF THE GENITOURINARY TRACT

Pain

1. Pain is not always a symptom of some of the most severe forms of urinary tract lesions.
2. Urologic pain is generally seen in more *acute* conditions.
3. Pain in flank radiating to lower abdomen, upper thigh, testis or labium may be from renal colic (kidney stones).
   a. Often accompanied by nausea, vomiting, paralytic ileus.
   b. Pain is produced from distention of ureter and pelvis by retained urine beyond point of obstruction or a blood clot.
4. Pain over suprapubic area (bladder pain) due to infection and urinary retention.
5. Urethral pain from irritation of bladder neck, from foreign body in canal or from urethritis due to infection or trauma.
6. Pain in scrotal area from inflammatory swelling of epididymis or testis, torsion of testis.
7. Testicular pain due to injury, mumps orchitis, torsion of spermatic cord.
8. Perineal or rectal discomfort from acute prostatitis, prostatic abscess.
9. Back and leg pain from cancer of prostate with metastases to pelvic bones.

Changes in Micturition (Voiding)

1. Hematuria (red blood cells in urine)
   a. Hematuria is considered a serious sign.
   b. Color of bloody urine dependent upon pH of urine and amount of blood present.
      (1) Acid urine is dark, smoky color.
      (2) Alkaline urine is red color.
   c. Hematuria may be from systemic causes such as blood dyscrasias, anticoagulant therapy, neoplasms.
   d. Painless hematuria may indicate neoplasm in the urinary tract.
   e. Hematuria from renal colic (stones in kidney).
   f. Bloody spotting reveals bleeding from urethra, bladder neoplasms.
   g. Hematuria also seen in renal tuberculosis, polycystic disease of kidneys, septic pyelonephritis, thrombosis and embolism involving renal artery.
2. Proteinuria (albuminuria)
   a. Normal urine does not contain persistent protein in significant quantities.
   b. Proteinuria characteristically seen in all forms of acute and chronic renal disease (more characteristic of glomerulonephritis than pyelonephritis).
      (1) The protein is mainly albumin but globulin is also present.
      (2) Albumin and globulin escape through damaged glomerular capillaries in a greater amount than can be reabsorbed by the tubules, or damaged tubules fail to reabsorb normal amount filtered.
   c. Proteinuria occurs in systemic diseases where there are varying degrees of renal anoxia such as in cardiac decompensation, diabetic glomerulosclerosis.
   d. Mild proteinuria may occur from other sources—urethritis, prostatitis, cystitis.
3. Dysuria (painful or difficult voiding)—seen in wide variety of pathological conditions.
4. Frequency—from acutely inflamed bladder or neurogenic bladder.

5. Urgency (strong desire to urinate)—due to inflammatory lesions in bladder, prostate or urethra, acute bacterial infections, chronic prostatitis in men and chronic posterior urethrotrigonitis in women.
6. Burning upon urination—as seen in urethral irritation.
7. Enuresis (involuntary voiding during sleep)—may be physiologic to age of 3; after this may be functional or symptomatic of renal disease (usually of lower tract).
8. Nocturia (voiding at night)—may indicate renal disease with decrease of functioning renal parenchyma and loss of concentrating power, obstructed bladder, systemic disease (congestive heart failure, diabetes).
9. Strangury (difficult, painful voiding associated with spasms)—seen in severe cystitis.
10. Incontinence (inability of bladder to retain any urine)—from injury to external urinary sphincter, acquired neurogenic disease.
11. Stress incontinence (intermittent leakage of urine from sudden strain)—indicates weakness of sphincteric mechanism.
12. Polyuria (large volume of urine voided in given time)—demonstrated in diabetes mellitus, diabetes insipidus.
13. Oliguria (small volume of urine voided in given time)—may be from acute renal failure, shock, dehydration, fluid-ion imbalance.
14. Anuria (no urine in bladder)—from acute renal failure and bilateral ureteral obstruction.
15. Pneumaturia (passage of gas in urine during voiding)—caused by fistulous connection between bowel and bladder, rectosigmoid cancer, regional ileitis, sigmoid diverticulitis (most common) and gas forming urinary tract infections.

Gastrointestinal Symptoms Related to Urologic Disease

1. Gastrointestinal symptoms may occur with urological conditions because of:
   a. Renal-intestinal reflexes.
   b. Anatomic relation of right kidney to colon (hepatic flexure), duodenum, head of pancreas, common bile duct, liver and gallbladder.
   c. Anatomic relation of left kidney to colon (splenic flexure), stomach, pancreas, spleen.
   d. Peritoneal irritation—anterior surface of kidneys covered by peritoneum which is affected by renal inflammation.
2. Gastrointestinal symptoms related to urologic conditions include nausea, vomiting, diarrhea, abdominal discomfort, paralytic ileus, gastrointestinal hemorrhage with uremia.

DIAGNOSTIC EVALUATION FOR UROLOGIC DISEASE

Roentgenography

A. *Roentgenogram* (flat plate)—is used to delineate size, shape and position of kidneys.
   1. Gives a base line of reference for subsequent films.
   2. Shows the position, number and size of radiopaque urinary tract calculi (stones).

B. *Infusion Drip Pyelography*—is an intravenous infusion of a large volume of dilute solution of contrast material to produce opacification of the renal parenchyma and complete filling of urinary tract. Films taken at intervals to demonstrate the filled and distended collecting system.

1. Patient preparation is same as for excretory urography *except the patient is not dehydrated* (see below).
2. Infusion drip pyelography is now almost replacing standard intravenous pyelography; used when regular urographic techniques fail to show drainage structures satisfactorily.

C. *Excretory Urography* (intravenous pyelogram or intravenous urogram)—introduction of a radiopaque contrast material intravenously which visualizes the kidneys, ureter and bladder. The contrast media is cleared from the bloodstream by renal excretion.
   1. Excretory urography is used in:
      a. Initial investigation of any suspected urologic problem, especially in diagnosis of lesions in kidneys and ureters.
      b. To provide a rough estimate of renal function.
   2. Patient Preparation
      a. See that patient is not overhydrated—will dilute contrast material causing inadequate visualization.
      b. Remove obstructing intestinal content if possible.
      c. See that nothing is taken by mouth after evening meal until after the examination is completed the next day.

NURSING ALERT: Elderly patients with poor renal reserve may not tolerate dehydrating procedures and should be given water to drink.

---

      d. Give laxative (usually castor oil) the night before the test to eliminate feces and gas in intestinal tract.
      e. Administer enemas by order of radiologist; this procedure may increase gas in intestinal tract.
      f. Ascertain if patient has history of allergies—to find the high-risk patient.
         (1) Evaluate for anaphylactoid reaction (rare) to intravenous dosage of contrast material. (No contrast media is completely innocuous.)
         (2) Watch patient during procedure so that reactions are recognized immediately.
            (a) Mild reaction (relatively common)—flushing, metallic taste, nausea, vomiting, faintness, tingling
            (b) Severe reaction—urticaria, edema, asthma, hypotension, convulsions, cyanosis, shock and cardiac arrest
         (3) Have emergency drugs (epinephrine, vasopressors, corticosteroids, etc.), oxygen and tracheostomy equipment ready to restore cardiac activity and maintain adequate respiration and blood pressure. Have equipment available to treat cardiac arrest (see p. 246).
         (4) Some clinics add antihistamine to the contrast media to abort allergic reactions.

D. *Retrograde Pyelography*—injection of opaque material through ureteral catheters which have been passed up ureters into renal pelvis by means of cystoscopic manipulation. The opaque solution is introduced by gravity or syringe.
   1. Retrograde pyelography usually done when nonfunctioning kidney is suspected.
   2. Performed with decreasing frequency due to danger of infection and trauma.

E. *Cystogram*—instillation of radiopaque fluid through catheter into bladder for purpose of outlining the bladder wall and most importantly to evaluate ureterovesical valves for reflux.

F. *Cysturethrogram*—visualization of urethra and bladder either by retrograde injection o: by voiding of contrast material.

G. *Radioisotope Studies of Urinary Tract* (renogram)—delineates structure and function o: kidneys without disturbing their normal physiologic processes.

    1. Intravenous radioiodine (Hippuran ^{131}I) is given.

    2. Sites over both kidneys are monitored with radiation counters to reveal difference: between the 2 kidneys with respect to blood flow, tubular function and excretion.

H. *Isotopic Localization of Renal Pathology* (renoscan)—delineates the kidney by externa scanning.

    1. Neohydrin labeled with radioactive mercury (^{197}Hg) is given intravenously.
        A lesion (tumor, infarct) is detected by absence of radioactivity in the involvec area and resultant defect in scan.

    2. Technetium scan for renal blood flow used to show vascular tumors.

I. *Renal Aortography*—visualization of renal arterial supply which may be performed by ε number of different techniques.

    1. Contrast material may be injected:

        a. Via translumbar route (needle placed directly into abdominal aorta).

        b. Via femoral route (needle and catheter injected into femoral artery up the iliac vessel into abdominal aorta).

        c. Intravenously into antecubital veins of arm(s) (rarely used).

    2. Useful in diagnosing renovascular hypertension and pheochromocytoma and in dif ferentiating renal cyst from renal tumor.

        a. Give cathartic in evening before examination to eliminate fecal material from colon and small intestine to ensure unobstructed radiographs.

        b. Procedure is usually done with preoperative medication and local anesthesia.

        c. Determine if patient has any allergies or previous minor reactions before test.

        d. Watch for reactions to contrast media (see p. 457).

Cystoscopic Examination

A *cystoscopic examination* involves visualization of urethra, prostatic urethra, and bladder by means of a tubular lighted telescopic lens.

A. *Uses*

    1. To inspect bladder wall directly for tumor, stone, ulcer, etc.

    2. To obtain a separate specimen from each kidney and evaluate renal functior separately.

    3. To see configuration and position of ureteral orifices.

    4. To remove calculi from urethra, bladder and ureter.

    5. To treat lesions of bladder and urethra and prostate.

B. *Patient Preparation*

    Give prescribed oral fluids and preoperative medication.

C. *Nursing Support Following Procedure*

    1. Expect patient to have some burning upon voiding, blood-tinged urine and urinary frequency from trauma to mucous membrane.

2. Watch patients with prostatic hypertrophy for urinary retention from edema from instrumentation.
3. Give warm sitz baths or apply heat to abdomen for pain relief and promotion of muscle relaxation.
4. Utilize indwelling catheter if urinary retention persists.

D. *Complications Following Cystoscopy*
1. Urinary retention
2. Urinary tract hemorrhage
3. Infection within prostate or bladder

Needle Biopsy of Kidney

Needle biopsy of the kidney is performed by percutaneous needle biopsy through renal tissue or open biopsy through a small flank incision.

1. Platelet study, C.B.C., prothrombin, clotting and bleeding and clot retraction times done before biopsy.
2. Intravenous pyelogram precedes biopsy to specifically locate kidney as guide for needle insertion.
3. Postbiopsy nursing management
   a. Place patient prone for at least 1 hour after procedure; the patient is to remain on bedrest for 24 hours.
   b. Take the vital signs every 5 minutes for first hour and then with decreasing frequency if stable to assess for hemorrhage which is a major complication.
   c. Keep the fluid intake at 3000 ml. daily if tolerated.
   d. Inspect and measure each voiding for bleeding; save urine for laboratory examination of sediment if indicated.
   e. Prepare for transfusion and surgical intervention for control of hemorrhage which may necessitate a nephrectomy (removal of kidney).

Tests of Renal Function

General Information

1. There is no single test of renal function. Best results are obtained by combining a number of clinical tests.
2. During tests of renal function the patient should lie quietly in bed.

Renal Concentration Test

1. Evaluates the ability of kidneys to concentrate urine.
2. Concentration ability is lost early in kidney disease; hence this test detects early defects in renal function.
3. *Procedure*
   a. Patient eats a dry supper and fasts after 6 P.M.
   b. Urine samples are collected in separate containers at 9, 10 and 11 A.M. the following day.
   c. Concentration measured primarily by specific gravity readings.
   d. Normal range of specific gravity: 1.022–1.035.

Phenolsulfonphthalein Excretion Test

1. A test of renal blood flow and tubular secretion.
2. *Procedure*
   a. Instruct the patient *not* to void during the hour preceding test.
   b. Phenolsulfonphthalein (6 mg.) is given I.V. (If intramuscular medication given, 10 minutes extra should be allowed for absorption of dye.)
   c. Give patient 2 glasses of water to drink 30 minutes before test. Patient should remain in bed during test.
      (1) Record exact time dye is administered.
      (2) Instruct patient to void 15 minutes after dye administration; collect at least 50 ml. of urine for test to be reliable.
3. Interpretation
   a. At least 25% excreted in 15 minutes, 40% in 30 minutes and 60% in 120 minutes (after injection).
   b. After I.V. injection: 55–75% excreted in urine in 2 hours.
   c. Delayed excretion in renal disease. Low in nephritis, cystitis, pyelonephritis and heart failure, and when kidneys are obstructed by benign prostatic hypertrophy.

Serum Urea Nitrogen (Blood Urea Nitrogen)

1. Serves as an index of renal excretory capacity.
2. Serum urea nitrogen is dependent on the body's urea production and on urine flow.
3. Normal range is 10–20 mg./100 ml. of blood.
   a. Increased in acute glomerulonephritis, obstructive uropathy and nephrotic syndrome.
   b. Also increased by nonrenal conditions such as gastrointestinal bleeding and dehydration.

Serum Creatinine Determination

1. Measures nitrogen retention in renal insufficiency.
2. Amount of creatinine excreted varies and is dependent on muscle mass.
3. Test results may be altered during exercise and in certain diseases.
4. Normal reading is 1–2 mg./100 ml. of blood.
   Elevated in nephritis and chronic renal disease.

Endogenous Creatinine Clearance

1. Measures glomerular filtration plus some tubular excretory activity. Is a useful test for following renal function quantitatively.
2. Is considered more accurate than the urea clearance test.
3. *Procedure*
   a. Collect all urine over a 24-hour period.
   b. Draw 1 sample of blood within the period.
   c. Normal values:
      Men: 140–200 liters/day (97–140 ml./minute)
      Women: 120–180 liters/day (85–125 ml./minute)

Urea Clearance

1. Clearance indicates the amount of blood that is cleared of a substance in a given amount of time.

2. Urea is the principal end product of protein metabolism. Urea clearance measures glomerular filtration rate.
3. *Procedure*
   a. Encourage the patient to drink several glasses of water before and during the test to ensure adequate urine volume.
   b. Have the patient remain in bed until the test is completed.
   c. Ask the patient to void at beginning of test; discard urine but record the time of voiding.
   d. Collect urine sample at the end of the 1st and 2nd hour. Measure and label the time of voidings.
   e. Draw blood samples at the mid-points of the 1st and 2nd urine collection.
   f. Normal urea clearance is 75 ml./minute.

Urine Examination

Factors Affecting Composition of the Urine

1. Nutritional status
2. Metabolic processes
3. Status of kidney function

Amount

1. 1200–1500 ml./24 hours; less than 600 ml. is considered oliguria.
2. Day volume 2 to 3 times more than night volume.

Odor

1. Normal—faint aromatic odor.
2. Characteristic odors produced by ingestion of asparagus, thymol.
3. Cloudy urine with ammonia odor—urea-splitting bacteria such as *Proteus,* causing urinary tract infections.
4. Offensive odor—bacterial action in presence of pus.

Color

1. Color shows degree of concentration and depends on amount voided.
2. Normal urine is yellow-amber—due to pigment urochrome.
3. Color varies with specific gravity:
   a. Dilute urine is straw-colored.
   b. Concentrated urine is highly colored.
4. Abnormally colored urine:
   a. Turbid or smoky colored—may be from hematuria, spermatozoa, prostatic fluid, fat droplets, chyle.
   b. Red or red brown—is due to blood porphyria and blood pigments, transfusion reaction, bleeding lesions in urogenital tract.
   c. Yellow-brown or green-brown—may reveal obstructive lesion of bile duct system or obstructive jaundice.
   d. Orange-red or orange-brown—from urobilin or from Pyridium, a urinary antiseptic.
   e. Dark brown or black—due to malignant melanoma, leukemia.

Appearance

1. Normal urine is clear.
2. Abnormally cloudy urine—from pus, blood, epithelial cells, bacteria, fat, colloidal particles, phosphate, urates.
3. Turbid urine is not always pathological.

Reaction (pH)

1. Reflects the ability of kidney to maintain normal hydrogen ion concentration in plasma and extracellular fluid; indicates *acidity* or *alkalinity* of urine.
2. Normal pH is 6 (acid); may vary from 4.6 to 8.
3. Urine acidity or alkalinity has relatively little clinical significance unless patient is on special diet or therapeutic program or is being treated for renal calculous disease.
4. Alkaline urine is cloudy.

Specific Gravity

1. Measures density of particles in urine; reflects concentrating and diluting power of kidneys.
2. Normal specific gravity ranges from 1.005 to 1.025.
3. Specific gravity fixed at 1.010 in chronic renal failure.

Osmolarity

1. A measure of the number of particles in a solution.
2. Normal—after a 14-hour fast is 850 mOsm or higher.

Basic Principles for Collecting Urine Specimens

1. The early morning urine specimen is most concentrated—it reveals sediment abnormalities.
2. Urine should not be left standing at room temperature as it becomes alkaline due to contamination of urea-splitting bacteria from the environment.
3. Microscopic examination should be done within 1 hour after collection—standing causes dissolution of cellular elements and casts and bacterial overgrowth unless obtained under sterile conditions.
4. Urine specimens should be collected from the patient by means of the clean-catch midstream technique (see p. 463).
5. Collection of 24-hour specimen:
   a. Ensure that the patient understands the procedure. *All* urine must be collected within a 24-hour period via clean-catch midstream technique.
   b. Have patient empty the bladder at specified time (Ex. 8:00 A.M.). *Discard urine.*
   c. Collect all urine voided during the next 24 hours.
   d. Collect last specimen at 8:00 A.M. on following day (or 24 hours after collection was started).
   e. Keep collected urine in the refrigerator in a clean bottle to which a preservative has been added (preservative prescribed by laboratory).

GUIDELINES: *Technique for Obtaining Clean-catch Midstream Voided Specimen*

A clean-catch midstream specimen is the only clinically effective method of securing a voided specimen for urinalysis. It is not a simple procedure and requires patient education and active assistance of the female patient.

Equipment

Antiseptic solution (benzalkonium chloride)
Cotton sponges
Disposable gloves for nurse in assisting female patient
Sterile specimen container

Procedure

Nursing Action	Rationale/Amplification
Male Patient	
1. Instruct the patient to expose glans and cleanse area around meatus. Wash area with a mild antiseptic solution (benzalkonium chloride).	1. The urethral orifice is colonized by bacteria. Urine readily becomes contaminated during voiding.
2. Allow the initial urinary flow to escape.	
3. Collect the midstream urine specimen in a sterile container.	
4. Avoid collecting the last few drops of urine.	4. Prostatic secretions may be introduced into urine at the end of the urinary stream.
Female Patient	
1. Ask the patient to separate her labia to expose the urethral orifice.	1. Keeping the labia separated prevents labial or vaginal contamination of the urine specimen.
2. Cleanse the area around the urinary meatus with cotton sponges liberally soaked with benzalkonium chloride. If pHisoHex is used, rinse well with sterile water.	2. The urethral orifice is colonized by bacteria. Urine readily becomes contaminated during voiding. pHisoHex can cause hemolysis of red blood cells in the urine thus making the specimen analysis inaccurate.
3. While the patient keeps her labia separated, instruct her to void forcibly.	3. This helps wash away urethral contaminants.
4. Allow initial urinary flow to drain into bedpan (toilet) and then catch the midstream specimen in a sterile container.	
5. Send the specimen to the laboratory immediately.	5. Too long a lapse of time between collection and analysis produces unreliable results.

CATHETERIZATION

GUIDELINES: *Catheterization of the Urinary Bladder*

Purpose

To empty contents of bladder.
To obtain a sterile urine specimen.
To determine amount of residual urine in bladder after voiding.

TYPES OF CATHETERS

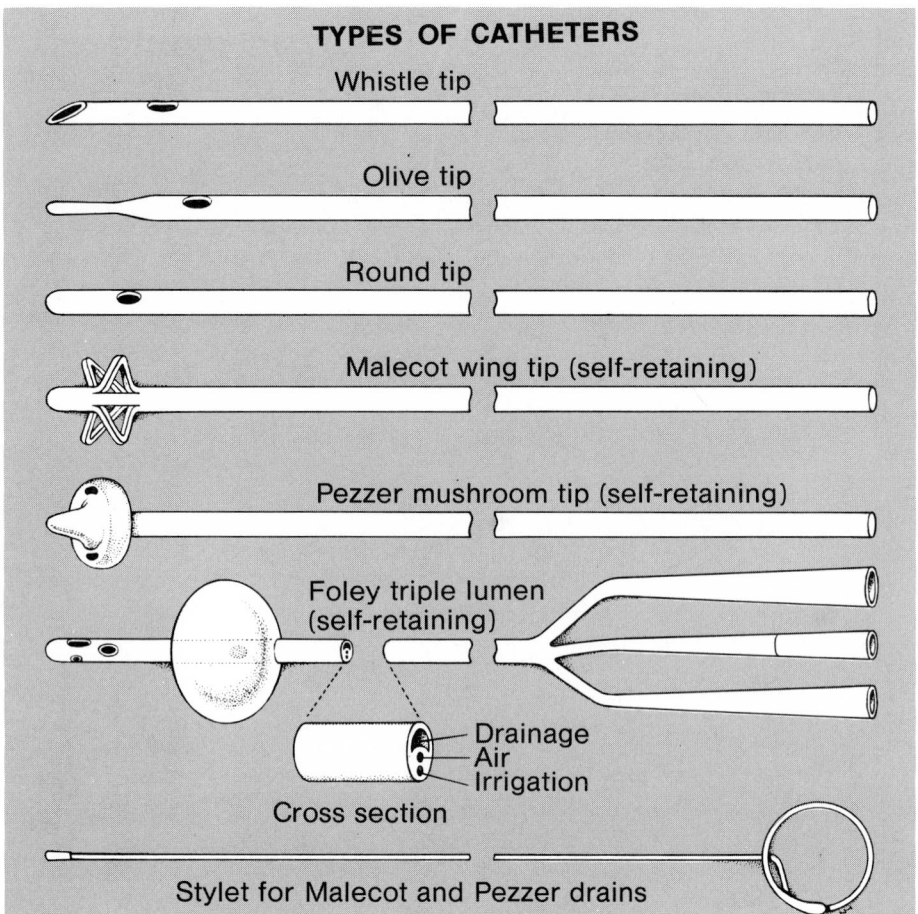

Whistle tip

Olive tip

Round tip

Malecot wing tip (self-retaining)

Pezzer mushroom tip (self-retaining)

Foley triple lumen
(self-retaining)

- Drainage
- Air
- Irrigation

Cross section

Stylet for Malecot and Pezzer drains

Figure 7-1. Types of catheters.

Equipment

Disposable sterile catheter set with water-soluble lubricant (See Fig. 7-1 for different types of catheters.)
Bath blanket/sheet for draping purposes
Standing lamp (preferred) or flashlight

Procedure for Catheterizing Female Patient (Fig. 7-2)

Nursing Action	Rationale/Amplification
Preparatory Phase	
1. Place patient at ease.	1. Patient will feel reassured if the procedure is explained and if she is handled gently and considerately.
2. Open catheter tray using aseptic technique. Place waste receptacle in accessible place.	2. Catheterization should require the same aseptic precautions as a minor surgical procedure.
3. Direct light for visualization of genital area.	
4. Place patient in a supine position with knees bent, hips adducted and feet resting about 2 feet apart. Drape the patient.	

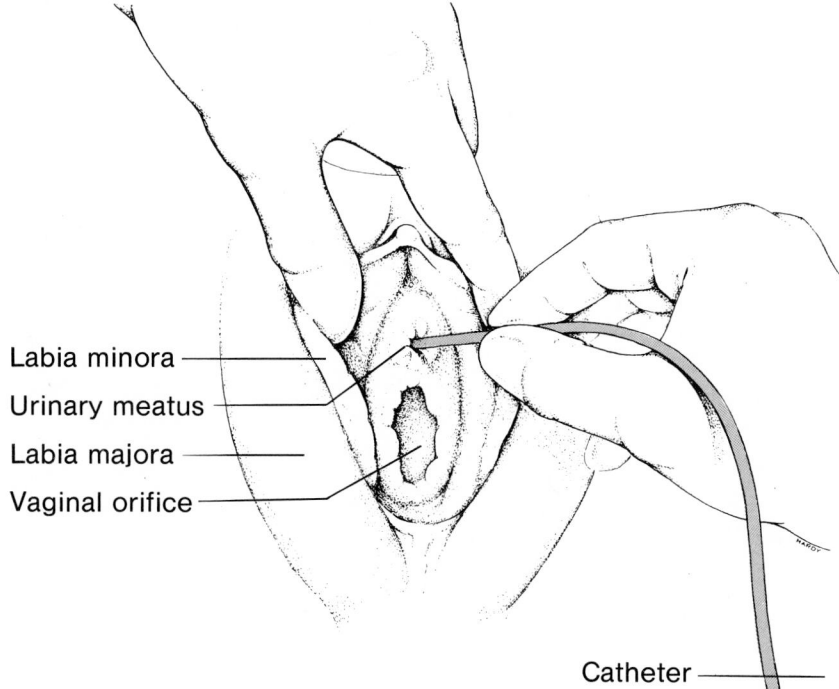

Labia minora
Urinary meatus
Labia majora
Vaginal orifice

Catheter

Figure 7-2. Catheterization of urinary bladder in female.

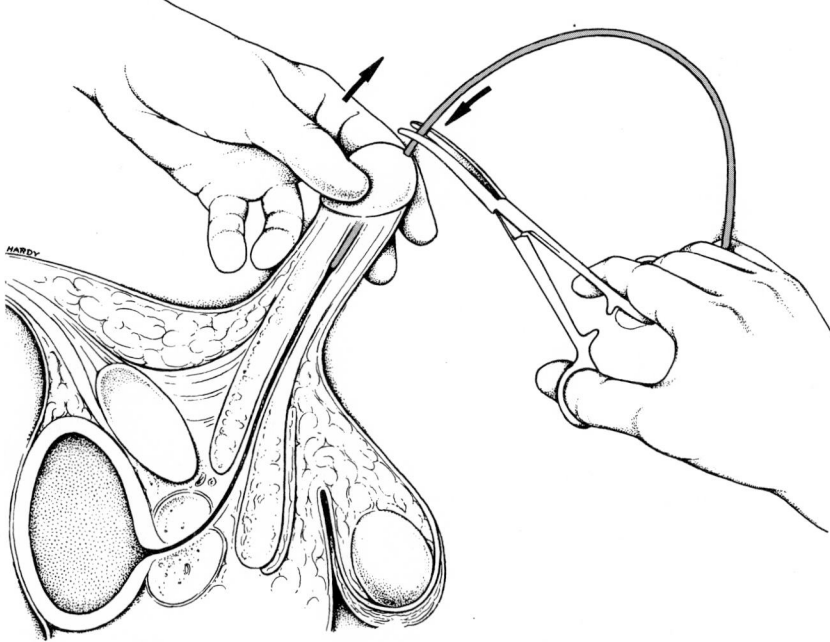

Figure 7-3. Technique for catheterization in male.

Nursing Action	**Rationale/Amplification**
5. Position moisture-proof pad under patient's buttocks.	
6. Wash hands. Put on sterile gloves.	

Performance Phase

Nursing Action	**Rationale/Amplification**
1. Separate labia minora so that urethral meatus is visualized; one hand is to maintain separation of the labia until catheterization is finished.	1. This maneuver helps prevent labial contamination of the catheter (Fig. 7-2).
2. Cleanse around urethral meatus washing outward from meatus with aqueous benzalkonium chloride (1:750). a. Manipulate cleansing sponges with forceps. b. Dispose of cotton sponge after each use.	2. Benzalkonium chloride is an adsorbing agent which leaves a bacteriostatic film over the area thus helping to prevent bacterial growth. Inadequate preparation of the urethral meatus is a major cause of infection.
3. Introduce well-lubricated catheter 5–7.5 cm. (2–3 inches) in an upward and backward direction into urethral meatus using strict aseptic technique. a. Avoid contaminating surface of catheter. b. Ensure that catheter is not too large or too tight at urethral meatus.	3. A well-lubricated catheter reduces friction and trauma to the meatus. The female urethra is a relatively short canal measuring 3.0–4 cm in length. b. Too large a catheter may cause pressure necrosis of the meatus.
4. Pinch catheter and remove gently when urinary flow ceases.	

Follow-up Phase

1. Make patient comfortable.
2. Measure urine and dispose of equipment.
3. Send specimen to lab as indicated.
4. Record time, procedure, amount and appearance of urine.

Procedure for Catheterizing Male Patient (Fig. 7-3)

Nursing Action	**Rationale/Amplification**
1. Carry out all of "preparatory phase" as for female patient except:	
2. Place the patient in a dorsal recumbent position with legs extended. Place the moisture-proof pad across upper thighs.	
3. Position the perineal drape.	
4. Lubricate approximately 17.5 cm (7 inches) of catheter.	4. A well-lubricated catheter prevents urethral trauma thereby decreasing the opportunity for bacterial invasion .
5. Wash off glans penis around urinary meatus with benzalkonium chloride using forceps to hold cleansing sponges. Maintain sterility of right hand.	

Nursing Action	**Rationale/Amplification**
Grasp shaft of penis (with left hand) raising it almost straight up. Maintain grasp on penis until procedure is ended.	6. This maneuver straightens the penile urethra and facilitates ease of catheterization. Maintaining a grasp of the penis prevents contamination and retraction of penis.
Using a sterile forcep, insert catheter into the urethra along the anterior wall; advance catheter 17.5–25 cm. (7–10 inches) until urine flows.	7. The male urethra is a canal extending from the bladder to the end of the glans penis. The length varies within wide limits; the average length is about 21 cm.
If resistance is felt at the external sphincter, slightly increase the traction on the penis and apply steady gentle pressure on the catheter.	8. Some resistance may be from spasm of external sphincter. If an impassable stricture is encountered, the urethra may have to be dilated with sounds by a urologist.
When urine begins to flow, advance the catheter another 2.5 cm. (1 inch).	9. Advancing the catheter ensures its position in the bladder.

or Indwelling Catheter

Advance catheter almost to its bifurcation.	1. This prevents the balloon from becoming trapped in the urethra.
Inflate the balloon according to manufacturer's directions.	
Withdraw catheter slightly and connect to drainage system.	
Tape tubing (not catheter) to shaved inner aspect of thigh.	4. Taping the tubing to the thigh prevents tension and traction on the bladder.
Reduce (or reposition) the foreskin.	5. Paraphimosis (retraction and constriction of the foreskin behind the glans penis), secondary to catheterization, may occur, if the foreskin is not reduced.

ollow-up Phase
ame as for female patient.

GUIDELINES: *Management of the Patient with Indwelling Catheter and Continuous Bladder Drainage*

Purpose

1. To empty urine from the bladder.
2. To rinse the bladder with a continuous solution of antibacterial fluid to prevent infection.
3. To clear an obstructed catheter.

Equipment

1. Use a completely closed system with plug-in bottles (see Fig. 7-4).
2. Catheter tray with triple lumen catheter.
3. Drainage solution as prescribed (usually sterile normal saline or neosporin solution).
4. Gauze squares.
5. Benzalkonium chloride.

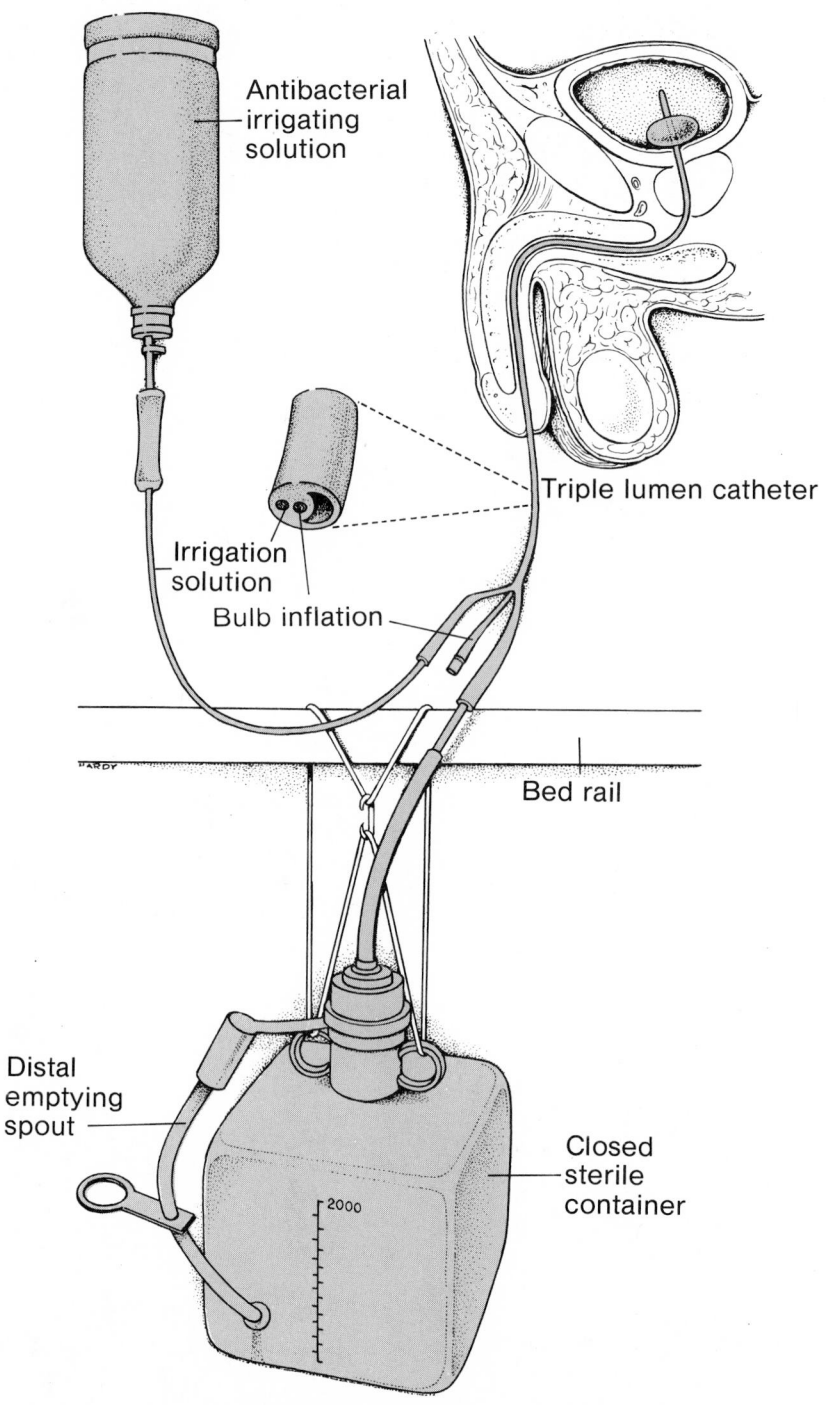

Figure 7-4. Closed sterile drainage system.

Procedure

Nursing Action	Rationale/Amplification

Performance Phase

1. Catheterize the patient (p. 463).
2. Prevent introduction of organisms where catheter enters urethral meatus
   a. Wash area around catheter several times daily with benzalkonium chloride.
   b. Place gauze square soaked in aqueous benzalkonium chloride (or hydrogen peroxide) around the catheter at the urinary meatus twice daily.
   c. Teach patient how to cleanse around catheter if he/she is able.
3. Prevent introduction of organisms through the lumen of the catheter
   a. Keep catheter sterile when introducing it into an aseptically prepared urinary meatus (p. 466).
   b. Avoid separating connecting tube and catheter.
      (1) If catheter has to be separated, wrap alcohol-soaked gauze around junction to disconnect catheter from tube.
      (2) Pinch catheter and irrigate with benzalkonium chloride before reconnecting catheter to tube. (Do not allow the benzalkonium chloride to drain into the bladder.)
4. Prevent introduction of organisms through the distal end of the drainage system:
   a. Do not allow drainage tube to contact urine in collecting bottle. Utilize a drip chamber.
   b. Do not disconnect tubing from drainage bottle; use a distal emptying valve to empty bottle.

2. Suppurative drainage and encrustation occur at the exit of any tube. Catheter care helps prevent exudate from entering urethra. Encrustations arising from urinary salts may enter bladder when catheter is removed and serve as a nuclei for stone formation. Benzalkonium chloride leaves a bacteriostatic film. The catheter must be cleansed of blood or pus to maintain antibacterial protection.

(1) This is a portal of entry for bacteria.

(2) This bathes the end of the catheter and connecting tube with bactericidal solution and prevents bacterial entry into the bladder via these sites.

Management of Continuous Irrigating System

A. *A 3-way (or triple lumen) catheter.*
   1. One lumen—inflates the bag holding the catheter in place.
   2. Second lumen—for outflow of urine and outflow of drainage solution.
   3. Third lumen—for inflow of drainage solution (antibacterial rinse) into bladder.

B. *Flow of Irrigating Solutions*
   1. For continuous irrigation:
      a. If drainage is bright red, allow irrigating solution to run in rapidly until drainage becomes lighter.
      b. If drainage is clear, allow irrigating solution to run at rate of 40–60 drops/minute.
   2. For P.R.N. irrigation with a syringe:
      a. Sponge the catheter and tubing connections with benzalkonium chloride.
      b. Disconnect catheter and allow urine to drain into emesis basin.

    c. Sponge the catheter with benzalkonium chloride.

    d. Insert tip of syringe into catheter and apply *gentle pressure* to the bulb.

        (1) Irrigate with 20–30 ml. of drainage solution every 2–4 hours if drainage i
clear.

        (2) If drainage is bloody, the patient may have to be irrigated every 5 minutes o
as frequently as necessary to keep clots from forming in the catheter, etc.

        (3) Allow the irrigating solution to drain by gravity into the emesis basin.

        (4) Sponge the catheter and connecting tube with benzalkonium chloride befor
reconnecting to drainage tubing.

C. *Other Measures to Prevent Infection*

    1. Ensure copious fluid intake—to produce mechanical flushing and to dilute urinar
elements producing encrustation.

    2. Keep the urine acid—to prevent tube obstruction and encrustation of urinary san
and calculus deposits.

      a. Oral intake of potassium acid phosphate

      b. Acid-ash diet

      c. Cranberry juice, 200 ml., 4 times daily

      d. Ascorbic acid.

GUIDELINES: *Assisting the Patient Undergoing Suprapubic Drainage (Cystostomy)*

Purpose

    1. To drain the bladder via a tube placed in the bladder from the suprapubic area.

    2. To divert the flow of urine from the urethra.

Clinical Usefulness

Injuries to the urethra—stricture, trauma
Following gynecological procedures (vaginal hysterectomy; vaginal repair)
Following bladder surgery
Prostatectomy
Neurogenic bladder

Equipment

Sterile suprapubic drainage system package (disposable)
Skin germicide for suprapubic skin preparation
Local anesthetic agent if needed

Procedure

Nursing Action	*Rationale/Amplification*
Preparatory Phase	
1. Place patient in a dorsal recumbent position with one pillow under head.	
2. Expose the abdomen.	

Nursing Action	**Rationale/Amplification**

Performance Phase (by physician)

3. The bladder is distended with 300–500 ml. of sterile saline via a urethral catheter which is removed.

3. Makes it easier to locate bladder.

4. The suprapubic area is surgically prepared. After the skin is dried the needle entry point is located.

4. The needle entry point is approximately 5 cm. (2 inches) above the symphysis.

5. The procedure may be performed in several ways:
   a. By open operation.
   b. By puncture with needle or trocar.
      (1) The catheter is threaded through the needle or trocar well into the bladder.
      (2) The needle or trocar is withdrawn leaving the catheter in place.
      (3) The catheter is secured with sutures, tape or a body-seal system.

      (3) Aseptic technique is employed in the area around the cystostomy tube.

      (4) Cover the area around the catheter with a sterile bandage.
      (5) Attach the drainage tubing to a closed sterile system.

6. Secure drainage tubing to lateral abdomen with tape (Fig. 7-5).

6. Prevent undue tension on the catheter.

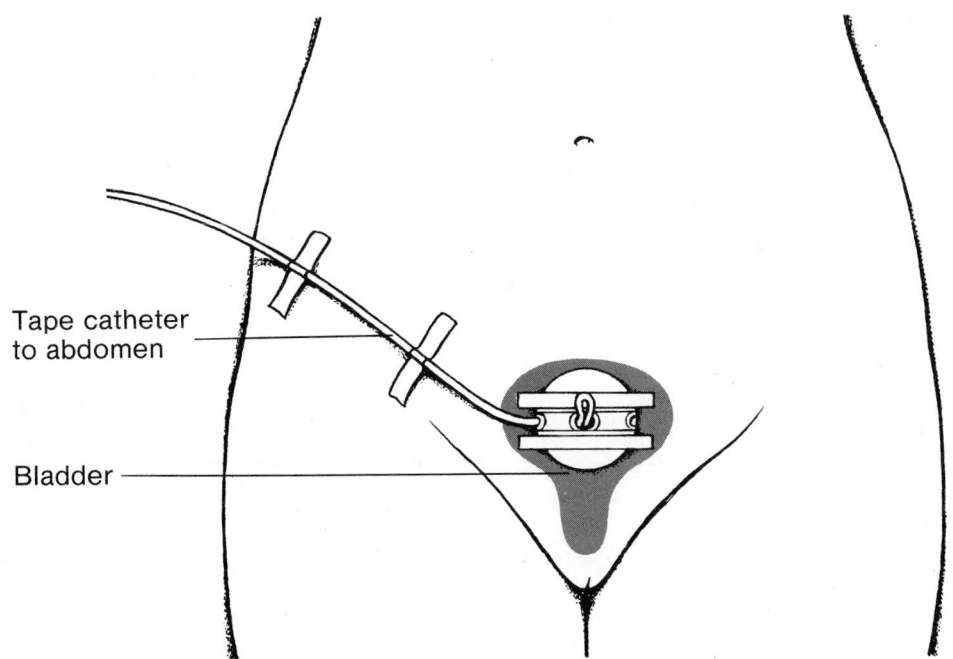

Tape catheter to abdomen

Bladder

Figure 7-5. Location of suprapubic bladder drain.

Nursing Action	**Rationale/Amplification**
7. Vent the collection system by placing a No. 18 gauge needle through the cap of the bag.	7. Some systems are already vented.
8. If it is necessary to disconnect the collecting system be sure there is a column of urine in the catheter. (Close the 3-way stopcock before disconnecting in order to maintain a column of urine in the catheter.)	8. The cystostomy tube acts as a siphon and must be kept full of fluid.
9. If the catheter is not draining properly, withdraw the catheter in 2.5-cm. (1-inch) increments until urine begins to flow. Do not dislodge catheter from bladder.	
10. The drainage is maintained continuously for several days.	
11. Upon order the catheter is clamped for 4 hours and released 15–30 minutes at a time.	
12. Have the patient attempt to void while the catheter is clamped. When the patient is able to void on his own, the catheter remains clamped.	12. Usually patients will void earlier after surgery with suprapubic drainage than with indwelling catheters.
13. The catheter is removed upon order and a sterile dressing is left over the needle or trocar or stab site.	13. Suprapubic drainage is considered more comfortable than an indwelling urethral catheter and there is less risk of bladder infection.

ACUTE RENAL FAILURE

Acute renal failure is a sudden and almost complete loss of kidney function caused by failure of the renal circulation or glomerular or tubular damage. The substances normally eliminated in the urine accumulate in the body fluids.

Precipitating Factors

1. Shock
2. Trauma
3. Septicemia
4. Dehydration
5. Hypersensitivity (allergic disorders)
6. Kidney stones
7. Nephrotoxic agents
8. Mismatched blood transfusion.

Altered Physiology

Hypotension or nephrotoxins → decrease in renal flow → decreased glomerular filtration rate → renal ischemia → tubular necrosis → tubular obstruction → oliguria.

Clinical Phases

1. Period of oliguria (urine volume less than 400–600 ml./24 hours). (However, there can be decrease in renal function with increasing nitrogen retention with the patient excreting 2–3 liters of urine daily—called high output failure.)
   a. Accompanied by rise in serum concentration of elements usually excreted by kidney (urea, creatinine, uric acid, organic acids and the intracellular cations—(potassium and magnesium).
   b. Clinical manifestations—scant bloody urine, lethargy, nausea.

2. Period of diuresis—gradually increasing urinary output reaching 2–6 liters or more daily.
3. Period of convalescence—restoration of renal function may take 6–12 months.

Preventive Measures

1. Initiate adequate hydration before surgical procedures, during intraoperative period and following operative procedures.
2. Avoid exposure to various nephrotoxins.
3. Monitor urinary output hourly in sick patients to detect onset of renal failure at the earliest moment. Give furosemide (Lasix), mannitol, etc. if necessary to maintain output around 60 ml./hour.
4. Treat hypotensive states promptly with steroids, fluid, blood, antibiotics, etc.
5. Schedule diagnostic studies requiring dehydration so that there are "rest days" especially in aged who may not have adequate renal reserve.
6. Avoid infections which may produce progressive renal damage.
7. Ensure that the patient has serial renal function tests while taking nephrotoxic antibiotics for prolonged periods (kanamycin, colistin, cephaloridine, etc.).

Objectives of Treatment and Nursing Management

A. *To remove the cause of renal failure if possible.*
   1. Rule out and treat urinary tract obstruction
      a. Plain film of abdomen
      b. Infusion pyelography to demonstrate kidney size, morphology, patency, and configuration of lower urinary tract
      c. Cystoscopy and retrograde study if necessary
      d. Arteriogram or radioisotope renogram or renoscan to evaluate arterial blood supply and detect kidney masses.
   2. Stop drugs that may be nephrotoxic.

B. *To prepare for peritoneal dialysis or hemodialysis to prevent metabolic deterioration (p. 476).*

C. *To restore adequate blood flow to the kidneys.*
   1. Give intravenous fluids and furosemide (Lasix) as directed to improve renal plasma flow, decrease intrarenal vascular resistance and increase blood flow to the renal cortex.
   2. Restore circulating blood volume.
   3. Control shock.
   4. Eliminate infection.
   5. Debride necrotic tissue.

D. *To maintain fluid and electrolyte balance.*
   1. Carry out biochemical studies as ordered. (Electrolyte administration is guided by serial measurements of central venous pressure, serum and urine electrolyte concentrations, fluid losses and the clinical status of the patient.)
   2. Give only enough fluids to replace current losses during oliguric phase (usually 400–600 ml./24 hours).
      a. Monitor the urinary output and urine specific gravity.
      b. Measure and record intake and output (include urine, gastric suction, stools, wound drainage, perspiration, etc.).

    c. Weigh patient daily to provide an index of fluid balance—expected weight loss 0.227–0.454 kg. (½–1 lb.) daily.

3. Limit dietary protein during oliguric phase to minimize protein breakdown. (See Diet for Renal Disease, below.)
    a. Give high caloric foods since carbohydrates have a greater protein-sparing power
    b. Give multivitamin supplements.

4. Measure and replace sodium losses especially if large losses occur from the gastrointestinal tract via vomiting or diarrhea.

5. Restrict sodium intake as ordered.

6. Observe fluid excess by assessing patient's clinical status—dyspnea, tachycardia, pulmonary edema, distended neck veins, peripheral edema.

7. Control potassium balance (protein catabolism causes release of cellular potassium into body fluids resulting in serious potassium intoxication).
    a. Evaluate for hyperkalemia (potassium intoxication) by assessment of blood determinations and elevation of P waves in ECG.
    b. Give potassium exchange resins—sodium polystyrene sulfonate (Kayexalate).
        (1) Orally
        (2) By retention enema as the colon is the principal site for potassium exchange.
            (a) Use catheter with balloon to facilitate retention if necessary.
            (b) Assist the patient to retain the resin 30–60 minutes to remove the potassium.
    c. Be prepared for cardiac arrest as increased potassium elevations lead to cardiac arrhythmias.
    d. Intravenous glucose and insulin is sometimes used as an emergency and temporary measure for potassium intoxication.

E. *To prevent infection.*
  1. Utilize environmental asepsis.
  2. Pay special attention to draining wounds, burns, etc. which may develop sepsis.
  3. Avoid use of indwelling urethral catheters if possible.
    a. Give meticulous catheter care to prevent cystitis and ascending pyelonephritis (p. 467). Obstructed catheter may lead to pyelonephritis.
    b. Utilize 3-way closed bladder irrigation system to decrease incidence of systemic infection if patient has to have indwelling catheter.
  4. Turn, cough and exercise the patient to prevent pulmonary infections.

F. *To anticipate and forestall complications.*
  1. Infection
  2. Potassium intoxication
  3. Acidosis
  4. Congestive heart failure; pulmonary edema
  5. Hypertension

Diet for Renal Disease

Objectives: to reduce the protein intake to a minimum in order to reduce the amount of nitrogenous waste products (which the damaged kidneys may not be able to eliminate).

       to provide enough calories for energy needs and protein-sparing effect.

       to restrict sodium intake to depress glomerular tubular imbalance as much as possible.

1. Protein-free diet is advocated during the initial stage of acute glomerulonephritis and acute renal failure.
2. Fruit juices fortified with sugar or dextrose are given to add calories and spare tissue protein.
3. The amount of juices given should not exceed the 24-hour fluid allowance. Give potassium-free juices if patient has oliguria.
4. A low protein diet is given when the patient's status improves.

LOW PROTEIN DIET

Foods to Avoid	Foods Allowed
Meat	Eggs (1–2 daily)
Fish	Milk (6½ ounces)
Cheese	Fruits
Vegetable proteins	Vegetables
Flour in any form	Meat is added gradually according to clinical response of patient

CHRONIC RENAL FAILURE

Chronic renal failure is a progressive deterioration in renal function which ends fatally in uremia (an excess of urea and other nitrogenous wastes in the blood) and its complications (unless hemodialysis or a kidney transplant is performed).

Reversible Causes

1. Urinary tract obstruction and infection
2. Infectious diseases which cause increased catabolism with retention of metabolites and hyperkalemia
3. Hypertension
4. Subacute bacterial endocarditis
5. Nephrotoxic (poisonous to kidney cells) agents

Clinical Manifestations

1. Gastrointestinal manifestations—anorexia, nausea, vomiting, hiccoughs, ulceration of gastrointestinal tract and hemorrhage.
2. Cardiopulmonary manifestations—hypertension, fibrinous pericarditis, pleuritis.
3. Nervous system manifestations—anxiety, irritability, delusions, hallucinations, drowsiness, muscle twitching, convulsions, coma.
4. Anemia
5. Skin discoloration (from retained urinary chromogen)
6. Uremic frost on face
7. Ammonia odor on breath

Diagnostic Evaluation

1. Anemia
2. Elevated serum creatinine
3. Elevated serum phosphorus
4. Decreased serum calcium
5. Low serum proteins, especially albumin
6. Usually low CO_2 and acidosis (low blood pH)

Treatment and Nursing Management

1. Treat reversible causes of chronic renal failure (see above).
2. Offer diet according to blood chemistry levels and clinical status of patient.
   a. Give 20–40 gm. of protein (high biological value) per day to reduce accumulation of protein-metabolic end products.
   b. Give additional amino acids.
   c. Offer supplementary B-complex vitamins as needed.
   d. Increase protein intake if patient is on a dialysis program.
3. Prevent water and electrolyte disturbances.
   a. Weigh patient daily to assess fluid overload or depletion. (Weight should not increase or decrease over 0.45 kg. [1 lb.] per day.)
   b. Treat acidosis if patient is symptomatic.
      (1) Assess patient for stupor, deep rapid breathing of Kussmaul type, shortness of breath on exertion, weakness, unconsciousness.
      (2) Replace bicarbonate stores by infusion or oral administration of sodium bicarbonate.
      (3) Give daily sodium requirements as ordered (determined by sodium balance studies and daily weights).
   c. Restrict or supplement potassium intake to prevent hyperkalemia and hypokalemia.
   d. Give fluids to maintain adequate urinary volume and avoid dehydration.
   e. Avoid restricting fluids for laboratory and radiologic examinations as dehydrating procedures are hazardous to these patients who cannot elaborate a concentrated urine.
4. Treat patient's discomforts symptomatically.
5. Treat associated cardiac conditions with digitalis, diuretics and antiarrhythmic agents to reverse congestive heart failure and to improve renal hemodynamics.
6. Prepare the patient for a chronic intermittent dialysis program if he is a candidate for this type of therapy.
7. Give special attention to "little things" as these chronically ill individuals become weary, discouraged and despondent.

GUIDELINES: *Assisting the Patient Undergoing Peritoneal Dialysis*

Peritoneal dialysis is a substitute for kidney function during renal failure. The peritoneum is used as a dialyzing membrane.

Purposes

1. To aid in the removal of toxic substances and metabolic wastes.
2. To remove excessive body fluid.
3. To assist in regulating the fluid balance of the body.

Equipment

Dialysis administration set (disposable)   Suture set
Peritoneal dialysis solution as ordered   Sterile gloves
Supplemental drugs as ordered   Skin germicide
Local anesthesia (2% procaine solution)

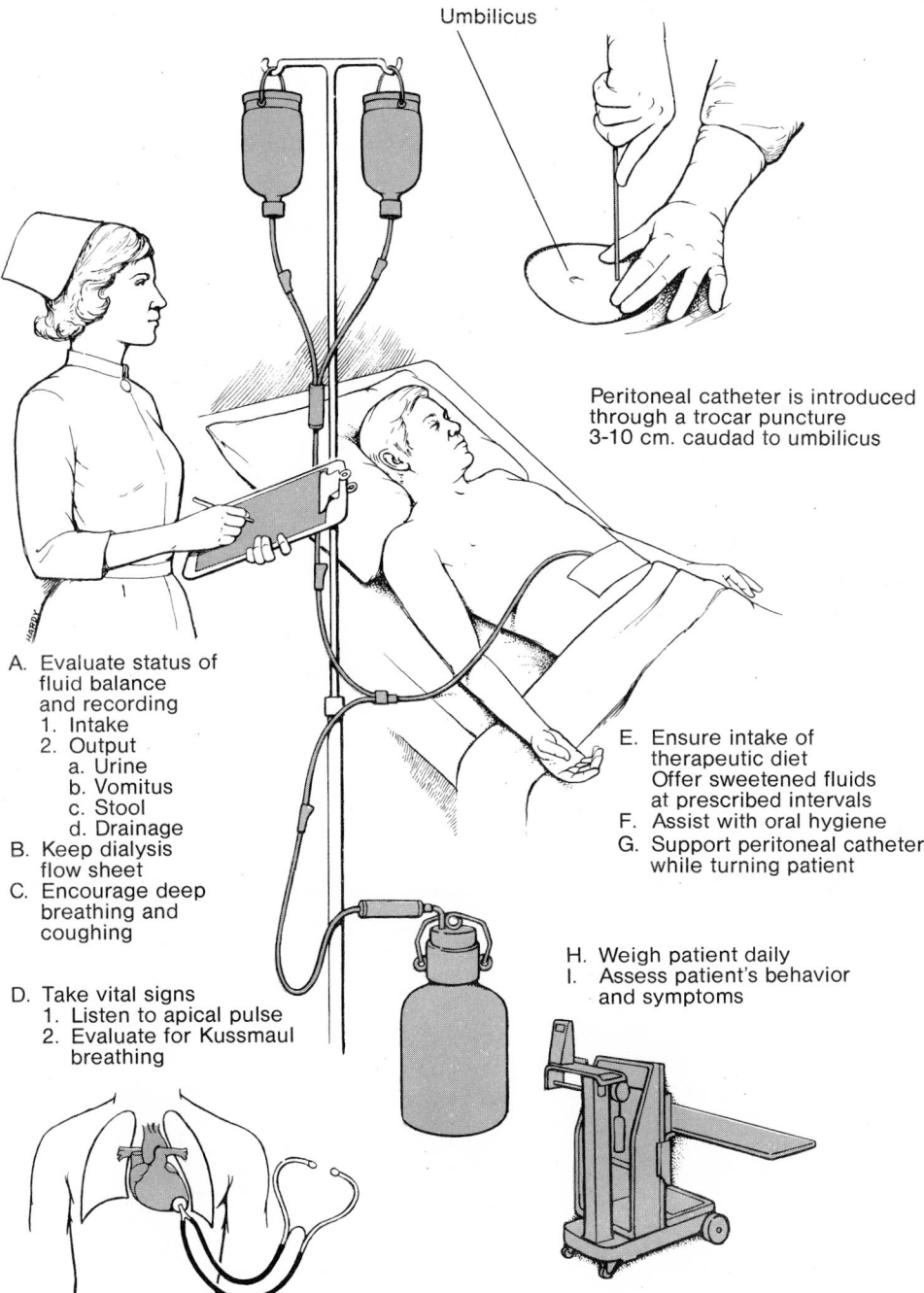

Umbilicus

Peritoneal catheter is introduced
through a trocar puncture
3-10 cm. caudad to umbilicus

A. Evaluate status of
   fluid balance
   and recording
   1. Intake
   2. Output
      a. Urine
      b. Vomitus
      c. Stool
      d. Drainage
B. Keep dialysis
   flow sheet
C. Encourage deep
   breathing and
   coughing

D. Take vital signs
   1. Listen to apical pulse
   2. Evaluate for Kussmaul
      breathing

E. Ensure intake of
   therapeutic diet
   Offer sweetened fluids
   at prescribed intervals
F. Assist with oral hygiene
G. Support peritoneal catheter
   while turning patient

H. Weigh patient daily
I. Assess patient's behavior
   and symptoms

Figure 7-6. Nursing management of patient undergoing peritoneal dialysis.

Procedure (Fig. 7-6)

Nursing Action	Rationale/Amplification
Preparatory Phase	
1. Prepare the patient emotionally and physically for the procedure.	1. Nursing support is offered by explaining procedure mechanics, providing opportunities for the patient to ask questions, allowing him to verbalize his feelings, and giving expert physical care.
2. Secure a signed operative permit.	
3. Weigh the patient before dialysis and every 24 hours thereafter, preferably on an in-bed scale.	3. The weight at the beginning of the procedure serves as a base line of information. Daily weight is helpful in assessing the state of hydration.
4. Take temperature, pulse, respiration and blood pressure readings prior to dialysis.	4. A knowledge of vital signs at the beginning of dialysis is necessary for comparing subsequent changes in vital signs.
5. Have the patient empty his bladder.	5. If the bladder is empty there is less likelihood of perforating it when the trocar is introduced into the peritoneum.
6. Make the patient comfortable in a supine position.	

Performance Phase

The following is a brief resumé of insertion of the peritoneal catheter which is done under strict asepsis.

Nursing Action	Rationale/Amplification
1. The abdomen is prepared surgically and the skin and subcutaneous tissues are infiltrated with a local anesthetic.	1. A surgical preparation of the skin minimizes or eliminates surface bacteria and decreases the possibility of wound contamination and infection.
2. A small midline stab wound is made 3-5 cm. below the umbilicus.	2. The midline area is relatively avascular.
3. The trocar is inserted through the incision with the stylet in place, or a thin stylet cannula may be inserted percutaneously.	
4. The patient is requested to raise his head from the pillow after the trocar is introduced.	4. This maneuver tightens the abdominal muscles and permits easier penetration of the trocar without danger of injury to the intra-abdominal organs.
5. When the peritoneum is punctured, the trocar is directed toward the left side of the pelvis. The stylet is removed, and the catheter is inserted through the trocar and maneuvered into position. After removal of the trocar, the skin is closed with purse-string suture that is looped around the catheter. A sterile dressing is placed around the catheter.	
6. Take blood pressure and pulse every 15 minutes during the first exchange and every hour thereafter.	6. A drop in blood pressure may indicate excessive fluid loss from the glucose concentrations of the dialyzing solutions. The heart rate is monitored for signs of arrhythmias. Changes in the vital signs may indicate impending shock or over-hydration.
7. Take patient's temperature every 4 hours, especially after catheter removal.	7. An infection is more apt to become evident after dialysis has been discontinued.

Nursing Action	**Rationale/Amplification**
8. Connect the catheter to the Y-tubing and allow 2 liters of warmed 37°C. (98.6°F.) dialyzing solution to run in rapidly (10–20 minutes).	8. The solution is warmed to body temperature for patient comfort and to prevent abdominal pain. Heating also causes dilation of the peritoneal vessels and increases urea clearance. The inflow solution should flow in a steady stream. If this does not occur, it may indicate displacement of the catheter or occlusion by a blood clot.
9. Allow the fluid to remain in the peritoneal cavity for the prescribed time period (30–45 minutes). Prepare the next exchange while the fluid is in the peritoneal cavity.	9. In order to remove potassium, urea and other waste materials, the solution must be in the peritoneal cavity for the prescribed time period.
10. Unclamp the outflow tube. Drainage should take approximately 20 minutes, although the time varies with each patient.	10. The outflow drainage should run by gravity in a free-flowing stream. A closed sterile connecting system is desirable to prevent ascending infection.
11. If the fluid is not draining properly move the patient from side to side and/or elevate the head of the bed to facilitate removal of peritoneal drainage.	
12. Keep an exact record of the patient's fluid balance during the dialysis.	12. Complications may arise if most of the fluid is not recovered.
13. When the outflow drainage ceases to run, clamp off the drainage tube and infuse the next exchange.	13. The amount of drainage should closely approximate or be slightly more than the amount administered.
14. The process is repeated until the blood chemistry levels approach normal. The usual time is 24–36 hours, but patients with high urea blood levels may require much longer periods. (The catheter may be left in situ and the dialysis done intermittently. This requires a special type of catheter that can be sealed to prevent bacterial contamination.)	
15. Heparin and an antibiotic may be added to an exchange when ordered.	15. The addition of heparin prevents fibrin clots from occluding the catheter. An antibiotic is used as prophylaxis against infection.
16. Promote patient comfort during dialysis: a. Give frequent back care and massage pressure areas. b. Change the dressing around the catheter, using *strict* asepsis.	a. The patient becomes fatigued during prolonged periods of dialysis.
17. Observe the patient for the following: a. Respiratory difficulty Elevate the head of the bed	a. This is caused by pressure from the fluid in the peritoneal cavity and upward displacement of the diaphragm producing shallow respirations. In severe respiratory difficulty, the fluid from the peritoneal cavity should be drained immediately and the physician notified.

Nursing Action	Rationale/Amplification
b. Severe abdominal pain (usually occurs at end of inflow or outflow period)	b. Pain may be caused by the dialyzing solutions not being at body temperature, incomplete drainage of solution, or as a fore warning of possible peritoneal infection. If severe pain persists, 10 ml. of 0.5% procaine may be instilled through the dialysis tubing immediately before each exchange. Patients sometimes develop peritonitis.
c. Bleeding	c. A small amount of bleeding around the catheter is not significant if it does not persist. During the first few exchanges, blood-tinged fluid from subcutaneous bleeding is not uncommon. The outflow drainage is usually straw-colored.
d. Shock	d. Symptoms of shock may occur due to excess fluid loss. If a sudden drop in blood pressure occurs, drain the peritoneal cavity, clamp the tubing and notify the physician.
e. Protein loss	e. There may be a significant protein loss because most serum proteins pass through the peritoneal membrane during dialysis. Serum albumin determinations are done frequently throughout the dialysis.
f. Leakage	f. If leakage occurs around the catheter, change the dressing frequently and use sterile plastic drapes to prevent contamination.

18. Keep accurate records.
    a. Amount of solution infused and recovered.
    b. Exact time of beginning and ending of each infusion.
    c. Fluid balance
    d. Number of exchanges
    e. Medications added to dialyzing solution
    f. Pre- and postdialysis weight of patient
    g. Assessment of patient's condition.

INFECTIONS OF THE URINARY TRACT

Predisposing Factors

1. Urinary stasis and obstruction—slowing of urinary flow causes kidney to be more susceptible to bacterial infection.
2. Presence of foreign body—indwelling catheter, stone
3. Neurogenic bladder dysfunctions
4. Diseases of blood vessels—(diabetes mellitus, arteriosclerosis)
5. Lowered body resistance

Pathways of Infection Within Urinary Tract

1. Kidney—from ureterovesical reflux (incompetence of ureterovesical valve which allows urine to regurgitate into ureters, usually at time of voiding)
2. Bladder—from bacteria ascending from urethra (or less commonly descending from kidney)
3. Prostate—from ascending urethral flora
4. Urethra—from ascending bacteria
5. Epididymis—from infected prostate
6. Testis—from bacteria via the blood stream

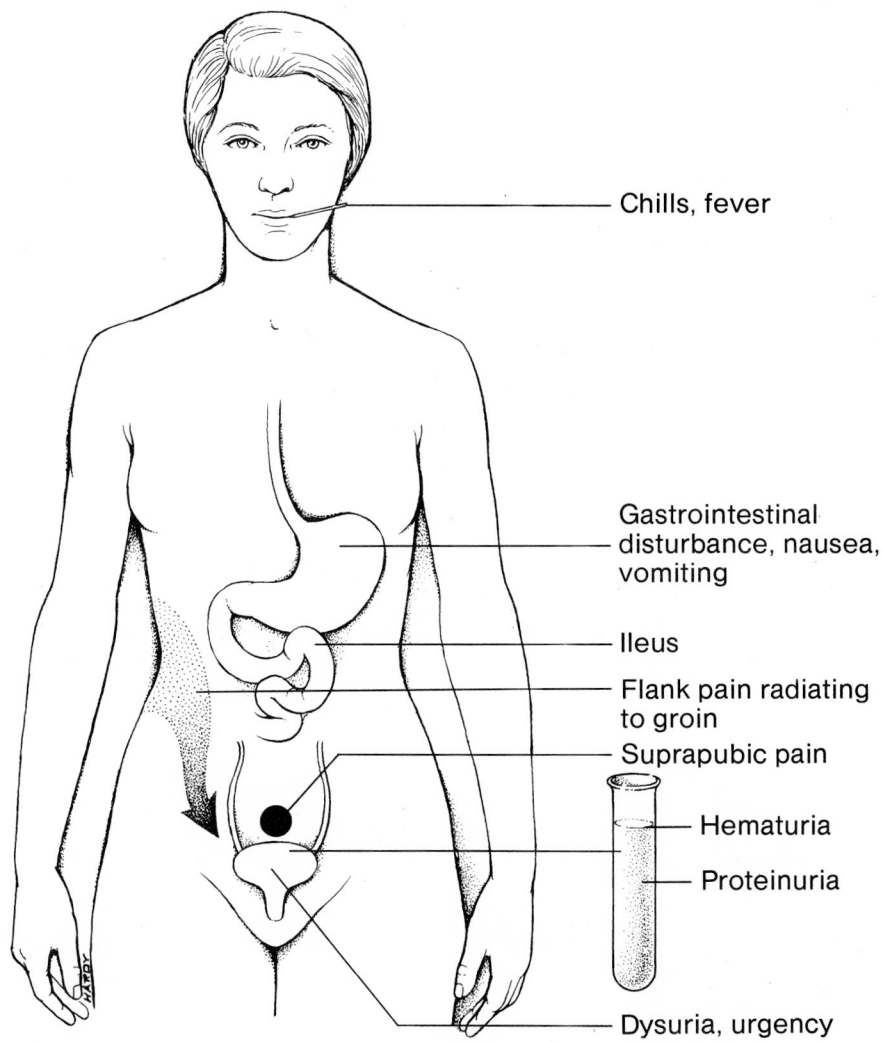

Figure 7-7. Assessment of patient with infection of genitourinary tract.

Cystitis

Cystitis is inflammation of the bladder.

Etiology

1. Urethral obstruction (most common)
2. Acute infections usually caused by *Escherichia coli*
3. Women more prone to develop acute cystitis due to length of urethra and anatomic proximity to vagina and periurethral glands
4. Upper urinary tract disease may produce recurrent bladder infection.

Clinical Manifestations

1. Frequency and urgency
2. Burning in the urethra
3. Pain in the region of the bladder
4. Changes in the composition of urine (pus and blood)

Treatment and Nursing Management

1. Do evaluation studies to determine if infection is secondary to a functional or structural abnormality (p. 456).
2. Remove the contributing cause(s) and source of obstruction if found (neoplasm of kidney or bladder calculus, prostatism, mechanical stricture, etc.).
3. Obtain uncontaminated urine specimen for culture and sensitivity studies so that appropriate drug may be determined (p. 463).
4. Give prescribed antibiotic or chemotherapeutic drug since urinary infections respond effectively to drugs that are excreted in the urine in high concentrations.
5. Encourage patient to drink adequate fluids to promote renal blood flow and to flush out bacteria in urinary tract. (But forcing of fluids may produce dilution of antimicrobial drugs.)
6. See that patient maintains an adequate urinary output (1000 ml. daily).
7. Give analgesic, antispasmodics and heat to the perineum to relieve pain, spasm and urgency.
8. Encourage bedrest during the acute phase.
9. Maintain an acid urine (pH 5.5) as invading organisms are not as viable in acid urine.

Prevention and Patient Teaching

1. Encourage patient to have follow-up urine studies (up to a year) to determine if asymptomatic infection is present—there is marked tendency for infection to recur.
2. Inform patients who have had urinary tract infections during pregnancy to have follow-up studies.
3. Remember that acute pyelitis in childhood may produce gastrointestinal symptoms.
4. Infections in any part of the urinary tract may persist for months or years without symptoms and eventually cause serious irreversible kidney damage.

Pyelonephritis

Pyelonephritis is an inflammation of the renal pelvis, tubules and interstitial tissue of one or both kidneys with variable manifestations. (Pyelonephritis may be acute, relapsing or chronic.)

Causes

1. Usually secondary to ureterovesical reflux (incompetence of ureterovesical valve which allows urine to regurgitate into ureters, usually at time of voiding).
2. Urinary obstruction
3. Renal disease
4. Trauma
5. Pregnancy
6. Metabolic disorders

Altered Physiology

Swelling of renal parenchyma→patchy distribution of acute infectious processes throughout kidney→swelling and scarring→kidney atrophy→renal failure.

Complications

1. Hypertension
2. Chronic infection (usually silent)
3. Renal insufficiency and renal failure

Clinical Manifestations

1. Symptoms vary from none to severe.
2. The patient may be asymptomatic for many years although renal damage may be extensive.
3. Scarring of kidneys may follow each acute infection causing the kidney to become atrophied.

Acute Pyelonephritis

1. Frequency, dysuria, burning on urination
2. Chills and fever with aching and malaise
3. Dull aching in back or pain over costovertebral angle
4. Pyuria and bacteriuria and casts in the urine sediment

Chronic Pyelonephritis
(caused by injury to kidneys)

1. Fatigue
2. Headache
3. Anorexia
4. Polyuria, excessive thirst
5. Weight loss
6. Symptoms of uremia

Objectives of Treatment and Nursing Management

A. *To find and treat factors known to produce urinary tract infection.*

B. *To obtain permanent eradication of bacteria from urinary tract.*

1. Obtain urine specimen for culture and sensitivity studies (under aseptic conditions) as choice of drug is based on sensitivity studies.
2. Give organism-specific antibiotic therapy. Antibacterial agent is maintained in urine at all times to prevent reseeding of residual foci of infection.

3. Obtain urine for repeat cultures to determine patient's response to treatment and to search for secondary organisms.
4. If patient has chronic or recurring infections:
    a. Employ continuous treatment with urine-sterilizing agents after initial antibiotic treatment has been employed.
    b. Advise patient to keep up this regimen for months to years until (1) there is no evidence of inflammation, (2) causative factors have been treated or controlled and (3) there is evidence of stability of renal function.
    c. Emphasize to patient that serial urine cultures and evaluation studies must be done for an indefinite period of time.
    d. Encourage patient to have blood counts and serum creatinine determinations if he is on long-term therapy.

Tuberculosis of the Kidney

Tuberculosis of the kidney (and urinary tract) is caused by the organism *Mycobacterium tuberculosis* and usually disseminates from the lungs via the bloodstream to the kidney and to other organs of the genitourinary tract.

Clinical Manifestations

1. Hematuria (microscopic or gross)
2. Bladder irritation—burning on urination, frequency, nocturia
3. Manifestations from infection of prostate and epididymis

Diagnostic Evaluation

1. Urine culture for tubercle bacilli (smears of urinary sediment also stained for acid-fast bacilli)
2. Excretory urogram—to reveal renal and ureteral lesions
3. Cystoscopic examination—to determine extent of bladder involvement, for biopsy purposes and for ureteral catheterization of each kidney to determine if one or both kidneys is affected.
4. Acid urine with persistent symptoms of cystitis and pyuria may yield a negative "routine" culture; it may take special culture media and up to 6 weeks to grow acid-fast bacillus.

NURSING ALERT:
1. The urine of the patient with renal tuberculosis is infectious.
2. A search for tuberculosis elsewhere in the body must be conducted when tuberculosis of the kidney or urinary tract is found.
3. Be alert for patient who has had previous contact with tuberculosis.

Treatment

1. Multiple drug regimen is more effective than single drugs.
    a. Isoniazid 100 mg., 3 times daily
    Sodium PAS 5000 mg., 3 times daily   (may produce skin rash)
    Cycloserine 250 mg, 2 times daily   Watch for bloating and loose stools

b. Ethionamide may be used instead of isoniazid
   (1) Watch for jaundice, particularly with the alcoholic patient.
   (2) Monthly liver function studies usually ordered for patient taking ethionamide.
c. Ethambutal may be combined with isoniazid and cycloserine.
2. Recently it has been found to be effective to give all medications together in a single daily dose.
3. The general health of patient should be promoted since renal tuberculosis is a manifestation of a systemic disease.
   a. Adequate rest
   b. Nutritious diet
   c. Avoidance of excessive exertion
4. Surgical intervention may be necessary to prevent obstructive problems and to remove severely infected organ. However, emphasis is on medical treatment.
5. Follow-up examination for lifetime—to detect reactivation of disease.
   a. Periodic urine cultures
   b. Excretory urograms as indicated

ACUTE GLOMERULONEPHRITIS

Acute glomerulonephritis is an inflammatory disease involving the renal glomeruli of both kidneys. It is thought to involve an antigen-antibody reaction which produces damage to the glomerular capillaries.

Etiology
1. Antecedent infection of pharynx and tonsils due to beta-hemolytic streptococci—certain strains are nephritogenic (capable of initiating nephritis).
2. May follow pneumococcal or staphylococcal infection.
3. Pyoderma (impetigo) is a common antecedent in children under 6.

Altered Physiology
Inflammation and swelling of glomeruli→narrowing of glomerular tufts→obstruction of blood flow through capillaries→interference with glomerular filtration→atrophy and disappearance of nephrons→renal failure.

Clinical Manifestations
1. The disease may be so mild that it is discovered accidently through a routine urinalysis.
2. History of preceding pharyngitis or tonsillitis with fever (7–20 days previously)
3. Scant smoky or bloody urine
4. Facial edema and edema of extremities
5. Fatigue and anorexia
6. Mild hypertension
7. Tenderness at costovertebral angle
8. Anemia—from azotemia (nitrogen retention in blood)

Diagnostic Evaluation
1. Urinalysis—hematuria (microscopic or gross), proteinuria (2+ to 4+), red cell casts, white cells, renal epithelial cells and various casts in the sediment.

2. Blood—elevated blood urea nitrogen and serum creatinine, low total serum protein level, Anti-streptolysin O (ASO) and CRP (C-reactive protein) titer rises during course of disease.
3. Needle biopsy—reveals obstruction of glomerular capillaries from proliferation of endothelial cells.

Clinical Course

1. Diuresis usually starts 1–2 weeks after onset of symptoms.
   a. Renal clearances and blood urea concentration return to normal.
   b. Edema decreases and hypertension lessens.
   c. Microscopic proteinuria or hematuria may persist many months.
2. Recovery is usual in children and young adults; in older person the disease may progress to chronic glomerulonephritis.

Objectives of Treatment and Nursing Management

A. *To protect the poorly functioning kidneys.*
   1. Encourage bedrest during the acute phase. (Rest also facilitates diuresis.)
      a. Keep patient at rest until urine clears and BUN and blood pressure are normal.
      b. Restrict normal activities until proteinuria and hematuria clear as increasing activity may increase urinary abnormalities.
      c. Allow patient to resume activity on a gradual basis.
   2. Restrict dietary protein moderately if there is oliguria and the BUN is elevated.
      a. Give carbohydrates liberally to give energy and to reduce catabolism of protein.
      b. Restrict protein more drastically if acute renal failure develops (see p. 474).
   3. Measure and record intake and output.
   4. Give fluids according to patient's urinary output and body weight.

B. *To recognize and treat complications promptly.*
   1. Explain to patient that he must have follow-up evaluations of blood pressure, urinary protein and BUN concentrations to determine if there is exacerbation of disease activity.
   2. Recognize and treat intercurrent infections promptly.
      a. Long-term penicillin therapy may be required to prevent recurrent streptococcal infections.
   3. Watch for symptoms of renal failure—oliguria, increasing azotemia and acidosis—(see p. 472).
   4. Evaluate patient for:
      a. Hypertensive encephalopathy
      b. Cardiac failure and pulmonary edema

NEPHROTIC SYNDROME

The *Nephrotic Syndrome* is a clinical disorder characterized by (1) marked proteinuria, (2) hypoalbuminuria, (3) edema and (4) hypercholesterolemia.

Etiology

Seen in any condition that seriously damages the glomerular capillary membrane.
1. Chronic glomerulonephritis
2. Diabetes mellitus (intercapillary glomerulosclerosis)

3. Amyloidosis of kidney
4. Systemic lupus erythematosus
5. Toxins
6. Renal vein thrombosis
7. Primary lipoid nephrosis in children (see p. 1244)

Clinical Manifestations

1. Insidious onset of edema; easily pitting edema
2. Proteinuria (4–5 gm. daily)
3. Extensive depletion of body proteins (hypoalbuminemia) from extensive urinary protein losses.
4. Hypercholesterolemia (high blood cholesterol level)

Diagnostic Evaluation

1. Needle biopsy of kidney—for histologic examination of renal tissue to confirm diagnosis.
2. Serum electrolyte evaluations (protein, albumin, etc.)
3. Triglyceride profile—to evaluate degree of hyperlipemia
4. Urinary tests—for microscopic hematuria, granular and epithelial cell casts
5. Renal function tests

Treatment and Nursing Management

1. Keep on bedrest for a few days—to mobilize edema.
2. Utilize dietary treatment—to replace protein losses.
   a. Low sodium diet (500 mg./day)—to control severe edema.
   b. High protein diet—to replenish wasted tissues and restore body proteins.
   c. High caloric diet (25–50 cal./kg. body weight/day)
3. Give diuretics—if renal insufficiency is not severe.
4. Give adrenocorticosteroids (prednisone)—to reduce edema and proteinuria.
5. Protect patient from infection—which causes exacerbation of symptoms.
6. See page 485 for nursing the patient with acute glomerulonephritis, and page 475 for care of patient with chronic renal failure.

HYDRONEPHROSIS

Hydronephrosis is distention of the pelvis and calyces of one or both kidneys due to obstruction of urinary flow. (A partial block may occur at any level in the urinary tract.)

Causes

1. Congenital causes—aberrant vessels, stenosis of ureter
2. Progressive changes in bladder, ureters and kidneys from:
   a. Obstruction from enlarged prostate
   b. Obstructing calculus
   c. Malignant lesion (cancer of prostate, bladder or cervix)
   d. Obstruction of ureter—from calculus, stricture, etc.
   e. Neurogenic causes

Altered Physiology

Interference with passage of urine from kidney→chronic infection→increasing pressure→ distention of renal pelvis and calyces→atrophy of renal parenchyma (as one kidney undergoes gradual destruction, the contralateral kidney gradually enlarges [compensatory hypertrophy]).

Clinical Manifestations

1. Often asymptomatic and insidious onset.
2. Aching in flank and back (present with acute obstruction)
3. Bladder irritability—fever and dysuria if infection is present
4. Gastrointestinal disturbances
5. Chills, fever, tenderness, pyuria—from infection
6. Hematuria—hydronephrotic kidney may bleed from congestion
7. Uremia—if condition is bilateral and advanced.

Diagnostic Evaluation

Complete urographic survey:

1. Excretory urography—gives information regarding cause, duration and reversibility of hydronephrosis
2. Total creatinine clearance
3. Isotope renography
4. Renal scan
5. Retrograde pyelography (done occasionally)

Treatment and Nursing Management

Objectives: to achieve complete relief of urinary stasis.
          to treat the patient's infection.
          to restore and conserve renal function.

1. Relieve obstruction, etc.
     Urine may have to be diverted by nephrostomy.
     (1) Place ureteral catheter to decompress kidney—if patient is having severe flank pain.
     (2) See page 496 for care of patient having a nephrostomy.
2. Eradicate infection as residual urine in calyces produces infection and pyelonephritis.
3. Prepare for surgical intervention to correct obstruction.
     a. Nephrectomy—if one kidney is severely damaged.
     b. Operations to improve drainage of kidney, including pyeloplasty—plastic operation to remove and correct results of obstruction at ureteropelvic junction.
     c. See page 494 for care of patient having urological surgery.

NEPHROPTOSIS

Nephroptosis refers to the downward displacement or falling of the kidney.

Causes

1. Congenital defects
2. Loss of musculature of abdominal wall
3. Underweight, poor posture (lack of perirenal fat)

Clinical Manifestations

1. Pain; dull dragging pain in lumbar area; however nephroptosis is a rare cause of backache.
   a. May be acute or chronic
   b. Dietl's crisis—severe pain as a result of kinking of ureter or torsion of renal pedicle
2. Fatigue
3. Gastrointestinal disturbances

Diagnostic Evaluation

1. History and physical examination.
2. Retrograde pyelography—to determine degree of renal mobility and rotation and presence of distortions of ureters and pelvis.

Treatment and Nursing Management

1. Exercises to improve posture and strengthen abdominal muscles.
2. Use of a supporting kidney belt (helpful to some, of questionable value to others).
   a. Adjust belt with patient lying down with hips elevated.
   b. Tighten belt from below and then upward.
3. Rest in bed with foot of bed elevated during painful episodes.
4. Surgical intervention: nephropexy—surgical elevation and fixation of a ptosed (fallen) kidney (rarely used unless there is associated hydronephrosis).
5. See page 494 for nursing management of patient following urological surgery.

UROLITHIASIS

Urolithiasis refers to the presence of stones in the urinary system.

Causes

1. Obstruction and urinary stasis
2. Infection—particularly of urea-splitting organisms (*Proteus vulgaris* and some staphylococcus strains)
3. Dehydration and urine concentration—produces colloid precipitation
4. Immobilization—produces slowing of renal drainage and altered calcium metabolism
5. Hypercalcemia (abnormally high concentration of blood calcium compounds) and Hypercalciuria (abnormally large amounts of calcium in urine)
   a. Hyperparathyroidism
   b. Excessive intake of vitamin D
   c. Excessive intake of milk and alkali
   d. Myeloproliferative disease (unusual proliferation of blood cells derived from bone marrow—leukemia, polycythemia vera)
6. Excessive excretion of uric acid (gout)
7. Vitamin A deficiency
8. Heredity plays a part in calcium oxalate stones (most common type)

Clinical Features

1. The problem occurs predominantly in the 3rd to 5th decade, affecting men more than women.
2. The majority of stones contain calcium or magnesium in combination with phosphorus or oxalate.

3. Infection and obstruction may cause destruction of renal tissue; large nonobstructive stones may cause serious kidney damage from ischemia and necrosis.
4. Most renal stones migrate downward and are discovered in the lower ureter.

Preventive Measures

1. Encourage a high fluid intake to keep solutes diluted.
2. Give appropriate antibiotic therapy for infections.
3. See that patient avoids periods of recumbency.
4. Advise patients to avoid excessive ingestion of vitamins and minerals, especially vitamin D.
5. Correct obstruction and stasis in urinary tract promptly.
6. Change acidity of urine depending on stone type.
7. Give special medications as prescribed for chronic stone-formers. The drug depends on the stone type (methylene blue, magnesium oxide, pyridoxine, phosphates, penicillamine, allopurinol).

Clinical Manifestations

Dependent upon presence of obstruction, infection, edema.

1. Pain
   a. Discomfort in renal region with sudden sharp pain radiating down ureter.
   b. Renal colic—severe pain caused by obstruction or passage of stone in the renal pelvis or ureter.
   c. Pain may be referred to testicle in male and radiate to vulva in female.
2. Gastrointestinal symptoms
   a. Due to renal-intestinal reflexes and anatomic relation of kidneys to stomach, pancreas, colon, etc.
   b. Includes nausea, vomiting, diarrhea, abdominal discomfort.
3. Hematuria
4. Symptoms of urinary tract infection—chills, fever, dysuria

Diagnostic Evaluation

1. Roentgenography of entire urinary tract—the majority of stones are radiopaque.
2. Cystoscopy.
3. Serum protein concentration, blood urea, serum concentrations of calcium, phosphorus, chloride, carbon dioxide combining power, alkaline phosphatase, uric acid.
4. Urinalysis for:
   a. Red cells
   b. Gram stain of sediment—for evidences of infection and to determine predominant crystals
   c. Urine culture—to identify bacteria and to provide spectrum of sensitivity to antimicrobial agents
   d. Urinary pH—to determine acidity or alkalinity
5. Urinary excretory studies for calcium, phosphorus, uric acid, cystine and oxalate.

Treatment and Nursing Management

1. Encourage patient to drink large quantities of water to ensure high urinary output.
2. Strain all urine to obtain the crystals or calculus for chemical analysis to establish the etiology of stone formation.

3. Employ principles of diet therapy (Table 7-1) and pharmacology if stone composition is known—to reduce the cause of stone ingredient from the diet.
   a. Calcium oxalate lithiasis and calcium phosphate lithiasis
      (1) Acidify the urine.
      (2) Give diet low in calcium and phosphorus and oxalate.
      (3) Encourage high input of fluids to keep solutes diluted.

TABLE 7-1 MODERATELY REDUCED CALCIUM AND PHOSPHORUS DIET

(This diet will contain from 500–700 mg. of calcium and from 1000–1200 mg. of phosphorus[*])

Foods Allowed	Foods to be Avoided
Beverages Coffee, Postum, Sanka, tea, ginger ale	*Beverages* Carbonated "soft" drinks; cocoa.
Milk Limited to 1 cup (½ pint) a day. Cream may be substituted for part of the milk.	
Cheese Pot or cottage cheese only. Limited to 2 ozs.	*Cheese* All except pot or cottage cheese.
Fats As desired	
Eggs Limited to 1 a day; egg whites as desired.	
Meat, fish, fowl Limited to 4 ozs. daily of beef, lamb, pork, veal, chicken, turkey, fish. See those to be avoided.	*Meat, fish, fowl* Brains, heart, liver, kidney, sweetbreads. Game (pheasant, rabbit, deer, grouse). Sardines, fish roe.
Soups and broths All. Cream soups made with milk allowance only.	
Vegetables At least 3 servings besides potato. One or 2 servings of deep green or deep yellow vegetables to be included daily.	*Vegetables* Beet greens, chard, collards, mustard greens, spinach, turnip greens. Dried beans, peas, lentils, soybeans.
Fruits All except rhubarb. Include citrus fruit daily.	*Fruits* Rhubarb
Breads, cereals, macaroni products White, enriched bread, rolls and crackers except those made from self-rising white flour. Farina (not enriched), cornflakes, corn meal, hominy grits, rice, Rice Krispies, Puffed Rice. Macaroni, spaghetti, noodles.	*Breads, cereals, macaroni products* Whole-grain breads, cereals and crackers. Rye bread. All breads made with self-rising flour. Oatmeal, brown and wild rice. Bran, Bran Flakes, wheat germ. All dry cereals except those allowed.
Desserts Fruit pies, fruit cobblers, fruit ices, gelatin. Puddings made with allowed milk and egg. Angel food cake. (Do not use packaged mixes.)	*Desserts* All except those allowed.
Condiments Sugar, jellies, honey, salt, pepper, spices.	*Miscellaneous* Nuts, peanut butter, chocolate, cocoa. Condiments having a calcium or a phosphate base. (Read labels.)

[*] Adapted from Anderson, L., et al.: Nutrition in Nursing. Philadelphia, J. B. Lippincott, 1972.

   b. Uric acid lithiasis
      (1) Offer low purine diet to reduce output of uric acid in urine.
      (2) Give allopurinol (Zyloprim) to reduce serum uric acid and urinary uric acid excretion.
      (3) Alkalinize the urine.
   c. Cystine lithiasis
      (1) Offer low protein diet
      (2) Alkalinize urine
      (3) Give oral administration of sodium bicarbonate, citrate mixtures or penicillamine as directed.
4. Treat infection (if present) with appropriate drugs.
5. Correct obstructive process to prevent impairment of tubular function, atrophy of nephrons, reduced renal blood flow and increased susceptibility to infection.
6. Prepare for surgical intervention if patient's condition indicates.

Surgical Procedures

Objective: to remove stone with a minimum of trauma to the kidney.
   1. Cystoscopic for stone extraction from distal ureter.
   2. Ureterolithotomy—removal of a stone lodged in the ureter.
   3. Pyelolithotomy—removal of a stone from kidney pelvis.
   4. Nephrolithotomy—incision into kidney for removal of stone.
   5. Nephrectomy—removal of kidney indicated when kidney is extensively and irreparably damaged and is no longer a functioning organ.

Diet Therapy for Kidney Stones

Objective: to encourage high input of fluid to keep solutes diluted.
            to reduce calcium intake.
Since 95% of kidney stones contain calcium combined with phosphate or another substance the diet selected is a moderately reduced calcium and phosphorus diet (Table 7-1).

TUMORS OF THE KIDNEY

Types of Kidney Tumors

   1. Tumors of the renal parenchyma
   2. Tumors of the renal pelvis
   3. Tumors of the renal parenchyma of children; usually of embryonal origin (Wilms' tumor)

General Considerations

   1. All renal tumors should be considered malignant until proven otherwise.
   2. Adenocarcinoma is the most common malignant renal tumor and occurs more frequently in males; it metastasizes early.
   3. Many renal tumors produce no symptoms and are discovered on routine physical examination as an abdominal mass.

Clinical Manifestations

1. Hematuria (intermittent, microscopic or gross)
2. Low grade fever, anemia, weight loss
3. Palpable mass in flank (late); dull ache in flank
4. Gastrointestinal symptoms—due to reflex action or encroachment on intraperitoneal organs.
5. Metastatic manifestations (such as severe bone pain, etc.) may be first indication.

Diagnostic Evaluation

1. I.V.P. and I.V. drip nephrotomogram.
2. Cystoscopic examination—for visualization of tumor
3. Exfoliative cytology of urinary sediment for exfoliated cells (tumors of renal pelvis)
4. Assessment of urinary lactic dehydrogenase activity; this enzyme may be elevated in carcinoma of the kidney, bladder, prostate, infection, etc.
5. Renal angiogram

Treatment

1. Radical nephrectomy (removal of kidney) perirenal tissue, lymph nodes and adjacent organs if involved (spleen bowel, tail of pancreas) if tumor is operable. (See p. 497 for nursing management following renal surgery.)
2. Radiation therapy if tumor is radiosensitive, or as palliative measure for patients with inoperable tumor. (See p. 882 for nursing management of patient with cancer.)
3. Chemotherapy or regional chemotherapy (Cytoxan and 5-fluorouracil) injected in tumors of solitary kidney or inoperable neoplasms.
4. Hormone therapy—medroxyprosterone acetate (Provera) or testosterone propionate.

INJURIES TO THE KIDNEY

Types of Injuries

1. Simple bruising and ecchymosis (contusion)
2. Lacerations of kidney
3. Rupture or renal vascular pedicle injury—produces massive bleeding

Major Problems Following Kidney Trauma

1. Control of hemorrhage—may be persistent or recurring
2. Injuries to other organs
3. Injuries vary from contusion to complete avulsion (tearing away)

Clinical Manifestations

1. Pain—costovertebral, flank, upper abdomen
2. Hematuria—usually gross
3. Nausea, vomiting, abdominal rigidity—from ileus (seen when there is retroperitoneal bleeding)
4. Shock if injury is severe.

Diagnostic Evaluation

1. History of injury
2. Urine studies for hematuria
3. Plain film of abdomen—to determine presence of other fractures (pelvis, ribs, transverse processes of lumbar vertebrae)
4. Excretory urograms—to define extent of injury of involved kidney and establish location and condition of contralateral kidney
5. Renal scanning—to evaluate renal blood flow and tubular function
6. Arteriographic visualization—to assess vascular integrity, outline renal parenchyma

Complications

1. Hemorrhage
2. Perinephritis infection

Treatment and Nursing Management

1. Place patient on bedrest.
2. Take blood pressure and pulse frequently—to assess for bleeding and impending shock.
3. Save, inspect and compare each urine specimen—to follow the course and degree of hematuria.
4. Carry out serial hematocrit and hemoglobin determinations—to assess degree of anemia as progressive anemia indicates hemorrhage.
5. Evaluate the patient frequently during the first few days following injury.
   a. Assess for flank and abdominal pain, muscle spasm and swelling over flank.
   b. Watch for any *sudden* change in patient's condition. This may indicate hemorrhage and require surgical intervention.
6. Avoid narcotic analgesia—may mask accompanying abdominal symptoms.
7. Prepare for surgical exploration if patient has increasing pulse rate, hypotension or shock (drainage of kidney region, repair of kidney, nephrectomy).
8. Give antibiotics as directed to discourage infection—from perirenal hematoma and/or urinoma (cyst containing urine).
9. Encourage patient to have follow-up examinations after discharge—to detect late developing complications (post-traumatic hypertension, destruction of renal function)

NURSING MANAGEMENT OF
THE PATIENT UNDERGOING UROLOGICAL SURGERY

Preoperative Nursing Care

Objective: to restore the patient to as normal a physiological state as possible with as little psychological trauma and physical morbidity as possible.

A. *To recognize the fear and anxiety of the patient concerning the threat of impending surgery.*
   1. Keep in mind that most patients entering the hospital with urological conditions have pain, fever, hematuria, difficulty in voiding, etc.
   2. Encourage the patient to recognize and express his feelings of anxiety.
   3. Obtain patient's confidence by establishing a relationship of trust and by giving gentle and considerate care.

4. Increase the patient's understanding of what to expect during the pre- and post-operative periods.
5. Assess for alertness, appetite and general well-being of the patient.
6. Avoid physical inactivity.
7. Give preoperative medications as prescribed to allay worry and fear.

B. *To assess anatomic and functional status of urinary tract and kidneys.*
   1. Diagnostic evaluation studies:
      a. Serum electrolyte studies
      b. Serum creatinine or blood urea nitrogen determinations
      c. Fractional determination of phenolsulfonphthalein excretion to assess tubular function
      d. Intravenous urogram
      e. Radioisotope renography
   2. Give antibacterial agents as indicated before surgery especially in following instances:
      a. Prostatic operations
      b. Surgery upon infected kidneys, ureters, bladder

C. *To assess cardiopulmonary status of the patient.*
   1. Do an electrocardiogram on all patients over 50. The preoperative cardiogram also serves as a base-line reference in event of postoperative cardiopulmonary complications.
   2. Secure a chest x-ray.
   3. Ensure that the blood volume is as normal as possible.
      a. Carry out total blood volume determination preoperatively when indicated.
      b. Give transfusions of whole blood, packed red cells, plasma when indicated.
   4. Assess status of vascular system of lower extremities (especially varicosities).
      a. Elevate patient's leg and apply elastic stockings to minimize stasis in superficial veins.
      b. Encourage patients to do leg exercises.
   5. Inquire if patient has any bleeding tendencies.
   6. Teach the patient deep breathing exercises and an effective cough routine (p. 148).
   7. Manage co-existing diseases (diabetes, congestive heart failure).

D. *To discover and correct any abnormalities of fluid and electrolyte balance.*
   1. Weigh patient daily to determine status of fluid balance.
   2. Assess state of tongue and skin turgor; maintain the hematocrit at optimal level as possible (normal—45%).
   3. Measure and record intake and output as an index of hydration.

E. *To determine the drug and allergy history of the patient in order that therapeutic corrections be made if necessary.*
   1. Antihypertensives and tranquilizers—predispose to refractory hypotension during general anesthesia
   2. Anticoagulants—depress prothrombin activity; can produce hemorrhagic complications especially in prostatic surgery and operations on retroperitoneal area.
   3. Adrenal cortical steroids—produce adrenal insufficiency during periods of stress
   4. Anticholinergics and antihistamines—may impair emptying of bladder
   5. Alcohol—previous overuse may precipitate onset of delirium tremens

Postoperative Nursing Care

Objective: to reduce factors that cause complications.

A. *To promote the safety and comfort of the patient.*
1. Employ frequent and close observation of blood pressure, pulse and respiration in order to recognize symptoms of shock, hemorrhage and early atelectasis.
2. Give postoperative sedation and pain control on an individual basis to reduce spliting of respiratory movements and to permit coughing.
3. Be alert for symptoms of postoperative ileus (fairly common following renal surgery).
   a. Assess for abdominal distention, pain and lack of intestinal peristalsis (determined by stethoscope auscultation).
   b. Avoid oral intake for patient until active bowel sounds are heard (auscultation) or passage of flatus is noted.
   c. Give adequate and appropriate fluid replacement intravenously.
   d. Give enema or rectal tube with neostigmine methylsulfate (Prostigmin) if patient is uncomfortable from gas (rectal tube may be contraindicated in prostatism); encourage moving and turning.
   e. Encourage patient to use bedside commode as soon as possible.
4. Weigh patient daily to determine status of fluid balance; adjust fluid intake to maintain patient's weight within 2% of preoperative level.
5. Give inhalation therapy (IPPB) (p. 134) to encourage deep respiratory movements and aid in expectoration of tracheobronchial secretions.
6. Give antibiotics as necessary on the basis of culture identification of causative organism.
7. Employ early ambulation techniques as an aid in preventing thromboembolic episodes and improving patient endurance.
   a. Ambulation contraindicated in prostatic patients with bleeding and with some types of plastic reconstruction surgery.
   b. Encourage patient to do leg exercises in bed.
8. Make certain that drainage tubes are functioning as almost all urological patients have tissue drains, tubes or catheters.
   a. Make sure indwelling catheter is dependent and draining.
      (1) Tape catheter to thigh to relieve traction on bladder.
      (2) Give meticulous catheter care (see p. 467).
   b. Change dressings as indicated when patient has profuse drainage.
   c. Observe patients with prostatic drainage as they have a tendency to bleed.
      (1) Irrigate catheter as often as every 30 minutes to flush out clots, or use continuous bladder irrigation at sufficiently rapid rate to keep drainage clear.
      (2) Institute straight drainage as soon as drainage is clear.
   d. Employ care with patient with nephrostomy tube drainage (intubation of kidney used as a method of temporary or rarely permanent diversion of urine).
      (1) Purpose of nephrostomy drainage:
         (a) To provide drainage from kidney after surgery.
         (b) To conserve and permit physiological restoration of renal tissue that has been traumatized by obstructive disease.
         (c) To provide drainage when ureter is no longer functioning.
      (2) Evaluate for bleeding from nephrostomy site (main complication of nephrostomy).
      (3) Do not clamp the nephrostomy tube.
      (4) Irrigate nephrostomy tube only by direct order of physician.

(5) Place gauze moistened with benzalkonium chloride around opening of nephrostomy tube to prevent bacterial growth in this area.

e. Assess patient with indwelling ureteral catheter (utilized to permit drainage from affected kidney).

(1) Ureteral catheters are inserted through a cystoscope and left in place for a period of time.

(2) Tape catheter to thigh to reduce pulling on catheter.

(3) Make notation on nursing care plan that catheter is a *ureteral* catheter.

(4) Do not irrigate a ureteral catheter; this is done by the urologist.

3. *To assess patient constantly for complications.*

1. Hemorrhage (and shock)—chief danger following renal surgery.

a. Evaluate patients who have had prostatic surgery, nephrostomy or nephrectomy especially for hemorrhage.

b. Employ adequate blood transfusion therapy before surgery.

c. Replace blood loss with fresh whole blood.

2. Acute renal failure

a. Watch patients who have prolonged surgery, shock or arterial hypotension for a period of time.

b. Measure urinary volume to determine if oliguria is present.

c. See page 472 for treatment of renal failure.

3. Infection

4. Postoperative atelectasis

a. Utilize preventive techniques of deep breathing, exercise and coughing.

b. Stimulate coughing by tracheal suctioning (p. 101) if necessary to dislodge mucous plug.

c. Prepare for bronchoscopic aspiration if necessary.

d. Give intermittent positive pressure breathing treatments as directed.

5. Pulmonary embolism

a. Prevent embolic episodes by early ambulation, passive and active leg exercises and elastic compression bandages.

b. Examine and measure circumference of calves of legs daily.

c. Examine for positive Homan's sign—pain in calf on dorsiflexion of the foot (see p. 80).

d. Assess patient for low grade fever and elevation of pulse rate.

e. See page 155 for treatment.

INJURIES TO THE BLADDER

Types of Bladder Injuries

1. Contusion of bladder
2. Intraperitoneal rupture
3. Extraperitoneal rupture } or combination of both

Problems Associated with Bladder Injury

1. With injury there is a rise in intravesical (within bladder) pressure which produces extravasation of urine into the peritoneal cavity or perivesical space.

2. Rupture of the bladder requires immediate treatment.

Clinical Manifestations

1. Shock and hemorrhage—pallor, rapid and increasing pulse rate
2. Suprapubic pain and soreness
3. Rigid abdomen—indicates intraperitoneal rupture
4. Gross hematuria
5. Failure to void

Diagnostic Evaluation

1. Cystogram—to detect and localize perforation of urinary bladder
2. Plain film of abdomen—may show associated pelvic fracture
3. Excretory urogram—to survey the kidneys for injury

Treatment

1. Catheterize patient to ascertain if there is urethral continuity.
   a. Indwelling catheter serves as a means of continuous urinary drainage.
   b. Catheter also serves as a splint to urethra if urethra has been injured.
2. Treat for shock and hemorrhage.
3. Prepare for surgical intervention if bladder rupture has occurred.
   a. Bladder tears will be sutured.
   b. Extravasated blood and urine will be drained and urine diverted with suprapubic cystostomy and indwelling catheter.
4. Observe drainage systems after surgery.
   a. Suprapubic cystostomy drainage—until healing of bladder is complete (p. 470)
   b. Indwelling urethral catheter drainage—to divert urine drainage and permit suprapubic incision to heal.
   c. Perivesical areas drained with Penrose drain (will be brought out through suprapubic incision).

Nursing Management

See page 494 for nursing management of patient with urological surgery.

TUMORS OF THE BLADDER

Causes

1. Cigarette smoking (now thought to be one of principal causes)
2. Prolonged exposure to certain dyes (aromatic amines)
3. Chronic bladder irritation
4. Bladder schistosomiasis (rare in U.S.)

Incidence

1. Bladder tumors comprise 2% of all malignancies and account for 3% of all cancer deaths.
2. They are seen 3 times more frequently in males, occurring after the 5th decade.
3. These tumors usually affect the base of the bladder and may obstruct one or both ureteral orifices.

Clinical Manifestations

1. Painless gross hematuria (most characteristic presenting sign)
2. Symptoms of bladder infection—dysuria, frequency, urgency, chills
3. Pelvic or back pain from distant metastasis

Diagnostic Evaluation

1. Cystoscopic examination for visualization and biopsy of lesion
2. Bimanual examination of pelvis
3. Urinalysis—shows blood and bacteria
4. Cytology study of fresh urinary sediment to assess for malignant transitional cells shed from tumor
5. Intravenous urogram to rule out ureteral obstruction
6. Enzyme studies—urinary lactic dehydrogenase and alkaline phosphatase which may or may not be elevated (a nonspecific test)
7. Chest x-ray and bone survey to demonstrate distant metastasis

Treatment

A. *Underlying Rationale*

1. There is no single method of treatment. The procedure of choice depends upon the characteristics of the tumor and whether or not bladder-wall infiltration and local or distant metastasis has occurred.
2. The patient is usually considered incurable if gross extension of the tumor beyond the bladder wall has occurred.

B. *Modalities for Treatment*

1. Transurethral and transvesical electroexcision done for simple papillomas.
2. Chemotherapy—usually injected into bladder tumor (as topical Thio-TEPA for low grade multiple tumors).
3. Intravesical application of radium or implantation of radioactive materials into tumor.
4. External radiation for undifferentiated types of tumors.
5. Segmental resection of bladder (partial resection).
6. Urinary diversion procedures to relieve frequency and reduce hemorrhage in patients with inoperable disease.
7. Cystectomy (removal of bladder) or radical cystectomy for invasive and poorly differentiated tumors.
   a. Radical cystectomy in male—removal of bladder, pelvic peritoneum, prostate and seminal vesicles with regional node dissection.
   b. Radical cystectomy in female—removal of bladder, pelvic peritoneum, urethra, uterus, broad ligaments, vagina, tubes, ovaries and regional lymphadenectomy (iliac and pelvic nodes).

Nursing Management (for cystectomy)

1. Cystectomy requires diversion of the urinary stream (anastomosing the ureters into an isolated loop of ileum which is brought out through the abdominal wall as an ileostomy).
2. Observe for complications following a cystectomy.
   a. Peritonitis
   b. Pyelonephritis

      c. Adynamic ileus
      d. Atelectasis
      e. Disturbances of vascularization of ileal loop (turns dark blue to black color)
      f. Leak from ureterointestinal anastomosis; urine may leak through wound
      g. Intestinal obstruction
      h. Wound dehiscence or evisceration
      i. Postoperative hemorrhage
  3. See below for nursing management of patient with a urinary diversion procedure.

URINARY DIVERSION

Urinary diversion refers to diverting the urinary stream from the bladder so that it exits via a new avenue.

Clinical Conditions Requiring Urinary Diversion

  1. Malignancy of bladder or ureters
  2. Pelvic malignancy
  3. Stricture and trauma to ureters and urethra
  4. Neurogenic bladder
  5. Severe ureteral and renal damage due to reflux.

Methods of Urinary Diversion

  1. *Cutaneous Ureterostomy*—anastomosis of ureters to the skin usually high on the abdominal wall, slightly medial to the spine of the ileum.
  2. *Ileal Conduit (ureteroileostomy)*—implantation of ureters to a section of the terminal ileum, one end of which is brought to the abdominal wall as an ileostomy opening. The loop of ileum acts as a conduit (passageway) for urine.
  3. *Ureterosigmoidostomy*—diversion of the ureter(s) into the sigmoid colon. This allows urine to flow through the colon and out of the rectum. The patient should have adequate control of the anal sphincter.
  4. *Nephrostomy*—insertion of catheter into renal pelvis via incision in the flank (see p. 496).
  5. *Cystostomy*—opening of bladder and drainage by catheter through an abdominal wound (see p. 470).

Preoperative Considerations for Patients Having Intestinal Urinary Diversion Procedures (Ileal Conduit and Ureterosigmoidostomy).

  1. See page 494, patient undergoing urological surgery, for general aspects of preoperative care.
  2. Prepare patient for sigmoidoscopy and barium enema if ureterosigmoidostomy is to be performed.
        Assess patient's ability to retain enema as a means of evaluating adequacy of rectal sphincter.
  3. Carry out renal function studies to determine kidney status and renal reserve.
  4. Apply several types of skin adhesives or cement to abdomen preoperatively to determine contact allergies and to facilitate management of ostomy appliance postoperatively.

5. Prepare the bowel for surgical intervention.
   a. Give low residue diet.
   b. Administer antibacterial agents (Sulfathalidine or neomycin)—for bowel disinfection to reduce pathogenic bacterial flora.
   c. Give enemas as directed for mechanical cleansing of lower bowel.
6. Assist patient undergoing nasogastric intubation on morning of surgery (p. 383).
7. Employ adequate hydration procedures including intravenous infusions to ensure urine flow during surgery.
8. Encourage patient to express his feelings about his situation.

Postoperative Nursing Emphasis

A. *General Considerations*

1. See page 399 for nursing management of patient following intestinal surgery and page 494 for nursing management of patient following urological surgery.
2. Watch for any abnormal signs and symptoms (wound infections, leaking at anastomosis site, peritonitis, paralytic ileus, intestinal obstruction, stenosis of stoma). These operations are extremely taxing and patients have little or no reserve.
3. Assure adequate circulating volume with blood and plasma.
4. Keep nasogastric tube in place until patient passes gas via rectum.
5. Accept the depression of the patient which usually follows any surgery which interferes with body integrity.
   a. Accept the patient's irritability and lack of motivation to learn.
   b. Give the patient extra support until he can cope with his situation.

B. *Following Cutaneous Ureterostomy*

1. Patient will have indwelling ureteral catheters for 7–10 days.
2. Following removal of ureteral catheters, uterostomy cups are fastened on the abdominal wall with special cement.
   a. The cemented-on appliance is worn at all times.
   b. Ureteral dilatation with sterile catheter is performed at regular intervals to assure patency and prevent ureteral stricture.
3. See page 502, nursing considerations for patient having ileal conduit, for general aspects of care.

C. *Following Ureterosigmoidostomy*

1. Patient will have rectal tube draining the urine for approximately 10 days.
   a. Tape the tube to the buttocks.
   b. If the tube must be removed for defecation reinsert the tube approximately 10 cm. (4 inches) into rectum to prevent trauma to site of ureteral anastomosis.
2. Following removal of the tube (per order) the patient voids through his rectum.
   a. In time, patient will be able to differentiate between the sensation to void and the urge to defecate.
   b. Reinsert the tube at night (attached to drainage bottle) to permit uninterrupted sleep.
   c. Do not give enemas or cathartics.
3. Evaluate patient for hyperchloremic acidosis, potassium loss, pyelonephritis due to bacterial absorption from colon and reflux of bacteria from sigmoid.

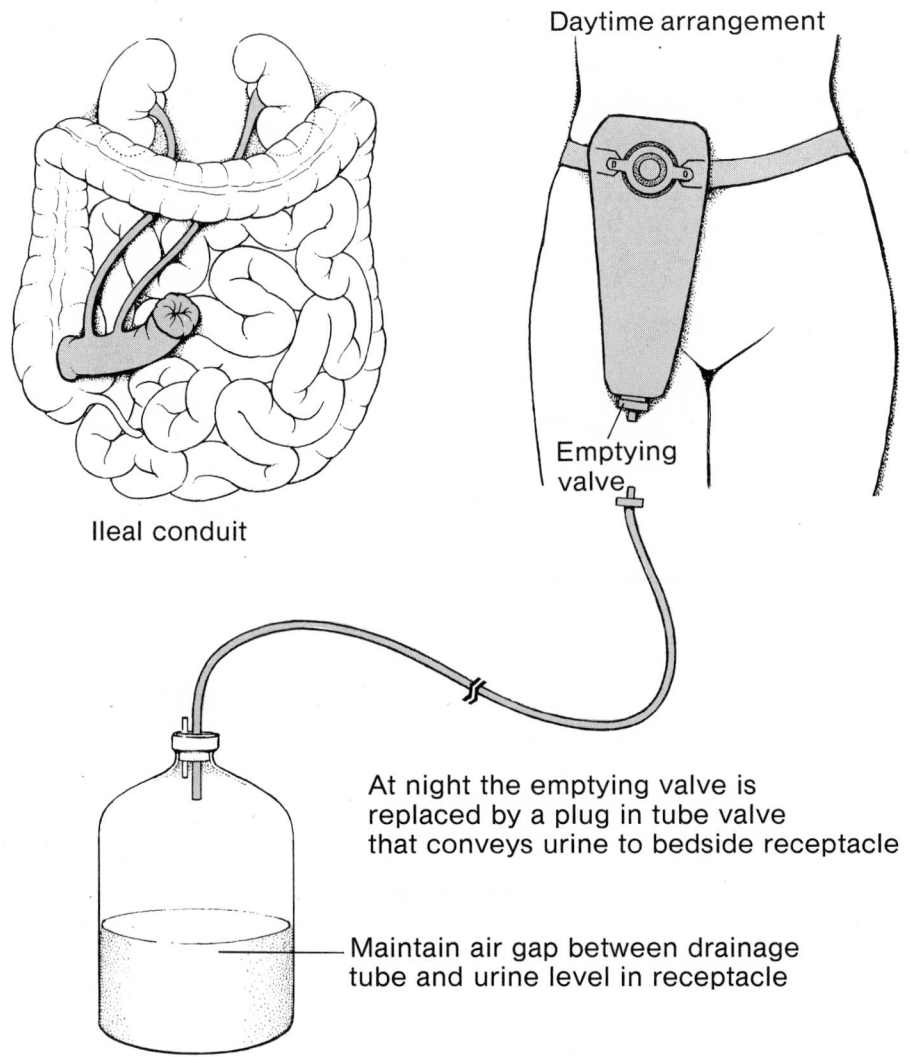

Daytime arrangement

Ileal conduit

Emptying valve

At night the emptying valve is replaced by a plug in tube valve that conveys urine to bedside receptacle

Maintain air gap between drainage tube and urine level in receptacle

Figure 7-8. Urinary diversion.

D. *Following Ileal Conduit* (Fig. 7-8)
1. Patient wears transparent disposable urinary drainage bags until edema subsides and stoma shrinks to normal size. (Some patients prefer using disposable bags permanently.)
2. The patient with an ileal conduit wears a cemented-on appliance day and night. The ileal bladder drains urine constantly but not feces. The appliance has an outlet valve for ease of emptying.
3. *Determining Stoma Size* (for ordering correct ostomy appliance)
    a. Measure widest part of stoma with a ruler after edema subsides.
    b. Order an appliance 1.0–1.25 cm. (⅜–½ inch) larger than the diameter of the stoma

4. *Changing the Appliance*
   a. Assemble all equipment; have patient sit in front of a mirror until this technique is mastered.
   b. Moisten the edge of the appliance plate with adhesive solvent or soap and water and gently remove it.
   c. Instruct the patient to bend over quickly and remain in that position for a minute to allow conduit to empty before the skin is washed and dried.
   d. Clean all cement from the skin with adhesive solvent. Wash skin with mild soap and water. Pat dry.
      (1) Inspect the skin for signs of irritation.
      (2) Keep the skin free from direct contact with the urine.
      (3) A gauze or tissue wick may be inserted in the stoma to absorb urine while the appliance is being changed.
   e. Apply the cement to the plate and skin. When they are both tacky to the touch, place the appliance directly over the stoma making sure the plate is centered over the stoma. The appliance should fit closely over the urinary stoma leaving very little skin exposed to urine.
   f. As soon as the appliance is secured, have the patient stand upright or lie flat to prevent the skin from stretching before the appliance becomes tightly adhered.
   g. An appliance with a karaya ring may be used for patients with an allergy to adhesive or solvents or those having an uneven or scarred peristomal skin surface.
   h. The skin under the appliance may be dusted with karaya powder or other soothing powder and protected with a bib or special appliance cover to absorb perspiration.
   i. Attach belt to appliance according to manufacturer's directions.
5. *Controlling Urinary Odor*
   Instruct the patient as follows:
   a. Avoid foods and medication that give strong odor to urine—patient will have to observe his reaction to food and drugs.
   b. Drink 250 ml. of cranberry juice 4 times daily—cranberry juice increases urine acidity and reduces bacterial action and fermentation thus suppressing urine-odor problems.
   c. Put aspirin tablet or other deodorizing tablets into ostomy bag.
6. *Managing the Ostomy Appliance*
   Instruct the patient as follows:
   Empty the appliance every 2 hours or when it contains 100 ml. of urine; urine ostomy appliances are closed with a drain valve (spigot) for periodic emptying.
      (1) Do not allow appliance to become over-distended with urine as the weight of appliance will loosen the plate from the skin.
      (2) Some patients prefer wearing a leg urinal attached with an adapter to the drainage apparatus.
7. *Assuring Uninterrupted Sleep*
   a. Attach tubular outlet on appliance to a collecting bottle with plastic tubing for nighttime drainage.
   b. Have at least 1.5 m. (5 ft.) of tubing to allow for turning.
8. *Cleaning and Deodorizing the Appliance*
   a. Clean appliance with detergent solution and soak in *distilled* vinegar, washing-soda solution, a few drops of clorox or lysol solution or any commercial deodorizing solution.
   b. After soaking the appliance, air-dry it overnight.

      c. Rinse plastic pouches with cold or lukewarm water (hot water loosens the seams)
      d. Instruct patient to experiment with various deodorizing solutions until he finds the one that meets his requirements.

9. *Rehabilitation and Patient Education for Wearing Urinary Ostomy Appliances*
      a. Help the patient to realize that ostomy care is not difficult or complicated and should be regarded as part of personal dressing and grooming routine.
      b. Patients using urinary ostomy appliance need
          (1) 2 well-fitting appliances; one to be worn while the other is air-drying; or he may use disposable appliances
          (2) Skin cement or liquid adhesive or double-faced adhesive disks
          (3) Karaya powder and karaya washers
          (4) Belt
      c. Successful ostomy management requires
          (1) Well-fitting appliance and belt
          (2) Meticulous skin care
          (3) Control of urinary odor
      d. Instruct patient to always carry spare bags and cement in a small case in handbag or pocket.
      e. If patient cannot tolerate skin cement there are appliances available which adapt to curved surfaces without cement. Contact United Ostomy Association for product manufacturers (address below).
      f. Encourage patient to contact local ostomy association for visits, reassurance and practical information from ostomy visitor.
      g. For further information and valuable periodical materials:
          United Ostomy Association, Inc., 1111 Wilshire Boulevard, Los Angeles, California 90017.

PROBLEMS AFFECTING THE URETHRA

Urethral Stricture

Urethral stricture is a narrowing of the lumen and loss of distensibility of the urethra from scar tissue formation and contraction.

Etiology

1. Urethral injury
      a. Urethral instrumentation—transurethral surgical procedures, indwelling catheters, cystoscopic procedures
      b. Straddle injuries, automobile accidents
2. Untreated gonorrheal urethritis
3. Congenital abnormalities (p. 1250).

Clinical Manifestations

1. Diminution in force and size of urinary stream
2. Urinary infection and retention—dysuria and urgency
3. Symptoms of complication from stricture—back pressure produces cystitis; prostatitis; pyelonephritis, etc.

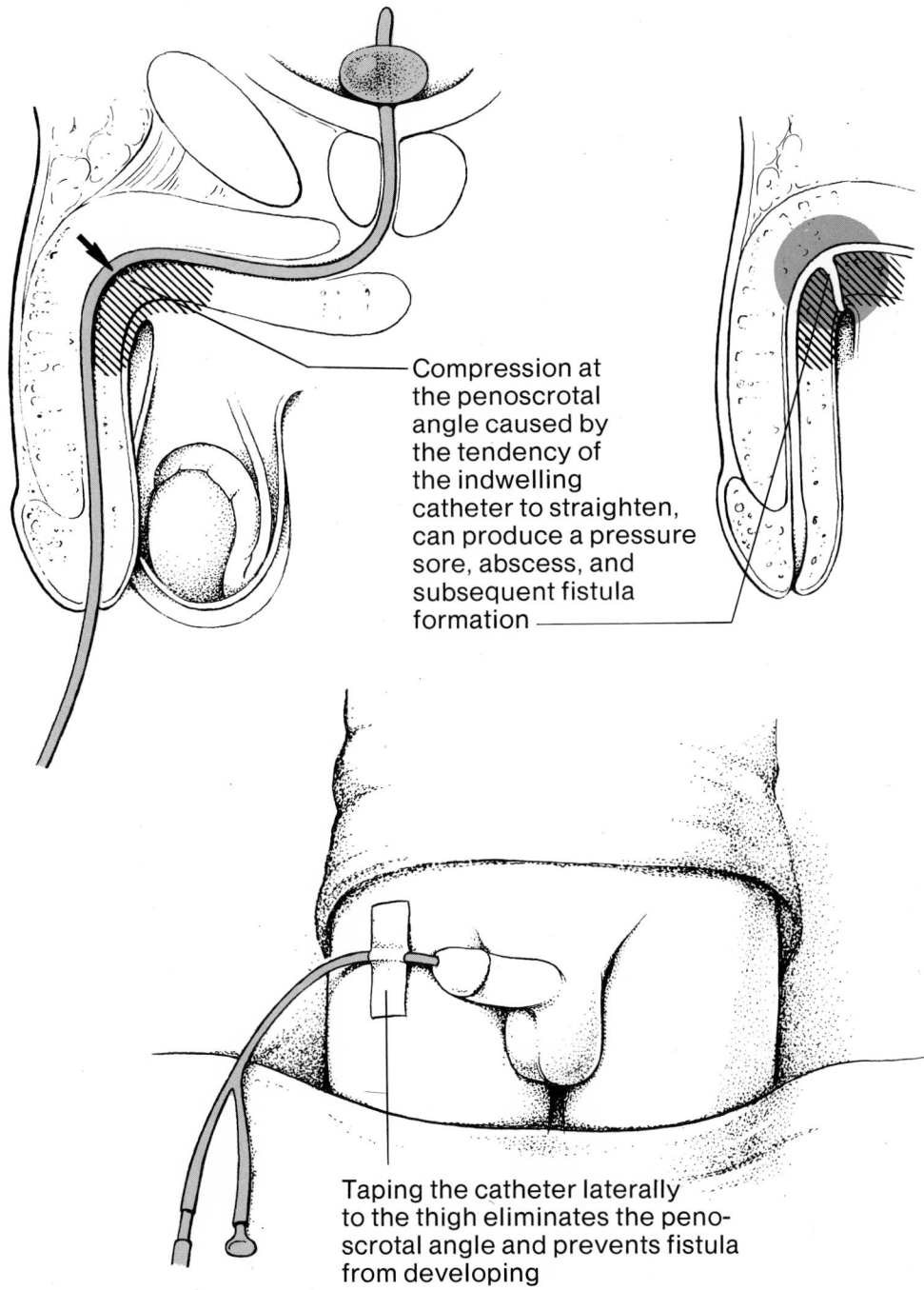

Compression at the penoscrotal angle caused by the tendency of the indwelling catheter to straighten, can produce a pressure sore, abscess, and subsequent fistula formation

Taping the catheter laterally to the thigh eliminates the penoscrotal angle and prevents fistula from developing

Figure 7-9. Tape the penis laterally (or on the abdomen) to eliminate pressure on the penoscrotal angle which is a source for infection, periurethral abscesses and urethral fistula formation.

Diagnostic Evaluation

1. Urethrogram and voiding cystogram—to locate site and degree of stricture
2. Elevated W.B.C. and pus and bacteria in urine—if urinary tract infection present
3. Passing of catheter or sounds (bougies)—to determine the diameter and location o urethral narrowings

Complications

1. Periurethral abscess, infection of bladder and kidneys
2. Hydroureter, hydronephrosis and pyelonephritis
3. Urethrocutaneous fistula
4. Chronic prostatitis

Prevention

1. Treat urethral infections promptly.
2. Utilize utmost care in urethral instrumentation (catheterization, etc.) (Fig. 7-9).
3. Avoid prolonged urethral catheter drainage.

Treatment

1. Dilatation of urethra with urethral sounds.
   a. Sounds of increasing size are used.
   b. Sounds are passed at increasing intervals (2 weeks, 1 month, 3 months) for a indefinite period depending on how long the strictured lumen is patent.
   c. Hot sitz baths and non-narcotic analgesics—to control pain after instrumentation
   d. Sulfonamides may be given several days after dilatation—lessens discomfort and minimizes infectious reaction.
2. Surgical excision or urethroplasty may be necessary for severe cases.

Urethritis

Urethritis is inflammation of the urethra.

Etiology

1. Nonspecific—urethritis not caused by gonococcus.
   a. From trauma—passage of urethral sounds, repeated cystoscopy, indwelling catheter.
   b. May be bacterial or viral; ascending infection or descending infection from prostate.
2. From gonorrhea (treatment below).
3. Reiter's syndrome—urethritis, conjunctivitis, arthritis of unknown etiology.

Clinical Manifestations

1. Urethral discharge—profuse or scanty, thick and purulent or thin and mucoid
2. Itching and burning around area of urethra

Diagnostic Evaluation

1. Study of stained urethral smear.
2. History and physical findings.
3. Culture (routine and on special media) for gonorrhea.

Treatment

1. Give antimicrobial therapy which may or may not be helpful.
2. Treat associated prostatitis (p. 508).
3. Advise patient to temporarily discontinue sexual intercourse and ingestion of alcohol. These activities prolong the acute phase of urethritis.

Urethritis from Gonorrhea

Etiology

1. *Neisseria gonorrhoeae*—the specific organism.
2. Transmitted through sexual contact.

Clinical Manifestations

Male

1. Purulent urethral discharge (4–10 days or longer after sexual exposure)
2. Inflammation of meatal orifice; burning on urination

Female

1. Purulent urethral discharge
2. Frequency, urgency, nocturia
3. Red, swollen urinary meatus
4. Pelvic inflammatory disease (P.I.D.) with abdominal pain
5. Often is essentially asymptomatic, so that disease is not diagnosed

Complications (local)

1. Male—periurethritis, prostatitis, epididymitis, urethral stricture, sterility due to vaso-epididymal duct obstruction
2. Female—pelvic inflammatory disease, abscess of greater vestibular glands (Bartholin's glands) urethral stricture

Treatment

1. Penicillin (see p. 835).
2. Tetracycline antibiotic (for patients with penicillin sensitivity).
3. Instruct patient to return for follow-up examination weekly for at least 3 weeks.
4. Instruct patient to refrain from sexual intercourse until after a cure has been verified.

CONDITIONS OF THE PROSTATE

Benign Prostatic Hypertrophy

Benign prostatic hypertrophy is enlargement of the periurethral glands from an overgrowth of normal glandular and muscular tissue.

Clinical Manifestations

1. Enlargement of gland causes narrowing of prostatic urethra.
2. Prostatic enlargement is usually a slow but continuous process.

  3. *Bladder*
     a. Symptoms of recurring urinary infection and stasis—frequency, dysuria, nocturia.
     b. Symptoms of urethral obstruction—hesitancy, decrease in size and force of urinary stream, partial or complete urinary retention, nocturia, hematuria, dribbling.
  4. *Renal*
     Symptoms of renal complications from retrograde pressure of urine—ureteral dilatation, hydronephrosis, renal infection, azotemia, uremia.

Diagnostic Evaluation

  1. Cystoscopic examination—to view degree of prostatic enlargement and subsequent bladder-wall changes
  2. Cystourethrography—to view the posterior urethra and outline of prostate gland
  3. Excretory urogram—to demonstrate complications from back pressure or urine
  4. Catheterization after voiding—to determine amount of residual urine
  5. Cystometrogram—to evaluate the presence of a neurogenic bladder

Treatment and Nursing Management

  1. The plan of treatment depends upon the cause, the severity of obstruction and the condition of the patient.
  2. Conservative treatment—for patients with good kidney function and minimal residual urine
     a. Prostatic massage—to relieve congestion (gives limited improvement)
     b. Urinary antiseptics—to relieve symptoms of infection and frequency
     c. Advise patient to report every 6 months for re-evaluation
  3. Cystostomy drainage of bladder—for poor-risk patient or one acutely ill with uremia, retention, etc. (see p. 470).
  4. Prepare patient for prostatectomy. See page 511 for nursing management of patient having a prostatectomy.

Prostatitis

Prostatitis is an inflammation of the prostate gland.

Etiology

  1. Bacterial invasion of prostate
     a. From hematogenous (bloodstream) origin (tonsils, G.I. tract, G.U. tract)
     b. From ascent of bacteria from urethra
     c. Secondary to urethritis (p. 506)
     d. Secondary to gonorrhea (p. 834)
     e. Descending infection from kidneys
  2. Prostatic stones and urethral stricture
  3. Benign prostatic hypertrophy
  4. Alcohol
  5. Irregular sexual activity

Clinical Manifestations

(from infection and local inflammation)
  1. Chills and fever (moderate to high fever)
  2. Pain in perineum, rectum, lower back and lower abdomen

3. Pain in groin—if seminal vesicles involved
4. Bladder irritability—frequency, dysuria, urgency, hematuria
5. Urethritis and urethral discharge—may or may not be present

Diagnostic Evaluation

1. Rectal examination—reveals enlarged, edematous and painful prostate
2. Culture and sensitivity tests of urethral and prostatic fluid
3. Urinalysis—for evidences of infection

Complications

1. Urinary retention—from swelling of gland
2. Bacteremia
3. Epididymitis, prostatic abscess
4. Pyelonephritis

Treatment and Nursing Management

1. Treat with sulfonamides or antibiotics for specific bacterial infection.
2. Keep the patient on bedrest.
3. Promote comfort with:
   a. Analgesics—for pain relief
   b. Antispasmodics and bladder sedatives—to relieve bladder irritability
   c. Sitz baths—to relieve pain and spasm
4. Ensure adequate fluid intake. (Avoid "forcing fluids" as this merely increases patient's urinary frequency.)
5. Use *small* indwelling catheter for severe urinary retention—to avoid urethral trauma.

Cancer of the Prostate

Cancer of the prostate is a malignant tumor of the prostate gland. It arises from the parenchyma of the prostate usually in the most posterior part; therefore most prostatic cancers are palpable on rectal examination.

Clinical Features

1. Cancer of the prostate is the most frequently encountered cancer in men over 50.
2. It spreads into the seminal vesicles, bladder neck and metastasizes to the regional nodes and the bony pelvis and spine.
3. Early localized cancer of the prostate does not produce symptoms while the obstructive symptoms occur late in the disease.

Clinical Manifestations

1. Symptoms from obstruction to urinary flow
   a. Hesitancy and straining on voiding, frequency, nocturia
   b. Diminution in size and force of urinary stream.
2. Symptoms due to metastases
   a. Pain in lumbosacral area radiating to hips and down legs
   b. Perineal discomfort
   c. Anemia, weight loss, weakness, nausea, oliguria (from uremia)

Diagnostic Evaluation

1. Palpation by rectal examination—reveals "stony hard" fixed gland if lesion is advanced (there are indurated lumps without fixation if condition is found earlier)
2. Cystoscopy—helps evaluate degree of fixation
3. Prostatic biopsy
4. Laboratory studies
   a. Serum acid phosphatase—frequently increases when cancer extends outside prostatic capsule; this test reveals extent of tumor.
   b. Serum alkaline phosphatase—increases when there is bony metastases.
   c. Tests for anemia—advanced anemia is present when bone marrow is replaced by bone tumor.
5. Bone scan—to detect metastasis
6. Skeletal roentgenograms—to reveal osteoblastic metastases
7. Bone marrow aspiration for tumor cells
8. X-rays of pelvis, lumbar spine, femoral heads, skull, ribs
9. Excretory urogram—to demonstrate changes from ureteral obstruction
10. Urinary function tests—to evaluate degree of urinary obstruction

Treatment

A. *Curative* (if performed before metastasis)
   1. *Radical Prostatectomy*—removal of prostate and its capsule, seminal vesicles and portion of bladder neck; may include regional lymphadenectomy if done by retropubic approach. This procedure may be followed by orchiectomy or estrogen therapy.
      a. Done by perineal or retropubic approach.
      b. Sexual impotency follows radical procedure but urinary control is usually normal.
   2. *Supervoltage radiation* (external) showing increasing promise as primary and adjuvant therapy.
   3. *Estrogen therapy* may be given before surgery to reduce risk of tumor dissemination.
   4. See page 511 for care of patient with prostatectomy.

B. *Palliative*
   1. *Cryosurgery* (freezing of prostatic tissue via a cryoprobe) results in cellular death of obstructive tissue.
   2. *Radiation therapy* to local lesion or gross tumor extension; may also be used as primary treatment with hope of cure.
      Results in decrease in tumor size and regression of obstructive lesions and frequently relief of bone pain.
   3. Antiandrogen therapy to slow rate of growth and extension of cancer (tumor influenced by sex hormones; administration of androgen usually increases rate of growth while estrogen therapy slows rate of growth).
      a. Estrogen—Diethylstilbestrol—1–5 mg. daily
      b. Bilateral orchiectomy (removal of testis) and administration of Diethylstilbestrol —removes androgenic hormone upon which growth of malignancy depends.
         Patient may experience side effects (enlarged painful breasts).
   4. Interstitial radiation with [198]Au.

C. *Symptomatic Treatment for Patients with Recurring Symptoms*
   1. Larger doses of Diethylstilbestrol.
   2. Corticosteroids give symptomatic relief but do not affect tumor.
      a. Restrict sodium intake as corticosteroids produce considerable sodium retention.
      b. Add potassium to diet.

3. Transurethral resection to remove obstructing tissue.
4. Suprapubic cystostomy drainage for bladder outlet obstruction when transurethral resection cannot be done.
5. If tumor increases and metastases is widespread the following treatment may be used:
   a. Hypophysectomy or bilateral adrenalectomy
   b. Discontinuation of estrogens as tumors sometimes become androgen dependent
   c. Discontinuation of steroids
   d. Testosterone therapy (may be used)
   e. Blood transfusions to maintain adequate hemoglobin when bone marrow is replaced by tumor
   f. External skeletal radiation for pain relief produced by metastatic growth (However adrenalectomy or hypophysectomy are usually done in younger patients with widespread metastatic involvement.)
6. See page 888 for nursing management of patient with terminal cancer and page 891 for nursing the dying patient.

Management of the Patient Undergoing Prostatic Surgery

Surgical Procedures

A. *4 Approaches for Prostatectomy*
   1. Transurethral-removal of prostatic tissue by an instrument introduced through urethra.
   2. Open surgical removal of prostate.
      a. Perineal
      b. Retropubic
      c. Suprapubic

B. *Factors Influencing Choice of Surgical Approach*
   1. Size of gland and location of pathology
   2. Age and condition of patient
   3. Presence of associated disease(s)

C. *Bilateral Vasectomy*
   1. May be performed at time of prostatectomy to reduce risk of epididymitis—a complication frequently following prostatectomy.

Preoperative Objectives of Nursing Management

A. *To establish kidney function at the patient's optimum level.*
   1. Maintain adequate bladder drainage via indwelling catheter or suprapubic cystostomy—renal function usually improves with re-establishment of drainage.
      a. Introduce indwelling catheter if patient has continuing retention or if residual urine is more than 75–100 ml. and patient is azotemic. (See p. 467.)
      b. Give antibiotics (according to culture and sensitivity tests)—to combat and control infection.
      c. Utilize cystostomy drainage if patient cannot tolerate urethral catheter.
      d. Watch patient closely after drainage is instituted—blood pressure fluctuates and renal function may decline first few days after drainage is established.
      e. Ensure adequate hydration—patient is frequently dehydrated from self-limitation of fluids because of frequency.

(1) Encourage fluid intake of 2500–3000 ml. daily (if cardiac reserve is adequate —to help in overcoming azotemia.
(2) Weigh patient daily and monitor fluid intake and output.
(3) Give intravenous fluids according to need as indicated by clinical status and serum electrolyte determinations.
2. Carry out prescribed renal function studies—to determine if there is renal impairment from prostatic back pressure and to evaluate renal reserve.

B. *To ensure that patient is in best possible condition.* (Older people have diminishing functional reserves of vital organs and may have co-existing disease.)
1. Carry out complete hematologic investigation—to ascertain specific clotting defects as hemorrhage is a major postoperative complication.
2. Correct nutritional deficiencies, hypoproteinemia, vitamin deficiencies, and anemia.
3. Give cardiac supporting drugs when indicated—helps alleviate renal symptoms.
4. Prepare patient with pulmonary emphysema with antibacterial agent, tracheobronchial cleansing and intermittent positive pressure breathing (p. 134). Patient should stop smoking at least 2 days before surgery.

Postoperative Objectives of Nursing Management (Fig. 7-10)

A. *To evaluate for shock and hemorrhage.*
1. Watch for evidence of hemorrhage in drainage bottle, on dressings and at incision site.
2. Take blood pressure, pulse and respiration as frequently as clinical condition indicates. Compare with preoperative vital-sign readings to assess degree of hypotension present.
   a. Observe for cold, sweating skin, pallor, restlessness, fall in blood pressure, increasing pulse rate.
   b. Prepare for surgical intervention if bleeding persists (suturing of bleeders or transuretheral coagulation of bleeders).
3. Give blood transfusion as indicated.

B. *To promote adequate drainage of the bladder.*
1. Utilize a closed sterile gravity system of drainage—3-way system is useful in controlling bleeding; irrigating system keeps clots from forming (does not correct the *cause* of bleeding).
2. Watch drainage for evidence of increased bleeding.
3. Irrigate bladder (amount and time prescribed by urologist) to avoid clot formation in the bladder.
4. Re-explain to the patient the purpose of the catheter.
   a. Tell him that the urge to void is from the presence of the catheter and bladder spasm.
   b. Encourage him to refrain from pulling on catheter—will cause bleeding, clots, plugging of catheter and distention.
5. Be alert for blockage of urinary drainage tube by kinking, mucous plugs and blood clots.
6. Tape the drainage tubing (not the catheter) to shaved inner thigh—to prevent traction on bladder. (However, traction on the catheter by the urologist may control bleeding.)
7. Tape cystostomy catheter to lateral abdomen.

NURSING MANAGEMENT OF PATIENT FOLLOWING PROSTATECTOMY

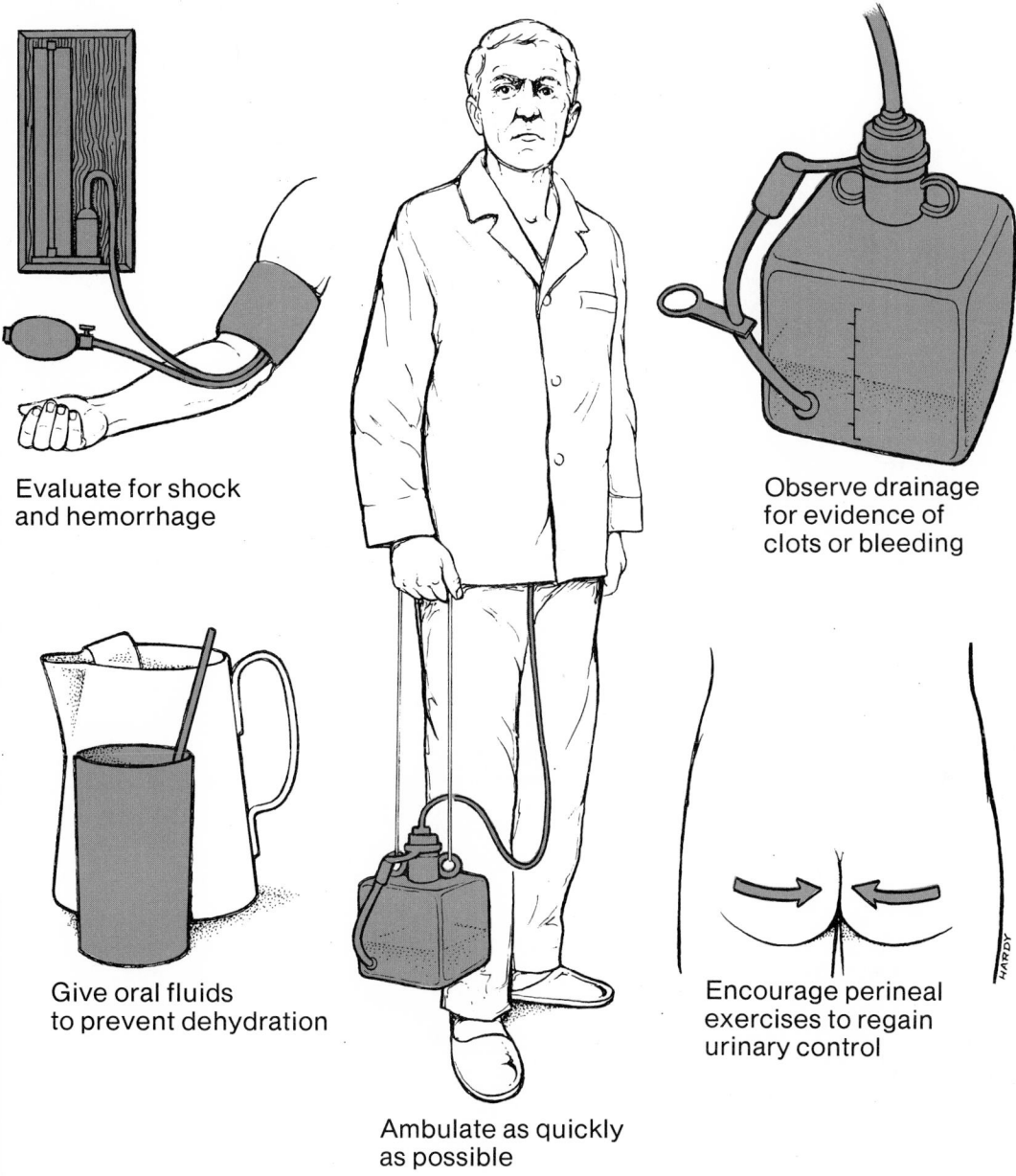

Evaluate for shock and hemorrhage

Observe drainage for evidence of clots or bleeding

Give oral fluids to prevent dehydration

Ambulate as quickly as possible

Encourage perineal exercises to regain urinary control

Figure 7-10. Nursing management of patient following prostatectomy.

8. Note time and amount of each voiding after removal of catheter.
   a. May be urinary leakage around wound several days after removal of catheter in perineal, suprapubic and retropubic surgery.
   b. Cystostomy tube may be removed before or after removal of urethral catheter.

C. *To anticipate postoperative complications.*
   1. Hemorrhage and shock
   2. Urinary infection
   3. Epididymitis

D. *To promote comfort and rehabilitation of the patient.*
   1. Keep patient quiet during *immediate* postoperative period to prevent episodes of bleeding.
   2. Use tranquilizers, sedatives, antispasmodics and appropriate analgesics for pain control.
      a. Elderly patients do not usually tolerate barbiturates.
      b. Take blood pressure before administering tranquilizers and analgesics.
   3. Give antibiotics as directed—to promote urinary antisepsis.
   4. Avoid rectal temperatures, rectal tubes and enemas following perineal prostatic surgery.
   5. Help the patient to ambulate as quickly as possible.
   6. Promote the comfort of the patient with perineal sutures.
      a. Wash perineum with surgical soap as directed.
      b. Use heat lamp to perineal area (cover scrotum with towel)—to promote healing.
      c. Assist patient with sitz bath as directed—to promote healing.
   7. Teach patient measures to gain urinary control—urinary incontinence may follow any type of prostatic surgery.
      a. Tense the perineal muscles by pressing the buttocks together; hold this position as long as possible; relax.
      b. Perform this exercise 10–20 times each hour.
      c. Expect "dribbling" immediately following catheter removal.

E. *To carry out effective patient teaching.*
   Instruct the patient as follows:
   1. Expect urinary dribbling for a period of time.
   2. Urinate as soon as the first desire to do so is felt.
   3. Avoid long automobile trips which increase tendency to bleed.
   4. Avoid alcohol which increases urinary burning.
   5. Drink enough fluids as dehydration increases tendency for clot obstruction.
   6. Do not take anticholinergics and diuretics unless by direct order of physician.
   7. Continue with perineal exercises until full urinary control is gained.

HYDROCELE

Hydrocele is an abnormal accumulation of fluid within the scrotum around the testicle and within the 2 layers of the tunica vaginalis.

Causes

(Caused by defective lymphatic drainage with inadequate readsorption of fluid)
1. Secondary to local injury including hernia operation
2. Secondary to infection

3. Following epididymitis or orchitis; torsion
4. As a complication of tumor of testicle.
5. In edematous states such as congestive heart failure, cirrhosis of the liver
6. Idiopathic

Clinical Manifestations

1. Enlargement of the scrotum
2. Usually painless until fluid accumulation is large enough to cause pressure

Treatment

1. No treatment is required unless complications are present.
   a. Circulatory complications to testicle
   b. Painful large hydrocele which is uncomfortable and cosmetically unacceptable to the patient
2. Surgical intervention—hydrocelectomy (excision of tunica vaginalis of testis) for removal of fluid and control of swelling.
   a. Periodic aspiration of hydrocele fluid in poor-risk patient
   b. Open operation for eversion of hydrocele sac or removal of hydrocele sac
3. Postoperative Nursing Emphasis—see below.

VARICOCELE

Varicocele is the dilatation, elongation and tortuosity of veins within the scrotum (varicosities usually of the left spermatic vein and its tributories due to incompetent venous valve where it takes off from the left renal vein).

Clinical Manifestations

1. Subfertility may occur with varicocele—may suppress spermatogenesis due to vascular and temperature changes or more likely reflux of left adrenal corticosteroids to both testes due to intercommunication of their venous circulations.
2. A dragging sensation in the scrotum is usually the patient's chief complaint.
3. Varicocele on the right may indicate retroperitoneal tumor.

Treatment and Nursing Management

1. Patient wears a scrotal support (or suspensory) to relieve discomfort (Fig. 7-11).
2. Operative intervention—ligation and excision of veins high (near or above) internal inguinal ring through hernia or McBurney's incision.
3. Postoperative nursing support
   a. Apply ice bag to scrotum first few hours postoperatively—promotes contraction of scrotal tissue and relieves edema.
   b. Apply scrotal support for comfort.

TUMORS OF THE TESTICLE

Clinical Features

1. Tumors of the testicle are usually malignant.
2. They usually develop in the 20–40 year age group.
3. Testicular tumors metastasize early to the periaortic lymph nodes and lungs.

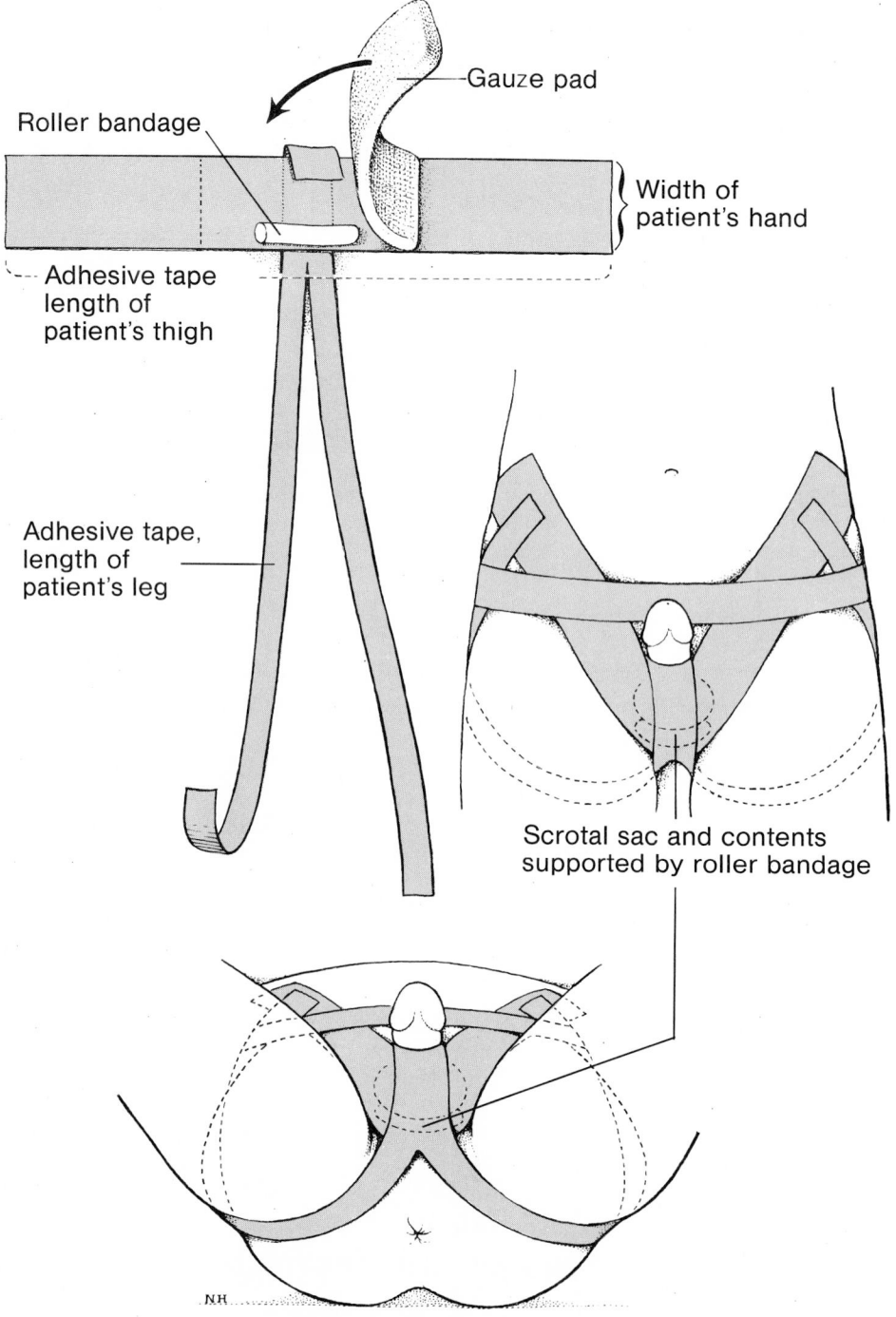

Gauze pad

Roller bandage

Width of patient's hand

Adhesive tape length of patient's thigh

Adhesive tape, length of patient's leg

Scrotal sac and contents supported by roller bandage

Perineal view of scrotal support bandage

Figure 7-11. Scrotal support.

Clinical Manifestations

1. Enlargement of the testes (swelling, hardness, lump)
2. Pain in the testes (if patient has epididymitis or bleeding into tumor)
3. Gynecomastia (enlargement of the breasts) from elaboration of chorionic gonadotropins from testicular tumor (considered a serious prognostic sign)
4. Symptoms of metastases
   a. Left supraclavicular or abdominal mass
   b. Abdominal pain
   c. Cough (lung metastases)

Diagnostic Evaluation

1. Assay of urinary chorionic gonadotropins
2. Intravenous urogram to evaluate presence of enlarged lymph nodes as manifested by ureteral displacement
3. Chest film to seek pulmonary or mediastinal metastases

Treatment and Nursing Management

1. Orchiectomy—removal of testicle (or testes) and spermatic cord to internal inguinal ring (usually through an inguinal incision).
   a. Removal of both testes (castration) renders the patient sterile and lacking in male hormones: this is rare since tumors of the testicle are usually unilateral.
   b. Resection of iliac and lumbar lymph nodes is carried out in certain histological types.
2. Radiation therapy is used in most cases of testicular neoplasm; may be curative or palliative.
3. Chemotherapy with cancerocidal agents (given in combination)
   a. Agents
      Chlorambucil—an alkalating agent
      Methotrexate—an antimetabolite
      Dactinomycin—antitumor antibiotic
      Mithramycin is effective in treatment of certain carcinomas
   b. Observe patient for toxic effects—nausea, vomiting and diarrhea, leukopenia, thrombocytopenia, skin eruptions, loss of hair.
   c. Drug(s) may have to be temporarily withheld in presence of serious toxic manifestations.
   d. See page 881 for nursing management of patient receiving chemotherapy.
4. Patient follow-up evaluation includes chest films, excretory urography and determination of urinary gonadotropins.

EPIDIDYMITIS

Epididymitis is an infection of the epididymis which usually descends from an infected prostate or urinary tract.

Causes

1. Prostatic infection (most common cause)
2. Urinary tract infection

3. Infection via the bloodstream with tubercle bacilli
4. Postoperative epididymitis—complication of prostatectomy and urethral catheterization
5. Reflux of sterile urine down the vas deferens

Clinical Manifestations

1. Pain in the groin and scrotum
2. Swollen, tender epididymis
3. Edema, redness and tenderness of scrotum
4. Chills and fever
5. Pyuria and bacteriuria

Diagnostic Evaluation

1. Elevated white blood count (may be as high as 20,000–30,000/cu. ml.)
2. Staining of urethral discharge if preceded by urethritis (either nonspecific or gonorrheal); usually no discharge is present with epididymitis

Treatment

1. Complete bedrest during the acute phase.
2. Antibiotic therapy (ampicillin and tetracycline)—until all evidence of acute inflammatory reaction has subsided (approximately 2 weeks).
3. Scrotal support for enlarged testicle—to relieve edema and discomfort.
4. Intermittent cold compresses to scrotum—for pain relief if heat increases pain.
5. Local heat or sitz bath later—to hasten resolution of inflammatory process.
6. Analgesics for pain relief.
7. Treatment for possible abscess formation.
8. Infiltration of spermatic cord with local anesthestic agent (1% procaine hydrochloride) —for pain relief if patient is seen 24 hours after onset.
9. Epididymectomy (excision of the epididymis from the testicle)—for patients with chronic painful condition or recurrent, incapacitating episodes.

ORCHITIS

Orchitis is infection or inflammation of the testes.

Clinical Features

1. Orchitis (relatively rare) is usually secondary to spread of inflammation in epididymis.
2. It may be pyogenic, viral, spirochetal, traumatic, etc. in origin.
3. Mumps is the main cause of pure orchitis that is not secondary to epididymitis.

Clinical Manifestations

1. Pain and swelling of the testicle with the scrotum becoming reddened and edematous
2. Fever and prostration

Treatment and Nursing Management

1. Treat underlying disease.
2. Keep the patient at bedrest with scrotum elevated and supported (see Fig. 7-11).
3. Give antibiotic therapy for specific etiologic agent.

4. Apply hot and cold compresses to scrotum for symptomatic relief.
5. Traumatic orchitis with rupture of the capsule (tunica albuginea) may require surgical repair and drainage as abscess may occur.

NURSING ALERT: A lump in the testis following minor trauma may call attention of the patient to a malignant testicular tumor.

VASECTOMY

Vasectomy is the ligation and transection of a section of the vas deferens; a bilateral vasectomy is a sterilization procedure for males.

Clinical Indications

1. Performed as a sterilization procedure.
2. Performed if the patient has recurrent acute epididymitis (p. 517).

Underlying Considerations

1. A vasectomy interrupts the transportation of the sperm. This procedure has no effect on sexual potency, erection, ejaculation or hormonal production.
2. Seminal fluid is mostly manufactured in the seminal vesicles and prostate which are unaffected by vasectomy.
   a. There will be no noticeable decrease in the amount of ejaculated fluid; the sperm accounts for less than 5% of the volume. The sperm cells are reabsorbed into the body.
      Some recent studies purport to show that vasectomy can lead to autoimmune disorders such as rheumatoid arthritis; this point is not yet settled.
   b. Psychological problems have been noted in an occasional patient following this procedure.
3. A vasectomy can be done on an out-patient basis.
4. The patient should be advised that he will be sterile but not sexually impotent following a bilateral vasectomy. Rarely is there a spontaneous re-anastomosis resulting in pregnancy.
5. A vasectomy may not be reversible and should be considered permanent.
6. A legal consent form must be obtained.

Postoperative Care

1. Apply ice bags intermittently to the scrotum for several hours after surgery to reduce swelling and relieve pain.
2. Advise patient to wear suspensory for added comfort and support.

Patient Education

1. Avoid strenuous activities for several days.
2. Sexual intercourse may be resumed as desired.
3. Contraceptives should be used until the sperm stored distal to the point of interruption of the vas is evacuated. *The patient is still fertile for a varying length of time after vasectomy.*

4. This evacuation of sperm may take approximately 10 ejaculations or up to 3–6 months
5. Absence of sperm must be demonstrated microscopically; laboratory tests confirm that no sperm are present in the seminal fluid.

Complications

1. Pain, swelling and scrotal edema
2. Infection
3. Nonbacterial epididymitis
4. Recanalization of vas deferens
5. Bleeding and hematoma

CONDITIONS AFFECTING THE PENIS

Ulceration of the Glans Penis

Causes

1. Cancer
2. Syphilis
3. Herpes progenitalis (virus existing in tissues of the glans and foreskin)
4. Chancroid
5. Lymphogranuloma venereum
6. Numerous benign skin lesions (ex. psoriasis)

Clinical Manifestations

Ulceration of the penis should be suspected as being venereal in origin until proved otherwise.

Diagnostic Evaluation

1. Dark field microscopic examination of smear for spirochetes
2. Serological (blood) test for syphilis

Treatment

Penicillin or tetracycline (see p. 840).

Carcinoma of the Penis

Carcinoma of the penis is a rare tumor usually involving the prepuce or glans.

Clinical Manifestations

1. Painless, warty growth; ulcer on glans or foreskin
2. Masses in inguinal region

Preventive Measures

Circumcision in infancy

Diagnostic Evaluation

Biopsy to secure diagnosis of malignancy and to differentiate from syphilitic chancre, etc.

Treatment
1. Local excision of lesion and irradiation therapy to small early lesions
2. Partial or complete amputation of penis for extensive lesions; usually done with bilateral groin (node) dissections.

Other Conditions

Chancre
Is a venereal ulcer caused by *Treponema pallidum* (syphilis).
1. Is the primary lesion of syphilis; appears 3–4 weeks after infection.
2. Begins as a dull red, hard and insensitive papule on or near the glans penis.
3. Persists 1–5 days or longer, then heals spontaneously.
4. The treatment of syphilis is outlined on page 841.

Balanitis
Is inflammation of the glans penis.

Phimosis
Is a condition in which the foreskin is narrowed and cannot be retracted over the glans. The treatment is circumcision.

Circumcision

Circumcision is the excision of the foreskin (prepuce) of the glans penis.

Clinical Indications
1. Usually done in infancy for hygienic purposes
2. Phimosis (inability to retract foreskin over the glans)
3. Paraphimosis (condition in which the foreskin cannot be reduced from a retracted position)
4. Recurrent infections of glans and foreskin

Postoperative Nursing Management
1. Watch for bleeding.
2. Change petrolatum (vaseline) gauze dressing as directed.
3. Give analgesia as patient's condition indicates; circumcision can be quite painful in the adult male.

NOTE: *Circumcision is an important preventive measure against carcinoma of the penis.*

2. Gynecologic Conditions
MENSTRUATION

Menstruation is a physiologic process in the female of child-bearing age.
1. If conception does not occur, the ovum dies; the mucous membrane lining the endometrium, which has become thickened and congested, becomes hemorrhagic.

2. Upper layer of cells in the lining and the blood that appears in the uterine cavity are discharged via the cervix and vagina.
3. The process, whereby blood is discharged along with mucus and cells, is called menstruation and usually occurs every 28 days.
4. Period of blood flow usually lasts 4–5 days with 50–150 ml. of fluid discharged.

Menarche or onset of menstruation occurs between 11 and 14 years.

Ovulation is the process in which an ovum is discharged from an ovary, usually midway in a 28- to 30-day cycle, 14 days after the onset of menstruation.

After cessation of menstrual flow, the endometrium returns to an inactive state until stimulated again by ovulation.

Disturbances of Menstruation

A relationship exists between the hormonal secretions of the ovary, the thyroid and the pituitary glands. An increase or decrease in the function of one or more glands can cause a disturbance in menstruation.

Dysmenorrhea

Dysmenorrhea is painful menstruation.

A. *Occurrence*

Common in unmarried women and women who have not borne children.

B. *Cause*
  1. May involve emotional and psychologic factors.
  2. Not completely understood.

C. *Symptoms*
  1. Pain may be due to uterine spasm caused by a narrowing of cervical canal.
  2. Pain may also be a result of endocrine-gland dysfunction.
  3. Cramp-like pain may occur in the lower abdomen—often associated with chills, headache, possible vomiting.

D. *Treatment and Nursing Management*
  1. Selective to meet needs of individual and severity of problem.
     a. Proper preparation of young women before menarche.
     b. Good posture; use special exercises to improve posture and correct weak musculature imbalance.
  2. Since emotional make-up may accentuate discomfort, psychotherapy or pharmacotherapy may be necessary.
  3. Complete physical examination to rule out other physical abnormalities.
  4. Instructions to patient:
     a. Avoid fatigue and overexertion.
     b. Lie down and use heat to lower abdomen.
     c. Control premenstrual edema by reducing salt intake and by taking a diuretic.
     d. Suppress ovulation by hormonal therapy.
     e. Ingest mild analgesics to control discomfort.

5. For more severe dysmenorrhea, the condition may be treated with "the pill." If this is unsuccessful, surgery may be necessary.
    a. Conditions causing narrowing of cervical canal and displacement may need to be corrected.
    b. Presacral neurectomy (cutting nerve fibers) may be done.
6. Pelvic exercises may be recommended.
7. Psychiatric therapy may be useful for some patients.

Amenorrhea

Amenorrhea is absence of menstrual flow.

A. *Primary*—when a young girl of 16 or 17 has not yet begun to menstruate.
    1. May be caused by variations in anatomic development.
    2. Treatment is according to etiology.

B. *Secondary*—menstruation has begun but is now stopped.
    1. Normal during pregnancy and lactation
    2. *Causes:* moderate to extreme anxiety, acute or chronic disease, anemia, disease of ductless glands and certain ovarian tumor (arrhenoblastomas)
    3. *Treatment:* directed to correction of cause

Menorrhagia

Menorrhagia is excessive bleeding during the regular menstrual flow.

A. *Causes*
    1. May be due to endocrine disturbances.
    2. In later life, may be due to inflammatory disturbances or tumors of uterus.
    3. Emotional disturbances may be responsible.

B. *Treatment*
    1. Search for underlying cause.
    2. Correct blood deficiency problem by replacement.
    3. Provide supportive care.

Metrorrhagia

Metrorrhagia is bleeding from the uterus between regular menstrual periods and after menopause.
    1. Significant because it is usually always a symptom of some problem—often cancer or benign tumors of uterus.
    2. Occasionally it may be due to a lost tampon.

Oligomenorrhea

Oligomenorrhea is infrequent menstruation occurring at intervals of less than 3 weeks.

Polymenorrhea

Polymenorrhea is frequent menstruation occurring at intervals of less than 3 weeks.

DIAGNOSTIC STUDIES FOR GYNECOLOGIC CONDITIONS

Pelvic Examination

A *pelvic examination* is an inspection of the external genitalia for signs of inflammation, swelling, bleeding, discharge or local skin and epithelial changes. A speculum is inserted to permit the gynecologist to visualize the vagina and cervix.

A. *Patient Preparation*
  1. Provide psychological support—patient needs reassurance, understanding and skillful consideration of her emotional as well as physical problems.
  2. Instruct patient to avoid douching before examination which might wash away cellular deposits.
  3. Encourage patient to go to bathroom before examination—voiding and bowel evacuation before the examination provide more relaxation of perineal tissues.
  4. Advise patient to remove sufficient clothing to permit adequate exposure of genitalia and allow for examination of the abdomen.
  5. Avoid undue exposure of the patient.

B. *Positioning of Patient* (best done on an examining table but can be achieved on a bed)
  1. *Lithotomy*—knees and hips flexed; heels resting on foot rests.
      a. Drape sheet diagonally over patient so that corner may be grasped and pulled upward to expose perineal area.
      b. When examination is done in bed, the patient is positioned across the bed with hips extending slightly over the edge (dorsal supine position); feet placed on examiner's knees or on 2 chairs placed next to the bed.
  2. *Sims' position*—the patient lies on one side, usually the left with the left arm behind her back. The right (uppermost) thigh and knee are flexed as much as possible; left leg is partially flexed.
      Drape sheet over lower extremities and hips to permit easy exposure of genitalia.
  3. *Knee-Chest*—Patient kneels on table with feet extending over the end.
      a. Separate knees and maintain thighs at right angles to the table.
      b. Turn patient's head to one side and allow face and chest to rest on a soft pillow.
      c. Patient's arms may grasp sides of table.

C. *Procedure for Examining the Pelvis*
  1. A speculum is inserted so that the vaginal tissues and nature of cervix can be visualized.
  2. *Cytology Smear* (Papanicolaou) can be made by aspirating the vaginal contents or obtaining scrapings directly from the cervix. (See below.)
  3. *Bimanual examination*—by inserting 1 or 2 gloved fingers of the left hand in the vagina and palpating the abdomen with the right hand, it is possible to further examine the uterus and adnexa.
  4. *Rectal Examination*—to detect abnormalities of contour, motility and placement of adjacent structures and tissues.

D. *Nursing Support*
  1. Attend and support the patient by encouraging her to relax, by holding her hand, etc.
  2. Focus the light and uncover examining tray with speculum, swabs, cytology necessities, etc.
  3. Assist physician by providing gloves, lubricant, etc.
  4. At conclusion of examination, wipe discharge from patient before assisting her from the table.

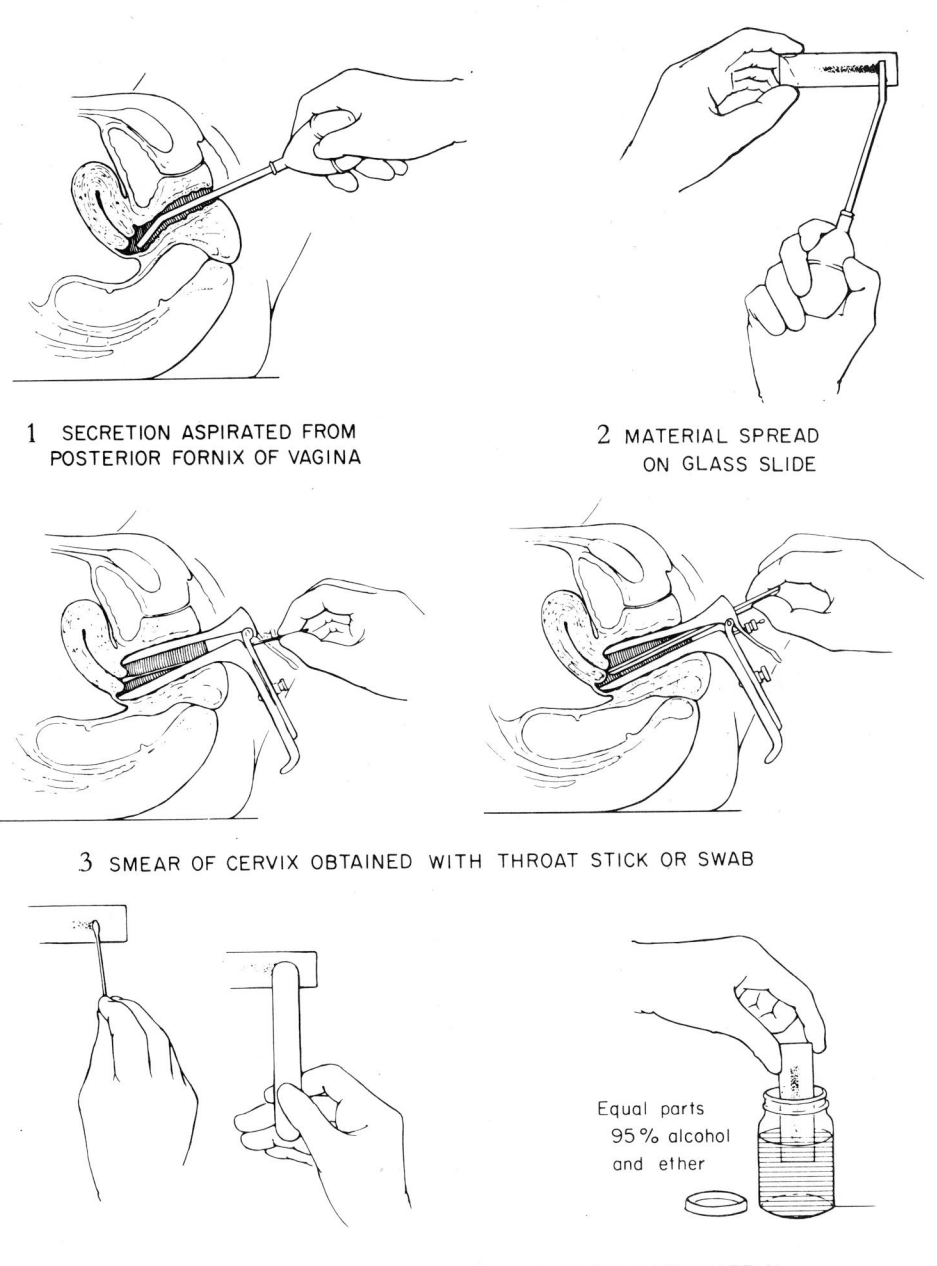

1 SECRETION ASPIRATED FROM POSTERIOR FORNIX OF VAGINA

2 MATERIAL SPREAD ON GLASS SLIDE

3 SMEAR OF CERVIX OBTAINED WITH THROAT STICK OR SWAB

4 MATERIAL SPREAD ON GLASS SLIDE

5 SLIDE IMMEDIATELY DROPPED INTO FIXATIVE

Equal parts 95% alcohol and ether

Figure 7-12. Methods of making cervical and vaginal smears for cytologic study. (From Dunphy, J. E., and Botsford, T. W.: Physical Examination of the Surgical Patient. Philadelphia, W. B. Saunders, 1964.)

5. Remove both legs from stirrups at same time and bring lower third of table into horizontal position.
6. Allow time for older patient to adjust to sitting position before helping her off the table.
7. Answer any questions patient may have; elaborate on physician's instructions.
8. Assist patient with dressing if necessary.

Cytology Test for Cancer (Papanicolaou)

A. *Purpose*—to diagnose cervical cancer by aspirating or swabbing vaginal secretions from posterior fornix and making a smear on a glass slide.
B. *Procedure*—See Figure 7-12.
    1. Examination and interpretation of cytologic smear as done by the pathologist.
    2. Classification of cytologic findings (after Papanicolaou)
        Class 1—Absence of atypical or abnormal cells.
        Class 2—Atypical cytology but no evidence of malignancy.
        Class 3—Cytology suggestive of, but not conclusive for, malignancy.
        Class 4—Cytology strongly suggestive of malignancy.
        Class 5—Cytology conclusive for malignancy.
    3. If the patient has an abnormal smear of Class 2, 3 or 4, explain to her that this is not conclusive but requires additional testing such as biopsy, D & C, etc.

Schiller Iodine Test

A long applicator stick is used to paint the cervix with Schiller's iodine solution.
    1. *Negative results*—a mahogany brown color covering entire surface indicates a reaction between iodine and glycogen of normal cells.
    2. *Positive results*—tissues are not stained brown indicating that immature cells are present.

Cervical Biopsy and Cauterization

A. *Purpose*—to remove cervical tissue for laboratory study; cauterization is done to control bleeding.
B. *Patient Preparation*
    1. To be done, preferably at a time cervix is least vascular (usually a week after the end of the menstrual flow).
    2. Explain the nature of the procedure to the patient.
    3. Place her in lithotomy position and properly drape her.
    4. Explain to her that no anesthesia is required since the cervix does not have pain receptors.
C. *Procedure*
    1. After the speculum is positioned in the vagina, and the cervix properly exposed, the surgeon uses a biopsy forceps to take bits of cervical tissues as specimens.
    2. Tissue is preserved in 10% formalin, labeled and sent to the laboratory.
    3. If bleeding occurs, packing may be inserted.
    4. If cauterization is necessary to control bleeding or to obtain additional tissue:
        a. Place a lubricated lead plate under the patient for grounding purposes.
        b. Explain the reason for doing so to the patient.
    5. Explain also that there may be an odor of burnt tissue but this will be over quickly.

D. *Aftercare of Patient*
1. A brief rest after the procedure is usually necessary before the patient leaves.
2. Instructions for home care:
   a. Rest, avoid heavy lifting and other work for 24 hours.
   b. Packing will remain in place for 12–24 hours depending upon physician's orders.
   c. There may be some bleeding; however, excess bleeding must be reported to the physician.
   d. Several days after a cauterization, a discharge and odor from sloughed tissue may be noted; a daily bath should control this.
   e. Obtain physician's orders regarding douching and sexual relations.

Culdoscopy

A *culdoscopy* is an operative, diagnostic procedure in which an incision is made into the posterior vaginal cul-de-sac through which a culdoscope is inserted for the purpose of visualizing the uterus, tubes, broad ligaments, uterosacral ligaments, rectal wall, sigmoid and even the small intestines.

1. The patient is prepared as for any vaginal operation (see p. 528).
2. Anesthesia may be local, general, or regional.
3. The knee-chest position is best for a culdoscopy.
4. Following the examination, the scope is withdrawn and rarely are sutures required; the patient is returned to her room.

X-Ray Studies—Hysterosalpingogram

A *hysterosalpingogram* is an x-ray study of the uterus and fallopian tubes following the injection of a contrast media.

A. *Purpose*
1. To study sterility problems.
2. To determine extent of tubal patency.
3. To note the presence of pathology in the uterine cavity.

B. *Procedure*
1. Patient is placed in lithotomy position.
2. The bivalve speculum is introduced to expose cervix.
3. Radiopaque dye is injected into uterine cavity.
4. X-rays are taken to determine configuration of pelvic area.

DILATATION AND CURETTAGE (D & C)

Dilatation and curettage is a widening of the cervical canal with a dilator and the scraping of the uterine endometrium with a curette.

Purposes

1. To secure endometrial and endocervical tissue for cytologic examination.
2. To control abnormal uterine bleeding.
3. To serve as a therapeutic measure for incomplete abortion.

Nursing Management

A. *Preoperative Care*

1. Acquaint the patient regarding the nature of the operation to be done (usually done by the gynecologist).
2. Answer questions patient may have regarding D & C.
3. Ascertain whether patient has been informed regarding expectation of postoperative discomfort, drainage or incapacity following the D & C.
4. Check with physician regarding perineal shave (some prefer no shave).
5. Prepare bladder and intestinal tract by having patient void and by giving a small enema.

B. *Postoperative Care*

1. Check that perineal pad is held in place with a sanitary belt.
2. Replace each perineal pad with a sterile pad as required during the time packing is in place.
3. Report excessive bleeding.
4. Recommend bedrest for the remainder of the day with bathroom privileges.
5. Offer mild analgesics for low back pain and pelvic discomfort.
6. Offer meals as desired.

GUIDELINES: *Using the Gravlee Jet Washer for Endometrial Cytology*

The *Gravlee Jet Washer* is an intrauterine washing device that uses the principle of negative pressure to obtain cytologic and tissue-fragment specimens.

Equipment

Gravlee Jet Washer sterile disposable unit (Upjohn) (Fig. 7-13).
Sterile gloves for gynecologist.
Antiseptic solution.

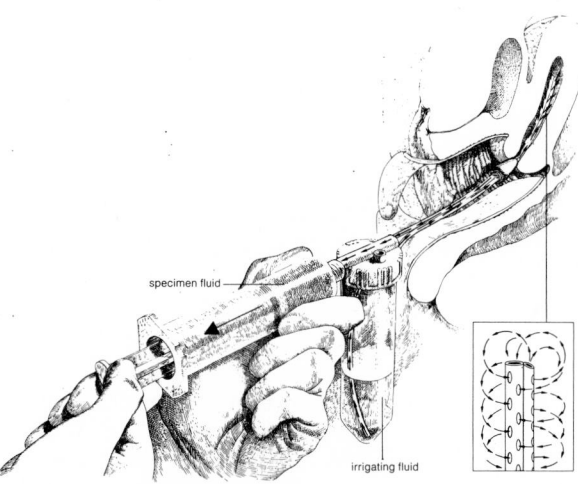

specimen fluid

irrigating fluid

Figure 7-13. Pulling on the plunger of a 30-ml. syringe in the Gravlee Jet Washer creates a negative pressure in the uterine cavity causing sterile saline from the vertical receptacle to be drawn into the uterine cavity for irrigation. Since no more than 1–4 ml. are in this cavity at one time, and since there is negative pressure, fluid does not get out into the fallopian tubes. Note the rubber plug at the cervical os which assists in creating an airtight system. The boxed diagram at the lower right demonstrates how the fluids circulate in the uterine cavity. (Courtesy Upjohn.)

Vaginal specula, tenaculum forceps, sterile uterine probes, water-solvent lubricant, long swab sticks.

Perineal drape.

Pap smear equipment.

Procedures

Preparatory Phase

1. Similar to that for a pelvic examination.
   a. Have patient empty bladder immediately before procedure.
   b. Place patient in lithotomy position (legs in stirrups).
2. Explain to the patient that a specimen of tissue lining the uterus will be taken by a flushing out process that is relatively painless; the patient may experience menstrual-like cramps during the procedure and for a day or so after.

Action	Rationale/Amplification
Performance Phase (by gynecologist)	
1. Insert speculum into vagina; perform Papanicolaou smear of cervix and vagina.	1. Cytology studies of tissue from the vagina and cervix can be done.
2. Remove speculum; perform bimanual examination.	2. Size and position of uterus can be noted.
3. Reintroduce speculum. Cleanse vaginal vault and cervix with antiseptic solution.	3. To minimize number of organisms in the area preparatory to entering uterine cavity.
4. Grasp cervix with tenaculum forceps and apply traction.	4. To reduce the amount of displacement of the uterus.
5. Introduce a sterile probe into cervical canal using extreme caution because of danger of perforating uterine wall.	5. To determine depth and angle of uterine cavity.
6. Prepare cannula from tray by adjusting rubber stopper; bend cannula to conform to curvature of uterine cavity.	6. To indicate length of cannula which can be safely introduced into the uterus and to serve as a water-seal plug at the cervical os.
7. Pour 30 ml. of sterile isotonic saline into reservoir (Fig. 7-13).	
8. Attach cap to receptacle after directing small tube into solution of receptacle; twist receptacle counterclockwise to screw cap in place.	8. To assemble equipment in working order.
9. Introduce cannula into uterine cavity and secure rubber plug into cervical opening.	9. To produce an intact irrigating system.
10. By drawing on the plunger of the syringe, irrigating fluid flows into the uterus and out into the barrel of the syringe.	10. Saline bathes the endometrial cavity and dislodges cells and small tissue fragments. This negative-pressure lavage system prevents the possibility of reflux into the fallopian tubes.
11. When the syringe is filled, remove the device from the uterus.	
Follow-up Phase	
1. Disconnect syringe, expel its contents into saline reservoir through port hole on top of cap.	1. This forms the handy receptacle which will be sent to the laboratory.
2. Expel any tissue collected along cannula into collecting receptacle.	
3. Apply unused screw cap, attach identification label, and send to laboratory immediately for block cytology.	3. If specimen does not go to laboratory immediately, a formalin or alcohol preservative must be added. (5 ml. of 10% buffered formalin or equal parts of 50% ethyl alcohol).

CONDITIONS OF THE EXTERNAL GENITALIA AND VAGINA

Pruritus

Pruritus is an itching of the vulva which often accompanies chronic infections of genital tract such as trichomoniasis, gonorrhea, or yeast infection—particularly in young women.

Clinical Manifestations
1. Itching followed by scratching and a thickening of tissues.
2. Patient often appears nervous.

Treatment
1. Real cause may be difficult to discover.
2. Cleanliness must be scrupulous.
3. Glycosuria and urinary incontinence must be controlled.
4. Temporary relief is obtained from soothing lotions and ointments.

Condylomata

Condylomata are warty papillary excrescences on the external genitalia.

Cause
1. Irritation and infection.

Types
1. Pointed type associated with gonorrhea.
2. Flat type considered syphilitic.

Clinical Manifestations
Leukorrheal discharge causing irritation.

Treatment
Directed to venereal problem.

Kraurosis and Leukoplakia

Kraurosis is a disease of the vulva; the skin becomes thin, dry, white and easily fissured.

Leukoplakia is similar to kraurosis; grayish-white patchy thickening and hardening of vulvar tissues with itching and burning. Treated like kraurosis.

Clinical Manifestations
1. With progress of the disease, vulva appears shrunken and leathery.
2. Marked itching.
3. May lead to cancer of the vulva.

Treatment
1. Ovarian extract, antihistaminics, vitamin A.
2. Advanced problem may require a vulvectomy (p. 534).

Vulvitis and Abscess of Greater Vestibular Gland (Bartholin's Gland)

Vulvitis is an inflammation of the vulva; the cause may be infection possibly caused by uncleanliness. Common offending organisms are *Escherichia coli*, staphylococcus, streptococcus, gonococcus and *Trichomonas vaginalis*.

Clinical Manifestations

1. Burning pain which is worse on urination and defecation.
2. Red and edematous tissue with profuse purulent exudate.
3. Acute throbbing pain and swelling between labia indicating vulvovaginal abscess (infection of Bartholin's glands).
4. When the acute infection subsides, the problem tends to become chronic.

Treatment and Nursing Management

1. Broad spectrum antibiotics to combat infection
2. Hot packs and sitz baths for comfort
3. Analgesics for the relief of pain
4. Bartholinectomy when there are painful recurrences, obstruction at introitus or fear of cancer
   a. Ice packs are applied intermittently for 24 hours to reduce edema and provide comfort.
   b. Thereafter, warm sitz baths or a perineal heat lamp are comforting.

Vaginal Fistula

A *fistula* is an abnormal, tortuous opening between 2 internal hollow organs, or an internal hollow organ and the exterior of the body.

Ureterovaginal fistula is an opening between the ureter and vagina.

Vesicovaginal fistula is an opening between the bladder and vagina.

Rectovaginal fistula is an opening between the rectum and vagina.

Clinical Manifestations

1. Patient with vesicovaginal fistula will experience continuous trickling of urine into vagina.
2. Patient with rectovaginal fistula will experience fecal incontinence and flatus passed through vagina, a malodorous condition.

Treatment and Nursing Management

1. Maintain cleanliness by encouraging frequent soothing sitz baths and deodorizing douches.
2. Use perineal pads and plastic or rubber pants if required.
3. Provide optimum skin care to prevent excoriation; bland creams or a light dusting of cornstarch may be soothing.
4. Recognize value of meeting psychosocial needs, such as feminine morale boosters (attractive hair-do, nail polish, perfume, new bed jacket etc.); encourage visitors, diversion, recreation, activities, etc.

SURGICAL TREATMENT
1. Surgery is recommended if tissues are healthy.
2. Maintain adequate nutrition and increase intake of vitamin and protein content of meals.
3. Promote local cleanliness by vaginal flushing and rectal enemata.
4. Administer chemotherapeutic agents to reduce pathogenic flora in intestine.

SPECIFIC POSTOPERATIVE NURSING MANAGEMENT
1. Rectovaginal fistula
   a. Limit bowel activity by keeping patient on clear fluids for several days; progress to a low residue, then a full diet.
   b. Give warm perineal irrigations and perhaps controlled heat lamp treatments to assist the healing process.
   c. Encourage rest because of the high degree of debilitation.
2. Vesicovaginal fistula
   a. Maintain proper drainage from indwelling catheter—otherwise, pressure may build up and be exerted against newly sutured tissues.
   b. Employ gentleness in administering bladder or vaginal irrigations because of tenderness of the operative site.

Vaginal Infections

Leukorrhea is a whitish vaginal discharge; it is considered normal to have a slight discharge at the time of ovulation or just before menstruation.

Simple Vaginitis
1. Normally, the vagina is acid (pH 3.5–4.5) in its secretions; Döderlein's bacilli are present.
2. *Escherichia coli,* staphylococci and streptococci usually are the invading organisms which cause a vaginitis.
3. Urethritis often accompanies vaginitis because of the proximity of the urethra to the vagina.
4. Symptoms
   a. Itching, redness, burning and edema
   b. Voiding and defecation aggravate the above symptoms.
5. Objectives of treatment
   a. To enhance the natural vaginal flora by administering a weak acid douche, 15 ml. of vinegar to 1000 ml. water (1 T. white vinegar to 1 qt. water).
   b. To stimulate the growth of Döderlein's bacilli, administer beta-lactose vaginal suppository; this dissolves with body heat and the sugar then acts.
   c. To foster cleanliness by meticulous care after voiding and defecation.
   d. To initiate chemotherapy by inserting medication into the vagina via applicator or by using a chemotherapeutic cream locally as prescribed.

Trichomonas Vaginalis
A condition produced by a protozoan which infects the vagina and is evident as a profuse bubbly white irritating leukorrhea.
1. Characteristics
   a. Caused by a pear-shaped mobile flagellate that thrives in an alkaline medium.

   b. *Trichomonas vaginalis* is persistent and resistant.
   c. Vulvar edema and hyperemia occur secondary to irritation of discharge.
   d. Remissions may occur; the organism meanwhile remains inaccessible to treatment in the urinary tract.
   e. The male partner may carry the organism in his urogenital tract and reinfect his mate.
2. Objectives of Treatment
   a. To destroy infective protozoa give metronidazole (Flagyl) for 10 days (by mouth)
      If above cannot be tolerated or is contraindicated, insert vaginal suppositories containing trichomonocidal compounds (Tricofuron, Vagisec, Devegan).
   b. To counteract alkaline-preferred environment of infecting organisms, administer acidic vaginal douches (Massengill, Nylmerate, white vinegar 15–1000 ml. (1 T. to 1 qt. of water).
   c. To prevent reinfection, instruct patient to avoid intercourse until cure is effected; treat male (if he has infection) with Flagyl also.

Monilial Vaginitis

A fungal infection caused by *Candida albicans*.
1. Characteristics
   a. *Candida albicans* is a normal inhabitant of the intestinal tract and therefore a frequent contaminant of the vagina.
   b. Since this fungus thrives in an environment rich in carbohydrates, it is seen commonly in patients with poorly controlled diabetes.
   c. This infection observed in patients who have been on antibiotic or steroid therapy for a while which reduces natural protective organisms in vagina.
2. Manifestations
   a. Vaginal discharge is thick and irritating; white patchy cheese-like particles adhering to vaginal walls.
   b. Itching is common.
   c. Vulva and vaginal appearance varies from normal to that of an acute inflammation.
3. Objectives of Treatment
   a. To eradicate the fungus, apply gentian violet by swabbing vagina; advise patient to wear perineal pad to prevent staining of clothing.
   b. To detect and control diabetes if present.
   c. To avoid intercourse until cure is effected.

Atrophic (Senile) Vaginitis

This is a common postmenopausal occurrence. Because of atrophy of vaginal mucosa, the woman is prone to infection.
1. Signs—Vaginal discharge causing itching and burning.
2. Treatment
   a. Similar to simple vaginitis (see p. 532).
   b. Estrogenic hormones taken orally or applied locally as an ointment are effective in restoring epithelium.

Cancer of the Vulva

Incidence

1. Occurs in elderly women over 60 years of age; cancer represents 5% of all malignancies of female reproductive system.
2. Women seem reluctant to seek medical attention in early phases when ulcer is small on the skin surface; they wait until the ulcer becomes infected and painful.
3. Early treatment may be curative; later treatment is in jeopardy because of inguinal lymph node involvement—metastasis beyond this to femoral, intrapelvic and iliac nodes.

Clinical Manifestations

1. In orderly progression, symptoms appear to be: ulcer on vulva, severe vulvar pruritus, "tumor" of vulva, pain, genital bleeding.
2. A concomitant and most annoying symptom—burning on urination.
3. Frequent site
   a. Labia majora—mid- or anterior portion
   b. Clitoris
   c. Encroachment upon urethra in larger lesions
4. Less frequent sites—fourchette and posterior labial areas.

Diagnostic Evaluation

1. A biopsy is taken after procaine is injected. The entire lesion when it is small may be excised, but final treatment is reserved until laboratory studies are completed.
2. Superficial lymph nodes on both sides are observed for enlargement and possible metastasis.
3. A pelvic examination is done.

Treatment

Choice of method depends upon extensiveness of lesion.

A. *Radiation therapy*—not tolerated as well as surgical excision
   1. Removable platinum needle implants
   2. Plaques containing radium or its isotopes
   3. Roentgen therapy

B. *Operative Intervention—Vulvectomy*
   1. Cancer of the vulva is treated by radical vulvectomy and superficial bilateral inguinal lymphadenectomy.
   2. Circular incisions are made around urethra to maintain its position.
   3. Plastic drainage tubes are inserted through stab wounds in each inguinal area attached to suction to facilitate closing of tissues and to prevent accumulation of serum.
   4. Compression dressings are usually applied in the form of hip spica bandaging.

Nursing Management

A. *Preoperative Care*
   1. Prepare a wide area to include perineal, pubic and inguinal areas.
   2. Encourage the patient to talk about her condition and to ask questions.
      a. Concerns occur regarding fear of mutilation and loss of sexual function.

b. Possibility of becoming pregnant again may be important to the woman of child-bearing age.

c. The possibility of metastasis and results concern the cancer patient regarding prognosis, suffering, relation to others in the family, etc.

3. Cleanse the vulva thoroughly 2 or 3 days prior to surgery by using sitz baths twice daily.

4. Evacuate the intestinal tract before surgery to allow for the advantage of no bowel movements for 2 to 3 days postoperatively.

5. Determine blood needs during surgery and have proper amount and correct type available in the event of need.

B. *Postoperative Care*

1. To maintain proper drainage and compression of tissues, connect drains to suction.

2. To promote comfort, place patient in low Fowler's position with knees slightly elevated with a pillow to lessen tension on sutures.

3. To minimize postoperative complications, mobilize patient on the day after surgery.

4. To prevent infection of wound and bladder, clean the wound daily with warm sterile solutions as prescribed (dilute hydrogen peroxide, saline, antibacterial solution) to be followed with a warm water spray. Later after the stitches are removed, a heat lamp to the vulva for 5 minutes twice a day may be required.

5. To facilitate wound healing, some physicians prefer dry heat such as provided by a heating lamp until the stitches are removed; this to be followed by perineal packs or soaks.

6. To prevent straining on defecation and wound contamination, offer a low residue diet.

7. To prevent bladder infection, give meticulous care to the vagina and urethral orifice.

8. To encourage social adjustment, maintain a relationship conducive to allowing the patient to voice her concerns.

9. To promote tissue repair, sitz baths of pHisoHex solution may be prescribed after the 10th day.

10. To maintain continuity of care upon discharge from the hospital, a follow-up plan is devised to provide for family care, visits by the community nurse, and return visits to the surgeon.

GUIDELINES: *Vaginal Irrigation*

Purpose

1. To cleanse or disinfect the vagina and adjacent tissues both before or after operation.
2. To soothe inflamed tissue.

Equipment

1. Sterile reservoir for irrigating fluid—can or bag
2. Sterile irrigating fluid as ordered (1000–4000 ml.) at 40.5°–43.3°C. (105°–110°F.)
3. Tubing, connecting tubes and clamp (sterile)
4. Irrigating vaginal nozzle (sterile)
5. Bedpan or douche pan
6. Plastic or rubber sheet with cloth protection
7. Sterile cotton balls, cleansing solution
8. Sterile rubber gloves

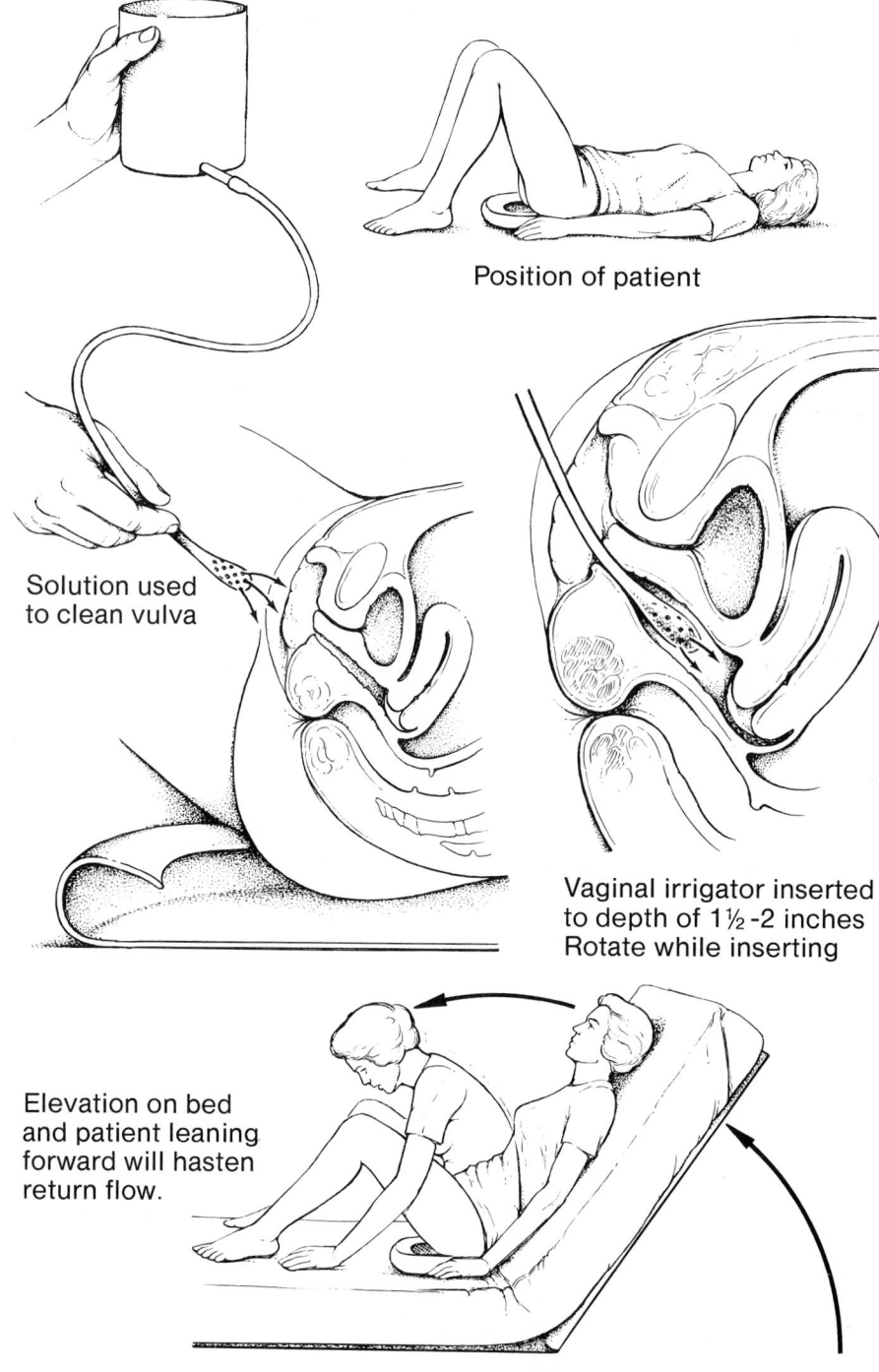

Position of patient

Solution used
to clean vulva

Vaginal irrigator inserted
to depth of 1½-2 inches
Rotate while inserting

Elevation on bed
and patient leaning
forward will hasten
return flow.

Figure 7-14. Vaginal Irrigation.

Procedure (Fig. 7-14)

Nursing Action	**Rationale/Amplification**

Preparatory Phase

1. Have patient void before beginning irrigation.

    1. A full bladder would prevent adequate distention of vagina by solution.

2. Place patient in dorsal recumbent position.

    2. To permit gravity to assist in allowing fluid to reach distal areas of vagina.

3. Drape patient.

    3. To prevent chilling and undue exposure.

4. Arrange irrigating receptacle at a level just above patient's hips (not more than 2 feet above hips) so that fluid flows easily but gently.

    4. The higher the fluid source, the greater the pressure.

Performance Phase

1. Cleanse vulva by separating labia and allowing solution to flow over area; if insufficient, use cotton balls saturated in soap solution cleansing from front toward anal area.

    1. Materials found around vaginal meatus may be introduced into vagina and cervix.

2. Allow some solution to flow through tubing and out over nozzle to lubricate it.

    2. Moisture provides lubrication and less resistance when one surface is moved against another.

3. Insert nozzle gently into vagina in a downward and backward direction.

    3. With the patient in a dorsal recumbent position, the natural anatomical position of the vagina is in the downward-backward direction.

4. Rotate nozzle gently in the vagina during inflow.

    4. All surfaces are irrigated when nozzle is rotated.

5. Clamp tubing when solution is almost all used; remove nozzle and permit patient to sit on bedpan for return flow.

    5. Gravity will assist in allowing return flow to drain from vaginal tract.

Follow-up Phase

1. Wipe patient dry using cotton balls in a front-to-back direction.

    1. Drying the area prevents skin excoriation and promotes comfort.

2. Remove bedpan from patient and apply sterile perineal pad.

3. Cleanse equipment with soap and water; dry before being stored in well-ventilated area.

    3. This will prolong life of equipment.

GUIDELINES: *Vulvar Irrigation*

Purpose

To cleanse the perineal area after urination or a bowel movement in order to minimize infection.

Equipment

Sterile pitcher with irrigating fluid (300–500 ml.) 40.5°–43.3°C. (105°–110°F.)
Sterile sponge forceps and cotton pledgets
Bedpan
Plastic or rubber sheet with cloth protection
Paper bag for cotton pledget disposal

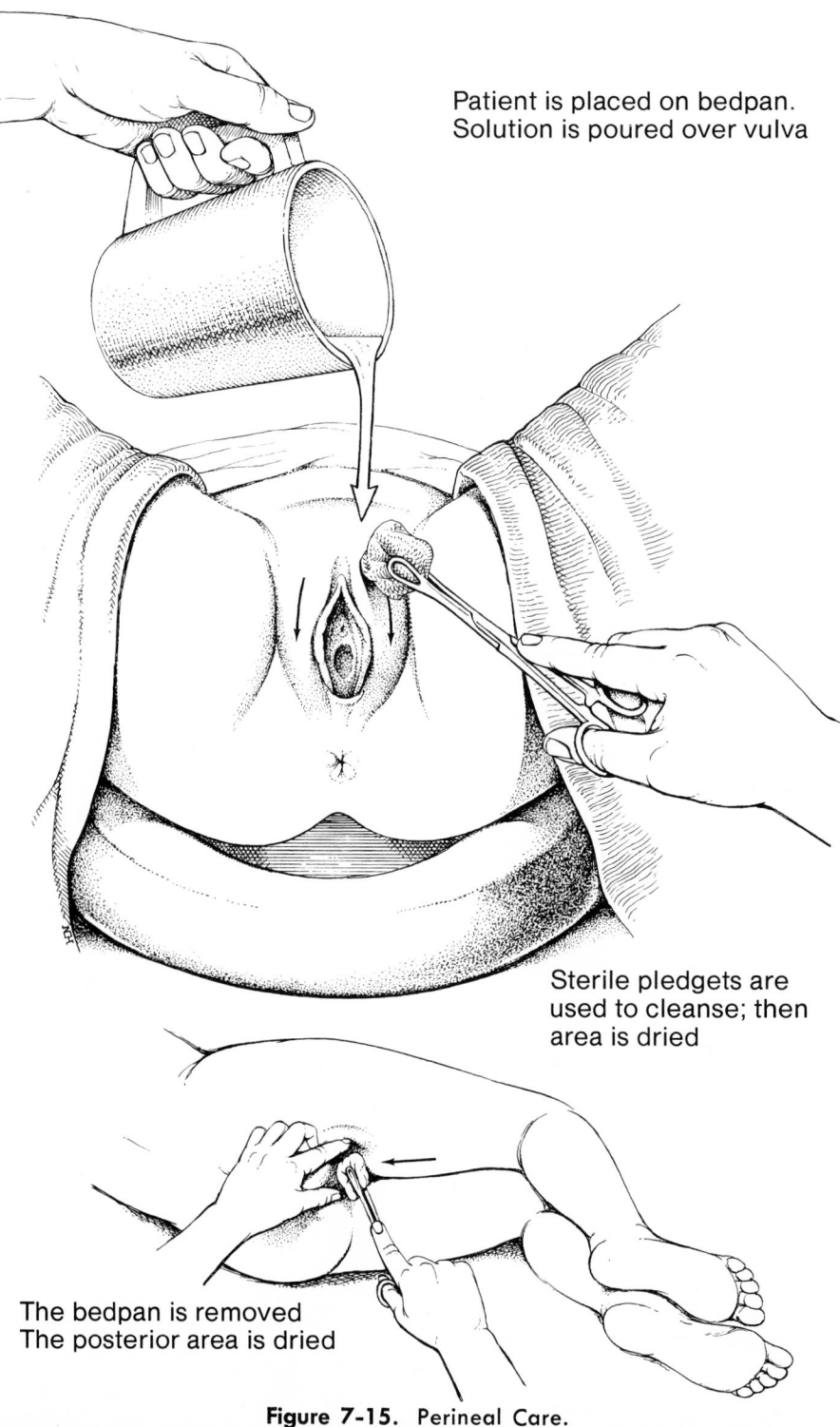

Patient is placed on bedpan.
Solution is poured over vulva

Sterile pledgets are
used to cleanse; then
area is dried

The bedpan is removed
The posterior area is dried

Figure 7-15. Perineal Care.

Procedure (Fig. 7-15)

Preparatory Phase
1. Place patient in dorsal recumbent position with legs flexed and separated.
2. Place protecting sheet under patient.

Nursing Action	Rationale/Amplification
Performance Phase	
1. Pour warmed irrigating solution gently over vulva from a sterile pitcher.	1. Materials will be flushed from perineal area into bedpan.
2. Cleanse perineal area with cotton pledget held in a sponge holder; use a top-down direction and discard each sponge in a plastic or paper bag after one use.	2. Friction facilitates cleansing process and the removal of soil.
3. Dry perineal area using dry cotton pledgets in same fashion as for cleansing.	3. Cleansing from front to back assists in preventing intestinal organisms from entering vaginal area.
Follow-up Phase	
1. Apply sterile perineal pad and hold in place with a T-binder.	1. To maintain cleanliness and provide comfort for patient.

PROBLEMS WHEN PELVIC MUSCLES RELAX

Cystocele

Cystocele is a downward displacement (protrusion) of the bladder into the vagina.

Etiology
1. Associated with obstetrical trauma to fascia, muscle, and ligaments during childbirth which results in poor support.
2. Often becomes apparent years later when genital atrophy associated with aging occurs.

Clinical Manifestations
1. Fatigue and pelvic pressure
2. Urinary symptoms—urgency, frequency, incontinence
3. At times a marked protrusion of anterior wall outside the vulva
4. Interference with coitus (intercourse)
5. Residual urine and urinary infection

Treatment
A. *Surgical*
    1. Anterior colporrhaphy—repair of anterior vaginal wall
    2. Perineal exercises to strengthen weakened muscles

B. *Nonsurgical*
    1. A pessary is fitted when surgery is contraindicated or refused.
    2. Pessary is removed periodically and cleansed thoroughly to prevent irritation.
    3. Douching with mildly acidic solutions is beneficial.
    4. Estrogen cream is applied locally for comfort.

Rectocele

Rectocele is displacement (protrusion) of the rectum into the vagina.

Etiology

Similar to cystocele, however, posterior vaginal wall is weakened in a rectocele

Clinical Manifestations

1. Constipation
2. Incontinence of gas and feces (in patients with a complete tear between rectum and vagina)

Treatment

Posterior colporrhaphy (perineorrhaphy)—repair of posterior vaginal wall

Objectives of Nursing Management

A. *To encourage women who have problems resulting from relaxed pelvic muscles to see a gynecologist. Patient may tend to:*
   1. Procrastinate and feel embarrassed.
   2. Expect that time will take care of it.
   3. Be resigned to the fact that this is a normal result of child-bearing.

B. *To enable the patient to relax during preoperative preparation phase*
   1. Promote rest particularly in a patient who has been working hard.
   2. Suggest low Fowler's position in bed to lessen edema and congestion.
   3. Recognize that this problem often occurs in older women.
   4. Prepare intestinal tract by administering a cathartic and enema.

C. *To prevent pressure on the suture line postoperatively, and prevent infection*
   1. Encourage voiding to reduce pressure; every 4–8 hours so that more than 150 ml. do not accumulate in bladder—catheterization or use of an indwelling catheter may be required.
   2. Administer perineal care to the patient after each voiding and defecation.
   3. Employ a heat lamp to help dry the incision line and enhance the healing process.
   4. Utilize available sprays for anesthetic and antiseptic effects.
   5. Apply an ice pack locally to relieve congestion and discomfort.

D. *To recognize the special care required by patients following operations for a complete perineal laceration*
   1. Encourage voiding (catheterization if necessary) to prevent pressure on suture line due to a full bladder.
   2. Avoid the use of enemas or a rectal tube for several days to permit wound healing.
   3. Provide liquid diet (no milk) for several days to prevent necessity of a bowel movement.
   4. Give tincture of opium (paregoric) to reduce peristalsis and inhibit bowel function.
   5. Administer mineral oil by about the 6th day and follow with an oil retention enema at sign of a possible bowel movement.

Displacement of the Uterus

Normally the uterus lies with the cervix at right angles to the long axis of the vagina; the body of the uterus is inclined slightly forward.

Backward Displacements (Retroversion and Retroflexion)

A. *Symptoms*
   1. Backache
   2. Easy fatigue
   3. A feeling of pelvic pressure
   4. Leukorrheal discharge

B. *Treatment* (Nonsurgical)
   1. Pessary—an S-shaped hard rubber, inflatable or Plexiglas device that keeps the uterus forward by exerting pressure on ligaments attached to the posterior wall of the cervix.
   2. A pessary must be removed and cleaned by the gynecologist at frequent intervals.

Prolapse and Procidentia

Uterine prolapse is a herniation of the uterus through the pelvic floor with a resultant protrusion into the vagina (prolapse) and at times even beyond the introitus (procidentia).

A *Factors Aggravating the Condition*
   1. Overstretching, which is allowed by pelvic fascia
   2. Standing, straining, coughing, lifting a heavy object
   3. Obstetrical trauma.

B. *Treatment*
   1. Surgical correction is the recommended treatment—a vaginal hysterectomy, Fothergill operation, or LeFort operation.
   2. When surgery is contraindicated or refused, a pessary provides partial relief to the problem.
      a. Douching is usually recommended 3 times weekly.
      b. Pessary removed, cleaned and checked monthly.

TUMORS OF THE UTERUS

Incidence and the Importance of Patient Education

   1. In the U.S., malignant tumors of the female reproductive system (excluding the breast) ranks as the 2nd cause of death.
   2. The death rate for uterine cancer has been showing a steady decline attributed to the unremitting education of women, which stresses the importance of annual check-ups, including the cytology smear.
   3. Nurses need to seek out the reasons why millions of women have not had Pap tests—lack of information, no transportation, inconvenient time of clinics, fear of results.

Cancer of the Cervix

Etiology

1. Cancer of the cervix is the most common cancer of the reproductive system in women.
2. It is most common between the ages of 30 and 50, but it can occur at any age.
3. Early cancer of the cervix is usually asymptomatic; it is almost always curable in its preinvasive stage.
4. Sexual activity appears to have some relationship to the incidence of this cancer.
5. Chronic infections and erosions of the cervix appear to be significant in the development of cancer.

Clinical Manifestations

1. Two chief symptoms of early carcinoma of the cervix are
   a. Leukorrhea—increases in amount, becomes dark and foul-smelling because of necrosis and infection of tumor mass.
   b. Irregular vaginal bleeding or spotting—between periods (metrorrhagia) or after the menopause; at first it may be very slight but as disease progresses, bleeding becomes more constant.
2. With advancing cancer there is excruciating pain in back and legs relieved only by large doses of narcotics.
3. Later, extreme emaciation and anemia occur; occasionally there is irregular fever due to secondary infection and abscesses in ulcerating mass.

Diagnostic Evaluation

1. Physical and gynecological examination plus a complete history are done initially.
2. Laboratory studies include cytology smear, routine blood examinations plus fasting blood sugar to detect diabetes, total plasma proteins for nutritional status evaluation, and bleeding and clotting time.
3. Roentgen studies should include chest x-ray, intravenous pyelogram and bone studies if indicated.
4. Electrocardiogram.

Treatment

Plan of treatment is for either surgery or radiation or a combination of both (see pp. 543–546).

Cancer of the Fundus

Incidence

1. One-third to one-fourth as often as cancer of the cervix
2. In postmenopausal women who have bleeding, one-half the cases are cancer of the fundus.

Clinical Manifestations

1. Irregular vaginal bleeding
2. Slow-growing malignancy

Diagnostic Evaluation

1. Early diagnosis is essential.
2. Encourage women over 40 especially, to have annual pelvic examinations. (See procedure on using a Gravlee Jet Washer, p. 528.)

Treatment

1. Hysterectomy (see p. 545)
2. Radiation (see below)

Myomata or Fibroid Tumors

Incidence and Clinical Manifestation

1. A benign muscle tumor of the uterus.
2. Occurs in about 40% of women.
3. Develops slowly until about age 40; larger size after this age.
4. Menorrhagia is most common symptom.
5. Pain, constipation, backache, urinary difficulties occur due to pressure of tumor.
6. Metrorrhagia and sterility may develop.

Treatment

1. If patient is of child-bearing age and desires children, treatment is conservative.
   a. If small tumor—myomectomy
   b. If large tumor—hysterectomy
   c. Ovaries are preserved
   d. If tumor is large with excessive bleeding—hysteromyomectomy (tumor and uterus removed)
2. For medical and nursing management, see page 545.

Nursing Care of the Patient Receiving Radiation Therapy of Uterus

Radiation Therapy (see also p. 882)

1. Radium, radioactive cobalt or iridium is introduced into the endocervical canal for a prescribed time.
2. Such therapy may be supplemented by external radiation with supervoltage machines directed over the pelvis in an effort to eliminate cancer spread via lymphatic system.
3. Therapy is individualized according to stage of disease and patient's response and tolerance for radiation.

Patient Preparation

1. Physician explains to the patient the reason such therapy is advocated.
2. Prepare the patient for various preliminary tests (may be done on an out-patient basis)—blood studies, biopsies (endometrial and cervical), chest x-ray, electrocardiogram, cystoscopy.
3. Be available for questions and conversation with the patient regarding any phase of the preliminary studies or treatment.
4. Following admission to the hospital, prepare the patient for surgery and, in addition, prepare the intestinal tract by enemata and the vaginal tract by a cleansing douche.

Radium Application

A. *Applicator, such as Ernst*
   1. Types
      a. Uterus—a tandem containing 1–3 radium tubes
      b. Vaginal vault surrounding cervix—ovoids, radium-loaded capsules
   2. Such an applicator is loaded in the radiotherapy department and transported to the operating room in a lead cart.
   3. An indwelling catheter is inserted to keep the bladder empty.
   4. Cervix is dilated, tandem is inserted and ovoids are positioned (without radium).
   5. Vaginal packing is inserted to maintain the position of the applicator.
B. *After-loading Technique*
   1. In surgery, the tandem and ovoids are positioned (without radium).
   2. Upon recovery from anesthesia, x-rays are taken in various positions in the x-ray department.
   3. Surgeon then inserts radium into prepositioned apparatus.

Nursing Management

> NURSING ALERT: It is imperative to keep the radium applicator in the uterine canal and to prevent a change of position. Adjust all nursing measures to meet this objective.

A. *While Radium Is in Place*
   1. Maintain patient on a low residue diet to prevent bowel movements which might dislodge apparatus.
   2. Inspect catheter frequently to insure proper drainage—a distended bladder may be in the path of radiation.
   3. Observe for symptoms of radiation sickness—nausea, vomiting, elevated temperature.
   4. Encourage patient to eat by offering a variety of small rather than large servings and present meals attractively to offset poor appetite.
   5. Offer citrus fruit juices because vitamin C is valuable in tissue repair.
   6. Permit patient to turn to either side; head of bed may be elevated 30 degrees.
   7. Provide back care but spend a minimum amount of time at the bedside.
   8. Relieve patient of anxiety and fear by utilizing wisely the contact time with the patient—engage in profitable conversation about her medical and nursing problems.
B. *Radium Removal*
   1. Notify surgeon when it is time to remove radium.
   2. Provide sterile gloves, long forceps and a large waste basin.
   3. Note on the chart the number of tubes applied so that this number is accounted for on removal.
   4. Practice radium precautions in handling and returning radium to the radiotherapy department.
   5. Administer a cleansing enema before the patient gets out of bed.
C. *Postirradiation Patient Care*
   1. Keep the patient's skin (exposed to radiation) dry; avoid use of soap since it irritates.
   2. Apply a soothing powder such as cornstarch to relieve itching and discomfort.
   3. For erythematous areas, apply a bland ointment such as A & D ointment to relieve irritation.

4. Nausea or vomiting may occur following large doses of radiation.

NURSING ALERT: Do not tell the patient nausea and vomiting may occur, since the power of suggestion may initiate these symptoms.

---

5. Observe for any symptoms which might suggest radiation injury to the intestine—diarrhea, tenesmus; report these if they occur.

HYSTERECTOMY

Hysterectomy is the surgical removal of the uterus.

Types of Abdominal Hysterectomy

1. *Subtotal hysterectomy*—fundus of uterus is removed but cervical stump remains.
2. *Total hysterectomy*—entire uterus is removed including cervix; tubes and ovaries remain.
3. *Panhysterectomy*—entire uterus, tubes and ovaries are removed.

Psychosocial Considerations

1. Patient may have deep-seated fears that cancer or venereal disease may be discovered.
2. There may be a conflict between recommended medical treatment and her personal religious beliefs.
3. Concerns may be raised regarding the possibility that all phases of her reproductive process may be disturbed.
4. She may be disappointed particularly if she never had children.
5. The patient may feel that she will no longer be able to fulfill her role and needs as a woman.
6. Depression and heightened emotional sensitivity to people and situations may need to be assessed.
7. The complexity of problems which are a mixture of physical, emotional and social factors need to be considered by the nurse as she assists this patient.
8. The relationship of this woman to her mate and family should be determined.

Postoperative Objectives of Nursing Management

A. *To reduce the possibility of bladder problems (which occur due to the proximity of the bladder to the surgical site).*
   1. Insert an indwelling catheter, if prescribed, because edema or nerve trauma may cause temporary bladder atony. A suprapubic catheter may be used (see p. 470).
   2. Remove catheter with physician's permission after the 3rd or 4th day.
   3. Catheterize patient if no catheter is in place and the patient has not voided after 8 hours.
   4. Determine whether there is pooling of residual urine; catheterize patient after each voiding; otherwise bladder infection may develop.

B. *To relieve the discomfort of abdominal distention.*
   1. A nasogastric tube may be inserted while the patient is in the operating room.
   2. Fluids and food may be restricted until peristalsis has resumed.

  3. Apply heat to the abdomen and insert a rectal tube to relieve abdominal flatus.
  4. Permit the patient to sit on edge of bed with feet supported and to get out of bed and ambulate.
  5. Serve additional fluids and soft diet as peristalsis returns.
C. *To prevent vascular disorders.*
  1. Change patient's position frequently.
  2. Avoid high Fowler's position and pressure under the knees which might cause stasis and pooling of the blood.
  3. Evaluate legs for positive Homan's sign (tenderness, pain in calf upon dorsiflexion of foot).
  4. Observe legs for the presence of varicosities; promote circulation with special leg exercises.
D. *To counteract effects resulting from removal of a large tumor or unusual blood loss.*
  1. Administer high protein diet with iron supplement to combat anemia.
  2. Recommend a girdle or apply an abdominal binder following removal of a large tumor to provide support for relaxed abdominal muscles.
E. *To instruct and inform the patient regarding any limitations imposed on her, following her hospitalization.*
  1. A subtotal hysterectomy does not stop menstruation; a total hysterectomy produces a surgical menopause.
  2. Explain to her the importance of hormonal replacement if she has had a total hysterectomy (according to the age of the patient).
  3. Remind her to ask the physician regarding resumption of physical activities including sexual relations.
  4. Emphasize the importance of follow-up physical and gynecological examinations for peace of mind and detecting pathology early.

ENDOMETRIOSIS

Endometriosis is a disease characterized by displaced groups of cells resembling those cells lining the uterus, but growing aberrantly in the pelvic cavity outside of the uterus.

Incidence
  1. Frequency of occurrence is about 25–30% in white women.
  2. It is rarely encountered in women of the black race.

Characteristics
  1. Pelvic endometriosis attacks many areas. Order of frequency is—the ovary, uretero-sacral ligaments, the cul-de-sac, ureterovesical peritoneum, cervix, umbilicus, laparotomy scars, hernial sacs and appendix.
  2. Misplaced endometrium responds to ovarian hormonal stimulation and even depends on this for survival.
     a. When uterus goes through the process of menstruation, this misplaced tissue also bleeds; because there is no outlet for accumulated blood, pain and adhesions result.
     b. At surgery, concealed bleeding is in evidence because lesions are brown or blue-black.
     c. Ovarian cysts in which such bleeding has occurred are referred to as "chocolate cysts."

Etiology

1. Backflow of menses causing endometrial tissue to be transported to ectopic sites through fallopian tubes.
2. Endometrial tissue, during surgery, may accidentally be transferred by way of instruments.
3. Such tissue may be spread via lymphatic or venous channels.
4. Embryonic tissue remnants may cover pelvic peritoneum and ovaries.

Clinical Manifestations

1. Abnormal uterine bleeding, backache, rectal pain and dyspareunia (painful intercourse).
2. Symptoms are more acute during menstruation and subside after menstruation.
3. When a cyst ruptures, symptoms mimic acute appendicitis or ruptured ectopic pregnancy.

Diagnostic Evaluation

1. Manual rectal and pelvic examinations reveal fixed tender nodular structures, ovarian abnormalities and uterus fixed by retraining adhesions.
2. X-ray studies, such as barium enema, may demonstrate constrictions indicative of endometriosis.

Treatment and Nursing Management

1. It is necessary for the patient to be included in treatment plans so that she knows why a particular method of treatment has been selected and how her role is a vital one in the success of the team effort.
2. Encourage the patient to express her concerns; often false ideas emerge such as "perhaps I have endometriosis because I used tampons."
3. Hormonal therapy is initiated to interrupt ovulation—relieves dysmenorrhea and temporarily postpones surgery.
4. Surgery when indicated is directed toward resection of cysts and lysis of adhesions.
5. Likelihood of recurrence of endometriosis is high; conservative and minor surgery is done during child-bearing years.
6. Ultimate treatment requires more radical procedures: total hysterectomy.

PELVIC INFLAMMATORY DISEASE (P.I.D.)

Pelvic inflammatory disease is an inflammation of the pelvic cavity that may involve the fallopian tubes (salpingitis), ovaries (oophoritis), pelvic peritoneum, or pelvic vascular system.

Etiology

1. Disease may be caused by staphylococcus, streptococcus or venereal organisms and may be acute or chronic.
2. Pathogenic organisms normally are introduced from outside; they pass through the cervical canal and uterus and into the pelvis via lymphatic channels, uterine veins or fallopian tubes.
3. When P.I.D. is caused by tubercle bacillus, it is usually transmitted via the bloodstream from the lungs.

Clinical Manifestations

1. Abdominal pain, nausea and vomiting, temperature elevation, malaise.
2. Leukocytosis.
3. Malodorous purulent vaginal discharge.

Treatment and Nursing Management

Objectives: to control the spread of infection within the patient.
to prevent the spread of infection to others, including the nurse.

1. Place patient in a semi-Fowler's position to facilitate drainage.
2. Avoid the use of tampons and do not catheterize this patient in order to minimize spread of infection.
3. Support patient nutritionally with attractive well-balanced meals.
4. Administer appropriate antibiotics and chemotherapeutic agents as prescribed.
5. Control spread of infection by the following safeguards:
   a. Handle perineal pads with extreme precautions:
      (1) Use an instrument or gloves.
      (2) Deposit pad in paper bag for proper disposal.
   b. Wash hands carefully before and after patient contacts.
   c. Disinfect utensils, bedpans, toilet seats and linen.
      Adopt procedure appropriate for specific organism.
   d. Instruct patient in procedure to protect herself from reinfection and to prevent spread to others.
6. Apply heat to the abdomen externally and hot douches vaginally as prescribed to improve circulation.
7. Record vital signs, patient responses (physical and mental) to therapy and nature and amount of vaginal discharge.
8. Recognize the depressing nature of the disease and that the patient needs support and understanding particularly when she has discomfort and vague symptoms.

Complications from Untreated P.I.D.

1. Chronic pelvic discomfort and disease becomes rampant.
2. Sterility occurs because of closing of fallopian tubes with scar tissue.
3. Ectopic pregnancy is possible if fertilized egg is unable to pass stricture.
4. Adhesions may develop, eventually requiring removal of uterus, tubes and ovaries.

ABORTION

Abortion is the interruption of a pregnancy or the expulsion of contents of a pregnant uterus before the fetus is viable.

Miscarriage is a lay term for abortion.

Spontaneous Abortion

Occurs naturally with no known cause.

1. *Threatened*—cervix does not dilate; it can be prevented with bedrest and conservative treatment.
2. *Inevitable*—when a threatened abortion cannot be prevented and is imminent.
3. *Incomplete*—when some of the tissue but not all is passed during an abortion.
4. *Complete*—the fetus and all related tissue are passed.

Habitual Abortion

When successive abortions of unknown cause occur 3 times.

1. Attempts are made to prevent this by ultra conservative measures.
   a. Complete bedrest.
   b. Administration of stilbestrol and progesterone to prevent sloughing of endometrium.
   c. Thyroid extract therapy.
   d. Psychotherapy.
2. For patients with "incomplete cervical os" (the cervix dilates painlessly in second trimester of pregnancy), a spontaneous abortion may occur.
   Treatment—Shirodkar operation (placing a purse-string suture of nylon or fascia in submucous layer)

NURSING ALERT: It is very important to know when a patient has this problem and that a suture is in place.
1. As soon as labor occurs, notify the physician.
2. Suture is cut to allow labor to proceed normally.
3. Otherwise, the uncut suture may cause uterus to rupture.

Therapeutic Abortion

According to U.S. Supreme Court ruling of January 22, 1973, pregnancy may be terminated as follows:

1. In the first trimester of pregnancy, the abortion decision is to be left to the woman and her physician.
2. During the next trimester, the state may not prohibit abortion but may regulate its practice in the interest of protecting the woman's health.
3. During the final weeks of pregnancy, the state may choose to protect the potential life of the fetus by prohibiting abortion except where necessary to preserve the life or health of the woman.
4. The religious beliefs of the patient are always respected.

Induced Abortion

Termination of a pregnancy by the patient or others.

1. Estimated that approximately a million a year occur in the U.S.
2. Approximately 10,000 deaths occur due to infection, rupture of uterus or drug overdosage.
3. The nurse should encourage a woman contemplating such an abortion to seek medical advice and counseling; many agencies are set up to assist in such situations.

Treatment and Nursing Management

1. Note the signs of a threatened abortion—vaginal discharge or bleeding and abdominal cramps.
2. Have patient see a physician: bedrest, light diet, no straining on defecation.
3. Save all tissue passed vaginally for physician's examination.
4. Give sedatives or tranquilizers as prescribed to permit the patient to relax.
5. Administer antibiotics as ordered to reduce the possibility of infection.
6. Be prepared to assist with blood transfusion if there is much blood loss.

7. Record numbers of pads in an effort to estimate blood loss.
8. In the event of an incomplete abortion, administer ergot to promote contraction of the uterus; usually a D & E (dilatation and evacuation) or ERS (evacuation of retained secretions) will be done. Nursing care is similiar to that required for a D & C (p. 527).
9. Recognize the severe emotional reaction such a patient is likely to experience. She needs understanding, to be 'cared' for and someone to talk to.

Ectopic Pregnancy

An *ectopic pregnancy* is a pregnancy in which the fertilized ovum does not reach the cavity of the uterus but becomes lodged and embedded in the fallopian tube or, less frequently, in the ovary or abdomen.

Clinical Course

The tube becomes more and more distended as fertilized ovum increases in size; rupture occurs and ovum is discharged into abdominal cavity.

Clinical Manifestations

1. Colicky pain on affected side.
2. With rupture—agonizing pain, faintness, shock, air hunger, signs of hemorrhage.
3. By vaginal examination, surgeon is able to feel a large mass of clotted blood behind uterus.

Treatment and Nursing Management

Always surgical: salpingectomy (removal of tube) and if necessary, an ovariectomy.

1. It may be necessary to treat shock and hemorrhage before surgery is attempted.
2. Recovery rate is high with surgery; without surgery, mortality rate is high (60–70%).
3. Postoperative care similar to care in postlaparotomy; transfusions may be necessary to treat acute anemia.

FERTILITY CONTROL

Basic Principles

1. The nurse should be familiar with the application, advantages and disadvantages of the various methods of contraception available.
2. The most effective method is the one a woman selects for herself and will use consistently.
3. Women are entitled to contraceptive advice as part of good medical care without the burden of moral judgment.
4. No one has the right to encourage a patient to use birth control if it is contrary to her religious or moral beliefs.

Mechanical Methods

A. *Intrauterine Devices*
1. Types—Lippes Loop, Hall-Stone Stainless Steel Ring, Birnberg Bow, Margulies Spiral.

2. Indications
   a. When hormonal medications are contraindicated.
   b. When woman has no preference for any one method.
   c. For a woman whose family is complete but who is not desirous of having permanent sterilization.
3. Contraindications
   a. Inflammation or infection of cervix, uterus, or uterine tubes.
   b. Objections on the part of the woman to a foreign device in her uterus.
   c. Severe dysmenorrhea.
4. Procedure for Insertion and Follow-up
   a. A pelvic examination and a (Pap) cytology smear.
   b. Caliber of interior of the uterus determined by means of sounding.
   c. Insertion of IUD with the aid of a plastic inserter.
   d. Patient instruction as to the nature of the device and detection of nylon thread to determine its placement.
   e. Need to be checked by a physician in a month and at yearly intervals.
5. Undesirable Effects
   a. Excessive staining or bleeding.
   b. Excessive cramps which persist.
   c. Expulsion of device spontaneously. (This accounts for 20–30% for a combination of expulsion and patient request for removal.)
6. Failure Rate (Pregnancy) is determined by the experience of 100 women for 1 year and is expressed as . . . pregnancies per 100 woman years.

B. *Diaphragm*
   1. Indications—preferred by women who
      a. Object to a device in utero.
      b. Object to hormonal or chemical contraceptives.
      c. Do not object to insertion of the diaphragm immediately prior to intercourse.
   2. Procedure for Insertion and Follow-up
      a. Bimanual pelvic examination and cytology smear.
      b. Measure depth of vagina; select largest diaphragm that can be retained comfortably.
      c. Teach the patient how to insert diaphragm behind lower edge of pubic bone; use spermicidal jelly or cream for additional contraceptive action.
      d. Instruct her to retain diaphragm for 6–8 hours after intercourse.
      e. Remind patient of annual gynecological examination.
      f. Inform patient that a larger diaphragm may be necessary after a pregnancy.
   3. Failure Rate (Pregnancy)
      15 undesired pregnancies per hundred woman years of using diaphragm.

C. *Condom*
   1. Indications—Rubber sheath worn by male when other contraceptive measures are impractical.
   2. Procedure for Use and Precautions
      a. Place condom over erect penis.
      b. Avoid leaving condom in vagina during withdrawal.
   3. Failure Rate (Pregnancy)
      Approximately 20 per hundred woman years of using condom.

D. *Oral Fertility Control—the 'Pill'*
  1. Basis of Operation of Oral Contraceptives
      Oral synthetic steroid preparations of estrogen and progesterone tend to block the stimulation of the ovary by the central nervous system thereby preventing the release of the follicle-stimulating hormone (FSH) from the anterior pituitary. With no FSH, a follicle does not ripen and ovulation does not take place.
  2. Indications
      a. For those desirous of a highly effective contraceptive with no special preparation immediately before intercourse.
      b. For women who will conscientiously adhere to a daily plan of pill-taking.
  3. Preliminary Concerns and Contraindications
      a. A complete physical examination is required prior to taking the "pill" and 6-month check-ups thereafter.
      b. Known or suspected malignancy, history of thrombophlebitis, pulmonary embolism or cerebrovascular accident, undiagnosed vaginal bleeding, fluid retention.
  4. Methods
      a. Combined—estrogen and progestogen
          Ovulation inhibited by hypothalamic-pituitary effect.
          Cervical mucus is changed thereby becoming a barrier to sperm.
      b. Sequential—estrogen suppresses pituitary gonadotropin and inhibits ovulation during first part of cycle. Then with combined hormones, a more physiologic endometrium results.
  5. Failure rate (Pregnancy)
      a. Combined—less than 1 pregnancy per hundred woman years.
      b. Sequential—approximately 5 per hundred woman years.

Sterilization Procedures

A. *Indications*
  1. The patient's desire
      a. Socioeconomic reasons
      b. Therapeutic or eugenic reasons to prevent a pregnancy that might endanger the mother's life
  2. Legal considerations
      a. Laws much less rigid than those governing therapeutic abortion.
      b. Written consent required from a legally responsible and informed person.
      c. Must be compatible with state laws.
  3. Incidence and indications
      a. About 100,000 are performed annually in U.S.
      b. Done for multiparity, 2 or more previous cesarean sections, hypertensive cardiovascular disease.
      c. Done for other reasons: vaginal plastic procedures, for inheritable life-threatening diseases.

B. *Tubal Sterilization*
  1. Types:
      a. Tubal ligation with or without resection
      b. Tubal ligation with or without crushing
      c. Tubal transection and burying of stumps

      d. Cornual resection

      e. Cornual occlusion utilizing cautery.

  2. Approaches

      a. Abdominal

      b. After a cesarean section

      c. Vaginally

      d. Intrauterine

  3. Evaluation

      a. There are advantages and disadvantages to each of the above—the individual situation must be considered.

      b. Reversible methods of tubal occlusion or semipermanent sterilization using metal clips or chemical injections are still experimental.

  4. Laparoscopy:

      a. A relatively new procedure in which coagulation and transection of the isthmic tubal segments is done through a laparoscope (an electrical current is passed for 3–5 seconds to cut and coagulate tube).

      b. The procedure is considered rapid, safe and effective.

      c. The patient is discharged from the hospital about 3 hours postoperatively with minimal discomfort; it can be done on an outpatient basis.

      d. Effectiveness

         (1) Hysterosalpingography done 12 weeks postoperatively confirms tubal occlusion in 98% of patients.

         (2) No adverse effects occur in sex relations, menstrual function, or outward bodily appearance.

      e. Hazards:

         (1) Pulmonary embolism, hemorrhage, infection

         (2) Tubal pregnancy

         (3) Some women are disturbed emotionally by procedure; however, 90% of patients who request this have no subsequent regret.

C. *Vasectomy* (See p. 519.)

3. Conditions of the Breast

CONDITIONS OF THE NIPPLE

Fissure of the Nipple

A *fissure of the nipple* is a longitudinal type ulcer that occasionally develops in the breast of the nursing mother.

Clinical Manifestations

  1. Irritated and sore nipple; aggravated by sucking of infant.

  2. Bleeding from nipple.

Preventive Measures

  1. Keep the nipple clean by washing and drying after each nursing period.

  2. In prenatal period, wash, dry and lubricate nipples in preparation for nursing.

Treatment

1. Wash with sterile saline solution.
2. Use artificial nipple for nursing.
3. If above does not initiate healing process, stop nursing and use a breast pump.

Bleeding from the Nipple

Clinical Manifestations

Bloody discharge—usually on edge of areola.

Causes

1. Most commonly due to wart-like papilloma in one of the larger collecting ducts at the edge of areola.
2. Occasionally a malignancy is responsible.

Surgical Treatment

Duct is identified; papilloma can be excised through a small periareolar incision.

Paget's Disease of the Breast

Incidence

1. Noted frequently in women over 40.
2. Is usually unilateral.

Clinical Manifestations

1. Begins as a mild eczema of nipple; spreads from nipple to areola to part of breast and then ulcerates.
2. Later, retraction of nipple—a malignant manifestation.

Treatment

Early and total mastectomy.

INFLAMMATION OF THE BREAST

Acute Mastitis

Incidence

1. May occur at beginning or end of lactation.

Source of Infection

1. Hands of patient; personnel caring for her.
2. Infection from baby.
3. Blood-borne.

Clinical Manifestations

1. Infection attacks duct causing stagnation of milk in lobules.
2. Dull pain occurs in the area affected.
3. Breast feels doughy and tough.
4. May also have a discharging nipple.

Treatment and Nursing Management

1. Have patient stop breast feeding.
2. Apply heat or cold (depending upon stage of the infection).
3. Administer chemotherapeutic agents.
4. Give progesterone to relieve congestion.
5. Have patient wear firm breast support.
6. Encourage patients to practice meticulous personal hygiene.

Mammary Abscess

Incidence

Often follows acute mastitis.

Clinical Manifestations

1. Area is very sensitive, appears dusky red.
2. Pus may be expressed from nipple.

Treatment

1. Administer antibiotics and chemotherapy.
2. Incise and drain.
3. Apply hot wet dressings to increase drainage and hasten resolution.

Chronic Cystic Mastitis

Cause and Incidence

1. Overgrowth of fibrous tissue around ducts
2. Occurs in women between 30 and 50

Clinical Manifestations

1. Patient complains of an uncomfortable feeling in the breast.
2. Small nodules (like buckshot) are palpable.
3. Pain may be of the "shooting" type.

Diagnosis

See page 556, Cancer of the Breast.

FIBROCYSTIC DISEASE

Retention Cyst

1. With advancing age, a mammary duct may become obstructed by fibrosis.
2. Secretion of duct beyond the obstruction collects and dilates the duct to form a cyst.
3. Retention cysts occur in women near menopause.
4. Cysts appear as firm, smooth round masses; tender on palpation or pressure.
5. Treatment consists of aspiration under local anesthesia.
6. Such a breast is more prone to develop cancer than is a normal breast.

TUMORS OF THE BREAST

Fibroadenomata

Clinical Manifestations

1. Firm, round movable, benign tumors of the breast.
2. Appear in breasts of girls in their late teens or early twenties.
3. No pain or tenderness

Treatment

Removal through a small incision

Prognosis

No malignant potential

Cancer of the Breast

Incidence

1. Breast cancer is the leading cause of cancer incidence and death in women today.
2. 74,000 new cases are predicted yearly and it is estimated that there will be 33,000 deaths.
3. Despite all efforts to date, breast cancer death rate remains high.
4. Survival rate for all breast cancer patients, treated or untreated, is roughly 50%.
5. About 95% of patients discover their condition themselves through breast self-examination:
   a. 60% will have spread to axillary lymph nodes; 5-year survival rate is 40–45%.
   b. 40% will be localized to breast; 5-year survival rate is 80–85%.

Underlying Factors

1. Cause is unknown.
2. Classification of women in whom breast cancer occurs more frequently.
   a. Those having a family history of breast cancer (5-fold increase).
   b. Those in the higher socioeconomic levels.
   c. Those having a late menopause.
   d. Those without children.
   e. Those who have not breast-fed.

3. Researchers in the U. S. and India have found high concentrations of virus-like particles in the milk of women with family histories of breast cancer.
4. Injuries, it is believed, do not lead to breast cancer.

Clinical Manifestations (Fig. 7-16)

1. Early signs are insidious.
2. A nontender lump appears in the breast, most frequently in the upper outer quadrant; it may be movable and isolated.
3. Pain usually is absent except in the late stages.
4. 'Orange-peel' skin or a dimpling of the skin may be noted.
5. On mirror examination, asymmetry may be observed with the affected breast appearing more elevated.
6. Nipple retraction or nipple bleeding may be apparent.
7. Later, the breast becomes more fixed to the chest wall.
8. Nodular axillary masses may appear.
9. Ulceration, cachexia and weight loss appear in late stages.
10. Breast cancer occurs more on left than right side—110:100

Diagnostic Evaluation

A. *Breast Self-examination*
   1. Clinical value
      a. Experience has verified that 90% of breast cancers are found by women themselves.
      b. When women discover lumps in their breasts at a very early stage, surgery can save 70–80% of proven cases.

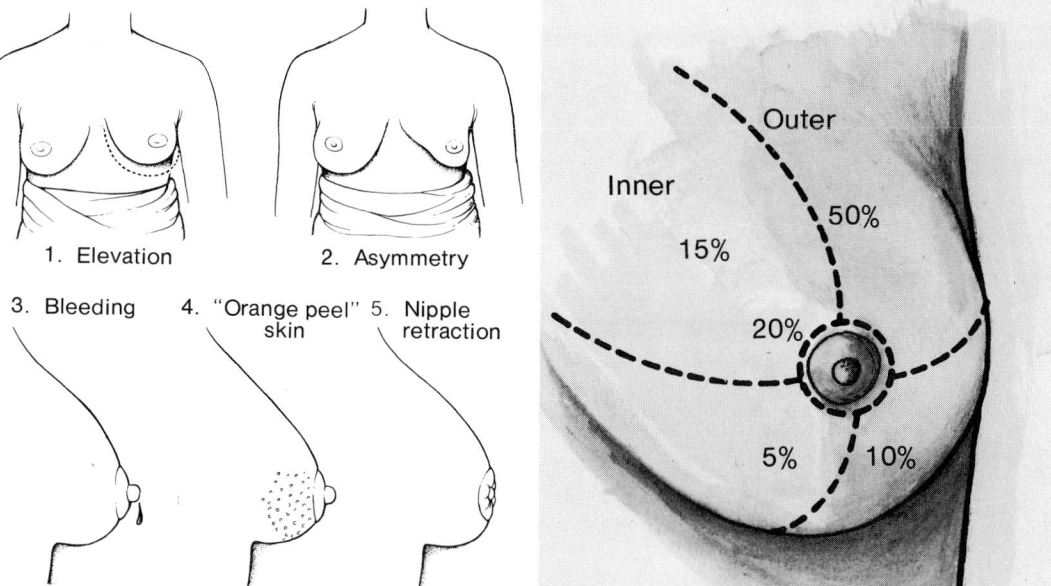

1. Elevation   2. Asymmetry

3. Bleeding   4. "Orange peel" skin   5. Nipple retraction

Outer

Inner

50%

15%

20%

5%   10%

Figure 7-16. Signs of cancer of the breast.

Figure 7-17. Distribution of carcinomas in different areas of breast.

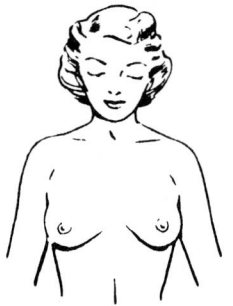 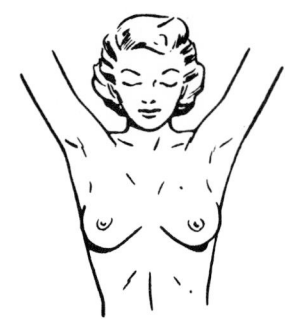 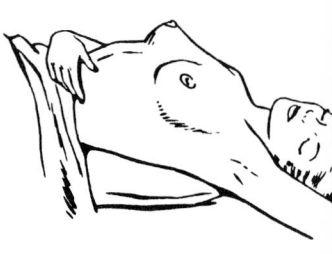

1. Careful examination of the breasts before a mirror for symmetry in size and shape, noting any puckering or dimpling of the skin or retraction of the nipple.

2. Arms raised over head, again studying the breasts in the mirror for the same signs.

3. Reclining on bed with flat pillow or folded bath towel under the shoulder on the same side as breast to be examined.

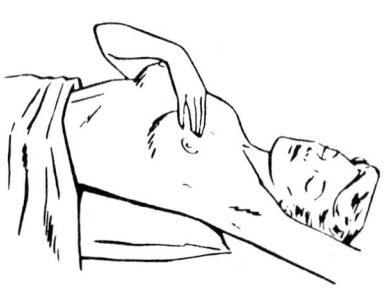 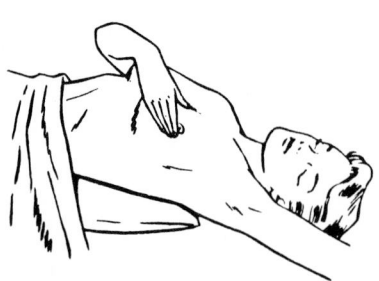 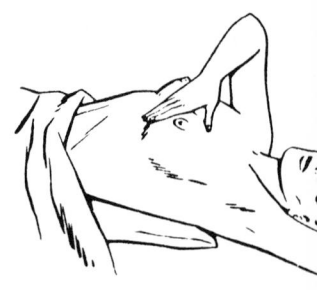

4. To examine the inner half of the breast the arm is raised over the head. Beginning at the breastbone and, in a series of steps, the inner half of the breast is palpated.

5. The area over the nipple is carefully palpated with the flat part of the fingers.

6. Examination of the lower inner half of the breast is completed.

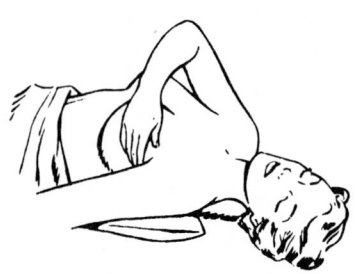 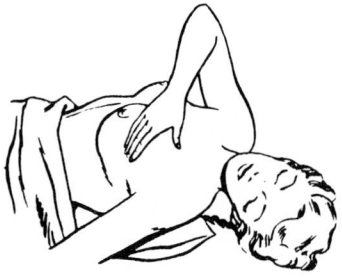 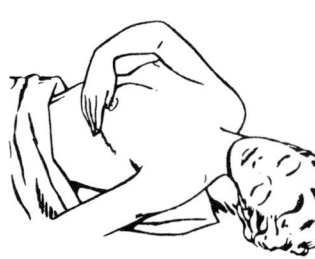

7. With arm down at side self examination of breasts continues by carefully feeling the tissues which extend to the armpit.

8. The upper outer quadrant of the breast is examined with the flat part of the fingers.

9. The lower outer quadrant of breast is examined in successive stages with flat part of the fingers.

Figure 7-18. Breast self-examination. (Courtesy American Cancer Society.)

2. Primary nursing care

   a. Encourage women to examine their breasts once a month. just after the menstrual period and, equally important, at regular monthly intervals after the cessation of menses (Fig. 7-18).

   b. Tell women's organizations about the breast self-examination film and advise them to see it.

   c. Arrange for local showings of the film.

   d. Take part in the discussion of the film. Be prepared—know the signs that may mean breast cancer.

   e. Help to create healthy psychological attitudes.

   f. Know the resources within the community where medical help is available, the physicians' offices, nearby hospitals, cancer clinics or cancer hospitals.

B. *Physical Examination by Physician*

   1. Annual physical check-up should include breast palpation.
   2. Twice-a-year examination recommended for women with a family history of cancer.

C. *Mammography*—roentgenography of breast without injection of contrast medium; 3 views; (1) craniocaudal, (2) mediolateral and (3) axillary.
   Indications

   a. Breast disease evident
   b. Family history of breast cancer
   c. Previous breast biopsy
   d. Lumpy or very large breasts which are difficult to examine
   e. Cancerophobia (fear of cancer)

D. *Thermography*—infrared photography which may detect abnormal circulating signs.

   1. By using heat sensing equipment, minute amounts of heat generated in and around areas of increased blood supply may be detected.
   2. Requires a skilled radiologist to interpret abnormal patterns.
   3. Not used exclusively but in context of physical examination and patient's history.

E. *Xerography*—a special x-ray in which a selenium-coated plate is subjected to an electrical charge; after the x-ray exposure is made, the plate is carefully developed. The xerogram portrays all tissue in bas-relief.

F. *Biopsy*

   1. *Aspiration*—A syringe and No. 18 needle is used to aspirate tissue from the site which is under local anesthesia. The specimen is spread on a glass slide, fixed, stained and sent to the laboratory.
   2. *Incisional*—A piece of tissue is obtained in the operating room, sent to the laboratory for frozen section which is then stained and examined under the microscope.

Classification of Breast Tumors and Preferred Method of Treatment

Clinical Anatomic Observation	Treatment
Stage I Breast mass localized; all nodes negative.	Radical mastectomy preferred by most U. S. surgeons. Some prefer simple mastectomy plus irradiation. Others prefer simple mastectomy without irradiation.
Stage II Breast mass localized; axillary nodes positive.	Radical mastectomy preferred with or without postoperative irradiation.
Stage III Breast mass locally extensive; axillary supraclavicular and internal mammary nodes positive.	Variable depending on extensiveness: 1. Simple mastectomy with radiation. 2. Simple mastectomy with excision of large axillary nodes. 3. Radiation therapy alone if tumor is fixed to chest wall.
Stage IV Distant metastasis.	Variable, depending upon nature of metastasis, such as to bone, soft tissue, etc. 1. Radiation therapy to primary lesion or metastasis 2. Hormonal therapy, hypophysectomy, adrenalectomy 3. Chemotherapy 4. Oophorectomy

Treatment and Nursing Management

Objective: to remove or destroy whole tumor
1. When malignancy is confined to breast—cure rate = 70%
2. When malignancy has spread to axilla—cure rate = 40%

A. Seek optimal physical and psychosocial approach in preparing patient for surgery.
1. Begin emotional support when patient is told that hospitalization and biopsy may be required.
2. Dispel fear by
   a. Listening to patient's concerns and dispelling misconceptions.
   b. Emphasizing successful program of rehabilitation and use of prosthesis.
   c. Having a patient who made a satisfactory postoperative adjustment visit present patient.
   d. Soliciting support of the husband.
   e. Providing encouragement and reassurance.
3. Minimize delay before operation.
   a. Determine physical and nutritional needs.
   b. If radical surgery is anticipated, have blood replacement available.
   c. Administer hypnotic to minimize concerns of patient.
4. Prepare skin adequately (see p. 45).
   When skin graft is anticipated, shave and clean donor area (usually anterior aspect of thigh).

B. Select a surgical approach to remove malignancy, minimize disfiguration, and prevent spread of cancer cells.
  1. *Simple mastectomy*—removal of breast without lymph node dissection.
  2. *Radical mastectomy*—removal of breast and underlying muscles down to chest wall; also removal of nodules and lymphatics of axilla.
  3. Pressure dressings usually applied to reduce serum collection, prevent hemorrhage, lessen edema and enhance wound healing.
  4. For drainage, a drainage tube may be placed in the axilla; portable suction may be used (see p. 70).
C. When radiation therapy is utilized, follow principles of care, page 882.
D. Initiate postoperative surveillance to minimize complications and hasten recovery.
  1. Assess blood pressure and pulse status since they are valuable indices in detecting shock and hemorrhage.

Table 7-2. Exercises for the Rehabilitation of the Patient Following Radical Mastectomy

Exercise	Equivalent Daily Activities
1. Stand erect. Lean forward from waist. Allow arms to hang. Swing arms from side to side together; then in opposite direction. Next, swing arms from front to back together; then in opposite direction.	Broom sweeping Vacuum cleaning Mopping floor Pulling out and pushing in drawers Weaving Playing golf
2. Stand erect facing wall with palms of hand flat against wall; arms extended. Relax arms and shoulders and allow upper part of body to lean forward against hand. Push away to original position. Repeat.	Pushing self out of bath tub Kneading bread Breast stroke—swimming Sawing or cutting type of crafts
3. Stand erect facing wall with palms of hand flat against wall. Climb the wall with the fingers; descend; repeat.	Raising windows Washing windows Hanging clothes on line Reaching to an upper shelf
4. Stand erect and clasp hands at small of back; raise hands, lower, repeat. Clasp hands back of neck; reach downward; upward; repeat.	Fastening brassiere Buttoning blouse or dress Pulling up a dress zipper Fastening beads Washing the back
5. Toss a rope over the shower curtain rod. Hold the ends of the rope (knotted) in each hand and raise arms sideways. Using a see-saw motion and with arms outstretched, slide the rope up and down over the rod.	Drying the back with a bath towel Raising and lowering a window blind Closing and opening window drapes
6. Flex and extend each finger in turn.	Sewing, knitting, crocheting Typing, painting, playing piano or other musical instrument

2. Inspect dressings for bleeding under axilla and shoulder.
3. Upon recovery from anesthesia, administer analgesic for relief of pain.
4. Encourage turning and deep breathing to prevent pulmonary complications.
5. Check dressings for constriction so that lung expansion is not hampered.
6. Connect drainage tubes to suction machine or portable suction to release serum and blood and to allow skin flap to adhere to chest wall.
7. Position patient in semi-Fowler's position; if arm is free, elevate on a pillow; gravity aids in removal of fluid via lymphatic and venous pathways.
8. Ambulate patient 2nd or 3rd day; diet as preferred and tolerated.

E. Plan a purposeful rehabilitative program; prepare for posthospital convalescence.
1. Talk to and listen to patient; encourage questions and provide helpful answers.
2. Prepare the husband for his role in providing the necessary emotional support.
3. Initiate active exercise on the affected side 24 hours postoperatively; this will increase daily with the patient doing more of her own activities such as hair combing, teeth brushing, etc. (Table 7-2).
   a. Exercise should not be painful.
   b. Bilateral activity should be emphasized.
   c. Proper posture should be maintained.
   d. If the patient has had a skin graft or the skin was approximated under tension, exercises will be limited.
4. Care of Wound
   a. Explain how the wound will gradually change.
   b. The newly healed wound may have less sensation due to severed nerves.
   c. Bathe gently and blot carefully to dry.
   d. Recognize signs of infection—pain, tenderness, redness, swelling, and if these are present, report to physician.
   e. Massage gently the healed incision with cocoa butter to encourage circulation and increase skin elasticity.
5. Use of a prosthesis—sponge rubber, air-filled or fluid-filled.
   a. Type and style are suggested on an individual basis; skilled fitters from reliable companies are most helpful.

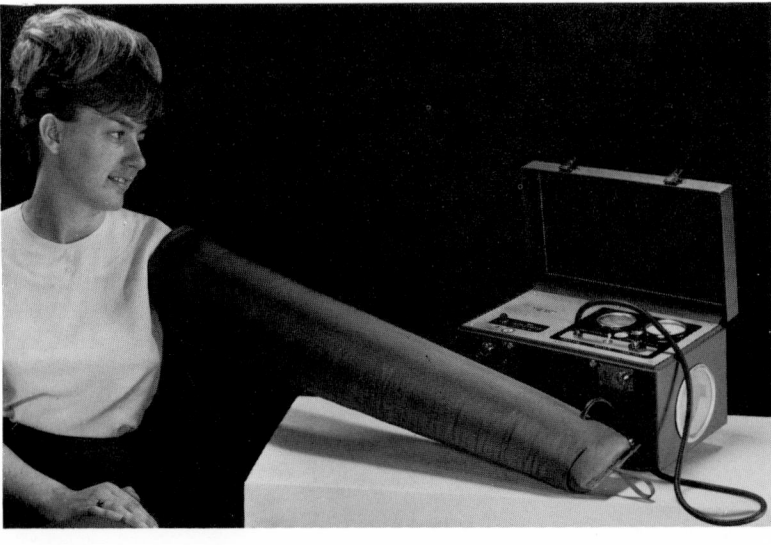

Figure 7-19. A home model of an intermittent compression unit which gently forces lymphatic fluid back into the venous system, thereby greatly reducing the size of the extremity. (Courtesy Jobst.)

    b. Observe effect of prosthesis on incision; to prevent irritation, lamb's wool padding may be used.

    e. A prosthetic should not be worn unless authorized by the physician.

6. *After Mastectomy,* a film from the American Cancer Society, is often helpful for post-mastectomy patients.

Complication—Lymphedema of the Arm

Lymphedema is an obstruction to the lymph flow in the arm on the operated side producing a chronic swelling of the part particularly if it is in a dependent position.

A. *Prevention*

1. Exercises should be done as indicated above.
2. The affected arm should be massaged 3 or 4 months postoperatively to increase circulation and lessen edema.
3. The affected arm should be elevated frequently.
4. The arm and operative site should be kept scrupulously clean.
5. Nonconstricting clothing should be worn.
6. The suggestions in the accompanying hand care chart should be followed diligently.

B. *Treatment*

1. May include a diuretic.
2. An intermittent compression unit may be used to force fluid back into venous system (Fig. 7-19).

HAND CARE°

After a radical mastectomy, an arm may swell because lymph nodes and lymph vessels were necessarily removed and the body is therefore less able to combat infection in this extremity.

Make every effort to avoid all cuts, scratches, pin pricks, hangnails, insect bites, burns, and the use of strong detergents as these can lead to serious infection with increased swelling.

Some "DO NOT'S":

DO NOT hold a cigarette in this hand.

DO NOT carry your purse or anything heavy with this arm

DO NOT wear a wristwatch or other jewelry on this arm

DO NOT cut or pick at cuticles or hangnails on this hand

DO NOT work near thorny plants or dig in the garden

DO NOT reach into a hot oven with this arm

DO NOT permit injection in this arm

DO NOT permit blood to be drawn from this arm

DO NOT allow your blood pressure to be taken on this arm

Some "DO'S":

DO wear a loose rubber glove on this hand when washing dishes

DO wear a thimble when sewing

DO apply a good lanolin hand cream several times daily

DO wear your "Life-Guard Medical Aid" tag engraved with "CAUTION—LYMPHEDEMA ARM—NO TESTS—NO HYPOS"

DO contact your doctor if your arm gets red, warm or unusually hard or swollen

DO return for a check-up and re-measurement for a new sleeve in two months

DO show this Hand Care Sheet to your surgeon

Reprinted through the courtesy of the CLEVELAND CLINIC Department of Physical Medicine and Rehabilitation.

Importance of Follow-up Visit

1. Incision healing evaluated
2. Rehabilitative effort assessed
3. Effectiveness of prosthetic determined
4. Patient's psychosocial adjustment evaluated
5. Possible recurrence detected

BIBLIOGRAPHY

Renal and Genitourinary Conditions

Books

Bauer, K. M.: Cystoscopic Diagnosis. Philadelphia, Lea and Febiger, 1969.

Beeson, P. B., and McDermott, W. (eds.): Cecil-Loeb Textbook of Medicine. Philadelphia, W. B Saunders, 1971, pp. 1139–1232.

Blandy, J. P., et al.: Tumours of the Testicle. New York, Grune and Stratton, Inc., 1970.

Brunner, L., et al.: Textbook of Medical-Surgical Nursing, 2nd ed. Philadelphia, J. B. Lippincott 1970, pp. 540–584.

Campbell, M. F., and Harrison, J. W. (eds.): Urology. Philadelphia, W. B. Saunders, 1970.

Dodson, A. I., Jr.: Urological Surgery. St. Louis, C. V. Mosby, 1970.

Emmett, J. L., and Witten, D. M.: Clinical Urography. Philadelphia, W. B. Saunders, 1971.

Gilette, P. J.: The Vasectomy Information Manual. New York, Outerbridge and Lazard, Inc., 1972

Glenn, J. F., and Boyce, W. H. (eds.): Urologic Surgery. New York, Harper and Row, 1969.

Keuhnelian, J. G., and Sanders, V. E.: Urologic Nursing. London, Macmillan, 1970.

Kintzel, C. K. (ed.): Advanced Concepts in Clinical Nursing. Philadelphia, J. B. Lippincott, 1971 pp. 277–320.

Krupp, M. A., et al.: Current Diagnosis and Treatment. Los Altos, Lange Medical Publications 1971, pp. 471–496.

Muehrcke, R.: Acute Renal Failure. St. Louis, C. V. Mosby, 1969.

Smith, D. R.: General Urology. Los Altos, Lange Medical Publications, 1969.

Sunderman, F. W., and Sunderman, F. W., Jr.: Laboratory Diagnosis of Kidney Diseases. St. Louis Warren H. Green, 1970.

Whitehead, S. L.: Nursing Care of the Adult Urology Patient. New York, Appleton-Century Crofts, 1970.

Winter, C. C.: Practical Urology. St. Louis, C. V. Mosby, 1969.

Winter, C. C., and Barker, M. R.: Nursing Care of Patients with Urologic Diseases. St. Louis C. V. Mosby, 1972.

Articles

Atkins, R., et al.: Management of chronic renal failure. Disease-A-Month, 3–38, March 1971.

Birum, L. H., et al.: Catheter plugs as a source of infection. Amer. J. Nurs., 71:2150–2152, Nov 1971.

Carter, C. B., et al.: Renal failure in the elderly. South. Med. J., 63:805–808, July 1970.

Clark, C. L.: Catheter care in the home. Amer. J. Nurs., 72:922–924, May 1972.

Davis, J. E.: Vasectomy. Amer. J. Nurs., 72:509–513, March 1972.

Delehanty, L., and Stravino, V.: Achieving bladder control. Amer. J. Nurs., 70:312–316, Feb 1970.

Desautels, R. E.: The causes of catheter induced urinary infections and their prevention. J. Urol 101:757–760, May 1969.

Hodson, J. M.: Vasectomy for voluntary sterilization. Postgrad. Med., 52:99–103, July 1972.

Kark, R. M.: Symposium on diseases of the kidney. Med. Clin. N. Amer., 55: (entire issue), Jan 1971.

Lange, K.: Nutritional management of kidney disorders. Med. Clin. N. Amer., 55:513–520, March 1971.

Langford, T. L.: Nursing problem: Bacteriuria and the indwelling catheter. Amer. J. Nurs., 72:113–115, Jan. 1972.

Langley, I.: Suprapubic cystotomy. Postgrad. Med., 50:171–173, Oct. 1971.

Lattimer, J. K., et al.: Current treatment for renal tuberculosis. J. Urol., 102:2–6, July 1969.

Merrill, J. P.: Acute renal failure. JAMA, 211:289–291, Jan. 12, 1970.

Moyer, J. H., and Swartz, C. D. (eds.): Treatment of pyelonephritis. Mod. Treat., 7:253–362, March 1970.

Murray, B. S., et al.: The patient has an ileal conduit. Amer. J. Nurs., 71:1560–1565, Aug. 1971.

Papper, S.: Renal failure. Med. Clin. N. Amer., 55:335–357, March 1971.

Read, M., and Mallison, M.: External arteriovenous shunts. Amer. J. Nurs., 72:81–85, Jan. 1972.

Tucker, R. M.: Management of renal insufficiency in surgical patients. Surg. Clin. N. Amer., 49:1095–1104, Oct. 1969.

Gynecologic Conditions

Books

Brunner, L. S., et al.: Textbook of Medical and Surgical Nursing, 2nd ed. Philadelphia, J. B. Lippincott, 1970, pp. 585–614.

Green, T. H., Jr.: Gynecology, 2nd ed. Boston, Little, Brown and Co., 1971.

Greenhill, J. P.: Office Gynecology, 9th ed. Chicago, Year Book Medical Publishers, Inc., 1971.

Novak, E. R., et al.: Novak's Textbook of Gynecology, 8th ed. Baltimore, Williams and Wilkins, 1970.

Articles

Celano, P. J., and Sawyer, J. R.: Vaginal fistulas. Amer. J. Nurs., 70:2131–2134, Oct. 1970.

Fitzpatrick, G.: Care for the patient with cancer of the cervix. Bedside Nurse, 4:11–18, Jan. 1971.

Gibbs, G. E.: Perineal care of the incapacitated patient. Amer. J. Nurs., 69:124–125, Jan. 1969.

Gravlee, L. C.: Jet-irrigation method for the diagnosis of endometrial adenocarcinoma. Obs. & Gyn., 34:168–173, Aug. 1969.

Guttmacher, A. F.: Family planning. Amer. J. Nurs., 69:1229–1234, June 1969.

Higgins, J. R.: More hysterectomies—fact, fantasy or fad? Canad. Nurse, 67:33–35, July 1971.

Hofmeister, F. J.: Guide to the complete gynecologic examination. Hosp. Med., 7:9–29, July 1971.

Holm, L. A.: Nursing care of patients having a hysterectomy. Canad. Nurse, 6:36–37, July 1971.

Keith, L. G., and Poma-Herrara, P.: Aggressive treatment of septic abortion. Amer. Fam. Phys., 3:99–103, June 1971.

Keller, C., and Copeland, P.: Counseling the abortion patient is more than talk. Amer. J. Nurs., 72:102–109, Jan. 1972.

Shah, C. A., and Green, T. H.: Evaluation of current management of endometrial carcinoma. Obs. & Gyn., 39:500–508, April 1972.

Siegler, A. M.: A review of tubal sterilization. J. Obs., Gyn. & Neonatal Nursing, 1:23–28, July-Aug. 1972.

Vlasis, G.: Treatment of bartholin cyst. Amer. Fam. Phys., 3:85–86, June 1971.

Conditions of the Breast

Books

Brunner, L. S., et al.: Textbook of Medical and Surgical Nursing, 2nd ed. Philadelphia, J. B. Lippincott, 1970, pp. 615–628.

Haagensen, C. D.: Diseases of the Breast, 2nd ed. Philadelphia, W. B. Saunders, 1971.

Lasser, T., and Clarke, W. K.: Reach to Recovery. New York, Simon and Schuster, 1972.

Articles

Bailey, A. G., and Geller, S. A.: Paget's disease of the nipple. Hosp. Med., *8*:7–16, May 1972.

Crile, G., Jr.: Results of simplified treatment of breast cancer. *In* Edgahl, R., and Mannick, H. A. (eds.): Modern Surgery. New York, Grune and Stratton, Inc., 1970, pp. 162–163.

Cronin, T. D., and Brauer, R. O.: Augmentation mammaplasty. Surg. Clin. N. Amer., *51*:441–452, April 1971.

Fitzpatrick, G.: Caring for the patient with cancer of the breast. Bedside Nurse, *3*:20–24, Part I, Feb. 1970; *3*:19–28, Part II, Mar. 1970.

Gribbons, C. A., and Aliapoulios, M. A.: Treatment for advanced breast carcinoma. Amer. J. Nurs., *72*:678–682, April 1972.

Harrel, H. C.: To lose a breast. Amer. J. Nurs., *72*:676–677, April 1972.

Owen, M. L.: Special care for the patient who has a breast biopsy or mastectomy. Nurs. Clin. N. Amer., *7*:373–382, June 1972.

Ravdin, R. G., et al.: Results of a clinical trial concerning the worth of prophylactic oophorectomy for breast carcinoma. Surg., Gyn. & Obs., *144*:1055–1064, Dec. 1970.

Seidman, H.: Cancer of the Breast: Statistical and epidemiological data. Amer. Cancer Soc., 1972.

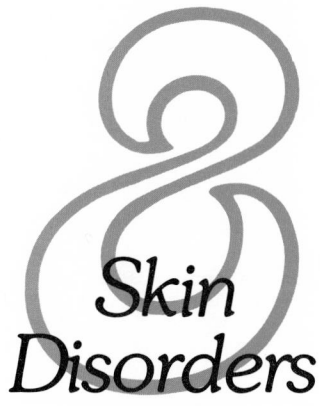

Skin Disorders

1. Dermatology

NURSING RESPONSIBILITIES IN DERMATOLOGY

Psychological Insights

1. Patients with dermatological problems can see and feel their problems and are more disturbed by their complaints than many patients with other conditions.
2. Skin eruptions evoke feelings of shame, disgust and fear which compound the problems of management of patients with skin conditions.
3. Irritation is a constant feature of skin disease and produces loss of sleep, anxiety and depression which reinforces discomfort and fatigue.
4. Cosmetic needs constitute the underlying motive that brings the patient to treatment.
5. Nursing support requires understanding, unending patience and continuing encouragement for these patients.

Clinical Observations

1. Be aware that many systemic conditions may be accompanied by dermatologic manifestations.
2. Describe the dermatosis (abnormal condition of the skin) clearly and in detail.
    a. What is the color(s) of the lesion?
    b. Is there redness, heat, pain or swelling?
    c. Is the eruption macular, papular, scaling, oozing, discrete, confluent?
    d. How large an area is involved and where?
3. Obtain a dermatological history.
    a. How long has the patient had the skin condition?
    b. What site was first affected?
    c. How did it spread?
    d. What is the distribution of the lesion—symmetrical, linear, circular?
    e. Is there itching? burning?—is it worse at a particular time?
    f. Is there history of hay fever, asthma, urticaria? These problems are associated with eczema.

g. Was the appearance of the eruption related to the intake of food?
h. What medications is the patient taking?
i. What is the patient's occupation?

Description of Skin Lesions

A. *Primary Lesions*—that do not break the skin.
1. Macule—nonelevated discoloration of the skin of various sizes, shapes and colors.
2. Papule—a solid elevation of the skin.
3. Vesicle—a small elevation of the skin that is filled with clear fluid.
4. Pustule—an elevation of the skin that contains pus; may form as a result of purulent changes in a vesicle.
5. Wheal—transient elevation of the skin caused by edema of the dermis and surrounding capillary dilatation.

B. *Secondary Lesions*—that break the skin.
1. Scales—heaped up horny layer of dead epidermis; may develop as a result of inflammatory changes.
2. Crusts—formed from serum, blood or pus drying on the skin.
3. Excoriations—linear scratch marks or traumatized area of skin, usually self-produced.
4. Fissure—a crack in the skin usually from marked drying and long-standing inflammation.
5. Ulcer—superficial loss of surface tissue due to death of cells.

DERMATOLOGIC THERAPY

Wet Dressings

Solution and Material	Desired Effect	Nursing Action
Solution Cool tapwater Physiologic saline Boric Acid Burow's Solution (aluminum acetate solution) Magnesium sulfate *Material* Soft toweling Diapers Soft cotton sheeting Kerlix (Bauer and Black)	Effective in treating oozing dermatosis or swollen, infected dermatitis (furunculitis, cellulitis). Relieves inflammation, burning and itching. Has cooling effect. Useful for removing crusts.	Keep dressing cool or at room temperature. Moisten compress to the point of slight dripping. Resoak compress every 5 minutes; compresses reach body temperature in 5 minutes. Compresses may be remoistened with asepto syringe. Add ice cubes to solution if coolness is desired. Apply for 15 minutes every 2–3 hours unless otherwise indicated. Keep patient warm if extensive areas are to be compressed. CAUTION: Avoid burns.

Baths (Balneotherapy)

Bath Solution and Medication	Desired Effect	Nursing Action
Water Saline Colloidal—Oatmeal or Aveeno (1 cup of oatmeal to a tub of water) Sodium bicarbonate—(1 box to tub of water) Starch (1 box starch to tub of water) Medicated tars (follow package directions) Alma-Tar, Ar-Extar bath, Balne-tar Bath oils Alpha-Keri, Aveeno-oilated, Domol, Lubath, Mellobath	Same effects as wet dressings. Used for widely disseminated lesions. Antipruritic and drying. Cooling Tar baths are used for psoriasis and chronic eczematous conditions. Bath oils are used for antipruritic and emollient actions.	Fill the tub half full (approximately 20 gallons). Keep the water at a tepid temperature—about 24–33.5°C. (75–92°F.). Do not allow the water to cool excessively. Use a bath mat—medications may cause tub to be slippery. Apply a lubricating agent to wet skin after bath if emollient action is desired—increases hydration. Dry by blotting with a towel. Keep room warm to minimize temperature fluctuations. Encourage patient to wear light, loose clothing after the bath.

Topical Medications

Type of Medication	Desired Effect	Nursing Action
Lotions Liquid vehicles for carrying medication; act by evaporation; May be protective, antiparasitic, antifungal, antipruritic; may act as sunscreen	Lubricates Cools through water evaporation Offers protective action Is antipruritic or drying	Apply with a soft paintbrush every 3–4 hours Do not wash off between applications
Ointments and Creams Have greasy, nongreasy or penetrating base depending on nature of lesion and drug applied	Retards water loss Lubricates Serves as a vehicle for medications Protects the skin Used in chronic or localized skin conditions	Apply ointments with a wooden tongue depressor Creams are rubbed into the skin by hand Teach patient to apply his own ointment or cream Ointments may have to be covered with a dressing to prevent soiling of clothing
Topical Adrenocorticosteroid Agents (many preparations available)	Has profound anti-inflammatory action	Apply to localized area requiring medication Use only a small amount and rub in thoroughly Use with occlusive dressing as directed

Type of Medication	Desired Effect	Nursing Action
Intralesional therapy Injection with a tuberculin syringe of sterile suspension of medication (usually suspension of corticosteroid) into or just below a lesion	Has anti-inflammatory action	Be aware that local atrophy may result Check patient for anaphylactoid reaction which may occur

Systemic Medications
    Adrenocorticosteroids
    Antibiotics
    Antihistamines
    Sedatives and tranquilizers
    Analgesics
    Antineoplastic

Dressings for Skin Conditions

A. *Occlusive dressing*—an airtight plastic film is applied to cover medicated skin (usually corticosteroid) (Fig. 8-1).
1. Enhances absorption of topically applied medication.
2. Increases penetration of corticosteroids in the skin thus enhancing its anti-inflammatory effect.
3. Produces moisture retention; prevents medication from evaporating.

NURSING ALERT: Prolonged use of occlusive dressings may cause skin atrophy and systemic absorption of corticosteroids.

B. *Other Dressings*
1. Fingers and toes—gauze or cotton cloth; held in place with small size tubular material

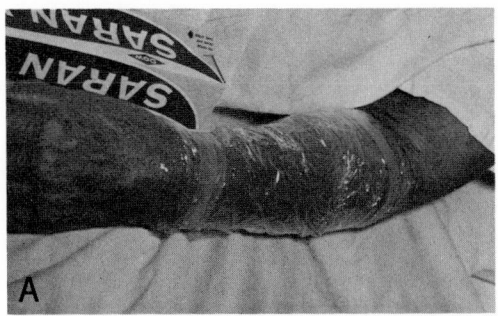 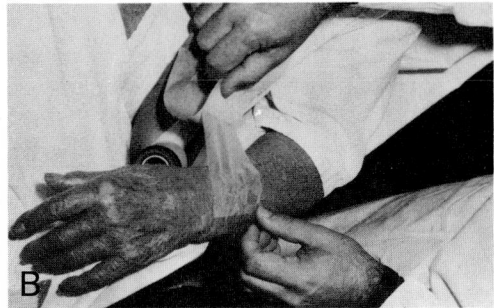

Figure 8-1. A. Occlusion of treatment area with plastic film greatly enhances the effectiveness of topical corticosteroid. Sealing the ends with tape adds air tightness and humidity. B. Plastic surgical tape containing corticosteroid in the adhesive layer can be cut to size and applied to individual plaques. (From Weinstein, G. D.: Postgraduate Medicine, *52*(5): 193, 1972.)

  2. Hands—disposable polyethylene gloves; sealed at wrists
  3. Feet—cotton socks or disposable plastic bags
  4. Extremities (arms and legs)—cotton cloth covered with tubular material
  5. Groin, perineum—disposable diapers; cotton cloth folded in diaper fashion
  6. Axillae—cotton cloth taped in place or held by commercial dress shields
  7. Trunk—cotton or light flannel pajamas
  8. Scalp—turban or plastic shower cap

DERMATOSIS (Abnormal Skin Condition)

Objectives of Treatment and Nursing Management

A. *To control itching and relieve pain.*
  1. Examine area of involvement.
     a. Attempt to discover the cause of discomfort.
     b. Record observations in detail, using descriptive terminology.
  2. Encourage rest and immobility to reduce stimuli of pain and itching and to raise the threshold of discomfort.
  3. Encourage patient to eliminate foods and beverages that produce flushing, e.g., condiments, coffee and alcohol.
  4. Advise patient to employ measures that produce vasoconstriction.
     a. Maintain cool environment.
     b. Reduce excess bedding or personal clothing.
     c. Provide tepid, cooling baths.
     d. Apply cool wet dressings.
  5. Treat dryness (xerosis) with lubricating creams or lotions applied after bathing (before drying) to enhance hydration.
  6. Apply anesthetic lotions or ointments.
  7. Supply analgesic and antipruritic medications as indicated.
  8. Administer tranquilizing agents or sedative drugs, as necessary.
  9. Instruct patient to refrain from self-medication with salves or lotions that are commercially advertised.
  10. Assist the anxious patient to improve his insight and to identify and cope with his problems.

B. *To treat an inflammatory lesion.*
  1. Apply continuous or intermittent wet dressings to reduce intensity of inflammation.
  2. Remove crusts and scales before applying topical medications.
  3. Use topical applications containing corticosteroid drugs, as indicated.
     a. Rub topical medicaments well into skin to enhance penetration.
     b. Observe lesion periodically for changes in response to therapy.

C. *To control oozing and prevent crust formation.*
  1. Provide tub baths and wet dressings to loosen exudates and scales.
  2. Remove medications with mineral oil before re-applying.
  3. Use mildly astringent solutions to precipitate proteins and decrease oozing.
  4. Supply a high protein diet if oozing is voluminous and serum loss substantial.
  5. Administer antibiotics by topical application or by mouth, as indicated.

D. *To avoid damage to skin.*
  1. Protect healthy skin from maceration when applying wet dressings.
  2. Remove moisture from skin by blotting gently and avoiding friction.

3. Guard carefully against risk of thermal trauma from excessively hot wet dressings.
4. Advise patient to use sun-screening agents to prevent actinic damage (chemical changes from ultraviolet light).

E. *To ensure efficacy of topical applications.*
  1. Use occlusive dressings, as needed, to retain medication in constant contact with affected skin.
  2. Elicit the patient's cooperation by having him perform his own dermatologic treatments.
  3. Instruct patient clearly and in detail to ensure that treatments are carried out as prescribed.

SEBORRHEIC DERMATOSES

Dermatoses refers to abnormal skin conditions.

Seborrhea is excessive production of sebum (secretion of sebaceous glands) in those areas where glands are normally found in large numbers (face, scalp, scrotum).

Seborrheic dermatitis is a chronic inflammatory disease of the skin with a predilection for areas that are well supplied with sebaceous glands or lie between the folds of the skin where the bacterial count is high.

Clinical Features

1. Characteristic lesion (remarkably varied)
   a. Dry moist or greasy scales
   b. Crusted pinkish yellow or yellowish patches of varying shapes and sizes
   c. Possible erythema (redness), fissuring (cracking) and secondary infection
   d. Dry flaky desquamation on scalp with profuse amount of fine powdery scales (dandruff)
2. Sites
   Scalp, eyebrows, eyelids, nasolabial crease, lips, ears, axillae, under breast, groin, gluteal crease.
3. Seborrheic dermatitis has a genetic predisposition; hormones, nutrition, infection and emotional stress influence its course.
4. There is a tendency to life-long recurrences lasting for weeks, months or years.

Treatment

Objective: to control the disorder (no known cure at this time)
1. Advise patient to remove external irritants and avoid excess heat and perspiration—rubbing and scratching will prolong the disorder.
2. Suggest local remedies
   Instruct the patient as follows:
   a. *For Scalp*—to control dandruff
      (1) Give the hair an initial cleansing shampoo to remove accumulated scale.
      (2) Use shampoo with selenium sulfide suspension (Selsun); leave shampoo on scalp 10 minutes; rinse thoroughly.
      (3) Shampoo daily, once or twice weekly depending on condition of the scalp.

   CAUTION: Observe precautions on container.

   b. *For Body and Face*
         Apply thin layer of corticosteroid cream—triamcinolone acetonide. (Aristo-
         cort, Kenalog), fluocinolone acetonide (Synalar, Fluonid).
         (a) Apply twice daily to face, scalp, ears or body folds.
         (b) Use with caution on the eyelids—can induce glaucoma in predisposed
             individuals.
   3. Give ACTH and corticosteroids for acute and severe seborrhea dermatitis.
   4. Use antibacterial measures if exudation and crusting occur—usually from
      staphylococcus.
      a. Give tetracycline 250 mg. 1 time daily or apply an antibiotic cream or ointment.
      b. Systemic antibiotic may be required for a spreading infection, especially of the
         scalp or ears.
   5. Combat yeast infection (moniliasis) that may occur in body creases or folds.
      a. Advise patient to cleanse intertriginous areas carefully; ensure maximum aeration
         of the skin.
      b. Suggest use of nystatin (cream or lotion) for complicating moniliasis.
      c. Patient with coincident candidiasis should be evaluated for diabetes.
   6. Encourage patient to eat a well-balanced diet.
         Diet may be supplemented with B complex and B_{12}.
   7. Advise patient to avoid systemic aggravating factors—overwork, lack of sleep,
      infection, emotional stress.

Acne Vulgaris

Acne vulgaris is a chronic disorder of the sebaceous (oil) glands, characterized by the presence of blackheads (comedones), whiteheads, pustules, nodules and cysts; it mainly affects
adolescents.

Predisposing Factors
   1. Genetic predisposition—strong genetic overtones
   2. Hormonal changes of adolescence—size and activity of sebaceous glands influenced
      by production of testosterone or progesterone
   3. Anxiety, stress, emotional tension

Altered Physiology
   Increase in amount and thickness of oil secretion → obstruction of sebaceous glands by
blackheads (comedones) → development of sebaceous cysts which may or may not become
secondarily infected → pustules → scarring.

Treatment
Objectives: to prevent follicular obstruction
              to reduce inflammation and combat secondary infection
              to eliminate factors that may predispose to acne

A. Prevent obstruction of the oil glands.
   1. Instruct patient as follows:
      a. Wash face 3 times daily with soap and water or special mildly abrasive cleansers.
      b. Shampoo scalp twice weekly with medicated shampoo.
      c. Use bath brush if back is involved.

2. Encourage regular and careful removal of comedones with comedone extractor. Instruct patient to:
   (a) Avoid mirror gazing and "picking" at skin.
   (b) Avoid squeezing the lesions—secondary infection with scarring may ensue.
3. Suggest topical remedies that degrease and cleanse the skin surface and encourage peeling of skin so that follicular orifices are kept open for proper drainage of their contents (Acne-Dome Medicated Cleanser, Fostex, etc.).
4. Give anovulatory drug in cyclic fashion if prescribed—thought to decrease sebum production.

B. Reduce inflammation and combat secondary infection.
   1. Advise patient to obtain sunlight whenever possible.
   2. Give tetracycline (1000–2000 mg. daily decreasing to maintenance dose of 250–500 mg. daily)—for pustular acne.
   3. Give corticosteroids for anti-inflammatory effect if ordered.
      Corticosteroids may be injected into or below chronic pustular lesions (intra-lesional injection).

C. Eliminate factors that may predispose patient to acne.
   1. Instruct patient to avoid excess consumption of carbohydrates and fat.
   2. Advise against eating chocolate and pork or other dietary fats if these foods make patient's acne worse.
   3. Give adolescent patient understanding, reassurance and support—acne may become source of power struggle between teenager and parents.

D. Other forms of treatment (by dermatologist)
   1. Intralesional corticosteroid injections
   2. Carbon dioxide slush treatment—produces redness and peeling
   3. Ultraviolet light treatment—stimulates growing epithelial cells and causes capillary hyperemia; increases cellular metabolism and vascular engorgement which enhances the skin's defenses against bacterial infections
   4. Surgical removal of pustules and cysts when necessary
   5. Dermabrasion—surgical planing of damaged skin
   6. Vitamin A applied topically

BACTERIAL INFECTIONS

Furuncles

A *furuncle* or boil is an acute inflammation arising deep in one or more hair follicles.

Clinical Features

1. Initial occurrence—usually begins around a hair follicle
2. Sites of predilection—back of neck, axillae, buttocks
3. Causative factors—irritation, pressure, friction, excessive perspiration, shaving of axillae (especially in persons with lowered resistance)
4. Symptoms—tenderness, pain and surrounding cellulitis; after furuncle localizes, the center becomes yellow or black.

Treatment

1. Protect area from irritation, squeezing and trauma.
2. Apply hot wet compresses—to hasten suppurative process and reduce discomfort.
3. Apply bacitracin or neomycin ointment—to limit surface spread of infection.
4. Give systemic antibiotic (erythromycin, dicloxacillin).
5. Prepare for surgical drainage—when furuncle has become localized and shows fluctuation (wave-like motion upon palpation).

NURSING ALERT: Take special precautions with boil on face as the skin area drains directly into the cranial venous sinuses.
1. Place patient with boils on nose, lip, groin, perineal or perianal region on bedrest.
2. Give course of systemic antibiotic therapy—to control spread of infection.

Carbuncles

A *carbuncle* is an abscess of the skin and subcutaneous tissues representing an extension of a furuncle invading multiple follicles; usually caused by staphylococcal infection.

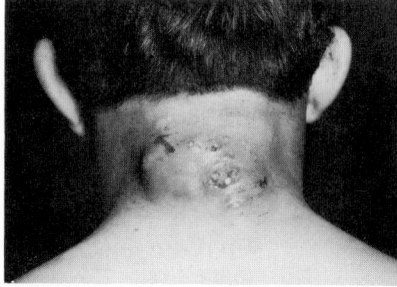

Clinical Features

1. Seen most frequently within the thick fibrous inelastic skin of the back of the neck and upper back.
2. More apt to occur in older and debilitated persons; especially frequent in diabetics.

Figure 8-2. Carbuncle on back of neck. (Courtesy Armed Forces Institute of Pathology.)

NURSING ALERT: Every patient past middle age with a carbuncle should be suspected of diabetes until it is disproved.

---

3. Symptoms
   a. Fever, leukocytosis, extreme pain and prostration.
   b. Bacteremia is common because the extensive inflammation makes it difficult to completely wall-off the infection, so that absorption of toxins takes place.

Treatment

1. Administer antibiotic (according to sensitivity studies)—antibiotic is continued until infective process is controlled.
2. Determine whether there is an underlying disease condition (diabetes, hematologic disease, etc.).
3. Prepare for surgical incision and drainage if there is pus formation, etc.
4. Use supportive modalities (infusions, fever sponges, etc.) for the toxic patient.

Impetigo

Impetigo (impetigo contagiosa) is a superficial infection of the skin caused by streptococci, staphylococci or both.

Clinical Features

1. Lesion appears as discrete thin-walled vesicle that ruptures and becomes covered with a loosely adherent, honey-yellow crust.
2. Tends to spread in circles, arcs or in serpiginous (creeping) manner.
3. Areas affected—exposed parts of body—face, hands, neck and extremities.
4. Is easily transmissible; occurs most frequently in early childhood during summer months in hot, humid weather.
5. Sources of infection—children's pets, dirty fingernails, other children, adults; barber shops, beauty parlors, swimming pools.
6. May be secondary to pediculosis capitis, scabies, herpes simplex, insect bites, poison ivy, eczema.

Treatment

1. Give systemic antibiotic (benzathine penicillin, erythromycin, tetracycline)—*glomerulonephritis is a complication of impetigo.*
2. Treat lesion with topical antibiotic (bacitracin, neomycin, polymycin).
3. Remove crusts with antiseptic soap and hot compresses—so that ointment will reach infected site.

FUNGAL INFECTIONS

Fungi are plant-like organisms feeding on organic matter. (See also page 854.)

Tinea Pedis (Athlete's Foot)

Tinea pedis (athlete's foot) is a superficial fungal infection which may manifest itself as an acute, inflammatory, vesicular process or as a chronic rash involving the soles of the feet and the interdigital web spaces.

Clinical Features

1. Tinea pedis is the most common fungal infection.
2. Causes intense inching and burning.
3. Lymphangitis and cellulitis may occur when bacterial superinfection is present.

Diagnostic Evaluation

1. Direct examination of scrapings (skin, nails, hair)
2. Isolation of the organism in culture

Treatment

1. Drain the vesicular lesions, using aseptic technique.
2. Use soaks (potassium permanganate, Burow's solution, saline) to remove scales, crusts, debris and residual medications; also has mild anti-inflammatory effect.

3. Apply fungistatic creams or lotions such as tolnaftate (Tinactin) to involved skin.
4. Give systemic antibacterial agents if there is superimposed infection.
5. Encourage bedrest and elevation of feet.

Preventive Measures

Instruct the patient to keep feet dry—moisture encourages the growth of fungi.
1. Dry carefully between the toes.
2. Alternate shoes—to permit adequate drying of shoes.
3. Change socks frequently.
4. Wear light cotton socks or hosiery with cotton feet—synthetic material does not absorb perspiration as well as cotton.
5. Wear perforated shoes—to permit aeration of feet.
6. Apply foot powder twice daily—to keep feet dry.
7. Use rubber or wooden clogs in community showers or bathing places.
8. Place small pieces of cotton between toes at night—to absorb moisture.

Tinea Capitis (Ringworm of the Scalp)

Tinea capitis (ringworm of the scalp) is a fungal disease of the scalp.

Clinical Features

1. Lesions appear as round, gray, scaly bald patches on the scalp.
2. Sometimes boggy swelling (kerion) occurs in an area of involvement; this may be followed by scarring.
3. Tinea capitis is contagious; usually occurs in prepubertal children.

Treatment

1. Give Griseofulvin (a fungistatic) 0.25–0.5 gm. by mouth in divided doses.
2. Instruct the patient as follows:
   a. Shave or clip the scalp around infected areas twice weekly.
   b. Apply topical fungicides to involved area.
   c. Shampoo scalp 2–3 times weekly.
      Wash the scalp after haircuts.
   d. Wear a cap—to protect other people.
      (1) Wash and disinfect cap frequently.
      (2) Avoid exchanging head gear.
3. Treat all infected individuals and household pets.

Tinea Corporis or Tinea Circinata

Tinea corporis or *Tinea circinata* is ringworm of the body.

Clinical Features

1. Appearance—rings of vesicles with central clearing; appear in clusters.
2. Lesions usually appear on exposed areas of body; may extend to scalp, hair or nails.
3. An infected pet is a common source of infection.
4. Ringworm of the body causes intense itching.

Treatment

1. Give Griseofulvin (0.5 gm. orally for children; 1 gm. orally for adults).
   Griseofulvin may cause phototoxicity, urticaria, headache and nausea.
2. Have patient apply topical antifungal medication to lesions as directed.
   Apply sparingly, 3 times daily.

PARASITIC SKIN DISEASES

Pediculosis Capitis

Pediculosis capitis is an infestation of the scalp by head louse, *Pediculus humanus* var. *capitis* (Fig. 8-3A).

Clinical Features

1. Appearance—minute white nits (eggs) (Fig. 8-3B) attached in hair shaft in series; usually on occipital and temporal areas.
2. Found most often in persons wearing long hair.
3. Saliva of the louse produces marked itching with resultant excoriation.
4. Secondary infection with crusting may occur—posterior occipital nodes may be enlarged and tender.
5. May be transmitted by direct physical contact or contact with infested combs, brushes, wigs, hats and bedding.

Treatment

1. Instruct the patient as follows:
   a. Use a shampoo containing gamma benzene hexachloride (Kwell, Kwellada).
   b. Shampoo the scalp at least 4 minutes with this preparation; rinse.
   c. Comb hair with a fine-toothed comb—to remove remaining nits.
   d. Disinfect comb and brushes with Kwell shampoo; sterilize all washable fomites.
   e. Repeat in 24 hours if necessary.
2. Treat all family members and close contacts.
3. Treat complications—severe pruritus, pyoderma (pus forming infection of the skin) and dermatitis with antipruritics, systemic antibiotics and topical corticosteroids.

Pediculosis Corporis

Pediculosis corporis is an infestation of the body by body louse, *Pediculus humanus* var. *corporis* (Fig. 8-3C and D).

Clinical Features

1. The body louse lives in the seams of undergarments but feeds on the skin.
2. The nits may remain viable for 1 month.
3. Appearance—long pruritic excoriations on the body; bites from body lice cause characteristic minute hemorrhagic points on the skin.
4. May produce secondary lesions—hyperemia, parallel linear scratches, eczema, hyperpigmentation in persistent cases.
5. Areas of skin involved are those that come in closest contact with the undergarments (trunk, extremities).

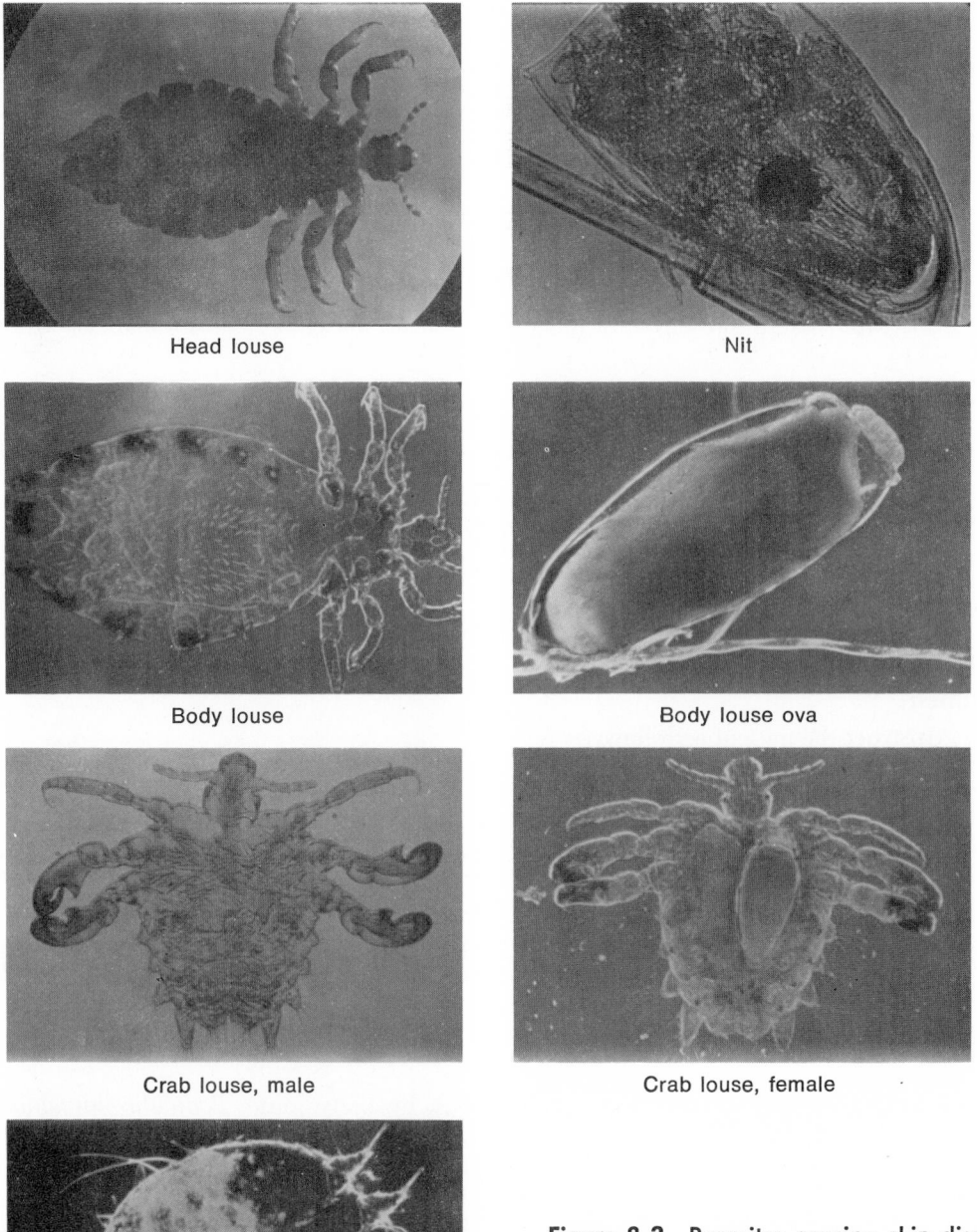

Head louse

Nit

Body louse

Body louse ova

Crab louse, male

Crab louse, female

Scabies

Figure 8-3. Parasites causing skin disease. (Courtesy Reed and Carnrick Research Institute.)

Treatment

1. Instruct the patient as follows:
    a. Bathe with soap and water.
    b. Apply gamma benzene hexachloride (Kwell) cream or lotion to trunk and extremities—leave medication on skin 24 hours.
    c. Eliminate parasites and nits from clothing, bedding and sleeping bags.
        Launder, dry clean, press with hot iron.
2. Examine and treat all family members and contacts.
3. Treat pruritus, secondary bacterial infections and dermatitis.

NURSING ALERT: Body lice are vectors for rickettsial disease; epidemic typhus, relapsing fever, trench fever. The causative organism may be in the gastrointestinal tract of the insect and excreted on the skin surface.

Pediculosis Pubis

Pediculosis pubis is an infestation by *Phthirus pubis* (crab louse) (Fig. 8-3E and F) which is chiefly transmitted by sexual contact and is generally localized to the genital region.

Clinical Manifestations

1. Chief symptom is itching.
2. Reddish brown "dust" (formed from the excretion of the insects) may be found on the underclothing.
3. Lice may infest chest, axillary hair, beard and eyelashes.
4. Gray-blue macules (1–3 cm. in diameter) may be seen on the trunk, thighs, and axillae—as a result of the reaction of the insects' saliva on bilirubin, converting it to biliverdin.

Treatment

1. Instruct the patient as follows:
    a. Bathe with soap and water.
    b. Apply gamma benzene hexachloride (Kwell) cream or lotion to areas of involvement.
        (1) Leave on for 24 hours.
        (2) Treat again in 4–7 days for heavy infestations.
        (3) Do not apply Kwell to eyebrows.
            (a) Remove nits manually from eyebrows or eyelashes with cotton-tipped applicator or toothpick.
            (b) Apply yellow oxide of mercury or physostigmine ophthalmic ointment before removing nits.
    c. Machine wash all clothing and bedding.
2. Treat all sexual contacts and family members.
3. Schedule patient for workup for coexisting venereal disease.
4. Treat secondary bacterial infection, itching and dermatitis.

Scabies

Scabies is an infestation of the skin by *Acarus scabiei* (itch mite) (Fig. 8-3G). It is a disease due to overcrowding and poor hygienic conditions.

Clinical Features

1. Infestation with mites from dogs, cats and small animals may occur.
2. *Symptoms*—intense itching more pronounced at night—usually occurs 1 month after initial infection.
3. *Primary lesion*—the burrow, produced by the female mite as it penetrates upper layers of the skin; burrows are short, wavy, brownish or blackish, thread-like lesions.
4. *Sites*—between the fingers, on the flexor surfaces of the wrists and palms and around the nipples.
5. Secondary lesions include vesicles, papules, pustules, excoriations and crusts; bacterial superinfection or eczematization may complicate the picture.

Treatment

1. Instruct patient as follows:
   a. Bathe or shower at bedtime.
   b. Apply benzyl benzoate (scabicide) topically over skin surface from neck downward; allow to remain 48 hours; or apply gamma benzene hexachloride (Kwell, Kwellada).
   c. Put on clean pajamas and sleep between freshly washed bed linens.
   d. Put on *all* clean clothing in morning.
   e. Repeat procedure as directed.
   f. Apply bland ointment to the skin after completion of treatment.
2. Advise patient that he may be uncomfortable for some weeks—the solution is irritating to the skin and pruritus may remain for a time.
3. Treat all infected family members.

Bedbug Infestation

Two species of bedbugs, *cimex lectularius* and *cimex hemipterus* invade human habitations. These are nocturnal blood-sucking insects.

Clinical Features

1. Appearance—bites are grouped in a straight line and consist of hemorrhagic spots associated with papular or wheal-like lesions; there may be a tiny red point marking the original site of the bite.
2. Sites—buttocks, back and extremities are most frequently bitten—patient experiences itching and burning; urticaria (hives) may accompany the lesions.
3. Secondary infection and pyoderma may occur.

Treatment

1. Advise patient to eliminate insect by spraying DDT in crevices of furniture, walls, floors, mattresses and beds.
2. Direct patient to apply lotions containing menthol and phenol to local areas of bites.

HERPES ZOSTER

Herpes zoster (shingles) is an inflammatory condition in which the virus produces a painful vesicular eruption in the distribution of the nerves from one or more posterior ganglia.

Etiology

Virus—appears to be identical with the causative agent of varicella (chickenpox).

Clinical Manifestations

1. Fever.
2. Severe pain occurs over the affected nerve.
3. Vesicles appear within 12 to 24 hours.
   a. Eruption appears in patches of various sizes.
   b. Early vesicles contain serum—then appear purulent and rupture to form crusts.
   c. Some vesicles dry up without scarring.
4. Eruption appears unilaterally along the distribution of the nerves from one or more posterior ganglia.
   Inflammation usually is unilateral involving the thoracic, cervical or cranial nerves in a band-like configuration.
5. Eruption usually accompanied by itching, tenderness and pain which may radiate over entire region supplied by the nerves.
6. Clinical course varies from 1–3 weeks; healing time varies between 7–26 days.
7. The disease is considered infectious only for the first 2–3 days.

Treatment

Objectives: to make the patient comfortable
to prevent postherpetic pain

1. Control the pain—controlling the pain may reduce incidence of postherpetic neuralgia.
   a. Pain is burning with stabbing overtones.
   b. Give analgesics—acetylsalicylic acid, codeine, propoxyphene hydrochloride (Darvon).
   c. Give barbiturates—to control nervousness associated with neuralgia.
   d. Give antihistamines—to control itching.
2. Restrict physical activities.
3. Give systemic corticosteroids as directed for patients with severe herpes—may be helpful in promoting healing and reducing the incidence of postherpetic neuralgia.
4. Give vitamin B_{12} injections daily (or every 2 days).
5. Treat secondary bacterial infection of skin lesions—culture and sensitivity studies will indicate appropriate antibiotic.
6. Apply local treatment to skin lesions.
   a. Apply cool wet dressings to pruritic lesions
   b. Apply topical steroid—triamcinolone acetonide (Kenalog) etc.—to give relief and promote healing.
      Do not apply topical steroids if secondary infection is present.
7. Support the patient undergoing diagnostic studies.

NURSING ALERT: Herpes zoster may indicate the presence of serious internal disease, especially in persons past middle age (Hodgkin's disease, leukemia, malignancy).

8. Watch for complications.
   a. Persistent pain (neuralgia) of affected nerve following healing, especially in the elderly.
   b. Ophthalmic herpes zoster—pain in the orbit radiating up over the forehead; constant boring pain.
      (1) Pain particularly severe in elderly following ophthalmic herpes zoster.
      (2) Patient with ophthalmic herpes zoster should be examined by ophthalmologist to avoid serious ocular complications and blindness.
   c. Facial nerve paralysis
   d. Encephalitis
9. Treatment of severe postherpetic pain.
   a. Procaine or alcohol injection to nerve ganglia
   b. Radiation therapy

CONTACT DERMATITIS

Contact dermatitis (dermatitis venenata) is a common inflammatory, often eczematous condition caused by a skin reaction due to contact with a variety of irritating or allergenic materials. There is damage to the epidermis by repeated physical and chemical insults.

Causes

1. Poison ivy
2. Cosmetics
3. Soaps, detergents and scouring compounds
4. Industrial chemicals
5. Hairdye, nickel, rubber additives

Predisposing Factors

1. Extremes in heat and cold
2. Frequent immersion in soap and water
3. Pre-existing skin disease

Clinical Manifestations

1. Skin eruptions begin at point of contact with causative agent.
2. Itching, burning, erythema, vesiculation and eczema.
3. Weeping, crusting, drying, fissuring and peeling.
4. Thickening of skin and pigmentation changes if repeated reactions occur or if there is continual scratching by patient.
5. Secondary bacterial invasion may occur—prevention of normal sweating produces vesicles, itching and inflammation.

Treatment

Objective: to protect and rest the involved skin.

1. Instruct the patient as follows:
   a. Identify and remove the offending irritant.
      (1) Avoid the use of soap until healing occurs.
      (2) Avoid exposing skin to the causative agent after recovery.
   b. *Topical Treatment*
      (1) Use bland unmedicated lotion for small patches of erythema.
      (2) Use cool wet dressing for small areas of acute, vesicular dermatitis.
         (a) Allow compresses to remain 2–3 hours twice daily.

(b) Apply calamine lotion or cortisone lotion after applying compresses.

(c) Apply thin layer of corticosteroid cream or lotion to patients with mild to moderate involvement.

(3) Use medicated baths at room temperature for generalized areas of dermatitis.

(4) Take oral antihistamines to allay itching.

2. Administer corticosteroids (cortisone, hydrocortisone, prednisone, prednisolone) to patients with acute and extensive dermatitis; use with caution.

3. Give systemic antibiotics if secondary bacterial infection is present.

Patient will have purulent exudate and systemic symptoms (fever, lymphadenopathy).

Poison Ivy

Poison ivy grows in the form of climbing vines or as upright shrubs; the leaves grow in clusters of 3, one at the end of the stalk and the other 2 opposite one another. Poison ivy has a sticky sap which contains an active ingredient known as *urushiol*, an oleoresin (a combination of plant resin and volatile oil). This urushiol can cause an allergic skin reaction (contact dermatitis).

Clinical Manifestations

1. Eruption may develop in hours or days after contact.
2. Eruption occurs in a streak or line and burns and itches.
3. Small weeping areas may form (papules, vesicles, blisters)—in more severe cases large blistered areas with inflammation and swelling may appear.

Exposure to Urushiol

1. Urushiol must make contact with the skin—contact is usually made by touching the plant leaves or stems.
2. Contact with urushiol may be made indirectly—clothing, tools or pets touching the plant can pick up the sap and pass it to a person indirectly.
3. Urushiol is present in all parts of the plants including dead stems and roots.
4. Smoke from burning plants carries droplets containing urushiol which can get on the skin or enter the nose, throat and lungs.

Prevention and Treatment

1. Advise patient as follows to avoid contact with urushiol (poison ivy, poison oak or sumac).
   a. Do not pull, chop or burn vines and brush—sap-carrying smoke may produce outbreak in a sensitive person.
   b. Wear protective clothing (long sleeves, gloves, slacks) in heavily wooded areas—to guard against exposure.
   c. Apply protective ointments before working in the vicinity of the plants.
   d. Take off contaminated clothing carefully and wash clothing immediately—urushiol on clothing can cause outbreak of poison ivy.
   e. Wash skin immediately with strong soap suds and rinse well—to remove the sap.
2. Treat severe reactions with corticosteroids.
   a. Give systemic corticosteroids (prednisone) as directed.
      (1) Dosage is adjusted according to severity of reaction and then tapered off gradually.

(2) Buffer the drug with milk or antacid if patient has peptic ulcer.
   b. Direct patient to apply cortisone cream locally.
3. Give supportive treatment for itching and burning of rash.
   a. Apply calamine lotion.
   b. Use tepid water compresses to relieve itching.
   c. Give tepid tub baths for generalized rash (see p. 570).

NONINFECTIOUS INFLAMMATORY DERMATOSES

Psoriasis

Psoriasis is a chronic inflammatory dermatosis of unknown etiology with a strong hereditary tendency and extreme variability in age of onset, course and severity.

Clinical Features

1. *Appearance*
   Small scaly papules develop into confluent patches of deep red thickly scaling lesions all of which are covered by profuse silvery scales (Fig. 8-4); the removal of the scale reveals punctate bleeding points.
   a. Psoriasis of the ears—scaling and dryness.
   b. Psoriasis of palms and soles—vesicular and pustular pruritic lesions.
   c. Psoriasis of nails—thickening, discoloration, crumbling beneath the free edges; pitting of nails.
   d. Psoriasis between skin folds—smooth shiny red lesions, easily fissured.
2. *Sites*
   Bony prominences (knees, elbows, sacrum), scalp, external ears, genitalia, perianal area, nails and dorsa of hands.
3. Psoriasis usually does not affect the general health; remissions and exacerbations occur unpredictably. However, arthritis and systemic reactions do occur.

Treatment

Objective: to reduce scaling and itching; the goal is control since no cure is known.

1. Removing scales.
   Instruct the patient as follows:

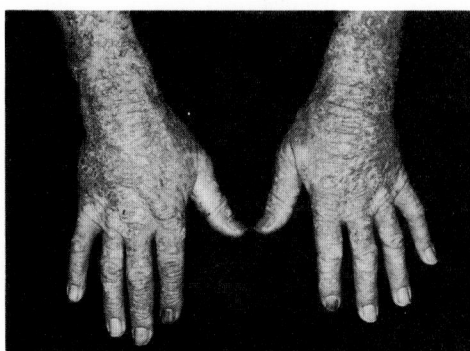

Figure 8-4. Psoriasis of the hands. (Courtesy Armed Forces Institute of Pathology.)

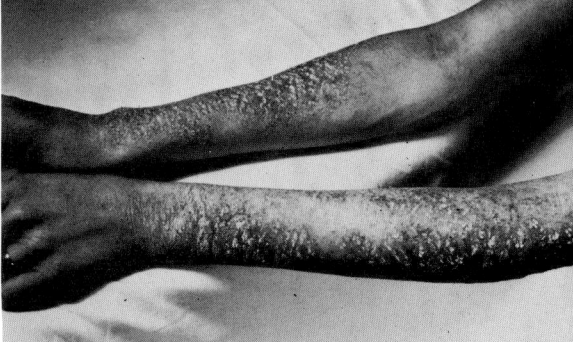

Figure 8-5. Exfoliative dermatitis of arms. (Courtesy Armed Forces Institute of Pathology.)

    a. Take daily tub bath—to help soak off scales.

    b. Gently remove excess scales with a soft brush while bathing.

    c. Apply prescribed ointment after removal of scales—to enhance penetration of ointment.

2. Topical medications

    a. Corticosteroids

    Instruct the patient as follows:

      (1) Apply wet dressings to irritated areas of psoriasis.

      (2) Apply corticosteroid preparations—triamcinolone (Kenalog)—to skin.

      (3) Cleanse area once daily and reapply medication to skin.

      (4) Hold dressing in place with shower cap or turban (head), with plastic gloves (hands) and with articles of clothing (body).

NURSING ALERT: After the use of corticosteroids there may be a rebound (rapid recurrence) of psoriasis more extensive than the original psoriasis.

---

    b. Anthralin preparations

      (1) Direct patient to apply anthralin medication as directed; do not apply to normal skin.

      (2) Instruct patient to wash hands thoroughly after application—medication can produce a chemical conjunctivitis.

    c. Coal tar mixture

      (1) Apply 10–20% solution of coal tar in hydrophilic cream.

      (2) This is followed by carefully graded doses of ultraviolet radiation. (Coal tar on the skin increases its sensitivity to ultraviolet rays.)

        (a) Begin ultraviolet radiation with low dose (10 seconds) and build up gradually to 10 minutes.

        (b) Ultraviolet produces mild redness and slight desquamation.

3. Chronic thickened patches of psoriasis may be treated with intralesional injections (triamcinolone acetonide).

4. Encourage patient to sun bathe—patients with psoriasis improve in summer months.

5. Systemic medication—methotrexate (Amethopterin)—a folic acid antagonist, may be used in patients with extensive psoriasis that is resistant to all other forms of treatment.

    a. Is given to prevent cell replication—in psoriasis the epidermal cells have a rapid rate of proliferation.

    b. May depress bone marrow to a dangerous degree.

      (1) Preliminary laboratory studies should be conducted to ensure adequate function of hepatic, hematopoietic and renal systems—CBC (including platelets), BUN, urinalysis, liver function tests.

      (2) These parameters should be monitored during course of drug treatment.

NOTE: Methotrexate is a potent abortive or teratogenic agent and should be used with extreme caution in women of childbearing age.

Exfoliative Dermatitis

Exfoliative dermatitis is characterized by an explosive and progressive inflammatory skin disease associated with chills and fever, prostration, severe toxicity and an itchy scaling of the skin.

Clinical Features

A. *Appearance*
1. Starts acutely as either a patchy or generalized erythematous eruption (Fig. 8-5) accompanied by fever, malaise and occasionally gastrointestinal symptoms.
2. The skin color changes from pink to dark red; then after a week the characteristic exfoliation (scaling) begins usually in the form of thin flakes which leave the underlying skin smooth and red, new scales forming as the older ones exfoliate (cast off).

B. *Multiplicity of Causes*
1. May arise as a primary condition.
2. May follow a previous skin condition (eczema, psoriasis) that had become generalized.
3. May appear as a part of the lymphoma group of diseases and may precede the appearance of lymphoma or leukemia.
4. Also appears as a severe reaction to a wide number of drugs, including penicillin and phenylbutazone.

Treatment

1. The treatment is individualized and supportive and depends on the cause.
2. Stop all drugs.
3. Hospitalize the patient and place him on bedrest.
4. Maintain fluid and electrolyte balance—considerable water and protein loss from skin surface; generalized vasodilation and fluid loss causes electrolyte imbalance.
   Give plasma expanders to replace protein losses.
5. Give systemic adrenocorticosteroid compounds as directed.
6. Apply compresses and soothing baths—to treat acute extensive dermatitis.
7. Prevent intercurrent (pneumonia) or cutaneous infections—give antibiotic therapy; pyoderma is a common complication.
8. Advise patient to avoid all irritants, particularly drugs.
9. Watch for symptoms of heart failure (p. 274)—hyperemia and increased cutaneous blood flow can produce a cardiac failure of high output origin.

Pemphigus

Pemphigus is a serious disease of the skin characterized by the appearance of variously sized blisters (bullae) on apparently normal skin and mucous membranes.

Clinical Features

1. Available evidence indicates that pemphigus is an autoimmune disease.
2. Appearance
   a. Asymptomatic large bullae appear on apparently normal skin and mucous membranes.
   b. The bullae enlarge and rupture forming painful raw and denuded areas.
   c. Bullae and erosions occur on the skin, mouth and vagina; large areas of skin may be denuded.
   d. Bacterial superinfection is common.

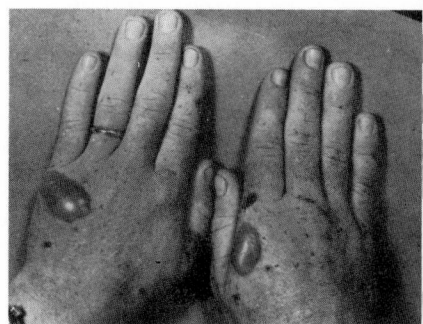

Figure 8-6. Bullous dermatitis of hand (vesicles). (Courtesy Armed Forces Institute of Pathology.)

Treatment

Objective: to bring the disease under control as rapidly as possible.

1. Administer corticosteroids (prednisone) in large doses (80–150 mg. daily) as prescribed to keep skin free of blisters.
   a. High dosage level is maintained until remission is apparent.
   b. Dosage is reduced to minimum daily maintenance dose as soon as possible.
2. Provide intravenous fluids and blood transfusions—there is a large amount of protein, fluid and blood lost from the denuded epithelial surfaces.
3. Watch for evidences of secondary infection—bullae susceptible to infection, and septicemia may follow.
4. Utilize cool wet compresses and baths for vesicular bullous and ulcerative lesions.
5. Give antibiotic treatment if secondary bacterial complications occur.
6. Give soft diet to patients with oral, pharyngeal or esophageal involvement—patients with painful oral involvement have difficulty in maintaining their nutrition.
   a. Encourage patients to drink enough fluids.
   b. Offer soothing mouthwashes frequently—to soothe ulcerative areas of the mouth.
7. Immunosuppressive agents (methotrexate or cyclophosphamide) may be given to help control disease and reduce maintenance dose of steroid. (See discussion of methotrexate, p. 874.)

ULCERS AND TUMORS OF THE SKIN

Ulcers of the Skin

Ulceration is a superficial loss of surface tissue due to death of cells.

Causes

Ulcers of the skin usually arise from (1) infection or (2) an interference with the blood supply.

1. Infection as cause of skin ulcers.
   a. Usually develop from an infection with anaerobic streptococci or from combination of infections (hemolytic streptococci and staphylococci).
   b. Tend to progress peripherally—characterized by an overhanging edge.
   c. Treatment
      (1) Infection tends to resist ordinary form of treatment.
      (2) Application of zinc peroxide (which liberates oxygen over a long period of time) converts the anaerobic portions of the wound into an aerobic area.
      (3) Penicillin, locally or parenterally, is also effective.
      (4) Healing occurs rapidly owing to inability of the anaerobic streptococci to live in an unfavorable environment.
2. Deficient circulation as cause of skin ulcers—see page 337.

Tumors of the Skin

Cysts

Epidermal cysts are common, slowly-growing, firm elevated tumors formed by a mass of epidermal cells; frequently found on the back.

Sebaceous cysts are rounded tumors of variable size due to retention of the excretion in the sebaceous follicles; also referred to as a *wen*.

Benign Tumors

A. *Verrucae (warts)*—common benign skin tumors caused by a virus
1. Many times warts do not need treatment as they tend to disappear spontaneously.
2. Treatment
   a. Freezing with liquid nitrogen—liquid nitrogen has a somewhat destructive action while tending to spare the epidermis.
   b. Area may be injected with lidocaine and the wart removed with a curet.
   c. Application of 3–5% salicylic acid in isopropyl alcohol—causes dryness and superficial peeling.

B. *Angiomas (birthmarks)*—benign vascular tumors involving the skin and subcutaneous tissues
1. May occur as flat, violet red patches (port-wine angiomas) or as raised, bright-red nodular lesions (strawberry angiomas). Strawberry angiomas may involute spontaneously.
2. Port-wine angiomas usually persist indefinitely.

C. *Pigmented nevi (moles)*—common skin tumors of various sizes and shades ranging from yellowish to brown to black
1. May be flat macular lesions or elevated papules or nodules that occasionally contain hair.
2. Majority of pigmented nevi are harmless; however, in rare cases malignant changes supervene and a melanoma develops at the site of the nevus.
3. Treatment
   a. Nevi at sites of repeated pressure should be removed—as a preventive measure against possible malignant changes.
   b. Excised nevi should be examined histologically.

D. *Keloids*—benign overgrowths of fibrous tissue at site of scar or trauma
1. More prevalent among black race.
2. Usually asymptomatic—may cause disfigurement and cosmetic concern.
3. Treatment—Irradiation or intralesional injection with corticosteroids.

Cancer of the Skin

Clinical Features

1. Skin cancer has a greater incidence than cancer of any other organ; comprises 22% of all cancers in men and 12% of all cancers in women.
2. There is a 95% cure rate due to early diagnosis, the slow progression of most skin cancers and the effective methods of treatment available.

Causes

1. Exposure to sun over a period of time (outdoor workers).
   Greater incidence of skin cancer in tropics and subtropics.
2. Texture of skin and its pigment content—persons with ruddy or light complexions seem to develop skin cancer more frequently than those with coarser or darker skin.
3. Exposure to roentgen ray.
4. Exposure to certain chemical agents (arsenic, nitrates, tar and pitch, oils and paraffins).
5. Cancer of skin may develop on scars of severe burns 20–40 years later.

Diagnostic Evaluation

1. Biopsy
2. Histologic evaluation

Types of Skin Cancer

A. *Basal Cell Carcinoma*
1. Most common skin cancer.
2. Lesions are small nodules with a rolled, pearly translucent border with telangiectasia (dilatation of end blood vessels), crusting and occasionally ulceration (Fig. 8-7).
3. These tumors may be pigmented, multiple, superficial or cystic.
   a. Basal cell carcinoma is chiefly caused by prolonged skin exposure to irritants.
   b. Characterized by invasion and erosion of continuous tissues—rarely metastasizes.
   c. Lesions appear most frequently on face and between the hairline and the upper lip.

B. *Squamous Cell (Epidermoid) Carcinoma*
1. A malignancy that arises on sun-exposed areas of skin and mucous membrane and is considered a truly invasive carcinoma.
2. Appears as an infiltrated plaque-like or nodular rapid-growing tumor.
3. May be preceded by leukoplakia (premalignant lesion of mucous membrane), actinic keratoses, scarred or ulcerated lesions.
4. Seen most commonly on lower lip, tongue, head, neck and dorsa of hands.
5. Requires more aggressive approach (wider margin of normal skin included in excision)—greater chance of metastases from squamous cell carcinoma and significantly lower cure rate.

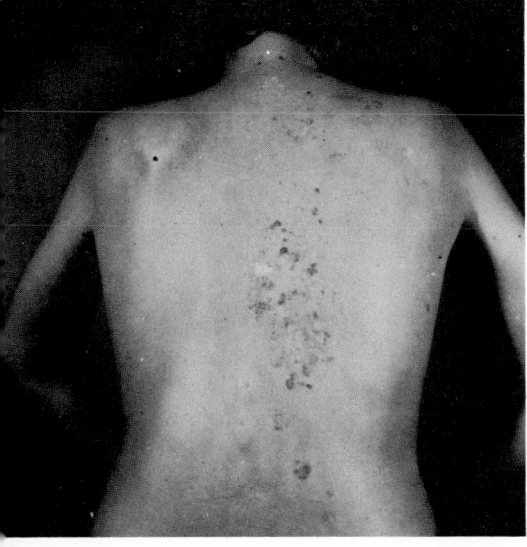

Figure 8-7. Basal cell carcinoma on skin of back. (Courtesy Armed Forces Institute of Pathology.)

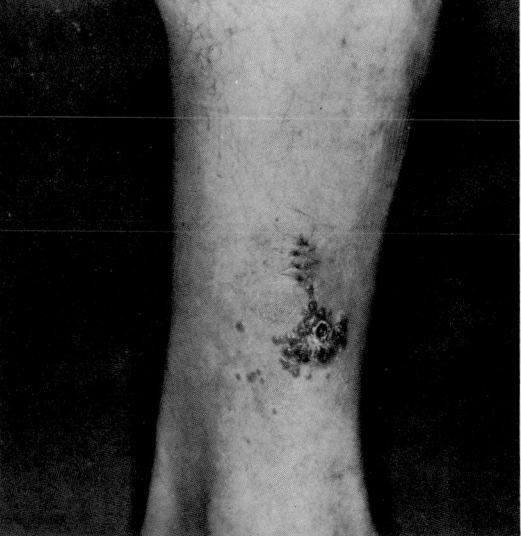

Figure 8-8. Melanoma. (Courtesy Armed Forces Institute of Pathology.)

Treatment

1. Method of treatment depends on tumor location, cell type (location and depth), cos metic desires of the patient, history of previous treatment and whether or not it i invasive and if metastatic nodes are present.

    Usual modes of treatment are (1) destruction by radiation and (2) surgica excision.

2. *Irradiation*

    Radiation is usually done for face and neck tumors of older patients and is useful for lesions of eyelids and nose.

    a. Reassure patient that treatment will not cause sterilization.

    b. Explain to patient that he may experience skin reddening and perhaps blistering of treated skin.

    c. Apply lanolin or other lubricant as directed—to keep skin soft after radiation therapy.

    d. Caution patient against exposure to the sun.

    e. Stress importance of follow-up care—there is always the possibility of recurrence or of a new primary lesion.

3. *Surgery*

    a. Wide surgical excision—adequacy of excision verified by microscopic study of sections of the specimen.

    b. Skin grafting may be necessary.

4. *Cryosurgery*—deep freezing to selectively destroy tumor tissue (analogous to irradiation).

    a. Thermocouple needles inserted into base of tumor.

    b. Liquid nitrogen ($-196°C.$) sprayed onto tumor until a temperature of $-20°C.$ is reached at tumor base.

    c. Site thaws naturally—then becomes gelatinous and heals spontaneously.

5. *Chemosurgery*—combined use of topically applied chemicals and the surgical knife to remove tissue.

6. *Electrodesiccation and curettage*—done on small tumors less than 1–2 cm.

    a. Wound is left open and kept dry by alcohol or antibiotics.

    b. Healing takes place in a few weeks.

7. Follow-up after treatment of skin cancer should be regular—should include palpation of the nodes through which the skin drains.

Patient Education

Instruct the patient as follows:

1. Avoid unnecessary exposure to the sun, especially during times when ultraviolet radiation light is most intense (10 AM to 2 PM).

2. Wear appropriate protective clothing (e.g., broad-rimmed hat, long-sleeved garments)

3. Use shading devices (e.g., umbrella over a tractor).

4. Apply a protective sunscreen cream or lotion if an activity requires long periods of exposure.

5. Have moles treated that are accessible to repeated friction and irritation (palms of hands and soles of feet).

6. Watch for indications of potential malignancy in moles (e.g., increase in size, ulceration, bleeding or serous exudation).

Malignant Melanoma

Malignant melanoma is a malignant tumor of the skin which occurs in 3 forms; lentigo-maligna melanoma, superficial spreading melanoma and nodular melanoma.

Classification

A. *Lentigo-maligna Melanoma*
  1. Slowly evolving pigment lesions; occur on exposed skin surfaces of elderly.
  2. First appears as tan, flat lesion—in time undergoes change in size and color.

B. *Superficial Spreading Melanoma*
  1. Occurs anywhere on body; usually affects persons of middle age.
  2. Tends to be circular with portion of its outline irregular (either protruding or indenting).
  3. Margins of lesion usually elevated and palpable (Fig. 8-8).
  4. Has combination of colors—hues of tan, brown and black admixed with gray, bluish-black or white.
  5. May be dull pink-rose color in a small area within the lesion.

C. *Nodular Melanoma*
  1. Spherical blueberry-like nodule with relatively smooth surface and relatively uniform blue black color.
  2. May be polypoidal with smooth surface or rose-gray or black color and may be present as elevated irregular plaque.

Clinical Features

  1. Skin of most persons has 15–30 nevi (moles), most of which are pigmented.
  2. Common sites of melanoma—skin of back, legs, feet, face, scalp.
  3. Etiology—unknown (ultraviolet rays are strongly suspected).

Diagnostic Evaluation

  1. Any change or alteration in size, color or other symptoms (itching, oozing, bleeding).
  2. Biopsy—excision of suspicious mole from both raised and invasive areas and from flat, noninvasive area.
  3. Prognosis—survival is related to depth of dermal invasion of malignant melanocytes in the primary lesion; melanoma is curable only when confined to primary site.

Preventive Measures

Educate people to observe their moles and report moles that *change* colors, *enlarge* or become raised or thicker.

Treatment

  1. Radical surgery—wide excision with regional node dissection followed by plastic repair or skin grafting.
  2. Regional isolation perfusion with appropriate cancer drugs (phenylanine mustard)—to protect against regional recurrence.

SYSTEMIC DISEASES WITH DERMATOLOGIC MANIFESTATIONS
Lupus Erythematosus

Systemic lupus erythematosus (SLE) is an inflammatory disease of unknown origin involving the vascular and connective tissues of many organs (primarily skin, joints, kidneys and serous membranes) with resultant multiple local and systemic symptoms.

Discoid lupus erythematosus is a chronic eruption of the skin which, although often disfiguring, does not pose a threat to life.

Clinical Features

1. Etiology is not understood—evidence indicates that it is an autoimmune disease.
2. Appears to be genetic and familial in nature.
3. Most frequently found in young women with signs and symptoms referable to the joints and skin.
4. May be drug-induced (procainamide-induced lupus).
5. Is characterized by remissions and exacerbations.

Clinical Manifestations

1. Vary greatly as they can affect every organ system
2. Weakness, malaise, weight loss
3. *Skin Manifestations*
   a. Malar rash, alopecia, dermal vasculitis, Raynaud's phenomenon, purpura.
   b. Possible skin rash with butterfly distribution over bridge of nose and malar bone prominences (butterfly distribution).
   c. Similar lesions over neck, chest, upper and lower extremities—may become pruritic and scaly.
4. Generalized lymphadenopathy
5. Long-continued low grade fever
6. Arthritis similar to rheumatoid arthritis
7. Anemia, leukopenia, thrombocytopenia
8. Musculoskeletal pains
9. Pericarditis, myocarditis, pleural effusion
10. Proteinuria, pyuria, nephritis—renal insufficiency and failure (primary cause of death)
11. Neuropsychiatric manifestations

Diagnostic Evaluation

1. Many laboratory abnormalities may be found.
2. Blood evaluation—shows evidence of anemia, leukopenia, thrombocytopenia.
3. Positive LE cell test—reaction of circulating proteins (LE factor) with white cells
4. Immunologic abnormalities
   a. ANA (antinuclear antibody test) positive—high titers of antibody to nuclear antigens
   b. Complement fixation test—decreased complement titers in patients with renal disease.
   c. Increased gamma globulins.

Treatment

Objective: to control the disease process by suppressing inflammation and relieving symptoms.

1. Treat intercurrent illness—exacerbations of SLE may follow infection, drug administration, emotional stress, surgical procedures.
2. Administer adrenal corticosteroids—used for suppressing inflammation.
   a. Prednisone—drug of choice.
   b. Observe patient carefully—may be difficult to distinguish between drug effects and those of SLE (steroids have multiple undesirable side effects).
3. Advise patient to avoid undue exposure to sunlight—can produce exacerbations and worsen dermal lesions.
4. Give salicylates for musculoskeletal pains.
5. Give antimalarials—chloroquine (Aralen) and hydroxychloroquine (Plaquenil)—to control the discoid and rheumatic manifestations.
6. Give immunosuppressive agents—to abrogate patient's immune response.
   a. Azathioprine (Imuran)
   b. Cyclophosphamide (Cytoxan)
   c. Immunosuppressive agents may have a steroid-sparing effect in some patients.
7. Administer iron salts and blood transfusions to correct the anemia.
8. Encourage the patient to eat a high caloric, high vitamin diet.
9. Treat the patient as his problem arises (depending on the organ system involved and its physiological consequences—(nephritis, congestive heart failure, central nervous system lupus).

Periarteritis Nodosa

Periarteritis nodosa (also polyarteritis) is a disease of unknown cause characterized by inflammation and necrosis of medium-sized and small arteries which results in altered function of the organ system in which the arterial supply has been impaired.

Clinical Manifestations

1. Varies according to organ(s) involved and amount of necrosis produced by obstructing vascular lesion.
2. Prolonged fever, hypertension, peripheral neuritis, palpable nodules along arterial trunks, renal disease, arthralgia.
3. Congestive heart failure, etc.
4. *Skin lesions*
   a. Papular eruptions, purpura, vesicles, bullae, subcutaneous nodules.
   b. Subcutaneous nodules vary in size and may be located in any part of the body.
5. Aneurysms may appear—result of focal weakening of the arterial wall.
6. Periarteritis is apt to run a course of a few years variation; recovery is unpredictable —death may ensue from renal decompensation and hypertension, congestive heart failure, etc.

Diagnostic Evaluation

1. Proteinuria, hematuria, casts—common urinary findings
2. Leukocytosis, eosinophilia, increased erythrocyte sedimentation rate
3. Elevated serum globulin rate
4. Biopsy of muscle section—may help establish diagnosis

Treatment

Objective: to give the patient symptomatic and supportive care.
1. Corticosteroids and immunosuppressive drugs may be given in combination.
   a. Corticosteroids (prednisone)—given to suppress manifestations of active inflammatory process. (Large doses given at first to bring prompt improvement in hypersensitivity reaction.)
   b. Immunosuppressive drugs—Azathiaprine (Imuran)
2. Treat intercurrent infection with antibiotics.
3. Advise patient to avoid drugs that may exacerbate symptoms.

DERMATOLOGIC SURGERY

Plastic Reconstructive Surgery

Reconstructive surgery (plastic surgery) is performed to repair extravisceral defects and malformations, both congenital and acquired, and to restore function as well as prevent further loss of function.

Cosmetic surgery involves reconstruction of the cutaneous tissues around the neck and face; done to restore function, correct defects and remove the marks of time (see Table 8-1).

Definitions

1. *Skin graft* (free graft)—a section of skin tissue which is separated from its blood supply and transferred as a free section of tissue to the recipient site.
2. *Skin flap* (pedicle graft)—a section of skin tissue used to cover or fill a defect; it is lifted from its bed but still has partial attachment by a pedicle from which it receives its blood supply until healing takes place in its new location.
   Flaps are used to cover defects in which there is poor vascularity; for reconstruction of eyelids, ears, nose and cheeks.
3. *Autograft*—transfers or transplants from same person.
4. *Allograft*—transfer or transplants from a different person.
5. *Split-thickness graft* (Thiersch's graft)—graft of approximately one-half the thickness of skin which is removed by a knife or dermatome; deeper layers of dermis are left behind. (Used for coverage and closure of skin defects.)
6. *Full-thickness skin graft*—contains the epidermis and all of the dermis.
   a. Used frequently for reconstruction of facial defects for it neither contracts nor develops unsightly pigmentation.
   b. Grafts may be further subdivided into thin and thick:
      (1) Thin (0.010–0.015 inch thick)—used to resurface contaminated granulations or recipient sites in which blood supply is jeopardized.
      (2) Thick (0.015–0.020 inch thick)—used where durability is the important factor.
7. *Pinch graft*—a small piece of skin graft obtained by elevating the skin with a needle or forceps and cutting it off with scissors or knife.
8. *Take*—refers to the appearance of the graft between the 3rd and 5th day after transfer, signifying that the vascular connections have developed between the recipient bed and the transplant.

TABLE 8-1. COMMON COSMETIC PLASTIC OPERATIONS

Operation	Purpose	Surgery	Postoperative expectations	Hospital discharge
Rhinoplasty (Nose)	To improve the shape of the nose in relation to the rest of the face	1–1½ hours. Excess bone or cartilage is removed; nose is reshaped	Nasal splint; soft intranasal packing; foam rubber dressings	1–5 days
Mentoplasty (Chin)	To improve the profile, such as is necessary with a receding chin	Incision approach is within the mouth. Silicone or plastic implant is positioned	Healing complete in a week	1–2 days
Rhytidoplasty (Face lift)	To remove excess skin due to elastosis and to tighten remaining skin	Incision is anterior to ear and extended down to nasolabial fold to the mental foramen near the chin and to the midline in the upper neck; the stretched subcutaneous tissues and fascia of the face are folded to provide a basic firmness	Improvement lasts up to 10 years	1 week
Glabellar rhytidoplasty	To remove 2 vertical furrows between eyebrows	Dermabrasion and excision; skin graft may be required		3–5 days
Otoplasty (Ear)	To correct deformed, flattened or protruding ears	1–1½ hours. Silicone or plastic implant may be used	Ear bandaged for a week; protection during sleep required for 3 weeks	1–2 days
Blepharoplasty (Eyelid)	To remove wrinkles and bulges caused by herniation of fat, aging or inheritance	1–1½ hours. Two incisions; one on upper lid and one on lower lid	Neosporin ointment applied around eyes and lids. Individual eye dressings are applied. Swelling and discoloration subsides in about 10 days	1–2 days

Causes of Graft Failure

1. Fluid beneath the graft
2. Hematoma—avoid by early inspection and removal of clots
3. Infection

Nursing Management (for Grafting Procedures)

A. *Preoperative Care*

Objective: to bring the patient to his optimal physical and emotional level.

1. Assess for nutritional status.
    a. Give vitamins and increase protein intake as directed—to facilitate healing.
    b. Note hemoglobin level and clotting time—these levels can affect healing process.
2. Prepare donor and recipient sites for surgical excision (see p. 599).
3. Inform the patient about what to expect postoperatively.
    a. Appearance of the wound—redness, distortion, swelling and unattractive suture lines are characteristics that will change with time.
    b. Pressure dressings, immobilization devices, etc.
4. Prepare the patient psychologically.
    a. Attempt to establish the reasons that the patient seeks surgery.
        (1) Patient's attitudes toward his disfigurement and his motivations for seeking surgery, his assessment of how his disfigurement has influenced his life and his psychosocial relationships are taken into consideration before surgery is considered.
        (2) Desirable to have unimpaired body image and realistic acceptance of surgical limitations.
        (3) Poor candidate for cosmetic surgery is one who has delusions concerning his deformity, unhealthy psychological responses and unrealistic expectations of results.
    b. Explain the limitations of the contemplated procedure, the possibility of complications and the unpredictability of the result (responsibility of the surgeon).

B. *Postoperative Care*

1. Inspect graft under dressing daily using a good light—to ensure that edema, blistering or hematoma has not formed and is jeopardizing successful graft.
    a. Surgeon carefully teases dressing away from wound—changing dressing may cause avulsion (tearing away) of recent graft around the margin of the wound.
    b. Surgeon will nick graft to evacuate blood clots.
        (1) Fluid may be rolled out of graft with cotton-tipped applicator or by aspirating with needle and syringe.
        (2) Seromas or hematomas may impede healing.
2. Apply mittens to patient if he is inadvertently scratching the graft during sleep—to protect graft and donor site from subconscious scratching.
3. Apply wet dressings to infected graft as directed.
4. Use prophylactic antibiotic therapy for patient with infected graft.
    Utilize sensitivity testing to identify organism.
5. Elevate grafted extremity for 7–10 days.
    a. Immobilize part—movement of body areas beneath graft may predispose to loss of graft.
    b. Apply cast or immobilizing bandages to restrict all regional movements of the extremity.
    c. Begin ambulation activities very gradually.
6. Inform the patient of the changing hues of the graft—to help him accept his situation.
    a. Free graft is at first pale, then pink and red—it then fades and appears similar to neighboring skin.

    b. Full-thickness grafts may remain deeply red for months.

    c. Anticipate skin scaling in full-thickness grafts.

    d. Teach the patient that the graft is vulnerable to sun; avoid over exposure to the sun.

  7. Instruct the patient to apply mineral oil or lanolin on wound after 2nd or 3rd week—to remove superficial crusts, moisten the graft and stimulate circulation to the wound area.

C. *Care of the Donor Site*

  1. The donor site is usually covered with lightly lubricated petrolatum or antibiotic-empregnated gauze and held in place with a gauze dressing to absorb blood and serum from the wound.

    a. The outer dressing may be removed in 24 hours.

    b. Area may be left exposed after 1st or 2nd postoperative day.

    c. Petrolatum dressing may be left in place until it loosens as epithelization becomes complete—prevents heavy crusting.

  2. Prevent area from coming in contact with clothing or bedding—to provide adequate circulation of air to the donor site.

  3. Apply wet dressing (as directed) if donor site becomes infected.

  4. Lubricate donor site with lanolin or cocoa butter after healing—to keep it soft and pliable.

  5. Donor sites heal by re-epithelization; healing should be complete in 2 weeks time.

Nursing Management (of Patient Undergoing Maxillofacial Surgery)

A. *Preoperative Care*

    See page 598 for nursing support.

B. *Postoperative Care*

  1. Maintain an adequate airway.

  2. Observe dressings for impairment of circulation and edema—pressure dressings are frequently used.

    a. Control oral hemorrhage by inserting gauze pad in the mouth and exerting pressure at bleeding point.

    b. Wipe blood from wound—blood under suture line may cause hematoma and infection and spoil the cosmetic result.

  3. Watch color of skin flaps—may appear blue and congested due to partial obstruction of the venous circulation.

    a. Surgeon may make small incisions in the flap to relieve the blood congestion and avoid gangrene of the flap.

    b. Moisten flap dressing with warm sterile solution as directed.

  4. Relieve pain—expect more pain on operations involving jaw and facial bones.

    a. Apply heat or cold according to direction.

    b. Give analgesics as ordered.

  5. Keep the patient well hydrated and nourished.

    a. Offer cracked ice and water as soon as nausea subsides.

    b. Give soft diet as tolerated.

      (1) Provide an adequate quantity and caloric quality to patient on prolonged liquid diet (following jaw surgery, etc.).

      (2) Give frequent feedings in order to obtain caloric equivalent of a full diet.

  6. Offer appropriate psychological support—numerous operations may be required.

Dermabrasion

Dermabrasion is surgical planing of the superficial portion of the skin.

Clinical Indications

1. Done on selected patients with facial disfigurements from scars resulting from acne, trauma, nevi, freckles, chickenpox or smallpox.
2. Removal of precancerous lesions (keratosis).

Surgical Procedure

The epidermis and some superficial dermis are removed, while enough of the dermis is preserved to allow re-epithelization of the dermabraded areas.

1. The patient is anesthetized.
2. The skin is sprayed with a topical anesthetic to stabilize and stiffen the skin.
3. The superficial layer of skin is removed by an abrasive machine (Dermabrader) or by sandpapering.
4. Copious saline irrigations are carried out during and after the planing procedure.
5. Petrolatum gauze or plastic-faced bandages are applied immediately after the procedure.

Nursing Management

Postoperative

1. Apply saline compresses over petrolatum dressings—to absorb oozing and clotting which are subject to infection.
   a. Mild oozing may be expected for 24 hours.
   b. Crusts then form; are shed in 7–10 days.
   c. Skin remains pink 6–12 weeks.
2. Discontinue saline compresses after 12–24 hours or as directed.
3. Assist with removal of dressing in 48 hours—patient will experience a "recent sunburn" sensation.
4. Apply lanolin, hypoallergenic cream, etc. as directed—to relieve the sensation of tightness when the crusts form.
5. Warn the patient to avoid exposure to direct sunlight for 3 to 4 months—planed area may become darker or lighter than surrounding skin due to sunlight.

2. *Burns*

CARE OF THE BURN PATIENT

Burns are wounds caused by excessive exposure to heat, heated objects, fire, steam, radiation, x-ray, electricity and certain chemicals.

Incidence

1. Over 2 million burn injuries occur annually in the U.S.
2. Approximately 75,000 burn victims require hospitalization each year in this country.
3. Over 8000 persons die from burns each year in the U.S.

4. Most burn accidents occur in the home and are caused primarily by carelessness or ignorance.
5. Authorities estimate that at least 75% of all burns could be prevented.
6. The nurse is in a prominent position to teach burn prevention and to promote legislation for safety practices.

Survival Prediction

1. Best survival expectancy occurs in young adult groups, age 15–45 years.
2. A burn of over 20% of the body endangers life.
3. Prognosis depends upon age of patient, depth and extent of burn, condition of patient and imminence of complications as well as dedication of the treating team.

Altered Physiology

A. *State of Neurogenic Shock*
1. First stage of a burn reaction—may be lethal.
2. Emotional reactions of the individual—fright, terror, hysteria.
3. Pain—irritation of thousands of nerve endings.
4. Fall in blood pressure.

B. *State of Fluid-loss Shock*
1. First effect of a burn—dilatation of capillaries and increasing permeability.
2. Plasma seeps into tissues causing blisters and edema.
3. Fluid loss → less blood volume (thicker) → hypovolemia → hypotension → renal perfusion and renal shutdown.
4. Increase in cell volume leading to increase in hematocrit.

C. *State of Burn Slough and Infection*
1. The third stage of a burn—eschar (burned necrotic tissue) separates from underlying viable tissue by formation of slough.
2. Resulting open wound may lead to infection—temperature elevation, local tenderness, tachycardia, lymphangitis.

D. *State of Repair*
1. Before repair of a large burn wound can take place, sloughed tissue must be removed.
2. Epithelization occurs if all the layers of the skin have not been destroyed.
3. With destruction of entire skin thickness, healing begins at edges of wound with the granulation (scar) of tissue—takes a long time.
4. To avoid excessive overgrowth of granulation tissue, skin grafts may be applied—healing is more rapid.
5. Debrided areas may be dressed with porcine skin while other areas are grafted with autografts.
6. To facilitate systemic repair, blood transfusions are given to reduce anemia, and high protein, high caloric diet is given to replace nutritional deficiencies.

Assessment of Patient's Burn Injury

A. Assess extent of body surface burned.
1. Anatomical location—greater morbidity and mortality for burns affecting hands, feet, face and perineum.

2. Determination is based on the use of tables for this purpose or the "Rule of Nine" Chart (Fig. 8-9). (For children, use Lund and Browder chart)—These tables or charts serve as a guide for fluid therapy.
3. Repeat assessment on 2nd and 3rd day inasmuch as demarcation may not be visible until then.

B. Assess depth of burn.
    1. Determine:
        a. Causative agent (boiling water, chemical, etc.)
        b. Duration of exposure
        c. Thickness of skin
    2. Classify:
        a. Major burns—Second-degree burns of over 30% of body
                       —Third-degree burns of over 10% of body.
        b. First-degree
            (1) Redness
            (2) Not serious unless large areas of body involved.
        c. Second-degree
            (1) Blisters form (vesicles).
            (2) Superficial layers of skin are destroyed.
            (3) Hospitalization required if large areas affected.
        d. Third-degree
            (1) Destruction of full thickness of skin and often underlying fat, muscles and bone.
            (2) Immediate hospitalization required.
        e. Differentiation between deep second- and third-degree is often difficult, and repeated evaluation over several days is necessary.

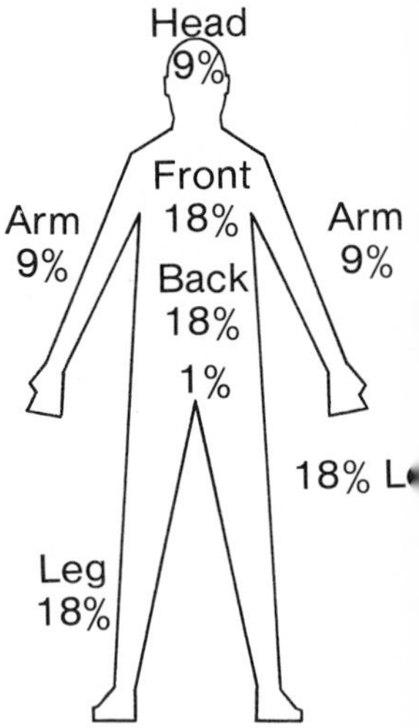

Figure 8-9. "Rule of Nine" chart.

Emergency First-aid Measures

> NURSING ALERT: Grease, ointment or antiseptic should *not* be applied to any large burn as an emergency measure.

1. Apply cold to the burn—immerse in ice water for 10 minutes (if pain present, repeat up to 3 times) or apply cold towels—relieves pain and reduces tissue edema and damage.
2. Get patient to treatment facility—do not delay.
3. Cover burn as quickly as possible with sterile dressings or any clean cloth—to prevent further wound contamination.
    a. Ointments and salves should not be used.
    b. Bacterial contamination is minimized.
    c. Pain is decreased by preventing air from contacting injured surface.
4. Irrigate chemical burns immediately.
    a. Flush eyes, if affected, with clean cool water.
    b. Consult physician.
5. When clothes catch on fire, have victim fall to floor or ground and roll him in a carpet or blanket.
    a. Standing would force him to breathe flames and smoke.
    b. Running would fan flames.

    c. After fire is extinguished, soak hot clothing with cold water.

    d. Get patient to treatment facility.

  6. Allow victim to lie down while awaiting transportation to hospital.

    a. Do not remove clothing unless it is hot or burning.

    b. Cover victim with a blanket to prevent loss of body heat.

    c. Place ice bottles or ice strategically to reduce pain.

  7. Evaluate patient as a whole.

    a. A history and a physical examination are required to determine priority of needs.

        (1) Maintenance of adequate oxygenation

        (2) Fluid replacement

        (3) Prevention of infection by cleansing of burn

        (4) Tetanus booster

        (5) Topical antibacterial medications

        (6) Treatment of associated injuries, such as digitalization, etc.

    b. Withhold oral fluids for the first day or two if the patient has a major burn—otherwise he may develop gastric dilatation and perhaps paralytic ileus.

Objectives of Medical and Nursing Management

Objectives: to prevent burns by initiating and promoting safety practices.

           to employ life-saving measures in the care of the severely burned person.

           to provide early specialized and individualized treatment of the burn victim in order to prevent disability and disfigurement.

           to promote rehabilitation of the burn patient through rehabilitative programs and reconstruction surgery if necessary.

A. *To remove burning agent, alleviate pain, and initiate plan of treatment.*

  1. Provide for immediate hospitalization.

  2. Observe for any breathing impairment; prepare for tracheostomy, if necessary.

  3. Remove burned clothing and assess extent of burned area.

  4. Make patient as comfortable as possible (morphine for pain, etc.) while history and physical examination progress.

B. *To prevent and treat for burn shock.*

  Prepare for fluid replacement immediately—blood, electrolytes, colloid and fluid.

    a. Weigh the patient (on admission) if possible; daily thereafter at the same time each day.

    b. Measure circumference of burned extremities; this may be useful later in determining edema formation (believed unnecessary by some authorities).

    c. Insert an indwelling catheter; measure hourly output and describe.

        Maintain urine output in range of 30–50 ml./hr.

    d. Assist with cannulization of vein for continuous intravenous therapy.

    e. Record intake and output conscientiously (Fig. 8-10).

    f. Observe for signs of dehydration or overhydration by use of hematocrit and urinary output; notify physician if signs occur.

    g. Note any untoward signs indicative of a transfusion reaction; if apparent, terminate transfusion and notify physician.

C. *To assess the physical and psychological reaction of the patient to his condition.*

  1. Take and record vital signs hourly.

  2. Note whether blood specimens are taken by the laboratory technician as requested.

I.V. MEDICATION AND FLUID THERAPY

	VITAL SIGNS					INTAKE				OUTPUT		
	B.P.	V.P.	T.	P.	R.	TYPE I.V. FLUID & MEDICATION ADDED	READING ON BOTTLE	AMOUNT ABSORBED	ORAL	URINE	SP. GR.	GASTRIC & STOOL
7:00 AM												
8:00												
9:00												
10:00												
11:00												
12:00 N												
1:00 PM												
2:00												
8 Hr. Total												
3:00 PM												
4:00												
5:00												
6:00												
7:00												
8:00												
9:00												
10:00												
8 Hr. Total												
11:00 PM												
12:00 M												
1:00 AM												
2:00												
3:00												
4:00												
5:00												
6:00												
8 Hr. Total												
24 Hr. Totals												

Figure 8-10. Twenty-four-hour flowsheet to monitor burn patients during initial treatment (The Burn Patient, Ethicon, 1969.)

    3. Obtain 24-hour urine specimen if ordered.
    4. Talk to the patient to determine his concerns.
    5. Observe patient for his reaction to his condition.

D. *To provide physical comfort and emotional support of the patient.*
    1. Administer sedatives and analgesics as prescribed for pain.
    2. Elevate the burned extremities for comfort and to lessen edema.
    3. Provide diversional therapy; allay fear and anxiety.
    4. Place patient in physiologically comfortable position.

E. *To meet nutritional needs and control gastrointestinal disturbances.*
    1. Administer oral fluids *slowly* so that patient's tolerance can be observed.
    2. If serum potassium levels drop, give fruit juices that contain potassium.
    3. After several days supplement the diet with high protein drinks.
    4. Offer more solid food toward the end of the first week as tolerance for food improves.
       a. Build up daily caloric intake to match daily caloric expenditures.
       b. Provide: 3 gm. of protein/kg. body weight; 20% of needed calories in form of fats; remainder in carbohydrates.
    5. Imagination and ingenuity may be required to stimulate a sluggish appetite. If patient does not maintain an adequate intake voluntarily, it may be necessary to pass a nasogastric tube for administration of high protein formula (Fig. 8-11).
    6. Be alert for evidence of Curling's ulcer—the incidence is in proportion to the extent of the burn.

a. Sudden drop in hemoglobin concentration may be diagnostic.
b. Note blood-tinged contents from nasogastric suction or in the stool. (Although not usual, be on alert for this.)

F. *To prevent complications*
1. *Infection*
   a. Assist in the cleansing and debridement of tissues.
   b. Practice rigid asepsis when wound is exposed.
   c. Wear mask and gown in addition to sterile gloves during change of dressings.
   d. Obtain wound culture when requested.
   e. Keep environment as clean as possible.
      (1) Maintain isolation precautions.
      (2) Restrict visitors.
   f. Administer antibiotics as prescribed (usually after first day since blocked capillaries at burn site will prevent medications from reaching the area).
   g. Recognize changes in vital signs that may indicate infection.
   h. Apply topical bacteriostatic substance as directed (silver nitrate, sulfamylon, etc.).
   i. Promote the best personal hygiene for the patient.
      (1) Cleanse unburned areas of the body with antibacterial soap or detergent-germicide; maintain clean nails.
      (2) Shave hairs from burned areas.
      (3) Provide meticulous mouth care.
      (4) Keep all orifices especially clean; give special attention to indwelling catheter and meatus.
   j. On admission administer tetanus toxoid (if immunized previously) or administer human antitetanus serum (if toxoid not given previously).
2. *Contractures and Deformities*
   a. Maintain proper body alignment using supports as necessary.
   b. Initiate active exercises where possible with physician's permission on first postburn day.
   c. Use a footboard to prevent footdrop.
   d. Splint hands at night *only*.
   e. Have patient feed himself with burned (second-degree) hands as early as first or second postburn day.
3. *Respiratory Difficulty*
   a. Assess respiratory rate, chest movement and any respiratory stress.
   b. Determine whether patient inhaled smoke, fumes, or flame—whether he has singed nasal hair, red pharynx, hoarse voice, cough, stridor, etc.
   c. Have tracheostomy and oxygen equipment easily accessible.

G. *To promote wound healing and rehabilitation.*
1. Recognize the importance of adequate nutrition.
   a. Entice patient's appetite with attractive servings.
   b. Encourage fluids when patient is able to take them by mouth.
2. Initiate treatment as prescribed, e.g., silver nitrate, sulfamylon, silver sulfadiazine, etc.
3. Prevent pneumonia, control edema, prevent decubiti.
4. Maintain proper body positions, turn frequently, encourage deep breathing.
   a. Encourage early ambulation of patient.
   b. Initiate passive, then active range of motion exercises.
5. Refer to page 609 for skin grafting.

METHODS OF TREATING BURNS

Open Air or Exposure Method

Exposing the burn to the drying effect of air, allows the exudate to dry, forming a hard crust in 3 days which then acts as a protection to the wound.

A. *Advantages and Mode of Action*
1. Effective during disaster when large numbers of persons must be cared for.
2. Most frequently used to treat burns of face, neck, perineum and extensive burns of the trunk.
3. There are no painful dressing changes; therefore, less equipment is used, and it is more comfortable for the patient.
4. Infection can be detected earlier.
5. Second-degree burns, beneath crust—regeneration of skin in 2–3 weeks.
6. Third-degree burns, beneath eschar—regeneration of skin in 4–5 weeks.
7. Eschar loosens and must be debrided.

B. *Imperative—Keep Immediate Environment Free of Organisms*
1. Everything that comes in contact with patient must be clean.
   a. Sterile linens on bed. (Sterility lost rather quickly.)
   b. Masks, sterile gowns and gloves for persons in contact with patient.
   c. Gowns and masks for visitors—instruct not to touch him or hand him anything.
   d. "Burn pack" desirable since it contains all linens for patient and gown and mask for attendant.
2. Room must be kept clean.
   a. Screens on windows.
   b. Dusting and mopping to be done with damp cloth or mop—not dry.
3. Humidity and temperature should be regulated—humidity (40–50%); temperature (preferably 24.4°C. or 76°F.).
   a. If too warm, patient may lose needed body fluids.
   b. Warmth encourages bacterial growth.
   c. Bed or partial cradle with cover can be used to prevent chilling.
   d. Electric dehumidifier can be used if necessary.

C. *Nursing Management*
1. Prevent burn area from sticking to the sheet—dust lower sheet with sterile cornstarch.
2. Avoid unnecessary trauma when changing linens by wetting those parts of tissue adhering to linen with sterile saline.
3. Have patient turn frequently to prevent cardiopulmonary complications and contractures.
4. Have patient feed himself if hand burns are not chiefly third degree.
5. Walk patient if complicating fractures are not present.

Occlusive (Pressure) Dressings

A. *Advantage*

Pain is less in first 48 hours postburn.

B. *Disadvantages*
1. High incidence of burn wound sepsis.
2. Discomfort and pain when changed.

C. *Nursing Management*
  1. Observe for signs of infection—temperature elevation, increased pulse, increased pain, perhaps an odor.
  2. Change dressings if exudate stain is noted; this may indicate the presence of moisture which may lead to bacterial growth.
  3. Elevate extremity to prevent edema.

Silver Nitrate (0.5%) Solution
  (Being used less because of its disadvantages)

A. *Advantages and Mode of Action*
  1. Silver nitrate is a bacteriostatic chemical and is effective in reducing colonization.
     a. Above 1% produces tissue necrosis.
     b. Below 0.5% solution is ineffective as an antiseptic.
  2. Cap, gown and mask are not required.
  3. An effective method for treating large numbers of burns as during war.
  4. Silver nitrate can be used over grafted areas and donor sites as well as burn surfaces.

B. *Disadvantages*
  1. Hyponatremia (loss of sodium ions) and hypochloremia (loss of chlorine ions) may occur. (For this reason, should not be used for children.)
  2. Methemoglobinemia (a modified form of oxyhemoglobin) may be caused due to the reduction of nitrates to nitrites, resulting in cyanosis.
  3. Silver nitrate turns black in sunlight.
     a. Clothes, hands, floor, etc. are stained black.
     b. Gloves must be worn by the nurse and her assistants.

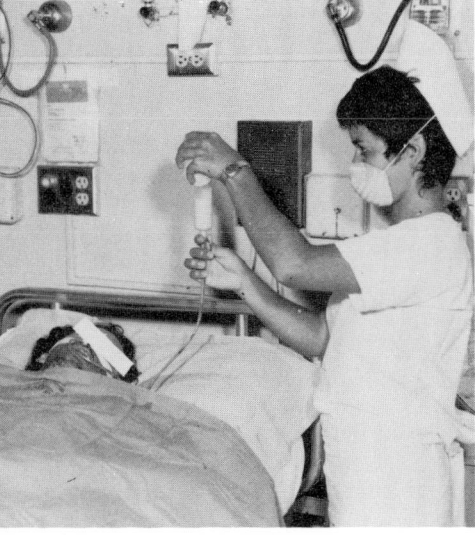

Figure 8-11. To maintain the nutritional needs of the burn patient, a nasogastric tube may be passed. (Courtesy Brooke Army Medical Center.)

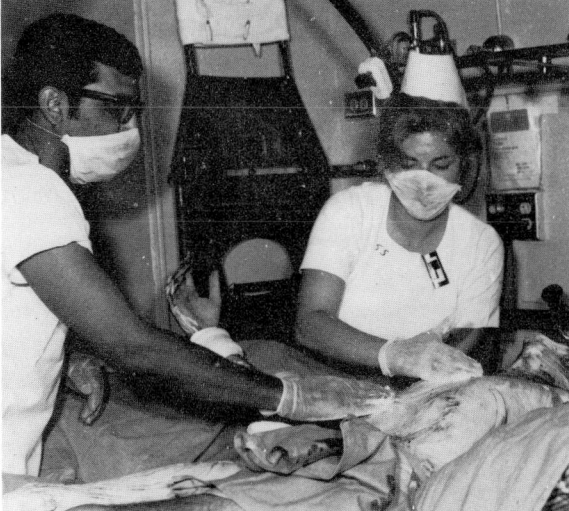

Figure 8-12. Nurses are applying a layer of sulfamylon cream, using sterile gloves to smooth the cream to the appropriate thickness. (Courtesy Brooke Army Medical Center.)

Silver Sulfadiazine (1%)

In a hydrophilic (readily absorbs moisture) petrolatum base.

A. *Advantages and Mode of Action*
1. Chlorides of the body are not readily precipitated as with silver nitrate. Therefore no electrolyte abnormality occurs and no acidosis develops.
2. Applied as a cream with tongue blades or in impregnated gauze.
3. Little pain experienced with application of cream.
4. Viscous dressings are easily and painlessly removed.
5. Silver sulfadiazine is odorless.
6. Action occurs by oligodynamic action (active in minute quantities) of silver and is dependent upon chloride and other anions in the wound exudate.
7. It utilizes the special antibacterial action of sulfonamide; it is particularly effective against infections due to Pseudomonas.

B. *Disadvantages*
Some patients develop skin rash.

C. *Mode of Application*
1. Silver sulfadiazine can be applied directly to the burn wound, spread thinly, 2–4 mm., and left exposed.
2. Some surgeons prefer that after ointment is applied, it should be covered with a single layer of mesh gauze.
3. Reapply as it rubs off; if occlusive dressings are used, change every 48 hours.

Gentamicin Sulfate (Garamycin cream) 0.1%

A. *Advantages and Mode of Action*
1. Useful against a wide variety of gram negative and gram positive organisms. (Even effective against *Providencia stuartii.*)
2. Application and use are similar to Sulfamylon acetate (see p. 609).
3. Ointment spreads easily and tends to become invisible.
4. No pain is associated with this cream.
5. Because of the tendency of organisms to become resistant to this antimicrobial, it is usually reserved for life-threatening manifestations.

B. *Disadvantages*
None

Mafenide Acetate (Sulfamylon Acetate)

A. *Advantages and Mode of Action*
1. Burn area is treated with an antibacterial agent that will penetrate the eschar (scar) to kill infecting organisms.
    Formerly, thrombosis and damage to vascular channels prevented systemic antibodies from reaching the wound of a burn.
2. In cream form, mafenide acetate diffuses rapidly through the burned skin and is relatively nontoxic.

B. *Disadvantage*
Causes a burning pain for the first few minutes following application.

GUIDELINES: *Application of Sulfamylon Ointment*

Equipment

Sulfamylon Acetate cream
Sterile gloves
Sterile scissors
Sterile forceps

Nonadherent absorbent pads
Fine mesh gauze strips
Stretch gauze bandage

Procedure

Nursing Action	Rationale/Amplification
1. Administer analgesic as prescribed.	1. To relieve burning pain which occurs during first few minutes following application of Sulfamylon cream.

2. Cleanse burn areas by most feasible method:
  a. Hubbard tub
  b. Bathtub
  c. Shower
  d. Local bathing in bed with nonirritating cleansing solutions
	2. To facilitate removal of necrotic tissue which at the same time provides relaxation for the patient.

3. Place nonadherent absorbent pad under patient's burned area.	3. To absorb exudate and provide a means of holding cream in contact with burn area.
4. Remove loose or necrotic tissue from wound using a sterile forceps and scissors.	4. To permit Sulfamylon cream to contact viable tissue and eliminate pressure areas where dried and dead tissue accumulate.
5. Apply a layer of Sulfamylon cream (2–4 mm.) to the burned area, using a sterile gloved hand (Fig. 8-12).	5. To provide adequate contact through diffusion of avascular burn tissue.
6. Cover creamed areas with a single-layer of fine mesh gauze; fasten with single-layer stretch gauze bandage. (Varies with clinics; some do not use this.)	6. To maintain contact with tissue—often cream rolls or slides off burned areas because of exudate.
7. Reapply Sulfamylon cream when absorbed; for first 2 to 3 days this may be required every 4–5 hours.	7. To maintain constant contact of ointment to burn area.
8. Assess for any unusual reaction such as increased redness, increase in pulse or respirations.	8. To detect allergic manifestations.
9. Place patient in Hubbard bath once every 24 hours (or as suggested by physician).	9. To remove dressings and loosen tissue. To permit motion of joints. To provide comfort and relaxation for the patient.
10. Reapply Sulfamylon.	
11. Check electrolytes.	11. To rule out metabolic acidosis or respiratory alkalosis.

SKIN GRAFTING OF BURN SITE

Removal of Eschar

This dead tissue is removed in preparation for skin grafting as soon as is feasible in the overall plan for grafting.

Effective Methods
1. Surgical excision.

2. Change dry dressings every 2 days; light anesthesia may be necessary to remove loose tissue; a scissors is used to cut strands that hold eschar.
3. Bathe daily in a Hubbard tank.
4. Apply wet soaks every 4 hours (saline) using coarse mesh gauze; frequent removal of gauze also facilitates pulling away dead tissue.

Autografts

Autografts are skin grafts taken from an uninjured part of the patient's body and applied elsewhere on his body where needed.

Types of Autografts

A. *Split thickness*—skin at thickness between 0.010–0.035 inches (useful for burn areas)

Free—a segment of skin completely removed from one area and transferred to the desired grafting area where it will be nourished by the capillary ingrowth from the granulating bed.

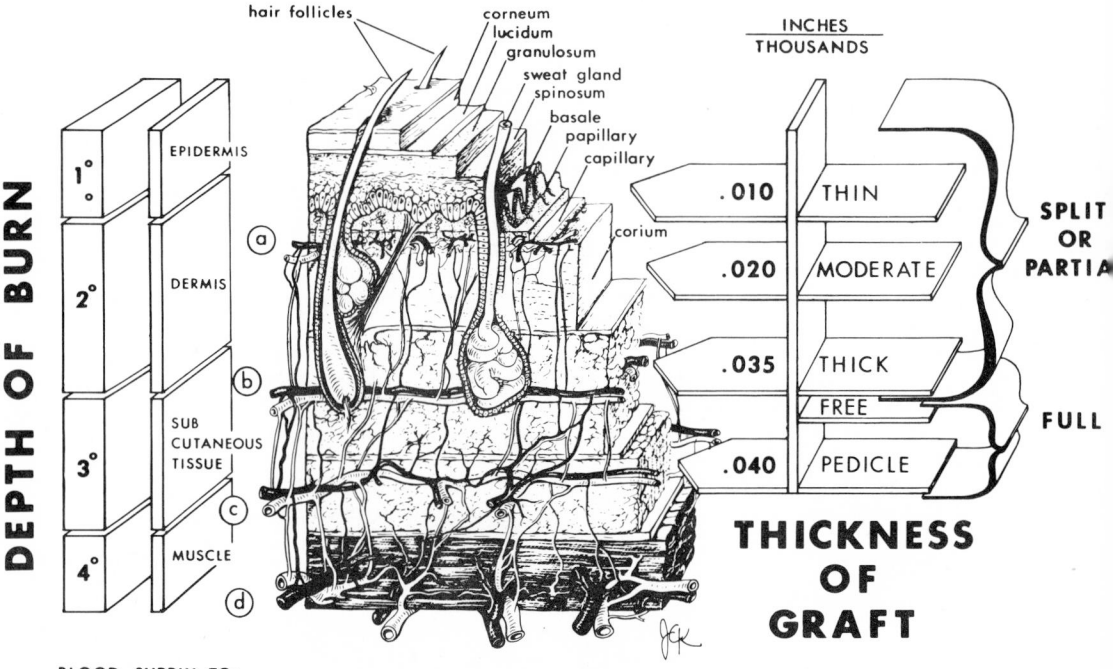

Figure 8-13. Cross section of skin depicting blood supply, depth of burn and relative thickness of skin grafts. (From Manteuffel, S. W., and Berkich, E. J.: The Burn Patient. Somerville, N.J., Ethicon, Inc., 1969.)

B. *Full thickness*—greater than 0.035 inch

Pedicle—a graft of skin in which 3 sides are freed from the donor site but the 4th remains attached through which blood supply is maintained.

Application of Autograft

1. Grafting may be done in 2 or more stages depending upon readiness of the burn surface and the condition of the patient.
   a. Priority areas in skin coverage (in order)
      (1) Hands   (3) Neck
      (2) Face   (4) Areas of motion: elbows, axillae, knees, lower leg.
   b. These areas should be grafted as soon as possible to lessen scarring and contracture formation.
2. Grafting is done in the operating room under aseptic conditions.

Care of Postgraft Recipient Site

A. *Methods of Initial Care*
   1. *Exposure Method*
      a. Note the progress of vascularization.
         Permits detection of hematomas and seromas—underneath such formation, graft will not take unless fluid is released and grafts are sutured.
      b. Roll out the graft using a sterile cotton applicator stick to flatten graft and permit fluid to escape.

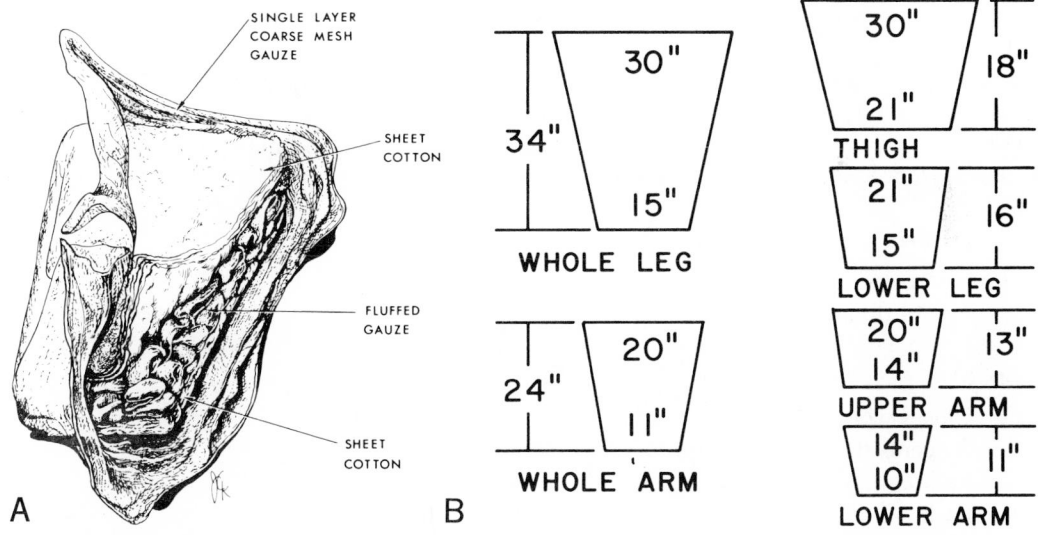

Figure 8-14. A. The preformed dressing showing construction with fluffed gauze, sheet cotton, and the covering of coarse mesh gauze. B. Sizes of frequently used preformed dressings for children and adults. (From Manteuffel, S. W., and Berkich, E. J.: The Burn Patient. Somerville, N.J., Ethicon, Inc., 1969.)

      c. Apply saline compresses for short intervals every 2–3 hours—this can provide the high humidity required for a graft to take.

      d. Immobilize the grafted area for 2–3 days by use of sand bags, trochanter rolls, etc.

  2. *Occlusive Dressing Method*

      a. Effective for young children or older persons who are irrational or uncooperative.

      b. Compression is desirable to lessen the formation of fluid beneath the grafts.

      c. Pressure dressings of the preformed variety (Fig. 8-14) are most effective.

        (1) Single layer of commercially prepared nylon fabric (Adaptic)

        (2) Preformed gauze pads

        (3) Fluffed gauze

      d. These dressings are removed after 3–5 days.

B. *Use of Hubbard Tank*

  1. About 4th day in exposure method

  2. When dressings are removed in occlusive dressing method

      a. Stimulates circulation.

      b. Keeps graft area clean.

C. *Care When Patient is Ambulatory*

  1. Have patient wear elastic rubberized bandages on lower extremities over graft sites for 3 months.

      a. Prevents epithelium breakdown.

      b. Eliminates burning sensation often felt when no supporting bandage is used.

  2. Provide diversional, recreational or occupational therapy.

Allografts (Homografts)

An *allograft* is a graft of skin taken from a person other than the burn victim and applied to a burn wound temporarily (a cadaver is most common source).

A *xenograft* or *heterograft* is a segment of skin taken from an animal such as a pig or dog. It is useful to prepare debrided area for grafting.

Donor Criteria

  1. Skin color unimportant since it is only a temporary graft.

  2. Age of donor should be adult under 60 years of age.

Purpose

  1. Closes wound temporarily.

  2. Prevents fluid and protein loss.

  3. Reduces risk of infection.

  4. Reduces pain.

Clinical Procedure

Graft is replaced about every 3 days, otherwise, there is too much trauma and bleeding when the homograft is pulled away.

BIBLIOGRAPHY

Dermatology

Books

Behrman, H. T., et al.: Common Skin Diseases. New York, Grune and Stratton, Inc., 1971.
Brunner, L., et al.: Textbook of Medical-Surgical Nursing, 2nd ed. Philadelphia, J. B. Lippincott, 1970, pp. 629–656.
Cohen, E. L., and Pegum, J. S.: Dermatology. Baltimore, Williams and Wilkins, 1970.
Domonkos, A. N.: Andrews' Diseases of the Skin. Philadelphia, W. B. Saunders, 1971.
Epstein, E. (ed.): Skin Surgery. Springfield, Charles C Thomas, 1970.
Maddin, S. (ed.): Current Dermatologic Management. St. Louis, C. V. Mosby, 1970.
May, H.: Plastic and Reconstructive Surgery. Philadelphia, F. A. Davis, 1971.
Pillsbury, D. M.: A Manual of Dermatology. Philadelphia, W. B. Saunders, 1971.
Stewart, W. D., et al.: Synopsis of Dermatology. St. Louis, C. V. Mosby, 1970.

Articles

Eaglstein, W. H., et al.: The effects of early corticosteroid therapy on the skin eruptions and pain of herpes zoster. JAMA, *211*:1681–1683, March 9, 1970.
Epstein, E.: Dermatologic surgery in aging skin. Geriatrics, *26*:94–99, March 1971.
Estes, D., and Christian, C. L.: The natural history of systemic lupus erythematosus by prospective analysis. Medicine, *50*:85–95, March 1971.
Flowers, R. S.: Unexpected postoperative problems in skin grafting. Surg. Clin. N. Amer., *50*:439–456, April 1970.
Hurwitz, A.: About faces. Amer. J. Nurs., *71*:2168–2171, Nov. 1971.
Medical Grand Rounds from the University of Alabama Medical Center: Lupus erythematosus. South. Med. J., *64*:839–846, July 1971.
Moschella, S. L.: The present status of chemotherapy in dermatology. Med. Clin. N. Amer., *56*:725–737, May 1972.
Sato, F. F.: Trials with cyclophosphamide in SLE. Amer. J. Nurs., *72*:1077–1079, June 1972.
Schragger, A. H.: Common childhood and adolescent skin problems. Amer. Fam. Phys., *5*:114–122, Jan. 1972.
Taylor, R. B.: Clinical study of ultraviolet in various skin conditions. Phys. Ther., *52*:279–282, March 1972.
Weatherley-White, R.C.A., and Mayer, A. W., Jr.: Skin grafting in the emergency room and outpatient department. Surg. Clin. N. Amer., *49*:1461–1468, Dec. 1969.
Zarem, H. A.: Current concepts in reconstruction surgery in patients with cancer of the head and neck. Surg. Clin. N. Amer., *51*:149–173, Feb. 1971.

Burns

Books

Artz, C. P.: The burned patient: Newer concepts of medical and nursing management. *In* Kintzel, K. C. (ed.): Advanced Concepts in Clinical Nursing. Philadelphia, J. B. Lippincott, 1971, pp. 321–349.
Artz, C. P., and Moncrief, J. A.: Burns, 2nd ed. Philadelphia, W. B. Saunders, 1969.
Brunner, L. S., et al.: Textbook of Medical and Surgical Nursing, 2nd ed. Philadelphia, J. B. Lippincott, 1970, pp. 657–673.
Jacoby, F.: Nursing Care of the Patient with Burns. St. Louis, C. V. Mosby, 1972.

Manteuffel, S. V., and Berkich, E. J.: The Burn Patient, Management and Operating Room Support. Somerville, New Jersey, Ethicon, Inc., 1970.

Moore, F. D.: Transplant. New York, Simon and Schuster, 1972.

Stone, N. H., and Boswick, J. A.: Profiles of Burn Management, Miami, Fla. Industrial Medicine Publishing Co., 1969.

Articles

Andreasen, N., et al.: Management of emotional reactions in seriously burned adults. New Eng. J. Med., *286*:65–69, Jan. 1972.

Boswick, J. A., Jr., and Pandya, N. J.: Emergency care of the burned patient. Surg. Clin. N. Amer., 52:112–123, Feb. 1972.

Bowden, M. L., and Feller, I.: Family reaction to a severe burn. Amer. J. Nurs., 73:317–319, Feb. 1973.

Cosman, B.: Management of the patient with burns. Hosp. Med., 7:29–45, Nov. 1971.

Crossman, A. R.: Silver sulfadiazine cream in the management of burns. Fam. Pract., *1*:69–75, Feb. 1970.

Evans, E. B., et. al.: Prevention and correction of deformity after severe burns. Surg. Clin. N. Amer., *50*:1361–1375, Dec. 1970.

Koepke, G. H.: The role of physical medicine in the treatment of burns. Surg. Clin. N. Amer., *50*:1385–1399, Dec. 1970.

MacMillan, B. G.: The use of mesh grafting in treating burns. Surg. Clin. N. Amer., *50*:1347–1359, Dec. 1970.

McDowell, A.: The burn problem today. Hosp. Med., 8:26–47, March 1972.

Minckley, B. B.: Expert nursing care for burned patient. Amer. J. Nurs., 70:1888–1893, Sept. 1970.

Pruitt, Lt. Col., B. A., Jr.: Current treatment of thermal injury. South. Med. J., *64*:657–662, June 1971.

Wiley, L.: Burn care. Nursing '72. 2:32–37, July 1972.

Williams, B. P.: The burned patient's need for teaching. Nurs. Clin. N. Amer., 6:615–639, Dec. 1971.

Zawacki, B. E., and Pruitt, B. A.: Emergency treatment of burns. Fam. Phys., 2:60–68, July 1970.

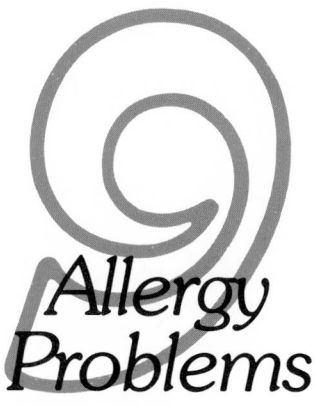

Allergy Problems

THE ALLERGIC REACTION

Definitions

1. *Antigen*—a substance which when it comes in contact with the body repeatedly causes it to produce a counteracting substance, a globulin "antibody."
2. *Antibody*—a globulin produced by the lymphoid cells as a result of stimulation of these cells by an antigen.
3. *Immunity*—a state of increased resistance to a particular substance.
   a. *Active-acquired immunization*—resistance brought about by the injection of an antigenic substance (ex., tetanus toxoid).
   b. *Passive-acquired immunization*—resistance brought about by the transfer of antibody-containing serum from an immunized donor to a normal recipient (ex., tetanus antitoxin).

Products of Antigen-antibody Union

(Chemical Mediator Products)
1. *Histamine*—released from tissue mast cells by the interaction of an antigen and its corresponding antibody.
   a. Causes contraction of smooth muscle of bronchioles, uterus, intestines.
   b. Dilates and causes increased permeability of capillaries of skin and mucous membrane.
   c. Lowers blood pressure.
   d. Stimulates secretion of nasal, lacrimal, salivary, and gastrointestinal glands.
   e. Produces itching of skin and mucous membrane.
2. *Serotonin*—an amine released at the same time as histamine.

615

3. *Bradykinin*—acts chiefly by increasing capillary permeability and contraction of smooth muscle.
4. *Acetylcholine*—acts to stimulate autonomic nervous system.

Antibody-antigen Reaction

1. These are not always protective and beneficial to the body.
   a. May cause tissue damage.
   b. May produce discomfort to the patient.
2. Under certain circumstances, an antibody is produced that reacts not only to a noxious agent but also to another harmless agent of similar chemical composition.

Hypersensitivity Phenomena

1. "Sensitivity" is a characteristic of a body when it reacts against substances in the environment to which most persons elicit no response.
2. Some authorities consider
   a. "Immunity" to be a manifestation when antigen and antibody benefit the individual.
   b. "Allergy" is a manifestation when antigen and antibody are harmful to the individual.
3. Inhaled allergens
   a. Plant pollens—ragweed, grasses, tree pollens
   b. Molds, fungi, spores, animal danders, house dust
4. Ingested allergens—cow's milk, egg white, fish, nuts, chocolate, certain fruits
5. Contact allergens—contact dermatitis (see p. 584)
6. Sensitivity reactions
   a. Local or systemic.
   b. Mediated by sensitized cells, not circulating globulins.
   c. Mediated by circulating immunoglobulin E (IgE).

HYPOSENSITIZATION
(Desensitization)

Hyposensitization is a procedure designed to increase a person's resistance to offending antigens by administration of small but increasing amounts of a specific antigen over a period of time.

Method

A skin test is done—an aqueous solution of an antigen is introduced into the dermis.
1. Scratch method—the skin is scratched with a needle through a drop of antigen-containing solution.
2. Intracutaneous method—allergen is injected between the outermost layers of the skin.

Reactions

1. A positive reaction—reddened, flushed area or a blanched wheal at skin site appearing within 20 minutes.

2. Systemic reactions may occur from a concentrated dose to a hypersensitized person.
   a. Apply a tourniquet proximal to the test site to retard absorption of the antibody.
   b. Administer epinephrine or antihistamines.
   c. Give hydrocortisone intravenously, if necessary.

Treatment

1. Therapy consists of injections of dilute allergenic extracts of such substances as pollens, dusts, mold spores and insects.
2. As injections are gradually increased, the body builds up a supply of blocking antibodies (mainly immunoglobulin G type—IgG).
3. When the patient comes in contact with allergens that previously caused allergic reactions, the blocking antibodies combine with them in a way to reduce or prevent symptoms.

RESPIRATORY HYPERSENSITIVITY

Hay Fever (Pollinosis)

Hay Fever (allergic coryza) is a rhinitis induced by airborne pollens (seasonal) which react to release histamine in the body, producing related symptoms.

Classification
(According to Season)

1. *Spring type*—March to early May.
   Stimulated by pollens of certain trees (oak, elm, poplar).
2. *Summer type*—May to early July.
   Stimulated by pollens of certain grasses (timothy, red top).
3. *Fall type*—August to the first frost.
   Stimulated by pollens of ragweed family.

Clinical Manifestations

1. Rhinitis—leading to edematous, closed nostrils
2. Nasal mucous membranes—itch, burn and secrete thin irritating discharge
3. Sneezing—violent paroxysms
4. Eyes—red, burning, lacrimating

Diagnostic Evaluation

Sensitivity Tests
Skin tests confirm patient's hypersensitivity to pollens.

Treatment

1. Advise patient to move to an area where pollen count is low; this, however, is often impractical.
2. Use antihistamines; this will not only control symptoms in 4 out of 5 patients but will also have an atropine-like drying effect.

3. Treat sinusitis and other otolaryngology infections during free seasons.
4. Administer prophylactic injections of extract of pollens (specific for the individual) begin several months before the attacks and administer once a week on through the peak season.
5. Utilize antihistamine therapy during active phase.
6. Resort to oral corticosteroids when antihistamines are not effective; these act by reducing the responsiveness of mucous membranes to histamine.

Vasomotor Rhinitis

Vasomotor rhinitis is a nonimmunologic, noninfectious chronic-type of rhinitis.

Etiology

Unknown

Altered Physiology

1. Nasal mucous membrane has a rich blood supply; the area is controlled by autonomic nerves.
2. Nonspecific stimuli act upon autonomic nerves, resulting in reflex changes in nasal mucosa, e.g., emotional stimuli, rapid changes in temperature or humidity, endocrine changes such as pregnancy, menstruation, menopause.

Clinical Manifestations

1. Chronic nasal congestion, rhinorrhea and sneezing occur.
2. Often the patient notes that nasal blockage alternates from side to side.
3. Symptoms do not change significantly with seasonal or geographic changes.
4. Physical factors and psychological stresses may trigger nasal symptoms.
5. Symptoms are triggered by exposure to drafts, high humidity, chemical fumes, tobacco smoke, emotional upsets.
6. Nasal mucosa will be edematous.

COMPARISON OF SYMPTOMS

Symptom	Allergic Rhinitis	Vasomotor Rhinitis
Seasonal variation	Yes	No
Nasal or ocular itching	Yes	Rarely
Discharge (rhinorrhea)	Watery	Mucoid
Nasal polyps	Occasionally	Occasionally
Other allergy	Often	Unusual (coincidental)

Treatment

According to symptoms—antihistamines, oral nasal decongestants and avoidance of precipitating factors.

Bronchial Asthma

See page 1140 for a discussion of asthma.

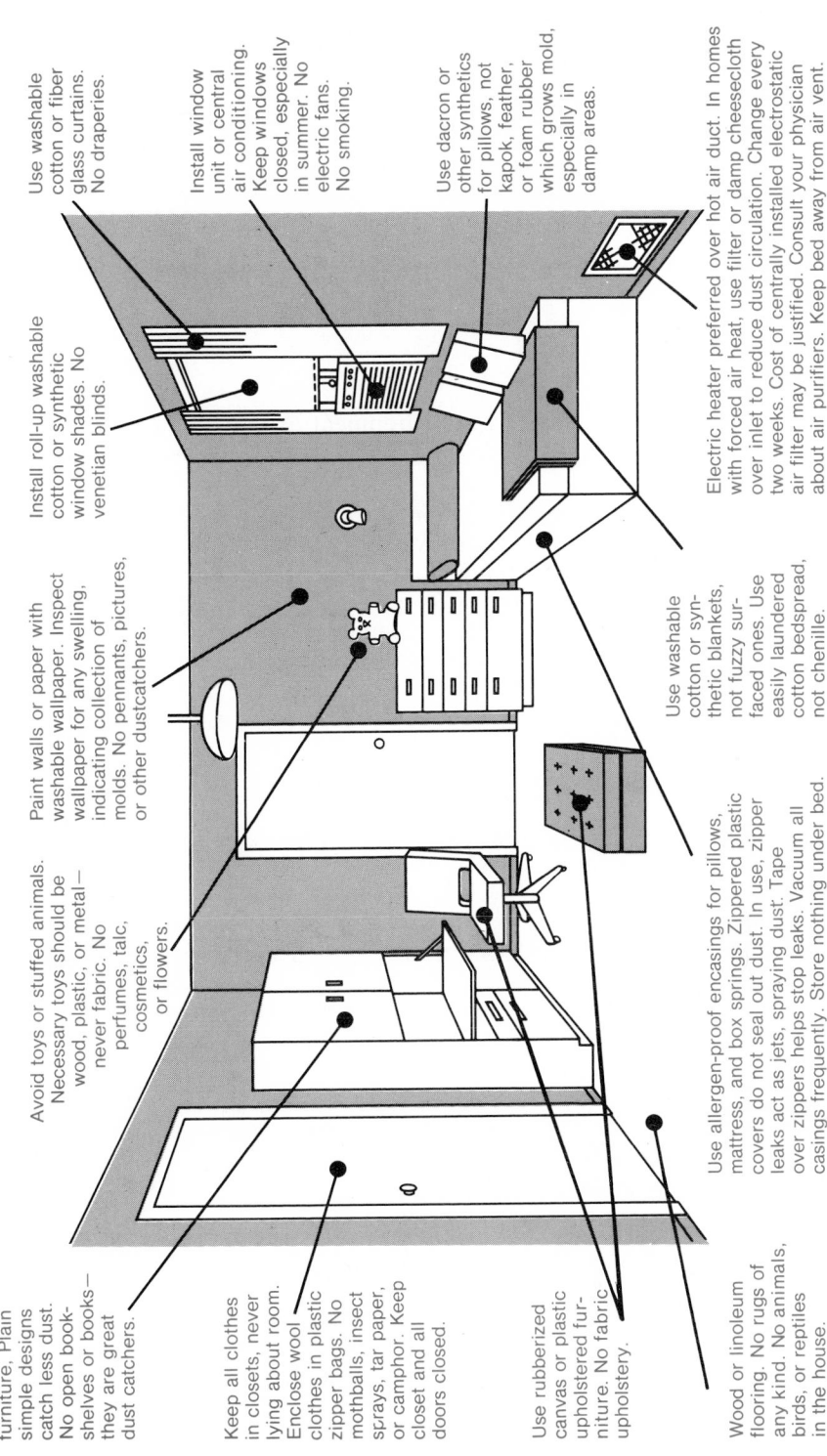

Use washable cotton or fiber glass curtains. No draperies.

Install window unit or central air conditioning. Keep windows closed, especially in summer. No electric fans. No smoking.

Use dacron or other synthetics for pillows, not kapok, feather, or foam rubber which grows mold, especially in damp areas.

Electric heater preferred over hot air duct. In homes with forced air heat, use filter or damp cheesecloth over inlet to reduce dust circulation. Change every two weeks. Cost of centrally installed electrostatic air filter may be justified. Consult your physician about air purifiers. Keep bed away from air vent.

Install roll-up washable cotton or synthetic window shades. No venetian blinds.

Paint walls or paper with washable wallpaper. Inspect wallpaper for any swelling indicating collection of molds. No pennants, pictures, or other dustcatchers.

Avoid toys or stuffed animals. Necessary toys should be wood, plastic, or metal—never fabric. No perfumes, talc, cosmetics, or flowers.

Use washable cotton or synthetic blankets, not fuzzy sur-faced ones. Use easily laundered cotton bedspread, not chenille.

Vacuum only if followed by airing of room. Use tank-type cleaner, vacuumed itself before using. Attach a second hose to outlet, placing end outside window or in hall to prevent redistributing allergens.

Avoid ornate furniture. Plain simple designs catch less dust. No open book-shelves or books—they are great dust catchers.

Keep all clothes in closets, never lying about room. Enclose wool clothes in plastic zipper bags. No mothballs, insect sprays, tar paper, or camphor. Keep closet and all doors closed.

Use rubberized canvas or plastic upholstered fur-niture. No fabric upholstery.

Wood or linoleum flooring. No rugs of any kind. No animals, birds, or reptiles in the house.

Use allergen-proof encasings for pillows, mattress, and box springs. Zippered plastic covers do not seal out dust. In use, zipper leaks act as jets, spraying dust. Tape over zippers helps stop leaks. Vacuum all casings frequently. Store nothing under bed.

Cleaning Tips: Wet-dust room twice daily. Damp-mop floor with solution containing disinfectant to prevent growth of mold spores. Oil-mop base-boards.

Figure 9-1. Controlling the environment of room. (Courtesy, A. H. Robins Company.)

MANAGEMENT OF THE PERSON WHO HAS AN ALLERGY

Objectives

1. To encourage the person with an allergy to find out what he is sensitive to.
2. To assist the patient in recognizing the importance of avoiding offending antigens whenever possible.
3. To seek relief for the patient when he has been exposed to an offending antigen.
4. To direct the patient to seek assistance in increasing his resistance to the offending antigen.

Measures to Control the Environment

A. *Respiratory Allergies*
   1. Encourage the patient to modify his environment as much as he can but not to the point of developing such a rigid regimen that it restricts his activities unduly.
   2. *In the Hospital unit*
      a. Restrict flowers and plants in patient's room since they introduce antigens or irritating vapors to which he is sensitive.
      b. Avoid dry-dusting and mopping while the patient is in the room.
      c. Do not flourish sheets or plump pillows excessively during bed-making.
      d. Recommend cake face powder rather than loose powder; limit the use of talcums.
      e. Replace feather pillows with dacron or hypoallergenic-filled pillows.
      f. Attempt to find acceptable replacements for those items removed from the patient's environment so that he will still be in a psychologically therapeutic environment.
   3. *In the Home* (primarily the bedroom)
      Advise the patient as follows:
      a. Use nonallergenic materials in bedding (blankets, comforters, bedpad, pillows).
      b. Enclose the mattress and box springs in plastic airtight covers.
      c. Avoid keeping the window open at night if allergy is due to a sensitivity to pollens and grasses.
      d. Replace carpeting with washable throw rugs; heavy draperies with easily laundered light curtains.
      e. Limit the number of dust-catching articles in the room (Fig. 9-1).
   4. *Room Air*
      Advise the patient as follows:
      a. Utilize a system of heating or cooling that can both humidify and filter the air.
      b. Avoid rapid changes in room temperature or variations in humidity that can aggravate or stimulate allergy symptoms.
      c. Weigh the benefits of air conditioning:
         (1) If it tends to circulate dust, it may be a source of irritation.
         (2) If it causes a marked change in temperature when the person moves from one part of the room to another, then it may be undesirable.
         (3) If it provides an evenness of temperature, humidity, etc., it may be most desirable.
   5. *Smoking*
      Encourage the patient as follows:

     a. Avoid smoking since this adds a pollutant likely to aggravate the respiratory passages.

     b. Make an effort to avoid areas where others are smoking.

B. *Dietary Allergies*

Advise the patient as follows:

1. Recognize the difficulties in trying to determine which food causes allergic reactions.
2. Develop a pattern of eliminating a certain food for a period of time.
   a. Keep a diary, indicating when food was eliminated from the diet.
   b. Record any allergic reactions or the fact that none occurred.
3. Begin with those foods commonly found to cause reactions—nuts, chocolate, milk, strawberries, eggs, etc.
4. Remember to note contents of prepared foods, canned foods, etc. for the specific ingredients one may wish to avoid.
5. Order those foods in a restaurant which are certain not to include the offending ingredients.

NOTE: Foods are considered a very rare cause of respiratory allergic symptoms.

C. *Contact Allergies*

Instruct patient as follows:

1. Exert extra effort to avoid household items likely to bring on allergic reactions.
   a. Use gloves to avoid skin contact with detergents, fabric dyes, strong soap powders, etc.
   b. Use liquid soaps rather than granules that might infiltrate the air breathed.
2. Avoid cosmetics unless they are known to be hypoallergenic.
3. Do not rub or scratch itchy skin. (Mild doses of barbiturate or tranquilizers may be necessary if this will assist the patient in such control.)
4. Eliminate those items of wearing apparel that irritate the skin, such as wool or nylon. Note that permanent press cottons may be a cause of dermatitis.
5. Avoid overexertion which will cause perspiration and itchiness.

Administration of Medications

1. Warn the patient that it may be dangerous for him to drive during the first few days of antihistaminic therapy inasmuch as these medications may cause drowsiness.
2. Advise patient to keep antihistamines out of reach of children—may cause serious accidental poisoning.
3. Utilize corticosteroids with caution because of their side effects when administered over a long period of time.
   a. For short-term use, apply drops or ointment form of eye medication effective in relieving conjunctivitis and swollen eyelids.
   b. Avoid long-term use of eye corticosteroids because they may cause an increase in intraocular pressure.
4. In instilling nose drops, have the patient lie on his back across the bed with his head hanging down; instill drops and have him remain in this position for 1 or 2 minutes; then have the patient turn over for another minute or two as though he were trying to look under the bed.
5. Caution the patient about the recurrent possibility of congestion when decongestants are used repeatedly; in such a situation, decongestants should be stopped.

BIBLIOGRAPHY

Books

Kintzel, K. C.: The immune reactions: Nursing intervention for the allergic patient. *In* Kintzel, K. C. (ed.): Advanced Concepts in Clinical Nursing. Philadelphia, J. B. Lippincott, 1971, pp. 350–367.

Patterson, R.: Allergic Diseases. Philadelphia, J. B. Lippincott, 1972.

Rapaport, H. G., and Linde, S. M.: The Complete Allergy Guide. New York, Simon and Schuster, 1970.

Sheldon, H., Lovell, R. G., and Mathews, K. P.: A Manual of Clinical Allergy. Philadelphia, W. B. Saunders, 1968.

Sherman, W. B.: Hypersensitivity—Mechanisms and Management. Philadelphia, W. B. Saunders, 1968.

Articles

Craven, R. F.: Anaphylactic shock. Amer. J. Nurs., 72:718–721, April 1972.

Lister, J.: Nursing intervention in anaphylactic shock. Amer. J. Nurs., 72:720–721, April 1972.

Norman, P. S. (interview): If you are allergic. U. S. News and World Report, pp. 40–44, Jan. 1, 1973.

Metabolic and Endocrine Disorders

1. Disorders of the Thyroid Gland
THE THYROID GLAND AND TESTS OF THYROID FUNCTION

Physiology

1. The thyroid gland affects the rate at which all tissues metabolize.
   a. Speed of chemical reactions
   b. Volume of oxygen consumed
   c. Amount of heat produced
2. The stimulating effect is through the production and distribution of 2 hormones:
   a. Levothyroxine (T_4)—contains 4 iodine atoms; maintains body's metabolism in a steady state: when there is a sudden need for a considerable increase in heat production, some of thyroxine is converted into the 2nd hormone, triiodothyronine
   b. Triiodothyronine (T_3)—contains 3 iodine atoms; approximately 5 times as potent as thyroxine; has a more rapid metabolic action and utilization than thyroxine. Probably some peripheral conversion of T_4 to T_3 occurs at the cellular level.

Diagnostic Evaluation

A. *Protein-bound Iodine (PBI)*
   1. A reasonably accurate index of thyroid function is the concentration of PBI in the blood.
   2. Normal values: 3.5–8.0 μg. (0.0035–0.0080 mg./100 ml. of plasma).
      a. Over 8.0—thyroid overactivity
      b. Under 3.5—hypothyroidism

NURSING ALERT: Certain factors impair the PBI test:
1. Ingestion of drugs or administration of dyes containing iodine
2. Mercurial diuretics, estrogens
3. Pregnancy

B. *Serum Thyroxine (T_4)*
   1. Elevated values found with estrogens and pregnancy.
   2. Normal values, 3.5–8.5 μg.

C. *T_3 Resin Uptake*
   1. Is an indirect measure of thyroid function based on the available protein-binding sites in a serum sample which can bind to radioactive T_3.

2. The radioactive triiodothyronine is added to the serum sample in the test tube.
3. The effect of estrogen and pregnancy is to produce an increase in binding sites, causing a lowered percentage of binding by the available thyroid hormones.
4. Rates.
   a. Normal binding (25–37%)
   b. High T_3 is associated with hyperthyroidism
   c. Low T_3 is associated with hypothyroidism

D. *Radioiodine* (^{131}I)
   1. *^{131}I Uptake*
      a. A solution of sodium iodide-131 is administered orally to the fasting patient.
      b. After a prescribed interval of time anywhere from 2 to 48 hours, but frequently by 24 hours, measurements are taken with a scintillator of radioactive counts per minute that are detected above the isthmus of the thyroid gland.
      c. Normal thyroid will remove 15–50% of the iodine from the bloodstream.
      d. Hyperthyroidism may result in the removal of as much as 90% of the iodine from the bloodstream.
   2. *Thyroidal Iodide Clearance*
      a. Radioiodine clearance test measures the amount of circulating blood that is completely cleared of iodide per unit of time.
      b. Radioiodine is injected intravenously; radioactivity over the thyroid gland is measured continuously for 30–60 minutes—total amount of ^{131}I concentrated in the gland per minute is computed.
      c. Also, plasma ^{131}I content is measured in samples of blood collected 45–70 minutes after injection; these values are averaged.
      d. Thyroid ^{131}I divided by the mean plasma ^{131}I equals thyroid clearance, i.e., ml. of plasma cleared of iodide per minute.
      e. Normal   25 ml./min.
         Hyperthyroidism   250 ml./min.
         Hypothyroidism   1.6 ml./min.
   3. *^{131}I Excretion*
      a. Urinary output of radioiodine is measured during 24- to 48-hour period after ingestion.
      b. Normal   40–80% of ingested iodine in 24 hours
         Hyperthyroidism   less than 40%
         Hypothyroidism   greater than 80%
   4. *Thyroid "Scan"*
      a. Patient ingests sodium iodide-131 and is scanned the next day; if medium given intravenously, patient may be scanned within ½ to 1 hour.
      b. A scintillator electromechanically maps the activity in the scanned area to produce a scintogram.
      c. A decrease of ^{131}I uptake in a particular area of the thyroid is considered suggestive of malignancy.
   5. *Nursing Responsibility in ^{131}I Thyroid Tests*
      Ascertain whether the patient has had an iodide salt before these tests, e.g., application of iodine to the skin, dye taken as a contrast medium for x-rays, iodine taken in cough medications. If iodine was taken by the patient prior to the planned test, the results would be inaccurate.

C. *Basal Metabolic Rate*
  1. B.M.R. refers to the oxygen consumption of a person at rest, whose body temperature is normal and who has fasted for at least 10 hours previously.
  2. It is possible to compute the rate at which heat is produced by the body from the volume of oxygen that is absorbed in a given period of time under resting conditions
  3. *Nursing Responsibility*
     a. Explain to the patient that this test will be done in the early morning when the patient is still quiet from the night's rest.
     b. Describe the procedure which involves breathing through a rubber tube for several minutes; explain the importance of not being stimulated or excited because it will affect test results.
     c. Recognize that this is one of several tests for the diagnostic work-up of the patient with a thyroid problem and is used less frequently.
  4. B.M.R. Values
     a. Normal   −15% to +15%
     b. Hypothyroidism   −15% and below
     c. Hyperthyroidism   +15% and above

HYPOTHYROIDISM

Hypothyroidism may be classified as primary or secondary. *Primary hypothyroidism* is a condition due to the inability of the thyroid gland to secrete a sufficient amount of hormone. *Secondary hypothyroidism* is due to a failure of the pituitary gland to secrete an adequate amount of TSH (thyroid-stimulating hormone).

Cretinism is a condition in which a person is born with a thyroid deficiency. The mother is likewise deficient.

Cause

The thyroid gland may have been removed surgically or damaged by disease.

Clinical Manifestations
  1. Temperature and pulse become subnormal.
  2. Patient begins to gain weight.
  3. Skin becomes thickened.
  4. The hair thins and falls out.
  5. Menorrhagia may develop.
  6. Facial expression becomes stolid and mask-like.
  7. Complaint of fatigue is most common.
  8. Mental processes become dulled.
  9. There is a tendency to rapid development of arteriosclerosis.

Treatment

Objective: to restore a normal metabolic state.
  1. Administer thyroid hormone: thyroid USP (desiccated thyroid), thyroglobulin (Proloid), liotrix (Euthroid, Thyrolar), levothyroxine (Synthroid).
     a. Give once a day

2. Anticipate such effects of treatment as:
   a. Diuresis, decreased puffiness
   b. Improved reflexes and muscle tone
   c. Accelerated pulse rate

Advanced Hypothyroidism

A. *Effects*
   1. May lead to *myxedema coma.*
   2. Causes increased susceptibility to all hypnotic and sedative drugs.
   3. Survival rate is 50%.

B. *Clinical Manifestations*

Hypotension, unresponsiveness, bradycardia, hypoventilation, hyponatremia, possible convulsions, hypothermia.

C. *Treatment*
   1. Maintain vital functions.
      a. Measure arterial blood gases to determine CO_2 retention.
      b. Provide assisted ventilation if needed to combat hypoventilation.
      c. Even though hypothermia exists, do not apply external heat since the resulting increased oxygen requirements and decreased peripheral vascular tone may compound the existing cardiac failure.
      d. Administer fluids cautiously even though hyponatremia is present.
      e. Give glucose in concentrated amounts to prevent fluid overload if hypoglycemia is in evidence.
   2. Replace thyroid hormone.
      a. Administer sodium levothyroxine (Synthroid) parenterally (until consciousness is restored) to restore thyroxine level.
      b. Later, continue patient on oral thyroid hormone therapy.
      c. Recognize that with rapid administration of thyroid hormone, plasma thyroxine levels may initiate adrenal insufficiency—hence, steroid therapy may be initiated.
   3. Treat precipitating factors.
      Treat initiating factors such as infection, stress from trauma or cold exposure.

HYPERTHYROIDISM

Hyperthyroidism (diffuse toxic goiter) is an excessive activity of the thyroid gland.

Incidence

More common in women than in men.

Etiology

1. Unknown
2. Possible causes
   a. LATS (long-acting thyroid stimulator) may be found in serum; it is capable of inducing iodine accumulation and thyroid hyperplasia independent of the pituitary.
   b. May appear after an emotional shock, infection or emotional stress.

Clinical Manifestations

1. Single or multiple adenomas
2. Nervousness, emotional hyperexcitability, irritableness, apprehension
3. Difficulty in sitting quietly
4. Rapid pulse, at rest as well as on exertion (ranges between 90 and 160); palpitation in evidence
5. Low heat tolerance; profuse perspiration; flushed skin (warm, soft, moist)
6. Fine tremor of hands; change in bowel habit—constipation or diarrhea
7. Bulging eyes (exophthalmos)—startled expression
8. Increased appetite—progressive weight loss
9. Muscle fatigability and weakness, amenorrhea
10. Atrial fibrillation possible (Cardiac decompensation is common in elderly patients.)

Clinical Course

1. Mild, characterized by remissions and exacerbations.
2. In rare instances, it may progress relentlessly—leading to emaciation, extreme nervousness, delirium, disorientation and eventual death.

Treatment

1. Hospitalize patient only if "thyroid storm" or other complications, such as heart failure, are impending.
2. Administer sedatives such as phenobarbital or tranquilizers such as chlordiazepoxide (Librium) or chlordiazepoxide plus clidinum bromide (Librax) to combat nervousness, hyperactivity and irritability.
3. Give vitamin supplements to offset demands of appetite which may continue after hyperthyroidism is controlled.
4. Administer digitalis if heart failure or atrial fibrillation occurs.
5. Give propranolol for sinus tachycardia and other supraventricular arrhythmias.

Modalities of Treatment

1. General Considerations
   a. Types of treatment—pharmacology, radiation and surgery.
   b. Treatment depends on causes, age of patient, severity of disease and complications
2. *According to Causes*
   a. Remission of hyperthyroidism (Graves' Disease) occurs spontaneously within 1–2 years; however, relapse can be expected in half of the patients.
      All 3 forms of therapy are appropriate.
   b. Nodular toxic goiter—excessive amounts of thyroid hormone secreted.
      Surgery or radioiodine is preferred.
   c. Thyroid carcinoma.
      Surgery or radiation.
3. *According to Age of Patient*
   a. Radioiodine therapy may be used in all patients, regardless of age, when other forms of therapy are inappropriate.
   b. Use radioiodine in older patients for whom surgery is contraindicated.

4. *According to Severity*
   Administer drug therapy before proceeding with radioiodine or surgery.
5. *According to Patient Preference*
   a. Suggest radioiodine or surgery to patient who does not take medication regularly.
   b. Recommend surgery to those who prefer it.

Pharmacotherapy—Drugs Which Inhibit Hormone Formation

Objective: to bring the metabolic rate to normal as soon as possible and maintain it at this level.

Anticipated Results
1. Diagnosis can be confirmed if patient responds to antithyroid therapy.
2. Autonomic nervous system is brought into balance and patient is more comfortable.
3. Opportunity is provided for getting to know the patient.

A. *Thiourea Derivatives*
1. Most commonly used.
2. Act by interfering with the formation of thyroid hormone.
3. Administered orally
   a. Detectable in blood in 15 minutes.
   b. 80% absorbed within 2 hours.
   c. Because half-life is short, must be given every 6–8 hours.
4. Preparations
   a. Propylthiouracil
   b. Methimazole (Topazole)
5. Assessment and duration of treatment determined by clinical criteria.
   a. Observe clinical course—thyroid gland usually gets smaller.
   b. Take PBI to determine adequacy of dose.
   c. Continue treatment for 1–20 years or until euthyroidism is maintained without therapy.
   d. Gradually withdraw therapy to prevent exacerbation.
   e. For continued relapses, shift therapy to radioiodine or surgery.
6. Toxicity
   a. Agranulocytosis is a most serious toxic condition, occurring with a sudden onset—therefore, patient should be apprized of this possibility and urged to report any signs of infection such as fever, sore throat, upper respiratory infection.
   b. Skin rashes, fever, urticaria, granulopenia, inflammation of the salivary glands are other possible side effects.
   c. Substitute an alternate drug if there are toxic manifestations.

B. *Potassium Perchlorate*
1. Inhibits transport of iodide into thyroid follicles.
2. Toxicity
   a. Severe gastric irritation sometimes occurs.
   b. Aplastic anemia has been reported.
3. Use
   Because of toxicity, use only when patient cannot take thiourea derivatives or other therapy.

Pharmacotherapy—Drugs Which Control Peripheral Manifestations of Hyperthyroidism

A. *Propranolol (Inderal)*
 1. Acts as a beta-adrenergic blocking agent.
 2. Abolishes tachycardia, tremor, excess sweating, nervousness.
 3. Controls hyperthyroid symptoms until antithyroid drugs or radioiodine can take effect.

B. *Guanethidine Sulfate (Ismelin)*
 Controls adrenergic manifestations of hyperthyroidism.

NURSING ALERT: Note that postural hypotension may occur with administration of Ismelin.

Radioactive Iodine

 1. Action
   a. Limits secretion of thyroid hormone by damaging and destroying thyroid tissue.
   b. Control dosage so that hypothyroidism does not occur.
 2. Considerations in Use
   a. Radiation thyroiditis, a transient exacerbation of hyperthyroidism, may occur as a result of leakage of thyroid hormone into the circulation from damaged follicles.
   b. Iodide should not be given prior to radioiodine since it interferes with the uptake of ^{131}I.

Psychotherapy

 1. Greater emphasis is being placed on the effect of psychogenic factors in the severity of this disease.
 2. A determination needs to be made in caring for each patient as to whether psychotherapy would be of value.

Surgery

A. *Subtotal Thyroidectomy*
 Effective in treating hyperthyroidism by removal of most of the thyroid gland.

B. *Preparation for Surgery*
 1. Patient must be euthyroid at time of surgery.
 2. Administer thiourea derivatives to control hyperthyroidism.
 3. Give iodide to increase firmness of thyroid gland and reduce its vascularity.

NURSING ALERT: Observe patient for evidence of iodine toxicity—swelling of buccal mucosa, excessive salivation, coryza, skin eruptions. If these occur, discontinue iodides.

C. *Complications*
 1. Damage to recurrent laryngeal nerve may occur (1–4%).
   a. Unilateral damage—results in minimal voice change.
   b. Bilateral damage—serious airway obstruction develops.
 2. Hypothyroidism
   a. Occurs in 10–15% of cases in first postoperative year.
   b. Give prophylactic doses of thyroid.

3. Hypoparathyroidism
   a. About 4% occurrence.
   b. Usually is mild and transient.
   c. Requires calcium supplements intravenously and orally when more severe.

Exophthalmos in Hyperthyroidism

Exophthalmos is abnormal protrusion of the eyeball.

Treatment

Objective: to protect eyes from irritation.

A. *Mild*
   1. Recommend wearing sunglasses.
   2. Instill methylcellulose eyedrops 0.5–1% (Tearisol) for comfort.
   3. Advise the patient to elevate his head while sleeping to improve drainage.
B. *Rapidly Progressive or Severe* (chemosis, conjunctivitis, proptosis, visual impairment)
   1. Tarsorrhaphy (suturing eyelids together) may need to be done to extend lid when proptosis is so marked that lid does not close during sleep.
   2. Administer corticosteroids in high doses to help arrest rapid progression of exophthalmos; with improvement, reduce dose.
C. *Orbital Decompression Procedures*
   1. Decompression of orbit into ethmoid sinus and maxillary antrum (Ogura procedure).
   2. Removal of lateral orbital wall (Krönleim operation).
   3. Decompression of orbit into cranial cavity (Naffziger operation).
D. *Muscle Surgery*
   1. Correction of imbalance of extraocular muscles.
   2. Lysis of adhesions.

Thyroid Storm

Thyroid storm (also called thyroid crisis) is characterized by tachycardia, vasomotor activity, agitation and, at times, delirium and heart failure. It is assumed to result from an increase in thyroid hormone.

Predisposing Factors

1. Decompensation of hyperthyroid state occurs spontaneously.
2. May be precipitated by infection or other stress (inadequate surgical preparation).

Clinical Manifestations

1. Hyperpyrexia, diarrhea, dehydration, tachycardia, arrhythmias
2. Coma, leading to shock and death

Objectives of Treatment and Nursing Management

A. *To control synthesis and release of thyroid hormone.*
   1. Administer sodium iodide intravenously—inhibits release of hormone from thyroid.
   2. Give methimazole or propylthiouracil orally or by nasogastric tube to prevent accumulation of hormone stores.

B. *To reverse peripheral effects of hyperthyroidism.*

Administer reserpine, guanethidine or propranolol.

C. *To restore and maintain vital functions.*
1. Give steroids.
2. Administer fluids, electrolytes and vasopressor agents to treat dehydration, electrolyte imbalance and hypotension.
3. Lower the temperature with hypothermia blanket and salicylates.
4. Try phenothiazines in large doses for hyperpyrexia, but watch for hypotension.
5. Sustain nutritional requirements with glucose intravenously; administer vitamin B.
6. Guard against infection; treat if infection is likely.

Medical and Nursing Management of the Patient Undergoing Thyroidectomy

Preoperative Objectives

A. *To provide a restful and therapeutic environment.*
1. Place the patient in a unit which is away from disturbing sights, very ill patients and noisy elevators or kitchens.
2. Provide, if possible, a pleasant window view.
3. Suggest radio music programs rather than exciting soap operas or movies.
4. Restrict visitors who may upset the patient with disturbing conversation or boisterous tendencies.
5. Administer soothing back massage at prescribed rest times during the day; draw the blinds for nap times.
6. Be selective in placing a suitable roommate with the patient, preferably one who is convalescing.
7. Gain the confidence of the patient and attempt to uncover anything which would cause aggravation or unhappiness; if a disturbance exists, it could thwart treatment efforts.

B. *To regulate his nutritional intake.*
1. Order an ample diet of carbohydrate and protein foods.
2. Recognize this patient's physiological need for a daily caloric intake of 4000–5000 calories caused by increased metabolic activity and rapid depletion of glycogen reserves.
3. Provide supplementary vitamins, particularly thiamine chloride and ascorbic acid.
4. Avoid tea or coffee because of their stimulating effects.

C. *To study the exact nature of the endocrine problem by supporting the patient undergoing various diagnostic tests.*
1. Explain the purpose and requirements of each prescribed test.
2. Inform the patient and visitors regarding precautions during radioisotope tests.
3. Remind the patient of his need to remain in his room until tests are completed.

D. *To prepare the patient for surgery.*
1. Shave the upper chest, neck (bedline to bedline), up to chin edge.
2. Exert a special effort to ensure that this patient has a good night's rest preceding surgery.

3. Explain to the patient that speaking is to be minimized immediately postoperatively and that oxygen may be administered to facilitate breathing.

4. Tell the patient that postoperatively, fluids may be given intravenously to maintain fluid, electrolyte and nutritional needs; glucose may also be given intravenously in the hours before the administration of anesthesia.

5. Proceed with usual preoperative preparation (see p. 47).

Postoperative Objectives

A. *To provide optimum immediate postoperative care in order to avoid complications.*

1. Move the patient carefully with adequate support to the head so that no tension is placed on the sutures.

2. Place the patient in semi-Fowler's position with the head elevated and supported by pillows.

3. Administer oxygen for a few hours if breathing is labored; check the infusion for prescribed flow rate and smooth flow into patient.

4. Avoid administration of epinephrine, norepinephrine, cholinergic depressants (atropine) because of patient's sensitivity to these drugs.

5. Discontinue antithyroid drugs as a more normal metabolic rate is attained (to continue such medication might cause a hypometabolism—hypothyroidism).

B. *To assess the patient's condition as he emerges from anesthesia.*

1. *Damage of laryngeal nerve*
   a. Observe for hoarseness or "whispery" voice suggesting possible nerve damage.
   b. Recognize that a bilateral flaccid paralysis may lead to cord paralysis → closure of glottis → suffocation, months after operation.

2. *Hemorrhage*
   a. Be alert for this possibility between 12 and 24 hours postoperatively.
   b. Watch for signs of irregular breathing, swelling and choking—signs pointing to the possibility of hemorrhage (see p. 81) and tracheal compression.
   c. Keep a tracheostomy set in the patient's room for 48 hours for emergency use.

3. *Tetany*
   a. The likelihood of tetany developing depends upon the number of parathyroid glands that have been removed or disturbed:
      1—no clinical tetany
      2—tetany mild and transient
      4—tetany within 24 hours and worsening within the next 24 hours.
   b. Progression of signs.
      (1) *First*—tingling of toes and fingers and around the mouth; apprehension
      (2) *Second*—positive Chvostek's sign (tapping the cheek over the facial nerve causes a twitch of the lip or facial muscles to occur)
      (3) *Third*—Trousseau's sign (carpopedal spasm induced by occluding circulation in the arm with a blood pressure cuff)
   c. Management
      (1) Determine calcium levels: If in 48 hours it falls below 7½ mg./100 ml. (3mEq.), replacement of calcium is done intravenously or intramuscularly.
      (2) Exert caution in intravenous administration of calcium in the patient who has renal disease or is receiving digitalis preparations.

OTHER THYROID-RELATED CONDITIONS

Subacute Thyroiditis

Thyroiditis is inflammation of the thyroid gland.

Incidence

Affects younger women predominantly.

Treatment

1. Patient should be placed on thyroid medications to maintain a normal level of circu lating thyroid hormone.
2. Steroids may be administered in active inflammatory stage.

Clinical Manifestations

1. Pain, swelling, thyroid tenderness which lasts weeks or months, then disappears
2. Pain referred to the ear, making swallowing difficult and uncomfortable
3. Fever, malaise, chills
4. Irritability, nervousness, insomnia and weight loss

Hashimoto's Thyroiditis (Chronic Thyroiditis)

Hashimoto's thyroiditis is a progressive disease of the thyroid gland caused by infiltration o lymphocytes and resulting in progressive destruction of the parenchyma and hypothyroidism

Incidence

1. Predominantly affects women in their 40's and 50's.
2. Possibly the most common cause of adult hyperthyroidism.
3. May be associated with antibodies in the serum.

Clinical Manifestations

1. Marked by slowly developing firm enlargement of the thyroid gland.
2. Hyperthyroidism develops in the later stages of the disease.

Treatment

1. Patient should be placed on thyroid medications to maintain a normal level of circu lating thyroid hormone.
2. Firm nodular thyroid enlargement may at times be associated with tracheal com pression, cough, hoarseness. Resection of isthmus of thyroid can produce relief o symptoms.

Cancer of the Thyroid

Incidence

It has been estimated that of the thyroid lumps which occur in 40,000 out of 1,000,00 persons, in any one year, only 25 will be cancerous.

Types

1. Papillary and well-differentiated adenocarcinoma
   a. Growth is slow and spread is confined to lymph nodes that surround thyroid area.
   b. Cure rate is excellent after removal of involved areas.
2. Rapidly growing, widely metastasizing type
   a. Occurs predominantly in middle-aged and elderly persons.
   b. Brief encouraging response may occur with x-ray irradiation.
   c. Progression of disease is rapid with a high mortality rate.

2. Disorders of the Parathyroid Glands
THE PARATHYROID GLANDS

The *parathyroid glands* are small bean-sized structures embedded in the posterior section of the thyroid gland.

Functions

1. Produces, stores and secretes parathormone.
2. Increases plasma calcium ions by acting on:
   a. The kidney to decrease elimination of calcium ions in the urine.
   b. The gastrointestinal tract to increase absorption of calcium ions from chyme.
   c. Bone to increase its contributions of calcium ions to the plasma.

HYPERPARATHYROIDISM

Hyperparathyroidism is overactivity of the parathyroids.

Cause

An overgrowth of parathyroid glands.

Clinical Manifestations

1. Decalcification of bones
   a. Skeletal pain, backache, pain on weight-bearing, pathologic fractures, deformities, formation of bony cysts
   b. Formation of bone tumors—overgrowth of osteoclasts
2. Formation of calcium phosphate stones in the kidneys
3. Depression of neuromuscular apparatus
   a. The patient may trip, drop objects, show general fatigue and experience blurring of the mind.
   b. Cardiac standstill may result.

Diagnostic Evaluation

1. Persistently elevated serum calcium
2. Lowered phosphate concentration
3. Skeletal changes—revealed by x-ray
4. Diagnosis often extremely difficult (Complications occur before this condition is diagnosed.)

Complications

1. Kidney disturbances
   a. Formation of renal stones
   b. Calcification of kidney parenchyma
   c. Renal shutdown
2. Gastrointestinal complications
   Ulceration of upper gastrointestinal tract (stomach, duodenum) leading to hemorrhage and perforation
3. Skeletal problems
   a. Simple demineralization
   b. Cysts and fibrosis of marrow—leading to fractures
   c. Collapse of vertebral bodies and fractures of the ribs

Objectives of Treatment and Nursing Management

A. *To offset the likelihood of impending complications.*
1. Provide adequate hydration—administer water, glucose and electrolytes by mouth or intravenously.

NURSING ALERT: A low specific gravity for urine does not necessarily mean adequate hydration.

---

2. Avoid calcium and alkalies in the diet to prevent stone formation and renal calcification.
   Obtain daily serum calcium and BUN determinations.
3. Limit operative procedures until primary metabolic disorder is treated.
   a. A rising serum calcium level may indicate increasing dehydration—impending crisis.
   b. A falling serum calcium indicates dehydration is being corrected.

B. *To treat complications as they arise.*
1. For ureteral stone—cystoscopic manipulation
2. For urinary tract infection—antibiotics, high fluid input
3. For upper gastrointestinal ulceration—aluminum hydroxide and proteins other than milk
4. For ulcer hemorrhage not stopped by conservative measures—surgical plication
5. For fractures—hyperextension for vertebral body fractures
                       —strapping for broken ribs
                       —fixation of other long bones
                       —continued hydration of patient
                       —earliest mobilization of fracture areas

C. *To operate and remove parathyroid tissue.*
   This is resorted to when diagnosis is established and clinical condition warrants definitive treatment.

D. *To develop priorities of care in the postoperative phase that will control concomitant possible complications.*
1. Assess fluid input and output.
2. Recognize that the patient will retain some fluid.
   a. This will be manifested by a low urinary output.
   b. Therefore, avoid overhydration for first day or two.

3. Avoid giving calcium until nature of the patient's calcium level is determined.
   a. To verify success of operation.
   b. To observe level to which calcium falls and the rate it falls.
      (1) If calcium level fails to fall surgery was inadequate.
      (2) If calcium level falls somewhat but not to normal and then rises, metastasis may have occurred.
   c. To determine patient's skeletal deficit and need for additional calcium.
4. Evaluate signs and symptoms which may lead to tetany.
   a. Observe calcium levels—if well below normal and the decline continues into the 2nd week, the skeletal system is absorbing calcium.
      If this was noted preoperatively (elevated alkaline phosphatase level), calcium should be administered.
   b. Administer calcium—usually lactate or gluconate.
      When gastrointestinal tract cannot absorb large amount, administer intramuscularly as gluconate, or intravenously, if it is a matter of avoiding spasm of the glottis.
   c. Give vitamin D to increase absorption of calcium.
5. Reassure patient regarding skeletal recovery.
   a. Bone pain diminishes fairly quickly.
   b. Cysts, brown tumors and osteoporosis resolve themselves.
   c. Fractures are cared for by usual orthopedic procedures.

HYPOPARATHYROIDISM

Hypoparathyroidism is a condition brought about by a diminution or absence of the secretion of the parathyroid glands.

Altered Physiology

1. Blood calcium falls to a low level—causing symptoms of muscular hyperirritability, uncontrolled spasms and hypocalcemic tetany.
2. Bood phosphate level is elevated. Phosphate excretion by renal tubules is decreased.

Clinical Manifestations

1. Due to deficiency of parathormone
   a. Accumulation of phosphorus in blood
   b. Decrease in amount of blood calcium
2. Tetany
   a. General muscular hypertonia; attempts at voluntary movement results in tremors and spasmodic or uncoordinated movements; fingers assume classic position.
   b. Chvostek sign—a spasm of facial muscles resulting when muscles or branches of facial nerve are tapped.
   c. Trousseau sign—carpopedal spasm induced by occluding circulation in the arm with a blood pressure cuff
   d. Reduced blood calcium level—to a low level (7.5 mg./100 ml. or less)
   e. Laryngeal spasm
3. Anxiety and apprehension are very marked.
4. Renal colic is often present if the patient has had stones; pre-existing stones loosen and fall down into the ureter.

Treatment and Nursing Management

1. Administer calcium.
   a. A syringe and ampule of a calcium solution is to be kept at the bedside at all times.
   b. Most rapidly effective calcium solution is ionized calcium chloride (10%).
   c. For rapid use to relieve severe tetany in 2 minutes:
      (1) Administer ionized calcium chloride (10%) slowly because it is highly irritating, stings and causes thrombosis; patient experiences unpleasant burning flush of skin and, more particularly, of the tongue.
      (2) Give 3–5 ml. intravenously.
   d. Less rapid use in a period of 10–20 minutes
      Administer calcium carbohydrate combination—gluconate or heptonate (10%); may be given rapidly when administered intravenously; not irritating.
   e. Continue a slow drip of intravenous saline containing calcium gluconate until control of tetany is assured; then switch to intramuscular or oral administration of calcium.
   f. Later, add vitamin D to calcium intake—increases absorption of calcium and also induces a high level of calcium in the bloodstream.
2. Control anxiety.
   a. It is difficult to reassure this patient who has a strong feeling of impending disaster.
   b. Administration of intravenous calcium seems to bring about rapid relief of anxiety.
3. Relieve renal colic.
   Stone may need to be removed cystoscopically or by surgery.

3. Diabetes Mellitus (Pancreatic Disorder)

DIABETES MELLITUS

Diabetes mellitus is a chronic hereditary disease characterized by hyperglycemia (abnormally high level of blood sugar) due to a relative insufficiency or lack of insulin which leads to abnormalities of the metabolism of carbohydrates, protein and fat.

Altered Physiology

1. In diabetes, insulin release is not proportional to portal vein blood sugar levels for the following reasons:
   a. Insufficient numbers of islet cells (juvenile diabetes)
   b. Delayed release (adult-onset diabetes)
   c. Excessive inactivation by chemical inhibitors or "binders" in the circulation
2. In the absence of sufficient or effective insulin, partial compensation is achieved by increasing the blood sugar in order to enhance glucose transfer into the cell.
3. Glucose in the blood comes from ingested carbohydrates or from conversion of amino acids and fatty acids to glucose by the liver (gluconeogenesis).
4. Gluconeogenesis is under the control of the adrenocortical hormones; therefore, protein and fats are mobilized rather than stored or deposited in the cells; the circulation of large quantities of fats may exert an influence upon blood vessels.

5. Excess ketone bodies (acid substances formed by incomplete metabolism of fats) appear in the circulation, causing acidosis.
6. Attempts by the body to compensate for the acidosis result in hyperventilation and the loss of sodium, potassium, chloride and water.
7. The net metabolic result is loss of fat stores, liver glycogen, cellular protein, electrolytes and water.
   a. If the intake of these substances is insufficient, acidosis and electrolyte imbalance develops.
   b. If the concentration of glucose in the blood is sufficiently high, the kidney does not reabsorb all of the filtered glucose—glucose appears in the urine (glucosuria).
   c. The sequelae of long-term diabetes leads to involvement of large vessels in the brain, heart, kidneys and extremities and of the small vessels in the eyes and kidneys (atherosclerosis, hemorrhage, edema), and neuropathy; the mechanism is not precisely determined.

Types of Diabetes
(differ in prognosis, treatment, causative mechanisms)

A. *Growth-onset or Juvenile Type*
   1. Usually begins in childhood but may occur at any age.
   2. Onset abrupt.
   3. Patient more prone to ketoacidosis and is *dependent upon insulin.*
   4. Diabetes is relatively unstable or "brittle" even with good management.
      (See p. 638 for fuller discussion.)

B. *Maturity-onset* (Adult Diabetes)
   1. Usually occurs after 40; onset usually insidious.
   2. Patient usually retains a capacity for endogenous insulin production.
   3. Patient not usually ketosis-prone.
   4. Control can be achieved if treatment is well-planned and the patient is cooperative.

C. *Nonhereditary*
   1. Damage to or removal of pancreatic islet tissue—tumors of pancreas, surgical removal of pancreas, pancreatitis
   2. Disorders of endocrine glands other than pancreas—pituitary, adrenal and thyroid disorders

Incidence
   1. Approximately 5% of world population has diabetes mellitus—estimated that 25% of persons are carriers.
   2. About 2% of U.S. population has diabetes—more than 4 million.
   3. Is 7th leading cause of death in U.S.; 3rd cause of blindness.
   4. Estimated that 4% of these persons have unrecognized diabetes.
   5. Estimated that 5 million additional persons in U.S. now living will develop diabetes.
   6. One-third of all patients have a known relative with the disease.

Individuals at Risk for Diabetes Mellitus
   1. Relatives of known diabetics
   2. Obese individuals

3. Mothers of large babies or those who have had an abnormal obstetrical history
4. Persons with early onset of arteriosclerosis
   a. Premenopausal women with myocardial infarction
   b. Men having myocardial infarctions before the age of 40
5. Persons with frequent or chronic infections (gallbladder disease, pyelonephritis pancreatitis)
6. Patients exhibiting temporary reduction in glucose tolerance during stress (myocardial infarction, infection, trauma, surgery)
7. Patients developing glucose intolerance during drug therapy (thiazides, glucocorticoids, ovulatory suppressants)
8. Persons with retinopathy, nephropathy or other vascular manifestations

Clinical Manifestations

A. *Growth-onset or Juvenile Diabetes* (see p. 1271)
   1. May occur in adults as well as children.
   2. Abrupt onset—weight loss, weakness, polyuria (excessive excretion of urine), polydipsia (excessive thirst), polyphagia (excessive ingestion of food) (Polyphagia may be short-lived as the metabolic imbalance worsens.)
   3. Patient prone to develop ketosis—may be brought into hospital with acidosis or in coma.

B. *Maturity-onset*
   1. Early adult diabetes exhibits postprandial hypoglycemia.
   2. Insidious onset—excessive fatigue, tendency to drowse after a meal, irritability, nocturia, pruritus (especially of vulva in the female), poorly healing wounds, blurring of vision, loss of weight, muscle cramps.
   3. Symptoms may be absent in mild cases.
   4. Metabolic stress (surgery, febrile illness, etc.) will evoke hyperglycemia.

Clinical Course

1. Intensity of diabetes mellitus, as measured by blood sugar levels, tends to wax and wane—depends upon patient's general state of health, life stresses, dietary control, weight control, physical activity and other factors.
2. Lifelong care is mandatory—poorly controlled diabetes contributes to incidence of heart disease, renal pathology, blindness, stroke and other peripheral vascular disease.
   a. However, these complications may develop in a well-controlled diabetic no matter what treatment he follows.
   b. *The threat of complications always exists.*

Diagnostic Evaluation

A. *Glucose Tolerance Test* (most sensitive test)
   1. Patient ingests a high carbohydrate diet (200–300 gm./day) for 3 days preceding test.
   2. Blood samples are drawn after overnight fast.
   3. Glucose load (65–100 gm.) is given and specimens of blood for glucose determination are taken at 1, 2 and 3 hours after glucose ingestion.

Carbonated sugar beverage—Glucola (Ames)—may be used as a carbohydrate load.
4. *Upper limits of normal for glucose tolerance:*
   1-hour value of 190 mg./100 ml. of serum (or more)
   2-hour value of 140 mg./100 ml. of serum
   3-hour value of 125 mg./100 ml. of serum

B. *Postprandial Blood Glucose Test*
   1. Blood sample taken 1–2 hours after a high carbohydrate meal.
   2. Levels over 120 mg./100 ml. of blood suspicious for diabetes.
   3. Blood glucose may not be elevated in mild cases of diabetes.

C. *Dextrostix test*
   Used in mass screening to estimate blood glucose levels.

Treatment and Nursing Management

Objectives: to correct the biochemical and metabolic abnormalities.
to attain and maintain optimal body weight.
to prevent the progression of the disease and complications.
to promote patient education.

Means of Accomplishing Objectives
1. Diet and weight control—the essential foundation of diabetic management, or
2. Diet and insulin injections, or
3. Diet and oral hypoglycemia drugs, and
4. Continuing program of patient education

Principles of Dietary Treatment

Objective: to meet the basic nutritional requirements of the individual so he may lead a normal life in comfort and good health.
1. The diet is planned according to patient's weight and activities and is adequate in all nutritional elements.
2. *The major dietary restriction is on concentrated sources of carbohydrates.*
3. The same number of prescribed calories are consumed daily—fluctuations in daily food intake lead to loss of tolerance for carbohydrates.
4. Calories are adjusted to attain or maintain optimal weight—there is a positive correlation between diabetes and obesity in maturity-onset diabetes.
5. To find caloric requirements:
   a. Determine ideal weight (Table 10-1).
   b. Multiply ideal weight in pounds by 10 = basic caloric allotment.
   c. Adjust for age and activity.
      (1) Light activity—increase calories by 20%.
      (2) Strenuous activity—increase calories by 40–50%.
   d. Reduce basic requirements by 10–20% if patient is obese.
   e. Increase basic requirements by 10–20% if patient is underweight.
   f. Adapt and modify diet according to patient's response.
6. Place obese patients on a weight reduction diet.
   a. *Obese individuals are more resistant to both endogenous and exogenous insulin.*
   b. Weight loss tends to restore insulin sensitivity.

TABLE 10-1. DESIRABLE WEIGHTS *

Weight in Pounds According to Frame (In Indoor Clothing)

	HEIGHT (with shoes on) 1-inch heels Feet Inches	SMALL FRAME	MEDIUM FRAME	LARGE FRAME
Men of Ages 25 and Over	5 2	112–120	118–129	126–141
	5 3	115–123	121–133	129–144
	5 4	118–126	124–136	132–148
	5 5	121–129	127–139	135–152
	5 6	124–133	130–143	138–156
	5 7	128–137	134–147	142–161
	5 8	132–141	138–152	147–166
	5 9	136–145	142–156	151–170
	5 10	140–150	146–160	155–174
	5 11	144–154	150–165	159–179
	6 0	148–158	154–170	164–184
	6 1	152–162	158–175	168–189
	6 2	156–167	162–180	173–194
	6 3	160–171	167–185	178–199
	6 4	164–175	172–190	182–204

	HEIGHT (with shoes on) 2-inch heels Feet Inches	SMALL FRAME	MEDIUM FRAME	LARGE FRAME
Women of Ages 25 and Over	4 10	92– 98	96–107	104–119
	4 11	94–101	98–110	106–122
	5 0	96–104	101–113	109–125
	5 1	99–107	104–116	112–128
	5 2	102–110	107–119	115–131
	5 3	105–113	110–122	118–134
	5 4	108–116	113–126	121–138
	5 5	111–119	116–130	125–142
	5 6	114–123	120–135	129–146
	5 7	118–127	124–139	133–150
	5 8	122–131	128–143	137–154
	5 9	126–135	132–147	141–158
	5 10	130–140	136–151	145–163
	5 11	134–144	140–155	149–168
	6 0	138–148	144–159	153–173

For girls between 18 and 25, subtract 1 pound for each year under 25.

* Courtesy of the Metropolitan Life Insurance Company.

7. Most clinicians now advise following some form of food-exchange groups from which patient may make selections for his diet—American Dietetic Association, American Diabetes Association and the U.S. Public Health Service have developed food-exchange lists.
   a. Foods are arranged in groups of exchanges (see Table 10-2).
   b. Patient modifies his prescribed diet by exchanging one item with another item on the same exchange list.

    c. The foods in each exchange list have approximately the same sugar content—facilitates individual meal planning and makes diet more acceptable.

8. The diabetic diet should fit the patient's food preferences and economic status, and *emphasis should be on what the patient is allowed* rather than on what is forbidden.

9. Foods should be measured to ensure correct portion sizes.

    a. Patient is not to omit meals or between-meal and bedtime snacks if ordered.

    b. Patient should weigh and record weight twice weekly.

TABLE 10-2. SAMPLE FOOD EXCHANGE LISTS FOR DIABETIC DIET*

1500 Calories	Daily Menu Guide		
	BREAKFAST	LUNCH	DINNER
carbohydrate	1 fruit exchange (List 3)	2 meat exchanges (List 5)	2 meat exchanges (List 5)
150 Gm.	2 bread exchanges (List 4)	2 bread exchanges (List 4)	1 1/2 bread exchanges (List 4)
protein	1 meat exchange (List 5)	Vegetable(s) as desired (List 1)	Vegetable(s) as desired (List 1)
70 Gm.	1 milk exchange (List 7)	1 fruit exchange (List 3)	1 vegetable exchange (List 2)
fat	2 fat exchanges (List 6)	1 milk exchange (List 7)	1 fruit exchange (List 3)
70 Gm.	Coffee or tea (any amount)	1 fat exchange (List 6)	1/2 milk exchange (List 7)
		Coffee or tea (any amount)	1 fat exchange (List 6)
			Coffee or tea (any amount)

List 1 allowed as desired
(need not be measured)

Seasonings: Cinnamon, celery salt, garlic, garlic salt, lemon, mustard, mint, nutmeg, parsley, pepper, saccharin and other sugarless sweeteners, spices, vanilla, and vinegar.

Other Foods: Coffee or tea (without sugar or cream), fat-free broth, bouillon, unflavored gelatin, rennet tablets, sour or dill pickles, cranberries (without sugar), rhubarb (without sugar).

Vegetables: Group A—insignificant carbohydrate or calories. You may eat as much as desired of raw vegetables. If cooked vegetable is eaten, limit amount to 1 cup.

Asparagus	Lettuce
Broccoli	Mushrooms
Brussels sprouts	Okra
Cabbage	Peppers, green
Cauliflower	or red
Celery	Radishes
Chicory	Sauerkraut
Cucumbers	String beans
Eggplant	Summer squash
Escarole	Tomatoes
Greens: beet, chard, collard,	Watercress
dandelion, kale, mustard,	
spinach, turnip	

List 2 vegetable exchanges

Each portion supplies approximately 7 gm. of carbohydrate and 2 gm. of protein, or 36 calories.

Vegetables: Group B—One serving equals 1/2 cup, or 100 gm.

Beets	Pumpkin
Carrots	Rutabagas
Onions	Squash, winter
Peas, green	Turnips

* Courtesy of Eli Lilly Company.

List 3 fruit exchanges
(fresh, dried, or canned without sugar)

Each portion supplies approximately 10 gm. of carbohydrate, or 40 calories.

	household measurement	weight of portion
Apple	1 small (2″ diam.)	80 gm.
Applesauce	1/2 cup	100 gm.
Apricots, fresh	2 med.	100 gm.
Apricots, dried	4 halves	20 gm.
Banana	1/2 small	50 gm.
Berries	1 cup	150 gm.
Blueberries	2/3 cup	100 gm.
Cantaloupe	1/4 (6″ diam.)	200 gm.
Cherries	10 large	75 gm.
Dates	2	15 gm.
Figs, fresh	2 large	50 gm.
Figs, dried	1 small	15 gm.
Grapefruit	1/2 small	125 gm.
Grapefruit juice	1/2 cup	100 gm.
Grapes	12	75 gm.
Grape juice	1/4 cup	60 gm.
Honeydew melon	1/8 (7″)	150 gm.
Mango	1/2 small	70 gm.
Orange	1 small	100 gm.
Orange juice	1/2 cup	100 gm.
Papaya	1/3 med.	100 gm.
Peach	1 med.	100 gm.
Pear	1 small	100 gm.
Pineapple	1/2 cup	80 gm.
Pineapple juice	1/3 cup	80 gm.
Plums	2 med.	100 gm.
Prunes, dried	2	25 gm.
Raisins	2 tbsp.	15 gm.
Tangerine	1 large	100 gm.
Watermelon	1 cup	175 gm.

List 4 bread exchanges

Each portion supplies approximately 15 gm. of carbohydrate and 2 gm. of protein, or 68 calories.

	household measurement	weight of portion
Bread	1 slice	25 gm.
Biscuit, roll	1 (2″ diam.)	35 gm.
Muffin	1 (2″ diam.)	35 gm.
Cornbread	1 1/2″ cube	35 gm.
Flour	2 1/2 tbsp.	20 gm.
Cereal, cooked	1/2 cup	100 gm.
Cereal, dry (flakes or puffed)	3/4 cup	20 gm.
Rice or grits, cooked	1/2 cup	100 gm.
Spaghetti, noodles, etc.	1/2 cup	100 gm.
Crackers, graham	2	20 gm.
Crackers, oyster	20 (1/2 cup)	20 gm.
Crackers, saltine	5	20 gm.
Crackers, soda	3	20 gm.
Crackers, round	6-8	20 gm.
Vegetables		
Beans (Lima, navy, etc.), dry, cooked	1/2 cup	90 gm.
Peas (split peas, etc.), dry, cooked	1/2 cup	90 gm.
Baked beans, no pork	1/4 cup	50 gm.
Corn	1/3 cup	80 gm.
Parsnips	2/3 cup	125 gm.
Potato, white, baked or boiled	1 (2″ diam.)	100 gm.
Potatoes, white, mashed	1/2 cup	100 gm.
Potatoes, sweet, or yams	1/4 cup	50 gm.
Sponge cake, plain	1 1/2″ cube	25 gm.
Ice cream (Omit 2 fat exchanges)	1/2 cup	70 gm.

10. The diet usually is planned so that snacks providing carbohydrate (10–20 gm.) are taken in midafternoon and at bedtime—food value of snacks is included in dietary prescription.

11. Patient should test urine at least 1 time daily, preferably 1–2 hours after supper (p. 658).

12. Exercise is encouraged since it usually facilitates the control of the disease.
    a. Exercise promotes metabolism and utilization of carbohydrates, thus diminishing insulin requirements of the body; enhances the effects of insulin.
    b. Encourage reasonable uniformity in the amount of exercise.

Principles of Insulin Therapy

1. *Insulin* is the active principle of secretion of beta cells in the islets of Langerhans.

2. Physiological effect of insulin—lowers the blood sugar by facilitating the uptake and utilization of glucose by the tissues; effects fat and protein metabolism as well as electrolytes.

List 5 meat exchanges

Each portion supplies approximately 7 gm. of protein and 5 gm. of fat, or 73 calories. (30 gm. equal 1 oz.)

	household measurement	weight of portion
Meat and poultry (beef, lamb, pork, liver, chicken, etc.) (med. fat)	1 slice (3" x 2" x 1/8")	30 gm.
Cold cuts	1 slice (4 1/2" sq., 1/8" thick)	45 gm.
Frankfurter	1 (8-9 per lb.)	50 gm.
Codfish, mackerel, etc.	1 slice (2" x 2" x 1")	30 gm.
Salmon, tuna, crab	1/4 cup	30 gm.
Oysters, shrimp, clams	5 small	45 gm.
Sardines	3 med.	30 gm.
Cheese, cheddar, American	1 slice (3 1/2" x 1 1/2" x 1/4")	30 gm.
Cheese, cottage	1/4 cup	45 gm.
Egg	1	50 gm.
Peanut butter	2 tbsp.	30 gm.

Limit peanut butter to one exchange per day unless allowance is made for carbohydrate in the diet plan.

List 6 fat exchanges

Each portion supplies approximately 5 gm. of fat, or 45 calories.

	household measurement	weight of portion
Butter or margarine	1 tsp.	5 gm.
Bacon, crisp	1 slice	10 gm.
Cream, light	2 tbsp.	30 gm.
Cream, heavy	1 tbsp.	15 gm.
Cream cheese	1 tbsp.	15 gm.
French dressing	1 tbsp.	15 gm.
Mayonnaise	1 tsp.	5 gm.
Oil or cooking fat	1 tsp.	5 gm.
Nuts	6 small	10 gm.
Olives	5 small	50 gm.
Avocado	1/8 (4" diam.)	25 gm.

List 7 milk exchanges

Each portion supplies approximately 12 gm. of carbohydrate, 8 gm. of protein, and 10 gm. of fat, or 170 calories.

	household measurement	weight of portion
Milk, whole	1 cup	240 gm.
Milk, evaporated	1/2 cup	120 gm.
*Milk, powdered	1/4 cup	35 gm.
*Buttermilk	1 cup	240 gm.

* Add 2 fat exchanges if milk is fat-free.

NURSING ALERT: There is a narrow margin between the therapeutic and toxic (hypoglycemia) effects of insulin. Exercise, illness and emotional stress can alter needs for insulin—can lower the blood sugar.

3. Obese patients with mild uncomplicated diabetes may control the disease solely by means of a low calorie diet without insulin.
4. The following individuals require regular injections of insulin.
   a. Patients with growth-onset or juvenile diabetes
   b. Diabetic adults who have lost an excessive amount of weight
   c. Diabetic individuals with acute complications
   d. Individuals with severe diabetes
   e. Patients (of any age) with febrile illness or those who are undergoing major surgery

Insulin Preparations

1. Insulin preparations are prescribed in units/ml. Units 40 (red label and red stopper) and units 80 (green label and green stopper) were most frequently used, but are now superseded by 100 μ/ml.
2. The preparation selected depends on onset of action desired, time of peak effect required and duration of action (Table 10-3).

TABLE 10-3. INSULIN PREPARATION

Action	Type of Insulin	Time of Onset (hr.)	Peak (hr.)	Duration (hr.)	Time when hypoglycemia most apt to occur
Rapid	Crystalline Zinc (regular)	Within hour or less	2–4	5–7	Before lunch
	Semi-lente	1	2–8	12–16	Before lunch
Intermediate	Globin	2–4	6–12	12–18	Late afternoon
	NPH	2–4	6–12	18–24	Late afternoon
	Lente	2–4	6–12	18–24	Late afternoon
Slow	Protamine Zinc	3–6	14–20	24–36	During night and early morning
	Ultralente	8	18–24	24–36	During night and early morning

3. Patient and nurse should know when insulin is having its effect—knowing when hypoglycemia is most apt to occur will assist nurse in assessing patient's symptoms and behavior.

Regulation of Insulin Dosage

1. The dosage of insulin is adjusted by the presence (or absence) and the degree of glucosuria and its time of appearance in relation to insulin injections and meals. Since some patients do not have glucosuria, the blood sugar is monitored in these cases.
2. Dosage of insulin is also adjusted according to determinations of blood glucose levels.
3. Most patients with maturity-onset diabetes require 1 injection of insulin daily before breakfast; other patients may require evening injections before supper or a small dose of NPH (or Lente) insulin at bedtime.
4. Instruct the patient to test his urine for sugar before each meal and at bedtime while insulin is being regulated—use the 2nd of 2 specimens voided one-half hour apart for greater accuracy.
5. Have the patient keep a record of results in a notebook—to facilitate subsequent insulin adjustments.

Hypoglycemia as a Complication of Insulin Treatment

1. Hypoglycemic reaction is an abnormally low level of glucose (sugar) in the blood; likely to occur when for any reason the blood sugar falls below 60 mg./100 ml. of blood.
2. Attack results from omission of a meal, from vomiting a meal after taking insulin, from undue exertion, or from an error in insulin dose.
3. Reactions begin 5–20 minutes following injection of regular insulin but not for several hours after NPH insulin—majority of attacks occur in morning and in early evening.

Signs and Symptoms of Hypoglycemia

Generalized muscular weakness
Sweating
Nervous instability, trembling
Faintness, hunger pangs in epigastrium
Headache, numbness or tingling of tongue or lips

Rapid heart action
Double vision; unsteady gait
Confusion

NURSING ALERT: Patients taking NPH insulin may not have typical symptoms of a hypoglycemia reaction but may have hot dry, flushing skin and show signs of disorientation or drowsiness.

NURSING ALERT: Some patients experience hypoglycemia so rapidly that the symptoms progress to epileptiform convulsions almost without warning.

Treatment of Hypoglycemia

1. Give some form of glucose orally if patient is conscious—orange juice, candy, lump sugar, corn syrup.
2. Give glucagon (subcutaneously or I.M.) (1.0 mg. in adults)—causes glycogenolysis in the liver which raises blood glucose level.
3. Give patient orange juice or ginger ale as soon as he regains consciousness—glucose level may fall faster than the transient rise produced by glucagon.
4. If patient is unconscious for period of time:
   a. Give 50% glucose solution I.V.—to restore normal blood glucose level quickly.
   b. Follow this with intravenous infusion of 5–10% glucose solution in water.
   c. Administer mannitol to combat cerebral edema if necessary—cerebral function may be compromised when patient has low level of blood glucose.
5. Once rapidly-absorbed carbohydrate is given, give a feeding with protein or fat.

Preventing Hypoglycemic Reactions due to Insulin

Instruct the patient as follows:
1. Prevent hypoglycemia with uniformity and timing of diet, insulin and daily exercise.
2. Recognize the early symptoms of hypoglycemia—lassitude, lethargy, hunger, inability to concentrate.
3. Take between meal and bedtime snack—to distribute the carbohydrate load over period of maximum insulin effect.
4. Test the urine so that changing insulin requirements may be anticipated.
5. Carry rapidly-absorbed carbohydrate (sugar/candy) and take at first warning of a reaction.
6. Carry an identification card or wear an identification bracelet:
   a. Card—American Diabetes Association, Inc., 18 E. 48th St., New York, New York 10017.
   b. Identification Bracelet—Medic Alert Foundation, Turlock, California 95380.

Other Complications of Insulin Therapy

1. *Insulin Allergy*
   a. Local reaction associated with redness, swelling, pain and nodule formation at site of injection.
   b. Occurs during first weeks of therapy and then disappears.
   c. Sensitization may be related to specific animal proteins from which insulin is derived.
2. *Insulin Lipodystrophy*
   a. Atrophy (large sunken areas at site of injection) and hypertrophy.
   b. Is harmless but cosmetically distressing in women.
   c. Reinforce patient teaching on changing sites of insulin injections (p. 657).
3. *Insulin Edema*
   a. Characterized by generalized retention of fluid.
   b. Usually appears with sudden restoration of diabetic control in a patient with uncontrolled diabetes over a period of time.
4. *Insulin Resistance*
   Term applied to a patient whose insulin requirement is at least 200 units daily over a period of weeks to months in the absence of infection.

Oral Hypoglycemic Agents

1. Oral hypoglycemic agents (Table 10-4) are advocated for a maturity-onset non-ketotic diabetic who cannot be controlled by diet and who is unable (or will not) take insulin.
2. Serious questions have recently been raised concerning effectiveness and safety of long-term use of oral hypoglycemic agents—increasing number of deaths reported among tolbutamide-treated patients over nontolbutamide-treated patients.
3. Patient should be placed on an effective dietary and weight control program before trying oral hypoglycemia agents.
4. Insulin is preferable to oral agents if dietary treatment fails to control diabetes.
5. Insulin is *required* when infection, trauma, major surgery or gangrene are present.

TABLE 10-4. ORAL HYPOGLYCEMIC AGENTS

Agent	Tablet Size	Usual Daily Dose
Sulfonylurea Group (stimulates insulin release from pancreatic beta cells; their action depends upon a functioning pancreas)		
Tolbutamide (Orinase)	500 mg.	500–2000 mg.
Chlorpropamide (Diabinese)	100 mg.; 250 mg.	100–500 mg.
Acetohexamide (Dymelor)	250 mg.; 500 mg.	250–1500 mg. (1.5 gm.)
Tolazamide (Tolinase)	100 mg.; 250 mg.	100–1000 mg. (1.0 gm.)
Biguanide Group (potentiates the action of insulin; lowers blood glucose in diabetic patients)		
Phenformin (DBI)	25 mg.	50–200 mg.
Phenformin, long-acting (DBI-TD)	50 mg. (capsule)	50–200 mg.

COMPLICATIONS OF DIABETES

Ketoacidosis and Coma

Ketoacidosis and *coma* are due to a lack of insulin resulting in a derangement of carbohydrate, fat and protein metabolism and dehydration and electrolyte imbalance. There is an increase in ketone bodies (blood acids) resulting from rapid breakdown of fat in the poorly regulated diabetic patient.

Precipitating Causes

1. Failure to take insulin, insufficient insulin, or resistance to insulin
2. Dietary indiscretions
3. Infections, vomiting, diarrhea
4. Physiologic stresses—injury, surgery, shock, pregnancy, emotional stresses

Clinical Manifestations

1. *Early Manifestations*
   Thirst, anorexia, vomiting
   Abdominal pain
   Headache, listlessness, drowsiness
   Hot, dry-flushed appearance
   Visual disturbances
2. *Later Manifestations*
   Coma
   Kussmaul breathing—very deep but not labored respiratory movements; a symptom of profound acidosis.
   Sweetish odor on breath
   Lowered blood pressure
   Drowsiness leading to coma

Laboratory Evaluation

1. *Blood*—high glucose concentration
   low CO_2 combining power
   Plasma ketones present
2. *Urine*—marked glycosuria and ketonuria

Treatment

Objective: to restore carbohydrate utilization and correct electrolyte imbalance.
1. Secure blood and urine samples immediately.
   a. Insert indwelling catheter.
   b. Obtain specimen at prescribed times.
   c. Report blood glucose, CO_2, pH, electrolyte, acetone, BUN and hematocrit levels.
   d. Use Ketostix to follow course of ketoacidosis if laboratory facilities are not available.
2. Look for evidence of infection.
3. Administer rapid-acting insulin: (⅓ of initial dose I.V. and ⅔ subcutaneously; all insulin thereafter, subcutaneously).
   a. Report blood glucose levels to the physician.
   b. Give doses of insulin as ordered.

4. Replace fluids and electrolytes.
   a. Give isotonic saline or sodium lactate solution I.V. to replace sodium loss.
   b. Give supplementary potassium if ordered.
   c. Measure and record input and output.
   d. Offer potassium-rich and sweetened fluids (orange juice) as tolerated.
   e. Give glucose infusion to prevent hypoglycemia, since carbohydrate metabolism will be accelerated by insulin and blood glucose will begin to decrease.

NURSING ALERT: There is danger of a hypoglycemic reaction occurring between 12–24 hours after treatment for ketoacidosis. Another danger is hypokalemia, especially if vomiting or diarrhea is present.

---

5. Treat for circulatory collapse if present.
   a. Give blood, plasma, plasma volume expanders as directed.
   b. Record vital signs as patient's condition indicates.
   c. Elevate the lower extremities.
   d. Administer vasopressors as ordered.
6. Prepare for gastric lavage if ordered (see p. 923).
7. Obtain electrocardiograms as directed.
8. Prevent the recurrence of diabetic ketoacidosis.
   a. Avoid infection.
   b. Make insulin and dietary adjustments during the periods of illness.
   c. See page 652 for other aspects of patient education.

Infection

Etiology

1. There is a complex interrelationship between diabetes mellitus and infections.
2. May be due to vascular disease and other host factors.
3. Diabetics are more susceptible to infections.
4. Infections remain a significant factor in morbidity and mortality in diabetes mellitus.

Types of Infection

1. Infections of urinary tract—probably from increasing frequency of catheterization, neuropathy with bladder paresis and renal vascular disease
2. Gram negative rod bacteremia
3. Soft tissue infection—probably from peripheral vascular insufficiency
4. Tuberculosis—diabetics are 2–4 times more susceptible to tuberculosis than the general population.
5. Fungal infections
   a. Candidiasis
      (1) Due to *Candida albicans* normally found on skin, oral cavity, gastrointestinal tract and vagina.
      (2) Local infection of these areas (particularly vagina and skin) may occur in poorly controlled diabetes.
   b. Phycomycosis
      (1) Due to Sacrophetic fungi commonly found in nature.
      (2) May cause disease of paranasal sinuses and central nervous system.

Treatment

1. Diabetes becomes temporarily more severe in the course of infections.
2. Usual insulin treatment may be ineffective in an acute spreading infection.
3. Infection must be treated aggressively—ketoacidosis frequently precipitated by infection.
4. Blood glucose determinations may have to be done every 12 hours to ascertain changing insulin requirements.

Long-term Complications of Diabetes

Cannot be prevented or adequately treated.

Vascular Complications

1. Diabetic person more prone to develop lesions of the small vessels (capillaries, arterioles and venules) of the renal glomerulus, retina, muscle and skin.
2. May cause major vessel occlusion—aorta, subclavian and innominate and extra-cranial arteries and the renal, iliac, femoral and popliteal systems.
3. Many patients have *advanced* cardiovascular disease before the diabetic condition is recognized clinically.

Diabetic Retinopathy

A disturbance in the retinal blood vessels leading to decreased vision and often blindness; seems to involve progressive impairment of retinal circulation.

1. Impairs vision (and causes blindness) from bleeding into the vitreous, from formation of scar tissue and from detachment of the retina.
2. Accounts for 12% of all blindness in U.S. and is rapidly becoming the leading cause of new adult blindness.
3. Incidence and severity of retinopathy is generally proportional to duration of disease.
4. No known way of preventing diabetic retinopathy.

Neuropathy

A disease of the nervous system primarily occurring as a consequence of diabetes mellitus; peripheral nerves most frequently involved.

1. Wide variety of manifestations—paresthesias, pain, weakness, paralysis, extraocular muscle palsies, pupillary changes, delayed gastric emptying, sexual impotence, atonic urinary bladder.
2. Treatment
   a. Ensure careful dietary control.
   b. Give supplementary vitamins, especially vitamin B_{12}.

MANAGEMENT OF THE DIABETIC PATIENT UNDERGOING SURGERY

Hazards

1. Patients with diabetes are usually considered poor operative risks due to early arteriosclerosis, vascular and neurologic complications, low resistance to infection and delayed healing.

2. Surgical stress may increase hyperglycemia because of increased secretion of epineph rine and glucocorticoids.
3. Diabetic ketoacidosis may simulate an acute surgical abdomen.
4. Diabetic patients are more prone to develop gangrene of foot, cholecystitis an cholelithiasis and cancer of pancreas.
5. Metabolic stress of anesthesia also accentuates problems of hyperglycemia an ketosis.

Treatment and Nursing Management

Objective: to achieve the best nutritional balance and optimal control of diabetes preoper atively

A. *Preoperative Preparation*
1. Have essential evaluation studies done preoperatively—urinalysis for sugar an acetone, postprandial blood glucose determination, blood urea nitrogen, serum cholesterol determination and ECG.
2. Give adequate carbohydrate intake (150–200 gm.) to prevent acetonuria.
3. Administer small dose of insulin to patient taking oral hypoglycemic agent the day before surgery; omit oral hypoglycemic agent.
4. Correct dehydration and electrolyte imbalance.

B. *Day of Surgery*
1. Have blood sugar determination within an hour before scheduled surgery—to guard against risk of hypoglycemic shock on the operating table.
2. Give 1000 ml. of 5% glucose in water (as directed)—given instead of breakfast i patient is in fasting state, is not well stabilized or is undergoing prolonged surgery
3. Give insulin as directed to cover glucose infusion.

C. *Postoperative Management*
1. Give adequate carbohydrate (200 gm.) daily and adequate insulin for utilization o carbohydrate calories—to maintain nutrition and prevent ketoacidosis and hypo glycemia.
   a. Carbohydrates may have to be furnished via I.V. glucose.
   b. Give insulin to cover infusions.
   c. Blood sugar levels may be disturbed due to intravenous glucose infusions.
2. Check blood glucose and serum ketone concentrations several times daily—to eval uate patient's diabetic control (patients receiving I.V. glucose may have marked glycosuria and only moderate hyperglycemia).
3. Carry out urine tests for sugar and acetone as guidelines to therapy.
4. Watch for signs and symptoms of ketoacidosis (see p. 649).

PRINCIPLES OF PATIENT EDUCATION FOR DIABETES MELLITUS

The person with diabetes mellitus must accept a major role in the management of his disease His education must be amplified, reinforced and updated continuously, since diabetes is life-long disease.

Objective: to maintain the best possible control of diabetes.

Patient's Objectives

A. To become familiar with diabetes and how it affects the body.

1. Visit the physician on a regular basis.
2. Study and review available literature from reputable sources (physician, AMA).
3. Secure booklets and pamphlets from the American Diabetes Association, Inc., 18 East 48th Street, New York, N.Y. 10017.
4. Attend available classes.

B. To maintain health at an optimal level.

1. Maintain a daily routine that is fairly consistent.
2. Get adequate rest and sleep.
3. Exercise regularly and consistently.
   a. Avoid "spurts" of arduous exercise before meals.
   b. Exercise 1½ hours after meals.
   c. Keep some form of carbohydrate (sugar, candy, orange juice) available during exercise periods.
4. Seek employment with regular hours.
5. Have an annual test for tuberculosis.

C. To follow the prescribed dietary regimen.

1. Consume a constant daily diet 3 times a day.
2. Become thoroughly familiar with the food exchange lists.
3. Learn how to follow a calculated diet.
4. Know the caloric value of foods frequently eaten.
5. Use household measures or a gram scale until serving sizes can be judged accurately.
6. Avoid concentrated carbohydrates.
7. Keep weight at optimal level; normalize body weight.
   a. Weigh weekly.
   b. Keep a weight record.
8. If taking insulin, eat extra calories when unusual physical activity is anticipated.
9. Eat a bedtime snack when taking insulin (if permissible).
10. Avoid foods high in cholesterol.

D. To be aware of the degree of diabetic control.

1. Test urine for both sugar and acetone at each testing.
2. Test urine upon arising, before lunch, in late afternoon and at bedtime while control is being attained or during periods of illness.
3. Test urine at least once daily during periods of good control.
4. Test only freshly voided urine.
5. Keep a daily record of urine sugar tests (date, hour, color reaction).
6. Take the record of urine tests to physician at appointed times.
7. Know that acetone in the urine indicates need for *more insulin.*
8. Avoid handling reagent tablets to prevent them from absorbing moisture; this may give a false interpretation to the test.
9. Protect test tapes from light, moisture and heat to prevent tape deterioration.

E. To become familiar with all aspects of insulin usage (see p. 655 for guidelines to teaching self-injection of insulin).

1. Know when the prescribed insulin is having its peak action.
2. Adjust insulin dosage according to urine sugar tests as prescribed.

3. Rotate the sites of insulin injections in a systematic manner.
4. Keep the sterile syringe and needle in the same place.
5. Keep a reserve supply of insulin in the refrigerator.
    a. Keep bottle in current use at room temperature.
    b. Avoid injecting cold insulin because it may contribute to tissue reaction.
6. Have an extra insulin syringe available.
7. Know the conditions that produce insulin reactions:
    a. Omission of a meal
    b. Unaccustomed or strenuous exercise
    c. Too much insulin
8. Know the symptoms of an insulin reaction.
    a. Any unfamiliar or peculiar sensation
    b. Hunger, perspiration, palpitation, tachycardia, weakness, tremor, pallor
9. Know how to combat an impending insulin reaction.
    a. Eat carbohydrates (orange juice, sugar, candy) when symptoms first occur.
    b. Test urine.
    c. Carry extra carbohydrate at all times (sugar lumps, candy).
    d. Eat extra carbohydrate before strenuous exercise and during periods of prolonge
       exercise.
    e. Eat a snack at bedtime.
10. Carry diabetic identification card or wear identification bracelet.

F. *To take prescribed oral hypoglycemic medication.*
    1. Adhere faithfully to the prescribed diet.
    2. Test the urine daily.
    3. Take the medication exactly as directed.

G. *To appreciate the importance of proper foot care to prevent infection, ischemia, an
   neuropathy which may lead to amputation and death.*
    1. Inspect the feet carefully and routinely for calluses, corns, blisters, abrasions and nai
       abnormalities.
    2. Bathe the feet daily in warm (never hot) water.
    3. Massage the feet with a lanolin preparation, except between the toes.
    4. Prevent moisture between the toes to prevent maceration of the skin.
        a. Insert lamb's wool between overlapping toes.
        b. Use powder in the web spaces.
    5. Wear well-fitting noncompressive shoes.
    6. Wear clean and nonrestrictive socks and stockings.
    7. Go to a podiatrist on a regular basis if corns, calluses and ingrown toenails ar
       present.
    8. Avoid heat, chemicals and injuries to the feet.
    9. If an injury occurs to the feet:
        a. Wash the area with soap and water.
        b. Cover with a dry sterile dressing *without* adhesive.
        c. Call the physician.
    10. Do foot exercises regularly.

H. *To maintain diabetic control during periods of illness.*
    1. Call physician when any unusual symptoms become evident.
    2. Make dietary adjustments during illness according to physician's directions.

3. Continue taking insulin.
4. Test urine for sugar and acetone more frequently.
5. Know the conditions that bring about diabetic acidosis.
   a. Nausea and vomiting
   b. Failure to increase insulin when urine sugar is increasing
   c. Failure to take insulin
   d. Dietary excesses
6. Know how to combat impending diabetic acidosis.
   a. Examine urine for sugar and acetone and report results to physician.
   b. Use Dextrostix to determine blood sugar abnormalities.
   c. Take additional insulin as advised by physician.
   d. Go to bed and keep warm.
   e. Alert someone to be in attendance.
   f. Drink a glass of liquid hourly if possible.

GUIDELINES: *Teaching Self-injection of Insulin*

Underlying Considerations

1. Insulin injection should be taught as soon as the need for insulin treatment has been established.
2. A member of the patient's family should also be taught how to administer insulin.
3. An optimistic approach will offer the patient encouragement.
4. Teach insulin injection *first* as this is the patient's major concern; then include loading the syringe and sterilization of equipment as the patient is able to grasp these concepts.

Equipment

Prescribed bottle of insulin	Medium size sauce pan
Insulin syringe*	Absorbent cotton and alcohol
Medium size tea strainer	Small tray for storage of supplies

Procedure

Teaching Action	Rationale/Amplification
1. Give the patient the prepared syringe containing the prescribed dose of insulin.	
2. Have patient prepare the skin with alcohol. (Nurse may do this at first.)	
3. Instruct the patient to hold the syringe as he would a pencil.	
4. Show the patient how to spread the skin taut on the anterior thigh (Fig. 10-1A). or Form a skin fold by picking up subcutaneous tissue between the thumb and forefinger if the patient is thin (Fig. 10-1B).	4. Either of the techniques ensures that the needle tip is inserted into subcutaneous tissue and outside the muscle. Avoid pressing the skin *tightly* between the fingers as this is a common cause of local induration and infection.

* Automatic injector available from Becton-Dickinson Company, Rutherford, New Jersey.

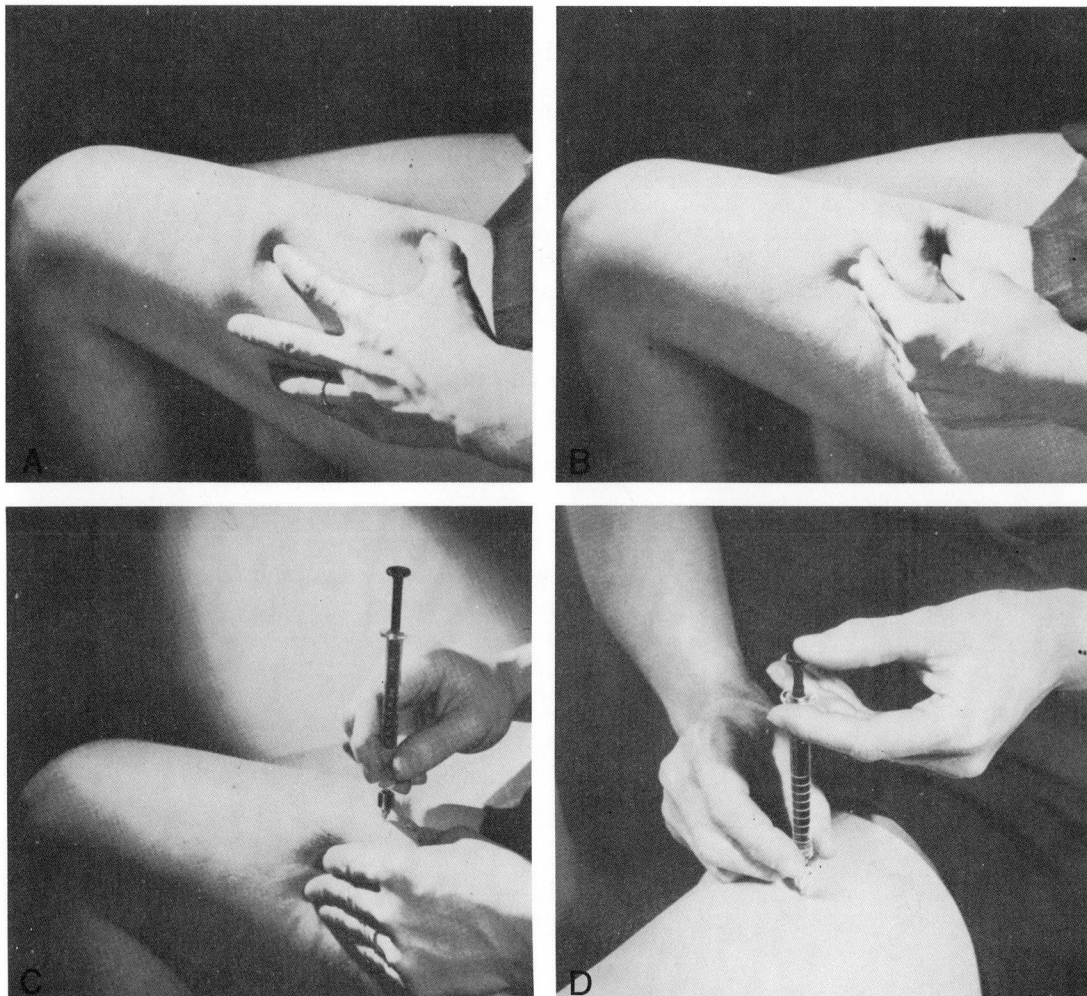

Figure 10-1. Self-injection of insulin.

A. The skin is spread taut.

B. If the patient is thin, a fold of subcutaneous tissue can be formed with the left hand.

C. The needle is injected at a right angle (straight, not slanted) to the leg. The syringe is held as one would hold a pencil, between the thumb and index finger of the right hand, and the needle is pushed firmly for its entire length into the skin. Once the needle is injected into the skin, it is not necessary to hold the flesh. The left hand is then used to gently pull the plunger of the syringe back. If blood is drawn into the syringe, the needle should be withdrawn and inserted elsewhere.

D. The right hand is used to hold the syringe steady while the left hand holds the syringe at the top, between the index and middle fingers, and thumb pushes the plunger to inject the insulin.
    (From Rosenthal, H., and Rosenthal, J.: Diabetic Care in Pictures, 4th ed. Philadelphia, J. B. Lippincott.)

Teaching Action	*Rationale/Amplification*

5. Select areas of upper arms, thighs, flanks and upper buttocks for injection after patient becomes proficient with needle insertion (Fig. 10-1*A*).

5. The skin is loose and there is more subcutaneous fat in these areas. The skin of the abdominal wall is a good site for women who develop atrophy of subcutaneous fat at sites of insulin injection.

6. Assist the patient to insert needle with a quick thrust to the hub at a right angle to the skin surface (Fig. 10-1*C*).

6. The insulin is injected into deep subcutaneous tissue.

7. Instruct the patient to release the skin fold and exert slight traction on the plunger (Fig. 10-1*D*). Push in plunger.

7. This ensures that the needle is not in a blood vessel.

8. Hold the alcohol sponge against the needle and withdraw needle. Rub the injection site gently with cotton sponge.

8. This maneuver prevents painful pulling of the skin as the needle is withdrawn.

9. Rinse syringe barrel, plunger and needle under cold running water.

10. Develop a systematic plan for insulin administration with rotation of sites in a clockwise fashion (Fig. 10-2).

10. Systematic rotation of sites will keep the skin supple, will favor uniform absorption of insulin and will prevent scar formation.

To Load the Syringe

1. Roll the bottle of insulin (Protamine Zinc, NPH and Lente) between the palms of the hands.

1. The rolling action mixes the insulin.

2. Wipe off the top of the insulin vial with an alcohol sponge.

3. Inject approximately the same volume of air into the insulin vial as the volume of insulin to be withdrawn.

3. This prevents the gradual production of a partial vacuum.

Figure 10-2. Setting up a rotation circle. The sketch shows that the right arm is marked A, the right side of the abdomen is B, and the right thigh is C. The left side of the body going upward is marked D, E, and F, counterclockwise.

Each of these areas can be marked as a rectangle and divided into 8 squares more than 1 inch on each side. These squares are numbered starting from the upper and outside corner (number 1) to the lowest corner (number 2). All even numbers are toward the body.

If you take the number 1 square and inject into it at each of the 6 areas through F, it will take you 6 days to reach area A again. Then you take square number 2 and inject each time on the squares so numbered in the areas A through F. And so on.

This provides 48 different places for an injection (6 x 8). At 1 injection daily, it will take 48 days or 7 weeks to cover each of the square. (From A. D. A. Forecast—the Diabetics' Own Magazine. January 1951, Vol. 4, No. 1. Courtesy, Becton, Dickinson.)

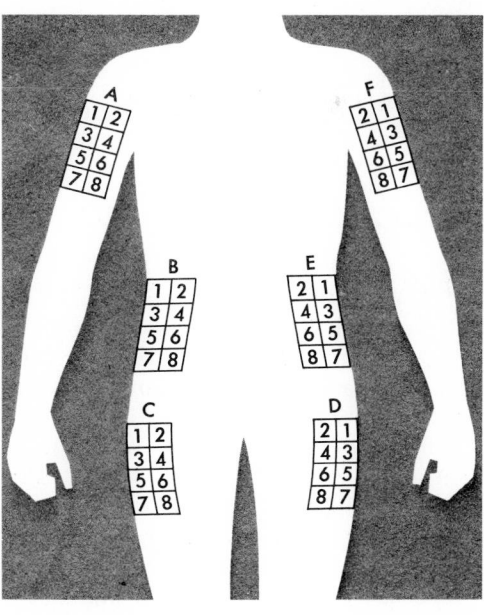

If Using 2 Varieties of Insulin in a Single Injection

1. Wipe off the vial tops with alcohol.
2. Inject air into the 1st vial; withdraw needle.
3. Inject air into the 2nd vial and withdraw prescribed amount of insulin.
4. Then withdraw prescribed amount of insulin from 1st vial.

To Sterilize Equipment

1. Take syringe apart and put in medium size strainer.
2. Put strainer in saucepan covered by 5 cm. (2 inches) of water. Boil 10 minutes.
3. Pick up strainer. Pour water out of pan.
4. Shake strainer and put back in pan.
5. Assemble syringe and attach needle.

Alcohol Method

1. Immerse syringe with needle attached into 4-ounce bottle of alcohol with cotton placed in bottom of bottle to protect the needle.
2. Prior to using, remove all traces of alcohol by pushing plunger back and forth before loading syringe. Alcohol may alter the effect of insulin and is also irritating when introduced under the skin.
3. Boil syringe and needle at least 1 time weekly.

Rapid Methods of Urine Testing
For Glucose (Sugar) and Ketones (Acetone)

Underlying Considerations

1. In diabetes, sugar may appear in the urine when the level of glucose in the blood rises above 160 mg./100 ml.
2. Urinary sugar (glycosuria) may appear when:
   a. Treatment is inadequate.
   b. Patient is not following his prescribed diet.
   c. Exercise is inadequate.
   d. Infection is present.
3. False negative tests may be obtained if:
   a. Deteriorated reagent tablets or reagent strips are used.
   b. The directions are not followed accurately.

Instructions to the Patient

Use the second-voiding technique to collect the urine specimen.

1. Void and discard the urine.
2. Drink several glasses of liquid.
3. Void into a clean container 30–45 minutes later—the second specimen reflects the status of glucose spillover into the urine more accurately.
4. Test this specimen.
5. Then agitate gently.

Tests for Sugar (Glucose)

A. *Clinitest**—uses a reagent tablet.
   1. *Two-drop method*—allows estimation of concentration of sugar up to 5%.
      a. Hold dropper vertically and place 2 drops (0.1 ml.) of urine in test tube.

* Clinitest is a product of Ames Company, Division Miles Laboratories, Inc., Elkhart, Indiana 46514.

b. Rinse dropper. Add 10 drops (0.5 ml.) of water in test tube.
c. Add 1 Clinitest reagent tablet. *Do not shake test tube.*
d. Wait 15 seconds after boiling stops.
e. Compare color of urine with appropriate color chart.
   Use only the 2-drop method color scale which has 7 colors ranging in value from 0–5%.

2. *Five-drop method*
   a. Hold dropper vertically and place 5 drops of urine in test tube.
   b. Rinse dropper. Add 10 drops of water in test tube.
   c. Add 1 Clinitest tablet in test tube.
      (1) Watch while reaction takes place.
      (2) Do not shake test tube during reaction nor for 15 seconds after boiling inside test tube has stopped.
   d. Observe the solution in the test tube *while the reaction takes place and during the 15-second waiting period to detect pass through color changes caused by glycosuria over 2%.*
      (1) If the solution passes through orange and dark shades of green-brown it indicates more than 2% (4+) urine sugar is present.
      (2) Record as such without reference to color scale.
   e. After 15-second waiting period, shake test tube gently and compare with the color scale.
   f. Record results.

B. *Diastix**—reagent strip
   1. Dip reagent end of strip in urine specimen for 2 seconds and remove (or wet end of strip for 2 seconds by passing through urine stream).
   2. Tap edge of strip against side of urine container or sink to remove excess urine.
   3. Exactly 30 seconds after removing from urine, compare reagent side of strip to closest matching color block on package label.

C. *Tes-Tape***—reagent tape
   1. Dip part of the Tes-Tape into the urine.
   2. Expose to air 60 seconds—the enzyme requires oxygen for color development.
   3. Compare the darkest area with the color chart.

Tests for Acetone (Ketone bodies)

A. *Acetest**—reagent tablets
   1. Use freshly voided specimen—prolonged standing of urine specimen encourages bacterial growth which can lead to changes in the number of ketone bodies.
   2. Place tablet on a piece of white paper.
   3. Place 1 drop of urine on tablet.
   4. Compare urine ketone test results to color chart after 30 seconds.

B. *Ketostix**—reagent strips
   1. Dip test area in freshly voided specimen or pass it briefly through the urinary stream.
   2. Remove immediately.
   3. Wait 15 seconds. Compare color of test strip with the color chart.

---

* Diastix, Acetest and Ketostix are products of Ames Company, Division of Miles Laboratories, Inc., Elkhart, Indiana 46514.
** Tes-Tape is a product of Eli Lilly and Company, Indianapolis, Indiana 46225.

Combined (Ketone-Glucose) Reagent Strip

Keto-Diastix*—combined ketone-glucose reagent strip

1. Dip reagent end of strip in urine specimen for 2 seconds and remove (or wet the end of strip for 2 seconds by passing through urine stream).
2. Tap edge of strip against side of urine container to remove excess urine.
3. Exactly 15 seconds after removing from urine, compare ketone test area on reagent side of strip to closest matching color block on package label; exactly 30 seconds after removing from urine, compare glucose test area on reagent side of strip to closest matching color block on the glucose section of the package label.

4. Disorders of the Adrenal Glands
THE ADRENAL GLANDS

Composition

A. *Medulla*
1. Is not necessary to maintain life but enables a person to cope with stress.
2. Secretes 2 hormones:
   a. Epinephrine
      (1) Acts on alpha and beta receptors.
      (2) Increases contractility and excitability of heart muscle, leading to increased cardiac output.
      (3) Facilitates blood flow to muscles, brain and viscera.
      (4) Enhances blood sugar—by stimulating conversion of glycogen to glucose in liver and decreasing uptake of glucose by muscle.
      (5) Inhibits smooth muscle contraction.
   b. Norepinephrine
      (1) Acts primarily on alpha receptors.
      (2) Increases peripheral vascular resistance leading to increases in diastolic and systolic blood pressure.

B. *Cortex*
1. Is essential to life.
2. Secretes adrenocortical hormones—originates in chemical, cholesterol.
   a. Cortisol (glucocorticoids): cortisone and hydrocortisone
      (1) Enhances protein catabolism and inhibits protein synthesis.
      (2) Antagonizes action of insulin.
      (3) Increases synthesis of glucose by liver.
      (4) Influences defense mechanisms of body and its reaction to stress.
      (5) Influences emotional reaction.
   b. Mineralocorticoids
      (1) Aldosterone—supplied by adrenal cortex.
      (2) Desoxycorticosterone—usually not present in significant amounts.
      (3) Regulates reabsorption of sodium cation.
      (4) Regulates excretion of potassium cation by renal tubules.
   c. Adrenosterones (adrenal androgens)

---

* Keto-Diastix is a product of Ames Company, Division Miles Laboratories, Inc., Elkhart, Indiana 46514.

HYPERFUNCTION OF THE ADRENAL MEDULLA

Pheochromocytoma

Pheochromocytoma is a neoplasm associated with hyperfunction of the adrenal medulla.

Clinical Manifestations

1. Variable symptoms depend upon whether the tumor secretes epinephrine or norepinephrine.
2. Hypertension may be paroxysmal or chronic.
   Chronic form may be difficult to differentiate from "essential hypertension."
3. Tachycardia, excessive perspiration, tremor, pallor or face flushing, nervousness and hyperglycemia.
4. Polyuria, nausea, vomiting, diarrhea and abdominal pain, paresthesia in extremities.

Diagnostic Evaluation

1. If there is sympathetic overactivity along with marked elevation of blood pressure, pheochromocytoma is strongly suspected.
2. Administration of certain drugs produces certain changes in arterial pressure.
   a. Provocative drugs—stimulate a sharp rise in arterial pressure: (histamine, tyramine, tetraethylammonium chloride).
   b. Adrenergic blocking drugs—produce a sharp fall in arterial pressure—phentolamine (Regitine).
3. Vanillylmandelic acid (VMA) determination:
   a. Determinations of catecholamines in urine and blood offer an effective test for overactivity of adrenal medulla.
   b. Normal urinary values: 2–6 mg./24 hrs.

Treatment

Surgery—excision of the tumor (adrenalectomy)—See page 666.

Cushing's Syndrome

Cushing's syndrome is a disease produced by hyperactivity of the adrenal cortex.

Etiology

1. Cushing's syndrome results mainly from the hypersecretion of cortisol.
2. The disorder may be caused by:
   a. An adenoma
   b. A neoplasm of the adrenal cortex
   c. Hyperplasia of both glands due to overstimulation of the adrenal cortex by ACTH

Diagnostic Evaluation

1. Excessive plasma cortisol levels
2. An increase in blood sugar—diabetes
3. A decrease in concentration of potassium in the blood
4. A reduction in the number of blood eosinophils

5. Elevation in the urine level of 17-hydroxycorticoids and 17-ketogenic steroids
6. Elevation of plasma ACTH in those patients having a pituitary tumor

Clinical Manifestations

A. *In children*
   1. Precocious puberty
   2. Affected growth rate

B. *Females*
   1. "Virilism" or masculinization
      a. Hirsutism—excessive growth of hair on the face
      b. Breasts—atrophy
      c. Clitoris—enlarges
      d. Voice—masculine
   2. In utero—possible hermaphrodite
   3. Menses—irregular and scanty; libido lost

C. *Adult* ("central type obesity")
   1. "Buffalo hump" in neck and supraclavicular area
   2. Heavy trunk; thin extremities
   3. Skin—fragile and thin; striae and ecchymosis, acne
   4. Face—rounded, plethoric, oily
   5. Muscles—wasted due to excessive catabolism
   6. Osteoporosis—characteristic kyphosis, backache
   7. Mental disturbances—mood changes, psychosis
   8. Increased susceptibility to infections
   9. Hypertension, edema

Objectives of Treatment and Nursing Management

A. *To remove the cause.*
   1. Tumor (adrenal or pituitary)—should be removed or treated with irradiation.
   2. Hyperplasia of adrenals—calls for an adrenalectomy.

B. *To administer replacement therapy.*
   1. Adrenalectomy patients require replacement therapy with the following:
      a. A glucocorticoid—cortisone
      b. A mineralocorticoid—fludrocortisone (Florinef)
      c. Extra salt
   2. Following pituitary irradiation or hypophysectomy, patients may require adrenal replacement plus thyroid and gonadal replacement therapy.
   3. Protein anabolic steroids may facilitate protein replacement—potassium stores are usually repleted rapidly.

C. *To observe the appearance and behavior of the patient.*
   Record all pertinent observations that may assist the physician in making the diagnosis.

D. *To assist with diagnostic tests.*
   1. Explain to the patient the necessity for the many blood and urine studies.
   2. Recognize the need for accurately recording input of food and fluid and output of urine.

E. *To encourage the patient to eat the prescribed diet.*

> Explain to the patient that his diet (low sodium and high potassium) is as significant to his treatment as his medications.

a. Foods high in potassium—meats, glandular meats, fish, most vegetables and fruits, legumes

b. Foods low in sodium—cereal, meat, fruits, squash, potatoes, lettuce, honey, unsalted butter

F. *To be aware of the psychological manifestations of this syndrome.*

1. Identify those situations which are disturbing to the patient; record these on the nursing care plan as situations to be avoided.
2. Be alert for evidence of depression; in some instances this has progressed to suicide; therefore, mood changes are most important.
3. Report when depression continues after surgery.
4. Understand the emotional stress in female patients who manifest masculinization tendencies.
5. Reassure the patient who has benign adenoma or hyperplasia that, with proper treatment, evidence of masculinization can be reversed.
6. Note that weakness is a frustrating experience in a patient who heretofore has been active.

G. *To prepare the patient for adrenalectomy when the diagnosis and treatment plan have been determined (see p. 666).*

ADDISON'S DISEASE

Addison's disease is a condition due to hypofunction of the adrenal glands.

Cause

A deficiency of cortical hormones due to:

1. Destruction of adrenal cortex
2. Atrophy—following prolonged steroid therapy or secondary to pituitary hypofunction

Clinical Manifestations

Due to (1) disturbance of sodium and potassium metabolism and (2) depletion of sodium and water—urine loss, severe chronic dehydration.

1. Muscular weakness, fatigue, weight loss
2. Gastrointestinal problems—anorexia, nausea, vomiting, diarrhea, constipation, abdominal pain
3. Low blood pressure, low blood sugar, low B.M.R., low blood sodium
4. High potassium
5. After a while, symptoms worsen and the patient is forced to go to bed.
   a. Skin color changes to tan, bronze or brown—diffuse or patchy, freckling.
   b. Mucous membranes also discolor—bluish black or gray.
   c. Mental changes occur—depression, irritability, anxiety, apprehension.
6. Normal responses to stress are lacking.

Diagnostic Evaluation

A. *Blood Studies*
1. Hypoglycemia—decrease in sugar concentration
2. Hyponatremia—decrease in sodium concentration
3. Hyperkalemia—increase in potassium concentration
4. Lymphoid hyperplasia
5. Low fasting plasma cortisol levels

B. *Urine Studies*

   24-hour specimen for 17-ketosteroids, 17-hydroxycorticoids and 17-ketogenic steroids —all values decreased

C. *Injection of a Potent Pituitary Adrenocorticotropic Hormone to Artificially Stimulate Adrenals*
1. Normal response—normal rise in plasma cortisol and urinary 17-ketosteroids
2. In Addison's disease
   a. Decrease in circulating eosinophils
   b. Increase in uric acid excretion in about 4 hours
   c. No rise in plasma cortisol and urinary 17-ketosteroids

Treatment and Nursing Management

1. Attempt to restore normal electrolyte balance.
   a. Administer high sodium, low potassium diet and fluids.
   b. Give hydrocortisone (17-hydroxycorticosterone).
      (1) Addisonian crisis—inject hydrocortisone 21-sodium succinate (Solu-Cortef) or hydrocortisone phosphate, 50–100 mg. via I.V.
      (2) Long-term basis—hydrocortisone in doses of 30–40 mg. plus DDCA or Florinef.
2. Detect early signs of *Addisonian crisis.*
   a. Nausea, vomiting, cyanosis
   b. Sudden drop in blood pressure
   c. Very high temperature
3. Recognize that circulatory collapse may result from the following:
   a. Overexertion
   b. Exposure to cold
   c. Acute infection
   d. Decrease in salt intake
   e. Excessive diarrhea
4. Be on guard for later signs of Addisonian crisis.
   a. Fall in systolic pressure to 40–50 mm. Hg
   b. Weak pulse and cold clammy skin
5. Initiate treatment immediately
   a. Administer blood transfusions to replace blood volume.
   b. Start intravenous flow of sodium chloride solution to replace sodium ions.
   c. Give hydrocortisone.
   d. Inject circulatory stimulants.
6. Assess vital signs frequently for deviation.
   a. Monitor vital signs and blood pressure; a drop in blood pressure may suggest impending crisis.
   b. Record the temperature hourly since an elevation may easily be precipitated.

7. Observe carefully the emotional status of the patient.
   a. Promote rest periods to avoid overexertion.
   b. Control the temperature of the room to avoid sharp deviations in patient's temperature.
   c. Maintain a quiet, peaceful environment; avoid loud talking and noisy radios.
8. Record conscientiously the salt intake and urine output.
   Inform the patient's family as well as all nursing personnel who come in contact with this patient that all urine must be saved for a 24-hour urine specimen.
9. Administer optimum physical nursing care.
   a. Do not allow the patient who is in adrenal crisis to do anything for himself.
   b. Assist him in moving and turning, in feeding, and in providing mouth care.
   c. Limit conversation to that essential to his care.
10. Protect the patient from infection.
    a. Control his contacts so that infectious organisms are not transmitted.
    b. Protect him from drafts, dampness, etc.
11. Be familiar with the nature of hormonal replacement required by the individual patient.
    a. Some are controlled with cortisol (via mouth: 5–15 mg. t.i.d.).
    b. Other patients require additional electrolyte-type medications to maintain homeostasis.
    c. Determine the method of administration of drug for the particular patient: most are taken by mouth, but some are administered intramuscularly.
    d. Note whether there is an effect on fluid retention—weigh patient frequently and record such weight.
12. Inform the patient of the nature of long-term therapy for adrenocortical insufficiency.
    a. Inform the patient that therapy must be continued for the rest of his life.
    b. Emphasize the importance of taking more hormones when he is under stress.
    c. Suggest that he carry an identification card on which is indicated the type of medication he is receiving and the phone number of his physician.

PRIMARY ALDOSTERONISM

Primary aldosteronism is a disorder caused by hypersecretion of the adrenal cortex.

Diagnostic Evaluation and Clinical Manifestations

1. A profound decline in blood levels of potassium (hypokalemia) and hydrogen ions (alkalosis)—results in muscle weakness and an inability of kidneys to acidify or concentrate urine leading to excess volume of urine (polyuria)
   a. Increase in pH
   b. Increase in CO_2-combining power
2. A decline in hydrogen ions (alkalosis)—results in tetany, paresthesias
3. An elevation in blood sodium (hypernatremia)—resulting in excessive thirst (polydipsia) and arterial hypertension
4. Hypertension

Treatment

Removal of adrenal tumor—adrenalectomy (see p. 666).

MANAGEMENT OF THE PATIENT HAVING AN ADRENALECTOMY

Preoperative Care

Similar to general surgery of the abdomen (see p. 47).

Postoperative Care

1. Similar to that of an abdominal operation (see p. 49).
2. May require temporary administration of hydrocortisone or similar compounds in large amounts.
3. For removal of pheochromocytoma:
   a. Because of manipulation of tumor during surgery, there may be extreme fluctuations of blood pressure.
   b. Upon ligations of vessels from tumor an abrupt fall of blood pressure may result. Administer large amounts of epinephrine intravenously.

NURSING ALERT: Be prepared to monitor blood pressure frequently for 24 to 48 hours and to regulate vasopressor intravenous medications in order to stabilize the blood pressure.

---

4. Monitor vital signs including blood pressure and central venous pressure up to 48 hours—to detect early changes which may lead to cardiovascular collapse.

STEROID THERAPY *

Classification of Steroids
(by major metabolic effects on body)

1. Mineralocorticoids
   a. Concerned with sodium and water retention and potassium excretion
   b. Example—fludrocortisone (Florinef)
2. Glucocorticoids
   a. Concerned with metabolic effects, including carbohydrate metabolism
   b. Examples—cortisol and corticosterone
3. Sex Hormones
   a. Important when secreted in large amounts or when the growth of hormone-sensitive cancers are stimulated
   b. Examples
      Androgens—dehydroepiandrosterone, testosterone
      Estrogens—estradiol
      Progestins—progesterone

Effects of Glucocorticoids

1. Antagonizes action of insulin—promotes gluconeogenesis which increases carbohydrate metabolism (increases glucose reserve).
2. Increases breakdown of protein (inhibits protein synthesis).

---

* Source acknowledgment: Hamdi, M. E.: Nursing intervention for patients receiving corticosteroid therapy. *In* Kintzel, K. C. (ed.): Advanced Concepts in Clinical Nursing. Philadelphia, J. B. Lippincott, 1971.

3. Increases breakdown of fatty acids.
4. Suppresses inflammation, inhibits scar formation, blocks allergic responses.
5. Decreases number of circulating eosinophils and leukocytes.
6. Exerts a permissive action on all effects caused by catecholamines.
7. Exerts a permissive action on functioning of central nervous system.
8. Inhibits release of adrenocorticotropin.

> IN SUMMARY: Glucocorticoids give an organism the capacity to resist all types of noxious stimuli and environmental change.

Uses of Steroids

1. Physiologically—to correct deficiencies or malfunction of a particular endocrine organ or system, e.g., Addison's disease.
2. Diagnostically—to determine proper functioning of the endocrine system.
3. Pharmacologically—to treat the following:
   a. Rheumatoid arthritis
   b. Acute rheumatic fever
   c. Blood conditions
      (1) Idiopathic thrombocytopenic purpura
      (2) Leukemia
      (3) Hemolytic anemia
   d. Allergic conditions—bronchial asthma, allergic rhinitis
   e. Dermatologic problems—drug rashes, giant hives, atopic dermatitis
   f. Ocular diseases—conjunctivitis, uveitis
   g. Collagen diseases—lupus erythematosus, periarteritis nodosa, rheumatoid arthritis
   h. Gastrointestinal problems—ulcerative colitis
   i. Organ-transplant recipients—as an immunosuppressive
   j. Other conditions—gout, multiple sclerosis

Preparing the Patient to Receive Steroid Therapy

1. Require a thorough physical examination and medical history.
2. Determine contraindications for such therapy.
   a. Peptic ulcer
   b. Diabetes mellitus
   c. Viral infections
3. Take a tuberculin test to determine need for antituberculin drugs.
   If this is not done prior to steroid therapy, the patient's hypersensitivity to tuberculin may be suppressed.
4. Assess the patient's own level of steroid secretion, if possible.
5. Explain the nature of the therapy, what is required of the patient, how long he is to be on steroid medications, what adverse signs to watch for, etc.

Choice of Steroid and Method of Administration (Table 10-5)

1. Determined by physician.
2. May be given for local effects or systemic effects.
3. May be given in a wide variety of methods.

TABLE 10-5. CORTICOSTEROID PREPARATIONS

USP Name	Structure of Synthetic Analog	Trade Names	Approx. Equiv. Dose (mg.)	Anti-infl. Potency	Mineralocort. Potency	Usual Starting Dose (mg./day) Life-threatening Illness	Usual Starting Dose (mg./day) Moderately Severe Illness
Hydrocortisone (cortisol)	—		20.0	1.0	1.0	—	80–120
Cortisone	—		25.0	0.8	0.8	—	100–150
Prednisone	delta-1-cortisone	Meticorten Deltasone	5.0	3.0–5.0	0.8	50–100	20–30
Prednisolone	delta-1-cortisol	Meticortelone Hydeltra Delta-Cortef	5.0	3.0–5.0	0.8	50–100	20–30
Triamcinolone	9-alpha fluoro-16-alpha-hydroxy-prednisolone	Aristocort Kenacort	4.0	3.0–5.0	0	40–80	16–24
Dexamethasone	9-alpha fluoro-16-alpha-methyl-prednisolone	Decadron Deronil Gammacorten Hexadrol	0.75	20.0–30.0	0	7.5–15.0	3.0–4.5
Methylprednisolone	6-alpha-methyl-prednisolone	Medrol	4.0	3.0–5.0	0	40–80	16–24
Fluprednisolone	6-alpha fluoro-prednisolone	Alphadrol	1.5	10.0–20.0	0	15–30	6–9
Betamethasone	9-alpha fluoro-16-beta-methyl-prednisolone	Celestone	0.6	20.0–30.0	0	6–12	2.4–3.6
Paramethasone	6-alpha fluoro-16-alpha-methyl-prednisolone 21-acetate	Haldrone	2.0	8.0–12.0	0	20–40	8–12

From Rosenfeld, M. G. (ed.): *Manual of Medical Therapeutics*, 20th ed. Boston, Little, Brown and Co. 1971, pg. 391.

Nursing Management of Patients Receiving Steroid Therapy

1. Know the routes by which steroids are given.
    a. Ascertain advantages of the method chosen for the particular patient.
    b. Determine what is expected of the medication in a particular situation.
    c. Be informed regarding side effects and untoward manifestations.
    d. NOTE:
        (1) Local medications to the skin using occlusive dressings over a prolonged period of time to a large area leads to decrease in plasma cortisol.
        (2) Local administration to the eye over a prolonged period leads to increased eye pressure, corneal ulceration.
    e. Recognize that it is necessary to understand pharmacologic action of a particular steroid before planning the scheduled doses.
        (1) How frequently it can be given.
        (2) How late in the day it may be administered.
        (3) Whether every other day is sufficient, etc.
            Patients on intermittent therapy have few side effects.
2. Be aware of the problems encountered during periods when steroids are being withdrawn or lowered in dosage.
    a. Associate symptoms of tiredness, muscular weakness and lethargy with drug withdrawal.
    b. Report any stress situations during this time, such as surgery, a family crisis, etc.
    c. Instruct the patient why it may be necessary to save all urine for 24 hours (for determination of 11-hydroxycorticosteroid level).
3. Monitor carefully the patient who is on intravenous corticosteroid therapy.
    a. Determine the flow rate of fluids necessary to give a precise amount of medication.
    b. Observe the tissues, catheter site, flow rate, fluid level and patient's response at frequent intervals to be sure the system is functioning well.
    c. Note signs and symptoms indicative of adrenal crisis—restlessness, weakness, headache, nausea, vomiting, diarrhea, and falling blood pressure.

Potential Side Effects of Steroid Therapy

A. *Classification*
    1. Mineralocorticoid
        a. Sodium and water retention
            Edema, weight gain, elevated blood pressure
        b. Potassium depletion
            Weakness, tiredness, alkalosis
    2. Glucocorticoid
        a. Masking of infections
        b. Osteoporosis
        c. Steroid diabetes
        d. Exacerbation of tuberculosis.

B. *Control or Avoidance of Side Effects*
    1. Mineralocorticoid
        Use triamcinolone or newer synthetic steroids. (Some of the newer synthetics have less sodium retention but have other side effects.)
    2. Glucocorticoid
        Difficult to separate anti-flammatory effects from sodium-retaining effects.

Acceptable and Expected Side Effects

Nature of Effect	Action
Facial mooning (Cushing's Syndrome)	May be minimized by restricted caloric intake.
Weight gain	Restrict caloric intake; may require a switch in steroid medication.
Edema	May require diuretics and potassium.
Potassium Loss	Prescribe diuretics and potassium.
	May require switch to a fluorinated synthetic. Administer potassium supplement.
Acne	Treat with topical medications.
Increased frequency and nocturia	Check for evidence of genitourinary infection or diabetes mellitus; urinalysis.
Insomnia, headache, fatigue	Treat symptomatically.

Undesirable and Unacceptable Side Effects

Nature of Effect	Action (Report to Physician)
Allergic reaction to ACTH or steroid	Withdraw drug promptly. Substitute synthetic ACTH or steroid.
Cardiovascular system effect: Hypertension Thromboembolic complications Arteritis	Suggest reduction in dosage of steroids.
Infection	Suggest antimicrobial medications as indicated.
Eye complications: Glaucoma Corneal lesions	Refer to ophthalmologist.
Musculoskeletal effects	Suggest sex hormones—synthetic estrogens and/or androgens. Suggest calcium supplement.
Adrenal insufficiency (after prolonged use) as manifested by peripheral circulatory collapse—in upright position.	Administer hydrocortisone promptly (intravenously). The following day give steroid replacement.

Advice and Admonitions for Patients on Long-term Steroids

1. Recognize that steroids are valuable and useful medications but if taken longer than 2 weeks, certain side effects may be noticed.
2. "Acceptable" side effects may include weight gain (perhaps due to water retention), acne, headaches, fatigue and increased urinary frequency.
3. "Unacceptable" side effects which are to be reported to the physician: dizziness when rising from chair or bed (postural hypotension indicative of adrenal insufficiency), nausea, vomiting, thirst, abdominal pain or pain of any type.
4. Additional side effect which are reportable are: convulsive seizures, feelings of depression or nervousness or development of an infection.

5. If the patient has a fall or is in an auto accident, his condition may precipitate adrenal failure. He requires an immediate injection of 100 mg. of hydrocortisone phosphate. (Long-term patients should wear a Medic Alert tag and have a kit with hydrocortisone.)

Careful Clinical Surveillance by the Nurse

Objective: to detect early signs of side effects from steroid therapy.
1. Because steroids may affect the circulating blood there is decreased eosinophils and reticulocytes, increased red cells and increased incidence of thrombophlebitis and infection.
   a. Encourage patient to avoid crowds and the possibility of exposure to infection.
   b. Utilize exercise schedules to prevent stasis.
   c. Be aware of the fact that cardinal symptoms of inflammation may be masked.
   d. Instruct all personnel coming in contact with this patient to wash hands thoroughly and practice asepsis meticulously.
2. Because steroids may cause weight gain and an increase in appetite determine whether the patient needs assistance in dietary control.
3. Because steroids affect the musculoskeletal system there is potassium depletion and muscular weakness. (Steroids cause increased output of calcium and phosphorus which leads to osteoporosis.)
   a. Be on the alert for the possibility of pathologic fractures; stress safety measures to prevent injury.
   b. Administer a diet high in calcium and protein.
   c. Recommend a program of activities of daily living, normal range of motion for the bedridden, etc.
4. Because mineralocorticoid differs from other steroids there is sodium retention and potassium depletion: edema, weight gain, potassium depletion.
   a. Restrict sodium intake and increase potassium intake.
   b. Check blood pressure frequently and weigh patient daily.
   c. Observe for evidence of edema.
5. Because steroids interfere with fibroblasts and granulation tissue there is altered response to injury, resulting in impaired growth and delayed healing.
   a. Admonish the patient to avoid injury; stress safety precautions.
   b. Observe daily the healing process of wounds, particularly surgical wounds, in order to recognize the potential for wound dehiscence.
6. Because steroids precipitate gluconeogenesis and insulin antagonism, this results in hyperglycemia, glucosuria, decreased carbohydrate tolerance.
   Check urine for evidence of glucose.
7. Because steroids affect protein metabolism, there may be negative nitrogen balance.
   Administer a high protein, high carbohydrate diet.
8. Because steroids cause an increase in secretion of gastric hydrochloric acid and have an inhibiting effect on secretion of mucus in the stomach they may aggravate an existing peptic ulcer or create an ulcer.
   a. Encourage patient to take steroids with milk or food.
   b. Be on guard for early evidence of gastric hemorrhage such as melena, blood in vomitus.
9. Because steroids may alter behavior patterns, increase excitability and affect the central nervous system, watch for convulsive seizures (especially in children).

      a. Avoid overstimulating situations.

      b. Recognize and report any mood deviation from the usual behavior patterns.

      c. Report unusual behavior, haunting dreams, withdrawal or suicidal tendencies.

10. Because steroids affect the hypothalamic-pituitary-adrenal system, this in turn affects the individual's ability to respond to stress.

      a. Recommend that the patient carry an identification card at all times indicating that he is on steroid therapy and including the name of his physician and instructions for emergency treatment.

      b. Advise the patient to avoid extremes of temperature, as well as infections and upsetting situations.

5. Disorders of the Pituitary

THE PITUITARY

The *pituitary gland* is called the master gland of the endocrine system because it controls hormone production of the other endocrine glands. It lies in the sella turcica at the base of the brain and is connected to the hypothalamus by the hypophyseal (pituitary) stalk.

1. *Anterior lobe*—produces at least 7 hormones, 6 of which have their primary action on other endocrine glands plus release hormones that control the posterior lobe.

2. *Posterior lobe*—believed to be responsible for storage of the antidiuretic, oxytocic and vasopressor hormones produced in the hypothalamus.

HYPERPITUITARISM

Hyperpituitarism results from an excessive amount of growth hormone secreted by the pituitary gland.

Predisposing Factors

1. Overactivity of the eosinophilic portion of the anterior lobe of the pituitary.
2. Effects of a benign adenoma (tumor).

Types of Hyperpituitarism

1. *Gigantism*

      Hyperfunction of the pituitary, causing a generalized increase in size, particularly in the long bones in children before the epiphyseal lines close.

2. *Acromegaly*

      a. Excessive secretion of growth hormone after epiphyseal closure, causing a chronic disease characterized by enlargement of bone, cartilage and soft tissues of the body.

      b. Causes

         (1) Increase in size and function of a portion of the anterior lobe of the pituitary gland.

         (2) Eosinophilic tumor of the pituitary gland.

HYPOPITUITARISM
(Simmonds' Disease, Pituitary Cachexia)

Hypopituitarism is pituitary insufficiency resulting from destruction of the anterior lobe of the pituitary gland.

Panhypopituitarism (Simmonds' Disease) is total absence of all pituitary secretions.

Clinical Manifestations

1. Severe asthenia
2. Emaciation
3. Reduced metabolism
4. Low temperature and blood pressure

Cause

Total destruction of the anterior lobe of the pituitary by trauma, tumor, hemorrhage.

PITUITARY TUMORS

Types of Pituitary Tumors

1. *Chromophobe Adenoma*—tumor of the anterior pituitary gland of adults.
   a. Comprises 90% of pituitary tumors.
   b. Produces failing vision, optic atrophy, bilateral hemianopsia, enlargement of sella turcica and endocrine disturbances.
2. *Eosinophilic Adenomas*—endocrine secretion of tumor produces gigantism in children and acromegaly in adults.
3. *Basophilic Adenoma*—rare.

DIABETES INSIPIDUS

Diabetes Insipidus is a disorder of water metabolism caused by deficiency of vasopressin, the antidiuretic hormone (ADH) secreted by the posterior pituitary.

Etiology

1. Unknown
2. Secondary causes—head trauma, neoplasm, surgical ablation or interstitial irradiation of pituitary gland.

Clinical Manifestations

1. Marked polyuria—daily output of 5–25 liters of very dilute urine; appearance of urine like that of water with a specific gravity of 1.001–1.005.
2. Polydipsia (intense thirst); 4–40 liters of fluid daily; patient has a craving for cold water.

Diagnostic Evaluation

Fluid Deprivation Test

Objective: to restrict water intake and observe changes in urine volume and concentration.

1. Fluids deprived for 8–12 hours or until 3% of body weight is lost.
2. Plasma and urinary osmolality studies are determined at beginning and end of test—inability to increase specific gravity and osmolality of urine are characteristic of diabetes insipidus.

Treatment and Nursing Management

Objectives: to replace vasopressin (usually a life-long therapeutic program).
  to search for and correct underlying intracranial pathology.

1. Give antidiuretic hormone, vasopressin tannate (Pitressin Tannate)—reduces urinar
   volume for 24–48 hours.
   a. Warm vial—medication is in oil and warming makes administration easier.
   b. Shake bottle vigorously before administering drug—active hormone settles to th
      bottom of the oil.
   c. Give in evening—maximum results obtained during sleep, or
2. Give synthetic lysine vasopressin as a nasal spray.
   a. Nasal insufflation administered every 3–6 hours.
   b. Watch for chronic rhinopharyngitis.
3. Administer chlorpropamide (Diabinese)—increases free water absorption.
   a. May be used as an antidiuretic in mild cases to potentiate action of vasopressin
   b. Warn the patient of possible hypoglycemic reactions.
   c. Give supplementary potassium—thiazides produce potassium depletion.
4. Weigh the patient frequently.
5. Support the patient undergoing studies for a cranial lesion (see p. 748).

HYPOPHYSECTOMY

Hypophysectomy is removal of the pituitary.

Indications

1. Primary neoplasms (tumors) of the pituitary gland
2. Diabetic retinopathy
   a. Used to halt progress of hemorrhagic diabetic retinopathy and to avoid blindness
   b. Also reduces insulin requirements.
3. Relief of bone pain secondary to metastasis of malignant lesions of breast and
   prostate
      Alters hormonal milieu of body to create a hormonal environment hostile to con-
      tinued growth of a neoplasm.

Methods of Pituitary Ablation (Removal)

1. Extirpative hypophysectomy—done by transfrontal, subcranial or oronasal-trans-
   sphenoidal approaches
2. Hypophyseal stalk section
3. Implantation of radioactive yttrium
4. Radiation x-ray—proton irradiation from a cyclotron
5. Destruction with stereotaxic radio frequency (heat) or cryosurgery (freezing)

Complications

The absence of pituitary gland alters function of many parts of the body.

1. Patient will need substitution therapy with adrenal steroids (hydrocortisone,
   20–30 mg. daily).
2. Patient will need substitution with thyroid (thyroxin, 0.2–0.3 mg. daily).

3. Pitressin is usually given for a week to months after operation.
4. Menstruation ceases and infertility occurs almost always after total or nearly total ablation. Testosterone or estrogen may be given.
5. See p. 732 for the nursing management of the patient undergoing cranial surgery.

6. Disorders of Purine Metabolism

GOUT

Gout is a metabolic disease of purine metabolism in which there is excessive accumulation of uric acid in the blood and eventual deposition of uric acid crystals in various tissues.

1. *Uric acid*—end product of purine metabolism
2. *Hyperuricemia*—persistent elevation of urates in the system
3. *Tophi*—deposits of urates in the tissues about the joints or on the ear; development of tophi related to duration of disease, degree of hyperuricemia and renal function status

Incidence

Affects chiefly men over 30.

Etiology

Hereditary factor present—mode of genetic transmission not established.

Types of Gout

1. *Primary*—basic problem appears to be a genetic defect in purine metabolism.
2. *Secondary*—hyperuricemia is produced by increasing breakdown of nucleic acids in certain diseases (blood dyscrasias) or because of interference with renal excretion of urate.
   Prolonged ingestion of thiazides (diuretic agents) may produce clinical gout.

Clinical Manifestations

1. Sudden onset of severe pain in one or more peripheral joints—may be accompanied by intense inflammation.
   a. Metatarsophalangeal joint of great toe is most susceptible.
   b. Joints of feet, ankles, knees, wrist and elbow commonly affected.
2. Fever 38.3–39.4°C. (101–103°F.).
3. Attacks, involving the same joints, tend to recur; variable lengths of time between attacks.

Diagnostic Evaluation

1. Sudden attack of severe pain in one or more peripheral joints in a previously healthy male.
2. Elevation of serum uric acid (above 7.0 mg.).
3. Sodium urate crystals become deposited in the joints, cartilage, subcutaneous and periarticular tissues, bone and kidneys.
4. Identification of urate crystals in synovial fluid—obtained by arthrocentesis (aspiration of fluid from a joint cavity).

5. Elevated erythrocyte sedimentation rate and white blood count—in acute attack.
6. X-ray findings—presence of tophi and roentgenographic evidence of urate deposits in bone (late manifestations).
7. Other diagnostic features
   a. Positive family history for gout
   b. Unexplained proteinuria and hypertension
   c. Passage of renal stones
   d. Patient taking thiazide for non-gouty conditions

Treatment and Nursing Management

Objective: to prevent the development of chronic gouty arthritis.

A. *Acute Attack of Gout*
   1. Give colchicine early in attack—suppresses inflammatory manifestations of acute gout; useful in establishing diagnosis since it gives dramatic relief if patient has gout.
      a. 0.5–0.65 mg. colchicine given hourly until pain is relieved or until there is onset of gastrointestinal disturbances (nausea, vomiting, abdominal cramping, diarrhea).
      b. *Colchicine produces diarrhea*—stop drug temporarily until diarrhea subsides. Give paregoric (4 ml.) after each loose stool.
      c. Give maintenance dose of colchicine as soon as diarrhea stops as a prophylactic agent against recurrent gouty arthritis.
   2. Consider alternative therapy
      Phenylbutazone (Butazolidin) or oxyphenbutazone or indomethacin (Indocin) are alternate drugs given during the acute stage of gout.
   3. Give analgesic (codeine, meperidine) for severe pain until specific drug is effective.

TABLE 10-6. LOW PURINE DIET *

Purines are derived from ingested food and from the breakdown of body proteins. Purines are also synthesized in the liver. A low purine diet is seldom used but it is advocated that patients with high blood uric acid levels avoid foods high in purine content.

Foods Highest in Purines	Foods High in Purine	Foods Lowest in Purines
Sweetbreads	Meat	Fruits
Anchovies	Poultry	Vegetables (except those
Sardines in oil	Fish	listed)
Liver (calf, beef)	Lobster, crabs, oysters	Most breads, cereals and
Kidneys	Meat soups and broth	cereal products
Meat extracts	Beans, dried	Milk
Gravy	Peas, dried	Cheese
	Lentils, dried	Eggs
	Spinach	Fish roe
	Oatmeal	Nuts
	Wheat germ and bran	Fats
		Sugars, sirups, sweets
		Gelatin
		Milk and fruit desserts
		Vegetable and cream soups

* Foods listed from Church, C. F., and Church, H. N.: Food Values of Portions Commonly Used. Philadelphia, J. B. Lippincott, 1970.

4. Encourage the patient to stay on bedrest for 24 hours after acute attack—early ambulation may precipitate a recurrence.
5. Advise the patient to avoid high purine foods (Table 10-6).
6. Encourage large fluid intake to maintain a high 24-hour urinary volume—urinary urate excretion increases 24 hours after introduction of uricosuric drugs and may lead to stone formation.

B. *Chronic Gouty Arthritis*
1. Give drug (uricosuric agent) to promote urinary acid elimination—acts on renal tubule to inhibit urate reabsorption and thereby increases urinary excretion of urate and lowers the serum urate level; prevents formation of new tophi and reduces size of those already present.
   a. Probenecid (Benemid)
      Side effects—headache, gastrointestinal disturbances, skin rash.
   b. Sulfinpyrazone (Anturane)
      Side effects—gastrointestinal disturbances (including peptic ulcer) skin rash, hematologic side effects.
   c. Give after meals or with antacids if there are gastric side effects.
2. Or give allopurinol (Zyloprim), a xanthine oxidase inhibitor—interferes with final stages of conversion of the products of purine metabolism to uric acid.
   Dosage based on serum urate determinations.
3. Encourage large fluid intake to maintain a high 24-hour urinary volume—urinary urate excretion increases 24 hours after introduction of uricosuric drugs and may lead to stone formation.
   a. Maintain an alkaline urine in patients with a history of stone formation.
   b. Give sodium bicarbonate or citrate solutions.

C. *During Prophylactic Period*
1. Give colchicine 0.5 mg. daily—as a prophylaxis against acute attack; suppresses joint symptoms.
2. Give uricosuric agent (see above) or allopurinol—to prevent further deposition of uric acid in joints.
   Colchicine and uricosuric agents are given in combination for indefinite periods of time.
3. Avoid specific foods or alcohol which the patient knows will precipitate an attack (see p. 676).
4. Give high fluid intake to maintain high urinary volume—minimizes urate precipitation in urinary tract.
5. Caution patient against fasting (to lose weight or when on alcoholic spree)—fasting has been found to increase the serum uric acid level.
   An obese patient should lose weight slowly—to avoid strain on involved joints.

BIBLIOGRAPHY

Thyroid

Books

Brunner, L. S., et al.: Textbook of Medical-Surgical Nursing, 2nd ed. Philadelphia, J. B. Lippincott, 1970, pp. 683–715.
Werner, S. C., and Ingbar, S. H. (eds.): The Thyroid, 3rd ed. New York, Harper & Row, 1971.

Articles

Ball, R.: Hypothyroidism. Nurs. Mirror, *135*:23–24, Oct. 6, 1972.
Becker, K. L.: Management of thyroid disorders. Postgrad. Med., *53*:60–65, Feb. 1973.
Grob, D.: Hypothyroidism. Hosp. Med., *8*:8–35, June 1972.
Hamburger, J. I., and Meier, D. A.: How to use modern thyroid function tests. Amer. Fam. Phys.,
    3:72–80, May 1971.

Endocrine, Diabetes Mellitus and Gout

Books

American Diabetes Association: Diabetes Mellitus: Diagnosis and Treatment. Vol. 3, New York,
    American Diabetes Association, 1971.
Boshell, B. R.: The Diabetic at Work and Play. Springfield, Charles C Thomas, 1971.
Brunner, L., et al.: Textbook of Medical-Surgical Nursing, 2nd ed. Philadelphia, J. B. Lippincott,
    1970, pp. 683–715.
Ellenberg, M., and Rifkin, H.: Diabetes Mellitus: Theory and Practice. New York, McGraw-Hill,
    1970.
Goldberg, M. F., and Fine, S. L. (eds.): Symposium on the Treatment of Diabetic Retinopathy.
    Washington, D.C., U.S. Government Printing Office, 1969.
Gormican, A.: Controlling Diabetes with Diet. Springfield, Charles C Thomas, 1971.
Lawrence, P. A.: Diabetes Mellitus. *In* Kintzel, K. C. (ed.): Advanced Concepts in Clinical Nurs-
    ing. Philadelphia, J. B. Lippincott, 1971, pp. 105–129.
Marble, A., et al.: Joslin's Diabetes Mellitus. Philadelphia, Lea & Febiger, 1971.
Traisman, H. S.: Management of Juvenile Diabetes Mellitus. St. Louis, C. V. Mosby, 1971.

Articles

Burke, E. L.: Insulin, injection—the site and the technique. Amer. J. Nurs., *72*:2194–2196, Dec.
    1972.
Cole, H. S., and Camerini-Davalos, R. N.: Diet therapy of diabetes mellitus. Med. Clin. N. Amer.,
    54:1577–1587, Nov. 1970.
Felig, P., and Bondy, P. K.: Symposium on diabetes mellitus. Med. Clin. N. Amer., *55*:791–1075,
    July 1971.
Ishmael, W. K.: Symposium: Gout. Clin. Orthop., *71*:3–98, July-Aug. 1970.
Johnson, E. S. B.: Understanding hyperuricemia: Nursing Implications. Nurs. Clin. N. Amer.,
    7:399–405, June 1972.
Klim, C. R., et al.: A study of the effects of hypoglycemic agents on vascular complications in
    patients with adult-onset diabetes. Diabetes, *19* (Suppl. 2), 747–830, Nov. 1970.
McFarlane, J., et al.: Two-drop and one-drop test for glycosuria. Amer. J. Nurs., *72*:939, May 1972.
Nickerson, D.: Teaching the hospitalized diabetic. Amer. J. Nurs., *72*:935–938, May 1972.
Randall, R. V. (ed.): Symposium on endocrine disorders. Med. Clin. N. Amer., *56*:841–1049, July
    1972.
Stuart, S.: Day-to-day living with diabetes. Amer. J. Nurs., *71*:1548–1550, August 1971.
Talbot, J. H.: Gout. Med. Clin. N. Amer., *54*:431–441, March 1970.

Adrenal Glands

Books

Brunner, L. S., et al.: Textbook of Medical-Surgical Nursing, 2nd ed. Philadelphia, J. B. Lippincott,
    1970, pp. 706–711.
Schneeberg, N. G.: Essentials of Clinical Endocrinology. St. Louis, C. V. Mosby, 1970.

Articles

Engelman, K.: Diagnosis and management of pheochromocytoma. Hosp. Med., 6:112–121, May 1970.

Gabrilove, J. L., and Nicolis, G. L.: Adrenocortical function and the glucocorticoids. Surg. Clin. N. Amer., 52:951–959, Aug. 1972.

Glenn, J. G.: Using corticosteroids. Amer. Fam. Phys., 3:96–100, May 1971.

Hamdi, M. E.: Nursing intervention for patients receiving corticosteroid therapy. *In* Kintzel, H. C. (ed.): Advanced Concepts in Clinical Nursing. Philadelphia, J. B. Lippincott, 1971, pp. 236–246.

Nursing care of patients with pheochromocytoma. A Nursing Clinical Conference, Dept. of Nursing, Bethesda, Md., Clinical Center, National Institute of Health, 1968.

Pittman, J. G.: Using corticosteroids. Amer. Fam. Phys., 3:96–100, May 1971.

Symposium, Right and wrong moves with corticosteroids. Patient Care, 3:14–63, Jan. 1969.

Thomson, J. A.: Acromegaly. Nurs. Mirror, 135:26–29, Oct. 6, 1972.

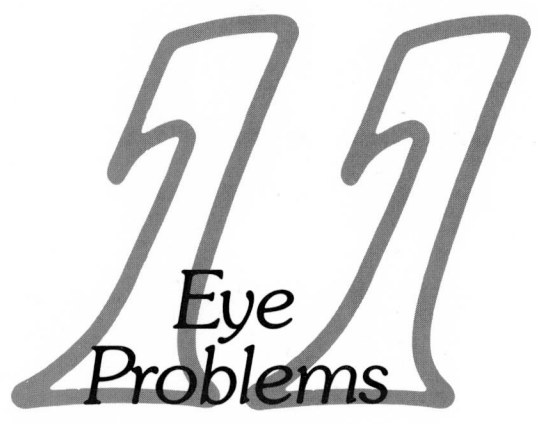

Eye Problems

EYE CARE SPECIALISTS

Definitions

1. *Oculist*
   Ophthalmologist
   Ophthalmic Physician } a physician (M.D.) who is skilled in the treatment of all conditions and diseases of the eye.

2. *Optician*—not a physician, but a technician who is able to grind, mount, fit and dispense lenses.

3. *Optometrist*—not a physician, but one licensed to examine the eye for refractive

errors by mechanical means and to provide appropriate corrective lenses. He does not use drugs in eye examinations.

4. *Ocularist*—not a physician, but a technician who makes artificial eyes and other prostheses used in ophthalmology.

NORMAL VISION AND REFRACTIVE ERRORS

Vision

Vision is the passage of rays of light from an object through the cornea, aqueous humor, lens and vitreous humor to the retina.

A. *Normal*—emmetropia

Rays coming from an object at a distance of 6 meters or more are brought to a focus on the retina by the lens.

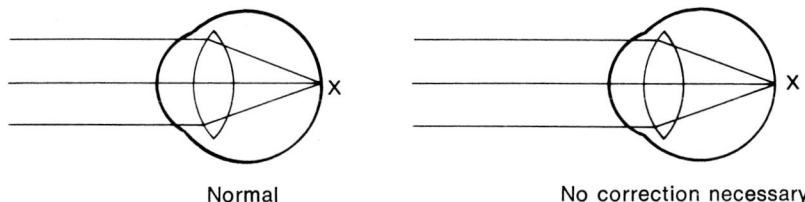

Normal   No correction necessary

B. *Abnormal*—ametropia

1. Nearsightedness (myopia)
   a. Rays of light coming from an object at a distance of 6 meters or more are brought to a focus in front of the retina.
   b. Correction—concave lens.

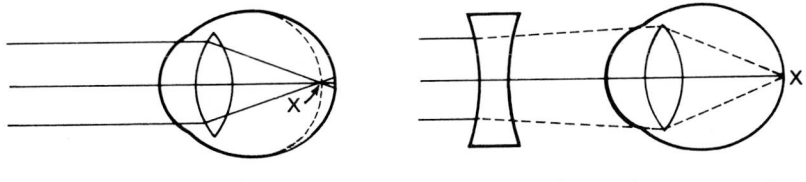

Myopic eye   Correction: concave lens

2. Farsightedness (hyperopia)
   a. Rays of light coming from an object at a distance of 6 meters or more are brought to a focus in back of the retina.
   b. Correction—convex lens.

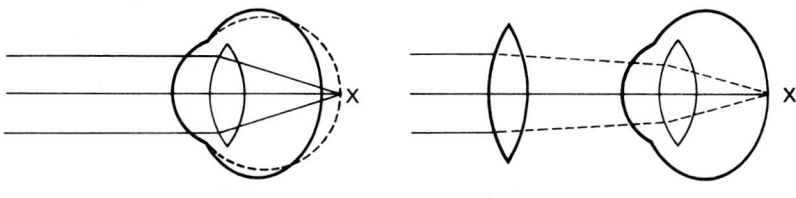

Hypermetropic eye   Correction: convex lens

Accommodation

In *accommodation* the focusing apparatus of the eye adjusts to objects at different distances by means of increasing the convexity of the lens (brought about by contraction of ciliary muscles).

    Abnormal Condition

        Presbyopia—the elasticity of the lens decreases with increasing age; a person with presbyopia will read a paper at arms length and requires prescription lenses to correct the problem.

Curvature of Cornea

A. *Normal*—equal curvature of cornea

B. *Abnormal*—astigmatism
1. Uneven curvature of the cornea causing the patient to be unable to focus horizontal and vertical rays on the retina at the same time.
2. Correction—cylinder lenses.

EXAMINATION AND DIAGNOSTIC PROCEDURES

External Examination

    Includes examination of eye and adnexa without special apparatus.

A. *Snellen Chart*
1. Each eye is tested separately with and without glasses.
2. Letters or objects are of the size that can be seen by the normal eye at a distance of 20 feet from the chart.
3. Letters appear in rows and are arranged so that the normal eye can see at distances of 30, 40, 50 feet, etc.
4. When a person can identify letters of the size 20 at 20 feet, his eye is said to have 20/20 vision.
5. The big "E" should be seen by a normal eye at 200 feet.

B. *Visual Fields*
1. With the eye fixed at a central point, peripheral and side vision is spot checked with an instrument called a perimeter.
2. A confrontation or target screen method may also be used.

C. *Color Vision*

    Colors in a color plate are identified.

D. *Refraction*

    When atropine or homatropine "drops" (or any mydriatic) are used in the eye, the lens is unable to accommodate, enabling the ophthalmologist to determine eye function with the lens completely at rest.

Internal Examination

A. *Ophthalmoscopic Examination*

    The interior of the eye is examined when a small beam of light is reflected through the pupil while the examiner looks through a small opening in the mirror.

B. *Gonioscopy*

　The juncture of the iris and cornea (angle of anterior chamber) is visualized by means of a contact glass, hand microscope and illuminator.

C. *Tonometry* (Schiotz)

　1. The tension of the eyeball can be measured with a tonometer (Fig. 11-1).
　2. Normal tension is approximately 11–22 mm.-Hg.

D. *Applanation Tonometry*

　1. Measures the force required to flatten rather than indent a small area of the central cornea.
　2. The tension measured is considered more accurate than Schiotz tonometry.

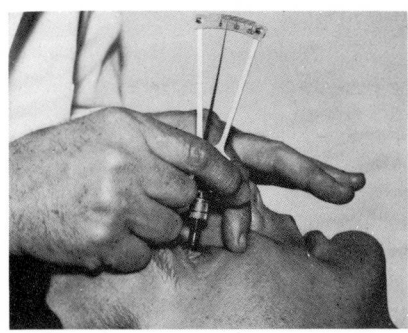

Figure 11-1. After a local anesthetic is instilled into the eye, the Schiotz tonometer is gently rested on the eyeball; the indicator measures in mm.Hg the ocular tension. (Courtesy, F. H. Roy, M.D.)

GUIDELINES: *Assisting the Patient Undergoing Tonometry*

Tonometry is the measuring of intraocular pressure by means of placing a sensitive instrument (tonometer) directly on the partially anesthetized eyeball. Normal reading: 11–22 mm.Hg.

Procedure

Preparatory Phase

1. The patient is placed in a tilt-type chair, tilted back and instructed to look upward.

Action	Rationale/Amplification
Performance Phase	
1. Physician:	
a. Instills a drop of Ophthaine 0.5% in each eye.	a. This will produce corneal anesthesia within a minute.
b. Place a sterile tonometer gently on the center of the cornea for a few seconds.	
c. Repeat for second eye.	
2. Nurse:	
a. Offer the patient an absorbent tissue.	
b. Instruct patient to pat the *closed* eyes dry.	
c. Caution the patient against rubbing his eyes.	c. The cornea is still anesthetized; painful lacerations can result from the natural tendency to rub the eyes because of the unusual numb sensation.

Follow-up Phase

1. Remind patient to have an eye-pressure check at least every 2 years if his pressure is normal.

GUIDELINES: Instillation of Eye Drops

Purposes

1. To dilate or contract the pupil.
2. To relieve pain and discomfort.
3. To act as an antiseptic in cleansing the eye.
4. To combat infection; to relieve inflammation.

Equipment

Sterile solution or medication
Tissue-wipes

Sterile eyedropper
(Most medications come in plastic bottles with built-in dropper.)

Procedure

Preparatory Phase

1. Inform the patient of the need and purpose of instilling eye drops.
2. Allow him to sit with head tilted slightly backward or lie in the dorsal recumbent position.

Nursing Action	Rationale/Amplification
Performance Phase	
1. Check orders and bottle or vial for correct medication and correct concentration.	1. To avoid medication error.
2. Check orders designating which eye requires medication: O.D. (oculis dexter)—right eye O.S. (oculis sinister)—left eye O.U. (oculis uterque)—both eyes	
3. Check glass eyedropper for defects. If plastic disposable dropper is used, squeeze plastic to allow medication to come to the tip.	3. Provides an effective and safe vehicle for transmission of medication.
4. Prevent medication from flowing back into bulb end.	4. Loose particles of rubber may slip into medication.
5. Using forefinger, pull lower lid down gently.	5. To expose inner surface of lid and cul-de-sac.
6. Instruct patient to look upward.	6. Prevents medication from hitting sensitive cornea.
7. Drop medication into center of lower lid (cul-de-sac).	
8. Instruct patient to close eyes but not to squeeze them.	8. Squeezing would express medication; closing allows medication to be distributed evenly over eye.
9. Wipe off excess solution with a tissue.	

NOTE: Eye ointments are frequently used—procedure is similar to instillation of eye drops. Ointment from tube is gently squeezed into cul-de-sac with care taken not to touch eye with end of tube.

Follow-up Phase

Record time, type, strength and amount of medication and the eye into which medication was instilled.

GUIDELINES: *Irrigating the Eye*
(Conjunctival Irrigation)

Purpose

To remove secretions from the conjunctival sac (conjunctival irrigation).

Equipment

1. For small amount of solution—an eyedropper
2. For larger amount of solution—asepto bulb syringe
3. For home use—a sterile eye cup

Procedure

Preparatory Phase

1. The patient may sit or lie in the dorsal recumbent position.
2. Have patient tilt head toward the side of the affected eye.

Nursing Action	**Rationale/Amplification**
Performance Phase	
1. Wash eyelashes and lids with the prescribed solution at room temperature; place a curved basin on the affected side of the face to catch the outflow.	1. Any materials on the lids or lashes can be washed off before exposing conjunctiva.
2. Evert the lower conjunctival sac.	2. The inner part of the lower lid is less sensitive than the cornea.
3. Allow irrigating fluid to flow from the inner canthus to the outer canthus along the conjunctival sac.	3. This prevents the solution from flowing toward the lacrimal sac, duct and nose, which would aid in transmitting the infection.
4. Use only enough force to flush secretions from conjunctiva.	4. Too much force may be injurious to eye tissues.
5. Occasionally have patient close his eyes.	5. This allows upper lid to meet lower lid with the possibility of dislodging additional particles.
6. Use prescribed amount of solution.	
Follow-up Phase	
1. Dry patient's face and pat eye dry with tissue.	1. Makes patient comfortable.
2. Record kind and amount of fluid used as well as its effect on the patient.	

EYE INJURIES
(Trauma to the Eye)

Preventive Measures

1. Appropriate glasses should be used for protection against very bright light, sun shining on snow, fumes of sprays or chemicals, etc.
2. Goggles should be worn if there is danger of flying gravel (power-mower lawn cutting), flying wood chips (while chopping wood), flying metal or glass bits (in a machine factory).
3. Children should be reminded of dangers of sling shots, BB guns, "sparklers," darts and arrows, etc.

Treatment

1. Irrigate eye with saline solution.
2. Have fluorescein solution available for physician to instill 1 drop in each eye; the greenish dye facilitates detection of abrasions or ulcers.
3. Irrigate eye again with saline.
4. Assist physician in determining extent of injury; treat accordingly.
5. Encourage follow-up care.

Types of Eye Injuries

A. *Acid or Alkali Burns*
1. Prevalence of hair sprays and other spray products have caused an increase in the incidence of chemical eye burns.
2. Acid or alkali on lids or in eye creates an emergency.
3. Action
   a. Copiously flush the lids, conjunctiva and cornea.
      (1) Immerse patient's head in a basin or sink filled with water.
      (2) Flush the eye using a syringe if available, or—
      (3) Hold patient's eye (head) under running water.
   b. Flush continuously for at least 15 minutes.

B. *Actinic Trauma*
1. Excessive sunlight (or other strong light such as a sun lamp, bright sun on snow) can cause ultraviolet-ray damage to cornea.
2. Damage may be superficial and resolve in 48 hours; however, punctate keratitis may develop.
3. An ophthalmologist should be consulted immediately.
4. Treatment
   a. Reassure patient.   c. Report to an ophthalmologist.
   b. Patch both eyes.   d. Instill anesthetic drops.

C. *Contusions and Hematoma*
1. Hemorrhage into orbit from trauma ("black-eye").
2. Bleeding into loose tissues of orbit produces discoloration of lids and surrounding skin, resulting in swelling.
3. Treatment
   a. Consult an ophthalmologist if hemorrhage is severe or if pain and double vision are noted—to rule out orbital fracture and hyphema (hemorrhage into anterior chamber).
   b. Apply cold compresses for the first 24 hours.
   c. Then hot compresses (at 15-minute intervals during the day).

D. *Corneal Laceration or Abrasion*
1. Can be detected through staining with sodium fluorescein.
2. Pain can be relieved with local anesthetic or by a patch over the eye for 24–36 hours.
3. Infection prevented by applying antibiotic eye drops.
4. Complication to be guarded against—corneal ulcer.

E. *Foreign Bodies*
   Dust particles, tiny bugs, etc., frequently cause considerable discomfort to the sensitive conjunctiva.

GUIDELINES: *Removing a Particle from the Eye*

Equipment

Local anesthesia	Eye spud
Hand lens	Saline (Irrigating)
Fluorescein	Antibiotic solution

Procedure

Nursing Action	Rationale/Amplification
1. As patient looks upward, evert lower lid to expose the conjunctival sac. (See A in illustration below.)	1. Dust particles are often washed downward by the upper lid.
2. With small cotton applicator dipped in saline, gently remove particle.	
3. If offending particle is not found, proceed to examine upper lid.	
4. Have patient look downward while you stand in front of him.	4. Serves as a safety measure since cornea is away from area of activity.
5. Place cotton applicator stick horizontally on outer surface of upper lid. (See B in illustration below.)	
6. Grasp eyelashes with fingers of other hand and pull the upper lid outward and upward over cotton stick. (See C in illustration below.)	6. Particles may be washed under the lid; visual exposure assists in detection.
7. With a cotton applicator moistened with saline, gently remove particle.	

NOTE: If particle cannot be removed by above method, it may have become embedded, in which case an ophthalmologist is required.

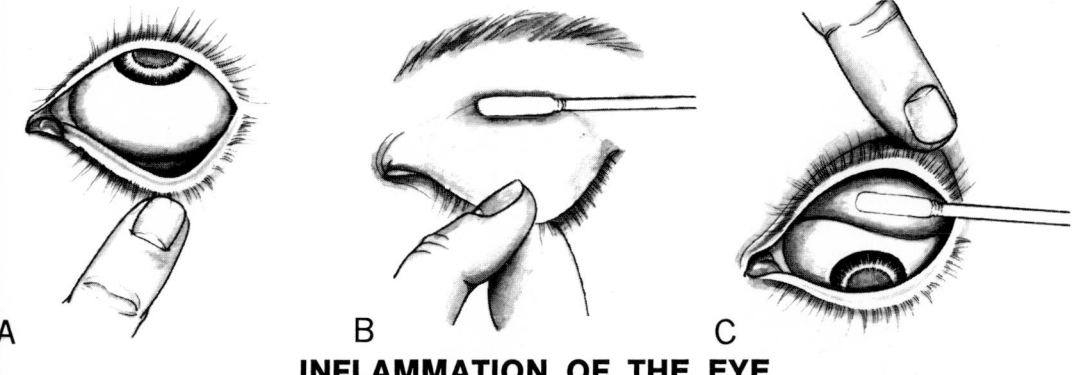

A   B   C

INFLAMMATION OF THE EYE

Conjunctivitis

Conjunctivitis is an inflammation of the conjunctiva, resulting from an allergy, a bacterial, viral or rickettsial infection or physical or chemical trauma.

Clinical Manifestations

1. Redness, pain, swelling, lacrimation
2. Discharge according to offending organisms
   Abundant purulence indicates infection caused by pneumococcus or gonococcus.

Treatment and Nursing Management

1. Administer frequent saline irrigations—to remove discharge.
2. Apply warm compresses—15 minutes, 3 or 4 times a day.
3. Instill chemotherapeutic ointments as prescribed—to clear infection in 1–3 days. (Without treatment infection subsides in 7–10 days.)
4. Prevent dissemination of infection to the other eye or other persons.
   a. Wash hands before treating eye.
   b. Restrict washcloth and towel to infected eye and change frequently.

Uveitis

Uveitis is an inflammation of the uveal tract (iris, ciliary body, choroid).

Classification

1. Location
   a. Anterior uveitis → iritis, iridocyclitis
   b. Posterior uveitis → choroiditis, chorioretinitis
   c. Panuveitis → entire uveal tract
2. Granulomatous or nongranulomatous

	a. *Granulomatous*	b. *Nongranulomatous*
Location:	Any portion, mostly posterior	Anterior
Onset:	Insidious	Acute
Pain:	None or minimal	Marked
Circumcorneal flush:	Minimal	Present
Course:	Chronic	Acute
Prognosis:	Fair to poor	Good

Complications

1. Anterior uveitis—adhesions impede aqueous outflow leading to glaucoma.
2. Posterior uveitis—adhesions impede aqueous flow from posterior to anterior uvea, causing metabolic disturbances of the lens and leading to cataracts.
3. Retinal detachment may result from traction exerted on retina by vitreous strands.

Treatment

1. Directed to specific type of uveitis.
2. Atropine—to reduce likelihood of adhesion formation.
3. Steroids, locally—for anti-inflammatory and anti-allergic action. Steroids, systemically, occasionally.
4. Analgesic—for pain.

Sympathetic Ophthalmia

Sympathetic Ophthalmia is a severe granulomatous bilateral uveitis that may occur after any surgical or traumatic perforation involving the uveal tract.

Clinical Manifestations

Photophobia, blurring vision and injection ("bloodshot") in sympathizing eye.

Treatment

1. Conservative
   Corticosteroids—locally and systemically
   Atropine—locally
2. Radical
   Preventive enucleation of originally injured eye before sympathetic ophthalmia occurs

Nursing Management

1. Understand the patient's condition and the objectives desired for him by the ophthalmologist.
2. Understand the difficult decision facing the patient if the radical approach is suggested.

CORNEAL ULCER

Keratitis is an inflammation of the cornea, which when combined with a loss of substance results in *corneal ulcer.*

Clinical Manifestations

1. Pain, marked photophobia and increased lacrimation
2. Injected ("bloodshot") eye
3. When a corneal ulcer progresses deeper to involve the iris, iritis develops; pus forms and collects as a white or yellow deposit (hypopyon) behind the cornea.
4. If corneal ulcer perforates, iris may prolapse through cornea.

Treatment and Nursing Management

1. Prevention is much easier than treatment.
   a. Foreign bodies must be removed quickly.
   b. Corneal abrasions must be treated promptly.
2. Suggest the wearing of dark glasses to relieve photophobia.
3. Explain to patient that physician will administer mydriatics preparatory to examining the eye and will instill tetracaine to relieve pain and fluorescein to outline ulcer.
4. Administer antibiotic or chemotherapeutic agent as prescribed for specific type of infection.
5. Apply warm compresses for comfort as ordered.
6. Administer systemic antibiotics when prescribed.

EYE CONDITIONS REQUIRING POSSIBLE SURGERY

Caring for the Patient Having Eye Surgery

Nursing Objectives and Management

A. *To understand the psychological effect of an eye problem on a patient.*
   1. Recognize that dependence on sight is exaggerated when one faces a possible diminution or loss of sight.
   2. Observe that the concern of the patient may be manifested as fear, depression, tension, resentment, anger and even rejection.

3. Encourage the patient to express his feelings in order to determine the underlying problems.
4. Provide diversional and occupational therapy to keep patient occupied mentally within the limits of his decreased vision so as not to accentuate his feelings of depression or despair over loss of vision.
5. Demonstrate interest, empathy and understanding, but try not to be oversolicitous.
6. Recognize individual differences which affect the method of dealing with patient anxiety.
7. Assure the patient that rehabilitative programs and personnel are available if his condition requires them.

B. *To assess the physical needs which have to be met while maintaining the highest level of self-sufficiency.*
1. Always orient the new patient who has diminished vision to his surroundings; his room and the people in his immediate environment.
2. Encourage patient to care for himself so that he will be self-sufficient and not feel that he is a burden.
3. Supervise him as he attempts to feed himself so that he does not become discouraged.
4. Promote proper elimination by an adequate diet, cathartics or an enema as required.
5. Provide a rest period daily if patient is ambulatory.
6. For safety reasons, discourage his reading, smoking or shaving.
7. Caution him against rubbing his eyes or wiping them with a soiled tissue or handkerchief.
8. Instruct him to wear dark glasses if he has had atropine instilled.
9. Maintain a safe environment that is free of obstacles such as footstools or loose rugs.

C. *To assist in the immediate preoperative preparation of the patient.*
1. In preparation for general anesthesia, evacuate lower bowel (enema) in the morning of the day of surgery; offer liquid diet only after this. (This is unnecessary for local anesthesia.)
2. Arrange the hair of female patients (braiding) so that it will be conveniently out of the way.
3. Cut eyelashes of the affected eye, using blunt scissors covered with petrolatum so lashes will adhere to it.
4. Check local hospital policy regarding preoperative skin preparation; in many hospitals, this is done in the operating room.
5. Remove dentures or artificial eye before patient goes to the operating room.
6. Caution patient to hold his head still during surgery if the operation is to be done under local anesthesia.
7. Instruct patient regarding postoperative restrictions—no reading, no showers, tub baths or shampoos; no bending from the waist or lifting of heavy objects, no sleeping on operated side. Tell him he will have a patch and shield on eye when he returns.

D. *To provide optimum care for the patient immediately following eye surgery.*
1. Place patient in the dorsal recumbent position with a small pillow under his head or permit him to lie on unoperated side.
2. Provide lateral pillows to the head if necessary to keep his head still.
3. Position bed rails so as to offer the patient a sense of security.
4. Place a call bell within reach of the patient; have him call the nurse rather than stress or strain in an attempt to be self-sufficient.
5. Direct anyone who enters his room to announce himself.

6. Notify physician if patient appears restless, has pain or disturbs his dressings.
7. Avoid disturbing the head with such activities as combing the hair; delay combing the hair until patient is allowed out of bed.

E. *To provide a relaxing convalescence.*
1. Consult ophthalmologist before recommending diversional or recreational therapy that is not fatiguing to the eyes—no reading; television in moderation.
2. Recognize the soothing and relaxing effect of soft pastels for the wall and ceiling colors.
3. Regulate lights so that they are not too bright or do not produce a glare.
4. Inform patient before he leaves hospital regarding medications, eye glasses, follow-up visits, type of work he can do and when he can do it.
5. Instruct the patient or family as follows on instillation of eye medications and proper cleansing of eyes:
   a. Wash hands before and after treating eyes.
   b. To clean around the eye, use sterile wet gauze and wipe gently across lid from inner corner to outer corner.
   c. To apply eye medications, pull down lower lid and place drop or ointment along lower lid margin.
   d. Tape protective shield over the operated eye at bedtime.
6. Inform patient of "Talking Book" records and machines that are available from most public libraries without charge.

Corneal Transplantation
(Keratoplasty)

Keratoplasty involves removing a circular segment of cornea from the patient and replacing it with a similar segment of cornea from a donor eye. For best results, graft should be removed from donor within 5–6 hours of his death and transplanted within 2 days.

Types of Grafts
1. Total penetrating (includes all layers of cornea)
2. Partial penetrating
3. Lamellar—includes only outer layers of cornea

Objectives of Treatment and Nursing Management

A. *To recognize and alleviate the concerns of the patient preoperatively.*
1. Psychological preparation for surgery is simplified because the patient is usually optimistic about the imminent transplant.
2. If cultural and spiritual concerns need to be voiced by the patient, the nurse should be available so that the patient faces surgery in the best frame of mind possible.

B. *To keep intraocular and external pressure on the operated eye at a safe level.*
1. Prevent sudden turning of the head.
2. Minimize those activities or sources of irritants which may cause sneezing (dusting or sweeping, heavily scented flowers, sprays).
3. Avoid conversation which annoys or disturbs the patient; caution visitors not to upset the patient since emotional disturbances may increase his intraocular pressure.
4. Instruct patient not to sleep on operated side.

C. *To provide rest for the operated eye in order to enhance the healing process.*
   1. Cover both eyes even though only 1 is involved; if 1 eye is left uncovered, both would move because of twin-like movements.
   2. Recognize that healing is slow due to the avascularity of the cornea.
D. *To utilize measures that will prevent infection of the eye.*
   1. Assist physician in practicing meticulous aseptic technique during dressing change to reduce the possibility of infection.
   2. Discourage the patient from touching the dressings.
E. *To recognize the differences in care of the patient having a penetrating corneal transplant as compared to a patient having a nonpenetrating transplant.*
   1. Penetrating type
      a. Emphasize the need for longer bedrest.
      b. Restrict the patient's activities according to physician's specifications: the patient must be fed, bathed and provided with bedpan service.
      c. Allow patient to raise his head slightly toward unoperated side.
      d. Initiate passive range of motion activities and deep breathing exercises to prevent circulatory and pulmonary complications.
   2. Nonpenetrating type
      a. With physician's sanction, help the patient out of bed and into a chair for short periods of time.
      b. Keep the patient's eyes bandaged, perhaps double patched, according to physician's order.
F. *To implement care that will prevent complications.*
   1. Avoid urinary retention by providing adequate fluids.
   2. Prevent constipation or straining on defecation by avoiding constipating foods and maintaining adequate hydration.
   3. Administer analgesics as necessary to relieve pain.
   4. Report unrelieved pain since it may indicate that dressings are too tight, that graft has slipped or that hemorrhage is occurring.
   5. Introduce additional activities gradually each day but continue to avoid those which will require straining.
   6. Emphasize the importance of follow-up visits to the ophthalmologist.

Detached Retina

Retinal detachment is the separation of the retina from the choroid.

Altered Physiology

1. The retina perceives light and transmits impulses from its nerve cells to the optic nerve.
2. Tears or holes in the retina may result rapidly from trauma or slowly from the aging process.
3. A tear in the retina allows vitreous humor and transudate from choroid vessels to seep behind the retina and separate it from the choroid.

Clinical Manifestations

1. Patient complains of flashes of light, or blurred, "sooty" vision.
2. He notes sensation of particles moving in his line of vision.
3. Delineated areas of vision may be blank.
4. A sensation of a veil-like coating coming down or coming up in front of the eye may be present.
5. Ultimately there is a loss of vision.
6. The effects of the above are frightening to the patient who is apprehensive about becoming blind.

Treatment and Nursing Management

A. *General*

1. Instruct the patient to remain in bed; both eyes may be bandaged (according to physician's orders).
2. Physician will determine proper position by the area of detachment; such an area must be in a dependent position if adherence is to take place.
3. Administer sedation and tranquilizing drugs for comfort and relief of anxiety; explain what to expect preoperatively and postoperatively.

B. *Surgical*

Surgery is called for to ensure that retina will adhere to choroid.

1. Types of Surgery
   a. *Electrodiathermy*—the passing of an electrode needle through the sclera to allow subretinal fluid to escape; an exudate forms from the choroid, adhering to the retina.
   b. *Cryosurgery* or *retinal cryopexy*—a supercooled probe is touched to the sclera causing minimal damage; as a result of scarring, the choroid adheres to the retina.
   c. *Photocoagulation*—a laser beam is passed through the dilated pupil, causing a small burn and producing an exudate between the choroid and retina.
   d. *Scleral buckling*—a technique whereby the sclera is shortened to allow a buckling to occur which forces the choroid closer to the retina.
2. Postoperative Nursing Management
   a. Keep patient in bed for several days with eyes bandaged.
   b. Take precautions to avoid bumping the patient's head and causing the retina to detach further.
   c. Allow additional activity as type of treatment permits; for example, scleral buckling is less confining than diathermy.
   d. Provide for diversional therapy since this patient often becomes depressed.
   e. In most instances, local anesthesia is used; patient is ambulatory postoperatively if condition permits (age, vision in other eye, other medical or physical problems).

Prognosis

1. For untreated retinal detachment, the prognosis is progressive detachment and eventual blindness.
2. The cure rate for patients having diathermy is about 75%.
3. Occasionally patients will require a second treatment if there is no improvement in 2 weeks.
4. Unilateral detachment becomes bilateral in 25% of situations.
5. See also nursing management of the patient having eye surgery. (See p. 689.)

Cataracts

A *cataract* is an opacity of the crystalline lens or its capsule.

Predisposing Factors

1. A cataract may occur at birth (congenital cataract).
2. Occasionally a cataract occurs in young individuals as a result of disease or trauma.
3. Most commonly, cataract occurs in adults past middle age (senile cataract).

Altered Physiology

1. Normally, the lens is a clear, transparent jelly-bean-like structure lying behind the iris; the lens possesses strong refractive powers.
2. Chemical change in the lens protein may cause coagulation; this produces a cloudiness of the lens.
3. Physical changes result in a swelling of the fibers which in turn causes a distortion of the image.
4. Metabolic changes which reduce vitamin C and B_{12} in the lens may be instrumental in forming opacities.
5. Although cataract may be readily diagnosed, the basic cause of senile cataract is unknown.

Clinical Manifestations

1. Alterations in vision are noted.
   a. Objects seem distorted and blurred.
   b. Glare annoys the patient when there are bright lights.
   c. Visual loss is gradual but eventually the opacity becomes complete.
2. The pupil, usually black, becomes gray and later, milky-white.

Treatment

1. Surgical removal of the lens is indicated.
2. Proper time for cataract removal is determined by the patient's eyesight, occupation, general health and his convenience.
3. Usually a patient with 1 cataract can manage without surgery.
4. If cataract occurs in both eyes, he need not suffer blindness before he can be helped by surgery.

Common Surgical Procedures

A. *Extracapsular Extraction*
1. This surgery is conservative, simple to perform and usually done under local anesthesia.
2. The lens capsule is incised and the lens is withdrawn.
3. Usually it is performed for congenital and traumatic cataract.
4. The posterior capsule is left in place. This may interfere with vision, necessitating a second operation, a capsulotomy, to produce a clear pupil.

B. *Intracapsular Extraction*

1. In this surgery, the lens as well as the capsule is removed.
2. Cryosurgery may be used as the technique for this operation; a pencil-like instrument with a metal probe is cooled to about $-35°C$.; when the lens capsule is available after dissection, the cryosurgical instrument touches the lens and freezes to it so that the lens is easily pulled out.

Objectives of Treatment and Nursing Management

A. *Preoperative Care*

1. To make the patient comfortable in his new surroundings.
   a. Explain the plan of care.
   b. Escort the patient as he walks around the unit.
   c. Provide bed rails if he is elderly.
   d. Encourage him to ask questions and then provide the answers.
2. To reduce the conjunctival bacterial count to minimize the chance of postoperative infection.
   a. Obtain a conjunctival culture if ordered.
   b. Administer local antibiotics as prescribed.
   c. Employ aseptic technique in any eye treatment or procedure.
   d. Instruct patient not to touch his eyes.
3. To introduce rehabilitative measures that the patient will practice postoperatively.
   a. Following general anesthesia, instruct patient to take deep breaths, move extremities and perform quadriceps muscle setting without moving his head.
   b. Point out the hazard of squeezing the eyelids shut: Teach him how to close his eyes slowly.
4. To prepare the eye to be operated upon in the immediate preoperative period.
   a. Instill mydriatic if prescribed.
   b. Note whether pupil dilates after instillation of mydriatic.
   NOTE: In some eye departments, only physicians instill mydriatics. Check local policy.

B. *Postoperative Care*

1. To prevent pressure build-up within the eye (intraocular) which may exert a stress on the fresh sutures.
   a. Caution patient to refrain from coughing or sneezing.
   b. Advise patient to avoid rapid movement but allow him to turn to the unoperated side or remain in the dorsal recumbent position.
   c. Admonish patient not to bend from the waist.
2. To promote comfort of the patient and reorient him to surroundings.
   a. Allow patient to turn on unoperated side to relieve back stress.
   b. Offer analgesics as prescribed to control pain; report severe pain to physician.
   c. Instruct those who enter room to announce themselves.
   d. Provide a quiet environment to promote patient's relaxation.
   e. Allow patient to be ambulatory as permitted by physician.

3. To control symptoms that may lead to serious complications.
   a. Sudden pain in the eye may be due to a ruptured vessel or suture and may lead to hemorrhage—notify physician immediately.
   b. Restlessness and increasing pulse rate may be indicative of hemorrhage.
   c. Nausea may lead to vomiting and increase intraocular pressure—administer antiemetic drugs as prescribed.

C. *Rehabilitative Phase*
   1. To encourage the patient to be independent.
      a. Assist patient in getting around his room.
      b. Gradually increase his activities each day.
   2. To demonstrate to patient and a responsible member of his family how to administer eye drops.
   3. To promote patient's interest in diversional activities as he recuperates.
   4. To acquaint patient with the step-by-step requirements of a healthy convalescence
      a. The use of dark glasses after the eye dressings are removed
      b. Hospitalization usually 7–10 days
      c. Fitting for temporary corrective lenses for the first 6 weeks if prescribed
      d. Application of plastic shield taped over the eye at night to avoid accidental injury during sleep
      e. Prescription for permanent lenses 6–8 weeks after surgery

Glaucoma

Glaucoma is a condition in which the pressure within the eyeball is higher than normal; if allowed to proceed uncorrected, the problem may lead to blindness.

Incidence
   1. It is estimated that 1 million Americans have undiagnosed glaucoma.
   2. Glaucoma is the cause of blindness in 1 of 10 persons who become blind.
   3. Two of every 100 persons over the age of 40 have glaucoma.

Altered Physiology
   1. Pressure within the eye is determined by the rate of input of aqueous humor as produced by the ciliary body and the resistance to output of aqueous humor.
   2. Inflow of aqueous humor is through the pupil; outflow is at the meshwork located at juncture of iris and cornea. Clogging at the meshwork by blood, fibrin or inflammatory cells accounts for the buildup of pressure which produces secondary glaucoma
   3. Thickening of the meshwork appears spontaneously in those older individuals who appear to have a hereditary predisposition; chronic simple glaucoma results and is the most common type.
   4. When the iris is abnormally anterior and exerts pressure against the meshwork, acute glaucoma results. (This is least frequent type.)

Classification

1. Primary: In the adult
   a. Chronic simple glaucoma (wide-angle)
   b. Congestive glaucoma (narrow-angle)
      (1) Acute
      (2) Chronic
2. Secondary
3. Congenital glaucoma
   a. Juvenile
   b. Infantile
4. Absolute glaucoma

Clinical Manifestations

1. Dull headache is frequently absent but may occur when pressure is high (chronic simple type).
2. Progressive loss of vision, beginning with periphery, is gradual over a number of years; patient is usually not aware of a problem until it begins to affect central vision (chronic simple type).

Diagnostic Evaluation

1. Because of relative ease of developing glaucoma, unless a person past 40 has a complete physical examination periodically, including the measurement of eye pressure (tonometry), he may not discover it until the disease is considerably advanced (chronic simple type).
2. Tonometry (Fig. 11-1).
   A reading of 24–32 mm.Hg suggests glaucoma.
3. Gonioscopy—a test to differentiate angle-closure from open-angle glaucoma.
4. Tonography—application of tonometer, usually electronic, with a special device which records intraocular tension over a 4-minute period.
5. Water Provocative Test—Breakfast is withheld and initial tonometer reading is recorded. The patient then drinks 1 liter of water, and intraocular pressures are recorded after 30, 45 and 60 minutes. 90% reliable in detecting open-angle glaucoma.

Acute (Closed-angle) Glaucoma

Clinical Manifestations

1. With pressure increasing rapidly, severe pain occurs in and around eye.
2. Artificial lights appear to have a rainbow of colors around them.
3. Vision becomes cloudy and blurred.
4. Pupils dilate; nausea and vomiting may occur.
5. If untreated, blindness may result.

Pharmacotherapy

A. *Parasympathomimetic Drugs Used as Miotic Drugs.*

1. Drug action—pupil contracts, iris is drawn away from cornea; aqueous humor may drain through lymph spaces (meshwork) into Canal of Schlemm.

2. Types:

Medication	*Action*	*Effect and Precautions*
Pilocarpine hydrochloride 1/2, 1, 2, 3, 4 and 6%	Acts directly on myoneural junction	Action lasts 6–8 hours; drug of choice in glaucoma.
Carbachol (Doryl) 1 1/2 to 3%	Acts directly on myoneural junction	Used if pilocarpine is ineffective.
Physostigmine salicylate (eserine) 1/4 to 1/2%	Cholinesterase inhibitor	Action lasts 6–8 hours; Allergenic, unstable, short in action.
Echothiophate iodide (Phospholine Iodide) 1/16, 1/8, 1/4%	Cholinesterase inhibitor	Water-soluble; produces less local irritation. Action lasts 24 hours.
Isoflurophate (DFP) (Floropryl) 1/10% (ophthalmic solution)	Cholinesterase inhibitor	Oil-soluble miotic. *Caution:* side effects — vomiting, diarrhea, tenesmus.

B. *Carbonic Anhydrase Inhibitor*
1. Drug action—restricts action of enzyme which is necessary to produce aqueous humor.
2. Kind frequently used.

Acetazolamide	Carbonic anhydrase inhibitor	Decreases production of aqueous humor. *Caution:* side effects —gastric distress, shortness of breath, dermatitis, tingling of extremities, acidosis, ureteral stones.

Surgical Treatment

1. *Iridectomy*—an incision through cornea so that a portion of the iris may be drawn out and excised—peripheral or total (keyhole).
    Result—Iris is prevented from bulging forward to cause the angle at cornea and iris to be crowded. Consequently drainage is facilitated and intraocular tension is reduced.
2. *Iridencleisis*—an opening is created between anterior chamber and space beneath the conjunctiva; this bypasses the blocked meshwork, and aqueous fluid is absorbed into conjunctival tissues.

Chronic (Open-angle) Glaucoma

Clinical Manifestations

1. Insidious—mild discomfort (tired feeling in eye).
2. Slowly developing impairment of peripheral vision.
3. Possible halos around lights.

Pharmacotherapy

1. Often treated with a combination of miotic and carbonic anhydrous inhibitors (p. 697).
2. Remission may occur; however patient should continue to see physician at 3- to 6-month intervals.

Surgery

Corneoscleral Trephine—making a permanent opening at the junction of the cornea and sclera through which aqueous humor may drain.

Postoperative Nursing Measures

    a. Patient may be ambulatory as physician prescribes.

    b. Provide a liquid diet to eliminate straining at defecation.

    c. Administer sedation or narcotics if required.

    d. Remind patient of periodic check-ups since pressure changes may occur.

Patient Education

1. Even though glaucoma cannot be cured, it can be controlled.
2. Activities which may increase intraocular pressure are to be avoided:
   a. Emotional upsets—worry, fear, excitement, anger
   b. Constricting clothing such as tight collar, belt or girdle
   c. Exertion such as snow shoveling, pushing, heavy lifting
   d. Upper respiratory infections
3. Recommended activities
   a. Exercise in moderation to maintain general well-being
   b. Moderate use of eyes for reading and watching television
   c. Maintenance of regular bowel habits (Straining on defecation causes increased intraocular pressure.)
   d. Continuous daily use of eye medications as prescribed
   e. Check-ups with ophthalmologist in order to keep condition under control
   f. Wearing a medical identification tag indicating patient has glaucoma

EMERGENCY CARE

GUIDELINES: *Removing Contact Lenses*

Purpose

Since contact lenses are designed to be worn while awake, if a person is injured and incapacitated due to accident, sickness or other cause, the lenses should be removed.

NURSING ALERT:

1. If the injured person is unconscious or unable to remove his lenses, an optometrist or ophthalmologist should be called.
2. If professional help is not available and the lenses must be removed:
   a. Determine the type of lens.
      (1) Small *corneal lenses* are most widely used. The diameter is less than the colored part of the eye (smaller than a dime).
      (2) Larger *scleral lenses* are worn by a few. These cover all the colored part of the eye and some of the sclera (about the size of a quarter).
   b. *When Not to Remove Lenses:* If the colored part of the eye is not visible upon opening the eyelids, await the arrival of an optometrist or ophthalmologist.

Procedure

Preparatory Phase

1. Since the patient will undoubtedly be in the recumbent position, it is acceptable to remove the lens while he is in this position.
2. Wash your hands thoroughly.

Nursing Action

Corneal Lens

1. For right eye, stand on right side of patient so hands will have easier access to eye.
2. Lightly place left thumb on upper eyelid; right thumb on lower eyelid close to the edge and parallel with lids (Fig. 11-2A). Thumbs are placed in a leverage position on the eyelids.
3. Gently pull lids apart and observe if contact lens is visible (Fig. 11-2B). If contact lens is not visible wait for an experienced practitioner.
4. If lens is visible, it should slide with the movement of the eyelids while thumbs are still kept at the edges of the eyelids.
5. Gently open the lids wider beyond the edge of the lens and maintain this position.
6. Press gently downward with right thumb on eyeball (Fig. 11-2C). This should cause the contact lens to tip up on one edge.
7. Then slide the eyelids and thumbs together gently (Fig. 11-2D). The lens should slide out between the lids where it can be taken off.
8. FORCE SHOULD NOT BE USED! Cornea may be irreparably damaged.
9. If lens can be seen but cannot be removed, gently slide it to the white sclera.
10. Move to left side of patient and repeat.

Scleral Lens

1. For right eye, stand on right side of patient.
2. Place left index finger parallel with and at the edge of the lower eyelid (Fig. 11-3A).
3. Press the lid downward and backward until the edge of the scleral lens becomes visible (Fig. 11-3B).
4. Maintain pressure but pull finger with lower lid toward the patient's right ear (Fig. 11-3C). This should cause the lid to slide under the lens. Avoid force.
5. Grasp scleral lens with right finger and thumb.

Disposition of Lenses

1. When lenses are found and removed, place in a case or bottle; label "right" and "left."

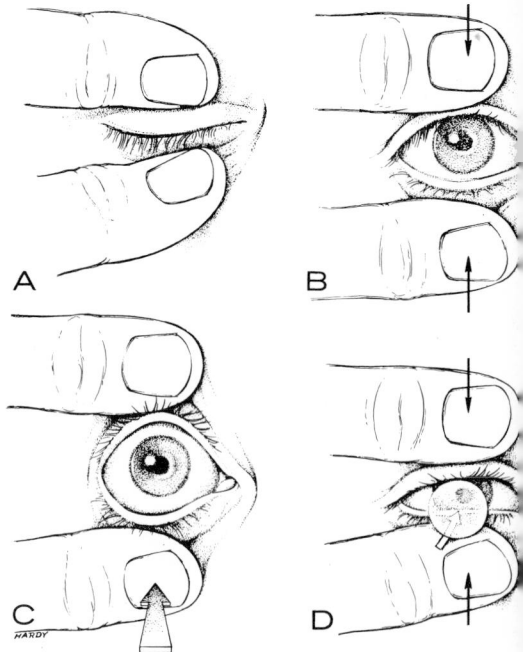

Figure 11-2. Removing corneal contact lens.

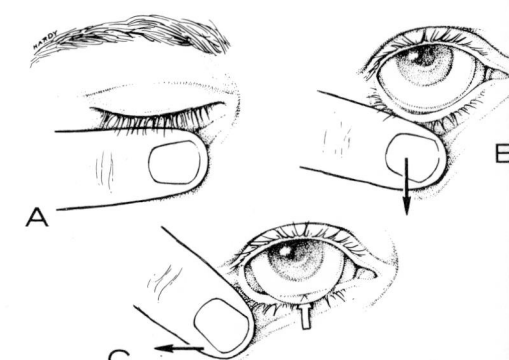

Figure 11-3. Removing scleral contact lens.

1. Since right and left lenses are often different storing them with proper labels will be appreciated by the patient.

BIBLIOGRAPHY

Books

Brunner, L. S., et al.: Textbook of Medical and Surgical Nursing, 2nd ed. Philadelphia, J. B. Lippincott, 1970, pp. 716–741.

Casset, A. R., and Kaufman, H. E.: Soft Contact Lenses. St. Louis, C. V. Mosby, 1972.

Girard, L. J. (ed.): Corneal Contact Lenses. St. Louis, C. V. Mosby, 1970.

Leopold, I. H. (ed.): Symposium in Ocular Therapy, Vol. 5. St. Louis, C. V. Mosby, 1972.

Vaughan, D., et al.: General Ophthalmology, 6th ed. Los Altos, California, Lange Medical Publications, 1971.

Articles

Condl, E. D.: Ophthalmic nursing: the gentle touch. Nurs. Clin. N. Amer., 5:467–476, Sept. 1970.

Fraunfelder, F. T., and Roy, F. H.: How to treat common external eye problems. Amer. Fam. Phys., 3:104–109, April 1971.

Gordon, D. M.: A guide to external examination of the eye. Hosp. Med., 6:41–51, April 1970.

Garrett, W. H., and Hagler, W. S.: Retinal detachment. Hosp. Med., 7:87–107, May 1971.

Hale, L. M.: Emergency eye care. Amer. Fam. Phys., 6:102–115, Sept. 1972.

O'Grady, R. B.: Glaucoma. Postgrad. Med., 51:69–72, March 1972.

Ohno, M. J.: The eye-patched patient. Amer. J. Nurs., 71:271–274, Feb. 1971.

Rabb, M. F.: The present status of corneal transplantation. Nurs. Clin. N. Amer., 5:477–482, Sept. 1970.

Roy, F. H., and Fraunfelder, F. T.: The red eye. Amer. Fam. Phys., 4:81–86, Sept. 1971.

Seamon, F. W.: Nursing care of glaucoma patients. Nurs. Clin. N. Amer., 5:489–496, Sept. 1970.

Stafford, T. J.: Disorders of the eyelids in the elderly. Postgrad. Med., 52:133–136, Oct. 1972.

Vaughan, D. G.: Common ocular emergencies. Hosp. Med., 7:22–51, Oct. 1971.

Weinstein, G. W.: Signs and symptoms of ocular disease. Occup. Health Nurs., 19:7–12, May 1971.

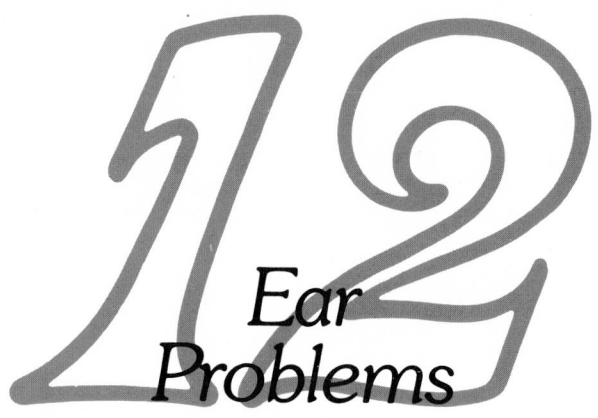

Ear Problems

EAR CARE SPECIALISTS

Definitions

1. *Otologist*—a physician who specializes in the diagnosis and treatment of problems of the ear.
2. *Otolaryngologist*—a physician who specializes in problems related to the ear, nose and throat.
3. *Audiologist*—an individual who specializes in nonmedical evaluation and rehabilitation of hearing disorders (usually not a physician).

CLASSIFICATION OF HEARING LOSS

1. *Conductive loss*—a hearing loss due to an impairment of the outer or middle ear or both. If causative problem cannot be corrected, a hearing aid may help.
2. *Sensorineural (perceptive) loss*—a hearing loss due to disease of the inner ear or nerve pathways; sensitivity to and discrimination of sounds is impaired. Hearing aids usually are helpful.
3. *Combined hearing loss*—a combination of the above.
4. *Psychogenic hearing loss*—usually a manifestation of an emotional disturbance and unrelated to evident structural changes in the hearing mechanisms. Loss is often total but without physical basis; thus patient may suddenly recover.

EXAMINATIONS AND DIAGNOSTIC PROCEDURES

Tuning Fork (nonquantitative)

A unique and inexpensive instrument that can differentiate between conductive and perceptive deafness.

1. *Conductive deafness*—caused by a disorder of the auditory canal, eardrum or middle ear (e.g., disruption of ossicles or fluid).
2. *Perceptive (sensorineural) deafness*—caused by a disorder of the organ of Corti or the auditory nerve.

A. *Weber test*

Place tuning fork on the forehead so that hearing in the 2 ears may be compared.
   a. If patient indicates he hears vibrations in the middle of his head:
      (1) This may be normal.
      (2) This may be deafness of equal quality in both ears.
   b. Variations imply hearing inequality.
      (1) In conductive hearing loss, bone-conducted sounds shift to poorer ear.
      (2) In sensorineural hearing loss, sounds are louder in the better ear.

B. *Rinne test**

1. After the fork is struck to set it in vibration, the handle is placed against the mastoid process.
2. Then the prongs are placed beside the ear.
3. The patient is asked to tell where he heard the sound better or longer.
4. "Rinne positive"—tone was heard longer by air conduction which may be normal or may indicate a perceptive loss.
5. "Rinne negative"—tone was heard longer by bone conduction which indicates conduction loss.
6. "Rinne equal"—tone heard the same by air and bone conduction and may indicate a loss, probably conductive.

Audiogram (Fig. 12-1)

A. *Types*

1. Pure-tone audiometry
   a. Sound stimulus consists of a pure (musical) tone.
   b. The louder the tone required before patient hears it, the greater the hearing loss.
   c. Decibel—unit of measuring loudness or intensity of sound.
2. Speech audiometry
   The spoken word is used to evaluate ability to understand and discriminate sounds.

B. *Procedure*

1. Test is performed in a soundproof room.
2. Patient is instructed to don earphones and signal when he hears the tone as well as later when the tone disappears.
3. Air conduction is measured by applying tone directly to external auditory opening.
4. Nerve conduction is measured when stimulus is applied directly to the mastoid process.

---

* Of limited value unless physician is certain clinically that the patient has a hearing loss.

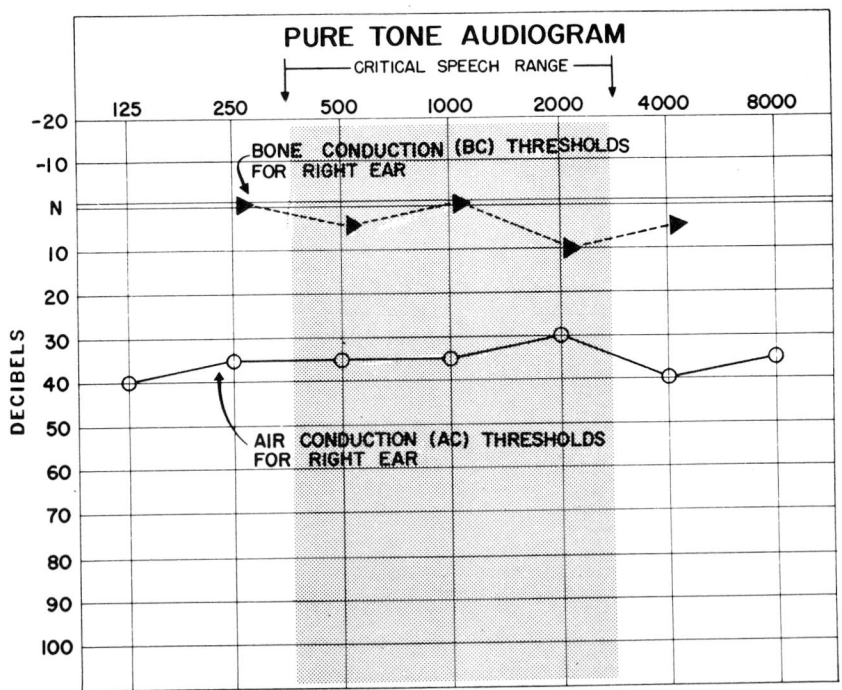

Figure 12-1. An audiogram presents a graphic outline of the individual's hearing as measured by tones of different pitches ranging from 125 through 8000 cycles per second (cps or Hz). Thresholds for these different tones as heard by air and bone conduction are plotted on this graph. The information is important for determining the type of hearing loss. Also, by testing through the critical speech range (approximately 300 to 3000 cps), one can predict how much difficulty there may be in hearing and understanding speech. (From Nilo, E. R.: Hearing Impairment. *In* Saunders, W. H., *et al.*: Nursing Care in Eye, Ear, Nose, and Throat Disorders. ed. 2. St. Louis, C. V. Mosby, 1968.)

C. *Evaluation*
  1. Normal human ear perception: 20 cycles per second (cps) or 20 Hz (Herz) to 20,000.
  2. Frequencies significant for speech range—500 to 2000 Hz.
  3. Clinical level of loudness: 30 decibels over threshold, i.e., the level at which speech discrimination is tested using phonetically balanced spoken words.

EAR HYGIENE

Hygienic Measures
  1. Avoid putting bobby pins, matches, toothpicks, etc. into the external auditory canal; the danger is possible infection and damage to the eardrum. Many physicians even object to the use of Q-tips.

2. To remove wax deposits, instill 3 or 4 drops of Debrox twice a day for 3 or 4 days; after the 4th day, irrigate gently with warm water.
3. During an upper respiratory infection, avoid vigorous blowing of the nose since middle ear infection can result.
4. In the presence of an ear infection, take precautions when swimming—either avoid this sport or insert a lamb's wool plug into the ear canal. It is preferable not to get the head wet.

Noise

1. Excess noise is detrimental to health and decreases work efficiency; conversely, elimination of noise or substitution of pleasant soft music increases work efficiency.
2. Decibels (dB) is the unit of measurement of sound intensity.
   a. Leaves rustling in a breeze—10 decibels
   b. Ordinary conversation—50 decibels
   c. Noisy subway—80 decibels
   d. Jet plane (100 feet away)—140 decibels
3. Frequency—Number of sound waves emanating from a source per second. This is described as cycles per second (cps or Hz).
4. Pitch is related to frequency.
   a. For example—100 cps or Hz is low pitch.
         10,000 cps or Hz is high pitch.
   b. A healthy young adult can distinguish frequencies from 16 cps to 20,000 cps.
5. Health Implications
   a. Individuals react differently to noise.
   b. The noise level in the home should not exceed 35–40 decibels.
   c. Very loud electrical music can damage hearing.
   d. Protective muffs are recommended in work areas where the noise level exceeds 80–85 decibels.

PROBLEMS AFFECTING THE EXTERNAL EAR

External Otitis

1. *Cause*
   Bacterial or fungal infections due to
      (1) Abrasion of ear canal
      (2) Swimming in contaminated water
2. *Clinical Manifestations*
   a. Pain—moving or even touching the auricle intensifies pain.
   b. Tissues may be edematous.
3. *Treatment*
   a. Administer codeine sulfate and acetylsalicylic acid for pain.
   b. Apply heat for comfort.
   c. Instill ear drops (antibiotic) for anti-inflammatory and anti-infection effect.
   d. Caution patient to avoid showering or swimming until infection is cleared.

Cerumen in Ear Canal

1. Accumulated earwax does not have to be removed unless it becomes impacted and interferes with hearing.
2. To irrigate ear canal, see *Guidelines*, page 706.

Foreign Bodies in External Canal

1. Inserted by young children or mentally retarded persons.
2. Insects
   Treat by instilling oil drops to smother insect which then will float out.
3. Vegetable foreign bodies (peas)
   a. Irrigation is contraindicated because vegetable matter absorbs water which would further wedge foreign body in ear canal.
   b. Unskilled persons should not attempt to remove foreign body because:
      (1) It may be forced into bony portion of the canal.
      (2) The canal skin may be perforated.
      (3) The ear drum may be perforated.
   c. Removal should be done skillfully with instruments; if the victim is very young, general anesthesia is required.

GUIDELINES: Irrigating the External Auditory Canal

Purposes

1. To remove discharge from the canal.
2. To facilitate removal of cerumen or foreign bodies.
3. To apply heat to the tissues of the ear canal.

NURSING ALERT: Ask the patient if he has a history of draining ears, or if he has ever had a perforation or other complications from a previous ear irrigation. If the reply is affirmative, check with the physician before proceeding with the irrigation.

Equipment and Solutions

Kind and amount of solution desired
Tray containing:
   Protective towels
   Cotton balls and cotton applicators
   Solution bowl and emesis basin
   Ear syringe or irrigating container with tubing, clamp and irrigating catheter
   Paper bag for disposable cotton

Procedure

Preparatory Phase

1. After explaining procedure to patient, place him in appropriate position, i.e., sitting or lying with head tilted toward affected ear.
2. Place protective toweling.

Nursing Action	**Rationale/Amplification**
Performance Phase	
1. Use a cotton applicator to remove any discharge on outer ear.	1. To prevent carrying discharge deeper into canal.
2. Place emesis basin close to the patient's head and under the ear.	2. To provide a receptacle to receive irrigating solution.
3. Test temperature of solution by allowing some to run on inner aspect of wrist. Should be 35 to 40.6°C. (95–105°F.).	3. Is more comfortable for patient; solutions that are hot or cold are most uncomfortable and may initiate a feeling of dizziness.

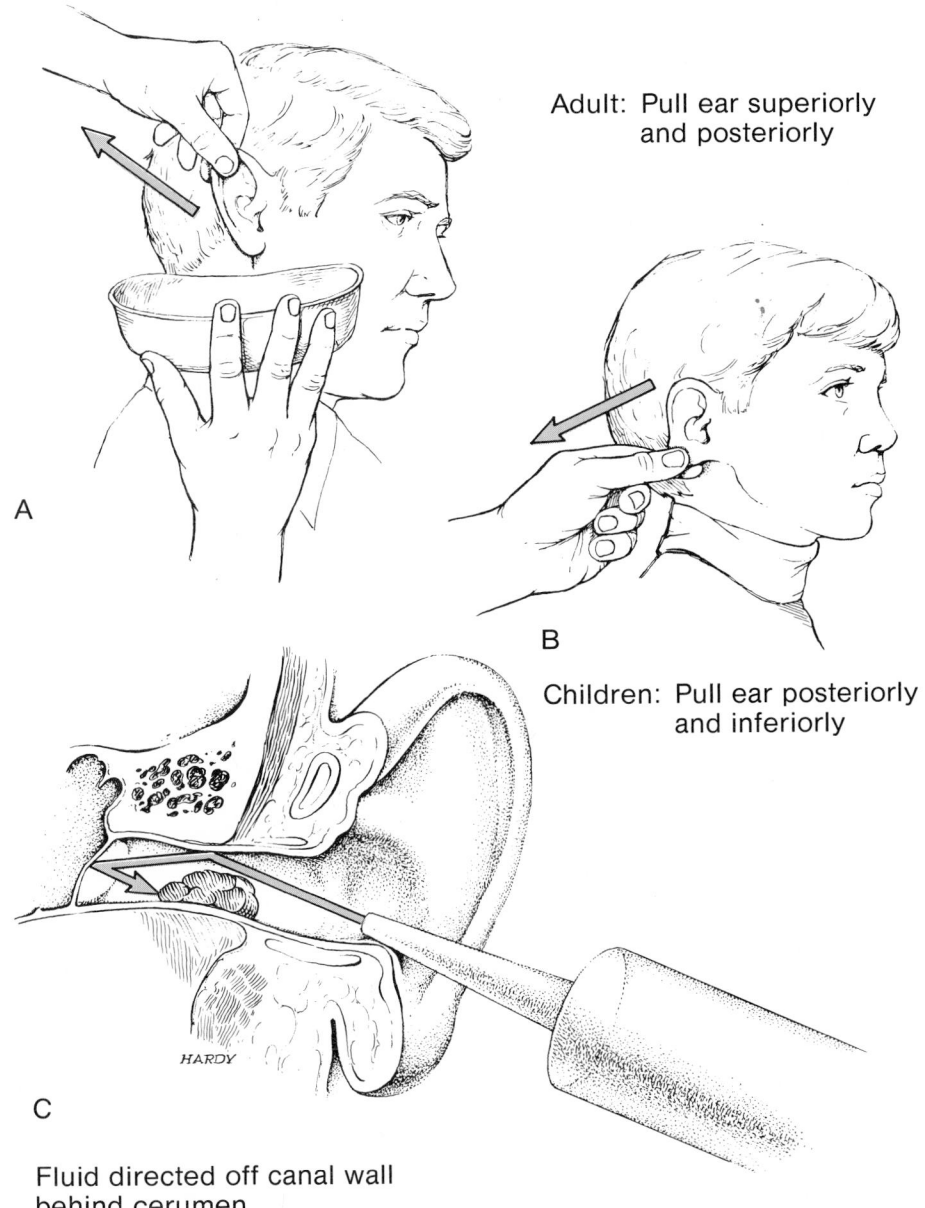

Adult: Pull ear superiorly
and posteriorly

A

B

Children: Pull ear posteriorly
and inferiorly

C

HARDY

Fluid directed off canal wall
behind cerumen

Figure 12-2. Ear irrigation. A. The external auditory canal in the adult can best be exposed by pulling the earlobe upward and backward.

B. The same exposure can be achieved in the child by gently pulling the auricle of the ear downward and backward.

C. An enlarged diagram showing the direction of irrigating fluid against the side of the canal. NOTE: This is more effective in dislodging cerumen than if the flow of solution were directed straight into the canal.

Nursing Action	***Rationale/Amplification***
4. Ascertain whether impaction is due to a foreign hygroscopic (attracts or absorbs moisture) body before proceeding.	4. If water contacts such a substance, it may cause it to swell and produce intense pain.
5. Gently pull the outer ear upward and backward (adult); downward and backward (child).	5. To straighten ear canal.
6. Place tip of syringe or irrigating catheter at opening of ear; gently direct stream of fluid against sides of the canal (Fig. 12-2).	6. To permit direction for inflow and outflow; if stream is directed forcefully against eardrum, it is possible to rupture it.
7. If an irrigating container is used, elevate not more than 15 cm. (6 inches).	7. To provide safe and effective pressure of fluid; if height is more than 6 inches, pressure will be too great and may damage tissue.
8. Observe for signs of pain or dizziness.	8. If they occur, discontinue treatment.
9. If irrigating does not dislodge the wax, instill several drops of glycerine, Debrox, or saturated solution of sodium bicarbonate, 2–3 times daily for 2–3 days.	9. To soften and loosen impaction.

Follow-up Phase
1. Dry external ear with cotton pledgets.
2. Remove soiled towels, etc. and make patient comfortable.
3. Record: Time of irrigation, kind and amount of solution used, nature of return flow, effect of treatment.

ACUTE OTITIS MEDIA

Acute otitis media is an inflammation of the middle ear caused by the entrance of pathogenic organisms. Normally the middle ear is sterile in its environs.

Etiology

Hemolytic streptococcus, pneumococcus, staphylococcus, influenza bacillus.

Mode of Entry

1. Auditory canal—if drum is perforated.
2. Eustachian tube—during indiscriminate use of nasal drops or nasal douching, or as a result of forcibly sneezing or blowing the nose.
3. Rarely, following a fracture of the skull.

Clinical Manifestations

1. Variable—may be mild or severe.
2. Pain is usually the first symptom—may be in and about the ear and it may be intense. May be relieved by spontaneous perforation of the drum or by myringotomy.
3. Fever—may be caused by a virus; in some patients temperature may rise to 40.0°–40.6°C. (104°–105°F.).
4. Headache, difficulty hearing, ear and head noises, anorexia, nausea and vomiting.

Treatment and Nursing Management

1. Varies with virulence of bacteria, efficiency of therapy and resistance of patient.
2. Usually the drug of choice is penicillin unless patient is allergic to it in which case erythromycin is used. Ampicillin is used for infants and small children.

3. Employ wide-spectrum antibiotic therapy.

NURSING ALERT:
1. With wide-spectrum antibiotic therapy, acute otitis media may become sub-acute with continued purulent discharge.
2. Healing may take place but the patient may be left with a residual deafness.
3. Recognize that such symptoms as headache, slow pulse, vomiting and vertigo are significant and should be reported.
4. Secondary complications may involve the mastoids or even the brain, producing meningitis or brain abscess.

---

4. *Myringotomy*—an incision made into the posterior inferior aspect of the tympanic membrane for draining purposes to relieve pressure and drain pus from middle ear infection.
   a. The incision heals rapidly.
   b. Hearing is not adversely affected.
   c. This procedure is done less frequently now because antibiotic therapy usually makes it unnecessary.

CHRONIC OTITIS MEDIA AND MASTOIDITIS

Chronic otitis media occurs as a result of repeated bouts of otitis media which causes perforation of the eardrum. This condition often begins in childhood and continues into adult life.

Causes

1. A strain of organism which is resistant to the antibiotic used
2. A particularly virulent strain of organism
3. Poor management of acute suppurative otitis media

Altered Physiology

1. Marginal perforation of drum membrane.
2. Presence of cholesteatoma (soft ball of dead skin) which erodes vital structures.
   a. Caused by an ingrowth of skin from the perforated drum.
   b. Fills area in the mastoid and middle ear.
   c. May encroach upon vital structures—facial nerve, labyrinth and brain.

Clinical Manifestations

Symptoms are minimal: mild deafness, foul-smelling discharge

Diagnostic Evaluation

1. Presence of above symptoms
2. X-rays to note mastoid pathology

Treatment and Nursing Management

A. *Antibiotic Therapy*
    1. Often effective in simple chronic otitis media.
    2. Sometimes disappointing when certain resistant organisms are involved.

B. *Surgery*
    1. Indicated when cholesteatoma is present.
    2. Indicated when there is pain or complications—profound deafness, dizziness, sudden facial paralysis, stiff neck (may lead to meningitis or brain abscess).
    3. *Simple Mastoidectomy*—removal of mastoid cells—indicated when there is persistent tenderness, fever, discharge from ear or headache.
    4. *Radical Mastoidectomy*—removal of all diseased tissue from mastoid area and middle ear.
    5. *Posteroanterior Mastoidectomy*—combines simple mastoidectomy with tympanoplasty.

C. *Nursing Concern*
    1. Shaving depends upon nature of the incision.
        a. Postaural—(incision behind the ear). Clip hair and shave scalp for 3–4 cm. around ear (only if desired by surgeon).
        b. Endaural—(incision through the ear canal). Shave is unnecessary.
    2. Provide for relief of pain preoperatively.
        a. Give acetylsalicylic acid or codeine sulfate.
        b. Apply ice cap to area.
    3. Postoperatively, administer sedatives for pain and restlessness.
    4. Assist with dressing change since area is packed with gauze for drainage; this may be done daily or every other day—packing is removed on 3rd or 4th day.
    5. Observe for possible complications:
        a. Facial paralysis may be indicative of facial nerve injury.
            (1) Immobility on side of face affected.
            (2) Eye cannot close, mouth droops.
            (3) Patient unable to whistle.
            (4) Patient unable to drink without dripping from mouth.
            (5) When patient speaks or smiles, immobility of affected side is noticeable.
            (6) Administer cortisone preparation as prescribed to assist in restoration of nerve function. (Not used if paralysis is caused surgically.)
        b. Infection
            (1) Observe for clinical signs of inflammation.
            (2) Administer antibiotics.
        c. Vertigo—may be apparent following radical mastoidectomy due to inner ear disturbance.
        d. Spread of infection to brain.
            Unusual rise in temperature, chills, stiff neck, nausea and vomiting.
    6. Note status of hearing.
        a. If stapes has been removed or dislodged then hearing is lost.
        b. If stapes or cochlea have not been removed or disturbed, then hearing is regained; may require a hearing aid.

PERFORATION OF EARDRUM

Etiology and Altered Physiology

1. Infection is the most frequent cause of permanent perforation of the tympanic membrane; often this is due to acute or chronic suppurative otitis media.
2. Trauma is the next cause of permanent perforation, caused by:
   a. A severe blow on the ear   d. Force of a stream of water
   b. Blast effect of high explosives e. Burns of face and head
   c. Foreign objects   f. Postmyringotomy defects

Treatment

A. *Medical*
   1. Most accidental perforations of the eardrum heal spontaneously.
   2. Cauterization of the perforation with trichloroacetic acid at frequent intervals and application of a prosthesis will produce a healed membrane with scar tissue.

B. *Surgical*
   Tympanoplasty, Type I—myringoplasty—(simple patching of drum). See below.

Tympanoplasty

Tympanoplasty is a reconstructive operation on the diseased or deformed components of the middle ear.
   1. Objective is to improve or preserve the conductive mechanisms in an effort to salvage or improve hearing
   2. Impetus for tympanoplasty has been aided by:
      a. Illuminated binocular microscope
      b. Use of antibiotics to prevent or control infection

Physiological Principles of Hearing

Why an intact drum is needed to hear.
   1. Sound waves are transformed from airborne vibrations to mechanical stimulation of endolymphatic lymph; this is accomplished by the conductive ability of the eardrum and ossicles.
   2. The ratio of the small oval window to the large tympanic membrane is 1:22; this combined with the vibratory action of the ossicles means a great increase in force from the air to the inner ear fluids.
   3. When there is a disturbance in the above relationships, the result is a loss of hearing.
   4. From the oval window, bordered by the annular ligament, impulses are received by the stapes footplate from the incus, malleus and drum membrane.
   5. A lag phase is normal after sound waves stimulate the oval window and before the final effect of the stimulus reaches the round window.

Altered Physiology

   1. With a perforation of the eardrum, the lag phase (described above) disappears, resulting in sound waves hitting the oval and round windows at the same time → diminished effect of labyrinth fluid motility → lessened stimulation of hair cells in the organ of Corti → diminished hearing.

2. Infections often produce fibrosis or necrosis of all or part of the ossicular chain.
3. Granuloma, polyps and fibrous or bony plaques may resist normal function of the oval and round windows.
4. In addition to sequelae from otitis media, otosclerosis may exist.
5. Obstruction of tympanic orifice of the eustachian tube may produce dysfunction.

Types of Tympanoplasty (Table 12-1)

TABLE 12-1. TYPES OF TYMPANOPLASTY

Type	Middle Ear Damage		Repair Process
	Tympanic Membrane	Ossicles	
I	Perforated	Normal	Close perforation—myringoplasty.
II	Perforated	Erosion of malleus and/or incus.	Close perforation; graft against incus or whatever remains of malleus.
III	Tympanic membrane destroyed or widely perforated.	Rest of ossicular chain destroyed BUT stapes are intact and mobile.	Grafts implanted to contact the normal stapes. "Tympanostapedopexy"
IV	Tympanic membrane destroyed or widely perforated.	Ossicular chain destroyed. Head, neck and crura of stapes destroyed. Stapes footplate mobile.	Expose mobile stapes footplate—graft implanted. Air pocket between graft and round window provides protection. "The Cavum minor operation"
V	Tympanic membrane destroyed or widely perforated.	Ossicular chain destroyed. Head, neck, and crura of stapes destroyed. Stapes footplate fixed.	Make opening in horizontal semi-circular canal; graft seals off middle ear to give sound protection for round window. "Tympanoplasty and fenestration of lateral semi-circular canal"

A. *Type I (Myringoplasty)*
1. *Purpose*—to close perforation by placing a graft over it in order to create a closed middle ear section which in turn will improve hearing.
2. *Indications*
   To avoid risk of contamination when patient bathes, swims or dives—this in turn prevents recurrence of chronic otitis media or mastoiditis.
3. *Contraindications*
   a. Ossicular involvement
      Prediction of surgical results can be made preoperatively by testing for improvement of hearing levels by placing a temporary patch over the defect. If no improvement noticed in audiometric testing, the ossicular chain may be involved.
   b. The presence of active infection
   c. The presence of chronic middle ear infection causing poor or absent drainage via eustachian tube
   d. Sinusitis or allergy which produces a chronic infectious discharge via nasopharynx
   e. History of acute exacerbations of otitis media.

4. *Surgical Repair*
   Perforation is closed using one of the following:
   a. Fascia from temporal muscle (in almost all cases)
   b. Vein grafts from hand or forearm (occasionally)

5. *Postoperative Management*
   a. Administer antibiotics for several days postoperatively to ensure freedom from infection.
   b. Reinforce external dressings if they become soiled; otherwise leave dressings intact.
   c. Remove gauze packing in canal at end of week; do not suction or probe canal.
   d. Gentle capillary suction may be attempted by end of 2nd week to remove debris and crusts (Gelfoam remains).
   e. Gently inflate canal to test efficiency of closed eardrums by new graft.
   f. Do not use ear drops because of danger of loosening graft.
   g. Dust lightly with antibiotic powder (Neosporin).

6. *Patient Instruction*
   a. Avoid shampooing or showering which could cause contamination of ear canal until permission is obtained from physician.
   b. Continue with antibiotics beyond first week if there is evidence of infection.
   c. Use antihistamine with an ephedrine derivative for at least 1 month postoperatively.
   d. Continue using an antihistamine if the patient experiences rhinologic allergy.

B. *Types II to V*
   1. *Purpose* (see Table 12-1). These procedures are modifications to correct middle ear problems.
   2. *Preoperative and Operative Treatment*
      a. Topical and systemic antibiotics are administered when infection is present.
      b. Suitable replacement (polyethylene tubing, stainless steel wire, bone, cartilage) is used to maintain continuity of conduction sound pathway.
      c. The necessity of a 2-stage procedure should be determined.
         (1) First stage—eradication of all diseased tissues; area is cleaned out to achieve a dry, healed middle ear.
         (2) Second stage—(performed 2–3 months after 1st stage) reconstruction using grafts.
   3. *Postoperative Nursing Management*
      a. Reinforce outer dressings as necessary but keep inner dressings intact.
      b. Assist patient in getting out of bed for the first time because he may become dizzy.
      c. Notify physician of any dizzy reaction by patient; medication will be prescribed for vertigo and nausea.
      d. Caution patient not to blow his nose with force and to avoid wetting dressings during bathing.
      e. Note that hearing improvement is achieved in indirect proportion to the amount of surgery required; the simpler the surgery, the better the chance for hearing to improve.

OTOSCLEROSIS

Otosclerosis is a form of deafness caused by the formation of new spongy bone in the laby rinth, fixation of the stapes, and prevention of sound transmission through the ossicles to the inner fluids.

Incidence and Clinical Manifestations

1. Cause is unknown.
2. It occurs more commonly in women than men; rare in the black race.
3. It has an hereditary basis.
4. Patient presents a history of slow, progressive hearing loss with no middle ear infection.
5. A frequent complaint is buzzing or ringing noises in the ears; both ears are usually affected equally.

Diagnostic Evaluation

1. Audiometry findings substantiate hearing loss.
2. Bone conduction is much better than air conduction. Reduced tuning fork trans mission by air, whereas there is intensification of bone conduction sound when tuning fork handle is placed over the mastoid bone.

Stapedectomy (Operation of Choice)

A *stapedectomy* is removal of otosclerotic lesions at the footplate of stapes and the creation of a tissue implant with prosthesis to maintain suitable conduction. To perform such delicate surgery, the otologic binocular microscope is used.

Types of Prostheses

1. Steel wire and fat implant
2. Gelfoam and stainless steel wire
3. Metal or teflon "piston"
4. Vein graft and polyethylene tubing (least frequent)

Nursing Management

1. Observe for unusual symptoms, such as:
   a. Fever—may indicate infection, external otitis, otitis media
   b. Headache—may indicate infection, nerve encroachment
   c. Vertigo—may indicate labyrinthitis or inner ear reaction
   d. Ear pain—may indicate infection or irritation of auditory nerve
2. Position patient postoperatively as desired by physician.
   a. Some surgeons prefer that the patient be positioned with operated ear uppermost to maintain position of graft and stability.
   b. Others prefer that patient be lying on operated ear to permit drainage.
   c. Still others advocate that the patient assume the most comfortable position.
3. Administer antimotion medications and sedatives if patient experiences vertigo, nystagmus or nausea.
4. Assist patient when he first tries to walk; he may feel dizzy for the first few days.

5. Instruct patient not to blow his nose for a week; air may be forced up the eustachian tube and disturb the operative site.
6. Encourage a restricted head position if the surgeon fears a misplacement of the prosthesis.
7. Replace soiled (bloody) cotton pledget in ear canal as necessary.
8. Administer meperidine or prescribed pain medication for first several hours.
9. Advise patient that it may be weeks before full effect of surgery is determined as far as hearing is concerned. At first, hearing may be impaired because of tissue edema, packing, etc.
10. Note that while patient may be ready for discharge in 4 or 5 days, packing is not removed until the 6th or 7th day in the physician's office.
11. Instruct patient as follows:
    a. Do not smoke.
    b. Do not blow nose.
    c. Protect ears when going outdoors for the first week.
    d. Avoid crowds or exposure to colds so that upper respiratory infection is prevented.

MENIERE'S DISEASE
(Endolymphatic Hydrops)

Meniere's Disease involves the inner ear and causes a triad of symptoms: vertigo, hearing loss and tinnitus.

Etiology
1. Meniere's syndrome stems from labyrinthine dysfunction.
2. Suggested theories as to the cause of this syndrome:
    a. Increase in pressure of endolymph
    b. Emotional or endocrine disturbance
    c. Vasomotor changes causing a spasm of the internal auditory artery
    d. Allergic manifestation

Clinical Manifestations
A. *During Attack*
1. Dizziness, tinnitus and reduced hearing occurs on involved side.
2. Patient complains somewhat of headache, nausea, vomiting, incoordination.
3. Sudden attacks occur in which patient complains that room appears to spin around.
4. Sudden motion of the head may precipitate vomiting.
5. Patient often presents a history of ear trouble, vasomotor rhinitis, and allergies.
6. The most comfortable position for the patient is lying down.
7. Personality changes manifest themselves in irritability, depression, withdrawal and refusal to eat.
8. Vertigo attacks may last several hours or all day.

B. *After or Between Attacks*
1. Patient behaves normally; may continue his work.
2. Only complaint may be tinnitus or impaired hearing.

Diagnostic Evaluation

Caloric Test

1. Useful in differentiating Meniere's syndrome from intracranial lesion.
2. Fluid, which is above or below body temperature, is instilled into auditory canal.
3. Reactions
   a. Normal patient—complains of dizziness
   b. Patient with acoustic neuroma—no reaction
   c. Patient with Meniere's syndrome—severe attack (as described on p. 715)
4. Nursing management
   a. Anticipate possibility of patient vomiting; have emesis basin and protective draping.
   b. Support patient as he walks after the test since he may be dizzy.

Surgical Treatment

1. *Destruction of the labyrinth*—recommended if the patient experiences progressive hearing loss and severe vertigo attacks and cannot assume normal tasks.
2. *Ultrasonic surgery*—semicircular canal reached through a mastoid incision; ultrasonic energy applied directly via a probe to the bone in the canal (may cause transient facial paralysis).
3. *Cryosurgery*—used infrequently; may cause residual dizziness.

Nursing Management

1. Recognize the need for encouragement and understanding; this is particularly true when the patient experiences symptoms of a subjective nature.
2. Remind the patient to slow down his bodily movements since jerking or making sudden movements may precipitate an attack.
3. Protect the patient who has an attack by placing him in a bed with side rails in position; if he is standing, help lower him to the floor to avoid injury.
4. Postoperatively, patient may experience vertigo; therefore, he may be more comfortable in bed for the first 2 days.
5. Assist patient when he gets out of bed since he may be unsteady; remind him to change his movements easily.
6. Inform him that dizziness may persist as long as 4–6 weeks.
7. Note that a possible complication is Bell's palsy (a peripheral facial weakness with noticeable pain near the angle of the jaw or behind the ear) (p. 735). This will clear up eventually.

COMMUNICATING WITH A PERSON WHO HAS A HEARING IMPAIRMENT

When the Person Is Able to Lip-read

1. Face the person as directly as possible when speaking.
2. Place yourself in good light for him to see your mouth.
3. Do not chew, smoke or have anything in your mouth when speaking.
4. Speak slowly and enunciate distinctly.

5. Provide contextual clues that will assist him in following your speech. For example, point to a tray if you are talking about the food on it.
6. To verify that he understands your message, write it for him to read. (That is, if you doubt that he is understanding you.)

When It Is Difficult to Understand the Person When He Speaks

1. Pay attention when the person speaks; his facial and physical gestures may help you understand what he is saying.
2. Exchange conversation with him where it is possible to anticipate his replies—this is particularly helpful in your initial contact with him and may help you become familiar with his speech peculiarities.
3. Anticipate context of his speech to assist in interpreting what he is saying.
4. If unable to understand him, resort to writing or include in your conversation someone who does understand him; request that he repeat that which is not understood.

BIBLIOGRAPHY

Books

Ballantyne, J., and Groves, J.: Scott-Brown's Diseases of the Ear, Nose, and Throat, 3rd ed., (Vol. 2). Philadelphia, J. B. Lippincott, 1971.
Brunner, L. S., et al.: Textbook of Medical and Surgical Nursing, 2nd ed. Philadelphia, J. B. Lippincott, 1970, pp. 742–758.
Council of Organizations Serving the Deaf: Medical Aspects of Deafness. Proceedings: National Forum IV., Atlantic City, N. J., 1971.
Saunders, W. H., et al.: Nursing Care in Eye, Ear, Nose and Throat Disorders. 2nd ed. St. Louis, C. V. Mosby, 1968.
Worrell, J. D.: Nursing implications in the care of the patient experiencing sensory deprivation. *In* Kintzel, K. C., (ed.): Advanced Concepts in Clinical Nursing. Philadelphia, J. B. Lippincott, 1971.

Articles

DeLancey, R. E.: Stapedectomy. Amer. J. Nurs., *69*:2406–2409, Nov. 1969.
Golub, S.: Noise, the underrated health hazard. R.N., *32*:40–45, May 1969.
Moore, M. V.: Diagnosis: Deafness. Amer. J. Nurs., *69*:297–300, Feb. 1969.
Myers, D., et al.: Otologic diagnosis and the treatment of deafness. Clinical Symposium. Summit, N. J., Ciba, Vol. 22, No. 2, 1970.
Nilo, E. R.: Needs of the hearing impaired. Amer. J. Nurs., *69*:114–116, Jan. 1969.
Rummerfield, P. S., and Rummerfield, M. J.: Noise induced hearing loss. Occup. Health Nurs., *17*:23–24, Nov. 1969.

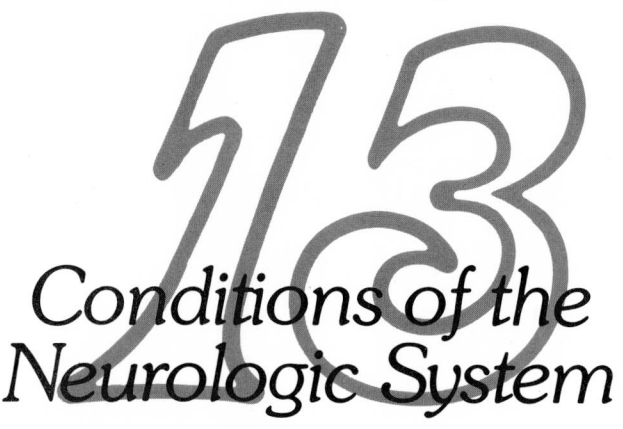

Conditions of the Neurologic System

DIAGNOSTIC EVALUATION OF NEUROLOGIC DISEASE

Radiologic Procedures

A. *Skull X-ray*—reveals configuration, density, vascular markings and intracranial calcification and tumor.

B. *Air Studies*—a gaseous replacement of the fluid within the ventricles and subarachnoid systems serves as a contrast medium because air is less dense than fluid to roentgen rays.
   1. *Pneumoencephalogram*—withdrawal of cerebrospinal fluid and injection of air or other gas by means of a lumbar puncture.
      a. Demonstrates ventricular system and subarachnoid space overlying the hemispheres and basal cisterns.
      b. Useful in diagnosing degenerative cerebral atrophy and in detecting mass lesions at the base of brain.
   2. *Fractional pneumoencephalogram*—withdrawal of small amounts of fluid and injections of small amounts of air to visualize the ventricular system.
   3. *Ventriculogram*—withdrawal of cerebrospinal fluid and injection of air or gas directly into the lateral ventricles through openings in the skull.
      Used in presence of increased intracranial pressure or when tumor is suspected.
   4. *Nursing management following pneumoencephalogram or ventriculogram*
      a. Patient may complain of severe headache—assess for fever and signs of shock.
      b. Watch the patient for increasing intracranial pressure (p. 724).
         (1) Disturbances of intracranial pressure may cause serious complications.
         (2) Prepare for ventricular tap and prompt decompression.
      c. Take vital signs as frequently as clinical condition indicates and until stabilized.
      d. Treat patient's headache by placing ice cap to head (intermittently).
         (1) Give analgesics as directed—duration of headache depends on the speed with which the intracranial air is absorbed.
         (2) Nausea and vomiting may also follow these air studies.

C. *Angiogram*—injection of contrast media into the carotid or vertebral arteries in the neck to visualize by means of x-rays the blood vessels of the head and neck.
   1. Tumors, abscesses, intracranial hemorrhages and occluded arteries may be demonstrated.
   2. Nursing support
      a. Observe patient for hypersensitivity reactions, seizures and hemiparesis.
      b. Apply an ice cap at injection site intermittently—to relieve swelling and discomfort.

D. *Myelogram*—injection of radiopaque oil into the spinal subarachnoid space through a lumbar puncture needle.
   1. Outlines the spinal subarachnoid space and shows distortions of the spinal cord or dural sac caused by tumors, cysts, herniated intervertebral disks or other lesions.
   2. Nursing implications
      a. Same as for lumbar puncture (p. 720).
      b. Observe for headache, nausea and general malaise after examination.

E. *Discogram*—injection of a radiopaque substance directly into the intervertebral disk. This study can be used in patients suspected of having a herniated nucleus pulposus but is infrequently done.

Brain Scan

Intravenous injection of radioactive compound and the application of a scintillation scanner of the patient's brain—there is an increased uptake of radioactive material at the site of pathology. (No special preparation or aftercare required.)

Echoencephalogram

1. Recording of echoes derived from the deep structures within the skull by transmission of ultrasound waves.
2. A rapid and useful technique for detecting a shift of the cerebral midline structure precipitated by subdural hematoma, intracerebral hemorrhage, massive cerebral infarction and neoplasms.
3. Used in combination with other procedures; no special nursing implications.

Electromyogram

Introduction of a needle electrode into muscle to study muscle action potentials. Helps distinguish the weakness of neuropathy from that of other causes.

Lumbar Puncture

Insertion of a needle into lumbar subarachnoid space and withdrawal of cerebrospinal fluid for diagnostic and therapeutic purposes.

GUIDELINES: Assisting the Patient Undergoing a Lumbar Puncture

Purposes

1. To obtain cerebrospinal fluid for examination.*
2. To relieve cerebrospinal pressure.
3. To determine the presence or absence of blood in the spinal fluid.

Equipment

Sterile lumbar puncture set	Skin antiseptic
Sterile gloves	Band-aid
Xylocaine 1–2%	

Procedure

Nursing Action	*Rationale/Amplification*
Preparatory Phase	
1. Position the patient on his side with a pillow under his head.	
2. Instruct the patient to arch the lumbar segment of his back and draw his knees up to his abdomen, clasping his knees with his hands.	2. This posture offers maximal widening of the interspinous spaces and affords easier entry into the subarachnoid space.

* See Appendix for characteristics of normal cerebrospinal fluid.

Nursing Action	**Rationale/Amplification**

3. While standing on the opposite side of the physician, assist the patient in maintaining his position by supporting him behind his knees and neck. Assist the patient to maintain the posture throughout the examination.

3. Supporting the patient helps prevent sudden movements which can produce a traumatic (bloody) tap and obscure the correct diagnosis.

Performance Phase (by the physician)

1. The skin is prepared with antiseptic solution and the skin and subcutaneous spaces are infiltrated with local anesthetic agent. The site is draped.

2. A spinal puncture needle is introduced between L3–L4 or L4–L5 interspace. The needle is advanced until the "give" of the ligamentum flavum is felt and the needle enters the subarachnoid space.

2. L3–L4 or L4–L5 interspace is *below* the level of the spinal cord.

3. After the needle enters the subarachnoid space, help the patient to slowly straighten his legs.

3. This maneuver prevents a false increase in intraspinal pressure. Muscle tension and compression of the abdomen give falsely high pressures.

4. Instruct the patient to breathe quietly; not to hold his breath or strain.

4. Hyperventilation may lower a truly elevated pressure.

5. The manometer is attached to the spinal puncture needle and the initial pressure reading is obtained by measuring the level of the fluid column after it comes to rest.

5. With respiration there is normally some fluctuation of spinal fluid in the manometer. Normally the initial pressure does not exceed 180 mm. of spinal fluid.

6. About 1 ml. of spinal fluid is placed in each of 3 test tubes for observation, comparison and laboratory analysis.

6. Spinal fluid should be clear and colorless. Bloody spinal fluid may indicate cerebral contusion, laceration or subarachnoid hemorrhage.

Queckenstedt test

1. A blood pressure cuff is placed around the patient's neck and inflated to a pressure of 20 mm.Hg (or an assistant compresses jugular vein or veins for 10 seconds).

2. Pressure readings are made at 10-second intervals.

3. After the needle is withdrawn, a Band-aid is applied to the puncture site.

The Queckenstedt test is made when spinal tumor is suspected. In normal persons there is a rapid rise in pressure of cerebrospinal fluid in response to compression of the veins of the neck with a rapid return to normal when the compression is released. If the pressure rises and falls slowly there is evidence of a block due to a lesion compressing the spinal subarachnoid pathways.

Follow-up Phase

1. Record (a) procedure, (b) appearance of spinal fluid, (c) whether or not specimens were sent to laboratory, (d) spinal pressure readings and (e) condition and reaction of patient.

2. Keep the patient flat in bed (small pillow under head) for 6–12 hours. Encourage liberal intake of fluid. Administer glucose or saline I.V. to patient with severe headache.

2. Some patients suffer from postpuncture headache which is thought to be due to leaking of cerebrospinal fluid into the epidural space with resultant settling of the brain against the base of the skull, causing traction on pain-sensitive intracranial vascular structures.

SPECIAL NEUROLOGIC NURSING CONSIDERATIONS
Nursing Management of the Patient with a Head Injury

Clinical Manifestations

Unconsciousness or disturbance in
   consciousness
Headache
Vertigo
Confusion or delirium

Changes in body temperature
Respiratory irregularities
Symptoms of shock—coldness, pallor,
   sweating, falling blood pressure
Pupillary abnormalities

Immediate Management in the Emergency Department

> NURSING ALERT: Regard every patient who has a head injury as having a potential spinal cord injury.

1. Maintain an open airway and ensure maximum respiratory function—oxygen deprivation and an excess of carbon dioxide may produce cerebral hypoxia and cause cerebral edema with subsequent irreparable damage.
   a. Employ adequate suctioning procedures (p. 115)—patient may have aspirated blood and mucus from face or head injuries and the nasopharynx may be flooded with gastric contents—leads to pneumonitis which contributes to respiratory acidosis.
   b. Ensure adequate oxygenation and humidification.
   c. Assist with endotracheal intubation if patient is comatose.
   d. Place patient in a semiprone head-level position to transport him from the emergency room to the clinical unit. (Place a small support under patient's head when he is in a lateral position.)
2. Determine the base-line condition of the patient; start Neurological Observation Record (see p. 725).
   a. Assess level of responsiveness.
   b. Determine presence of headache, double vision, nausea or vomiting.
   c. Evaluate pupil size and reaction to light.
   d. Measure blood pressure, pulse, respirations.
   e. Evaluate motion and strength of extremities.
   f. Assess for injuries to other organ systems.
3. Obtain as accurate a history as possible from patient or observer.
   a. What caused the injury? A high velocity missile? Object striking the head? A fall?
   b. What was the direction and force of the blow?
   c. *Was there loss of consciousness?* How long? Could the patient be aroused?
   d. Was there any bleeding from eyes, ears, nose, mouth?
   e. Was there paralysis or flaccidity of the extremities?
4. Give intravenous medication for immediate convulsive seizures.

Treatment and Nursing Management*

Objective: to observe the patient constantly for the development of focal or generalized deficits of function that indicate need for surgical intervention.

1. Support the airway—small degrees of anoxia rapidly increase cerebral dysfunction and brain swelling.

---

* See also nursing management of the unconscious patient, page 728.

    a. Carry out blood gas studies—to determine respiratory adequacy.

         pO_2 levels less than 80 mm.Hg $\Big\}$ indicate need for ventilatory assistance.
         pCO_2 levels of more than 50 mm.Hg

    b. Prepare for tracheostomy if there is labored breathing or pooling of secretions (p. 98).

    c. Give intermittent positive pressure breathing treatments as directed (p. 134).

    d. Position the patient in a semiprone, three-quarters prone or prone position with his head level—improves oxygen and carbon dioxide exchange and prevents aspiration of secretions or blood.

    e. Turn from side to side—to prevent stasis of secretions in lungs and pressure on skin.

2. Observe and evaluate and carry out repeated clinical examinations to determine minute-to-minute, hour-to-hour changes in patient's status. (See Neurological Observation Record, p. 725).

    a. Observe and record:

        (1) Level of responsiveness   (3) Motor strength
        (2) Changes in vital signs   (4) Pupillary changes

    b. See page 724 The Patient with Increasing Intracranial Pressure.

3. Give fluids and electrolytes in physiological proportions—to ensure fluid balance and an adequate urinary output.

    a. Do not give fluids by mouth to an unconscious patient.

    b. Weigh daily and keep intake and output record—to determine fluid loss.

    c. Carry out serial blood and urine electrolyte and osmolality studies—head injuries may be accompanied by disorders of sodium regulation.

    d. Give nasogastric feedings (or gastrostomy feedings) if patient is unable to swallow after several days.

    e. Give intravenous solutions fairly slowly—overhydration tends to cerebral edema.

    f. Insert indwelling catheter if patient is unconscious—for assessment of urinary volume and to prevent restlessness from distended bladder.

4. Control rising temperature with hypothermia blankets, fever sponges—to lower the metabolic requirements of the brain.

5. Give medications to control brain edema (steroids). In selected patients mannitol or urea may be used.

6. Support the patient during episodes of restlessness.

    a. Avoid restraints.

    b. Give small doses of chloral hydrate, paraldehyde or tranquilizing drugs.

    c. Be aware that restlessness may be caused by shock, respiratory obstruction, pain from fractured extremities, extradural hematoma, distended bladder.

7. Give diphenylhydantoin (Dilantin) or phenobarbital as ordered—for control of seizures (see p. 731).

8. Protect the eyes from corneal irritation (see p. 731).

9. Carry out rehabilitation techniques.

    a. Put all extremities through range of motion exercises.

    b. Position the patient correctly to prevent contractures.

    c. Keep the skin dry, clean and free of pressure—to prevent decubitus ulcers.

    d. Begin a program of graded exercises—exercise restores fitness and flagging motivation and assists in elevating the patient's mood to one of optimism.

    e. Ensure a well-balanced diet.

    f. Gradually increase physical and mental activity (including returning to increasingly difficult mental tasks).

10. Be aware of aftereffects of head injury—usually directly related to the severity of the injury.
    a. Headache
    b. Dizziness or vertigo
    c. Emotional instability or irritability
    d. Posttraumatic epilepsy
    e. Posttraumatic neuroses and psychoses

Nursing Management of the Patient with Increasing Intracranial Pressure

Causes

Head injury
Cerebral edema
Abscess or inflammation

Hemorrhage
Brain tumor
Cranial surgery

> NURSING ALERT: As intracranial pressure increases, the brain substance is compressed. A sudden increase may produce an emergency situation in a few minutes. This condition may lead rapidly to death or produce a vegetative existence for the patient.

Clinical Manifestations

1. Change in level of responsiveness (consciousness)
   a. *The level of responsiveness is the most important measure of the patient's condition.*
   b. Look for lethargy, delay in response to verbal suggestions, slowing of speech.
   c. Watch for sudden changes in condition—quietness to restlessness, orientation to confusion, increasing drowsiness, stupor, coma.
   d. *Progressive deterioration is a serious sign* that may require immediate surgical intervention.
2. Changes in vital signs
   a. Pulse changes—slowing rate to 60 or below; increasing rate to 100 or above.
   b. Respiratory irregularities; slowing of rate with lengthening periods of apnea; Cheyne-Stokes or Kussmaul breathing.
   c. Rising blood pressure or widening pulse pressure (the difference between systolic and diastolic blood pressure).
   d. Moderately elevated temperature.
3. Headache
4. Vomiting
5. Pupillary changes—increasing pressure or an expanding clot can displace the brain against the oculomotor or optic nerve.

Treatment and Nursing Management

A. *Assessment of Patient's Level of Responsiveness*
   1. Response to commands:
      a. Answers questions readily and correctly.
      b. Can perform a complex maneuver.
      c. Responds to simple command.
      d. Gives delayed or unequal response.
      e. Reacts only to loud voice.
      f. Does not respond.

TABLE 13-1. NEUROLOGICAL OBSERVATION RECORD*

	Time 7/14 9³⁰ AM	10⁰⁰ AM	
Spontaneous behavior	Quiet. lies in bed; little activity; complains of headache	No spontaneous activity	
Level of responsiveness to stimulation	Drowsy; can be aroused. Responds to voice	Less response; more difficult to arouse but does respond to deep pain (supra-orbital pressure)	
Orientation (time/place)	Oriented to place, knows year but not day or month	—	
Movements: Rt. and left arm Rt. and left leg	Moves all 4 extremities but left less than right	Moves right side in response to pain. left side gives decerebrate response	
Pupil size (draw) Rt. Left reaction	Rt O Left O Rt reacts sluggishly to light	Rt O Left O Fixed Slight reaction	
Speech Clear Rambling Incoherent Aphasic	Slightly slurred	No speech	
Vital Signs — Blood pressure	150/60	200/60	
Pulse	60	48	
Respirations	18	12	
Temperature	37°C. (98.6°)	37°C.	

* Based on following case study:
Mr. Elliott Smith, a 36-year-old computer-programmer, sought the services of an ophthalmologist because he had been having generalized headaches for a period of "several months." Moderate papilledema and a left hemianopsia field defect (loss of vision in one-half of the visual field of one or both eyes) was noted upon examination. He was admitted immediately to the hospital with a possible brain tumor and increasing intracranial pressure. These nursing observations were part of a continuing assessment record and were made 36 hours after admission.

2. Assessment of spinal motor reflexes (pinch Achilles tendon, arm or other body site):
   a. Prompt purposeful withdrawal.   c. Facial grimace.
   b. Sluggish or nonpurposeful movement   d. Involuntary voiding.
      of extremities.   e. No response.
3. Observation of patient's spontaneous activity:
   a. Verbal or other communication.   d. Retching, vomiting.
   b. Changes in posture (frequency).   e. Restlessness, twitching, tremors,
   c. Breathing pattern.   convulsions.

B. *General Treatment of Increasing Intracranial Pressure*
   1. Keep a Neurological Observation Record (see Table 13–1, p. 725).
      Purpose: To provide a continuing assessment of the patient so that a *change* in condition may be noted immediately. All observations should be compared and evaluated from the *base-line* (initial) condition of the patient.
      a. Know the patient's base-line condition.
      b. Carry out *repeated* nursing assessments—to determine clinical improvement or deterioration.
   2. Give intravenous mannitol, urea, steroids, etc. as ordered—to reduce brain swelling.
      a. Watch for extravasation of I.V. solution since hyperosmolar solutions can produce a skin slough.
      b. Give antacids and systemic anticholinergic agents as directed—to prevent gastrointestinal bleeding.
   3. Insert an indwelling urinary catheter (p. 467)—to measure urinary volume as dehydrating agents produce diuresis.
   4. Use hypothermia methods—hypothermia blanket, fever sponges (See Guidelines, below), aspirin—if patient has elevated temperature—to assist in controlling anoxic changes to the brain by reducing its oxygen requirements.
   5. Prepare for surgical intervention if patient's condition deteriorates.

GUIDELINES: *Administering a Fever Sponge*

Fever is any abnormal elevation of body temperature.

A *fever sponge* is the bathing of the body with tepid water (or alcohol and water) for a period of time to reduce fever. It is particularly effective in neurological conditions in which there is a disturbance of the temperature-regulating center.

Causes

Infection or inflammation   Extravasation of blood in the tissues
Disturbance of temperature-regulating center   Drugs or toxins
   (trauma, central nervous system, hemorrhage)

Purpose

To reduce body temperature.

Equipment

Basin of tepid water 21.1–29.1 C. (70–85°F.).
   or
Basin of alcohol (25% saturated with tepid water)
Bath blanket/plastic sheet

Hot water bottle with cover
Ice bag with cover
Towels
7 washcloths and wash mitts

Procedure

Nursing Action	Rationale/Amplification

Preparatory Phase

1. Place plastic sheet under patient and bath blanket over patient.
2. Remove top bedding.

Performance Phase

1. Take temperature, pulse and respiration before starting sponge.

1. This serves as a base line for comparison of effectiveness of treatment.

2. Give antipyretic medication as ordered 15–20 minutes before starting sponge.

2. There is a more rapid reduction of fever when sponging is combined with administration of antipyretic medication.

  a. Acetaminophen or
  b. Acetylsalicylic acid

  b. Salicylates lower a raised body temperature but increase oxygen consumption and metabolic rate.

  c. Phenobarbital

  c. Phenobarbital decreases heat production and this partially reduces body temperature.

  d. Chlorpromazine

  d. Controls shivering.

3. Apply ice bag to head.

3. Relieves headache and promotes patient comfort.

4. Apply hot-water bottle to feet.

4. Aids in combating chilliness and shivering.

5. Use the same sequence for sponging as for giving a bed bath.
6. Place a cold wet compress (washcloth) on neck and in each groin and axilla.

6. The application of cold over superficial large blood vessels aids in lowering body temperature.

7. Expose the body area to be sponged. Place a towel under area.
8. Using 2 wet washcloths or mitts alternately, in water or alcohol and water solution; pat each area so that solution is uniform over skin surface.

8. Vaporization of water removes heat from the surface of the skin. Alcohol vaporizes at a lower temperature and removes heat from the skin more rapidly. Tepid water and alcohol are highly effective in producing vasodilation and evaporation of heat from skin.

9. If the patient's skin feels cold to the touch, apply skin friction to bring the blood to the surface.

Nursing Action	**Rationale/Amplification**
10. Bathe each extremity 5 minutes; bathe entire back and buttocks, 5–10 minutes; bathe trunk and abdomen 5 minutes.	10. The fever sponge should not exceed 30 minutes.
11. Allow a fan to blow over the patient while sponging him if temperature is high.	11. Increased air movement augments heat loss.
12. Watch for extreme shivering. Cover the patient and wait a few minutes before proceeding with sponge.	12. Shivering may raise heat production.
13. Stop sponge if cyanosis, mottling, chilling do not stop when friction (rubbing) is applied to the skin.	13. These symptoms indicate a change in vasomotor tone.

Follow-up Phase

1. Remove bath blanket and plastic sheet. Place a dry gown on patient.	
2. Record T.P.R. 30 minutes after sponge is finished.	2. Postsponge temperature indicates whether or not treatment has been effective.

Nursing Management of the Unconscious Patient

Clinical Problems

There are 2 major threats to the unconscious patient:

1. The disease or trauma that produced unconsciousness.
2. The threat of the unconscious state.

Objectives of Treatment and Nursing Management

Nursing Goal: to assume the protective reflexes for the patient until he is aware of himself and can function in his environment.

A. *To establish and maintain an adequate airway* (Fig. 13-1).

   1. Place the patient in a three-fourths prone or semiprone position with his face dependent—prevents the tongue from obstructing the airway, encourages drainage of respiratory secretions and promotes oxygen and carbon dioxide exchange.
   2. Insert oral airway if tongue is paralyzed or is obstructing airway—an obstructed airway increases intracranial pressure.
   3. Prepare for insertion of cuffed endotracheal tube if patient's condition requires (see p. 107)—endotracheal intubation is more effective in permitting positive pressure ventilation. The cuffed tube seals off the digestive tract, thus preventing aspiration and allows efficient removal of tracheobronchial secretions.
   4. Utilize oxygen therapy, positive pressure assisted breathing techniques or artificial ventilation with a respirator when there is indication of impending respiratory failure (see p. 125).
   5. Keep the airway free of secretions with efficient suctioning—with the absence of the cough and swallowing reflexes, secretions rapidly accumulate in the posterior pharynx and upper trachea and can pave the way to fatal respiratory complications.
   6. Prepare for tracheostomy if coma is deepening and there is evidence of inadequate respiratory exchange (see p. 98).

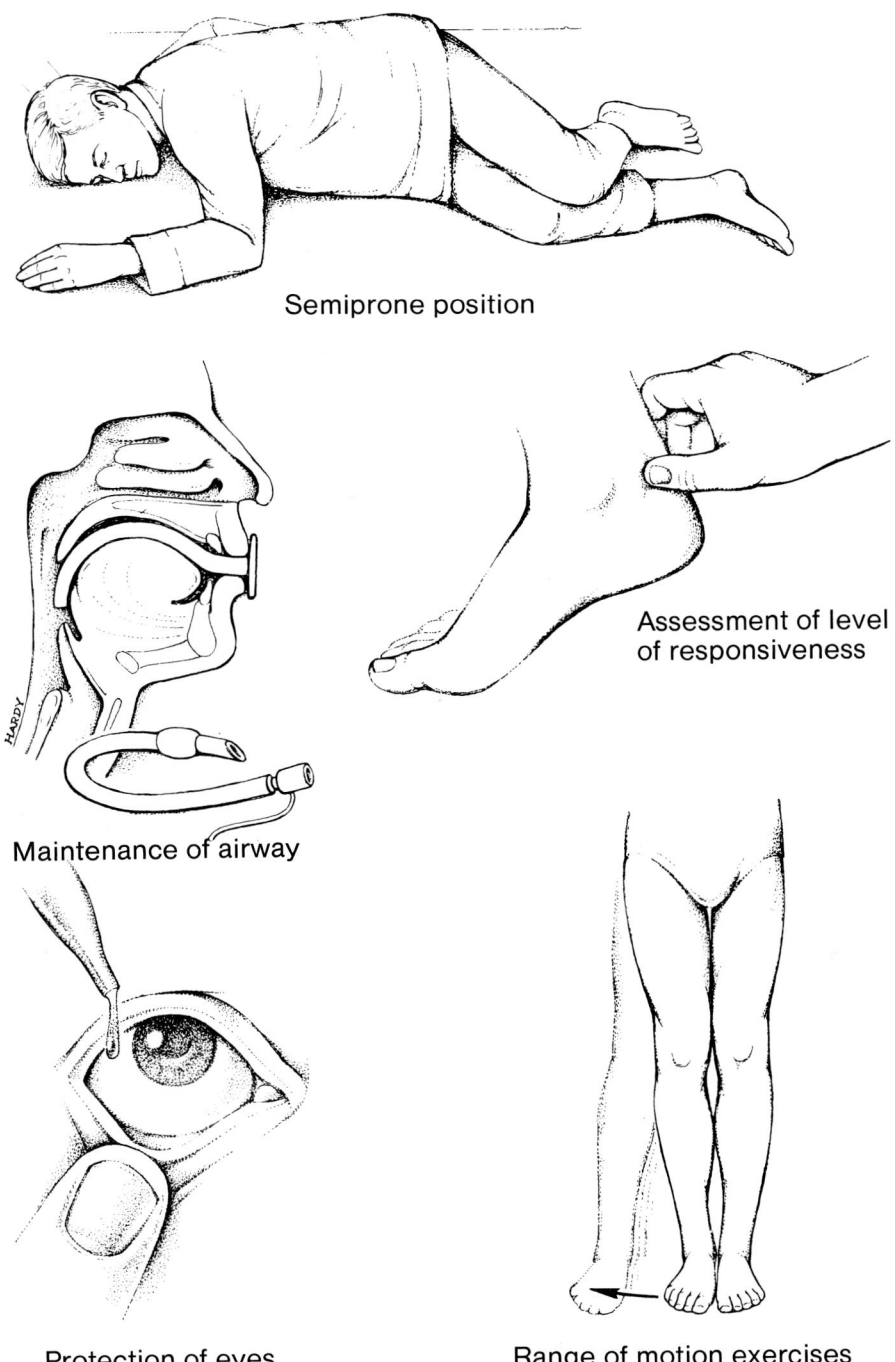

Semiprone position

Maintenance of airway

Assessment of level
of responsiveness

Protection of eyes

Range of motion exercises

Figure 13-1. Nursing priorities in the care of the unconscious patient.

B. *To assess the level of responsiveness.*

 1. Maintain a constant assessment of the patient's level of consciousness and changes in responsiveness—the level of consciousness is the most important measure of the patient's condition. Unconscious patients may deteriorate rapidly from numerous clinical causes.
 2. Record the patient's *exact reactions,* movements and quality of speech.
    a. Request the patient to speak.
    b. Ask the patient to perform some activity (raise arm, protrude tongue, etc.).
    c. Apply painful stimuli if there is no response (pinching skin of arms or thighs) and assess patient's perception of pain. No response or a delayed or unequal response is an unfavorable clinical sign.

C. *To evaluate the progression of vital signs.*

 1. Know the patient's base-line vital signs and alert the physician if there are significant fluctuations of blood pressure and instability of the pulse and respiratory cycle—fluctuations of vital signs indicate a change in intracranial homeostasis.
 2. Take blood pressure readings, pulse and respiratory rate and temperature at frequently specified intervals until there is evidence of stabilization.

D. *To maintain fluid and electrolyte balance.*

 1. Give intravenous fluids as indicated, using a vein in the hand—serial laboratory electrolyte evaluations are made when the patient is maintained on intravenous fluids to ensure proper balance.
 2. Initiate nasogastric feedings (see p. 383)—feeding through a gastric tube ensures better nutrition than does intravenous feeding. Paralytic ileus is fairly frequent in the unconscious, and a nasogastric tube assists in gastric decompression.

E. *To give nursing support as the patient's changing condition indicates.*

 1. Be aware of the varying phases of restlessness—a certain degree of restlessness may be favorable, as it may indicate the patient is regaining consciousness. However, restlessness is quite common in cerebral anoxia or when there is a partially obstructed airway, distended bladder, overlooked bleeding or fracture; it may be a manifestation of brain injury.
    a. Have adequate lighting in the room to prevent hallucinations as the patient regains consciousness.
    b. Pad side rails or use other devices to protect patient.
    c. Avoid oversedating the patient.
    d. Avoid restraints if at all possible.
 2. Keep the skin clean, dry and free of pressure—comatose patients are susceptible to formation of decubitus ulcers (p. 20).
 3. Put all extremities through range of motion exercises 4 times daily—contracture deformities develop early in unconscious patients.
 4. Turn the patient from side to side at regular intervals—turning relieves pressure areas and helps keep lungs clear by mobilizing secretions. Prolonged pressure on extremities produces nerve palsies.
 5. Observe the patient for indication of an overdistended bladder.
    a. Utilize external sheath catheter (condom catheter) for male patient.
    b. If patient is unable to void, insert 3-way indwelling catheter with continuous drainage—infection invariably follows prolonged use of an indwelling catheter that is attached to straight drainage.

    c. Tape the catheter horizontally to the side of the male patient (see p. 505) and to the inner thigh of the female to prevent urethral compression (male) and traction on the urethra.

6. Protect the eyes from corneal irritation—the cornea functions as a shield. If the eyes remain open for long periods, corneal drying, irritation and ulceration are apt to result.

    a. Inspect the size of pupils and condition of eyes with a flashlight.

    b. Remove contact lenses if worn (see p. 699).

    c. Irrigate eyes with sterile saline solution and instill sterile mineral oil drops in each eye.

    d. Prepare for temporary tarsorrhaphy (suturing of eyelids in closed position) if unconscious state is prolonged.

7. Protect the patient during convulsive seizures (see below)—a patient with head trauma is a potential candidate for convulsive seizures.

    a. Protect the patient from self-injury.

    b. Observe the patient during the seizure and record observations.

    c. Give prescribed anticonvulsant medications through the nasogastric tube.

8. Be alert for the development of complications.

    a. Respiratory complications (infection, aspiration, obstruction, atelectasis)

    b. Fluid and electrolyte imbalance

    c. Infection (urinary, decubitus ulcers, central nervous system)

    d. Bladder and gastrointestinal distention

    e. Convulsive seizures

Nursing Management of the Patient Having a Convulsive Seizure

A *convulsion* is involuntary contractions of muscles resulting from abnormal cerebral stimulation.

Nursing Management

Objective: to prevent injury to the patient.

1. Observe and record the progression of symptoms during the seizure.

    a. State whether or not the beginning of the attack was observed.

    b. Note the following:

        (1) The first thing the patient does in an attack—where the movements or stiffness starts; position of eyeballs and head

        (2) The type of movements of the part involved

        (3) The parts involved (turn back covers and expose patient)

        (4) Size of pupils

        (5) Incontinence of urine and feces

        (6) Duration of each phase of the attack

        (7) Unconsciousness, if present, and its duration

        (8) Any obvious paralysis or weakness of arms or legs after the attack

        (9) Inability to speak after the attack

        (10) Whether or not the patient sleeps after the attack

2. Support the patient during the convulsive seizure.

    a. Ensure an adequate airway.

    b. Give the patient privacy and protect him from curious onlookers.

    c. Protect the head with a pad to prevent head injury.
      (1) Remove the pillows if he is in bed.
      (2) Loosen constrictive clothing.
    d. When jaws are clenched in spasm do not attempt to pry open to insert a mouth gag.
        If aura precedes seizure, insert a folded handkerchief between the teeth—to reduce possibility of patient biting his tongue and cheek.
    e. Place patient on his side during convulsion (if possible)—to facilitate drainage of mucus and saliva.
    f. Reorient the patient to his environment when he awakens.

Nursing Management of the Patient Undergoing Intracranial Surgery

Craniotomy is a surgical opening of the skull to remove a tumor, relieve intracranial pressure, evacuate a blood clot or stop hemorrhage.

Craniectomy is excision of a portion of the skull.

Cranioplasty is repair of a cranial defect.

Treatment and Nursing Management

A. *Preoperative Management*

Objective: to determine the precise location of the lesion (clot, tumor, aneurysm).
    1. Assist the patient undergoing diagnostic tests and frequent neurologic examinations.
    2. Evaluate and record patient's symptoms and signs (paralysis, aphasia) preoperatively in order to make postoperative comparisons.
    3. Support the patient with neurologic motor and sensory defects.
      a. Position paralyzed extremities to prevent contracture deformities (see p. 5).
      b. Familiarize the blind patient with his environment.
        (1) Personnel entering room should announce themselves—helps patient understand incoming stimuli.
        (2) Help patient to assume an active role in his care.
      c. Assist the aphasic patient to communicate by means of picture cards, writing materials, etc.
      d. Protect the confused patient.
        (1) Remove disturbing environmental stimuli.
        (2) Keep patient oriented to time and place; place wall calendar and clock where patient can see them.
      e. Instruct and encourage the patient and family about the impending surgery—to relieve anxiety and tension.
    4. Prepare the patient physically for surgery.
      a. Shave entire scalp as directed—save the hair.
      b. Shampoo the scalp—report evidences of scalp infection.
      c. Give enemas only as directed—straining upon defecation raises intracranial pressure.
      d. Give medications and treatments as indicated.
        (1) Steroids—to decrease brain edema
        (2) Indwelling spinal catheter—to decrease brain edema
        (3) Indwelling urethral catheter—to assess urinary volume during dehydrating operative period

B. *Postoperative Management*

Objectives: to watch for life-threatening complications, namely increasing intracranial pressure from edema and bleeding.

to improve the functional status of the patient.

1. Establish proper respiratory exchange—to eliminate systemic hypercarbia and anoxia which increases cerebral edema.
   a. Keep the patient in a lateral or a semiprone position—to facilitate respiratory exchange.
   b. Employ tracheopharyngeal aspiration—to remove secretions.
   c. Carry out arterial blood gas studies—to determine respiratory adequacy.

   Ventilatory assistance (p. 137) is needed if:
   Arterial pO_2 level is less than 80 mm. Hg
   Arterial pCO_2 level is 50 mm. Hg or higher
   d. Elevate the head of the bed 30 cm. (12 inches) after patient is conscious—to aid venous drainage of the brain.
   e. See that the patient has nothing by mouth until an active coughing and swallowing reflex is demonstrated.

2. Assess patient's level of responsiveness.
   a. Response to commands:
   (1) Answers questions readily and correctly.
   (2) Can perform a complex maneuver.
   (3) Responds to simple command.
   (4) Gives delayed or unequal response.
   (5) Reacts only to loud voice.
   (6) Does not respond.
   b. Assessment of spinal motor reflexes (pinch Achilles tendon, arm or other body site):
   (1) Prompt purposeful withdrawal
   (2) Sluggish or nonpurposeful movement of extremities
   (3) Facial grimace
   (4) Involuntarily voiding
   (5) No response
   c. Observation of patient's spontaneous activity:
   (1) Verbal or other communication
   (2) Changes in posture (frequency)
   (3) Breathing pattern
   (4) Retching, vomiting
   (5) Restlessness, twitching, tremors, convulsions

3. Keep the patient normothermic during the postoperative period—temperature control may be lost in certain neurologic states; a higher temperature increases the metabolic demands of the brain.
   a. Take rectal temperature at specified intervals.
   Extremities may be cold and dry due to paralysis of heat-losing mechanisms (vasodilation and sweating).
   b. Employ measures to reduce excessive fever when present.
   (1) Remove blankets; place loin cloth over patient.
   (2) Give aspirin—however, high fever of central origin is less responsive to salicylates.
   (3) Apply ice bags to axilla and groin—application of cold over large superficial vessel helps lower body temperature.
   (4) Give tepid water or alcohol sponge (see p. 726).
   (5) Use a fan blowing on patient—to increase surface cooling.
   (6) Use hypothermia blanket.
   (7) Give chlorpromazine (I.M.)—controls hyperpyrexia and prevents shivering.

(8) Utilize ECG monitoring to detect arrhythmias during hypothermia procedures.
4. Evaluate for signs and symptoms of increasing intracranial pressure.
    a. Assess patient (minute by minute, hour by hour) for:
        (1) Decrease in response to stimuli
        (2) Fluctuations of vital signs
        (3) Restlessness
        (4) Weakness and paralysis of extremities
        (5) Increasing headache
        (6) Changes or disturbances of vision; dilated pupils
    b. Control postoperative cerebral edema.
        (1) Keep patient *slightly* underhydrated—to combat cerebral edema.
        (2) Record urinary specific gravity at intervals—indicated for surgery of the pituitary and hypothalamus.
        (3) Evaluate electrolyte status:
            (a) Early postoperative weight gain indicates fluid retention; a greater than estimated loss of weight indicates negative water balance.
            (b) Loss of sodium and chlorides will produce weakness, lethargy and coma.
            (c) Low potassium will cause confusion and decreased level of responsiveness.
        (4) Give steroids and osmotic dehydrating agents, in selected cases, in postoperative period.
        (5) Institute hypothermia procedures (see above) to decrease brain metabolism.
5. Perform supportive measures until the patient is able to care for himself.
    a. Change position frequently as pain and pressure responses are variable.
    b. Give analgesics that do not mask level of responsiveness—codeine, aspirin.
    c. Support the patient if convulsive seizures occur (see p. 731).
    d. Relieve signs of periocular edema.
        (1) Lubricate eyelids and area around eyes with petrolatum.
        (2) Apply light compresses in pliofilm (taped over eye) at specified intervals.
        (3) Watch for signs of keratitis if cornea has no sensation.
    e. Put extremities through range of motion exercises.
    f. Use aseptic measures in management of indwelling 3-way urethral catheter (see p. 467).
    g. Evaluate and support patient during episodes of restlessness.
        (1) Evaluate for airway obstruction, distended bladder, meningeal irritation from bloody cerebrospinal fluid.
        (2) Pad patient's hands and bed rails—to protect from injury.
    h. Watch for leakage of cerebrospinal fluid as there is ever present danger of meningitis.
        (1) Differentiate between cerebrospinal fluid (CSF) and mucus.
            (a) Collect fluid on Dextrostix—if CSF is present, indicator will have positive reaction as cerebrospinal fluid contains sugar.
            (b) Assess for moderate elevation of temperature and mild neck rigidity.
        (2) Keep cerebrospinal pressure low.
            (a) Lumbar puncture—pressure elevated with an increased white cell count.
            (b) Elevate head of bed.
            (c) Give antibiotics as indicated.
    i. Reinforce blood-stained dressing with sterile dressing—blood-soaked dressing acts as a culture medium for bacteria.

j. Evaluate patient with hypophysectomy (surgery upon pituitary) for diabetes insipidus.

(1) Weigh daily. (2) Keep intake and output record.

6. Assess for complications.

a. Intracranial hemorrhage—postoperative bleeding may be intraventricular, intracerebral, intracerebellar, subdural or extradural.

(1) Watch for progressive impairment of responsiveness—signs of increasing intracranial pressure.

(2) Prepare for cerebral angiography.

(3) Hematoma formation can cause progressive cerebral compression and death —requires reoperation and evacuation of hematoma.

b. Brain edema (see above).

c. Postoperative meningitis.

(1) Evaluate for deteriorating neurological status, wound swelling or drainage.

(2) Treat with appropriate antibiotics determined by culture and sensitivity studies.

d. Wound infections (scalp, boneflap).

e. Pulmonary complications.

f. Epilepsy—greater risk of epilepsy with supratentorial operations.

(1) Give anticonvulsants on a long-term basis.

(2) Status epilepticus (prolonged seizures without recovery of consciousness in the interval between seizures) may occur after any intracranial operation.

g. Gastrointestinal ulceration.

(1) There is an association between acute gastrointestinal ulceration and intracranial lesions.

(2) Watch for signs and symptoms of hemorrhage and perforation or both.

CRANIAL NERVE INVOLVEMENT

Bell's Palsy

Bell's Palsy (facial paralysis) involves the facial nerve (7th cranial nerve) on one side, producing weakness or paralysis of the facial muscles.

Clinical Manifestations

1. Feeling of numbness in face
2. Distortion of face—from paralysis of facial muscles
3. Speech difficulties
4. Inability to eat on affected side
5. Pain—behind ear or in face
6. Increased lacrimation (tearing); painful sensation in eye—causes exposure of cornea to potential injuries

Treatment and Nursing Management

Objectives: to maintain muscle tone of the face.
to prevent or minimize denervation.

1. Reassure the patient that spontaneous recovery occurs with the majority of patients; recovery usually takes place in 3–5 weeks.

2. Start facial massage (if no nerve tenderness present) several times daily—to help maintain muscle tone.
   a. Teach patient to massage his face with a gentle upward motion.
   b. Keep the face warm.
3. Promote pain relief.
   a. Give salicylates or codeine as indicated.
   b. Apply heat to involved side of face—to provide comfort and to stimulate blood perfusion through facial muscles.
4. Protect the involved eye—facial paralysis has abolished the blinking reflex; eye is vulnerable to dust and foreign particles.
   a. Use mild eyewash several times a day during acute stage (see p. 685).
   b. Instill a drop of sterile oil in eye—to keep cornea and sclera healthy.
   c. See that patient wears a protective eye patch, particularly at night.

NURSING ALERT: Keratitis is a major threat to a patient with Bell's palsy.

---

5. Use galvanic (electrical) stimulation to face (by physical therapist)—maintains nutrition of facial muscles by contracting them with an electrical current.
6. Give injection of adrenocorticotropic hormones (ACTH) I.M. as directed—to prevent or minimize denervation and permanent sequelae.
7. Teach patient facial exercises—to prevent facial muscle atrophy.
   Exercises to do while looking in a mirror.
   a. Wrinkle forehead.   d. Move mouth from side to side.
   b. Close eyes.   e. Blow out cheeks.
   c. Purse lips.   f. Whistle.

Trigeminal Neuralgia (Tic Douloureux)

Trigeminal Neuralgia (tic douloureux) is a condition of the 5th cranial nerve, characterized by paroxysms of lancinating or burning pain in the distribution of one or more branches of the trigeminal nerve and separated by periods of complete comfort.

Etiology
Unknown

Clinical Manifestations
1. Sudden and severe pain appearing without warning—in distribution in one or more branches of trigeminal nerve
2. Numerous individual flashes of pain, ending abruptly
3. Attacks precipitated by pressure on a trigger point, the terminals of the affected branches. (Shaving, talking, washing, cold wind may precipitate an agonizing attack.)

Treatment
1. Avoid serving food or fluid that is too hot or cold—may initiate an attack.
2. Drug therapy.
   a. Antiepileptic drugs—diphenylhydantoin (Dilantin)—gives pain relief in some patients.

   b. Carbamazepine (Tegretol)—relieves and prevents pain of trigeminal neuralgia.
      (1) Dosage individualized; patients tend to become resistant to drug.
      (2) Observe for evidences of hematologic and skin reactions.

NURSING ALERT: Do not give anticonvulsant drugs with narcotics to patient with trigeminal neuralgia—may have potentially dangerous interaction.

---

   c. Vitamin B$_{12}$ (I.M.)—in daily doses may prevent recurrence of pain.
3. Alcohol injection of ganglion of peripheral branches produces a chemical destruction of the affected nerves—pain returns after nerve regeneration.
4. Surgical intervention.
   a. Sectioning the preganglionic fibers to the area of pain—gives permanent relief but makes affected side of face permanently numb.
   b. Nursing surveillance
      (1) Watch for postoperative corneal infection (keratitis)—cornea insensitive if the ophthalmic division of the nerve has been sectioned.
      (2) Irrigate eye several times daily as directed (see p. 685).
      (3) Cover eye with eyeshield when necessary.
      (4) Teach patient to carry pocket mirror and inspect his eye for foreign bodies several times daily.

CEREBROVASCULAR DISEASE

Cerebrovascular disease refers to any functional abnormality of the central nervous system caused by a pathologic condition of the individual vessels or of the cerebral vascular system. It either causes hemorrhage from a tear in the vessel wall or impairs the cerebral circulation by a partial or complete occlusion of the lumen of the vessel.

Cerebrovascular Disease from Hemorrhage

1. *Extradural hemorrhage*—hemorrhage occurring outside the dura mater
   a. This is considered a life-threatening emergency.
   b. See care of the patient with a head injury for principles of immediate care (p. 722).
2. *Subdural hemorrhage*—hemorrhage occurring beneath the dura mater
      See care of the patient with a head injury (p. 722).
3. *Subarachnoid hemorrhage*—hemorrhage occurring in the subarachnoid space
      See nursing management of patient with cerebral hemorrhage (p. 746).
4. *Intercerebral hemorrhage*—hemorrhage occurring within the brain substance
      See nursing management of patient with cerebral hemorrhage (p. 746).

Cerebrovascular Disease from Impairment of Cerebral Circulation

1. *Transient ischemic attacks*—transient attacks of dysfunction of central nervous system, lasting for several minutes with the absence of neurologic disturbances between the attacks.
   a. Causes—transient impairment of the cerebral blood flow to a specific region from atherosclerotic involvement of the vessels supplying the brain.
   b. Therapy—reconstructive vascular procedures if the patient is a candidate for surgical intervention. Anticoagulant therapy.

2. *Cerebral thrombosis*—usually producing transient loss of speech, hemiplegia or paresthesia in one-half of the body which may precede severe paralysis. (See nursing management of the patient with a cerebrovascular accident.)
3. *Cerebral embolism*—caused by abnormalities of the left heart (subacute bacterial endocarditis, rheumatic heart disease, myocardial infarction) or pulmonary infections.
   a. Embolism usually lodges in middle cerebral artery or its branches where it disrupts circulation.
   b. Symptoms—sudden onset of hemiparesis or hemiplegia.
   c. See the nursing management of the patient with a cerebrovascular accident (see below).

STROKE OR CEREBRAL VASCULAR ACCIDENT (CVA)

Cerebral vascular accident (stroke) is a condition in which the blood supply to the brain is reduced as a result of intracerebral hemorrhage, thrombosis, embolism or vascular insufficiency.

Treatment and Nursing Management

A. *The Acute Phase:* The Unconscious Patient

Objectives: to keep the patient alive.
             to minimize cerebral damage by providing adequately oxygenated blood to the brain.

1. See the nursing management of the unconscious patient (p. 728).
2. Carry out a nursing assessment of the following:
   a. A change in the level of responsiveness as evidenced by movement, resistance to changes of position and response to stimulation.
   b. Presence or absence of voluntary or involuntary movements of the extremities; the tone of the muscles; the body posture and the position of the head.
   c. Stiffness or flaccidity of the neck.
   d. Comparison of pupils as to size and reaction to light.
   e. The color of the face and extremities; the temperature and the moisture of the skin.
   f. The quality and the rates of pulse and respiration; the body temperature and the arterial pressure.
   g. The volume of fluids ingested or administered and the volume of urine excreted each 24 hours.
3. Assure an adequate perfusion pressure so that oxygenated blood can reach the brain.
   a. Maintain blood pressure and cardiac output—to sustain cerebral blood flow.
   b. Watch for evidence of myocardial infarction, arrhythmias and congestive heart failure.
   c. Ensure hydration; rehydration may reduce blood viscosity and thereby improve cerebral blood flow.
4. Reorient the patient when he begins to regain consciousness.
   a. Expect some aphasia if patient has right-sided hemiplegia.
   b. Reassure patient that he has not lost his mind and that he will receive help with his communication (speech pathologist or therapist).
   c. *Talk* to the patient while caring for him.
   d. Make every effort to understand the patient.
   e. Employ a calm and accepting manner during periods of emotional lability.

Figure 13-2. Dorsal supine position for patient with cerebrovascular accident. (Dark side of pajamas represents affected or hemiplegic side.) Note the heels are suspended in the interspace between the mattress and the foot of the bed. A footboard is used to keep the feet at right angles to the legs. This prevents footdrop and heel-cord shortening caused by contracture of the gastrocnemius muscle. (Patient may wear shoes.) A pillow is placed in the axilla to prevent adduction of the affected shoulder. Pillows are placed under the arm which is in a slightly flexed position with each joint positioned higher than the preceding one.

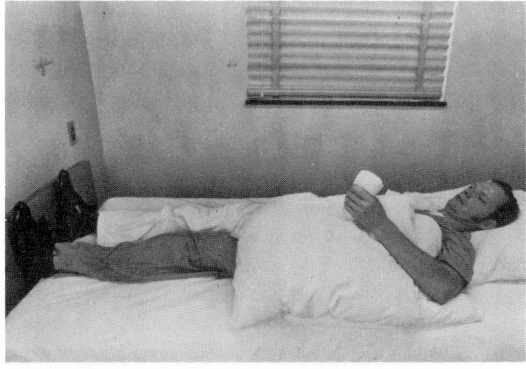

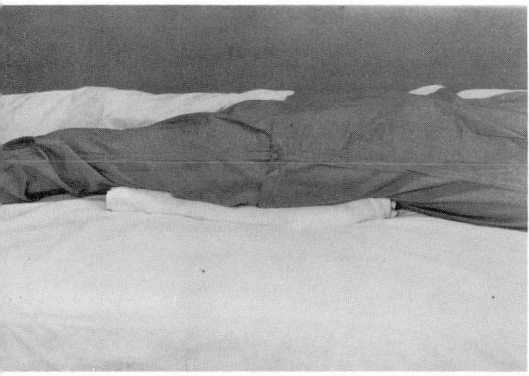

Figure 13-3. The trochanter roll should extend from the crest of the ilium to the midthigh since the hip joint lies between these 2 points. The trochanter roll acts as a mechanical wedge under the projection of the greater trochanter and prevents the femur from rolling.

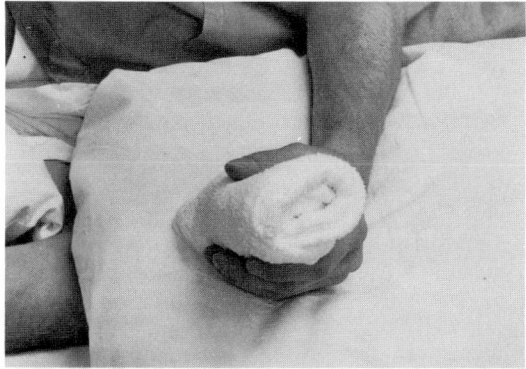

Figure 13-4. A hand roll (made of 2 washcloths) is used to keep the fingers in a slightly flexed position. The thumb is away from the hand in the position of apposition, and the hand is placed in slight supination.

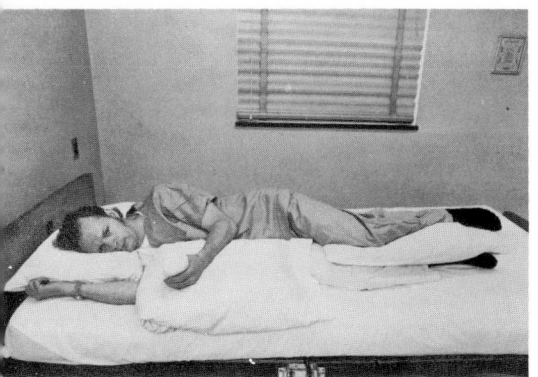

Figure 13-5. Lateral or side-lying position. The patient should be turned on his unaffected side. His upper thigh should not be acutely flexed.

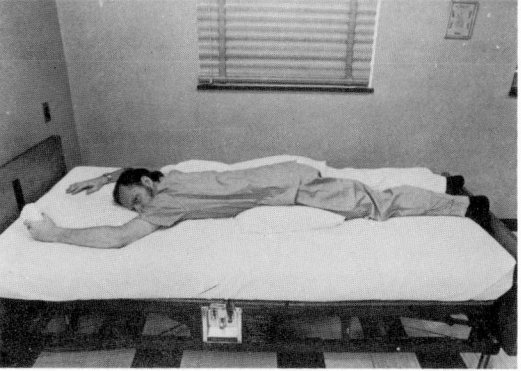

Figure 13-6. Prone position. A pillow is placed under the pelvis to help promote hyperextension of the hip joints which is essential for normal gait. Note the position of arms.

5. Remove indwelling catheter as soon as patient is conscious.
   a. Offer bedpan or urinal at scheduled short intervals.
   b. Increase time intervals as more bladder control is gained.
6. Prepare for surgical intervention if necessary—to halt potential occlusive lesions and restore circulation.

B. *Rehabilitation Phase*

Objectives: to prevent deformities.
            to retrain the affected arm and leg.
            to help the patient gain independence in personal hygiene and dressing and ambulation activities.

1. Position the patient in bed correctly—to prevent contractures, relieve pressure and maintain good body alignment. (These principles of positioning are also carried out during the unconscious phase.)
   a. Place a board under the mattress—to give the body firm support.
   b. Encourage patient to remain flat in bed except when engaged in activities of daily living—to prevent hip flexion deformities.
   c. Use a footboard to keep the feet at right angles to the legs when patient is in dorsal position (Fig. 13-2)—prevents footdrop, heel-cord shortening and plantar flexion.
   d. Use a padded posterior splint at night (if necessary)—to prevent flexion of the affected extremity.
   e. Apply a trochanter roll from the crest of the ilium to the midthigh (Fig. 13-3)— to prevent external rotation of the hip joint when the patient is in a dorsal position.
   f. Place a pillow in the axilla of the affected side—to keep arm away from the chest and prevent adduction of the affected shoulder.
   g. Place the affected arm on pillow supports with each joint positioned higher than the preceding one—to prevent edema and resultant fibrosis.
   h. Position the fingers around a small hand roll (Fig. 13-4)—to keep the fingers in the most functional (grasp) position.
   i. Use a dorsal hand splint if finger spasticity develops.
   j. Turn the patient on his *unaffected* side every 2 hours (Fig. 13-5).
   k. Place the patient in a prone position for 15 minutes to ½ hour daily (Fig. 13-6)— to promote hyperextension of hip joints which is essential to normal gait.

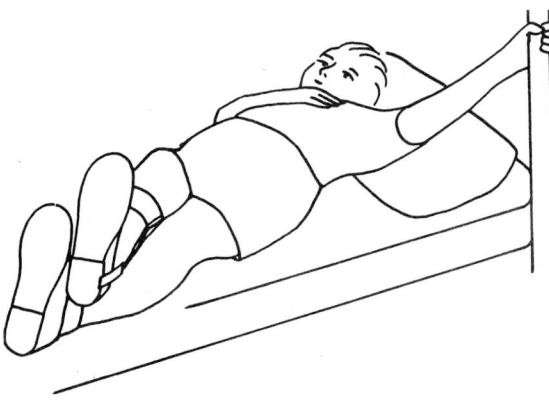

Figure 13-7. Bed exercise for the patient with hemiplegia: moving the legs over the side of the bed. The paralyzed leg is carried by the uninvolved leg. (From Hirschberg, G., Lewis, L., and Thomas, D.: Rehabilitation. Philadelphia, J. B. Lippincott.)

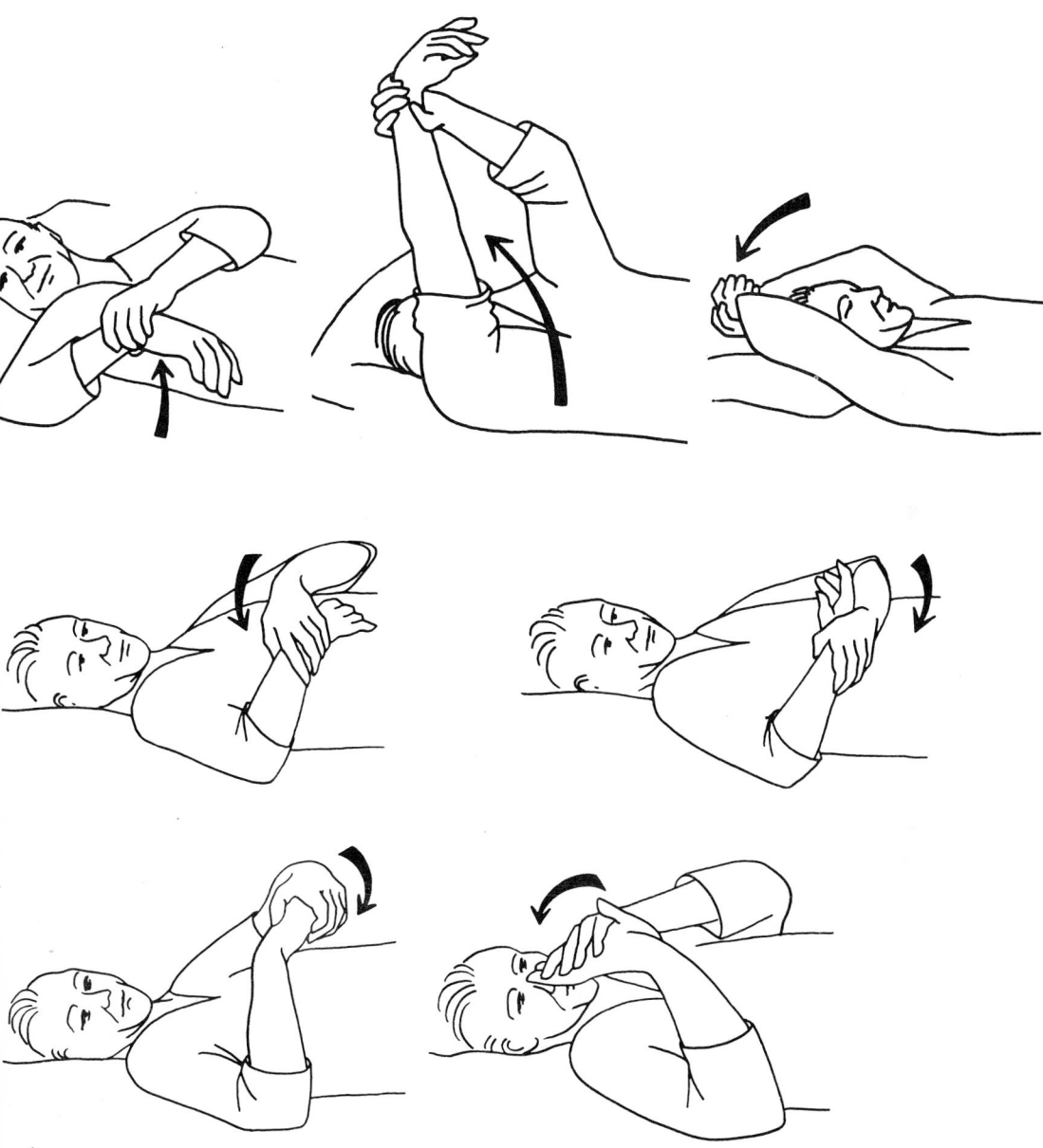

Figure 13-8. *A.* Exercise to maintain range of motion of the involved shoulder and the elbow in hemiplegia. *B.* Exercise to maintain range of motion of pronation and supination in affected hand. *C.* Exercise to maintain range of motion of the wrist and the finger in hemiplegia. (From Hirschberg, G., Lewis, L., and Thomas, D.: Rehabilitation. Philadelphia, J. B. Lippincott.)

2. Exercise the affected extremities passively and carry out range of motion exercises 4–5 times daily—to prevent contracture development in the paralyzed extremity.
   a. Remind the patient to exercise unaffected extremities at intervals throughout the day—to prevent contracture development in the normal extremities.
   b. Teach patient to put his unaffected leg under the affected one in order to move and turn himself (Fig. 13-7).
   c. Instruct the patient to move his affected arm (and hand) with his good hand (Fig. 13-8).
   d. Teach quadriceps muscle setting and gluteal exercises (5 times daily for 10 minutes)—to improve the muscle strength needed for walking.
      (1) *Quadriceps Setting* (to each extremity)
         Instruct the patient as follows:
         (a) Contract the quadriceps muscle (anterior portion of thighs) while raising the heel and attempting to push the popliteal space against the mattress.
         (b) Hold the muscle contracture for the count of 5.
         (c) Relax for the count of 5. Repeat.
      (2) *Gluteal Setting*
         Instruct the patient as follows:
         (a) Contract or "pinch" the buttocks together for the count of 5.
         (b) Relax for the count of 5. Repeat.
3. Assist the patient out of bed as soon as permitted.
   a. *To Develop Sitting Balance*
      (1) Slowly assist patient to a sitting position.
      (2) Place patient's feet on floor (or on the seat of a chair).

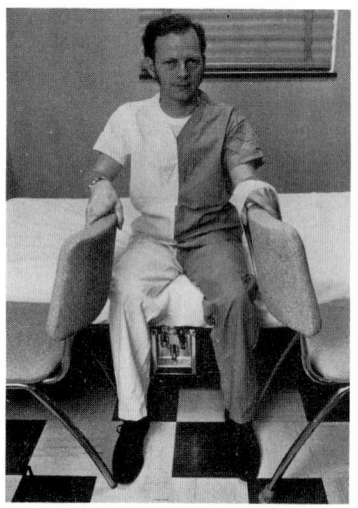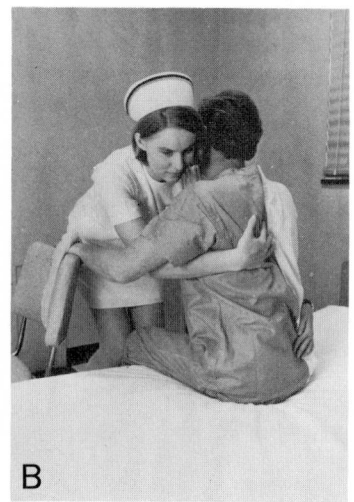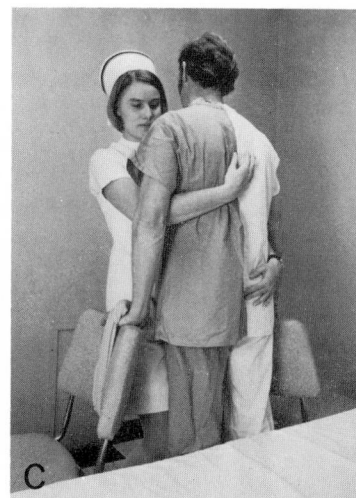

Figure 13-9. A. Getting the patient out of bed following a stroke. Place the bed in the low position so that the feet are resting on the floor. The affected hand may be tied to a chair for stabilization. Observe the patient's reaction and increase sitting time-as rapidly as the patient's condition permits. B. Arising to a standing position. Help the patient to come to a standing position while supporting his affected knee with the nurse's knees. This support will prevent the patient's affected knee from buckling. C. Stabilizing the patient as he assumes a standing position.

(3) Place the patient's unaffected hand behind him—to assist in maintaining balance.

(4) Stand in front of patient—to help him maintain this posture.

(5) Assess for change in color, shortness of breath, profuse perspiration—indications that patient should be placed back in dorsal position.

(6) Increase sitting time as rapidly as patient's condition permits.

b. *To Develop Standing Balance*

(1) Put walking shoes with strong shank on patient for all ambulation activities.

(2) Seat the patient on edge of bed and place a straight-back chair on each side of him (Fig. 13-9A).

    (a) Tie affected hand to the chair if patient lacks grasp strength.

    (b) Assist the patient to a standing position, supporting (locking) his affected knee with the side of your knee (Figs. 13-9B and C).

(3) Stand behind patient and stabilize him at his waist.

(4) Assess for dizziness, pallor and increasing pulse rate.

(5) Assist patient to achieve standing balance at frequent intervals throughout the day.

(6) Help the patient begin walking as soon as standing balance is achieved.

4. Encourage patient to perform his self-care activities as soon as possible.

a. Have the patient immediately transfer all self-care activities to the unaffected side.

b. Encourage him to brush his teeth, comb his hair and bathe and feed himself.

c. Help the patient to dress himself for ambulatory activities.

(1) Instruct family to bring clothing that is one size larger than usually worn.

(2) Have patient dress himself (with assistance if necessary) while seated—to achieve better balance.

(3) Use clothing with front fasteners preferably of stretch fabrics.

5. Assist in securing supportive devices if needed—most patients develop spasticity of lower extremity and will lack motor control.

a. Secure posterior knee splint if patient has a weakened or absent quadriceps muscle—gives better balance and helps prevent loss of position sense.

b. Secure an adjustable aluminum cane (with 3-prong support if necessary) when patient is able to walk alone.

c. Use a sling on the paralyzed arm—to prevent subluxation (incomplete dislocation) of the shoulder.

(1) Support the affected arm with a pillow when patient is seated.

(2) Instruct patient to flex his affected wrist and fingers (with unaffected hand) at frequent intervals.

d. Secure a wheelchair of the correct size with brakes that the patient can manage if he is unable to ambulate.

(1) Teach patient to propel chair by pushing with his uninvolved leg.

(2) Equip bed and wheelchair with an overhead sling to exercise affected arm.

6. Prepare the patient for discharge.

a. Some patients will have to be transferred to rehabilitation centers for further therapy.

b. Encourage patient to keep active, adhere to his exercise program and remain as self-sufficient as possible.

7. Instruct the family as follows:

a. Avoid doing those things for the patient that he can do for himself.

b. Be supportive and sympathetic but firm and direct.

    c. Expect some emotional lability and some degree of brain damage if the patient has had a more severe stroke.

    d. Install hand rails by the toilet and tub or shower and put safety rails on the bed

    e. Obtain self-help devices to assist in activities of daily living.

APHASIA

Aphasia is a disturbance of language function. It may also involve impairment of the ability to read and write as well as to speak and listen.

Causes
1. Traumatic head injury
2. Cerebral vascular accident

Types of Aphasia
1. *Auditory aphasia*—loss of ability to comprehend spoken language
2. *Conduction aphasia*—aphasia due to a lesion of the pathway between the sensory and motor speech centers
3. *Motor aphasia*—loss of ability to express one's thoughts in speech and writing; person understands what is said to him but he cannot produce sequence of movements necessary to utter words.
4. *Sensory aphasia*—inability to comprehend spoken (auditory aphasia) or written (visual aphasia) language
5. *Mixed aphasia*—combined motor and sensory aphasia
6. *Visual aphasia*—loss of ability to comprehend written language

Nursing Management
Principle: There are a variety of symptoms and disorders underlying aphasia. Therefore, the treatment is individualized.

Objective: to stimulate attempts at communication.
1. Determine the communication abilities of the patient—usually done by speech pathologist, ophthalmologist, otologist.
2. Give the patient as much psychological security as possible.
3. Employ a calm, accepting and deliberate manner especially during periods of emotional lability.
4. Keep the environment relaxed and permissive.
5. Keep distractions at a minimum—damaged input pathways cannot sort out distracting stimuli in the environment.
6. Accept the patient as he is now; avoid artificial praise.
7. Keep the patient in the social world.
    a. Talk to him while caring for him.
    b. Give directions and requests in a simple manner.
    c. Supplement speech with gestures when indicated.
    d. Give the patient plenty of time to speak and respond—he cannot sort out incoming messages and formulate a response under pressure.
    e. Encourage socialization of the patient with his family and friends.

8. Give support by assuring the patient that there is nothing wrong with his intelligence.
    a. Treat him as an intelligent adult; his basic intelligence and personality are usually not affected.
    b. Avoid shouting at the patient.
9. Be consistent by using the same wording each time instructions are given and questions are asked.
10. Watch the patient for clues and gestures if his speech is unintelligible or jargon-like.
    a. Continue to listen to him.
    b. Nod and make neutral statements occasionally.
    c. Shift the topic when appropriate to gain another point of interest and frame of reference.
11. Observe the patient during the course of his daily schedule for clues to evaluate and assess his progress.

CEREBRAL ANEURYSM
(Intracranial Aneurysm)

A *cerebral aneurysm* is a sac formed by dilation of the walls of an artery within the head.

Etiology

1. Congenital defect of vessel wall (most common)
2. Arteriosclerosis—reflects an acquired defect in vessel wall with subsequent weakness of wall
3. Mycosis
4. Syphilis (rare)
5. Trauma

Clinical Manifestations

1. Due to compression on cranial nerves or brain substance.
2. Due to leakage from or rupture of aneurysm.
    a. Headache or headpain, often associated with pain in eye—usually unilateral, frontal, recurrent and severe.
    b. Pain and rigidity in back of neck and spine
    c. Visual disturbances—visual loss, diplopia (double vision), ptosis (drooping of upper eye lid)
    d. Tinnitus (ringing in the ears)
    e. Dizziness
    f. Hemiparesis (muscular weakness affecting one side of body) or hemiplegia (paralysis of one side of body)

Underlying Principles

1. An aneurysm may cause pressure on the 3rd cranial nerve, producing a dilatation of the pupil on the same side.
2. Rupture of an aneurysm leads to subarachnoid hemorrhage.
3. Spontaneous subarachnoid hemorrhage is confirmed by lumbar puncture.

Treatment

A. *Before Rupture—Surgical Intervention*
    1. Ligation of carotid artery in neck—to reduce pressure in the aneurysm and reduce the danger of rupture and hemorrhage.

2. Intracranial procedures
   a. Clipping the aneurysm from its vessel wall.
   b. Clip-graft procedure—patching and reinforcing the defect in the media of the vessel wall.
   c. Wrapping aneurysm with muscle, gauze or other substance.
B. *After Rupture*
   See below for nursing management of the patient with cerebral hemorrhage.

CEREBRAL HEMORRHAGE
(Subarachnoid Hemorrhage; Intracerebral Hemorrhage)

Cerebral hemorrhage is bleeding into the intracranial cavity.

Causes

1. Hypertension with atherosclerosis
2. Ruptured aneurysm
3. Trauma
4. Angioma
5. Hemorrhagic disorders—leukemia, aplastic anemia, liver disease, anticoagulant therapy, etc.

Clinical Manifestations

May occur with or without premonitory signs
1. Abrupt onset of headache
2. Dizziness and vomiting
3. Unconsciousness (unfavorable prognosis)
4. Convulsions
5. Varying abnormalities in vital signs and neurologic impairment—depending upon severity of hemorrhage
6. Hemiplegia

Treatment and Nursing Management

1. Place on bedrest for approximately 3–4 weeks—high incidence of *recurrence of bleeding during first 3 weeks.*
   a. See nursing management of the unconscious patient, page 728.
   b. Elevate head—to reduce venous pressure inside head and to assist respirations.
   c. Avoid straining during bowel movement which increases intracranial pressure.
2. Treat headache with simple analgesics (aspirin and codeine).
3. Give hypotensive agents as directed—to treat underlying hypertension.
4. Administer steroids to reduce brain edema.
5. Prepare for surgical intervention if directed (see page 732).
6. Start rehabilitation measures as soon as patient recovers from the acute phase (see page 740).

BRAIN TUMOR

A *brain tumor* is a localized intracranial lesion which occupies space within the skull and tends to cause a rise in intracranial pressure.

Incidence

1. Tumors of the brain originate in the brain (including the roots of the cranial nerves and the meninges) in about 95% of all patients with this problem.
2. Tumors may be benign or malignant.
3. The greatest incidence of brain tumors occurs between the ages of 30 and 50 years.

Classification

1. *Tumors arising from covering of brain*
   Meningioma—encapsulated, well-defined, growing outside the brain tissue; compresses rather than invades brain
2. *Tumors developing in or on the cranial nerves*
   a. Acoustic neuroma—derived from sheath of acoustic nerve
   b. Optic nerve spongioblastoma polare
3. *Tumors originating in the brain tissue*
   Gliomas—infiltrating tumors that may invade any portion of brain; most common type of brain tumor
      Astrocytoma
      Glioblastoma multiforme } subclassified according to predominating
      Medulloblastoma   cells (histogenesis)
4. *Metastatic lesions*—most common primary site is lung or breast
5. *Tumors of the ductless glands*
   a. Pituitary   b. Pineal
6. *Blood vessel tumors*
   a. Hemangioblastoma   b. Angioma
7. *Tumors in children* (see pp. 1393–1397)

Clinical Manifestations

A. *General Symptoms*
   1. Brain tumor is usually characterized by a *progressive* course of symptoms over a period of time.
   2. Brain tumors manifest themselves by:
      a. *Symptoms due to increased intracranial pressure*
         (1) Headache—intensified by activity which increases intracranial pressure (stooping, straining)
         (2) Vomiting, unrelated to food intake—usually due to irritation of vagal centers in medulla
         (3) Papilledema (choked disk)—edema of optic nerve
         (4) Mental clouding, lethargy
      b. *Symptoms due to local effects of tumor interfering with specific regions of the brain*
         (1) Motor abnormalities—rigidity, lack of coordination, weakness, convulsive seizures
         (2) Sensory abnormalities—aberration in smell, vision, hearing
B. *Manifestations According to Site*
   1. *Frontal lobe tumor*
      a. Mental changes (memory loss, personality changes)
      b. Headache
      c. Failing or blurring vision
      d. Impairment of sphincter control
      e. Focal seizures
      f. Hemiparesis or aphasia

2. *Temporal lobe* (may be relatively silent)
    a. Focal epileptic seizures   c. Papilledema
    b. Dysphasia or aphasia   d. Headache
3. *Parietal lobe tumors*
    a. Motor seizures   c. Jacksonian convulsions
    b. Sensory loss or visual impairment
4. *Occipital tumors*
    a. Visual impairment and visual hallucinations
    b. Focal seizures
5. *Cerebellar tumors* (common brain tumors of childhood)
    a. Disturbances of equilibrium and coordination
    b. Early development of increasing intracranial pressure and papilledema
6. *Tumors of brain stem*
    Symptoms of cranial nerve palsies (dysphagia, dysphonia, nystagmus, ataxia in extremities
7. *Tumors of the 3rd ventricle*
    Symptoms arise from increasing intracranial pressure

Diagnostic Evaluation

Objective: to determine the precise location of the tumor.
1. X-ray of skull—to demonstrate intracranial calcification, displacement of calcified pineal gland, signs of increased intracranial pressure, bone destruction.
2. X-ray of chest—metastatic brain tumors are associated with many primary or metastatic lung tumors.
3. Lumbar puncture—to determine spinal fluid pressure (usually increased over 200 mm.); glucose, protein (usually increased); cytologic studies done to detect malignant cells.
4. EEG—abnormal brain waves can be detected in regions occupied by tumor.
5. Echoencephalography—demonstrates displacement of certain structures from the midline by a lesion in one hemisphere.
6. Cerebral angiography—shows displacement or obliteration of certain structures from the midline by a lesion in one hemisphere; has largely supplanted air studies in diagnosis of brain tumor.
7. Air studies (pneumoencephalogram)—to indicate obstruction, deformity, dilatation, shift in ventricular system caused by abnormal growth.
8. Brain scan—abnormal amount of radioactive material will be present in area of tumor and can be localized with scintillation counter.
9. Neurologic examination—to determine area(s) of involvement.
10. Audiometry or vestibular function studies—performed in suspected cases of acoustic neuroma.

Treatment

Objectives: to remove the tumor and cure the patient (if possible).
            to achieve palliation by partial tumor removal and decompression, radiation or chemotherapy.

A. *Problems Affecting Treatment*
1. Effectiveness of treatment depends on type and site of tumor; many tumors are in vital or inaccessible areas (brain-stem tumors).

2. Nonencapsulated and infiltrating tumors make complete removal almost impossible; resulting neurologic defects (blindness, paralysis) would be too severe.
3. Cures may be obtained in certain tumors (meningiomas, acoustic neuromas, pituitary adenomas, dermoids, astrocytomas) if treated early.

B. *Principles of Treatment*
   1. See nursing management of the patient undergoing intracranial surgery, page 732.
   2. Support the patient undergoing radiation.
      a. Give steroids (methyl prednisolone) or osmotic dehydrating agents (urea) as directed—to reduce cerebral edema associated with brain tumors.
      b. Watch for upsets in water and electrolyte balance—produced by osmotic dehydrating agents.
      c. See page 882 for management of patient undergoing radiation therapy.
   3. Support the patient undergoing palliation procedures.
      a. Patient may receive alkylating agents, systematically or by carotid injection in a single dose or by continuous infusion over a 2 to 3 week period.
      b. Ventricular shunting procedure may be done for irremovable tumor that blocks ventricular system. (Increasing intracranial pressure may be relieved by ventricular shunting of blocked spinal fluid.)
      c. See page 888 for the nursing management of patient with cancer.

BRAIN ABSCESS

A *brain abscess* is a localized collection of pus within the brain substance.

Etiology

1. By direct invasion of the brain
   a. Penetrating wound
   b. Spread of infection from otitis media, sinusitis, mastoiditis
2. By spread of infection from other organs (remote from the brain)
   a. From the lung (bronchiectasis, pneumonia)
   b. From the heart (bacterial endocarditis)
   c. From other organs—septicemia, pelvic abscesses

Clinical Manifestations

1. Headache
2. Focal neurologic signs (depending on site of abscess)—weakness of arm or leg, depression of vision, focal epileptic seizures
3. Fever and leukocytosis—may be subnormal with a thick-walled abscess
4. Change in patient's mental alertness

Treatment and Nursing Care

1. Observe patient for increased intracranial pressure (p. 724)—cerebral edema surrounds an acute brain abscess which may produce sudden increases of intracranial pressure.
2. Give antimicrobial therapy—to reduce the virulence or to eliminate the organism. Large doses of the appropriate antibiotic are given to penetrate the abscess cavity until the lesion becomes encapsulated.

3. Assist in making an accurate localization of abscess—nursing assessments, laboratory studies, brain scanning, angiography and repeated neurologic examinations.
4. Treat seizures if they occur (p. 731)—patient may receive antiseizure medication (diphenylhydantoin, phenobarbital) as a prophylaxis against convulsions.
5. Prepare for surgical intervention.
   a. Tapping and drainage of abscess.
   b. Craniotomy with elevation of bone flap and removal of abscess (see nursing management of the patient undergoing intracranial surgery, p. 732).
6. Support the patient during repeated x-rays after treatment—to ascertain if infection has been eradicated.
   a. Relapse is common.
   b. Mortality rate is fairly high.
   c. Neurologic defects following treatment of brain abscess include hemiparesis, seizures, visual defects and learning problems (in children).

PARKINSON'S DISEASE

Parkinson's disease is a progressive neurologic disorder affecting the brain centers responsible for control of regulation of movement.

Etiology
1. Unknown.
2. Unknown virus, cerebrovascular disease and certain metallic poisons have been suspected.
3. Theory advanced that there is an imbalance of 2 neurochemical systems, cholinergic and dopaminergic, and that the symptoms of parkinsonism are caused by overactivity or underactivity by one or the other of these systems.

Clinical Manifestations
1. Tremor (tends to decrease or disappear on purposeful movement)
2. Rigidity and slowness of movements, particularly of large joints
3. Bent posture; shuffling propulsive gait
4. Mask-like facial expression; unblinking eyes
5. Muscle weakness—affecting writing, speaking, eating, chewing and swallowing

Treatment and Nursing Management
Treatment is based on a combination of drug therapy, physical therapy and rehabilitation techniques and patient and family education.

Objective: to keep the patient functionally useful and productive as long as possible.

A. *Drug Therapy:* Levodopa (L-dopa) Therapy
   1. Levodopa (an amino acid which is depleted in the substance in the brain involved in nerve transmission in patients with parkinsonism) is given in increasing doses until the patient's tolerance is reached.
   2. Levodopa must be given in a large enough dose for a long enough time period to build up an effective and stable blood level—small amounts are metabolized into dopamine which will not cross the blood-brain barriers.

3. Dosage is increased gradually until side effects begin to appear—nausea, vomiting, anorexia, fluctuations in blood pressure, mental disturbances, cardiac arrhythmias, twitching.
4. Levodopa is not a cure for parkinsonism but is effective in controlling the patient's symptoms (improves dyskinesia and rigidity).
   a. Encourage patient to visit his physician regularly.
   b. Emphasize that patient should have blood chemistry evaluations, blood count and urinalysis as directed.
5. Pyridoxine (vitamin B_6) seems to cancel out the effectiveness of Levadopa and has to be taken out of the diet.

B. *Anticholinergic Agents*—counteracts the action of acetylcholine in the central nervous system.
   1. Anticholinergic agents are given when Levodopa is not effective or the patient is unable to tolerate it.
   2. Assess for side effects of anticholinergic agents—dryness of mouth, blurred vision, urinary retention, constipation, mental disorders.
   3. Frequently used anticholinergics:
      a. Trihexyphenidyl (Artane)   d. Benztropine mesylate (Cogentin)
      b. Cycrimine (Pagitane)   e. Diphenhydramine (Benadryl)—an antihistamine
      c. Procyclidine (Kemadrin)

C. *Physical Therapy*
   1. Encourage patient to continue with his physical therapy program—to treat rigid musculature and prevent contractures.
   2. Emphasize the importance of a daily exercise program—to maintain joint mobility.
   3. Encourage patient to take warm baths and massage with passive and active exercises—to help relax muscles and relieve painful muscle spasms that accompany rigidity.
   4. Advise patient to do stretching exercises—to loosen the joint structures.
   5. Encourage walking and postural exercises—to maintain normal gait.
      a. Use stationary bicycle.   b. Exercise each joint daily.
   6. Encourage the patient and family to get self-help devices (p. 25)—to keep him independent.

D. *Emotional Support*
   1. Offer realistic reassurance and psychological support.
   2. Tell the patient that his disease is *slowly* progressive and there is no mental or intellectual impairment.
   3. Re-emphasize that disability can be prevented or delayed.
   4. Try to dispell anxiety and fears of patient that may be as disabling as his condition.
   5. Keep the patient as socially active as possible.

E. *Surgical Intervention*
   1. Thalamotomy—the small area of the brain where the tremors originated is inactivated by heat, freezing or other methods—relieves contralateral tremor and rigidity of extremity.
   2. Thalamotomy does not alter course of progressive Parkinson's disease but can help some patients with the unilateral syndrome (tremor and rigidity on one side of body).
   3. See page 732, nursing management of the patient undergoing intracranial surgery.

MULTIPLE SCLEROSIS
(Disseminated Sclerosis)

Multiple sclerosis is a chronic progressive disease of the neurologic system characterized by the occurrence of small patches of demyelination and overgrowth of glial tissue throughout the white substance of the brain and spinal cord.

Clinical Manifestations

Patients with multiple sclerosis have a wide range of clinical symptoms and a great variability in the course of the disease with many remissions and exacerbations.

Weakness	Paresthesias
Abnormal reflexes; either absent or hyper	Sphincter impairment
Visual disturbances; nystagmus, diplopia	Impaired vibration and position sense
Tremor, ataxia, incoordination	

Incidence

Multiple sclerosis is one of the most disabling neurologic diseases striking young adults in this country. It maximizes the medical, psychologic, social and economic problems encountered by the patient and his family.

Objectives of Treatment and Nursing Management

Objectives: to keep the patient as active and functional as possible in order to lead a purposeful life.

to relieve the patient's symptoms and provide him with continuing support.

A. *To prevent and treat muscle spasticity—spasticity interferes with normal function.*
1. Do muscle stretching exercises daily—to minimize joint contractures.
    a. Give particular emphasis to hamstrings, gastrocnemius, hip adductors, biceps, wrist and finger flexors.
    b. Teach patient's family passive exercises and range of motion exercises for patients with severe spasticity.
2. Avoid muscle fatigue—stop physical activity just short of fatigue.
3. Prevent muscle contractures and loss of muscle power from lack of use—decreasing motor power is a significant problem in multiple sclerosis.
4. Encourage patient to sleep prone—to minimize flexor spasm at knees and hips.
5. Advise patient to participate in walking exercises—to improve gait affected by loss of position sense in legs.
6. Give muscle relaxants (diazepam) as directed.
7. Utilize braces, canes, crutches, walker when necessary—to keep patient ambulatory.
8. Prepare patients with severe spasticity and contractures for surgical intervention—to prevent further contractures and disability.

B. *To avoid skin pressure and immobility—sensory loss is usually present and decubitus ulcers accompany severe spasticity in a bedridden patient.*
1. Avoid skin trauma, heat, cold and pressure.
2. Change position at least every 2 hours if patient is immobile.
3. Teach patient to inspect pressure areas (using a mirror for posterior sites) for heat and redness.
4. Give careful attention to sacral and perineal hygiene.
5. Use flotation pad, sheepskin, alternating air pressure mattress and other modalities—to minimize skin pressure.

C. *To assist patient to overcome effects of incoordination—caused by motor dysfunction.*
1. Teach patient to walk with feet wider apart—to widen his base of support and increase his walking stability.
2. Use a cane or walker.
3. Utilize weighted bracelets, wrist cuffs, eating utensils—to help overcome incoordination of upper extremities.

D. *To support the patient with bladder disturbances—bladder dysfunction may lead to progressive renal failure.*
1. Assess for urinary retention.
   a. Catheterize patient; insert indwelling catheter only if absolutely necessary.
   b. Give urinary antiseptics—to reduce incidence of bacteriuria.
2. Ensure adequate fluid intake (3–5 liters daily)—to reduce urinary bacterial count, minimize precipitation of urinary crystals and stone formation and encrustation of the lumen of the indwelling urethral catheter.
3. Support the patient who has urinary incontinence (or frequency and urgency).
   Female Patient
   a. Set up a voiding time schedule; every 1½ to 2 hours initially with lengthening time intervals if regimen is successful.
   b. Encourage the patient to drink a measured amount of fluid every 2 hours.
   c. Have the patient try to void 30 minutes after drinking.
   d. For permanent urinary incontinence, urine may have to be diverted by means of ileal conduit (cutaneous uretero-ileostomy).
   Male Patient
   a. See a, b, c, under female patient.
   b. For permanent incontinence, patient may wear external sheath or condom appliance for urine collection (see p. 36).

E. *To place the patient on a bowel program if he has bowel incontinence.*
1. Establish a program of *regularity.*
   a. Have patient eat regularly scheduled meals.
   b. Establish bowel evacuation at *same time each day.*
2. Encourage patient to drink 120 ml. (4 ounces) of prune juice at bedtime (same time each night).
3. Insert a glycerine suppository into the rectum 30 minutes before scheduled bowel evacuation time—*after* eating a meal (preferably after breakfast).
4. Advise patient to attempt to have a bowel movement within 30 minutes of eating, using as normal a position for defecation as possible.
   a. Instruct patient to bear down and contract abdominal muscles.
   b. Teach patient to apply pressure to abdomen with his hands—to assist with defecation.
5. After this routine is established, mechanical stimulation with the suppository may not be necessary.

F. *To treat the patient with appropriate therapy during periods of exacerbation.*
1. Give ACTH or corticosteroids—in high dosages for short periods during acute exacerbations.
2. Take corrective action for each new problem as it arises.
3. Invent, adapt and modify equipment that can be used for self-help devices so that patient will not lose ground (see p. 25).

G. *To help patient with optic and speech defects—cranial nerves affecting sight and speech are affected by multiple sclerosis.*
   1. Utilize eye patch, frosted lens—to block visual impulses of one eye when patient has diplopia (double vision).
   2. Secure services of speech pathologist or therapist—to strengthen the muscles of speech.

H. *To train patient in activities of daily living—to keep patient as independent as possible*
   1. Teach transfer activities (see p. 25).
   2. Secure services of a knowledgeable wheelchair dealer to select correct wheelchair
   3. Use assistive and self-help devices.
      a. Toilet facilities—raised toilet seat or bedside commode
      b. Bathing facilities—use stool in shower or tub and hand rails
      c. Self-care aids—prism glasses, telephone modifications, long-handled combs, tongs, modified clothing (see p. 25)

I. *To help the family (and patient) understand the stresses imposed by multiple sclerosis.*
   1. Understand the problems faced by the patient.
      a. There are embarrassing and humiliating symptoms to which the patient may respond "inappropriately."
      b. Patient may have brain damage with resultant denial of his disease, euphoria or depressive and paranoid behavior.
   2. Understand that patients adapt to illness in many ways—denial, depression, withdrawal, inactivity, resentment, etc.
   3. Try to avoid physical and emotional stresses—may worsen symptoms and impair performance.
   4. Assist the patient to accept his new identity as a handicapped person and cope with the disruption in his life.
      a. Re-emphasize that the medical team understands the needs of the patient.
      b. Encourage him to learn about the services of the National Multiple Sclerosis Society* and meet others with his problems.
   5. Keep open the channels of communication.
   6. Encourage the patient to use and be on alert for new self-help devices.
   7. Offer meaningful and realistic short-term goals—to achieve a sense of purpose.

EPILEPSY

Epilepsy is a symptom-complex characterized by attacks of unconsciousness that may or may not be associated with convulsions, sensory phenomena or abnormalities in behavior. The basic problem is thought to be due to an electrical disturbance (dysrhythmia) in the nerve cells of the brain.

Causes

The underlying disorder of the brain may be structural, chemical or physiological or a combination of all three.

1. Congenital anomalies
2. Brain injury
3. Infection (meningitis, encephalitis)
4. Vascular disturbances
5. Metabolic or nutritional disturbances
6. Tumors
7. Degenerative diseases
8. Genetic disorders

* National Multiple Sclerosis Society, 257 Park Ave., New York 10010.

Clinical Manifestations

1. Loss of consciousness
2. Disturbances of the mind
3. Excess or loss of muscle tone or movement
4. Disorders of sensation or special senses
5. Disturbances of the autonomic functions of the body

Diagnostic Evaluation

Electroencephalograph (EEG)—finds and measures brain electrical discharge pattern

International Classification of Epileptic Seizures*

A. *Partial Seizures* (seizures beginning locally)
1. Partial seizures with elementary symptomatology (generally without impairment of consciousness)
    a. With motor symptoms (includes Jacksonian seizures)
    b. With special sensory or somatosensory symptoms
    c. With autonomic symptoms
    d. Compound forms
2. Partial seizures with complex symptomatology (generally with impairment of consciousness)
    (temporal lobe or psychomotor seizures)
    a. With impairment of consciousness only
    b. With cognitive symptomatology
    c. With affective symptomatology
    d. With "psychosensory" symptomatology
    e. With "psychomotor" symptomatology (automatisms)
    f. Compound forms
3. Partial seizures secondarily generalized

B. *Generalized Seizures* (bilaterally symmetrical and without local onset)
1. Absences *(petit mal)*
2. Bilateral massive epileptic myoclonus
3. Infantile spasms
4. Clonic seizures
5. Tonic seizures
6. Tonic-clonic seizures *(grand mal)*
7. Atonic seizures
8. Akinetic seizures

C. *Unilateral Seizures* (or predominantly unilateral)

D. *Unclassified Epileptic Seizures* (due to incomplete data)

Treatment and Nursing Management

Objectives: to determine and treat (if possible) the primary underlying cause of the seizures.
to prevent a recurrence of seizures.
to gain an understanding of the patient and his relationship to his environment.
1. See Nursing Management of the Patient with Convulsive Seizures, page 731.
2. Encourage the patient to study himself and his environment to determine what specific factors precipitate his seizures.

* Abstracted from: Gastaut, H.: Clinical and electroencephalographical classification of epileptic seizures: *Epilepsia, 11*:102–113, 1970.

3. Teach the patient to practice *regularity* and *moderation* in his daily activities—diet, exercise, rest, abstention from alcohol, avoidance of mental and physical stress.
4. Stress the importance of *activity,* both physical and mental. Activity tends to inhibit, not stimulate, epileptic seizures.
5. Emphasize the importance of regularity in taking the prescribed antiepileptic medication.
    a. The majority of patients are treated with a combination of phenobarbital (has selective anticonvulsive effect), diphenylhydantoin, primidone and trimethadione.*
       (1) Ethosuximide and phensuximide produce good results in the treatment of some seizures.
       (2) Diphenylhydantoin, mephenytoin, methsuximide and primidone show favorable results in treatment of partial seizures.
    b. Tranquilizers may be used to control associated behavioral disorders.
    c. Treatment is usually started with 1 drug; the drug is increased slowly until seizures are controlled or toxic symptoms develop.
    d. Warn the patient not to stop his medication. Not taking the medication may precipitate the development of status epilepticus.
    e. Watch for toxic effects from the antiepileptic medication; gum hypertrophy, nervousness, rash, ataxia, drowsiness, bone marrow depression leading to blood dyscrasias).
6. Emphasize the importance of having follow-up urinalysis and blood studies.
7. Instruct the patient to have a card or wear an emergency medical signal device identifying that he has epilepsy.
8. Reorient the attitude of the patient and his family to his disease.
    a. Epilepsy is a disease that can be controlled; it is not insanity or a supernatural condition.
    b. Advise the patient to learn of the services and publications of the National Epilepsy League, Inc., 116 S. Michigan Avenue, Chicago, Illinois 60603.

FRACTURES AND DISLOCATIONS OF THE SPINE

Underlying Considerations
1. Fractures of the spine are serious because of danger of injury to the spinal cord.
2. Fractures appear most frequently in the 5th, 6th and 7th cervical vertebrae, the 12th thoracic and the 1st lumbar vertebrae—there is a greater range of mobility of the vertebral column in these areas.

Causes
1. Trauma—automobile and motorcycle accidents, falls, diving and surfing injuries, trampoline injuries
2. Infections or inflammatory arthritis—producing spontaneous dislocations of cervical spine
3. Prior laminectomy

Clinical Manifestations
1. Severe pain in back, especially on movement
2. Tenderness directly over localized area of injury

* Reader is referred to a pharmacology text for a more complete description of antiepileptic drugs.

NURSING ALERT: Injury to the spinal cord may produce paralysis of the body below the level of the lesion.

Treatment and Nursing Management

Objectives: to reduce the fracture and obtain immobilization of the spine as soon as possible to prevent cord damage.

to observe for symptoms of progressive neurologic damage.

1. See page 910 for moving the patient from the scene of the accident.
2. Maintain the airway and ventilate the patient.
3. Evaluate the patient constantly for motor and sensory changes—motor and sensory loss occurs from cord edema, transection of cord.
   a. Direct the patient to move his toes or turn his feet.
   b. Pinch the skin, starting at shoulder level and progress down the sides of both extremities.
      (1) Ascertain when patient feels pinching sensation.
      (2) Record findings—for subsequent comparison.
      (3) Note presence or absence of level of sweating.
      (4) Note that any evidence of neurologic deterioration raises suspicion of cord edema or postoperative hematoma (in operative patients)—indicates need for immediate surgical intervention.
4. Transfer the patient to a Stryker frame or a CircOlectric bed. (If none is available, place on a firm mattress with a bedboard under the mattress.)
   a. Keep patient in an extended position—do not allow body to be twisted or turned.
   b. Place patient (who is strapped to a transfer board) directly on the posterior frame of a Stryker frame.
   c. Place a blanket roll between the patient's legs.
   d. Place anterior frame in position. Secure frame straps.
   e. Turn the patient to the prone position.
   f. Remove frame straps, head bandage and posterior frame. Remove transfer board.
5. For Patient with Fracture of Cervical Vertebrae
   a. Crutchfield tongs or Vinke tongs are inserted in the skull (on each side just above and in front of the ears)—usually done in emergency department under local anesthesia.
      (1) Initially 4.5–15.8 kg. (10–35 lbs.) of traction is applied, depending on patient's size and the degree of displacement.
      (2) The traction is gradually increased by addition of weights—as the amount of traction is increased the spaces between the intervertebral discs widen and the vertebrae slip back into position. Reduction will take place after correct alignment has been regained.
      (3) X-rays are made every few hours until the fracture is reduced.
      (4) When reduction is obtained the weights are reduced and x-rays again taken to verify reduction.
   b. Elevate head of bed (if patient is on regular bed)—patient's body serves as a counterweight to that applied by traction weight.
      (1) Keep traction tongs several inches from top of bed and allow weights to hang freely—to prevent interference with traction.
      (2) Give tranquilizers for apprehension and restlessness.

6. Observe for symptoms of progressive neurologic damage—symptoms of cord compression depend on level at which compression occurs. Clinical symptoms of cord compression are indistinguishable from those of cord edema.
    a. Loss of sensation
    b. Inability to move extremities
7. Prepare for laminectomy if progressive symptoms of cord compression occur—permits direct exploration and decompression of cord.
8. Evaluate for presence of spinal shock—spinal shock represents a sudden loss of continuity between spinal cord and higher nerve centers. Sensation, muscle tone and reflexes are absent below the level of the lesion.
    a. Falling blood pressure
    b. Paralysis of body below level of cord injury
    c. Bladder distention—from paralysis of bladder
    d. Bowel distention—caused by depression of reflexes; retroperitoneal hemorrhage may occur with fracture of low back, producing paralytic ileus
9. Maintain the patient's body defenses until shock remits and the system has recovered from the traumatic insult. (Spinal shock is temporary but may last several weeks.)
    a. Support the airway, especially in cervical cord injury.
    b. Support circulation—give blood transfusions as indicated.
    c. Avoid overdistention of bladder—after spinal injury the bladder may lack functional nerve supply; overstretching of bladder may produce permanent damage. (Urinary tract infection is common cause of death after spinal injury.)
        (1) Insert indwelling catheter early in acute phase.
        (2) Remove catheter as soon as possible.
        (3) Initiate bladder training regimen (see p. 764).
    d. Give neostigmine methylsulfate—for severe bowel distention.
        (1) Use intestinal decompression if indicated (see p. 383).
        (2) Give stool softeners.
        (3) Place patient on bowel training regimen as needed (see p. 38).
10. Prevent decubitus ulcers—bedsores with subsequent infection constitute a common cause of death after spinal injury; inadequate peripheral circulation from spinal shock can cause decubitus ulcer to develop within 6 hours.
    a. Turn patient at least every 2 hours on Stryker frame.
    b. Wash patient's skin with mild soap, rinse well and blot dry after each turning period.
    c. Lubricate sacrum, trochanters, ischia, iliac spines, knees and heels with emollient lotion at frequent intervals.
11. Maintain patient in proper alignment to prevent contracture deformities.
    Dorsal or Supine Position
    a. Position feet against padded footboard—to prevent footdrop.
    b. Be sure there is a space between end of mattress and foot of bed—to allow for free suspension of the heels.
    c. Apply trochanter rolls from crest of ilium to midthigh of both extremities—to prevent external rotation of the hip joints.
    d. Initiate passive range of motion exercises to affected extremities within 48–72 hours *upon order*—to preserve joint motion.
    e. Ambulate only upon order—if patient has partial cord function, activity may produce further cord injury.

12. Employ active rehabilitation procedures when patient's spine is stable enough to resume upright position.

   Period of immobilization determined by patient's condition (usually 6 weeks on a turning frame and 6 weeks of gradual mobilization with brace or cast).

HERNIATION OF INTERVERTEBRAL DISC
(Ruptured Disc)

Herniation of the intervertebral disc is a protrusion of the nucleus of the disc in the annulus (fibrous ring around the disc) with subsequent nerve compression. The herniation may occur in any portion of the spine.

Types of Disc Herniation

Lateral—compressing a single nerve root
Central—causing pressure on the spinal cord; can cause paralysis with sphincter involvement
Lumbar—causing pressure on the cauda equina

Causes

1. Degeneration
2. Trauma (accidents, strain, repeated minor stresses)

Clinical Manifestations

Depend on location, size, rate of development (acute or chronic) and effect on surrounding structures

A. *Cervical Disc*
   1. Pain and stiffness in neck, top of shoulders and in region of scapulae
   2. Pain descending to upper arms

B. *Lumbar Disc*
   1. Low back pain accompanied by varying degrees of sensory and motor impairment
   2. Pain in buttock and thigh radiating to calf and ankle—aggravated by actions that increase intraspinal pressure (sneezing, straining)

Diagnostic Evaluation

1. X-ray of spine—may show narrowing of disc space.
2. Myelogram—demonstrates area of pressure and localizes herniation of disc (see p. 719).

Treatment and Nursing Management

CERVICAL DISC

Objectives: to immobilize the cervical spine to allow for healing of soft tissues.

to reduce inflammation in supporting tissues and affected nerve roots in the cervical spine.

1. Immobilize the cervical spine by:
   a. Traction (Fig. 13-10)   c. Collars
   b. Bedrest   d. Braces

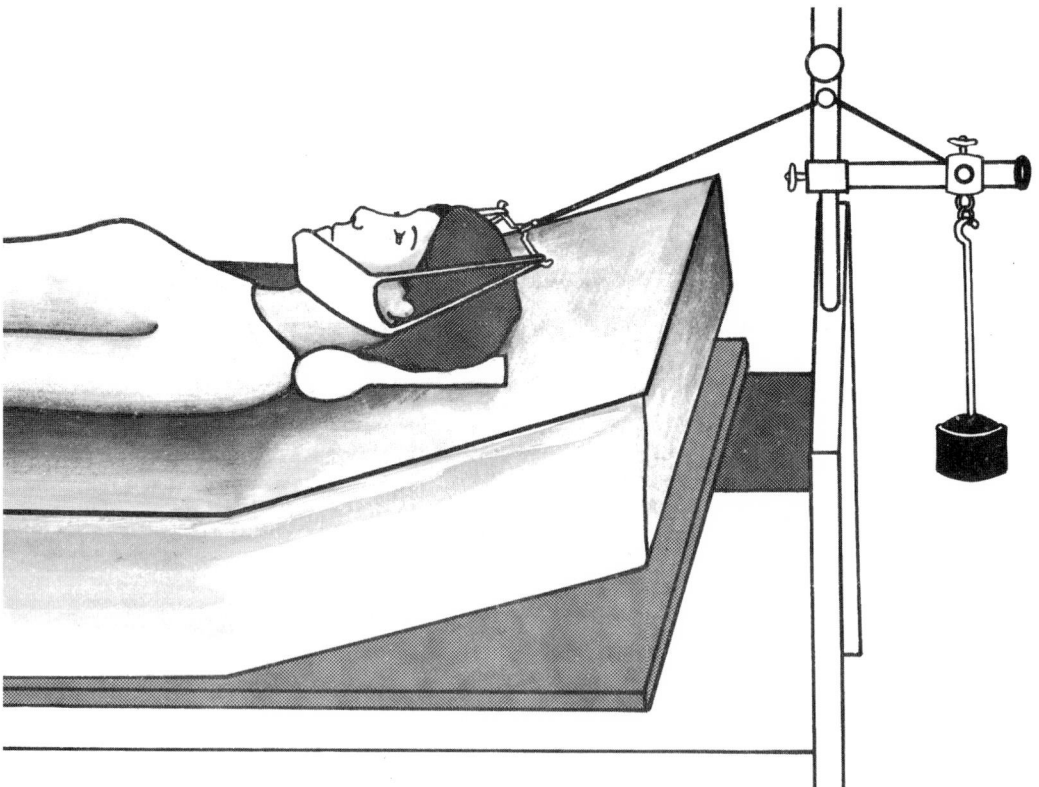

Figure 13-10. Traction.

2. Give muscle relaxant, e.g., carisoprodol (Soma)—to interrupt cycle of muscle spasm and allow for patient comfort; to increase range of motion in the cervical spine.
3. Administer anti-inflammatory medications, e.g., phenylbutazone (Butazolidin)—to treat inflammatory response.
   a. Give food or antacid with anti-inflammatory agents—to prevent gastrointestinal irritation.
   b. Take periodic blood counts—to watch for development of blood dyscrasias.
4. Give analgesics and sedatives—to control discomfort and anxiety often associated with cervical disc disease.
5. Apply moist hot compresses (10–20 minutes, several times daily) to back of neck— to increase blood flow to muscles.
6. *Patient Teaching Emphasis*
   Instruct the patient as follows:
   a. Avoid extreme flexion, extension and rotation of the cervical spine while working.
   b. Keep head in a neutral position while sleeping.
      (1) Pillow should be filled with feathers or down.
      (2) Sleep on side or back; do not sleep prone.

(3) Avoid excessive neck flexion—do not prop up in bed with several pillows.
  c. Avoid excessive automobile riding during acute phase—vibration has adverse effect on spine.

LUMBAR DISC

Objectives: to relieve the pain and slow the progress of the disease.
to increase the functional ability of the patient.

1. Encourage the patient to remain on bedrest—disc is freed from stress when the patient is horizontal.
    a. Place patient in a moderate Fowler's position with moderate hip and knee flexion.
    b. Place hinged bedboard under mattress—to limit spinal flexion.
    c. Help patient to ambulate (usually after 2 weeks bedrest) when inflammatory reaction and edema from disc herniation has subsided.
    d. Use corset or brace if necessary to mobilize patient (for obese patient with poor abdominal musculature).
2. Use appropriate drug therapy.
    a. Muscle relaxants—muscle spasm is prominent in acute phase.
        (1) Methocarbamol (Robaxin)
        (2) Carisoprodol (Soma)
    b. Anti-inflammatory drugs
        (1) Phenylbutazone (Butazolidin)
            (a) Give with food or milk—to prevent gastric irritation.
            (b) Have blood evaluations at periodic intervals—blood dyscrasias are an untoward effect of phenylbutazone.
        (2) Hydroxyphenylbutazone (Tandearil)
        (3) Systemic steroids (Dexamethasone)
    c. Analgesic agents—to relieve patient's acute pain.
3. Utilize heat and massage—to relax muscle spasm.
4. Watch for development of neurological deficit.
    a. Muscle weakness and atrophy
    b. Loss of sensory and motor function
    c. Unrelieved acute pain
5. Prepare for surgical intervention when indicated (hemilaminectomy with removal of ruptured disc).
    Patients with multilevel involvement may have recurrences of pain and require reoperations.
6. *Patient Teaching Emphasis*
    a. Encourage patient to do lumbar flexion exercises after acute symptoms subside—to strengthen abdominal muscles and flexors of the spine.
        (1) Start exercises gently and gradually.
        (2) Discontinue exercises if pain worsens.
    b. Advise patient to sleep on side with knees and hips in position of flexion (pillow between knees).
        (1) Do not sleep in prone position—hyperextends the spine.
        (2) Pick up loads correctly (bend knees, keep back straight, avoid lifting anything above the elbows).

PARAPLEGIA

Paraplegia is loss of motion and sensation in the lower extremities.
Quadriplegia—loss of motion and sensation involving both upper and lower extremities.

Causes

1. Trauma—accidents, gunshot wounds
2. Multiple sclerosis
3. Cerebral palsy
4. Tumors
5. Infections (epidural abscess, tuberculosis)

Nursing Management

1. See the nursing management of patient with spinal cord injuries for immediate management principles, page 757.
2. Understand the psychological significance of the disability.
   a. Support the patient undergoing a series of emotional reactions to a newly acquired disability—denial, depression and grief.
   b. Understand that patient may take 1 of 2 courses.
      (1) Acceptance of disability—leading to development of realistic goals for the future.
      (2) Rejection of disability—patient may require psychiatric assistance.
3. Prepare for weight-bearing activities—patient with complete cord severance should start early weight-bearing to decrease osteoporotic changes in long bones and to diminish urinary infections and the formation of renal calculi.
   a. Use tilt table—to help overcome vasomotor instability and tolerate upright posture (p. 33).
   b. Apply elastic hose from toes to thigh or a Jobst* counter-pressure leotard—to prevent pooling of blood in abdominal area; a patient with spinal-cord paralysis lacks vasomotor tone in the lower extremities and will become hypotensive in the upright position.
   c. Start with elevation of 45 degrees and gradually increase angle of elevation.
      (1) Take blood pressure immediately before and as soon as patient is positioned on tilt table.
      (2) Observe for nausea and excessive perspiration.
4. Initiate bladder training program.
   a. Give meticulous attention to indwelling catheter (see p. 467).
   b. See page 764 for principles of bladder training.
5. Start bowel training program (see p. 38).
6. Build the unaffected part of body to optimal strength—to prepare for ambulation with braces and crutches.
   Encourage patient to continue with muscle strengthening exercises for hands, arms, shoulders, chest, spine, abdomen and neck—patient must bear full weight on these muscles.
   Instruct patient as follows:
   (1) Do push-ups in prone position.
   (2) Do sit-ups in sitting position.
   (3) Extend and flex arms while holding weights.
   (4) Squeeze rubber ball to promote hand strength.

---

* The Jobst Institute, Toledo, Ohio 43601.

7. Prevent the complications of paraplegic disorders.
   a. Infection of urinary tract; urinary calculi; urethrocutaneous fistula.
      (1) Prevent overdistention of the bladder.
      (2) Maintain continuous urinary drainage using a 3-way system (p. 505).
      (3) Keep the urine acid; do frequent urinalyses.
      (4) Institute tidal drainage at earliest possible time—not later than 1 week after onset of paraplegia.
      (5) Encourage fluid intake to at least 4000 ml./24 hours; urinary output should be 2000 ml./24 hours.
      (6) Prevent periurethral abscess formation and urethrocutaneous fistula—in male patient tape the penis horizontally to the side to prevent pressure and kinking of the urethra on the catheter at the penoscrotal angle (Fig. 7-9).
   b. Development of decubitus ulcers
      (1) Position patient on Stryker frame—prevents pressure on heels and other bony prominences and facilitates turning.
      (2) Turn every 2 hours; give skin care immediately after turning.
      (3) Give special attention to the perineal area.
      (4) Prevent development of hypoproteinemia.
         (a) Give high vitamin, high protein, high caloric diet.
         (b) Give high protein formula as in-between-meal feedings.
      (5) Maintain normal hemoglobin and normal red blood count.
   c. Abdominal distention; reflex ileus; fecal impaction
      (1) Use rectal tube and intestinal decompression (see p. 409) for patients with high cervical and thoracic cord lesions.

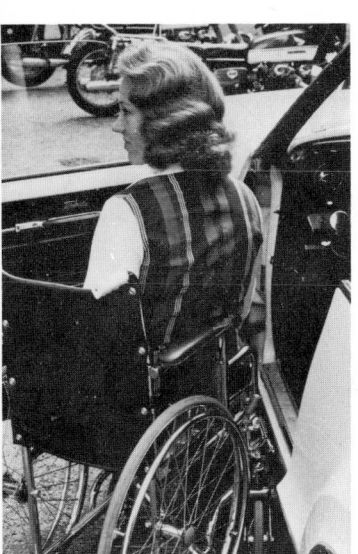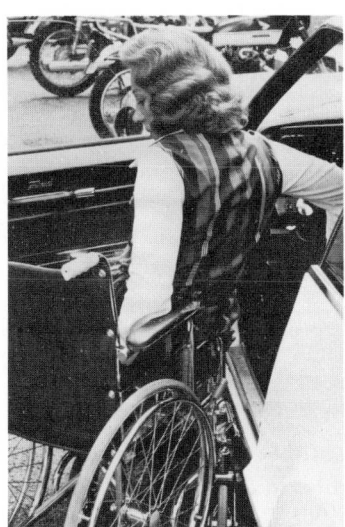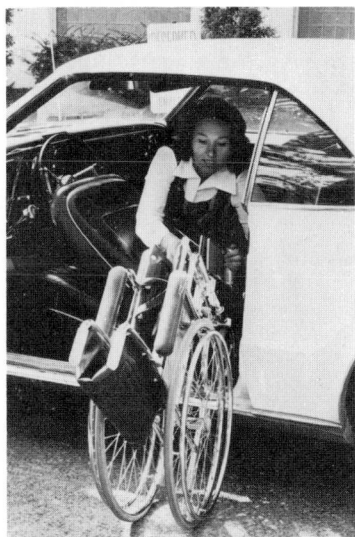

Figure 13-11. Rehabilitation of the paraplegic patient should be done as rapidly as possible to prevent secondary disabilities, including depression and loss of motivation. Mrs. D. W., shown here, has been a paraplegic for over 20 years. She successfully manages a home and family and a secretarial position. Here she accomplishes a transfer from the wheelchair to the car.

(a) Use prostigmine methylsulfate (neostigmine methylsulfate) whenever necessary.

(b) Omit gas-forming foods and liquids.

(2) Ensure total evacuation of fecal material from lower bowel every day.

(a) Give enemas or colonic irrigation.

(b) Employ regular digital examination of rectum—to determine presence of impacted fecal material.

(c) Keep patient on bowel training program (see p. 38).

d. Ankylosis of joints; contractures

(1) Start passive exercises and range of motion early in course of treatment.

(2) Position patient in functional positions (see p. 5).

(3) Use splints and supports for spastic joints as indicated by patient's condition.

NEUROGENIC BLADDER

Neurogenic bladder is any bladder disturbance due to a lesion of the nervous system.

Normal Physiology

1. Normal bladder action depends on intact sensory and motor nerve supply.
2. The bladder fills to approximately 500 ml.—triggers an emptying reflex.
3. This reflex initiates a contraction of the musculature inside the bladder wall forcing urine out through the urethra until the bladder is empty.

Causes

1. Spinal cord injury
2. Disease—multiple sclerosis, tabes dorsalis, diabetes mellitus
3. Spinal cord tumor or herniated intervertebral disc
4. Certain congenital anomalies (spina bifida, myelomeningocele)

Types of Neurogenic Bladder

A. *Spastic (reflex or automatic)*

1. A bladder disorder caused by any lesion of the cord above the voiding reflex arc (upper motor neuron lesion).
2. Most common type.
3. There is loss of conscious sensations and cerebral motor control.
4. Patient has reduced bladder capacity and marked hypertrophy of bladder wall.
5. Bladder behaves in reflex fashion with minimal or no controlling influence to regulate its activity.

B. *Flaccid (atonic, nonreflex or autonomous)*

1. A bladder disease caused by lower motor neuron lesion.
2. Bladder continues to fill until it becomes greatly distended—bladder musculature does not contract forcefully at any time.
3. When pressure reaches a breakthrough point, small amounts of urine dribble from urethra as bladder continues to fill (overflow incontinence).
4. Sensory loss may accompany flaccid bladder; patient is not aware of discomfort.
5. Extensive distention causes damage to bladder musculature, infection of stagnant urine and infection of kidneys by back pressure of urine.

Complications

1. *Infection*—bladder cannot empty itself; catheterization produces infection.
2. *Hydronephrosis*—from hypertrophy of bladder wall leading to vesicoureteral reflux.
3. *Calculus*—from demineralization of bone from bedrest; urinary stasis and infection.
4. *Renal failure*—major cause of death of patients with neurologic impairment of the bladder.

Treatment

Objectives: to empty bladder regularly, completely and easily.
to maintain urine sterility with no stone formation.
to maintain adequate bladder capacity without ureterovesical reflux.

A. *Initial Treatment*

There is temporary bladder paralysis immediately following spinal cord injury; there is a time of reorganization of the central nervous system which eventually leads to the development of spasticity.

1. Catheterize patient intermittently using strict aseptic technique.
   Fluids must be restricted if the intermittent catheterization method of treatment is used.
2. Or catheterize patient using continuous closed drainage and irrigation system (p. 469) to avoid overdistention and risk of contracture from bladder being constantly empty.
   Tape catheter to abdomen or lateral thigh (male)—to remove sharp angulation and pressure at penoscrotal angle (Fig. 7-9).
3. Encourage liberal fluid intake (3–5 liters daily)—there is reduction in urinary bacterial count with increase in urine flow; hydration reduces stasis and decreases concentration of calcium in urine and minimizes precipitation of urinary crystals and stone formation.
4. Keep patient as mobile as possible—to reduce incidence of calculosis (presence of calculi).
   a. Turn, move and exercise patient.
   b. Get patient up on tilt table (p. 33) or in wheelchair as soon as possible.
   c. Give low calcium diet—to prevent calculosis.
      Avoid dairy products.
5. Use acidifying agents (ammonium chloride)—to maintain urine pH below 6.0.

B. *Treatment After Removal of Catheter*

1. Start bladder training program—for spastic type bladder.
   a. Initiate voiding by manual stimulation; apply pressure with hands over suprapubic area or bend over to increase intra-abdominal pressure.
   b. Record time and amount of voiding.
   c. Record time and amount of fluid intake.
   d. Repeat voiding by manual compression every 2 hours—to prevent overdistention.
      (1) Set alarm clock for 2-hour intervals during day.
      (2) Have patient void twice during the night.
2. Give parasympathomimetic drugs, e.g., bethanechol (Urecholine)—to increase contraction of detrusor muscle.
3. Do vaginal and rectal contractions to strengthen periurethral tissue.
   a. Tighten the rectum or vaginal vault.

  b. Hold the contraction while counting slowly to 6; relax.
  c. Continue relaxing and tightening for a 5-minute period.
  d. Perform these exercises twice daily for 5 minutes over a 6- to 8-week period—success or failure of exercise program is then evaluated.

C. *Program for Patient with Diminished Functional Bladder Capacity*
   This patient may void every 15–30 minutes and is not a candidate for a bladder training program.
   1. Male patient—use condom collecting device (see p. 36).
   2. Female patient—there is no satisfactory appliance for female patient.
      a. *Indwelling catheter*
         Clinical problems
         (1) Gives rise to urinary infection which may spread to kidneys; also may cause bladder spasms.
         (2) Urethra dilates around indwelling catheter and there is urinary leakage (pericatheter incontinence).
      b. *Pads and waterproof pants* (obtain from medical supply houses)
         Clinical problems
         (1) Exposes perineal skin to irritation and maceration.
         (2) Is expensive.
      c. *Urinary diversion procedures* (see p. 500)
         May be most satisfactory method of bladder control for female patient.

MANAGEMENT OF THE PATIENT FOLLOWING A LAMINECTOMY

Laminectomy is removal of the lamina to expose the spinal cord.
Spinal fusion is removal of bone graft from the posterior iliac crest to fuse (blend together) the spinous processes. The spinal fusion bridges over the faulty disc and stabilizes the spine.

Indications for a Laminectomy

   1. As an emergency procedure to prevent irreversible neurologic damage.
   2. For progressive central nervous system involvement with muscular weakness and atrophy.
   3. For recurring episodes of pain or unrelieved acute pain.

Postoperative Nursing Management
(See the preoperative principles for patient undergoing orthopedic surgery, p. 792).

Objective: to provide a stable spine to meet the functional demands of the body.
   1. Keep the patient on bedrest for first few postoperative days.
      a. Use pillow under head and elevate the knee rest slightly (slight knee flexion to relax muscles of the back).
      b. Encourage the patient to move and turn from side to side to relieve pressure.
         (1) Turn patient as a unit (log rolling); place pillow between patient's legs while turning.
         (2) Place pillow between legs when patient is lying on his side.
         (3) Avoid extreme knee flexion when patient is on side.
   2. Give narcotics and sedatives to relieve pain and anxiety.

3. Explain to the patient that there may be varying degrees of pain and sensory manifestations in the legs (sciatica type pain)—due to temporary inflammatory changes, edema and swelling of compressed nerve.
4. Be alert for postoperative complication of infection.

Patient Teaching

Instruct the patient as follows
1. Increase activities as tolerated—move up to the point of individual tolerance.
2. Avoid activities that produce flexion strain to the spine—stair climbing, automobile riding.
3. Have scheduled rest periods.
4. Apply heat to back when indicated—helps absorb exudates in the tissues.
5. Avoid heavy work for 2–3 months after surgery.

INTRACTABLE PAIN

Intractable pain is pain that cannot be relieved satisfactorily by drugs short of drug addiction or incapacitating sedation.

Causes

1. Malignant disease (especially of cervix, bladder, prostate, lower bowel)
2. Trigeminal neuralgia
3. Uncontrollable ischemia or other forms of tissue destruction

Procedures for Management of Intractable Pain

Objective: to interrupt the pathways by which the painful sensations are perceived.
1. *Posterior spinal rhizotomy*—surgical interruption of selected posterior spinal nerve roots between the ganglion and the cord. This results in permanent sensory deficit (loss of sensation).
2. *Chemical rhizotomy*—injection of alcohol (phenol or mixture of phenol and Pantopaque) into subarachnoid spine; medication is maneuvered over affected nerve roots by tilting the patient to achieve desired level. The patient's perception of pain is absent but motor nerve roots sensations are not.
3. *Cordotomy*—division of anterolateral columns of the spinal cord for the relief of intractable pain.
   a. Procedure may be performed percutaneously rather than by open operation.
   b. Lesion is produced by radio-frequency generator with a percutaneously inserted needle.

Nursing Management

1. Be alert for signs of shock, respiratory distress, bladder dysfunction, paralysis, constipation.
2. Explain to the patient and the family the changes in sensation that will occur.
3. See Management of the Patient Following a Laminectomy, page 766 for principles of care relevent also to these operations.
4. Test motion, strength and sensation of each extremity every few hours during the first 48 hours.
   Hemorrhage may produce motor and sensory loss—immediate surgical intervention is indicated.

5. Feel patient's skin temperature at intervals—to ascertain skin temperature changes.
6. Watch for development of pressure sores.
   a. Teach patient to inspect his skin using a hand mirror to view hard-to-see areas.
   b. Place patient on bladder training program (p. 764) if high cervical procedure has caused loss of bladder control.
7. Turn the patient as a unit (log rolling)—produces less tension on the incision.
8. For postcordotomy care:
   a. Keep patient flat in bed for prescribed time period.
   b. Assist patient with bladder training program (p. 764) if he has high cervical incision.

Patient and Family Education

Instruct the family and patient as follows:
1. Protect patient against external temperature changes and extremes of weather—may not be aware of sunburn/frostbite.
2. Test bath water before getting in tub.
3. Avoid constricting clothing that impairs circulation.

BIBLIOGRAPHY

Books

Alpers, B. J., and Mancall, E. L.: Clinical Neurology. 6th ed. Philadelphia, F. A. Davis, 1971.
Brain, W. R., and Walton, J. N.: Brain's Diseases of the Nervous System. New York, Oxford University Press, 1969.
Brunner, L., et al.: Textbook of Medical-Surgical Nursing. 2nd ed. Philadelphia, J. B. Lippincott, 1970, pp. 759–833.
Carini, E., and Owens, G.: Neurological and Neurosurgical Nursing. St. Louis, C. V. Mosby, 1970.
Chusid, J. G.: Correlative Neuroanatomy and Functional Neurology. Los Altos, Lange Medical Publications, 1970.
DePalma, A. F., and Rothman, R. H.: The Intervertebral Disc. Philadelphia, W. B. Saunders, 1970.
Draper, I. T.: Lecture Notes on Neurology. Philadelphia, F. A. Davis, 1970.
Elliott, F. A.: Clinical Neurology. Philadelphia, W. B. Saunders, 1971.
Gurdjian, E. S., and Thomas, L. M.: Operative Neurosurgery. Baltimore, Williams and Wilkins, 1970.
Hitchcock, E. R., and Masson, A. H. B.: Management of the Unconscious Patient. Oxford, Blackwell Scientific Publications, 1970.
Jennett, W. B.: An Introduction to Neurosurgery. St. Louis, C. V. Mosby, 1970.
Logue, V.: Operative Surgery; Neurosurgery. Philadelphia, J. B. Lippincott, 1971.
Mayo Clinic and Mayo Foundation, Department of Neurology and Department of Physiology and Biophysics: Clinical Examinations in Neurology. Philadelphia, W. B. Saunders, 1971.
Mountjoy, P., and Wythe, B.: Nursing Care of the Unconscious Patient. London, Bailliere, Tindal and Cassell, 1970.
U.S. Department of Health, Education and Welfare: Literature Relating to Neurological and Neurosurgical Nursing. Washington, D.C., U.S. Government Printing Office, 1970.
Woodbury, D. M., et al.: Antiepileptic Drugs. New York, Raven Press, 1972.

Articles

Abramson, A. S.: Advances in the management of the neurogenic bladder. Arch. Phy. Med. Rehab., 52:143–148, April 1972.

Bouzarth, W. F.: The ABC's of emergency care of serious head injuries in industry. Ind. Med. Surg., 39:25–29, Jan. 1970.

Carozza, V. J.: Understanding the patient with epilepsy. Nurs. Clin. N. Amer., 5:13–22, March 1970.

Cassidy, F. M.: Adult hydrocephalus. Amer. J. Nurs., 72:494–499, March 1972.

Cooney, L. M., and Solitare, G. B.: Primary intracranial tumors in the elderly. Geriatrics, 27:94–104, Jan. 1972.

Dervitz, H. L., and Zislis, J. M.: A medical perspective of physical therapy and stroke rehabilitation. Geriatrics, 25:123–132, June 1970.

Elwood, E.: Nursing the patient with a cerebrovascular accident. Nurs. Clin. N. Amer., 50:47–53, March 1970.

Fox, M. J.: Talking with patients who can't answer. Amer. J. Nurs., 71:1146–1149, June 1971.

Griggs, W. L. (ed.): Advances in the treatment of some common neurologic disorders. Mod. Treat., 8:219–317, May 1971.

Henderson, G. M.: Teaching-learning for rehabilitation of the spinal-cord disabled individual. Nurs. Clin. N. Amer., 6:655–688, Dec. 1971.

Hull, J. T.: The prevalence and incidence of Parkinson's disease. Geriatrics, 25:128–133, May 1970.

Jacobansky, A. M.: Stroke. Amer. J. Nurs., 72:1260–1263, July 1972.

Kay, E., et al.: Stereotactic surgery for Parkinson's Disease. Amer. J. Nurs., 72:2200–2205, Dec. 1972.

Kinney, A. B., and Blount, M.: Systems approach to myasthenia gravis. Nurs. Clin. N. Amer., 6:435–453, Sept. 1971.

Kott, H. S.: The treatment of multiple sclerosis. Med. Clin. N. Amer., 56:711–716, May 1972.

Lehrer, G. M.: Etiology, diagnosis and treatment of multiple sclerosis. Mod. Treat., 7:879–968, Sept. 1970.

Liverani, L., and Osserman, R. S.: Myasthenia gravis: A nursing care plan. Nurs. Clin. N. Amer., 7:185–195, March 1972.

Parsons, L. C.: Respiratory changes in head injury. Amer. J. Nurs., 71:2187–2191, Nov. 1971.

Perrine, G.: Needs met and unmet. Amer. J. Nurs., 71:2128–2133, Nov. 1971.

Pitts, F. W., and Stauffer, E. S.: Spinal injuries in multiple injured patient. Orth. Clin. N. Amer., 1:137–149, July 1970.

Massell, T. B., et al.: Surgery for stroke. Geriatrics, 27:106–113, Feb. 1972.

Raskind, R., et al.: Common carotid artery ligation for intracranial aneurysm in patients over 50. Geriatrics, 27:87–93, Jan. 1972.

Schulz, D.: Myasthenia gravis: surgical and anesthesiological considerations. J. Amer. Assoc. Nurse Anesth., 39:285–289, Aug. 1971.

Suggs, K. M.: Coping and adaptive behavior in the stroke syndrome. Nurs. Forum, 10:100–111, 1971.

Tate, G.: Assessment and direction of nursing care for patients with acute central nervous system insult. Nurs. Clin. N. Amer., 6:165–171, March 1971.

Todd, J. (ed.): Intensive care of the patient with central nervous system disease. Med. Clin. N. Amer., 55:1233–1248, Sept. 1971.

Torres, H., and Ferguson, L.: Acute head injuries. Amer. Fam. Phys., 2:88–98, Dec. 1970.

Trigiano, L. L.: Independence is possible in quadriplegia. Amer. J. Nurs., 70:2610–2613, Dec. 1970.

Wanger, S. L.: The management of Parkinson's syndrome. Med. Clin. N. Amer., 56:693–707, May 1972.

Whitehouse, F. A.: Stroke: the present challenge. Nurs. Forum, 10:90–99, 1971.

Whiteman, M.: Bell's palsy. Amer. J. Nurs., 71:2139–2140, Nov. 1971.

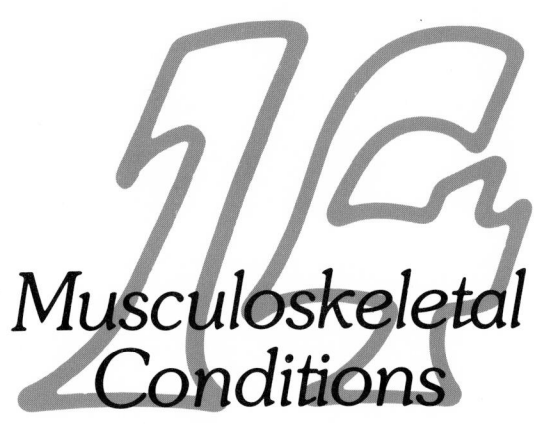

Musculoskeletal Conditions

SPECIFIC PROBLEMS ASSOCIATED WITH ORTHOPEDIC CONDITIONS

Pain

Types of Pain

1. Sharp pain—may be from bone infection with muscle spasm or pressure on sensory nerve
2. Soreness and aching—due to muscular pain
3. Increasing pain—progression of an infectious process or malignant tumor
4. Pain increasing with activity—may indicate joint strain
5. Pain that is worse in bad weather, felt in more than one part of body—may be arthritis
6. Radiating pain—rupture of intervertebral disc and pressure on the nerve root

Nursing Assessment

1. What activities precipitated the pain?
2. Is the body in proper alignment?
3. Is there pressure from traction, splints, cast, other appliances?
4. How does the patient describe the pain? Can he localize it?
5. Does it radiate?
6. What relieves the pain? Makes it worse?

Nursing Management

1. Position the patient in correct alignment.
2. Support the painful parts under the joints.
   a. Move the patient slowly and steadily.
   b. Avoid bumping the bed.
3. Apply heat to relieve muscle spasm.
4. Apply cold to relieve pain in inflammatory conditions.

Deformity

Types of Deformity

1. Contracture deformities are caused by limitation of motion and disuse.
2. Pain and muscle spasm produce limitation of motion.
3. Inflammation limits joint motion and causes fibrous tissue to form, producing fibrous or bony ankylosis (abnormal rigidity of joint).

Nursing Assessment

1. When was the deformity noted?
2. Was the onset accompanied by injury?
3. Is the deformity increasing? Decreasing?
4. Is paralysis present?
   a. What was the time and mode of onset of paralysis?
   b. Are there sensory disturbances?
   c. Where is the paralysis located?
   d. Are there trophic changes?
   e. Are there any disturbances in control of bladder and bowel?

Nursing Management

1. Position the patient in accordance with principles of body mechanics.
2. Place a hinged bedboard under a firm mattress.
3. Avoid semirecumbent positions for prolonged periods—such a position promotes flexion deformities of the hip.
4. Encourage and assist patient to perform passive and active exercises—to maintain and improve muscle strength, maintain and restore optimal joint function, prevent deformities, stimulate circulation and build endurance.

Psychosocial Problems

Types of Psychosocial Problems
(From Prolonged Periods of Disability)

1. Immobility. (Patients tend to become depressed when mobility is restricted, and tend to improve when the treatment program is modified to permit some movement.)
2. Economic problems
3. Despondency

Nursing Management

1. Encourage and reassure the patient.
2. Keep the patient busy—action absorbs anxiety.
3. Schedule a program of activity to include exercise program and occupational therapy —to promote feelings of independence.

DIAGNOSTIC EVALUATION OF MUSCULOSKELETAL DISORDERS

A. *Patient's History*

B. *Physical Examination*
   1. Observation for muscle atrophy or swelling
   2. Observation of gait and posture
   3. Examination of joints—shape, alignment, circumference, range of motion, stability, instability, presence of abnormal joint fluid
   4. Palpation for skin temperature, local swelling, tenderness
   5. Measurement of muscle strength, length of extremities, circumference of extremities
   6. Neurologic evaluation—including cranial nerve testing, motor and sensory nerve testing, reflexes of extremities (frequently have orthopedic significance)

C. *X-ray*
   1. Of bone—to determine bone density, texture, erosion, changes in bone relationships
   2. Of cortex—to detect any widening, narrowing, irregularity
   3. Of medullary cavity—to detect any altered density
   4. Of involved joint—to show fluid, irregularity, spur formation, changes in joint contour

D. *Special X-ray Techniques*
   1. Laminography—shows in detail a specific plane of involved bone
   2. Myelography—injection of radiopaque dye into subarachnoid space at lumbar spine —to determine level of disc herniation or site of tumor

3. Arthrography—injection of radiopaque substance or air into joint cavity—outlines soft tissue structures and contour of joint

E. *Electromyography Nerve Condition Studies*
   See page 720.

F. *Bone Scanning*—injection of bone-seeking radioactive isotope; increased concentration of isotope uptake revealed in metastatic bone lesions or osteomyelitis

MUSCULOSKELETAL TRAUMA

Contusions

A *contusion* is an injury to the soft tissue produced by a blunt force, blow, kick or fall.

Clinical Manifestations

1. Hemorrhage into injured part (ecchymosis)—from rupture of small blood vessels
2. Pain, swelling and discoloration

Treatment

1. Elevate the affected part.
2. Apply cold compresses—to diminish edema formation.
3. Apply pressure bandage (elastic or elastic adhesive)—to reduce swelling and edema.
4. Apply heat to affected area after 6 hours—to promote absorption.

Strains

A *strain* is an injury to muscles or tendons.

Treatment

Same as for contusions.

Sprains

A *sprain* is an injury to ligamentous structures surrounding a joint and is usually caused by wrenching or twisting

Clinical Manifestations

1. Rapid swelling—due to extravasation of blood within tissues
2. Pain upon joint movement

Treatment

1. X-ray injured area—to ensure there is no bone injury.
2. Elevate and rest affected part.
3. Apply cold compresses (or ice bag) intermittently for 12–36 hours—vasoconstricting effects of cold retard extravasation of blood and lymph (edema) and suppress pain.
4. Apply mild heat after 36 hours if indicated.

Joint Dislocation

A *dislocation of a joint* is a condition in which the articular surfaces of the bones forming the joint are no longer in anatomic contact (bones are "out of joint").

Classification

1. Congenital; (most often noted with hip)
2. Pathologic or spontaneous—from disease of articular or periarticular structures
3. Traumatic—from injury

Clinical Manifestations

1. Change in contour of the joint
2. Change in the length of the extremity
3. Loss of normal movement
4. Change in axis of dislocated bones.

Treatment

1. X-ray affected part—to rule out associated fracture.
2. Immobilize part while patient is transported to emergency room or clinical unit.
3. Reduce (bring displaced parts to normal position) dislocation (usually under anesthesia).
4. Essentials of nursing management are the same as for reduction of fractures (see p. 775).

Fractures

A *fracture* is a break in the continuity of bone.

Classification of Fractures (Fig. 14-1)

A. *General Classification*
1. *Complete*—a fracture involving the entire cross section of the bone.
2. *Incomplete*—a fracture involving only a portion of the cross section of bone.
3. *Open*—the wound of fracture extends through the skin and mucous membrane (formerly called compound fracture).
4. *Closed*—the fracture does not communicate with outside area (formerly called simple fracture).

B. *Specific Types of Fractures* (Fig. 14-1)
1. *Greenstick*—a fracture in which one side of a bone is broken, the other side being bent.
2. *Transverse*—the fracture is straight across the bone.
3. *Oblique*—a fracture occurring at an angle across the bone (less stable than transverse).
4. *Spiral*—a fracture twisting around the shaft of the bone.
5. *Comminuted*—a fracture in which bone has splintered into fractures.
6. *Depressed*—a fracture in which a fragment(s) is in-driven (seen frequently in fractures of skull and facial bones).
7. *Impacted*—a fracture in which one bone fragment is driven firmly into the other by the force producing the fracture.

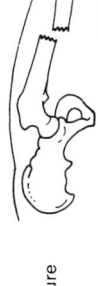
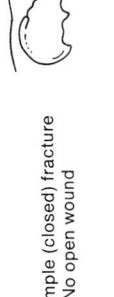
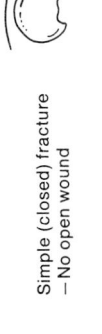

Transverse fracture—Break runs across bone

Oblique fracture—Break runs in slanting direction on bone

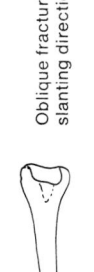
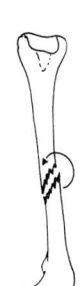

Spiral fracture—Break coils around bone

Pathologic fracture—Break is at site of bone disease

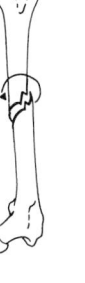
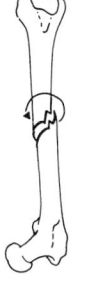
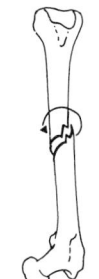

Impacted fracture—Bone broken and wedged into other break

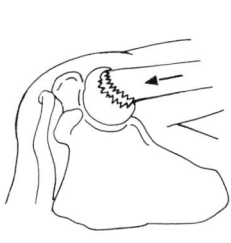
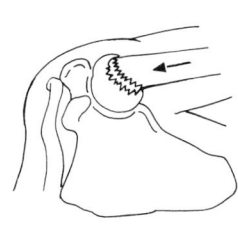
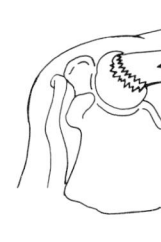

Depressed fracture—Broken skull bone driven inward

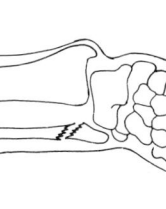
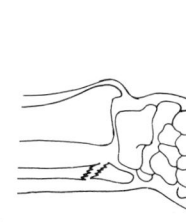

Fracture dislocation—Break complicated by bone out of joint

Simple (closed) fracture—No open wound

Compound (open) fracture—Wound in skin communicates with fracture

Extracapsular fracture—Bone broken outside joint

Intracapsular fracture—Bone broken inside joint

Comminuted fracture—Bone splintered into fragments

Greenstick fracture—Bone broken, bent but still securely hinged at one side

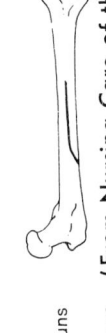

Longitudinal fracture—Break runs parallel with bone

Figure 14-1. Types of fractures. (From Nursing Care of the Patient in the O.R. Somerville, New Jersey, Ethicon, Inc., 1972.)

8. *Compression*—a fracture in which the fractured bone has been compressed by another bone(s) (seen in vertebral fractures).
9. *Pathologic*—a fracture that occurs through an area of diseased bone (bone cyst, bony metastasis).

Clinical Manifestations

1. Pain—continues with increasing severity until bone fragments are immobilized
2. Inability to use the part (except in impacted or incomplete fracture)
3. Localized swelling and discoloration of the skin—from trauma and hemorrhage that follows
4. Visible or palpable deformity
5. False motion
6. Crepitation—grating sensation felt upon examination due to rubbing of the fragments upon the other. (Testing for crepitation can produce further tissue damage)

Emergency Management

See page 915.

Treatment

A. *Reduction* (Setting the Bone)

    Objectives: to regain the function of the involved part.
                    to regain correct alignment.
                    to maintain the alignment.

1. Restores, as nearly as possible, the fracture fragments into anatomic rotation and alignment.
2. Methods
   a. *Closed reduction*—bringing the bony fragments into apposition (ends in contact) by *manipulation* and *manual traction* (most commonly used to restore alignment).
   (1) Usually done under anesthesia—to relieve pain and relax muscles.
   (2) Cast is usually applied—to immobilize extremity and maintain reduction.
   b. *Traction*—applying force in 2 directions to obtain reduction and regain normal length and alignment.
   (1) May be used for fractures of long bones.
   (2) Traction applied to extremity by:
       (a) Skin traction—by means of adhesive or moleskin strips.
       (b) Skeletal traction—by means of wires, pins or tongs placed through bone.
   (3) For nursing management see under Traction, pages 782–785.
   c. *Open reduction* (open operation)—operative intervention to achieve fracture reduction.
   (1) Bone fragments are replaced under direct visualization.
   (2) Internal fixation devices (metallic pins, wires, screws, plates, nails, rods) may be used to hold bone fragments in position until solid bone healing occurs (may or may not be removed after bony union has taken place).
   (3) For nursing management following open reduction, see Nursing Management of the Patient Undergoing Orthopedic Surgery, pages 792–794.
   d. *Prosthetic replacement*

B. *Immobilization*
1. Maintains reduction in place until healing occurs.
2. Methods
   a. *External fixation*
      (1) Plaster cast fixation
      (2) Splints
      (3) Continuous traction
   b. *Internal fixation*
      (1) Pin and plaster technique
      (2) Internal fixation devices
         (nails, plates, screws, wires, rods)
3. Assess patient for increasing pain—usually indicates an ill-fitting cast or splint.

C. *Rehabilitation* (Regaining normal function of the affected part)
1. Instruct the patient to actively exercise joints above and below the cast at frequent intervals.
   a. Isometric exercises of muscles covered by cast—start exercise as soon as possible after cast application.
   b. Increase isometric exercises as fracture stabilizes.
2. After removal of cast, have patient start active exercises.
   a. Recommend that patient start moving affected extremity under water if necessary, as water supports extremity and provides warmth which helps promote muscle relaxation.
   b. Instruct patient in methods of ambulation—walker, crutches and cane (see pp. 28–33).

Treatment of Open Fractures

Objective: to minimize chance of infection of wound and bone.
1. Cleanse and debride the wound—to minimize chance of infection, debridement should be done as soon as possible.
2. Protect patient from tetanus.
   a. For patients not previously immunized:
      (1) Give human tetanus immune globulin (according to severity and duration of wound).
      (2) Start tetanus toxoid series—for active immunization
         (a) 2nd dose given 4 weeks after initial dose.
         (b) 3rd dose given 6–12 months later.
   b. For patients previously immunized with tetanus toxoid:
      Give booster dose if previous dosage given within 6–10 years.
3. Give antibiotics as directed—to avoid and treat serious infection.

Complications of Fractures

A. *Immediate Complications*
1. Shock
   a. May be fatal within a few hours after injury (see p. 78).
   b. Treatment
      (1) Replace depleted blood volume.
      (2) Relieve patient's pain.
2. Fat embolism
   a. May occur after severe multiple fractures, particularly in the long bones.
   b. After injury innumerable fat globules appear in the bloodstream and act as emboli; abnormalities may develop in any part of the body, producing lethal changes in brain, lungs, heart.

    c. Evaluate for increasing pulse rate without apparent cause.

    d. Watch for petechiae from fat embolism over chest, anterior axillary fold—Inspect the conjunctival sacs, buccal membranes and hard palate for petechiae.

  3. Thromboembolism (see pp. 80–81).

  4. Infection—all open fractures are considered contaminated.

B. *Delayed Complications*

  1. Delayed union—signifies that a specific fracture has not healed in the time considered as being average for this fracture.

  2. Nonunion—failure of the ends of a fractured bone to unite.

  3. Avascular necrosis of bone—may occur when bone loses its blood supply following fracture or dislocation, notably in the hip.

CASTS

Purposes

  1. To immobilize and hold bone fragments in reduction.

  2. To apply uniform compression of soft tissues

  3. To permit early weight-bearing activities

Complications

A. *Constriction of Circulation*

Vascular insufficiency due to unrelieved swelling; can progress to the point of gangrenous necrosis.

  1. *Symptoms*

    a. *Unrelieved pain*

    b. Swelling

    c. Blanching or discoloration

    d. Tingling or numbness

    e. No pulse

    f. Inability to move fingers or toes

    g. Temperature change of skin

  2. *Nursing Management*

    a. Bivalve the cast; split cast on each side over its full length into 2 halves.

    b. Cut the underlying padding—blood-soaked padding may shrink and cause constriction of circulation.

    c. Spread cast sufficiently to relieve constriction.

B. *Pressure of Cast on Tissues, especially on Bony Parts*

  1. Causes necrosis and decubitus ulcers.

  2. Causes nerve palsies from prolonged pressure on nerve trunk.

  3. Symptoms

    Unrelieved pain—Pain over bony prominence is a warning symptom of an impending pressure sore.

  4. *Pressure Sites*

    a. *Lower extremity*—heel, malleoli, dorsum of foot, head of fibula, anterior surface of patella.

    b. *Upper extremity*—medial epicondyle of humerus, styloid of the ulna.

    c. When plaster jackets or body spica casts are used—sacrum, anterior and superior iliac spines, vertebral borders of scapulae.

  4. *Nursing Management*

    a. Cut the cast at the pain point (over bony prominence) in a criss-cross fashion.

    b. Elevate each flap of plaster.

Types of Casts

1. *Forearm cast*—extends from below the elbow to the proximal palmar crease.
2. *Gauntlet cast*—extends from below the elbow to the proximal palmar crease, including the thumb.
3. *Long-arm cast*—extends from upper level of axillary fold to proximal palmar crease; elbow usually immobilized at right angle.
4. *Boot or short-leg cast*—extends from below knee to base of toes.
5. *Long-leg cast*—extends from junction of the upper and middle third of thigh to the base of toes; foot is at right angle in a neutral position.
6. *Spica or body cast*—incorporates the trunk and an extremity
   a. *Shoulder spica cast*—a body jacket that encloses trunk and shoulder and elbow
   b. *Hip spica cast*—encloses trunk and a lower extremity
      (1) Single hip spica—extends from nipple line to include pelvis and one thigh
      (2) Double hip spica—extends from nipple line or upper abdomen to include pelvis and extends to include both thighs and lower legs
      (3) One and a half hip spica—extends from upper abdomen and includes one entire leg and extends to the knee of the other.

Applying a Cast

1. Skin is protected with sheet wadding, stockinette, felt (smoothly and evenly arranged).
2. The plaster bandage is applied, turn upon turn, with the open hand.
3. Places of strain (back of knee, etc.) are reinforced with plaster splints.
4. The finished cast should be well molded and without wrinkles.

Care of Patient While Cast Dries

A. *Extremity Cast*
   1. Explain to the patient that he will experience the feeling of heat under the plaster.
   2. Leave area enclosed in cast uncovered until the cast is dry—covers restrict escape of moisture and make cast musty.
   3. Elevate extremity on pillow after the cast has cooled and started to harden.
   4. Avoid weight-bearing on cast for 48 hours.

B. *Spica or Body Cast*
   1. Place a bedboard under the mattress—prevents sagging of bed from pressure of cast.
   2. Support the curves of the cast with small plastic-covered flexible pillows—prevents cracking while cast is drying.
   3. Avoid placing a pillow under head and shoulders while cast is drying—causes pressure on the chest.
   4. Handle moist cast with palms of hands.

Observation of the Patient in a Cast

1. Listen to the patient's complaints (see complications).
2. Ask the patient to localize the exact site of pain.
3. Avoid giving analgesics for pain. Do not mask the pain until the cause has been determined.
4. Watch for signs of pressure and constriction of circulation (see p. 778).
5. Notify physician if symptoms persist.
   a. Reassure the patient that the cast cutter will cause vibration but is not painful.
   b. Loosen or bivalve the cast (see p. 782).

Care of Patient After Cast Dries

A. *Spica Cast* (Fig. 14-2)

   1. Keep the cast level by elevating the lumbar sacral area with a small pillow when the head of the bed is elevated or when the patient is placed on the bedpan.

   2. Protect the toes from the pressure of the bedding.

   3. Encourage the patient to maintain physiologic position by:
     a. Using the overhead trapeze.
     b. Placing good foot flat on bed and pushing down while lifting himself up on the trapeze.
     c. Avoiding twisting motions.
     d. Avoiding positions that produce pressure on groin, back, chest and abdomen.

   4. Provide hygienic care of the patient.
     a. Cover perineum with a towel and spray perineal area with spray (laquer-type). Tuck 4-inch strips of thin polyethylene sheeting under perineal area of cast and tape to cast exterior. Replace when soiling occurs.
     b. Clean outside of cast with dry cleanser on almost dry cloth.
     c. Pull stockinette taut, trim and fasten to cast edges with adhesive.
     d. Inspect skin for signs of irritation:
       (1) Around cast edge.
       (2) Under cast—pull skin taut and inspect under cast, using a flashlight for illumination.
     e. Massage accessible skin with an emollient lotion.

   5. Turn the patient.
     a. Move the patient to the side of the bed, using a steady even pulling motion.
     b. Place pillows along the other side of the bed; 1 for the chest and 2 (lengthwise) for the legs.
     c. Instruct the patient to place his arms at his side.
     d. Turn the patient as a unit. Avoid twisting the patient in the cast.
     e. Turn the patient toward the leg not encased in plaster or toward the unoperated side if both legs are in plaster.
       (1) One nurse stands at other side of bed to receive patient's shoulders.
       (2) Second nurse supports leg in plaster while the third nurse supports the patient's back as he is turned.
       (3) DO NOT GRASP CROSS BAR OF SPICA CAST TO MOVE PATIENT.

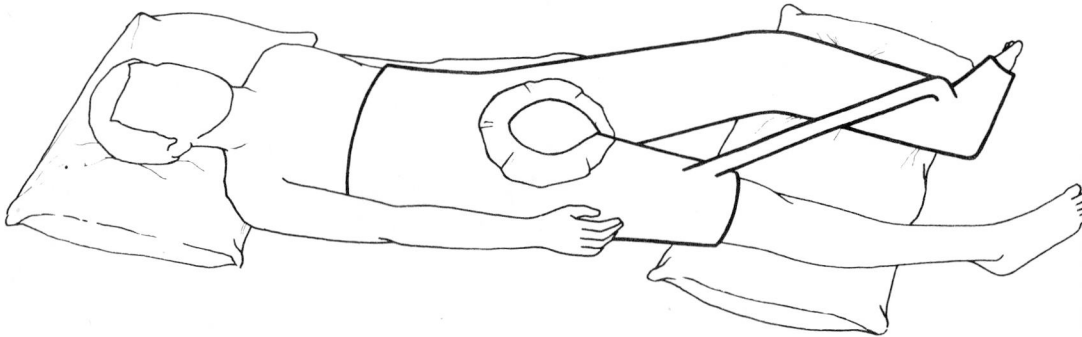

Figure 14-2. Spica cast. Single hip spica. The polyethyl sheeting around perineal area helps keep the cast clean.

NURSING ALERT: Watch for symptoms *(nausea)* of cast syndrome (acute obstruction of duodenum after spica or body cast is applied). (See intestinal obstruction, p. 407.)

If symptoms occur

1. Place patient prone to relieve pressure symptoms.
2. Remove patient from cast if necessary.
3. Employ nasogastric suction.
4. Maintain normal electrolyte balance.

Surgical intervention (duodenojejunostomy) may be necessary when conservative measures fail to relieve duodenal obstruction.

B. *Leg Cast*

1. Prevent or reduce swelling.
   a. Elevate the extremity in the cast.
   b. Apply ice bags to each side of the cast.
   c. After patient begins ambulation, encourage him to elevate the cast when he is seated.
2. Prevent irritation at cast edge—pad edges of cast with moleskin.
3. Examine toes and foot for:
   a. Blanching or cyanosis
   b. Swelling
   c. Inability to move toes
4. Ascertain if patient is experiencing sensory disturbances to foot (numbness, tingling, burning, cold)—peroneal nerve injury from pressure at the head of the fibula is a common cause of footdrop.

C. *Arm Cast*

1. Watch for symptoms of circulatory disturbance in hand (blueness or cyanosis, swelling, inability to move fingers).
2. Reduce and control swelling.
   Elevate arm with each joint positioned higher than preceding joint (i.e., elbow higher than shoulder, hand higher than the elbow).

NURSING ALERT: Guard against Volkmann's contracture—a severe fibrosis with resulting contracture of muscles which have become ischemic by obstruction of the arterial flow to the forearm and hand. This complication is prevented by proper care; if allowed to develop the results are disastrous.

Exercising the Patient in a Cast

1. Teach the patient to perform isometric exercises—contracting the muscles without moving the joint to maintain muscle strength and prevent atrophy.
2. Leg cast—"Push down on the popliteal (knee) space, hold it, relax, repeat."
3. Arm cast—"Make a fist, hold it, relax, repeat."
4. Actively exercise joints that do not move bone fragments.

Removing a Cast

1. Remove cast by using electric cast cutter or shears.
2. After cast is removed, support the part with pillows—maintain the same position that existed in the cast.
3. Move the extremity gently.
4. Wash skin with mild soap followed by application of oil or lanolin.
5. Encourage patient to do his prescribed muscle strengthening exercises.
6. Treat edema of foot following removal of leg cast.
   Instruct the patient as follows:
   a. Wear shoes.
   b. Elevate foot when sitting.
   c. Wrap leg with an elastic compression bandage or use elastic stocking.

TRACTION

Traction is force applied in 2 directions. To apply the needed force a system of ropes, pulleys and weights is used.

Purposes

1. To regain normal length and alignment.
2. To reduce and immobilize fracture.
3. To lessen or eliminate muscle spasm.
4. To prevent fracture deformity.

Methods

A. *Skin Traction*

1. Traction applied to the skin using adhesive or moleskin strips fastened with elastic bandage (Fig. 14-3).
   a. Skin traction is accomplished by a weight that pulls on the tape, sponge rubber or plastic materials attached to the skin; traction on the skin transmits traction to the neuromusculoskeletal structures.
   b. Used in form of Buck's extension when the pull is exerted in one plane and when partial or temporary immobilization is desired.
2. Shave the part and apply tincture of benzoin to the skin—makes traction strip adhere better and prevents skin itching.
3. Inspect for skin irritation and pressure on peripheral nerves.
   a. Achilles tendon about the heel
   b. Peroneal nerve (as it passes around the neck of the fibula, just below the knee)

B. *Skeletal Traction*

1. Traction applied to bone, using wires, pins or tongs placed through bones (most effective means of traction).
   Skeletal traction is used most frequently in treatment of fractures of femur, humerus and tibia.
2. Watch for signs of infection, especially around pin tract.

C. *Cervical Traction*

   See page 757.

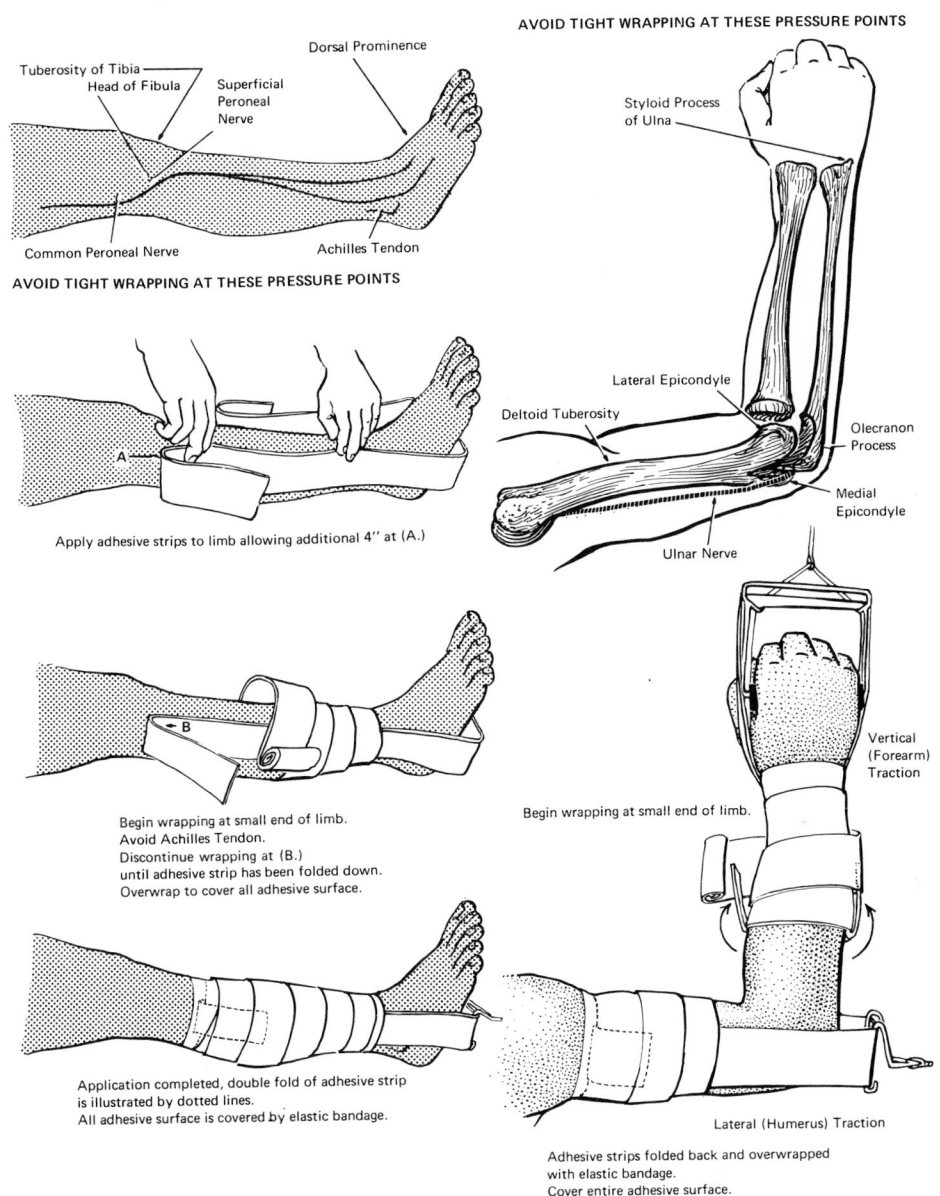

AVOID TIGHT WRAPPING AT THESE PRESSURE POINTS

Tuberosity of Tibia
Head of Fibula
Superficial Peroneal Nerve
Dorsal Prominence
Common Peroneal Nerve
Achilles Tendon

AVOID TIGHT WRAPPING AT THESE PRESSURE POINTS

Apply adhesive strips to limb allowing additional 4" at (A.)

Styloid Process of Ulna
Lateral Epicondyle
Deltoid Tuberosity
Olecranon Process
Medial Epicondyle
Ulnar Nerve

Begin wrapping at small end of limb.
Avoid Achilles Tendon.
Discontinue wrapping at (B.)
until adhesive strip has been folded down.
Overwrap to cover all adhesive surface.

Begin wrapping at small end of limb.

Vertical (Forearm) Traction

Application completed, double fold of adhesive strip
is illustrated by dotted lines.
All adhesive surface is covered by elastic bandage.

Lateral (Humerus) Traction

Adhesive strips folded back and overwrapped
with elastic bandage.
Cover entire adhesive surface.

Figure 14-3. Method of applying adhesive strips for traction. (Courtesy Zimmer Manufacturing Co.)

Nursing Management

1. The patient is placed on a firm mattress, often with a hinged bedboard beneath it.
2. The ropes and the pulleys should be in straight alignment.
3. The pull should be in line with the long axis of the bone.
4. Any factor that might reduce the pull or alter its direction must be eliminated.
   a. Weights should hang free.
   b. Ropes should be unobstructed.
5. The amount of weight applied in skin traction must not exceed the tolerance of the skin. The condition of the skin must be inspected frequently.
6. There is always the possibility of bone infection when skeletal traction is used. Be alert for odors, signs of local inflammation or other evidence of osteomyelitis.
7. The patient's skin should be examined frequently for evidences of pressure or friction over bony prominences.
8. Provision should be made for supplying additional countertraction by increasing the pull in the opposite direction, i.e., by raising the bed in such a manner that the weight of the patient's body tends to oppose the pull of the traction.
9. Active motion of all unaffected joints should be encouraged.
10. Every complaint of the patient in traction should be investigated.

Principles of Balanced Suspension Traction

Balanced suspension traction is produced by a counterforce other than the patient's body weight. The extremity balances or floats in the traction apparatus. The line of traction on the extremity remains fairly constant despite changes in the patient's position. Example: Russell's leg traction for treating fractures of the femoral shaft.

A. *Activities Permitted the Patient*
   1. The patient may sit, turn slightly and move as desired.
   2. The affected heel must remain free of the bed to maintain the traction.

B. *Nursing Management*
   1. The angle of hip flexion is 20 degrees (the angle between the thigh and the bed).
   2. A pillow may be used under the thigh to maintain this angle, with a second pillow placed under the calf to support the lower leg.
   3. The ropes and the pulleys should be freely movable, and the traction should be applied securely to the leg.
   4. Observe for skin irritation around the traction bandage.
   5. Check the patient for signs of odor and infection.
   6. Observe for pressure under the sling at the popliteal space.
   7. Provide foot supports to prevent footdrop.
   8. The traction must be continuous to be effective.

Principles of Running Traction

Running traction is a form of traction in which the pull is exerted in one plane. It may utilize skin or skeletal traction, and it may be either unilateral or bilateral. Example: Buck's extension.

A. *Activities Permitted the Patient*
   1. The head of the bed may be elevated to the point of countertraction (e.g., if the countertraction is 20.3 cm. (8 inches), the head of the bed may be elevated 20.3 cm.

2. The patient may not turn from side to side because the position of the leg on the bed will cause the bony fragments to move against each other.

B. *Nursing Management*
 1. The foot should be inspected for circulatory difficulties within a few minutes and then periodically after the elastic bandage has been applied.
 2. Special care must be given to the back at regular intervals, because the patient maintains a supine position.
 3. Any complaint or burning sensation under the traction bandage should be reported immediately.
 4. Observe for wrinkling or slipping of the traction bandage.
 5. The patient should have foot supports to prevent footdrop.

FRACTURES OF SPECIFIC SITES*

Fracture of the Clavicle (Collar Bone)
 1. The clavicle helps hold the shoulder upward, outward and backward from the thorax.
 2. Aim of reduction—to hold the shoulder in the position described above.
 3. Accomplished by closed reduction and immobilization.
    a. Clavicular strap (Pad axilla to prevent nerve damage from pressure)
    b. Figure-of-8 bandage
    c. Plaster shoulder spica—gives more secure immobilization
    d. T-splint

Fractures of the Upper Extremity

Fractures of the Surgical Neck of the Humerus
 1. Most occur from falls in which the outstretched arm strikes the ground (impacted fracture).
    a. Most impacted fractures of the surgical neck of the humerus do not require reduction.
    b. Arm supported by sling and swathe (or Velpeau's bandage) for comfort.
    c. Start active motion of shoulder joint early—to prevent limitation of motion and stiffness of shoulder.
       Instruct patient to lean forward and allow affected arm to abduct and rotate (termed *pendulum exercise*).
 2. Displaced fracture of neck of humerus is treated with reduction under x-ray control. Reduction maintained with dressing and sling.

Fractures of the Shaft of the Humerus
 1. Fracture above deltoid insertion is reduced by manipulation.
    Hanging cast may be used to apply suspension traction.
 2. Reduction accomplished by traction on skin or skeletal traction with wire through olecranon.
    a. Cast is suspended from patient's neck by narrow bandage.

* For fracture of the skull, see page 722.

> Nursing Alert: Allow rest of cast to remain unsupported—continuous traction is made in long axis of arm by weight of the cast.

    b. See that patient sleeps in a fairly upright position—to maintain uninterrupted 24-hour traction.
    c. Start pendulum exercises as directed—to provide active exercise of shoulder muscle to prevent adhesions of the shoulder joint capsule.

Supracondylar Fracture (Above the Elbow)

1. Fragments usually maintained by holding elbow in an acutely flexed position after reduction.
2. Watch for signs of impaired circulation in forearm and hand.
    a. Observe hand for swelling or blueness of fingernails.
    b. Evaluate radial pulse—if it disappears it is a sign of circulatory failure.
3. If satisfactory reduction cannot be maintained with elbow in acute flexion, a traction method is indicated.
    Traction may be accomplished by Dunlop's traction or skeletal traction with Kirschner wire through olecranon. The forearm is thus held by suspension.

Fractures of the Lower End of the Humerus

1. *Undisplaced fracture*—immobilized in plaster cast extending from upper arm to proximal palmar crease of the hand. The elbow is immobilized at a right angle.
2. *Displaced fracture*—reduction by closed manipulation or open reduction with internal fixation.

Fractures of the Olecranon

1. Usually occur from direct fall on elbow
2. *Undisplaced fracture*—in elbow maintained at 90-degree angle and supported with a sling and pressure dressing to the elbow
3. *Separated fracture of olecranon*—open reduction and internal fixation

Fractures of the Head and Neck of the Radius

1. Usually produced by a fall on the outstretched hand with elbow in extension
2. *Undisplaced fracture*—no specific treatment except sling for symptomatic relief
3. *Displaced fracture*—open operation with excision of radial head

Fractures of the Shaft of Forearm

1. Closed reduction
    a. Long-arm cast is applied from upper arm to proximal palmar crease.
    b. A sling is pulled through a wire loop (incorporated in the cast) near the elbow to prevent cast sagging against the forearm (Fig. 14-4).
2. Open reduction—internal fixation accomplished by medullary nail, compression plate.
    a. Sometimes compression dressing is applied after surgery.
    b. Long-arm cast may be used for external fixation.

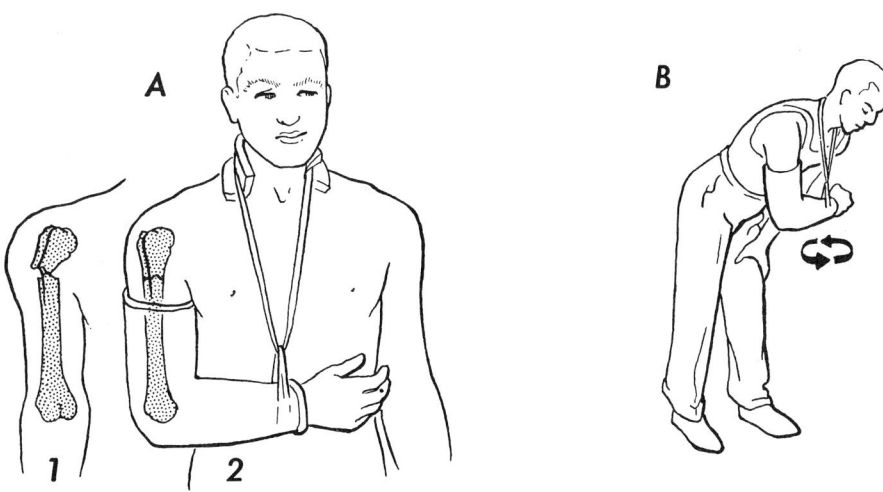

Figure 14-4. Treatment of fractures of the humerus with hanging cast. *(A)* Fracture of the proximal shaft showing abduction of the proximal fragment and kinking of long head of biceps (1) and effect of hanging cast (2). *(B)* Circumduction exercises as shown. Patient leans well forward. The arm is allowed to remain suspended by loop sling so that the alignment of the fracture is not disturbed. The shoulder is rotated in a circular motion to prevent stiffness. (From Rhoads, J. E., Allen, J. G., Harkins, H. N., and Moyer, C. A.: Surgery, Principles and Practice. Philadelphia, J. B. Lippincott, 1970.)

Fractures of the Wrist and Hand

1. Fractures of the wrist are immobilized with a short-arm cast.
2. Fractured fingers are placed in functional position.
3. Encourage the patient to exercise his fingers. Instruct him to "Do whatever the cast will permit."

Fractures of the Lower Extremity

Objectives: to obtain adequate bony union with full length and normal alignment and without rotational deformity.

to restore muscle power and joint motion.

Treatment and Nursing Management

1. Avoid placing extremity in dependent positions for prolonged periods—*edema is a common problem following all injuries of lower extremities.*
2. Encourage regular exercise of joints which do not move the bone fragments.
3. Have patient wear elastic bandage or hose after cast is removed to support venous circulation.
4. Elevate extremity intermittently when the patient becomes ambulatory to minimize recurrence of edema.

Fractures of the Shaft of the Femur

1. *Closed reduction*
   Balanced skeletal traction with Thomas leg splint with a Pierson attachment.
2. *Open reduction with intramedullary rod*
   a. Full weight-bearing not permitted for at least 6 months. (See nursing considerations, p. 792.)
   b. Instruct patient to exercise lower leg, foot and toes on a regular basis.

Fractures of the Tibia and Fibula

1. Fractures of the shaft of the tibia and fibula frequently occur in association with each other.
2. Reduction accomplished under x-ray guidance by traction and manipulation or by open reduction.
3. Plaster cast may be used to immobilize fracture. Elevate extremity to reduce edema.
4. Encourage patient to do quadriceps exercises (see p. 742).

Nursing Management Following Knee Surgery

1. Elevate affected extremity on pillow permitting slight flexion (bend) of the knee.
2. Evaluate for effusion into the knee—a common complication following knee surgery.
   a. Cut pressure dressing and reapply if pain is severe.
   b. Support patient undergoing aspiration of fluid from knee joint.
3. Encourage quadriceps exercise to prevent atrophy of the thigh muscles.

NOTE: Young adults frequently have difficulty in voiding after knee surgery. (reason obscure)

Fractures of the Lumbar and Dorsal Spine

Fracture of the vertebrae of the dorsal and lumbar spine include the vertebral body, lamina and articulating processes and spinous processes or transverse processes. (Fractures of the cervical spine are discussed on p. 757.)

Clinical Manifestations

Severe pain in back—may radiate

Clinical Problems

1. Fractures of the vertebral bodies are compression fractures; they are frequently multiple and comprise the most common types of fractures of the spine.
2. The majority of vertebral fractures seem to be related to osteoporosis.
3. A spinal cord injury may occur with dislocation of a vertebrae.

Treatment and Nursing Management

Objective: to determine if there is injury to the spinal cord.
1. Assess and treat the patient for spinal cord injury (see p. 757).
2. Evaluate for paralytic ileus and difficulty in voiding—may occur the first few days after compression fracture of the lower dorsal or lumbar spine. (See p. 407 for treatment of paralytic ileus.)
3. Treat the vertebral fracture.

For uncomplicated fracture:

a. Place patient on a firm mattress and keep on bedrest until pain subsides (usually 2–3 weeks).

b. Support the region of the fracture with a full-length back brace or back support when the patient is ambulatory; remove the brace when the patient is in bed.

c. Encourage the patient to do the prescribed back exercises—to increase and maintain the strength of the back muscles.

For moderate or severe fracture:

a. Patient may be placed in a position of hyperextension of spine—to reduce compression of affected vertebral bodies.

b. Hyperextension may be accomplished by a hyperextension brace which may be tightened to maintain its effectiveness.

For fracture of transverse processes:

a. The back may be strapped and the patient permitted to ambulate if the fracture is not severe.

b. If patient has displacement and soft tissue injury, place patient on bedrest followed by support in a corset or brace while ambulating.

4. Mobilize the patient when physical examinations and x-ray examinations determine there is no displacement or neurologic deficit.

5. Prepare patient for laminectomy (see p. 766) when cord or cauda equina injury has occurred.

Fractures of the Pelvis

Clinical Manifestations

1. Inability to bear weight without discomfort
2. Local swelling and tenderness at site of fracture

Treatment and Nursing Management

Objective: to assess for injuries of the bladder, intestine and iliac blood vessels.

1. Determine the extent of internal injuries.

   a. Catheterize the patient immediately (usually done by the physician)—to determine whether or not the bladder has been ruptured.

NURSING ALERT: 15% of all patients with pelvic fractures have associated bladder injuries.

---

   b. Assess and evaluate for intra-abdominal hemorrhage—pelvic fractures may produce death from local hemorrhage.

   c. Examine stools and urine for blood.

   d. Palpate peripheral pulses—absence of peripheral pulses may indicate possibility of a torn iliac artery.

   e. Observe for impending shock.

2. Treat the fracture.

   a. Undisplaced fracture requires no specific treatment.

(1) Have patient rest in bed with board under mattress until acute symptoms subside.
(2) Gradually mobilize patient, permitting weight-bearing as tolerated.
b. For anterior displacement of pelvic ring: these fractures have the highest incidence of associated injuries and mortality of all pelvic fractures.
    (1) Patient rests in pelvic sling—pelvic sling serves to exert a compression force against the iliac bones which helps mold the fracture back in place.
    (2) Pelvic sling lifts the weight of the pelvis very slightly off the mattress.
        (a) Adjust pressure by moving the ropes of the sling closer together or farther apart by direction of the physician.
        (b) Fold back sling over buttocks to enable patient to use the bedpan.
        (c) Reach under sling to give skin care—sheep skin may be used to line sling to prevent decubitus ulcers.
        (d) Loosen the sling only upon order.
c. For bilateral fracture of both rami:
    (1) Bilateral traction with lower extremities in abduction. Lateral compression and support is maintained by means of a pelvic sling.

Hip Fractures (Treated by an Internal Fixation Device)

Clinical Manifestations

Shortening, adduction and external rotation of affected leg
Pain

Types of Hip Fractures

Intracapsular—femur is broken inside the joint
Extracapsular—femur is broken outside the joint

Treatment and Nursing Management

Objectives: to prolong the patient's life.
           to prevent physical, psychological and social dependence.
           to restore the function of the hip joint.

A. *Preoperative Nursing Management*
  1. Alleviate the pain.
    a. Assist with the application of Buck's extension as indicated. Buck's extension is used to afford patient mobilization and to relieve pain until the operative procedure is performed.
    b. Handle the affected extremity gently.
    c. Give analgesics as patient's condition indicates.
    d. Keep the skin dry and relieve pressure areas—decubitus ulcers develop rapidly in the preoperative period. (See p. 20 for prevention of decubitus ulcers.)
  2. Ensure that the patient is in as favorable a condition as possible preoperatively.
    a. Coordinate ECG, blood chemistry studies and x-ray evaluation procedures preoperatively—mental alertness, bright facial expression and good skin turgor are considered favorable prognostic indications.
    b. Give intravenous infusions (if prescribed) *slowly*—patients with limited cardiac reserve cannot stand additional circulatory loading.

B. *Postoperative Nursing Management*
 1. Encourage the patient to move by himself as much as possible.
    a. Teach the patient to assist with turning by having him grasp the trapeze or bed-rails for support.
    b. Support the affected extremity in a position of abduction when the patient turns on his side.
 2. Get the patient out of bed as soon as possible.
    a. Wrap the lower extremities with elastic compression bandages or elastic hose—supports venous circulation and helps minimize dependent edema.
    b. Use the tilt table as soon as patient's condition permits (p. 33). With the use of the tilt table the patient becomes accustomed to the upright position, and circulation and respiratory functioning improve.
    c. Assist the patient into a wheelchair several times daily as ordered.
       (1) With the aid of the overhead trapeze, encourage the patient to move himself into the dangle position. (Use a Hi-low bed.)
       (2) Assist him to stand on the *unaffected extremity* and to transfer to a chair.
       (3) Allow the patient to get up at his own pace and avoid hurrying him.
    d. Encourage the patient to participate in activities of daily living (eating, bathing, hair care)—to condition patient for future ambulation activities and help to maintain a degree of independence.
 3. Watch for and prevent complications.
    a. Thrombophlebitis
       (1) Give prophylactic anticoagulants as directed.
       (2) Apply elastic stockings.
    b. Pneumonia—have the patient breathe deeply and cough to clear tracheobronchial tree of secretions.
    c. Fat embolism—characterized by fever, tachycardia, dyspnea and cough. (Fat embolism sometimes occurs after fractures of the long bones, particularly in elderly patients.)
    d. Knee contractures
       (1) *Maintain the knee in a position of extension while patient is in bed.*
       (2) *Flex the knee in a 90-degree angle while the patient is in the chair*—Avoid extending the knee when the patient is in a sitting position because extension produces undue strain on the fractured hip.
       (3) Move the knee through assisted range-of-motion exercises.
    e. Urinary tract infection
       (1) Avoid the routine use of an indwelling catheter—infection almost always follows the use of an indwelling catheter. (A urinary tract infection can cause a prolonged period of morbidity and incontinence in the elderly.)
       (2) Watch the color, odor and volume of urinary output.
       (3) Maintain a liberal fluid intake (within limits of cardiorenal function).
    f. Decubitus ulcers
       (1) Encourage the patient to move about freely using the overhead trapeze as an assistive device—peripheral arterial insufficiency, poor nutrition and lack of movement contribute to skin breakdown.
       (2) Use protective heel padding and massage reddened skin areas (see p. 20 for nursing prevention).
       (3) Use air and flotation mattresses when necessary.

4. Start active exercises as soon as pain and soreness subside to prepare the patient to walk.
5. Encourage quadriceps setting exercises hourly—the quadriceps femoris muscle extends the leg and is one of the major muscles necessary for ambulation.
   a. Do heel-cord stretching of both legs and abdominal and gluteal contractions (isometric contractions). Isometric muscle contractions strengthen the muscle but do not move the joint.
   b. Assist the patient to perform arm strengthening exercises (flexion and extension of the arms). The muscles in the shoulder girdle and upper extremities must be strong enough to bear the patient's weight while he is using the walker.
   c. Assist the patient to learn to use the walker—ambulating with a nonweight-bearing technique.
   d. Remind the patient *not* to bear weight on the affected extremity until the orthopedist gives permission and the x-rays reveal sufficient healing. Early weight-bearing before bony union occurs exerts too much stress and may cause bending or breaking of the pin or crushing of the bone.

SPECIAL NURSING CONSIDERATIONS

Nursing Management of the Patient Undergoing Orthopedic Surgery

Underlying Consideration

Orthopedic operations usually require a longer period of convalesence and rehabilitation than other surgical procedures.

Nursing Management

A. *Preoperative Care*
   1. Question patient to determine if he has had previous therapy with corticosteroids (especially patients with arthritis).
      a. Steroid therapy (current or past) may adversely affect patient's response to anesthesia.
      b. Steroids (hydrocortisone, prednisolone) should be administered per order to cover stress of surgery.
   2. Have patient practice voiding in bedpan or urinal in recumbent position before surgery. This helps reduce necessity of postoperative catheterization.
   3. Acquaint patient with traction apparatus, necessity for splints and cast—to familiarize him with his postoperative environment.
   4. Prepare skin according to institution's policy—may or may not be covered with sterile towels until the time of operation.

B. *Postoperative Care*
   1. Evaluate the blood pressure, pulse and respiratory rates frequently—rising pulse rate or slowly falling blood pressure indicates persistent bleeding or development of a state of shock.
   2. Assess changes in respiratory rate or in patient's color—may indicate obstruction of respiratory exchange or pulmonary or cardiac complications.
   3. Watch circulation distal to the portion of the extremity where cast, bandage or splint has been applied.

a. Prevent constriction leading to interference of blood or nerve supply.
b. Watch toes and fingers for normal temperature and healthy color.

NURSING ALERT: Abnormal coolness of skin, cyanosis, rubor or paleness indicates interference with circulation.

c. Notify surgeon and loosen cast or dressing at once.
4. Watch for excessive bleeding—orthopedic wounds have a tendency to ooze more than other surgical wounds.
5. Maintain sufficient pulmonary ventilation.
  a. Avoid or give respiratory depressant drugs in minimal doses.
  b. Change position every 2 hours—mobilizes secretions and helps prevent bronchial obstruction.
6. Maintain urinary output.
  a. Maintain adequate fluid intake.
  b. Watch for urinary retention—elderly men with some degree of prostatism may have difficulty in voiding.

Long-term Management

Orthopedic operations frequently require prolonged periods in bed; movement may be limited by pain, casts or splints.
1. Watch for development of decubitus ulcers (see also p. 20).
  a. Turn patient.
  b. Wash, dry and massage skin frequently.
  c. Expose skin to air.
  d. Maintain nutrition—administer plasma and vitamins as indicated to prevent hypoproteinemia and avitaminosis, conditions which make decubitus ulcers resistant to treatment.
2. Watch for complications of prolonged disability.
  a. Venous thrombosis
    (1) Mild swelling of extremity
    (2) Pain, tenderness and distention of veins
    (3) Positive Homan's sign (pain upon dorsiflexion of foot)
    (4) Tenderness
  b. Prevent venous complications.
    (1) Encourage the patient to exercise by himself with a planned program of exercise as soon as possible after surgery.
    (2) Have patient flex his knee, extend the knee with hip still flexed, and then lower the extremity to the bed.
    (3) Encourage patient to move fingers and toes periodically.
    (4) Advise patient to move joints which are not fixed by traction or appliance through their range of motion as fully as possible.
    (5) Suggest muscle-setting exercises (quadriceps setting) if active motion is contraindicated.
    (6) Wrap lower extremities with elastic bandages or apply elastic hose.
    (7) Treatment for venous thrombosis is discussed on page 333.
  c. Give prophylactic anticoagulants as directed (heparin, warfarin).

3. Give a normal balanced diet.
   a. Give supplemental vitamins (B and C) to elderly patients or those with chronic disease.
   b. Avoid giving large amounts of milk to orthopedic patients on bedrest—adds to calcium pool in the body and demands more calcium excretion by the kidneys, predisposing to the formation of urinary calculi.
4. Watch for signs and symptoms of anemia—especially after fracture of long bones.
   a. Hemoglobin determination usually done on 3rd postoperative day.
   b. Give iron supplements as directed.
   c. Blood transfusion may be given to raise level of hemoglobin to 10 gm or above.

Hip Arthroplasty (Cup or Prosthesis)

Arthroplasty is an operation to restore motion to a joint and function to the structures (muscles, ligaments, soft tissues) that control it. An inert substance is interposed between the re-shaped ends of the bone to mold or maintain joint function, or the joint is replaced. The procedure depends upon the anatomy and function of the joint.

Purposes

1. To restore, improve or maintain joint function.
2. To provide greater stability of arthritic hip.
3. To create a new joint in bony ankylosis.

Clinical Indications

1. Arthritis of the hip (rheumatoid or primary degenerative arthritis)
2. Complications of femoral neck fractures
3. Problems resulting from congenital hip disease

Nursing Management

A. *Preoperative Care*
   1. Educate the patient concerning his postoperative regimen.
      a. Extended exercise program lasting 6–12 months after surgery—atrophied muscles must be re-educated and strengthened after surgery.
      b. Crutch walking to last 6–12 months after surgery.
   2. Fit with crutches and instruct patient to walk with gait prescribed—to develop crutch-walking ability and facilitate patient's postoperative ambulation (see p. 29).
   3. Teach isometric exercises (muscle setting) of lower extremities.
   4. Teach deep breathing exercises—to assist in complete expansion of lungs.
      a. Do IPPB treatments as prescribed.
      b. Urge patient to stop smoking in preoperative period.
   5. Encourage patient to learn to use bedpan or urinal for voiding in the recumbent position—acquaints patient with procedure of voiding while lying down thus reducing probability of postoperative catheterization.
   6. Show patient balanced suspension apparatus—to acquaint him with his postoperative environment.
   7. See page 792 for other aspects of preoperative management.

B. *Postoperative Care*

Objectives: to maintain the affected extremity in a position of abduction and internal rotation.

to prevent and treat complications.

1. Place the patient in balanced suspension with traction (except in shaft-type of arthoplasty)—abduction of hip is used to keep the hip in a stable position and to relieve strain on transposed abductor muscles. (Patient maintained in balance suspension approximately 3 weeks.)
   a. Place pillow longitudinally between the knees—to decrease possibility of adduction.
   b. Place pillow beneath operated extremity—for comfort. (Pillow removed after several days.)
   c. Place trochanter roll on unaffected leg—to prevent external rotation.
   d. Keep the affected leg slightly abducted—to help keep the cup (or prosthesis) and the head of the femur in the acetabulum.
2. Ensure that suspension traction is correctly balanced—if patient is not aligned correctly, the operated extremity may become adducted.
3. Assist the patient to change position.
   a. Have the patient grasp overhead trapeze and place good foot flat on bed. Have him push with unoperated knee and hip flexed while raising himself off the bed.
   b. Place hand beneath patient's sacrum and lift while supporting the proximal thigh of operated leg (which is in suspension) with the other hand.
4. Help patient assume a sitting position.
   a. Instruct the patient to rock from side to side while using the trapeze to pull himself to an upright posture.
   b. See that the low part of back is as straight as possible.
5. Assist the patient to lie down from a sitting position.
   a. Instruct the patient to press his back against the bed while *slowly* lowering his body to a horizontal position.
   b. See that patient does not fall back against the bed.
6. Monitor suction and drainage apparatus—portable suction is used to decrease incidence of wound hematoma and swelling of thigh.
7. Encourage hourly deep breathing—to prevent atelectasis and pulmonary complications and to help relax muscle groups that can reduce muscle spasm.
8. Offer oral fluids after nausea is controlled and peristalsis is present (verified by intestinal auscultation with a stethoscope).
9. Assess patient frequently for complications.
   a. Thrombophlebitis or pulmonary embolism (common complications following hip surgery)
      (1) Give anticoagulants or low-weight dextran as prescribed.
      (2) See page 334 for nursing management of patient with thrombophlebitis.
   b. Infections
      (1) Watch for elevation of temperature.
      (2) Inspect wound daily.
   c. Subluxation (postoperative dislocation of hip)
10. Keep bed flat except during mealtime (45-degree elevation) and other prescribed times—to prevent recurrent hip flexion contraction. (Elevating and lowering head of bed produces flexion and extension of the hip joint.)

11. Encourage patient to carry out prescribed exercise program (usually under direction of physical therapist).
    a. Instruct him to think about the motion required to contract the appropriate muscles.
    b. Encourage patient to breathe deeply while exercising.
    c. See that patient does not perform exercises that are painful.
        (1) Active motion of affected foot and ankle—first postoperative day.
        (2) Isometric exercises of quadriceps, gluteals, abductors—started 2nd postoperative day.
        (3) Flexion, extension, abduction and internal rotation—started upon order of orthopedic surgeon.

Patient Education

Instruct the patient as follows:
1. Crutches (with partial weight-bearing) will be required:
    a. Unilateral operation—use 2-point gait.
    b. Bilateral operation—use 4-point gait.
2. Avoid prolonged sitting.
3. Carry out prescribed exercise program *faithfully* but exercise only up to the point of discomfort.
    a. Patient must have a daily program of stretching, exercise and rest—for a lifetime.
    b. Acquire a stationary bicycle if possible.
4. Use self-help devices.
    a. Handrails by toilet
    b. Raised toilet seat (if patient has some residual hip flexion)
    c. Bar type stool for shower and kitchen work

Above-the-knee Amputation

Indications

Congenital deformities	Infection
Vascular disease	Tumor
Trauma	Thermal, chemical, electrical injuries

Nursing Management

A. *Preoperative Care*

Objective: to have patient attain his highest physical, and emotional level in preparation for wearing a prosthesis (artificial limb).
1. Assist the patient undergoing circulatory patency tests (surface temperature, color changes, oscillometric readings, arteriography).
    a. The status of the sound limb is also evaluated.
    b. Heart studies are carried out. Cardiac decompensation in older patients may on rare occasions contraindicate a prosthesis after surgery.
2. Support the patient psychologically. Knowing what to expect helps reduce anxiety.
    a. Explain various phases of rehabilitation involved—active participation in rehabilitation is essential for a successful outcome.
    b. The physician will discuss the possibilities of obtaining and using a prosthesis—not all amputees can benefit from a prosthesis.

3. Build up the patient's nutritional status.
4. Have the patient strengthen the muscles of the upper extremity, trunk and abdomen as a preparation for crutch walking.
   Instruct the patient as follows:
   a. Flex and extend arms while holding traction weights.
   b. Do push-ups from a prone position.
   c. Do sit-ups from a seated position—to strengthen the tricep muscles which are necessary for crutch walking.
5. Teach the patient to crutch walk preoperatively (see p. 29)—to prevent complications of inactivity.
6. Site of amputation determined by:
   a. Circulation in the part
   b. Requirements of artificial limb or prosthesis

B. *Postoperative Care*
Objectives: to avoid complications.
          to prevent prolonged inactivity.
1. Watch for signs and symptoms of hemorrhage.
   a. Keep tourniquet (in view) attached to end of bed—to apply to stump if bleeding occurs.
   b. Raise foot of bed slightly to elevate stump. Do not flex patient's hips by elevating stump on pillow as this will produce a hip flexion contracture.
   c. Reinforce dressing as required using aseptic technique.
2. Prevent deformities in the immediate postoperative period. Contracture of the next joint above an amputation is a frequent complication.
   a. Deformities include:
      (1) Flexion deformities
      (2) Nonshrinkage of stump
      (3) Abduction deformities
   b. Encourage patient to turn from side to side.
   c. Place patient in prone position twice daily—to stretch the flexor muscles and prevent flexion contracture of the hip.
      (1) Keep patient's legs close together—to prevent abduction deformity.
      (2) Place pillow under abdomen and stump while patient is prone.
   d. Encourage patient to move stump—to avoid contractures.
   e. Start range of motion exercises—contracture deformities develop rapidly and cause serious problems in management of prosthesis.
3. Continue with muscle strengthening and balancing exercises—to strengthen muscles, mobilize joints and increase balance sense.
   Instruct patient as follows (stand behind patient and stabilize him at the waist, if necessary):
   a. Arise from chair and stand.
   b. Stand on toes while holding on to a chair.
   c. Bend the knees while holding on to a chair.
   d. Balance on one leg without support.
   e. Hop on one foot while holding on to a chair.
4. Condition the stump—so that prosthesis can be fitted properly in future.
   a. Shrink and shape the stump—to permit accurate measurement of prosthesis and maximum fit.

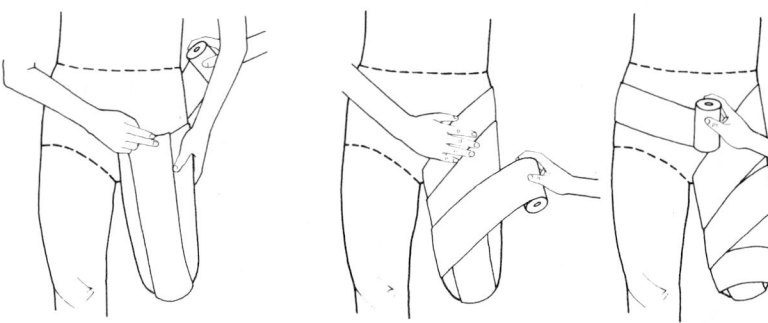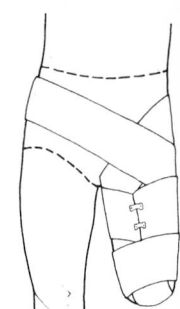

Figure 14-5. Bandaging stump.

          (1) Apply elastic stump shrinker, or
          (2) Use elastic bandages—to prevent edema and to shrink stump.
               (a) Apply bandage smoothly with no folds—creases will produce skin abrasions (Fig. 14-5).
               (b) Bandages are worn constantly; re-wrap when necessary.
    b. Prosthesis is measured and fitted when maximum shrinkage occurs.
    c. Have the patient do stump-conditioning exercises—to harden the stump.
          (1) The patient pushes the stump against a soft pillow.
          (2) Gradually he pushes stump against harder surfaces.
    d. Teach the patient to massage the stump—to soften the scar, decrease tenderness and improve vascularity.
          (1) Massage is usually started 1 week postoperatively.
          (2) Initially massage is usually done by physical therapist.
    e. Keep the stump clean.
          (1) Wash stump with mild soap and water.
          (2) Expose stump to air and sun.
  5. Keep the patient active—decreases occurrence of phantom-limb pain.
  6. Accept the frustrations and behavior of the patient.
    a. The self image has to be adjusted after amputation.
    b. It will take time for the patient to make this modification.

LOW BACK PAIN

Low back pain is characterized by acute pain in the low back associated with severe spasm of the paraspinal muscles.

Muscle spasm is a condition in which muscles are painfully contracted.

Etiology (multiple causes)

  1. Mechanical (joint strains, disc and muscle strain, spondylitis)
  2. Tension
  3. Lack of physical activity or not enough exercise
  4. Deviation from normal posture
  5. Predisposing endocrine and systemic diseases
  6. Diseases of bone (Paget's, metastatic carcinoma)

Diagnostic Evaluation

1. History—to determine when, where and how the pain occurs.
2. Neurologic evaluation—to spot localized weakness of extremities and reflex and sensory loss from ruptured disc.
3. Muscle testing—to evaluate strength and flexibility of key posture muscles.

Treatment and Nursing Management

Objectives: to relieve muscle spasm.
to gain normal elasticity of affected muscles.
to return normal joint motion.

1. Advise the patient to rest in bed in a Fowler's position (spine, hips and knees flexed)—to relax muscles, relieve tension on sciatic nerves and open the posterior part of the intervertebral spaces.
   a. Acute spasm should subside in 3–7 days if there is no nerve involvement.
   b. Do prescribed exercises hourly while on bedrest if possible.
2. Use heat to relax muscle spasm and relieve discomfort.
   a. Apply moist warm heat.
   b. Follow heat by massage.
3. Use appropriate medication to relieve pain.
   a. Give oral pain medication.
   b. Inject painful trigger points with hydrocortisone and Xylocaine for pain relief (by physician).

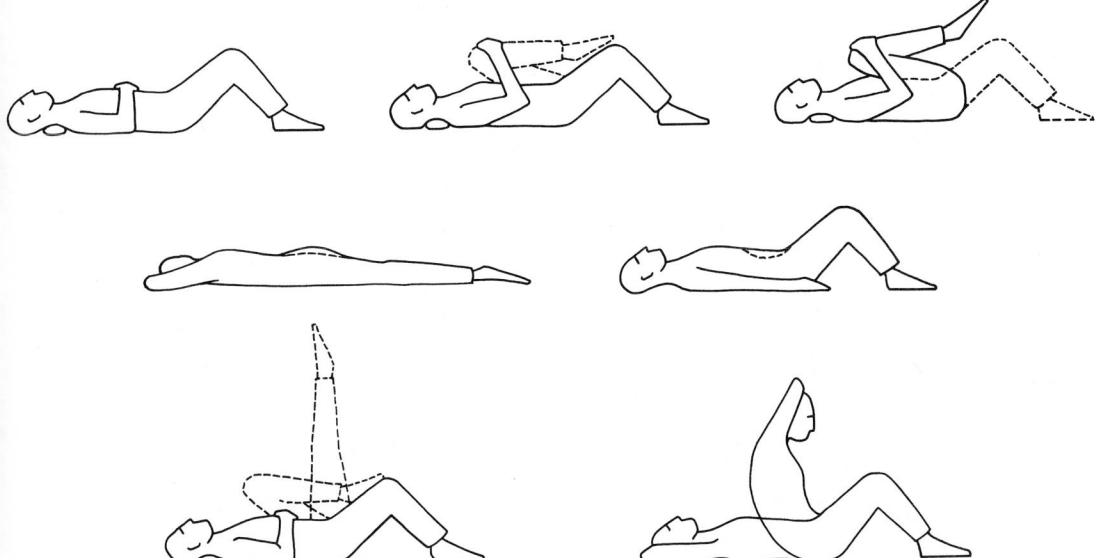

Figure 14-6. Back exercises are designed to strengthen abdominal muscles and stretch the contracted back muscles. They help keep posture muscles strong and flexible and aid in reducing nervous tension which increases low back pain.

    c. Surface anesthetics may be used (ethyl chloride spray).
       (1) Skin is sprayed with nozzle held 7.5–20 cm. (3–8 inches) from skin until white film appears on skin.
       (2) Active motion of involved part is carried out after anesthetic spray is used.
    d. Give tranquilizers and reassurance for tense patients.
    e. Give muscle relaxants for patients with muscle spasm.
4. Have patient start abdominal muscle strengthening exercises after acute symptoms subside—the abdominal muscles are the anterior supporting muscles of the spine.
5. Encourage patient to do prescribed back exercises (Fig. 14-6). Exercise keeps postural muscles strong and serves as an outlet for emotional tension.
6. Advise patient to start activity as soon as possible—activity speeds recovery and helps prevent loss of muscle function.
7. Psychiatric intervention may be needed for patient with chronic depression with low back syndromes.
8. Prepare patient for myelogram if he shows no improvement after 7–10 days of conservative treatment; operative intervention may be necessary. (See page 759 for treatment of herniated nucleus pulposus.)

Patient Education

Instruct patient as follows:
1. Explain that tension can contribute to spasm in the back muscles.
2. Avoid prolonged standing, walking, sitting and driving.
3. Rest at intervals throughout the day.
4. Avoid assuming tense cramped positions.
5. Use a hard plywood board under a firm mattress.
6. Stay with the exercise program which should be supervised and reviewed frequently.
7. Reduce weight if indicated.

RHEUMATOID ARTHRITIS

Rheumatoid arthritis is a chronic systemic disease affecting any or all of the body systems and is characterized most prominently by recurrent inflammation involving the synovium or lining of the joints.

Cause

Unknown

Clinical Manifestations

1. Easy fatigability and malaise
2. Fever
3. Weight loss, general weakness
4. Anemia
5. Painful joint swelling with stiffness, redness, warmth, tenderness and pain
6. Subcutaneous nodules over bony prominences, bursae and tendon sheaths
7. Enlarged lymph nodes

Pathophysiology Underlying Joint Destruction

Inflammation of joint (synovitis)→synovial effusion→joint capsular destruction→pain→loss of mobility of joint due to shortening of para-articular supporting tissues→muscular weakness about the joint→damage to tendons and ligaments→disuse→muscular atrophy and contracture deformity.

Diagnostic Evaluation

1. Blood count (most patients are anemic)
2. C-reactive protein (CRP) test (positive in rheumatoid arthritis) and erythrocyte sedimentation rate (ESR) (elevated during periods of active arthritis). These tests reveal disease actively and give guidelines for therapy.
3. Tests for rheumatoid factor in the serum; positive in 80% of patients with rheumatoid arthritis.
   a. Antinuclear antibodies
   b. Latex fixation test and sensitized sheep-cell test
4. Serum protein electrophoresis—increased globulins (gamma and alpha globulins); decreased albumin.
5. Roentgenograms of clinically involved joints—reveals osteoporosis of bone near the joint, swelling of soft tissue, erosions of bone at articular margins.
6. Examination of synovial fluid of joint (usually knee)—to distinguish between inflammatory, traumatic or degenerative arthritis.
7. Infrared thermography—pinpoints areas of inflammation and increased metabolic activity in the body by pictorially recording the increased heat emitted from the skin over the affected areas.

Objectives of Treatment and Nursing Management

Objective: to prevent crippling deformities by:
   1. maintaining joint mobility and muscle power
   2. promoting comfort
   3. halting the activity of the disease
   4. educating and helping the patient and family to adjust to a chronic disability

A. *To maintain joint mobility and muscle power; inflammation, scarring and mechanical damage to joint structures produce pain and disability.*
   1. Have regular rest at specified periods to control fatigue—arthritis affects the whole body.
      a. Complete bedrest for patients with active inflammatory disease.
      b. Have patient rest in a recumbent position (one pillow under head) upon a firm bed—to take the weight off the joints.
      c. Establish one or two daytime rest periods of 60–90 minutes.
      d. Encourage patient to rest in bed at least 10 hours at night.
      e. Turn in prone position twice daily to prevent hip flexion and knee contractures.
      f. Avoid placing pillows under painful joints—promotes flexion contractures.
   2. Rest painful joints with splints—to prevent flexion deformities.
      a. Support the joint in a good position.

   b. Splint the knee at full extension.
   c. Splint the wrist with slight dorsiflexion.
   d. Splints may need modifications with changes in joint structures.
   e. Support inflamed joints in their most functional positions. Use resting splints, sandbags, bivalved casts—to rest joints, reduce pain of acutely inflamed joint and prevent deformities.
3. Have patient do exercises to maintain function of all joints and strengthen muscles that support the joints.
   a. Encourage the patient to follow his prescribed daily program of exercise composed of conditioning exercises and specific exercises for particular joint problems (after inflammatory process is controlled).
   b. Carry out isometric exercises—to help prevent muscle atrophy which contributes to joint instability.
   c. Move joints through full range of motion 1 to 2 times daily to prevent loss of joint motion.
       (1) Assist patient to perform required joint motion if necessary.
       (2) Avoid grasping painful joints; grasp at belly of muscle.
   d. Do progressive resistive exercises—for muscle building.
   e. Evaluate for pain after exercise—pain lasting more than 15 minutes after exercise indicates patient's tolerance has been exceeded.
   f. Use self-help devices to help with daily activities.
       (1) Eating utensils with built up handles
       (2) Raised chair seats, toilets
       (3) Special fastening on clothing
   g. Use crutches or cane when joints are mechanically abnormal.
4. Control pain.
   a. Apply moist heat to reduce muscle spasm and post-rest stiffness and give as much relief from pain as possible so that exercise program can be carried out.
       (1) Take hot tub bath or shower upon arising—shortens period of morning stiffness.
       (2) Use hot paraffin baths for fingers, hands (see p. 805).
   b. Employ gentle massage to relax muscles.
   c. Take joints through range of motion after heat treatments.
   d. Advise rest to alleviate pain.
   e. Relieve foot pain with properly placed metatarsal bars.
   f. Give salicylates to alleviate pain (although primary function of salicylates in rheumatoid arthritis is anti-inflammatory).
   g. Give non-narcotic analgesic if patient has pain at night.

B. *To support the patient who is depressed and anxious due to the constant, unremitting nature of the disease.*
   1. Maintain a close patient-nurse-doctor relationship.
   2. Adopt a positive and optimistic attitude.
   3. Emphasize that something can and will be done to relieve the patient's pain and mobilize his joints.
   4. Give tranquilizers and mood-elevator drugs as prescribed.

C. *To educate patient and his family to adapt to a chronic disease.*
1. Re-emphasize that the primary goal is to maintain function of all joints.
2. Educate patient about the nature of his disease and the rationale of treatment.
3. Work with patient to achieve his goals of self-care and independence, using self-help devices and energy-saving methods.
4. Stress the need to avoid dietary fads and "quack" treatments.
5. Advise patient to have scheduled rest periods to reduce joint stresses.
6. Emphasize the need to take medication exactly as prescribed.
7. Encourage the use of heat treatments for muscle relaxation and relief of pain.
8. Advise patient to do prescribed exercises to preserve joint motion and to gain muscular strength and endurance.
   Review *Home Care in Rheumatoid Arthritis* put out by Arthritis Foundation, 1212 Avenue of the Americas, New York, New York 10036. (Has specific exercise instructions.)
9. Note the importance of a combined regular medical and functional re-evaluation to determine if there is loss of joint function.
10. Re-emphasize that the therapeutic program must be maintained for a lifetime; there is no cure at this time.

Drug Therapy

(Drug dosages depend upon patient's tolerance and response.)

Drug	Possible Toxic Effect
1. *Anti-inflammatory drugs* (to control synovial inflammation)	
Acetylsalicylic acid (aspirin)	Tinnitus
a. Should be taken with meals or antacid.	Gastrointestinal irritation
b. Periodic hematocrits and stool analysis for occult bleeding that may occur.	
Phenylbutazone (Butazolidin)	Gastrointestinal hemorrhage Salt and water retention Bone marrow depression
Oxyphenbutazone (Tandearil)	Nausea
Indomethacin (Indocin)	Peptic ulcer Headache; dizziness
2. *Antimalarial agents* Chloroquine (Aralen)	Retinal disease; blurring of vision, halos surrounding light, streaks and flashes of light.
Hydroxychloroquine (Plaquenil)	

NURSING ALERT: These drugs may cause permanent retinal changes. The patient should be assessed ophthalmologically every 6 months.

Drug	*Possible Toxic Effect*

3. *Gold Salts*
   Gold sodium thiomalate

   Aurothioglucose
     a. Requires careful clinical and hematological supervision.
     b. Patients should have laboratory monitoring during entire period of treatment.

Skin rash; renal disease
Bone marrow depression
Mucosal ulceration
Hepatitis

4. *Corticosteroids* (used in fulminating types of arthritis)
   Prednisone (Deltasone, Delta, Meticorten)

Osteoporosis; peptic ulcer; gastrointestinal hemorrhage; Psychoses.

NURSING ALERT: Corticosteroids interfere with normal tissue response to injury and inflammation. Patient may not show signs and symptoms of infection.

---

5. *Immunosuppressive drugs* (thought to affect the production of antibodies at the cellular level; suppresses autoimmune mechanism)
   Nitrogen mustard
   Cyclophosphamide (Cytoxan)
   Azathioprine (Imuran)

Highly toxic
Skin rash
Gastrointestinal manifestations
Bone marrow depression
Nephritis

NURSING ALERT: Immunosuppressive drugs have teratogenic (capable of producing fetal abnormality) potential. Patients should be advised of contraceptive measures.

---

6. *Intra-articular (into the joint) corticosteroid injections*
   Cortisone injected into joint when:
     a. only 1 or 2 joints affected
     b. to mobilize painful extremity with limited range of motion

Surgical Intervention

Objective: to halt the disease activity before crippling abnormalities occur.
1. *Synovectomy*—removal of the inflamed synovial membranes from affected joints
     a. Synovectomy helps prevent recurrence of inflammatory process.
     b. Performed mainly on knees, elbows, wrists and fingers.
2. *Arthroplasty*—an operation to restore motion to a joint and function to muscles, ligaments and other soft tissue structures that control it.
3. *Joint replacement*—total hip, knee, fingers.
4. *Arthrodesis* (fusion)—an operation to produce bony ankylosis in a joint in which motion is undesirable. It is performed to halt disease, relieve pain and provide joint stability.
5. *Soft tissue procedures*—include early repair of ruptured tendons (usually on hand), removal of nodules and median nerve decompression procedures.

GUIDELINES: *Paraffin Hand Bath for Rheumatoid Arthritis*

Purposes

1. To relieve pain.
2. To decrease duration of morning stiffness of fingers, hand and wrist.

Equipment

Double boiler
7 parts of canning grade paraffin
   mixed with 1 part mineral oil

Aluminum foil
Towel
Candy thermometer

Procedure

Nursing Action	Rationale/Amplification
Preparatory Phase	
1. Melt the paraffin and oil in a double boiler.	1. The addition of mineral oil lowers the melting point of the wax to 52.0°C. (125.6°F.).
2. Heat the mixture to 53°C. (126–130°F.).	
Performance Phase	
3. Dip the hand and wrist in warm paraffin rapidly (Fig. 14-7).	3. The heat is transferred from the paraffin to the skin by conduction.
4. Allow the wax to harden after each immersion.	
5. Immerse the hand in paraffin again; allow the wax to harden and re-immerse.	5. This builds up a glove of warm wax about 0.3-cm. (⅛-inch) thick which also acts as a splint.

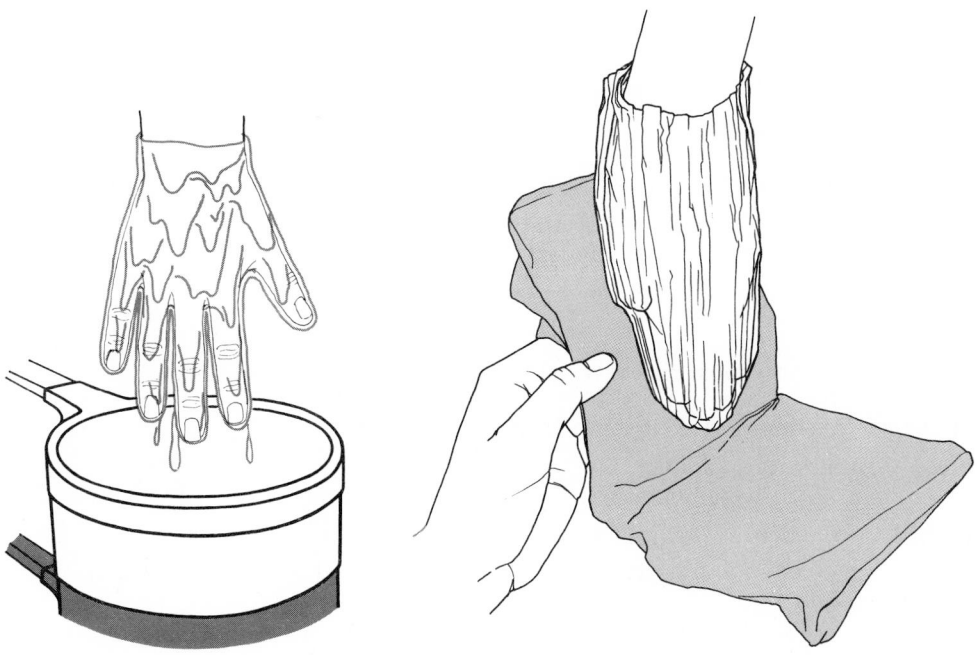

Figure 14-7. Paraffin hand bath.

Nursing Action	*Rationale / Amplification*
6. Wrap hand with aluminum foil and cover with a towel.	6. Wrapping with foil and a towel helps to retain the heat.
7. Allow paraffin to remain on hand 15–20 minutes.	
8. Peel off paraffin and replace in double boiler for next application.	
9. Put fingers and wrist through range of motion exercises after paraffin has been removed.	9. Heat relieves the patient of pain and enables him to exercise his fingers and wrists with greater mobility.

OSTEOARTHRITIS

Osteoarthritis, the most common of all joint diseases, is degeneration of the articular cartilage in the joints. It is characterized by spur formation at the edges of the joint surfaces and thickening of the capsule and the synovial membrane.

Underlying Principles

1. Osteoarthritis is to be regarded essentially as a senescent process—the result of prolonged wear and tear of the joint surfaces which has produced changes not only in the bony structures but also in the cartilaginous and soft tissue components of the joints.
2. The nature of the disease should be explained to the patient and he should be reassured that the disease is usually not progressive or incapacitating.

Predisposing Factors

1. Aging—occurs mainly in middle aged and elderly
2. Trauma—mild or continuous irritation
3. Obesity—places unnatural strain on joints
4. Excessive joint use—strenuous physical labor

Clinical Manifestations

1. Stiffness
2. Gradual development of aching type of joint pain
3. Limitation of joint motion
4. Heberden's nodes—nodular bony enlargements that grow on the distal joints of some or all of the fingers
5. Joints involved—hips, knees, vertebrae and fingers

Objectives of Treatment and Nursing Management

Objectives: to relieve discomfort.
           to protect the joints from undue strain and trauma.

A. *To relieve strain on the affected joints.*
1. Rest involved joints—excessive use aggravates the symptoms and accelerates degeneration.
   (a) Use splints, braces, cervical collars as necessary.
   (b) Have prescribed rest periods in recumbent position.
2. Advise the patient to avoid activities that precipitate pain.

3. Use heat—relieves pain, muscle spasm and stiffness and allows a more effective follow-up exercise program.
4. Give analgesics for pain control.
5. Give anti-inflammatory agents when synovial inflammation is present (see p. 804).
6. Assist the patient undergoing intra-articular (into the joint) injections of long-acting steroids.
7. Teach the patient to use correct body mechanics.
8. Advise patient to avoid emotional strain, which increases muscle tension and joint strain.
9. Have patient use crutches, braces or cane when indicated—to reduce weight on the joints.

B. *To avoid trauma and further degeneration of the weight-bearing joints.*
   Instruct the patient as follows:
   1. Use postural exercises to correct poor posture.
   2. Wear corrective shoes and metatarsal supports for foot disorders—also helps in treatment of osteoarthritis of the knee.
   3. Carry out weight reduction program under nursing and medical supervision.
   4. Stop excessive weight-bearing activities such as standing for prolonged period, lifting, carrying heavy loads, engaging in excessive vigorous overhead reaching.

C. *To restore function to the maximal extent.*
   1. Use range of motion exercises to prevent capsular and tendon tightening.
   2. Avoid flexion deformities.
   3. Use corrective and graded exercises to improve muscle strength around the involved joint.
   4. Support the patient undergoing orthopedic surgery for disabling arthritis of joints.

MALIGNANT BONE TUMOR

Osteosarcoma is a highly malignant neoplasm of bone usually occurring in the shaft at either end of the long bone.

Clinical Manifestations

1. Pain
2. Limitation of motion and joint effusion
3. Significant weight loss (an ominous finding)
4. *Physical findings*
   a. Palpable, tender fixed bony mass
   b. Increase in skin temperature over mass
   c. Venous distention
5. *Sites of occurrence*—lower end of femur, upper ends of tibia and humerus
6. *Sites of metastasis*—lung, other bone, local recurrence, brain

Diagnostic Evaluation

1. X-ray will usually reveal bone tumor.
2. Serum alkaline phosphatase—increases to 20 or more Bodansky units (normal, 2–4 Bodansky units per 100 ml. of blood).
3. Open biopsy of bone and permanent tissue section—to confirm suspected diagnosis.

Treatment and Nursing Management

Objective: to destroy or remove all obviously malignant tissue by the most effective method possible.
1. Support the patient undergoing irradiation therapy.
   a. Large doses of irradiation may be given before amputation.
   b. Radiation may be done for palliation (relieve but not cure).
2. Help the patient cope with the physical and emotional problems of surgical intervention.
   a. Amputation of involved extremity (see p. 796).
   b. Radical surgery; i.e., disarticulation of hip joint may be performed for lesions at lower end of the femur.
3. Encourage patient undergoing chemotherapy (see p. 874).
   a. Chemotherapy may be given initially when the tumor is first discovered.
   b. Chemotherapy may also be given as palliation.

NURSING ALERT: Osteosarcoma is usually highly malignant; early metastases is frequently seen.

OSTEOPOROSIS
(Osteopenia)

Osteoporosis (decreased density of bone) is a bone disorder in which there is an imbalance between bone formation and bone reabsorption. It is characterized by generalized loss of density and tensile strength throughout the skeleton.

Causes

1. Disuse atrophy—from immobilization
2. Diminution or loss of anabolic sex hormone, especially in postmenopausal women
3. Excess of catabolic hormones (in thyrotoxicosis and Cushing's syndrome or after therapeutic administration of large doses of cortisone)
4. Diet deficient in calcium, protein and other nutrients
5. Malabsorption syndrome (extensive diverticulitis)

Clinical Manifestations

1. Pain in lumbar spine
2. Tendency to kyphosis; loss of stature
3. Nephrolithiasis (kidney stones)—from hypercalciuria

Diagnostic Evaluation

Roentgenograms show decreased skeletal density; changes found in lower thoracic and lumbar vertebrae.

Treatment and Nursing Management

Objective: to keep the patient active.
            to provide optimal nutrition.
1. Provide estrogen therapy—provides positive calcium balance and stops bone destruction in postmenopausal or hypogonadal patients.

2. Give testosterone when ordered—has a protein anabolic effect and helps lay down bone matrix; testosterone does not induce skeletal remineralization.
3. Encourage a high protein diet with adequate milk and milk products for supplementary calcium. Give multivitamin pills (for vitamin D).
4. Give oral fluorides as directed.
5. Be aware that compression fractures of the vertebrae are a complication of osteoporosis.
6. Instruct patient to sleep with bedboard under mattress.
7. Encourage the patient to keep physically active—to strengthen muscles and prevent disuse atrophy and further bone destruction.
8. Teach the patient to weigh herself periodically—indicates whether or not the disease is stabilized.
9. Provide bracing and support when indicated.

OSTEITIS DEFORMANS
(Paget's Disease of the Bone)

Osteitis deformans is a bone disease of unknown cause which produces excessive bone destruction and repair.

General Features

1. Occurs mainly in middle-aged or older men.
2. May develop in any part of the skeleton—usually the skull, the tibia or vertebral column.
3. Eventually produces marked hypertrophy and bowing of the long bones and irregular deformities of the flat bones.

NURSING ALERT: Osteitis deformans predisposes to malignant bone tumors.

Clinical Manifestations

1. Bone pain; tenderness on pressure in the bones
2. Bone deformity:
   Bowing of femur and tibia
   Kyphosis—producing decreasing height
3. Enlargement of the skull
4. Deafness, blindness—from pronounced thickening of skull and bony overgrowth impinging on vital structures

Diagnostic Evaluation

1. Skeletal roentgenograms—involved bones appear expanded and more dense than normal.
2. Serum alkaline phosphatase (serves as index of bone absorption)—markedly elevated.

Treatment and Nursing Management

1. Provide symptomatic relief:
   a. Androgen therapy for men; estrogen therapy for women—these hormones reverse hypercalciuria when present.

     b. Give salicylates—to combat pain; may reduce hypercalciuria.

     c. Small fractional doses of x-ray irradiation—to relieve pain.

  2. Watch for occurrence of fractures—stress fractures occur with minimal trauma.

     a. Fractures usually treated with internal fixation.

     b. Avoid immobilization—increases hazard of hypercalciuria and stone formation.

     c. For temporary immobilization due to fracture, limit calcium intake and provide high fluid intake—to avoid serious hypercalcemia and the development of kidney stones.

  3. Watch for evidences of bone sarcoma (see p. 807).

MYASTHENIA GRAVIS

Myasthenia gravis is a disorder of neuromuscular transmission of the voluntary muscles of the body. The etiology is unknown.

Altered Physiology

Defect in transmission of impulses from nerve to muscle cells which may be due to inadequate synthesis or release of acetylcholine at the neuromuscular junction.

Clinical Manifestations

  1. Extreme muscular weakness.

  2. Sleepy mask-like expression—from involvement of facial muscles.

  3. Drooping of eyelids (ptosis) and diplopia—due to involvement of ocular muscles.

  4. Speech weakness and choking or aspiration of food—from weakness of laryngeal and pharyngeal muscles.

Diagnostic Evaluation

  1. Neostigmine methylsulfate injection—positive result evidenced by striking increase in muscular strength 5–10 minutes after injection.

  2. Edrophonium (Tensilon) test—intravenous injection of edrophonium may relieve weakness in 20–30 seconds.

Treatment and Nursing Management

A. *Drug Therapy*

  1. Give anticholinesterase drugs—will increase response of muscles to nerve impulses and improve strength; not a cure.

     a. Neostigmine bromide (Prostigmin)   c. Ambenonium chloride (Mytelase)

     b. Pyridostigmine bromide (Mestinon)   d. Edrophonium bromide (Tensilon)

  2. *Give drug according to fixed (exact time) and permanent schedule to control symptoms*—a delay in drug administration may result in patient losing his ability to swallow.

  3. Give anticholinesterase with milk, crackers or other buffering substance.

  4. Dosages may be increased gradually and time intervals shortened between doses if improvement is noted.

  5. Watch for side effects—abdominal cramps, nausea and vomiting.

B. *Crises in Myasthenia Gravis*
1. Watch for rapid development of myasthenic crisis—sudden inability to swallow or maintain a patent airway for adequate respiratory exchange.
2. *Types of Crises in Myasthenia Gravis*
   a. *Myasthenic crisis*—patient may be temporarily resistant to anticholinesterase drugs or may need increased dosage; may also be brought about by ACTH therapy.
   b. *Cholinergic crisis*—from overtreatment of these drugs.
   c. *Brittle crisis*—occurs with an unpredictable response to drugs and is not controllable by increasing or decreasing anticholinesterase therapy.
3. Tensilon may be given to differentiate type of crisis;
   Tensilon (2 mg.) I.V. improves patient in myasthenic crisis; temporarily worsens patient in cholinergic crisis and is unpredictable in brittle crisis.
4. *Nursing Management During Crisis*
   a. Give patient a tap bell to be used in emergency situations.
   b. Give neostigmine methylsulfate immediately if severe symptoms develop.
   c. Support respiration when muscles of respiration and swallowing become severely involved.
      (1) Suction patient as indicated—*aspiration is a common problem.*
      (2) Prepare patient for tracheostomy (see p. 98).
      (3) Place patient on assisted mechanical ventilation (see p. 139).
      (4) Give appropriate antibiotics as indicated.
   d. Determine the time of onset of symptoms in relation to the last dose of anticholinesterase—shows whether patient is undermedicated or having a mild cholinergic reaction.
   e. Place patient in intensive unit for constant monitoring—myasthenia gravis is a disease of rapidly fluctuating intensity.
   f. Keep in mind that myasthenic crisis may be precipitated by emotional upset, surgery, physical activity or failure to take anticholinesterase medication.
5. Avoid sedatives and tranquilizing drugs—may aggravate hypoxia and hypercapnia and cause respiratory and cardiac depression.

NURSING ALERT: Morphine, a respiratory depressant, is made more potent in its effect by anticholinesterase compounds and is strictly contraindicated in a patient with myasthenia gravis.

---

6. Feed patient with nasogastric tube if he is unable to swallow.
7. Prepare patient for thymectomy (removal of thymus gland) if patient has a tumor of thymus or is responding poorly to therapy.
8. Emphasize the following in patient education.
   a. Set alarm clock *to ensure taking medication on time.*
   b. Wear an identification band indicating myasthenia gravis.*
   c. Try to prevent emotional upsets and infection—may precipitate a myasthenic crisis.
   d. Utilize educational services of The Myasthenia Gravis Foundation, Inc., New York Academy of Medicine Building, 2 East 103 Street, New York, New York 10029.

* Medic Alert Foundation, Turlock, California 95380.

BIBLIOGRAPHY

Books

Adams, J. C.: Outline of Orthopaedics. Baltimore, Williams and Wilkins, 1971.

American Academy of Orthopaedic Surgeons: Symposium on the Spine. St. Louis, C. V. Mosby, 1969.

Brunner, L., et al.: Textbook of Medical-Surgical Nursing, 2nd ed. Philadelphia, J. B. Lippincott, 1970, pp. 834–890.

Crenshaw, A. H.: Campbell's Operative Orthopedics. St. Louis, C. V. Mosby, 1971.

Cruess, R. L., and Mitchell, N. S. (eds.): Surgery of Rheumatoid Arthritis. Philadelphia, J. B. Lippincott, 1971.

Gillis, L.: Diagnosis in Orthopaedics. New York, Appleton-Century-Crofts, 1969.

Kraus, H.: Clinical Treatment of Back and Neck Pain. New York, McGraw-Hill, 1970.

Larson, C. B., and Gould, M.: Orthopedic Nursing. St. Louis, C. V. Mosby, 1970.

Lenman, J. A. R., and Ritchie, A. E.: Clinical Electromyography. Philadelphia, J. B. Lippincott, 1970.

Lichtenstein, L.: Bone Tumors. St. Louis, C. V. Mosby, 1972.

————: Diseases of Bones and Joints. St. Louis, C. V. Mosby, 1970.

Meltzer, W. (ed.): Orthopedics. New York, Harper and Row, 1971.

Raney, R. B., et al.: Shands' Handbook of Orthopaedic Surgery. St. Louis, C. V. Mosby, 1971.

Salter, R. B.: Textbook of Disorders and Injuries of the Musculoskeletal System. Baltimore, Williams and Wilkins, 1970.

Articles

Baum, J., and Vaughan, J.: Immunosuppressive drugs in rheumatoid arthritis. Ann. Intern. Med., 71:202–204, July 1969.

Bennett, J. C.: Chronic arthritis. Mod. Treat., 8:753–858, Nov. 1971.

Bosanko, L. A.: Immediate postoperative prosthesis. Amer. J. Nurs., 71:280–283, Feb. 1971.

English, C. B., and Nalebuff, E. A.: Understanding the arthritic hand. Amer. J. Occup. Ther., 25:352–359, Oct. 1971.

Eyre, M. K.: Total hip replacement. Amer. J. Nurs., 71:1384–1387, July 1971.

Gerhardt, J. J., et al.: Immediate post-surgical prosthetics: rehabilitative aspects. Amer. J. Phys. Med., 49:3–105, Feb. 1970.

Johnston, R. C., and Larson, C. B.: Results of treatment of hip disorders with cup arthroplasty. J. Bone & Joint Surg., (A) 51:1461–1479, Dec. 1969.

Kitridow, R. C., and Solomon, S. D.: The patient with rheumatoid arthritis. Amer. Fam. Phys., 4:109–116, July 1971.

Loxley, A. K.: The emotional toll of crippling deformity. Amer. J. Nurs., 72:1839–1840, Oct. 1972.

Marmor, L.: Surgery for osteoarthritis. Geriatrics, 27:89–95, Feb. 1972.

Mooney, V., et al.: Comparison of postoperative stump management: plaster vs. soft dressings. J. Bone & Joint Surg., (A) 53:241–249, March 1971.

O'Connor, B. T., et al.: Rehabilitation in orthopaedics. Rheum. Phys. Med., 10:408–415, Nov. 1970.

Rothman, R. H. (ed.): Disease of the intervertebral disc. Orth. Clin. N. Amer., 2:309–592, July 1971.

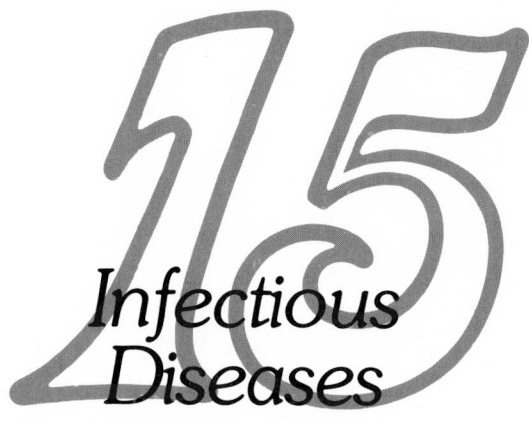

Infectious Diseases

THE INFECTION PROCESS

Causative Agent

1. Bacterial (includes cocci, bacilli and spirilla)
2. Viral
3. Rickettsial
4. Protozoal
5. Fungal
6. Helminthic (worm infestation)

Reservoir

(the environment in which the agent is found)

1. Human—man is the reservoir of disease most dangerous to himself rather than to other species.
2. Animal—responsible for infestations due to trophozoites and worms.
3. Nonanimal—street dust, garden soil, lint from bedding.

Mode of Escape from Reservoir

1. Respiratory tract (most common in man)
2. Intestinal tract
3. Genitourinary tract
4. Open lesions
5. Mechanical escape (includes bites of insects)

Mode of Transmission (to the next host)

1. *The Contact Route*
   a. Direct contact
   b. Indirect contact
   c. Droplet spread
2. *The Vehicle Route*
   a. Contaminated food (salmonellosis)
   b. Water—shigellosis
   c. Drugs—pseudomonas infections from contaminated ophthalmic ointment
   d. Blood—hepatitis
3. *Airborne*
   a. Residue of evaporated droplets that remain suspended in air
   b. Dust particles
4. *Vector borne*
   Mosquito—malaria

Mode of Entry of Organisms into Human Body

1. Respiratory tract
2. Gastrointestinal tract
3. Direct infection of mucous membranes
4. Break in the skin

Susceptible Host

Illness following entrance of infection into the body depends upon:

1. Dosage of organisms—number of organisms invading body of host
2. Duration of exposure
3. Individual's general physical, mental and emotional state
4. Inherent susceptibility
5. Nutrition, fitness, environmental factors

Table 15-1. Epidemiology, Therapy and Control of Communicable Infections

Disease	Infective Organism	Infectious Sources	Entry Site	Method of Spread	Incubation Period	Chemotherapy*	Prophylaxis
Amebiasis	Endamoeba histolytica	Contaminated water and food	Gastrointestinal tract	Patients and carriers; fecal-oral route	Variable	Metranidazole; emetine	Detection of carriers and their removal from food handling; plumbing safeguards
Bacillary Dysentery	Shigella group	Contaminated water and food	Gastrointestinal tract	Patients and carriers; fecal-oral route	24–48 hours	Ampicillin; cephalothin sodium; Kanamycin; Nalidixic acid; nitrofurantoin	Detection and control of carriers; inspection of food handlers; decontamination of water supplies
Brucellosis	Brucella melitensis and related organisms	Milk or meat from infected cattle, goats and pigs	Gastrointestinal tract	Oral ingestion of infective material	6–14 days	Sulfadiazine; streptomycin; tetracycline	Milk pasteurization; control of infection in animals
Chancroid	Ducrey bacillus	Human cases and carriers	Genitalia	Sexual intercourse	2–5 days	Sulfadiazine; streptomycin; tetracycline	Effective case-finding and treatment of infection
Chickenpox (Varicella)	Virus	Human cases	Probably nasopharynx	Probably respiratory droplets	14–16 days	None	Patient isolation
Diphtheria	Corynebacterium diphtheriae	Human cases and carriers; food; fomites	Nasopharynx	Nasal and oral secretions; respiratory droplets	2–5 days	Diptheria antitoxin; penicillin or erythromycin	Active immunization with diphtheria toxoid or toxinantitoxin mixture; quarantine; disinfection of carriers
Encephalitis, epidemic (Eastern and Western Equine)	Viruses	Chicken and wildbird mites; horses; hibernating garter snakes	Skin	Mosquitoes	Variable	None	Formalinized virus vaccines for persons at great risk
German Measles (Rubella)	Virus	Human cases (early)	Probably nasopharynx	Probably respiratory droplets	10–22 (aver. 18) days	None	Patient isolation when pregnant woman is in household. Rubella virus vaccine
Gonorrhea	Neisseria gonorrhoeae	Urethral and vaginal secretions	Urethral or vaginal mucosa	Sexual intercourse	3–8 days	Penicillin Spectinomycin; tetracycline	Chemotherapy of carriers and potential contacts; case-finding and treatment of patients
Granuloma Inguinale	Donovan body (bacillus)	Infectious exudate	External genitalia; cervix	Sexual intercourse	3–40 days	Chloramphenicol; tetracyclines; streptomycin	Chemotherapy of carriers and potential contacts; case-finding and treatment of patients
Type A Hepatitis	Hepatitis A virus	Contaminated food or water; parenteral inoculum	Gastrointestinal tract; skin	Fecal-oral route; parenteral injection	2–6 weeks	None	Enteric precautions applied to infected cases; passive immunization with gamma globulin
Type B Hepatitis	Hepatitis B virus	Infected blood donor; contaminated injection equipment	Skin	Oral and parenteral route	6 weeks to 6 months	None	Screening of blood donors; avoidance of unnecessary use of blood and blood derivatives; passive immunization of blood recipients with course of gamma globulin injections

Table 15-1. Epidemiology, Therapy and Control of Communicable Infections (continued)

Disease	Infective Organism	Infectious Sources	Entry Site	Method of Spread	Incubation Period	Chemotherapy*	Prophylaxis
Infectious Mononucleosis	Virus	Human cases and carriers	Mouth	Uncertain	30–50 days	None	None
Influenza	Virus (types A, B & C)	Human cases; animal reservoir	Respiratory tract	Respiratory	18–36 hours	None	Specific virus vaccine
Lymphogranuloma Venereum	Virus	Human cases	External genitalia; urethral or vaginal mucosa	Sexual intercourse	2–30 days	Sulfadiazine; tetracyclines	Case finding and treatment of infection
Measles	Plasmodium, vivax, falciparum, malariae and ovale	Human cases	Skin	Mosquitoes (Anopheles)	2 weeks	Chloroquine; primaquine; paludrine; atabrine Amodiaquine; quinine Amodia	Coordinated measures for wide-scale mosquito control; prompt detection and effective treatment of cases
Measles	Virus	Human cases	Respiratory mucosa	Nasopharyngeal secretions	11–14 days	None	Measles vaccine
Meningococcal Meningitis	Neisseria meningitidis	Human cases and carriers	Nasopharynx; tonsils	Respiratory droplets	Variable	Penicillin; chloramphenicol	Group chemotherapy with sulfadiazine (when strain is sensitive to sulfonamide)
Mumps	Virus	Human cases (early)	Upper respiratory tract	Respiratory droplets	8–30 (aver. 18) days	None	Live mumps vaccine
Paratyphoid Fever	Salmonella paratyphi A and B; S. typhimurium; S. choleraesuis and related organisms	Contaminated food and water, rectal tubes and barium enemas	Gastrointestinal tract	Infected urine and feces	7–24 days	Chloramphenicol; tetracycline; ampicillin	Control of public water sources, food vendors and food handlers; treatment of carriers; individual vaccination with S. paratyphi A and B vaccine
Pneumococcal Pneumonia	Pneumococcus	Human carriers; patient's own pharynx	Respiratory mucosa	Respiratory droplets	Variable	Penicillin; tetracyclines	Control of upper respiratory infections; avoidance of alcoholic intoxication; communicable disease precautions applied to cases
Poliomyelitis	Polioviruses (Types I, II, III)	Human cases and carriers	Gastrointestinal tract	Infected feces and pharyngeal secretions	4–7 days	None	Wide-scale application of parenteral (Salk) and oral (Sabin) poliovirus vaccines; case isolation
Rocky Mountain Spotted Fever	Rickettsia rickettsii	Infected wild rodents, dogs, wood ticks and dog ticks	Skin	Tick bites	3–12 days	Tetracyclines; chloramphenicol	Avoidance of tick-infected areas, or wearing of protective clothing in such areas; frequent search for, and prompt removal of, ticks from body; specific vaccination of exposed persons
Rubella	Virus	Human case	Respiratory mucosa	Nasopharyngeal secretions	14–21 days	None	Rubella virus vaccine; Immune serum globulin (human) given to contacts of Rubella. Rubella in early stages of pregnancy legally recognized as indication for abortion.

Table 15-1. Epidemiology, Therapy and Control of Communicable Infections (continued)

Disease	Infective Organism	Infectious Sources	Entry Site	Method of Spread	Incubation Period	Chemotherapy*	Prophylaxis
Scarlet Fever	Streptococcus hemolyticus	Human cases; infected food	Pharynx	Nasal and oral secretions	3–5 days	Penicillin	Case isolation; prophylactic chemotherapy with penicillin; asepsis during obstetrical procedures; specific chemoprophylaxis for persons with recurrent streptococcal infections
Syphilis	Treponema pallidum	Infected exudate or blood	External genitalia; cervix; mucosal surfaces; placenta	Sexual intercourse; contact with open lesions; blood transfusion; transplacental inoculation	10–90 days	Penicillin; Erythromycin	Case-finding by means of routine serologic testing and other methods, and adequate treatment of infected individuals
Tetanus	Clostridium tetani	Contaminated soil	Penetrating and crush wounds	Horse and cattle feces	5 days to 5 weeks (aver. 10 days)	Human tetanus immune globulin; tetracyclines Tetanus antitoxin; penicillin	Wound debridement; toxoid booster injections for patients previously immunized and tetanus antitoxin plus penicillin for nonimmune persons
Trichinosis	Trichinella spiralis	Infected pigs	Gastrointestinal tract	Ingestion of infected pork, undercooked	3–7 days	Thiabendazole	Regulation of hog breeders; adequate meat inspection; thorough cooking of pork
Tuberculosis	Mycobacterium tuberculosis	Sputum from human cases; milk from infected cows	Respiratory or gastrointestinal mucosa	Sputum; respiratory droplets; infected milk	Variable	Isoniazid; streptomycin; paraaminosalicylic acid Ethambutol	Early discovery and adequate treatment of active cases; milk pasteurization
Tularemia	Pasteurella tularensis	Wild rodents	Eyes; skin; gastrointestinal tract	Insect parasites of infected rodents; ingestion of undercooked infected meat	3–5 days	Streptomycin; tetracyclines	Avoidance of contact with potentially infected rodents; adequate cooking of wild rabbit dishes; vaccination of hunters, butchers and laboratory workers risking heavy exposure
Typhoid Fever	Salmonella typhi	Contaminated food and water	Gastrointestinal tract	Infected urine and feces	5–14 days	Chloramphenicol; ampicillin	Decontamination of water sources; milk pasteurization; individual vaccination; control of carriers
Typhus, endemic	Rickettsia typhi (mooseri)	Infected rodents	Skin	Flea bites	5–21 days	Tetracyclines; chloramphenicol	Delousing procedures; specific vaccination; case quarantine
Whooping Cough (Pertussis)	Hemophilus pertussis	Human cases	Respiratory tract	Infected bronchial secretions	12–20 days	Tetracycline chloramphenicol	Active immunization with H. pertussis vaccine; case isolation

* Research developments produce changes in drug therapy. The reader is referred to drug brochures and digests to keep abreast of changing dosages and uses.

[817]

10 Most Reported Cases of Specified Notifiable Diseases in U.S.*

1. Gonorrhea
2. Streptococcal sore throat and scarlet fever
3. Mumps
4. Syphilis
5. Infectious hepatitis
6. Rubella
7. Measles
8. Tuberculosis (newly reported active cases)
9. Salmonellosis
10. Shigellosis (bacillary dysentery)

Epidemiology, Therapy and Control of Communicable Infections

See Table 15-1. (pp. 815–817)

MANAGEMENT AND CONTROL OF INFECTIOUS DISEASES

Nursing Objectives and Management

A. *To assist in identifying the etiologic agent and establishing the diagnosis.*
   1. Obtain specimens of blood, urine, stools, sputum, throat swabbings, nasal secretions and pyogenic exudates for bacteriologic study.
   2. Secure or assist in securing smears of blood and other materials for microscopic examination.
   3. Assist with aspirations of spinal fluid, bone marrow and other body fluids or tissues for cytologic, serologic and bacteriologic tests.
   4. Carry out appropriate skin tests for specific diagnostic reactions as directed.

B. *To control the infection in patient.*
   1. Administer the appropriate antimicrobial agents as ordered.
   2. Assist in administering specific immune therapy, if available, employing immune antiserum, gamma globulin, antitoxin, toxoid, vaccine or an appropriate mixture of antigen and antibody, depending on the circumstances.
   3. Observe patient carefully for evidences of drug or serum sensitivity.

C. *To prevent spread of the infection to others.*
   1. Carry out isolation techniques as required by disease (see p. 820).
   2. Observe asepsis as indicated.
   3. Use mask technique effectively. (Masks are not currently being used as much as in the past.)
      a. Change masks frequently—a moist mask is ineffective.
      b. Refrain from handling mask while in use.
   4. Use gown as required by patient's disease (see p. 820).
      Use gown once and discard in appropriate receptacle.
   5. Use gloves when indicated by patient's condition (see p. 820).
      a. Use once and discard in appropriate container.
      b. Disposable single-use gloves are preferable.
   6. Handle needles and syringes carefully.
      a. Handle with extreme care.
      b. Rinse nondisposable needles and syringes in cold water and wrap using double bag technique—place in clean bag in contaminated area and then place in a second clean bag outside the patient's room.

* 1970

7. Wash hands immediately after contact with each patient and after every contact with material that may be contaminated and is potentially infectious.
8. Disinfect and handle wastes with all due precautions.
9. Avoid creating aerosols—example: shaking bedlinens.
10. Carry out concurrent disinfection of fomites.
11. Control dissemination of infectious droplets.
    a. Encourage patient to cover nose and mouth when coughing or sneezing.
    b. Wrap contaminated tissues and articles in paper before disposal.
12. Collect dirt and dust.
    a. Require damp dusting of furniture and wet vacuum cleaning of floors.
    b. Reduce to a minimum the activity of personnel in the patient's environment.
    c. Maintain cleanliness of surroundings.
13. Have mechanical devices for filtering, diluting or directing airflow; if not available, use a window fan that exhausts air from the room.
14. Ventilate patient's room properly.
    a. It is desirable that a fresh supply of air from outside be brought into the room.
    b. Some forms of air conditioning may present a problem where recirculation of air is used.
15. Keep room door closed.
16. Disinfect room air with laminar airflow system, if available.

D. *To provide physiologic support.*
    1. Ensure adequate hydration in the event of excessive fluid loss through vomiting, diarrhea or excessive sweating.
       a. Encourage liberal fluid intake.
       b. Prepare for the administration of intravenous fluids as required.
    2. Reduce the fever.
       a. Administer antipyretic drugs as prescribed.
       b. Employ cool sponges cautiously as indicated (see p. 726).
    3. Measure and record body temperature, pulse and respiratory rates frequently.
    4. Measure arterial pressure at regular intervals if patient exhibits a tendency to vascular collapse.
    5. Weigh patient periodically, preferably at same hour of the day.

E. *To provide symptomatic relief.*
    1. Combat generalized aching and malaise.
       a. Utilize warm applications and massage as indicated.
       b. Apply cold compresses for headache.
       c. Administer analgesic medications as ordered.
       d. Attend to oral hygiene.
       e. Limit physical activity.
    2. Relieve cough.
       a. Humidify inspired air.
       b. Administer hot gargles and throat irrigations.
       c. Supply expectorants or cough depressants as indicated and prescribed.
    3. Relieve anxiety and depression.
       a. Recognize loneliness of the isolated patient.
       b. Lend encouragement to patient faced with prospect of prolonged convalescence.

F. *To protect exposed individuals and public at large against infectious illness.*
   1. Make available, facilitate or perform whatever vaccination procedures are known to be effective and are indicated for the stimulation of active immunity in exposed and susceptible individuals (see p. 823).
   2. Furnish specific immune serum (heterologous or human convalescent) or human gamma globulin if indicated, to provide passive immunity and temporary protection to contacts who are particularly vulnerable.
   3. Isolate patients with communicable infections, as well as known carriers and contacts, when required.
   4. Educate the public with respect to:
      a. The availability and importance of prophylactic immunization
      b. The manner in which infectious illnesses are spread and methods of avoiding spread
      c. The importance of seeking medical advice in the event of a febrile illness or skin eruption
      d. The importance of environmental cleanliness and personal hygiene
      e. Means of preventing the contamination of food and water supplies:
         (1) Discipline, cleanliness and inspection of food handlers
         (2) The dangers of "perishable" foods; the identity of foods that tend to promote bacterial growth; and methods of food preservation
         (3) The significance of milk pasteurization
         (4) The indications for, and methods of, sterilizing food by means of heat
      f. Knowledge of insect, rodent and other animal vectors and reservoirs of human infections and the importance of eliminating them

*Classification of Infectious Diseases Requiring Isolation or Precautions**

Strict Isolation

Private Room—*necessary;* door must be kept closed.
Gowns—must be worn by all persons entering room.
Masks—must be worn by all persons entering room.
Hands—must be washed on entering and leaving room.
Gloves—must be worn by all persons entering room.
Articles—must be discarded or wrapped before being sent to Central Supply for disinfection or sterilization

Diseases Requiring Strict Isolation

1. Anthrax, inhalation
2. Burns, extensive, infected with *Staphylococcus aureus* or Group A streptococcus
3. Diphtheria
4. Eczema vaccinatum
5. Melioidosis, pulmonary, or extrapulmonary with draining sinus(es)
6. Neonatal vesicular disease (Herpes simplex)
7. Plague
8. Rabies
9. Congenital rubella syndrome
10. Smallpox
11. Staphylococcal enterocolitis
12. Staphylococcal pneumonia
13. Streptococcal pneumonia
14. Vaccinia, generalized and progressive

Respiratory Isolation

Private Room—*necessary;* door must be kept closed.
Gowns—not necessary.

* Courtesy, U.S. Public Health Service.

Masks—must be worn by all persons entering room if susceptible to disease.
Hands—must be washed on entering and leaving room.
Gloves—not necessary.
Articles—those contaminated with secretions must be disinfected.
Caution—all persons susceptible to the specific disease should be excluded from patient area;
if contact is necessary, susceptibles must wear masks.

Diseases Requiring Respiratory Isolation

1. Chickenpox
2. Herpes zoster
3. Measles (rubeola)
4. Meningococcal meningitis
5. Meningococcemia
6. Mumps
7. Pertussis (whooping cough)
8. Rubella (German measles)
9. Tuberculosis, pulmonary-sputum-positive (or suspect)
10. Venezuelan equine encephalitis

Enteric Precautions

Private Room—*necessary for children only.*
Gowns—must be worn by all persons having direct contact with patient.
Masks—not necessary.
Hands—must be washed on entering and leaving room.
Gloves—must be worn by all persons having direct contact with patient or with articles contaminated with fecal material.
Articles—special precautions necessary for articles contaminated with urine and feces. Articles must be disinfected or discarded.

Diseases Requiring Enteric Precautions

1. Cholera
2. Enteropathogenic *E. coli* gastroenteritis
3. Hepatitis, viral (infectious or serum)
4. Salmonellosis (including typhoid fever)
5. Shigellosis

Wound and Skin Precautions

Private Room—desirable.
Gowns—must be worn by all persons having direct contact with patient.
Masks—not necessary except during dressing changes.
Hands—must be washed on entering and leaving room.
Gloves—must be worn by all persons having direct contact with infected area.
Articles—special precautions necessary for instruments, dressing, and linen.

Diseases Requiring Wound and Skin Precautions

1. Burns, extensive, not infected with *Staphylococcus aureus* or Group A streptococcus
2. Gas gangrene
3. Impetigo
4. Staphylococcal skin and wound infections
5. Streptococcal skin infection
6. Wound infection, extensive

Protective Isolation

Private Room—*necessary;* door must be kept closed.
Gowns—must be worn by all persons entering room.
Masks—must be worn by all persons entering room.
Hands—must be washed on entering and leaving room.
Gloves—must be worn by all persons having direct contact with patient.

Conditions Requiring Protective Isolation

1. Agranulocytosis
2. Severe and extensive, noninfected vesicular, bullous, or eczematous dermatitis
3. Certain patients receiving immunosuppressive therapy
4. Certain patients with lymphomas and leukemia

Discharge Precautions

A. *Secretion Precautions—Lesions*

> Private Room—not necessary.
> Gowns—not necessary.
> Masks—not necessary.
> Hands—must be washed before and after patient contact.
> Gloves—not necessary.
> Articles—double bagging technique for soiled dressings and equipment.
>
> *Diseases*

1. Actinomycosis
2. Anthrax
3. Brucellosis
4. Burns and wounds
5. Coccidioidomycosis
6. Conjunctivitis
7. Cryptococcosis
8. Gonococcal ophthalmia neonatorum
9. Gonorrhea
10. Granuloma inguinale
11. Herpes simplex
12. Keratoconjunctivitis
13. Listeriosis
14. Lymphogranuloma venereum
15. Nocardiosis
16. Syphilis
17. Orf
18. Trachoma
19. Tuberculosis
20. Tularemia
21. Wound infection

B. *Secretion Precautions—Oral*

> Private Room—not necessary.
> Gowns—not necessary.
> Masks—not necessary.
> Hands—must be washed before and after patient contact.
> Gloves—not necessary.
> Articles—discard disposable handkerchiefs in impervious bags, which should be sealed before being discarded in trash.
>
> *Diseases*

1. Mycoplasma pneumonia
2. Q fever
3. Psittacosis
4. Scarlet fever
5. Streptococcal pharyngitis
6. Viral diseases

C. *Excretion Precautions*

> Private Room—not necessary.
> Gowns—not necessary.
> Masks—not necessary.
> Hands—careful handwashing following any patient contact and contact with secretions.
> Articles—no special precautions.
>
> *Diseases*

1. *Clostridium perfringens (Cl. welchii)* food poisoning
2. Hand-foot-and-mouth disease
3. Herpangina
4. Infectious lymphocytosis
5. Leptospirosis
6. Meningitis
7. Pleurodynia
8. Poliomyelitis
9. Staphylococcal food poisoning
10. Taeniasis
11. Viral diseases

Immunization

Immunity is resistance that an individual has against disease.

The Immune Mechanism

Antigens (substances which induce the formation of antibodies in the body) react with antibody, producing immunity (or immunologic disease).

Active Immunity

Active immunity is immunity produced by natural or artificial stimulation so that the body produces its own antibodies. It may be produced by an attack of the specific disease or by introduction of vaccines or toxoids by injection.

Agents Producing Active Immunity

A. *Toxoid*—a toxin (antigenic and harmful proteins elaborated by microorganisms) treated by a heat and chemical agent to destroy its harmful properties without destroying its ability to stimulate antibody production.

Preparation	*Dose* (see package insert or label)
Diphtheria toxoid	0.5–1 ml. subcutaneously; repeat in 4–6 weeks
Tetanus toxoid	0.5–1 ml. subcutaneously; repeat in 3–4 weeks (see p. 825)

B. *Vaccines*—a suspension of attenuated or killed microorganisms (viruses, bacteria or rickettsiae) administered for prevention, amelioration or treatment of infectious diseases.

Preparation	*Dose* (see package insert or label)
Smallpox vaccine	By multiple pressure technic into the skin (see p. 843)
Yellow fever vaccine	0.5 ml. subcutaneously
Rabies vaccine	1 ml. subcutaneously for 14 days (see p. 848)
Influenza virus vaccine, polyvalent or mono-valent, Type A	1 ml. subcutaneously
Mumps virus vaccine, inactivated	1 ml. subcutaneously; repeat in 1–4 weeks
Mumps virus vaccine, attenuated	0.5 ml. subcutaneously
Poliomyelitis virus vaccine	1 ml. subcutaneously or intramuscularly; repeat in 1, 6 and 12 months
Poliomyelitis vaccine, live, oral Types I, II, III	Orally administered according to directions
Measles virus vaccine, live attenuated Rubeovax (immunity to measles, rubeola)	0.5 ml. of reconstituted vaccine subcutaneously; may be followed by 0.02 ml.; kg./wt. of immune serum globulin (human), intramuscularly
Measles virus vaccine, inactivated, adsorbed	See package directions
Rubella live virus vaccine, attenuated	Single dose, subcutaneously. Not to be given to pregnant women or those who are likely to become pregnant within 3 months after vaccination
Epidemic typhus vaccine	Dose according to directions
Pertussis vaccine	0.5 ml. subcutaneously; repeat in 4 and 8 weeks
Typhoid vaccine and typhoid* and paratyphoid vaccine	0.5 ml. subcutaneously; repeat in 2 and 4 weeks (see p. 831)

* Many authorities now question the efficacy of typhoid vaccine, depending more on surveillance of known cases and carriers by means of periodic stool specimens.

Preparation	*Dose* (see package insert or label)
Typhus vaccine	According to directions
Cholera vaccine	0.5 ml. subcutaneously; then 1 ml. at 10 and 20 days
Plague vaccine	0.5 ml. subcutaneously; then 1 ml. in 7–10 days
Rocky Mountain Spotted Fever vaccine	1 ml. subcutaneously 7–10 days apart

Passive Immunity

Passive immunity is acquired immunity produced by administration of preformed antibody; protection is of short duration and is employed to protect individual against disease to which he has been exposed.

Agents Producing Passive Immunity

A. *Serums Prepared in Man* (found in patient recently convalescent from disease or acquired from donors who have been recently vaccinated).

PREPARATION (dose according to package insert or label)
Immune serum globulin (human)—antibodies against polio, measles, infectious hepatitis
Poliomyelitis immune globulin (human)—measles, infectious hepatitis or polio
Hyperimmunized gamma globulin—mumps, pertussis, rabies
Scarlet fever immune serum (human)—scarlet fever
Tetanus immune globulin (human)—tetanus

B. *Serums Prepared in Animals.*

> NURSING ALERT: The patient must be given skin tests for sensitivity before he is given preparations of animal antiserum.

PREPARATIONS (see package insert or label for dosage and route of administration)
Diphtheria antitoxin
Tetanus antitoxin (now being replaced with human tetanus immune globulin)
Gas gangrene antitoxin (bivalent, trivalent or pentavalent mixtures with tetanus antitoxin)
Antivenin (Lacrodectus mactans) (black widow spider bites)
Antivenin (Crotalidae) polyvalent (bites of crotaline snakes, including copperhead, water moccasin, rattlesnake and Asiatic and tropical crotalids)

BACTERIAL DISEASES
Tetanus (Lockjaw)

Tetanus is an acute disease caused by the *Clostridium tetani* (tetanus bacillus) whose spores are introduced into the body when an injury becomes contaminated with soil, street dust or animal and human feces. The bacillus is an anaerobe (cannot live in presence of oxygen).

Clinical Manifestations
(Caused by potent neurotoxins elaborated by *C. tetani* which have a special affinity for nervous tissue.)

1. Rigidity of muscles
   a. Trismus—painful spasms of masticatory muscles with difficulty in opening the mouth (lockjaw).
   b. Risus sardonicus—grinning expression produced by spasm of facial muscles.
   c. Recurrent tetanic spasms of almost every muscle group in body.
2. Hyperirritability
3. Hyperactive reflexes

Treatment and Nursing Management

Objective: to prevent the disease from developing.
   1. The treatment depends on the immunization status of the patient.
      a. For previously immunized patient:
         (1) Tetanus toxoid 0.5 ml.
         (2) Human tetanus immune globulin, as directed
         (3) Immediate debridement of wound
         (4) Antibiotic therapy—penicillin; tetracycline
   2. For patient with no previous immunization (or if immunization is in doubt):
      (1) Tetanus toxoid 0.5 ml. followed by second dose (0.5 ml.) in 4–6 weeks
      (2) Human tetanus immune globulin or antitoxin as directed
      (3) Immediate debridement of wound
      (4) Antibiotic therapy—tetanus organism sensitive to tetracycline and penicillin. (These antibiotics given promptly after injury may be a deterrent to the development of tetanus.)

NURSING ALERT: Tetanus-prone wounds are those in which there has been an invasion of soil or feces or those involving a severe traumatic injury. Tetanus may develop from an insignificant wound contaminated by soil.

---

   3. Equine or bovine antitoxin is not usually given because of high incidence of allergic and anaphylactic reaction.

Treatment of Tetanus

Objective: to prevent respiratory and cardiovascular complications.
   1. Maintain an adequate airway—tetanic spasm of larynx, pharynx and respiratory muscles usually occurs during convulsions and may lead to asphyxia and death.
      a. Insert a cuffed endotracheal tube (p. 107)—laryngeal spasms cause airway obstruction, inadequate pulmonary ventilation, hypoxia, cyanosis and death.
      b. Prepare patient for tracheostomy—relieves laryngeal dyspnea, reduces risk of aspiration and permits speedy application of controlled ventilation.
      c. Maintain patient on mechanical ventilation (see p. 137).
      d. Aspirate secretions as necessary—observe aspirate and keep a record of its appearance to assess for signs of pulmonary infection (e.g., sputum becomes colored).
   2. Carry out effective wound care; debride all necrotic tissue—necrotic tissue favors growth of tetanus bacillus.
   3. Give antibiotics (penicillin, tetracycline)—to eradicate persisting *Cl. tetani* and other pathogens from the wound.
   4. Give tetanus human immune globulin daily—in an effort to neutralize the toxins.

5. Maintain the fluid and electrolyte balance.
6. Support the patient during tetanic spasms and convulsions—due to the action of toxins in cells of central nervous system; mortality rate of patients with frequent and severe spasms is high.
   a. Provide for continuing observation of the patient.
   b. Place patient in a quiet room.
   c. Avoid sudden stimuli and light.
   d. Disturb the patient as little as possible—tactile stimuli often provoke spasms.
   e. Give muscle relaxants to keep patient quiet and relaxed.
   f. Be alert for the development of fractures of the vertebral bodies which may occur with severe spasm.
   g. See page 731 for management of the patient with convulsive seizures and page 728 for management of the unconscious patient.

> NURSING ALERT: The hearing of the patient with respiratory paralysis may be acute. Do not make unguarded comments in his presence.

7. After recovery, the patient should receive 3 doses of the primary immunization series plus booster dose every 10 years—recovery from tetanus does not imply immunity.

Nursing Isolation Procedure

No isolation or precautions are required.

Gas Gangrene

Gas gangrene is a severe infection caused by gram positive clostridia which may complicate compound fractures and contused or lacerated wounds. Several species of clostridia *(Cl. welchii, Cl. perfringens, Cl. septicum, Cl. novyi, Cl. histolyticum, Cl. sporogenes)* and others may produce gas gangrene. These organisms are anaerobes and spore-formers and are found normally in the intestinal tract of man and in soil.

Altered Physiology

Injury→bacteria *(clostridia)* invade devitalized tissue, especially where blood supply is compromised→bacteria multiply and produce toxins→toxins cause hemolysis, vessel thrombosis and damage to myocardium, liver and kidneys.

Clinical Manifestations

1. Sudden and severe pain at site of injury—caused by gas and edema in the tissues
2. Rapid feeble pulse progressing to circulatory collapse
3. Anemia—from hemolysis
4. Apathy—delirium and stupor
5. *Appearance of wound:*
   a. Skin is white and tense initially; the color then progresses to a dusky hue.
   b. Vesicles appear; are filled with red, watery fluid.
   c. Muscle is dark red, edematous and contains red, watery foul-smelling fluid.
   d. Gas bubbles seen emanating from tissues—toxins ferment muscle sugar and produce acid and gas which digest muscle protein. (Obvious gangrene is present.)

Treatment and Nursing Management

1. Place patient in hyperbaric oxygen chamber if available—increases the dissolved oxygen in the arterial system by increasing the partial pressure of the oxygen breathed by the patient.
2. Prepare for surgical removal and debridement of necrotic tissue—this is preventive as well as curative therapy; extensive incisions in affected part allow air to inhibit growth of anaerobic organisms.
3. Give antibiotic therapy (penicillin, chloramphenicol)—may prevent spread of infection.
4. Support the patient with toxemic manifestations—gas bacillus infection produces an intense toxemia.
   a. Monitor central venous pressure (p. 241) and urinary output.
   b. Give I.V. fluids to support cardiovascular system; maintain fluid and electrolyte balance.
5. Give antiserum (if ordered) if hyperbaric oxygen therapy is not available.

Isolation Nursing Procedure

Use wound and skin precautions (see p. 821).

Staphylococcal Disease

Staphylococci are responsible for a wide variety of infections. They cause most superficial infections, but they also produce serious infections of the lungs, pleural space, bones, kidneys and surgical wounds.

Examples of Staphylococcal Disease

1. *Skin infections*—furuncles (boils), impetigo, carbuncles, abscesses, infected lacerations
2. *Invasion of lymphatics*—axillary, cervical, mediastinal, retroperitoneal or subdiaphragmatic abscesses
3. *Invasion of bloodstream*—acute ulcerative endocarditis, staphylococcal pneumonia, empyema, perinephritic abscess, hepatic abscess, staphylococcal enteritis, pyogenic arthritis, meningitis, osteomyelitis, generalized sepsis

Infectious Agent

Various strains of coagulase-positive staphylococci *(Staphylococcus aureus)*

Mode of Transmission

Nasal secretions, draining wound, asymptomatic nasal carrier

Hospital Staphylococcal Infections

(Include all of the above infections)

A. *Susceptible Hospital Patients.*
  1. Chronically ill or debilitated patients
  2. Patients receiving systemic steroids or antimetabolite therapy
  3. Patient undergoing major or prolonged surgery
  4. Infants in the nursery

B. *Epidemiology of Hospital Infections.*
    1. Hospital personnel and patients have significantly higher carrier rate for staphylococci than the general population.
    2. Staphylococcal organisms remain viable in dust, bedlinens, clothing, etc., for long periods.

NURSING ALERT: In the majority of patients with hospital-acquired staphylococcal disease, the infecting organisms are resistant to penicillin or other commonly used antibiotics.

C. *Prevention and Control.*
    1. All hospitals should enforce aseptic techniques supervised by infection control committee of the individual hospital.
    2. Certain antibiotics should be reserved for staphylococcal infection—oxacillin, methicillin, vancomycin.
    3. Strict surveillance of patients undergoing parenteral injections and continuous intravenous therapy with indwelling cannulae should be carried out.

Specific Therapy for Staphylococcal Infections (Systemic)
    1. Penicillinase-resistant penicillin
    2. Semi-synthetic cephalosporin or vancomycin—when allergy to penicillin is present
    3. Gentamicin

Nursing Isolation Procedures Required for Staphylococcal Disease
    1. Burns—strict isolation (p. 820)
    2. Dermatitis—wound and skin precautions (p. 821)
    3. Enterocolitis—strict isolation
    4. Pemphigus—wound and skin precautions
    5. Pneumonia and draining lung abscess—strict isolation
    6. Wounds—wound and skin precautions

Preventive Measures
    1. Public should be educated concerning personal hygiene.
    2. Persons with draining lesions should be isolated from their group and treated.

Streptococcal Infections

Most *streptococcal infections* in man are caused by Group A hemolytic streptococci. Beta hemolytic streptococci gain entrance to the body primarily through the upper respiratory tract from persons with streptococcal infections or those who are asymptomatic carriers.

Beta Hemolytic Streptococcal Infections
    1. Streptococcal sore throat ("strep" pharyngitis, p. 267)
    2. Scarlet fever (streptococcal throat with a rash which occurs if infectious agent produces erythrogenic toxin and patient is not immune to toxin)
    3. Sinusitis, otitis media, mastoiditis, peritonsillar abscess
    4. Pericarditis, arthritis, peritonitis, meningitis
    5. Pneumonia and empyema
    6. Wound and skin infections—impetigo, puerperal infections, erysipelas

Poststreptococcal Diseases (sequel of Hemolytic Streptococci)

1. Rheumatic fever   2. Acute glomerulonephritis

Diagnostic Evaluation

1. Throat culture and sensitivity test   2. Culture from wounds

Treatment

1. All beta hemolytic streptococci are sensitive to penicillin G (Bicillin); several forms are available.
   a. Therapy should be continued for as least 10 days—to reduce frequency of suppurative complications, prevent majority cases of rheumatic fever (and to a lesser extent, acute glomerulonephritis) and help prevent further spread of streptococci.
   b. Erythromycin may be used for penicillin-sensitive patients.
2. Streptomycin or kanamycin may enhance the action of penicillin in destroying streptococci, particularly the enterococci.
3. Make sure the patient understands the importance of completing the course of antibiotic treatment.

Nursing Isolation Procedures

1. Burns (extensive)—strict isolation (p. 820)
2. Burns (minor)—secretions precautions (p. 822)
3. Cellulitis—wound and skin precautions (p. 821)
4. Endometritis—secretions precautions
5. Erysipelas—wound and skin precautions
6. Impetigo—wound and skin precautions
7. Pharyngitis—secretions precautions until 24 hours after initiation of effective therapy
8. Pneumonia—strict isolation
9. Scarlet fever—secretions precautions

Preventive Measures

1. Public should be educated concerning the relationship of streptococcal infections to heart disease and glomerulonephritis.
2. Pasteurize milk.
3. Food handlers should be instructed about hygienic procedures.
4. Obstetrical patients should be protected from personnel or visitors with respiratory or skin infections.
5. Long-term penicillin prophylaxis may be used for high-risk individuals (those who have had rheumatic fever, recurrent erysipelas).

Typhoid Fever

Typhoid fever is a bacterial infection transmitted by contaminated water, milk, shellfish or other foods, caused by *Salmonella typhi* which is harbored in human excreta. Its characteristic lesion consists of ulcers which form in the ileum and the colon, and its distinctive clinical features consist of long-continued fever, rose-spot rash, enlarged spleen, slow pulse and leukopenia.

Altered Physiology

Organism enters body by gastrointestinal tract; it invades the walls of gastrointestinal tract leading to bacteremia which localizes in mesenteric lymph nodes and in the masses of lymphatic tissue in the mucous membrane of the intestinal wall (Peyer's patches) and in small solitary lymph follicles in the ileum and colon; ulceration of the intestines may ensue.

Clinical Manifestations

A. *Gradual onset.*
   1. Headache, malaise, muscle pains
   2. Chills and fever
   3. Pulse is full and slow in comparison to height of fever
   4. Skin eruption—irregularly spaced small rose spots on abdomen, chest, back—each spot fades over a period of 3–4 days.

B. *Second week.*
   1. Fever ascending in a step-ladder fashion
   2. Abdominal distention and tenderness; constipation or diarrhea
   3. Delirium in severe infections—from severe toxemia

C. *Third week.*
   Gradual decline in fever and subsidence of symptoms

Diagnostic Evaluation

   1. White blood count—leukopenia is a distinctive hematologic feature.
   2. Blood culture—positive for organism after 1st week.
   3. Stool culture—positive for organism after 1st week.
   4. Urine culture—organism may or may not be present.
   5. Blood serum agglutination test usually becomes positive by the end of 2nd week.

Treatment and Nursing Management

Objectives: to give supportive care.
             to observe for hemorrhage and perforation.
   1. Give specific treatment for typhoid.
      a. Chloramphenicol as directed.
      b. Monitor blood count every 5 days to detect chloramphenicol toxicity.
   2. Give supportive care—typhoid fever is a nursing challenge.
      a. Support patient during period of toxemia—patient may be drowsy and partially incontinent.
      b. Give hydrocortisone (I.V.) or prednisone if ordered for toxic patients.
      c. Prepare for blood transfusions—has beneficial tonic effect on patient with toxemia.
      d. Take rectal temperature every 2–4 hours.
         (1) Give fever sponge (p. 726) for temperature of 40°C. (104°F.) or more.
         (2) Encourage a high fluid intake.
      e. Watch for bladder distention—patient may lose urge to void during toxic state.
      f. Observe for retention of feces.
      g. Give a high caloric, low residue diet during febrile stage.
   3. Watch for complications which can occur after an apparent clinical cure.

a. *Intestinal hemorrhage*—from erosion of blood vessel in ulcerated small intestine (occurs in 10% of patients).
  (1) Clinical manifestations

Apprehension, sweating, pallor	Hypotension
Weak rapid pulse; narrowing pulse pressure	Bloody or tarry stools

  (2) Treatment

Withhold food	Give blood transfusions

b. *Perforation of intestine*—from erosion of one of ulcers; most common during 3rd week.
  (1) Symptoms
      Sudden sharp abdominal pain—may stop suddenly
      Abdominal rigidity
      Shock
  (2) Treatment
      Prepare for intestinal decompression procedure (p. 409), intravenous fluids and surgical intervention if conservative measures do not produce clinical improvement.
4. Take preventive measures.
  a. Give typhoid vaccine—0.5 ml. subcutaneously followed by 2nd injection in 4–6 weeks; booster injection every 3 years.
  b. Patient must be followed with routine stool culture after recovery to detect the development of the carrier state—approximately 2–5% of typhoid patients become permanent carriers haboring the organism and excreting it in their urine and stools.
    (1) Carriers may be given ampicillin—to attempt to abolish carrier state.
    (2) Positive stool culture after 4 months indicates a carrier.
    (3) Carriers must not become food or milk handlers.
  c. Maintain environmental hygiene.
    (1) Protect and purify water supplies.
    (2) Employ sanitary waste disposal techniques.
    (3) Pasteurize milk and dairy products; refrigerate while transporting.
    (4) Supervise foods served, especially raw foods.
    (5) Ensure that food handlers use hand-washing facilities.

Isolation Nursing Procedure

Isolation nursing procedure. Use enteric precautions (p. 821) until 3 consecutive negative stool cultures (taken at least 24 hours apart) are obtained.

Salmonella Infections (Salmonellosis)

Salmonellosis is a form of food poisoning causing acute gastroenteritis due to certain species of the genus *Salmonella*. The patient is infected by the oral route from contaminated food or drink.

Infectious agent—1200 known serotypes of salmonella—most common in U.S. are *S. typhimurium, S. Heidelberg, S. Newport, S. infantis, S. enteritidis, S. derby* and *S. St. Paul.*

> NURSING ALERT: Common food offenders causing salmonella infections include commercially processed meat pies, poultry (especially turkey), sausage (lightly cooked), foods containing egg or egg products and unpasteurized milk or dairy products.

Clinical Manifestations

1. Diarrhea—sudden onset of frequent, bulky stools followed by profuse watery diarrhea
2. Abdominal pain
3. Nausea and vomiting
4. Fever
5. Other manifestations due to infectious agent localizing in any body tissue—abscesses, cholecystitis, arthritis, endocarditis, meningitis, pericarditis, pneumonia, pyelonephritis

Diagnostic Evaluation

Culture of feces, urine and blood

Treatment

The treatment is supportive:
1. Restrict food until abdominal pain subsides.
2. Offer clear liquids as tolerated.
3. Correct fluid and electrolyte depletion.
4. Give antispasmodics as directed.

Nursing Isolation Procedure

Use enteric precautions for duration of illness. (See p. 821.)

Preventive Measures

1. Raw eggs or egg drinks should not be eaten, nor cracked or dirty eggs used.
2. All foods from animal sources, especially fowl, egg products and meat dishes, should be thoroughly cooked.
3. Foods should be refrigerated during storage.
4. Any person handling food should be instructed to wash hands before and after food preparation and to protect food against insect or rodent contamination.
5. Chicks, ducklings and turtles (as well as other domestic animals and pets) are sources of salmonella infections.

Shigellosis (Bacillary Dysentery)

Shigellosis includes a group of enteric infections caused by bacilli of the *shigella* group of which there are 4 types: *Sh. dysenteriae, Sh. flexneri, Sh. boydii, Sh. sonnei.* The source of infection is feces from an infected person. The route of spread is fecal-oral.

Clinical Manifestations

Fever and headache
Abdominal cramps
Persistent diarrhea

Treatment and Nursing Management

Objectives: to provide aggressive treatment for the patient.
   to prevent the spread of shigellosis to the patient's contacts, i.e., eliminate the carrier state.
1. Determine the type of shigella—organism is recovered from the stool of the patient.

2. Do sensitivity testing for selection of antibiotic—resistance to commonly used antibiotics may occur.
3. Give ampicillin trihydrate—eliminates shigellae from intestinal tract 24–48 hours after treatment in majority of patients; significantly shortens duration of diarrhea, cramps and fever.
   Cephalothin sodium, kanamycin, nalidixic acid, nitrofurantoin are also used.
4. Maintain fluid and electrolyte balance—to prevent profound dehydration owing to an excessively great loss of salts in the diarrheic stools.
   a. Assess weight loss, skin turgor, dryness of mucous membranes, urinary volume, vital signs.
   b. Weigh daily and measure urinary volume.
5. Offer clear fluids during acute stage of illness.
6. Carry out epidemiology studies in every patient where the organism is found.
   a. Ask if patient has been recent traveler to Mexico or Central America or has had contacts with travelers from these countries.
   b. Notify local and state authorities.

Nursing Isolation Procedure

Use enteric precautions, p. 821.

Preventive Measures

1. Handwashing after defecation
2. Surveillance of water sanitation
3. Program of fly control

Botulism[*]

Botulism is a poisoning which affects the central nervous system and is caused by eating food in which *Clostridium botulinum* has grown and produced toxins. The organism is widely distributed in soil. Human intoxication usually follows ingestion of inadequately sterilized home-canned vegetables or vacuum-packed fish.

Clinical Manifestations

(Appear 12–36 hours after ingestion of toxin.)

1. Nausea and vomiting
2. Malaise, headache, dizziness
3. Dilated fixed pupils; diplopia and sometimes blindness—from cranial nerve involvement
4. Severe dryness of mouth and throat
5. Difficulty in speaking and swallowing
6. Respiratory paralysis with progressive muscle paralysis

Course

Variable; illness may be prolonged with *a high risk of superinfection and fatal outcome.*

[*] Botulism is an intoxication, not an infection. National Center for Disease Control, Atlanta, Georgia 30333, offers diagnostic consultation and laboratory testing services and support for epidemiological studies of botulism.

Treatment and Nursing Management

Objectives: to prevent respiratory failure.
            to give supportive care.

1. Maintain adequate ventilation—death is frequently due to acute onset of respiratory failure.
   a. Utilize suctioning, tracheostomy procedure and artificial ventilation as necessary. (See p. 137.)
   b. Carry out blood gas determinations as required.
2. Administer trivalent antitoxin, types A, B and E as soon as possible after skin testing for serum sensitivity.
3. Administer cleansing enemas—to remove unabsorbed toxin from colon.
4. Treat superimposed infections with antibiotics if necessary.

Prevention

1. Home-canned foods with bulging lids or jars should not be used.
2. Home-canned foods should be inspected before being eaten—foods contaminated with *Clostridium botulinum* look soft, contain gas bubbles and give off an odor of decay.
3. Canned vegetables should be boiled 10–20 minutes and stirred thoroughly before serving—toxin is heat labile and destroyed by proper cooking of foods.

Gonorrhea

Gonorrhea is an inflammation involving the mucous membrane of the genitourinary tract and is caused by the gonococcus, *Neisseria gonorrhoeae*. It is an infectious disease which is transmitted almost wholly by sexual intercourse.

Epidemiology

Incidence arises during:
1. Social unrest
2. War
3. Migration
4. Early maturity (Half of the cases occur in persons 25 years or younger.)
5. Changing standards of morality
6. Homosexual practices

Clinical Problems

1. Gonorrhea is the number 1 reported bacterial infection of adults. It is now considered to be epidemic in the U.S.
2. Gonorrhea has a short incubation period which permits rapid spread.
3. Syphilis and gonorrhea are frequently observed in the same patient.
4. Gonorrhea is becoming increasingly resistant to penicillin.

Complications

1. Sterility in women
2. Secondary foci of infection may develop in any organ system—gonococcal arthritis, tenosynovitis, endocarditis, pelvic inflammatory disease, meningitis, lesions of the skin, severe proctitis, postgonococcal urethritis (male)

Clinical Manifestations

NURSING ALERT: 80% of women who have the disease may be asymptomatic and unaware that they are infected.

Women (small percentage)	*Men* (incubation period 2–5 days)
Vaginal discharge	Painful urination accompanied by profuse mucopurulent urethral discharge
Urinary frequency and pain	Spread of infection to posterior urethra, prostate, seminal vesicles and epididymis
Pelvic inflammatory disease when gonococcus spreads through fallopian tubes:	Prostatitis
Fever	Pelvic pain and fever
Nausea and vomiting	Epididymitis
Lower abdominal pain	Severe pain, tenderness and swelling
Gonococcal septicemia	Postgonococcal urethritis becomes a major problem in male

Diagnosis

A. *Women.*

Culture specimen obtained from the cervix and anal canal and inoculated on separate Thayer-Martin (TM) culture plates or Transgrow medium

B. *Men*

Smear of urethral exudate for microscopic examination

In homosexuals: additional culture specimens obtained from anal canal and pharynx and inoculated on Thayer-Martin culture plates or Transgrow medium

Treatment

Objective: to obtain a high blood level of an effective antibiotic for a moderately short time.

1. Penicillin G or ampicillin is the preferred drug for *Neisseria gonorrhoeae.*
   a. *Parenteral* (men or women)
      Aqueous procaine penicillin G, 4.8 million units intramuscularly divided into at least 2 doses and injected at different sites at 1 visit, together with 1 gm. of oral probenecid, preferably given at least 30 minutes prior to the injection, *or*
   b. *Oral*
      Ampicillin, 3.5 gm., with probenecid, 1 gm., administered simultaneously.
2. Treatment of contacts: Same treatment as for gonorrhea.
3. For patients with allergies to penicillin or ampicillin:
   a. *Parenteral*
      Men: Spectinomycin, 2 gm. in 1 intramuscular injection.
      Women: Spectinomycin, 4 gm. *or*
   b. *Oral* (men and women)
      Tetracycline HCl, 1.5 gm. initially, followed by 0.5 gm. 4 times a day for 4 days (total dose, 9 gm.). Other tetracyclines are not more effective.
4. *Follow-up*
   a. Men: follow-up urethral cultures 7 days after completion of treatment.
   b. Women: follow-up cervical and rectal cultures 7–14 days after completion of treatment.

Nursing Isolation Procedure

Use secretion precautions until 24 hours after initiation of effective therapy (see p. 822)

Principles of Control

1. Each patient should be interviewed for names of contacts.
2. Contacts of known gonorrhea cases should be investigated; known contacts should be treated within 10 days.
3. The patient should be instructed to avoid re-infection by sexual intercourse with untreated previous sexual partners.

GUIDELINES: *Obtaining Culture Specimen for the Diagnosis of Gonorrhea**

Purpose

To obtain a specimen from the cervix and anal canal (women) and urethral specimen (men) for culture for *N. gonorrhoeae*.

Equipment

Vaginal speculum
Ring forceps
Cotton balls
Sterile, cotton-tipped swabs

Thayer-Martin medium plates
or
Transgrow medium bottles
Sterile wire loop
Sterile disposable gloves

Procedure

Nursing Action	Rationale/Amplification
Preparatory Phase	
1. Place patient in dorsal lithotomy position with adequate draping.	
2. Put on sterile disposable gloves.	
Performance Phase	
FOR FEMALE PATIENT:	
Cervical Culture	
1. Moisten vaginal speculum with warm water. Do not use any other lubricant.	
2. Separate labia. Depress the perineum and posterior vaginal wall with the finger of one hand.	2. This maneuver helps avoid uncomfortable pressure against the more sensitive anteriorly placed structures.
3. Gently insert a bivalve vaginal speculum.	3. The speculum is made self-retaining by adjusting one or more screws. The short blade should be uppermost. The tip of the posterior blade is pushed down into the posterior fornix.
4. Insert sterile cotton-tipped swab into endocervical canal (Fig. 15-1A). a. Move from side to side in the cervix. b. Allow several seconds for absorption of organisms by the swab.	4. The endocervical canal is considered the best culture site. Movement of the cotton swab ensures adequate sampling.

* Adapted from Criteria and Techniques for the Diagnosis of Gonorrhea, U.S. Department of Health, Education and Welfare.

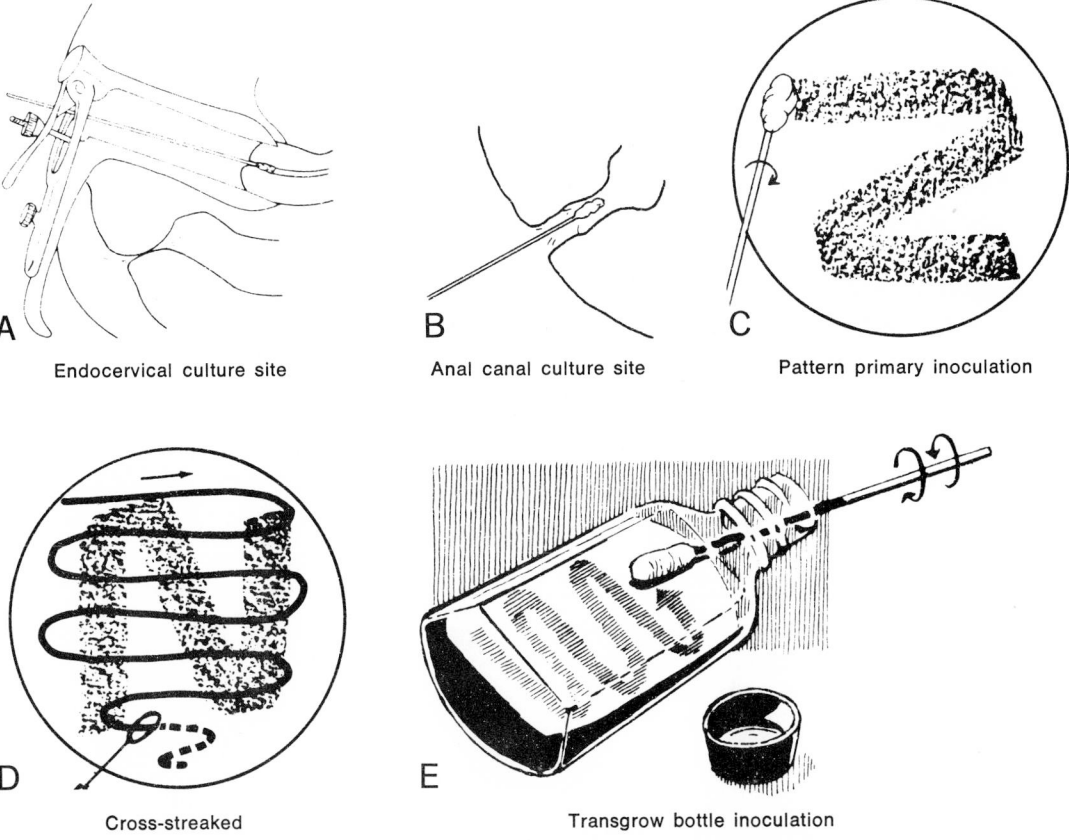

A Endocervical culture site

B Anal canal culture site

C Pattern primary inoculation

D Cross-streaked

E Transgrow bottle inoculation

Figure 15-1. Obtaining culture for specimen in diagnosis of gonorrhea.

Nursing Action	Rationale/Amplification
Anal Canal Culture (Rectal Culture)	
1. Obtain anal specimen *after* getting cervical specimen.	1. The anal canal is the most likely site to be positive when the cervix is negative.
2. Insert sterile cotton-tipped swab approximately 2.5 cm. (1 inch) into the anal canal (Fig. 15-1B).	2. Use another swab to obtain specimen if swab is inadvertently pushed into feces.
3. Move swab from side to side in anal canal.	3. Movement of the swab in anal canal permits specimen to be secured from anal crypts.
4. Allow several seconds for absorption of organism by the swab.	
FOR MALE PATIENT:	
Urethral culture	
1. Use bacteriological wire loop to obtain specimen from anterior urethra by gently scraping the mucosa.	1. A urethral culture of the male is indicated when the gram stain of urethral exudate is not positive in tests-for-cure or as a test for incubating gonorrhea.

Nursing Action	**Rationale/Amplification**

Anal Canal Culture
(Same as in women)

To Inoculate the Culture Medium

Thayer-Martin plates

Thayer-Martin plates are used when there is immediate access to the laboratory.

1. Roll swab directly on Thayer-Martin (TM) Medium in a large "Z" pattern (Fig. 15-1C).
   1. This pattern provides adequate exposure of swab to plate for transfer of organisms.
2. Cross-streak immediately with sterile wire loop. (This streak dilution can be done in laboratory.) (Fig. 15-1D)
   2. Streaking with a wire loop isolates colonies of *N. gonorrhoeae* from the few contaminants that occasionally grow on selective medium.
3. Place the culture plate in a candle jar as soon as possible.
   3. Placing the culture plate in a candle jar retards drying and provides an appropriate carbon dioxide environment. Successful recovery of *N. gonorrhoeae* requires an atmosphere enriched in carbon dioxide.
4. Send the plates to lab for incubation.
   4. Plates are examined by laboratory personnel after 20 hours' incubation.

For Transgrow Bottle Inoculation (Fig. 15-1E)

Transgrow, a selective medium for transport and cultivation of *N. gonorrhoeae*, is used for sending specimens to a central laboratory.

1. Remove cap of bottle only when ready to inoculate.
   1. Keep neck of bottle in elevated position to minimize loss of carbon dioxide.
2. Soak up all excess moisture in bottle with specimen swab and then roll swab from side to side across the medium, starting at the bottom of the bottle.
3. When possible, incubate the Transgrow bottle in an upright position at 35–37°C. for 16–18 hours before mailing. Note this on accompanying request form.
   3. Resultant growth survives prolonged transport and is ready for identification upon arrival at laboratory.
4. Package the capped Transgrow bottle and request form in a suitable container to prevent breakage. Transport immediately to a central bacteriologic laboratory by postal service or other convenient means.

Meningococcal Meningitis

Meningococcal meningitis is an acute bacterial infectious disease caused by the meningococcus, *Neisseria meningitidis*. It starts as an infection of the nasopharynx or the tonsils followed by meningococcal septicemia which extends to the meninges of the brain and the upper region of the spinal cord. There are several distinct immunologic strains of the meningococcus but the groups A, B, and C are the most important.

Clinical Manifestations

1. High fever
2. Nausea and vomiting
3. Headache, confusion, delirium, convulsions
4. Neck, shoulder and back stiffness

Positive Kernig's sign—when lying with the thigh flexed upon the abdomen, patient cannot completely extend his leg (a sign of meningeal irritation)

Positive Brudzinski's sign—when the patient's neck is bent forward, flexion of the ankle, knee and hip are produced.

When passive flexion of the lower extremity on one side is made, a similar movement will be seen in the contralateral (opposite) extremity.

5. Petechial rash

Infectious Source of Infection

Human cases and carriers

Method of Spread

Respiratory droplets

Diagnostic Evaluation

Organism usually demonstrated by smear and culture of cerebrospinal fluid, oropharynx and blood

Clinical Features

1. Meningococcus may localize in the brain, skin or joint synovia.
2. The disease occurs in winter and spring months; epidemics are most apt to occur when people live in crowded quarters.
3. Approximately 10% of patients with meningococcus meningitis die from overwhelming infection.

Treatment and Nursing Management

Objective: to observe and treat for vasomotor collapse and shock.

1. Support patient undergoing diagnostic lumbar puncture (p. 720)—cerebrospinal fluid will be cloudy (from pus) with elevated pressure.
2. Give specific drug therapy—penicillin (drug of choice) chloramphenicol, tetracyclines, erythromycin, sulfonamides as prescribed.
3. Maintain a clear airway—altered consciousness may lead to airway obstruction.
   a. Carry out arterial blood gas determinations.
   b. Provide oral airway or cuffed endotracheal tube or tracheostomy (p. 107) as patient's condition indicates.
   c. Administer oxygen to maintain arterial pO_2 between 55–65 mm. Hg.
4. Provide monitoring procedures and care for patient with fulminating (coming on suddenly with severity) disease.
   a. Assess patient for generalized vasoconstriction, circumoral cyanosis, cold extremities—may lead to coma.
   b. Monitor the patient's central venous pressure—to assess for incipient shock which precedes cardiac or respiratory failure.
   c. Monitor intake and output.
   d. Provide for rapid intravenous replacement.
5. Encourage a liberal fluid intake (at least 3000 ml. daily).
6. Watch for signs of increasing intracranial pressure (p. 724)—acute cerebral edema can occur.

   Use osmotic diuresis with I.V. mannitol, urea, etc.

7. Give diazepam (Valium) or diphenylhydantoin (Dilantin) to control convulsive seizures.
8. Employ measures to reduce temperature in patient with high fever (see p. 726).

Nursing Isolation Procedure

Use respiratory isolation precautions (p. 820) for 24 hours after initiation of effective therapy.

SPIROCHETAL INFECTIONS
Syphilis (Lues)

Syphilis is a chronic infectious disease caused by *Treponema pallidum* (a spirochete). It is congenital in origin or acquired by sexual contact.

Incidence

1. Syphilis is the 3rd most common reportable communicable disease.
2. Most prevalent in teenagers and young adults; 62% of cases in 15–25 age group.
3. More prevalent in males than females.
4. More prevalent in large urban centers.
5. Promiscuity and indiscretion—each person with infectious syphilis has an average of 4.6 recent contacts, 2 of whom were infected.

Epidemiology

Tracing the source and spread of infections by interviewing known patients for sex contacts.
1. Interviewing and re-interviewing every reported patient with syphilis for sex contacts.
2. Rapid investigation to identify contacts for examination within a minimal time period.
3. Identifying and conducting blood tests of other persons who by definition (suspect or associate) are possibly involved sexually in an infectious chain (cluster procedure). (Promiscuous persons behave sexually in somewhat similar patterns.)
4. Epidemiologic (preventive or prophylactic) treatment of sexual contacts and infectious syphilis cases.

Clinical Manifestations

Syphilis is capable of destroying tissue in almost any organ in the body thus producing a wide variety of clinical manifestations.

Stages of Untreated Syphilis

A. *Incubation period.*
   1. 10–60 days; average 21 days
   2. No symptoms or lesions
   3. Spirochetemia is present; patient's blood is infective.
B. *Primary (early) Syphilis.*
   1. Most infectious stage
   2. Manifestations include:
      a. Chancre or primary sore—appears at the site where the treponema enters the body (glans penis, cervix, labia, scrotum, anus, mouth, nipple)
      b. Enlargement of regional lymph nodes

C. *Secondary Syphilis.*
1. Lesion appears 3 weeks after onset of primary lesion; may involve any cutaneous or mucosal surface of the body as well as any organ.
2. Skin lesions—bilaterally symmetrical in distribution, polymorphous (macular, papular, follicular, pustular)
   a. Moist papules occur most frequently in anogenital region (condylomata lata) and the mouth.
   b. Lesions of mouth, throat and cervix (mucous patches) frequently occur in secondary stage.
   c. Hair may drop out during period of skin eruption.
3. Generalized lymphadenopathy
4. Arthritic and bone pain
5. Acute iritis
6. Hoarseness, chronic sore throat

D. *Late Syphilis.*
1. Manifestations may occur 10–30 years after exposure; recovery unpredictable.
2. Syphilis will mainly affect cardiovascular system (aneurysm of ascending aorta, aortic insufficiency), central nervous system and skeletal system.

Diagnostic Evaluation

There are 2 types of serologic tests:

A. *Nontreponemal or reagin tests*—to detect antibody-like substances called reagin found in serum of infected patient.
1. Flocculation tests—a reaction in which a suspension of antibody particles when added to serum, plasma or spinal fluid containing antibody will form small, usually visible, clumps or floccules.
   a. VDRL (Venereal Disease Research Laboratory)
   b. Kline
   c. Kahn
   d. Hinton
   e. Mazzini
2. Complement fixation tests—involves bringing together an active complement, an antigen and its antibody under proper temperature and time conditions.
   a. Kolmer
   b. Wasserman (no longer in wide clinical use)
3. Rapid reagin tests—specific-purpose tests using flocculation procedures on plasma or serum; used as a rough screening guide.

B. *Treponemal tests*—test for detection of treponemal antibody produced in response to syphilitic infection.
1. Treponema pallidum immobilization test (TPI)
2. Fluorescent treponemal antibody test (FTA)
3. Fluorescent treponemal antibody absorption test (FTA-ABS)

Treatment

The Public Health Service recommends the following treatment schedule according to the stage of syphilis:

A. *Primary, Secondary Syphilis.*
1. Benzathine penicillin—2.4 million units total (1.2 million units in each buttock) by intramuscular injection; or

2. PAM (procaine penicillin G. in oil with 2% aluminum monostearate) 4.8 million units total; usually given 2.4 million units at first session as above and 1.2 million units of each of 2 subsequent injections 3 days apart; or
3. Aqueous procaine penicillin G—600,000 units daily for 8 days to total 4.8 million units.

B. *Latent Syphilis.*
   1. Benzathine penicillin G
      a. If no spinal fluid examination is done, treatment must encompass the possibility of asymptomatic neurosyphilis. In this case, 6.0–9.0 million units total; given 3.0 million units (1.5 in each buttock each session) at 7 day interval.
      b. With nonreactive spinal fluid examination, 2.4 million units (as primary); or
   2. PAM—aqueous penicillin G—same as in primary syphilis.

C. *Alternate Antibiotics.*
   (for patients with penicillin sensitivity)
   1. Erythromycin and tetracycline are the best alternate drugs; 30–40 gm. of erythromycin or 30–40 gm. of tetracycline given orally over a period of 10–15 days.
   2. Treatment with alternate antibiotics must be accompanied by close follow-up of syphilitic patient since none of these drugs has had adequate evaluation in all stages of syphilis. Spinal fluid examination must be done as part of follow-up after this type of therapy.

Prevention

1. All patients known to have been exposed to the lesion of spyhilis should be treated.
2. Preventive treatment (2.4 million units of benzathine penicillin G) should be given before or after exposure.
3. Program of public health and sex education should be conducted.
4. Patient should be instructed to refrain from sexual intercourse with previous partners not under treatment.
5. Mass serologic examinations of special groups with known high incidence of venereal disease should be conducted.

VIRAL INFECTIONS

Smallpox (Variola)

Smallpox is an acute, highly contagious viral disease with a characteristic eruption on the skin and mucous membrane. The virus is transmitted in the skin lesions. Man is the only reservoir.

Clinical Manifestations

1. Prodromal illness—fever, backache, headache, prostration, sore throat, cough (lasting 2–4 days)
2. Characteristics of skin eruption:
   Rash appears on face, neck and upper extremities and spreads distally.
   Rash begins as macules and papules and progresses to vesicle and then to pustules and crusts (scabs) which fall off at the end of the 3rd or 4th week.
3. High mortality rate in the severe form of the disease

Diagnostic Evaluation

Isolation of virus from tissue culture from scrapings of lesions or from vesicular or pustular fluid.

Nursing Isolation Procedures

Strict isolation until all crusts are shed (see p. 820).

Treatment and Nursing Management

Objectives: to give supportive and symptomatic care.

to observe for complications.

1. Give supportive and symptomatic care.
   a. Keep the patient on bedrest.
   b. Control fever with fever sponges, aspirin, etc.
   c. Use analgesic medication to control the severe pains of onset.
   d. Give fluids and electrolytes—amounts, character, route of administration determined by degree or rate of dehydration.
2. Give careful attention to the skin and mucous membranes.
   a. Use antipruritic lotions to relieve itching.
   b. Give sedatives and antihistamine medications to reduce itching.
   c. Protect the skin from bright light.
   d. Employ meticulous oral hygiene measures.
3. Assess the patient for complications. (The treatment of complications is symptomatic.)
   a. Bacterial infections (abscesses, osteomyelitis, septicemia)
   b. Corneal variola—involvement of the cornea
   c. Laryngeal variola—extensive ulceration and edema of larynx
   d. Hemorrhagic smallpox

Preventive Measures

1. Vaccination—inoculation of virus into the skin. (See below.)
2. Methisazone (Marboran)—antiviral chemotherapeutic agent given to exposed individuals or to patients having vaccination reactions.

Smallpox Vaccination

A. *Methods.*
   1. Multiple puncture—a drop of vaccine is placed on the skin; 2–10 indentations (according to age of patient) are made on the skin with a needle.
   2. Scratch method—a 0.625-cm (¼-inch) scratch is made on the skin; a drop of vaccine is then placed over the scratch. (The vaccine can be placed on the skin before the scratch is made.)
   3. Simultaneous puncture—puncture and vaccine made at the same time (administered by means of a plastic device).

B. *Skin Preparation.*
   1. Prepare skin with acetone or ether. (No preparation is needed for clean skin.) (Alcohol may inactivate the virus.)
   2. Avoid traumatizing skin—may produce large lesion.

C. *Vaccination Site*—Place vaccination on outer aspect of left arm above the level of the insertion of the deltoid muscle—less subject to trauma, heat and moisture and protected from friction and scratching.

D. *Care of Vaccination.*
   1. Maintain dryness and free flow of air around site.
   2. Do not use a shield over site.
   3. Avoid washing over site after crust is formed.

E. *Successful Take*—umbilicated vesicle (Fig. 15–2) shows good assurance of immunity. (Fever and lymphadenopathy may accompany primary response.)

F. *Contraindications to Vaccination.*
   1. Eczema and other forms of chronic dermatitis in the person to be vaccinated or in someone in the house.
   2. Pregnancy.
   3. Altered immune states from disease or therapy.

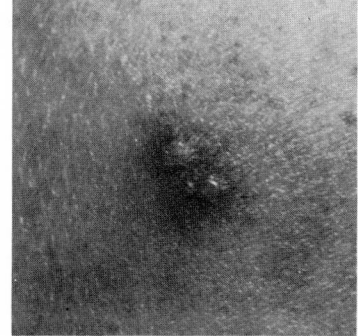

Figure 15-2. Positive reaction to smallpox vaccination.

NURSING ALERT: Smallpox vaccination has a definite, measurable risk of untoward reaction and death. The U.S. Public Health Service recommends that health officials in the U.S. consider discontinuation of compulsory smallpox vaccination. Vaccination should be routinely required only in special risk cases: travelers to and from countries where smallpox is still endemic and health services personnel who come into contact with patients with smallpox.

G. *Complications of Smallpox Vaccination.*
   1. Postvaccinal encephalomyelitis
   2. Allergic reaction
   3. Pyogenic infections
   4. Cutaneous and sometimes generalized reaction

Influenza

Influenza is an acute viral infection which is characterized by respiratory and constitutional symptoms. Epidemics of influenza develop rapidly and there is a fairly high mortality rate among the elderly and those debilitated by chronic disease.

Etiology

Myxovirus containing ribonucleic acid (RNA).
   1. Three crops have been identified: A, B and C.
   2. Group A is the most virulent and is responsible for the most recent epidemics.
   3. The Hong Kong virus is a variant of the A_2 strain.
   4. These 3 groups do not produce cross immunity.

Clinical Course

   1. The virus is airborne and multiplies in the upper respiratory tract—selected invasion of nasal, tracheal and bronchial mucosal cells.

2. Influenza virus damages the ciliated epithelium of the tracheobronchial tree, rendering the patient vulnerable to the development of pneumonia.

Clinical Manifestations

1. Headache and profound malaise
2. Muscular aches—especially in back and legs
3. Respiratory features—dry cough, sore throat, nasal obstruction and discharge
4. Fever—37.8°C. (100°F.)

Treatment and Nursing Management

Objectives: to offer the patient supportive therapy.
to observe for pulmonary complications.

1. Give aspirin or acetaminophen (Tylenol) every 4 hours for fever, headache and myalgia.
2. Offer cough syrup for dry hacking cough.
3. Use a vaporizer—to reduce irritation to respiratory mucosa.
4. Watch for dyspnea in early course of influenza—points to *influenzal pneumonia,* which is a potentially life-threatening disease.
   a. Pneumonia may also be of viral, mixed viral or bacterial origin.
   b. Treat pneumonia (see also p. 158).
      (1) Obtain cultures of throat, blood and sputum immediately.
      (2) Give antibiotic therapy as required—usually penicillin G or erythromycin.
      (3) Assess for vasomotor collapse.
      (4) Observe for acute respiratory failure.
      (5) Initiate tracheal suctioning, tracheal intubation and assisted ventilation as required.
   c. Assess for neurologic complications—from direct invasion of the nervous system or by autoimmune response (hypersensitivity) in the nervous system.

Prevention

1. *Vaccination*
   Active immunization consists of 2 doses (inactivated virus in aqueous suspension of formalin) administered subcutaneously 6–8 weeks apart.
2. Immunization should be reserved for patients at risk:
   a. Rheumatic heart disease (particularly mitral stenosis)
   b. Cardiovascular disorders (arteriosclerotic heart disease, hypertension)
   c. Chronic bronchopulmonary disease (asthma, chronic bronchitis, bronchiectasis, emphysema, advanced tuberculosis)
   d. Diabetes mellitus; Addison's disease
3. Selective use of antiviral chemoprophylactic agents
   a. Amantadine hydrochloride has been used prophylactically against the Asian strain of influenza; may be effective against Hong Kong strain
   b. Patients with high priority for antiviral therapy include:
      (1) Patients with chronic respiratory or cardiovascular disease
      (2) Patients hospitalized for treatment of other illnesses
      (3) Elderly persons residing in nursing homes or other institutions
4. Restrict visiting privileges within hospital or nursing home during epidemics—to minimize chance of introducing influenza.

Infectious Mononucleosis

Infectious mononucleosis (glandular fever; "mono") is an acute infectious disease characterized by sore throat, irregular fever, painful enlargement of the cervical lymph nodes and
prostration. The disease is presumed to be viral in origin although no infectious agent has
actually been isolated from "mono" patients.

Incidence

1. Occurs mainly between ages of 15 and 30.
2. No definite mode of transmission has been established but evidence suggests that
   mononucleosis is spread through the oropharyngeal route; kissing may facilitate the
   spread of "mono" among young adults.

Clinical Manifestations

(Usually are vague and masquerade as those of leukemia, hepatitis, meningitis.)

1. Fatigue
2. Headache, chilliness
3. Irregular fever and sore throat
4. Generalized lymphadenopathy
5. Enlargement of spleen

Diagnostic Evaluation

1. Blood smears—show many abnormal cells, especially lymphocytes.
2. Elevated sheep cell heterophile antibody test—blood from patient with "mono" will
   clump red blood cells of sheep or cow; highest heterophile antibody test found during
   2nd or 3rd week of illness.

Nursing Isolation Procedures

No isolation or precautions required.

Treatment

1. The treatment is symptomatic and supportive.
   a. Encourage patient to obtain additional rest and a well-balanced diet.
   b. Give aspirin for headache, muscle pains and chills.
2. Avoid strenuous exercise—exertion or trauma may cause rupture of spleen. (Competitive sports should be avoided until full recovery.)

Arthropod-borne Viral Encephalitis

Encephalitis (inflammation of the brain) may be caused by a number of agents including
viruses, bacteria and chemicals. The viral encephalitides comprise a group of acute infections
that affect predominantly the nervous system (brain, spinal cord and meninges). Each variety
is caused by a specific virus. For each of these viruses there exists a particular animal reservoir, and each finds its access to man through the bite of a particular species of blood-sucking
arthropod.

Occurrence

1. Eastern equine encephalitis—eastern and north central U.S.A.
2. Western equine encephalitis—western U.S.A.

3. California encephalitis—scattered east and west
4. St. Louis encephalitis—scattered throughout U.S.A.

Mode of Transmission

Bite of infective mosquitoes.

Clinical Manifestations (variable)

Acute onset:

High fever	Signs of meningeal and spinal cord irritation
Severe headache	Disorientation; coma—convulsions in infants

Diagnostic Evaluation

1. Lumbar puncture (p. 720)—reveals lymphocytosis in cerebrospinal fluid
2. Rising titer of complement-fixing or neutralizing antibodies

Treatment

1. Reduce the intracranial pressure.
   a. Assist patient undergoing repeated lumbar punctures if cerebrospinal fluid pressure is elevated.
   b. Give I.V. mannitol or a urea-invert sugar preparation to reduce intracranial pressure.
2. Maintain the airway.
3. Control convulsive seizures (see p. 731).
4. Support patient during periods of prolonged coma (see p. 728).
5. Ensure adequate nutrition.
   a. Give intravenous nutrition for 48–72 hours if patient is comatose.
   b. Feed via nasogastric tube if patient remains in coma (see p. 383).
6. There is no specific therapy for arthropod-borne viral encephalitis.

Nursing Isolation Procedure

No isolation or precautions are necessary.

Rabies (Hydrophobia)

Rabies is an acute severe viral infection of the central nervous system communicated to man from the saliva of infected animals, usually dogs, foxes, squirrels, skunks and bats.

Incubation Period

1. 30 to 60 days to a year in man.
2. Direct relationship between severity and location of bite and length of incubation period.

Clinical Manifestations

1. May occur weeks or months after exposure.
2. May appear in 10 days if head or face is severely bitten.

A. *Prodromal Stage.*

    1. Headache and nausea
    2. Fever
    3. Malaise; loss of appetite
    4. Sore throat
    5. Abnormal sensations around site of infection
    6. Unusual sensitivity to sound, light and changes in temperature
    7. Dilation of pupils; increased salivation

B. *Stage of Excitement.*

    1. Episodes of irrational excitement alternating with periods of alert calm
    2. Convulsions
    3. Severe and painful throat spasms when patient attempts to swallow (or even view) liquids (hydrophobia)
    4. Death usually occurs in this stage from cardiac or respiratory failure

C. *Paralytic Stage.*

    Fatal progressive paralysis

Diagnostic Evaluation

    1. History of exposure and development of characteristic symptoms
    2. Demonstration of rabies antibodies in patient's blood
    3. Demonstration of characteristic *Negri bodies* in samples of brain tissue

Prophylaxis: Management of Patient After a Bite

    1. Cleanse bite wounds immediately and thoroughly with soap and water—to remove saliva from area.
       a. Squeeze wound to promote bleeding—helps to cleanse wound.
       b. Use 70% alcohol or quaternary ammonium (Zephiran) as an antiseptic.
       c. Take patient to physician at once.
    2. Capture dog or animal inflicting the bite and keep under veterinary surveillance—this may enable bitten person to avoid undergoing rabies vaccination unnecessarily.
       a. If animal remains healthy 7–10 days, it is assumed that it was not infective.
       b. If animal becomes ill or dies, notify local health department.
    3. Kill wild animal that bites a person and send head to health department—brain examined immediately for rabies.
    4. If the biting animal escapes or is unknown, determination of the degree of risk is judged by following factors:
       a. Prevalence of rabies in the area   c. Severity of wound(s)
       b. Species of the biting animal   d. Whether attack was provoked or unprovoked
    5. Antirabies serum and vaccine is given if there is a significant likelihood that an individual has been exposed to rabies (not invariably successful). (Vaccination with virus grown in duck embryo and inactivated chemically—DEV.)
       a. Patient inoculated subcutaneously with 1 dose for 14 consecutive days followed by booster doses 10 and 20 days later.
          (1) Usual reactions are redness, itching, pain and tenderness at the site of injection.
          (2) If severe sensitivity appears, patient is given nervous tissue vaccine (NTV) prepared in rabbit brain.
       b. Passive immunization by administration of horse serum containing antibodies to rabies virus may be used along with vaccine treatment.

RICKETTSIAL INFECTIONS

Rocky Mountain Spotted Fever

Rocky Mountain spotted fever (tick-borne typhus fever) is characterized by a continuous fever of 3 weeks duration. It is caused by the bite of an infected tick, by an infected tick being crushed on the skin or via conjunctival contamination with infected tick juice.

Etiology

1. The organism responsible for Rocky Mountain spotted fever is *Rickettsia rickettsii*.
2. The infection has its reservoir in rabbits, small wild rodents and dogs; its principal or sole vector is the wood tick.

Incidence

1. Most prevalent in South Atlantic States
2. Also occurs in western Canada, Mexico, Panama, Colombia and Brazil

Clinical Manifestations

Sudden onset of:
  Shaking chills
  Prostration or lethargy
  Myalgia
  Abdominal pain
  Nausea and vomiting
  High fever—up to 42°C. (107°F.) in severe cases—subsides by lysis
  Rash—appears in 3–7 days (discrete maculopapular lesions appearing on wrists and
    ankles and spreading to other parts of the body; may progress to petechial or
    purpuric stages)

Diagnostic Evaluation

1. Patient's history
2. Positive Weil-Felix test and specific complement fixation test

Treatment and Nursing Management

1. Administer chloramphenicol or tetracyclines as directed—loading dose of 2000 mg. followed by 500 mg. every 6 hours until the temperature is normal.
2. Assist with transfusion of packed red blood cells, platelets, and Vitamin K; administer heparin and injections of albumin—to treat multiple coagulation defects and increase capillary permeability.
3. Give sedatives and analgesics as required for restlessness, insomnia and pain.
4. Utilize supportive nursing measures for combating fever (p. 726) and promoting patient comfort.

Nursing Isolation Procedure

No isolation precautions are required.

Prevention

1. Encourage immunization of high-risk persons (those who are apt to be in tick-infested areas)
2. In a tick-infested area:
   a. Tick repellents should be used.
   b. Body and clothing should be examined for ticks twice daily.
   c. Tick should be removed with a pair of forceps, it should be pulled gently and firmly without being crushed.
   d. Hands should be protected while the tick is being removed.

PROTOZOAN DISEASES

Malaria

Malaria is an acute infectious disease caused by protozoa which strongly resemble leukocytes. Their transmission is by way of an intermediate host, the bite of an infective female Anopheles mosquito. (Malaria has also been transmitted via the use of common needles in narcotic addicts.) The parasite has a complicated life cycle.

Etiology

4 species of malaria parasites—grouped under generic name, *Plasmodium,* each causing a different type of malaria.
1. *P. vivax*—causes benign tertian malaria with a 36- to 48-hour cycle of chills and fever
2. *P. malariae*—causes quartan malaria with fever and chills every 3rd day
3. *P. falciparum*—causes falciparum or malignant tertian malaria (36- to 48-hour cycle)
   a. This is the most serious type of malaria
   b. Infected red cells tend to agglutinate and form microemboli
4. *P. ovale*—less common form of malaria

Clinical Manifestations

1. Paroxysms of shaking chills
2. Rapidly rising fever
3. Profuse sweating
4. Paroxysms last about 12 hours after which cycle may be repeated daily, every other day or every 3rd day

Diagnostic Evaluation

Demonstration of malaria parasites in blood films by microscopic examination.

Clinical Problems

1. The parasite is becoming resistant to major synthetic drugs.
   a. The majority of falciparum cases from Vietnam, Thailand, Cambodia and Laos, and some from other areas of Southeast Asia are resistant. Therefore cases from Southeast Asia are usually assumed to be resistant.
   b. Some falciparum cases in northwest South America (mostly Colombia) are also resistant.
2. The use of antimalarial drugs depends on the stage of the life cycle of the parasite which is affected.

Treatment and Nursing Management

Objective: to destroy the blood trophozoites and schizonts of *Plasmodium* that cause the signs and symptoms and the pathologic effects that characterize the disease.
1. Determine the species of parasite infecting the patient by way of blood smear. The most favorable time for the discovery of the parasite is during and 12–18 hours after a chill.
2. Give specific therapy—the use of antimalarial drugs depends on the stage of the life cycle of the parasite which is to be attacked. See Table 15–2.
3. Make patient comfortable.
   a. Give medication to control headache.
   b. Use nursing measures to reduce fever (see p. 726).
   c. Prevent dehydration.

Nursing Isolation Procedures

1. Blood precautions for duration of hospitalization.
2. Screened rooms in tropical climate.

Preventive Measures

1. Mosquito bites should be prevented.
   a. Effective repellents can be used.
   b. Houses can be sprayed with insecticides.
   c. Bed netting should be used if necessary.
2. Mosquitoes should be destroyed by draining and filling breeding places.
3. All new cases of malaria should be treated.
4. Suppressive drugs can be used for persons temporarily residing or traveling in endemic areas.
   a. Chloroquine (Aralen)   c. Pyrimethamine (Daraprim)
   b. Amodiaquine (Camoquin)   d. Proguanil hydrochloride (Chlorguanide; Paludrine)

PARASITIC INFECTION

Amebiasis (Amebic Dysentery)

Amebiasis is a world-wide parasitic disease which is responsible for multiple medical-surgical problems and is caused by the protozoa, *Entamoeba histolytica*. It is acquired by ingestion of the cyst stage of *E. histolytica* in food or water contaminated by infected human feces.

Incidence

1. In the U.S. found in rural areas or in patients who have lived or traveled in the tropics.
2. Generally limited to warmer regions of the world.

Pathological Insights

1. *E. histolytica* lives in the large intestine feeding mainly on bacteria.
2. Ameba may be located in the bowel lumen, intestinal wall or outside the gastro-intestinal tract.
   a. Trophozoites develop from viable cysts in small intestine.

Table 15-2. Drugs for Malaria*

I. SUPPRESSION AND PREVENTION

	Drug of Choice	Adult Dosage	Alternative Drugs	Adult Dosage
—while traveler is in endemic area *and* for 6 weeks after departing from endemic area	chloroquine phosphate	500 mg. (300 mg. base) once a week	amodiaquine dihydrochloride	520 mg. (400 mg.) once a week
—for 14 days after leaving endemic area	primaquine phosphate[1,2]	26.3 mg. (15 mg. base) daily	none	

II. TREATMENT for infection with *Plasmodium vivax, P. ovale, P. malariae,* or *P. falciparum* (except resistant strains)

	Drug of Choice	Adult Dosage	Alternative Drugs	Adult Dosage
—uncomplicated attack	chloroquine phosphate[3,4]	1 gm. (600 mg. base) then 0.5 gm. in 6 hr. then 0.5 gm. daily for 2 days	amodiaquine dihydrochloride	780 mg. (600 mg.) first day, then 520 mg. (400 mg.) daily for 2 days
—severe illness	chloroquine hydrochloride[4] (parenterally)	250 mg. (200 mg. base) I.M. every 6 hrs. (maximum 1 gm. a day) until oral therapy can be given	none	
—to prevent relapses except *P. falciparum* ("radical" cure after "clinical" cure)	primaquine phosphate[1,2]	26.3 mg. (15 mg. base) daily for 14 days	none	

* The routine use of primaquine for chemoprophylaxis in all civilians who have been in a malaria endemic area is questionable. Intensity of exposure should determine its use.

[1] Dosages of primaquine in excess of 26 mg. (15 mg. base) per day for 14 days may cause hemolytic anemia, especially in patients whose red cells are deficient in glucose-6-phosphate dehydrogenase. This deficiency is more common in Negroes but more severe in Caucasians.

[2] Dosage is oral unless otherwise stated. The World Health Organization has suggested (1965) an initial dose of 10 mg. chloroquine base per kg. of body weight, and subsequent doses of 5 mg./kg.

[3] In falciparum malaria, if the patient has not shown a prompt response to conventional doses of chloroquine, parasite resistance to this drug must be considered.

Table 15-2. Drugs for Malaria* (continued)

III. *TREATMENT* for infection with resistant *Plasmodium falciparum*[5]

—uncomplicated attack	quinine sulfate[6]	650 mg. 3 times a day for 14 days	sulformethoxine[7,8] 1 gm. once
	plus pyrimethamine[9]	25 mg. 2 times a day for 3 days	*plus* pyrimethamine[9] 50 mg. once
	plus either sulfadiazine	500 mg. 4 times a day for 5 days	
	or dapsone	25 mg. daily for 28 days	
—severe illness	quinine dihydrochloride[10]	600 mg. in 300 ml. normal saline i.v. over at least 30 min., repeat in 6-8 hrs. until oral therapy is possible	none

[5] Chloroquine-resistant strains of *P. falciparum* have been reported from Brazil, Cambodia, Colombia, Guyana, Malaya, South Vietnam, and Thailand.

[6] Quinine alone will control an acute attack of resistant *P. falciparum*, but in a substantial proportion of infections, particularly strains from Southeast Asia, it fails to prevent recurrence. Addition of pyrimethamine, with either sulfadiazine or dapsone, substantially lowers the recurrence.

[7] Not available for clinical use in the United States (March 1969).

[8] A prolonged-action sulfonamide.

[9] To prevent hematologic toxicity from pyrimethamine, it is advisable to administer folinic acid or calcium leucovorin, about 10 mg./day intramuscularly.

[10] Intravenous administration of quinine dihydrochloride can be hazardous, but it is preferred in very seriously ill patients. Constant monitoring of the pulse and blood pressure is necessary to detect arrhythmia or hypotension. Oral quinine sulfate should be substituted as soon as possible.

* Reproduced with permission of the Center for Disease Control, Public Health Service, Atlanta, Georgia.

  b. Trophozoites may erode intestinal mucosa and invade the bloodstream and travel to the liver via the portal circulation.
  c. Amebas can produce abscesses and other serious complications.

Clinical Manifestations

  1. Diarrhea—watery, foul-smelling stools often containing blood-streaked mucus.
  2. Abdominal discomfort.

Diagnostic Evaluation

  1. Stool specimen for *E. histolytica.* (Trophozoites or cysts may be found in the feces.)
     a. Several stool specimens should be collected daily.
     b. Stool specimen should be examined *immediately* for trophozoites.
  2. Positive serological tests (indirect hemagglutination test and complement-fixation test).

Complications

  1. Liver abscess
  2. Lung suppuration
  3. Meningoencephalitis
  4. Intestinal obstruction, rupture of colon; peritonitis
  5. Ameboma (amebic granuloma found in cecum, rectum, transverse colon, sigmoid)

Treatment

Objectives: to give specific therapy.
               to support the patient's general condition.
  1. Specific therapy—metronidazole (Flagyl) is most effective and least toxic intestinal amebacide available.
     a. Single large dose (2.0–2.4 gm.) capable of curing majority of patients with amebic dysentery or with liver abscess.
     b. Metronidazole produces prompt cessation of diarrhea and discharge of parasite from stools in 24 hours.
     c. Serial follow-up of stools is necessary.
  2. Keep patient on bedrest if diarrhea is acute.
  3. Offer nonirritating, low residue, bland foods—weak tea, broth, rice, toast, soft-cooked eggs.
  4. Give infusions as indicated to correct fluid and electrolyte imbalance resulting from severe diarrhea.

Nursing Isolation Procedures

  No isolation or precautions are required.

FUNGAL INFECTIONS

Mycoses

Fungi are primitive organisms that take their nourishment from living plants and animals and decaying organic material. The 3 main types of mycoses (fungal infections) determined by the tissue level at which the fungus settles are:
  1. Systemic or deep mycoses—involving primarily the internal organs, usually centering in the lungs

2. Subcutaneous mycoses—involve the skin, subcutaneous tissue and sometimes the bone
3. Superficial or cutaneous mycoses—grow in outer layer of skin (epidermis), the hair and the nails

Histoplasmosis is a chronic systemic fungus infection caused by a spore-bearing mold called *Histoplasma capsulatum.* This highly infectious mycosis is transmitted by airborne dust which contains *H. capsulatum* spores. (Partially decayed droppings of pigeons, chickens, birds offer an excellent medium for growth of this fungus.)

Clinical Manifestations

(Fungal infections mimic symptoms of other diseases.)
1. Closely resembles pulmonary tuberculosis, including symptoms of fever, cough, dyspnea, anorexia and loss of weight and strength.
2. Patient may present findings of malignant lymphoma, including anemia, thrombocytopenia, splenomegaly, hepatomegaly.
3. Other patients may develop ulcerations at mucocutaneous junctions, e.g., the lip margins and the perianal area.
4. Histoplasmosis may produce bleeding gastrointestinal ulcers and the syndrome of Addison's disease.

Diagnostic Evaluation

1. X-ray—appearance of lesions scattered throughout the lung fields.
2. Positive sputum culture of *H. capsulatum.*
3. Skin test with histoplasmin—shows hypersensitive reaction.
4. Complement fixation titers for histoplasma yeast.

Treatment

1. Amphotericin B is the mainstay of therapy.
   a. Dosage is controlled by blood level studies. (Patient is assessed for renal toxicity, manifested by rising blood urea nitrogen and decreased creatinine clearance.)
   b. Severe toxic reactions to amphotericin B include nausea and vomiting, chills, fever, diarrhea, hypokalemia, phlebitis.
2. Surgery may be done for persistent lung cavitation.

Actinomycosis

Actinomycosis is a chronic suppurative granulomatous disease caused by the fungi of the actinomyces (ray-fungus) group. The characteristic lesions are firmly indurated granulomas which spread slowly to adjacent tissues and break down focally to form multiple sinus tracts which penetrate to the surface. The exudate from the sinus tracts contains the characteristic sulfur granules which are visible masses of the organism.

Portal of Entry

1. Portal of entry is probably the mouth since pathogenic actinomyces *(A. israelii)* inhabit the mouth and tonsillar crypts of apparently healthy individuals, especially those with carious (decayed) teeth.
2. It is not known how and why it becomes invasive.

Clinical Manifestations

1. *Cervicofacial type*—swelling about the teeth, submaxillary region and neck producing a flat, hard painless tumor mass which is fixed firmly to the jawbone. Granuloma ultimately breaks down and becomes riddled with abscesses which perforate externally.
2. *Abdominal type*—affects any visceral organ, especially the cecum and appendix, ovaries and tubes. Tumor mass, resembling carcinoma, develops. By extension it may involve the abdominal wall, discharging externally through open sinuses.
3. *Thoracic type*—acute and chronic inflammatory reaction may involve lungs, pleura, mediastinum or chest wall, producing chest pain, fever, cough and hemoptysis.

Treatment

1. Give penicillin (drug of choice)—large doses are given parenterally for 4–6 weeks until the disease is eradicated.
2. Give lincomycin or other antibiotic as ordered if the patient is allergic to penicillin.
3. Prepare for surgical excision of infected tissue as necessary.
4. Encourage good dental hygiene to reduce infection around teeth.

HELMINTHIC INFESTATIONS

Trichinosis

Trichinosis is infestation by the parasite *Trichinella spiralis*, one of the roundworms.

Clinical Course

1. Tiny embryos of the parasite *Trichinella spiralis* become encysted in the muscle fibers of an infected pig.
2. These calcified cysts appear in meat (pork) like tiny grains of sand.
3. If insufficiently cooked pork is eaten, the embryos are set free by the gastric juice and develop in the intestine during the following week, becoming adult worms, 3–4 mm. long.
4. These worms make their way into the mucous membranes and there produce myriad embryos (period of invasion).
5. The embryos, carried by the bloodstream and their own activity, migrate to all parts of the body (period of migration).
6. The embryos gradually become encysted, each in a muscle fiber, after which there are no symptoms.

Clinical Manifestations

Intestinal stage

1. Malaise
2. Gastrointestinal complaints, diarrhea
3. Mild fever
4. Nausea and vomiting

Muscular invasion (symptoms develop from inflammatory process developing in the muscles).

1. Edema of the eyelids; scleral hemorrhages
2. Generalized pain and soreness in the muscles (myalgia)
3. Cardiac irregularities (occasional)—from trichinae in the heart muscle; may be fatal
4. Difficulty in breathing, masticating, swallowing and speaking

Diagnostic Evaluation

1. Biopsy specimen of muscle—reveals embryos. (Deltoid, biceps gastrocnemius muscles are sites of biopsy.)
2. Positive serologic tests (precipitin, complement-fixation, flocculation, fluorescent-antibody)—demonstrable titers 3–4 weeks after infection.
3. Rising eosinophil count—appears in 2nd week.
4. Positive skin test.

Treatment

The treatment is symptomatic.
1. Thiabendazole (Mintezol) 20–25 mg./kg. of weight is given twice daily for 1 day; may be repeated in 7 days.
   a. Thiabendazole produces clinical improvement but its effect on larvae that have migrated to muscle is not conclusive.
   b. Adverse effects—nausea, vertigo, headache and weakness.
2. Steroidal anti-inflammatory agents may be given to relieve symptoms in the acute stage.
3. Keep the patient on bedrest.
4. Give analgesics to relieve muscle pain.
5. Carry out ECG evaluations to determine evidence of myocarditis.

Preventive Measures

1. Public should be educated regarding the importance of thoroughly cooking all pork and pork products, especially sausage. There should be no trace of pink in cooked pork.
2. Garbage intended for feed for hogs should be cooked.
3. Pork should be inspected to determine if disease is present.

Hookworm Disease

Hookworm disease (ancylostomiasis; ground itch) is the result of infestation of the upper part of the small intestine by one of 2 quite similar roundworms about 1.2 cm. (½ inch) long:
   Uncinaria americana (the New World hookworm)
   Ancylostoma duodenale (the Old World form)
The infection is usually contracted by persons walking with bare feet over contaminated soil.

Incidence

1. Southeastern U.S.
2. Endemic in tropical and subtropical countries

Clinical Course

1. Hookworm eggs are passed in human feces onto the ground (indiscriminate defecation habits). Eggs develop into infective larvae.
2. The larvae enter through the mouth if the individual eats with dirty hands, or they *bore through the skin of bare feet* ("ground itch").
3. After gaining access to the blood or lymph vessels, they are carried via the blood to the lungs, migrate from the pulmonary capillaries into the alveoli, reach the pharynx and are swallowed, maturing to adult forms in the bowel.

Clinical Manifestations

1. *Gastrointestinal symptoms*—maturation of worms in the intestine is usually marked by onset of diarrhea and other gastrointestinal symptoms:
   a. Diarrhea
   b. Nausea and vomiting
   c. Flatulence and constipation
   d. Intestinal cramps
2. *Severe anemia*—the worms attach to intestinal mucosa and suck blood; a single adult worm can extract 0.05 ml. of blood daily. Thus a patient with pronounced hookworm infestation may lose over 100 ml. of blood daily.
   Severe anemia may produce:
   a. Symptoms of heart failure
   b. Tachycardia
   c. Poor growth and development
3. *Dry cough and dyspnea*—from rupture of larvae through the capillary bed and their dissemination throughout bronchial tree.

Diagnostic Evaluation

1. History of anemia and malnutrition
2. Recovery and identification of eggs in feces

Treatment

1. Specific therapy: one of following drugs.
   a. Tetrachloroethylene (Perchloroethylene)
   b. Hexylresorcinol
      or
   c. Bephenium hydroxynaphthoate (Alcopar)

NURSING ALERT: Alcohol should not be ingested 24 hours before or after the use of these anthelminthics as it reduces their effect.

---

2. Ensure that the patient is eating a nutritious diet—hookworm disease occurs in persons suffering from malnutrition.
   a. Correct anemia prior to therapy for worms in patients with severe anemia.
   b. Give protein and iron supplementation—to aid in correction of anemia.
3. Instruct the patient to wear shoes at all times.
4. Dispose of excreta in a sanitary manner.

Ascariasis (Roundworm Infestation)

Ascariasis is an infection caused by *Ascaris lumbricoides* (intestinal roundworm) characterized by an early pulmonary invasion from larval migration and a later more prolonged intestinal phase.

Incidence

Occurs throughout the world in both temperate and tropical areas, particularly in areas of poor sanitation.

Clinical Course

1. Indiscriminate defecation in streets, fields and doorways provides a major source of infective eggs.
2. Eggs are swallowed and pass into intestine where they hatch into larvae.
3. Larvae reach liver and lungs via blood or lymphatic system.
4. After reaching the lungs, they pierce the capillary wall, crawl up the trachea and are swallowed to be returned to the small intestine where they grow, mature and mate.

Clinical Manifestations

1. *Pulmonary phase*—pneumonitis develops from invasion of lungs by large number of larvae.
2. *Intestinal phase*—masses of worms cause gastrointestinal discomfort, severe abdominal pain, vomiting.

NURSING ALERT: Large numbers of worms may migrate into various organs of the body and cause obstruction (to the trachea, bronchi, bile duct, appendix, pancreatic duct).

Diagnostic Evaluation

1. Stool specimen—for detection of ova and worms in stool.
2. Patient occasionally vomits a worm.

Treatment

1. Piperazine citrate—roundworm is susceptible to paralyzing action of this medication.
   a. Give drug daily for 1 week.
   b. Drug clears intestinal tract of worms without the aid of a laxative.
2. Pyrvinium pamoate is another roundworm anthelmintic.

Preventive Measures

1. All patients with infections should be treated.
2. Adequate toilet facilities should be provided.
3. The importance of personal hygiene should be taught.

Enterobiasis (Pinworm Disease; Oxyuriasis)

The pinworm *(Enterobius vermicularis)* is a small white thread-like worm, about 0.5 cm. long, commonly found in the rectum of children.

Clinical Problems

1. Enterobiasis (pinworm) is the most common helminthic infection in the U.S.
2. One pinworm may release over 10,000 eggs.
3. The gravid female worm migrates from the anus and deposits the eggs about the anus.
4. The infection cycle (from egg [ova] to larva to adult worm) requires 3–6 weeks.
5. Scratching leads to contamination of the hands and nails; hand to mouth contact results in reinfection.
6. Infective eggs may contaminate food and drink, bed linen, dust, etc.

Clinical Manifestations

1. Intense itching (nocturnal) about the anus—from nocturnal migration of gravid females from anus and deposition in eggs in perianal folds of skin
2. Restlessness; irritability

Diagnostic Evaluation

1. Anal impressions on cellophane tape for 7–10 days (Fig. 15-3).
2. Detection of characteristic eggs in freshly passed stool or about the anus.

Treatment

1. Give pyrvinium pamoate (Povan) (5 mg./kg. of body weight).
   a. A single dose is given when patient is in fasting state.
   b. This medication coats the stool a bright red; alert the patient and family to this fact.
2. Piperazine citrate (Antepar) may be an alternate drug which is given for 7 days.
3. All members of large families with repeated infestations should receive medication several times yearly.
4. Teach measures of personal cleanliness:
   a. Cut fingernails short—eggs may be obtained from beneath the nails of infected persons.
   b. Wash hands with soap and water after using toilet and before meals.
   c. Wash around anal area upon arising.
   d. Apply salve or ointment to anal area—to prevent dispersal of eggs.
   e. Infected child should wear tight fitting cotton pants—to discourage contact of hands with perianal region and contamination of bed linen.
   f. See that the infected person sleeps alone.
   g. Handle bedding and night wear carefully—there are large numbers of infective eggs in a contaminated house that cause reinfection.

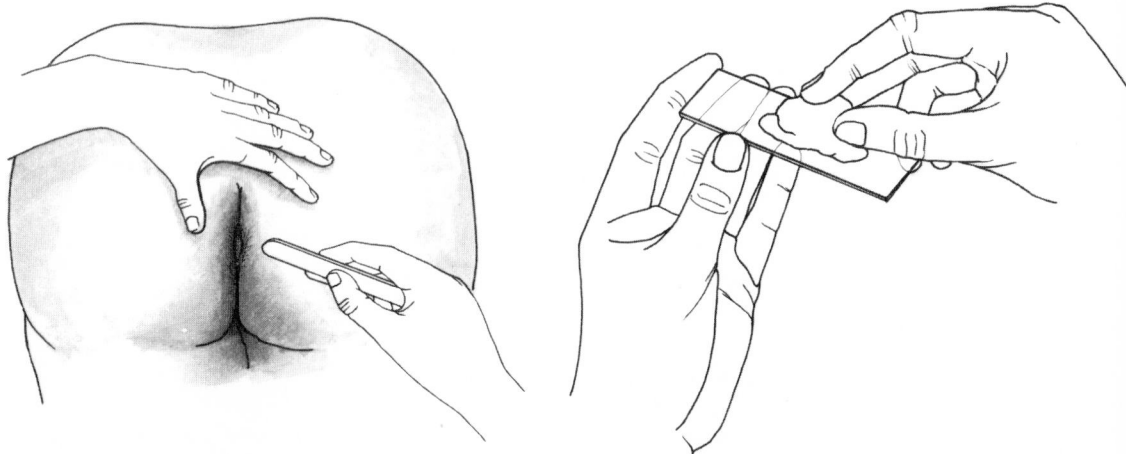

Figure 15-3. Collecting the eggs of the pinworm. Cover a tongue blade with clear tape with the adhesive side out. Blot around the anal area to pick up the eggs. Then place the tape on a glass slide. The slide is examined microscopically.

BIBLIOGRAPHY

Books

Beck, J. W., and Connor, E. B.: Medical Parasitology. St. Louis, C. V. Mosby, 1971.

Behbehani, A. M.: Human, Viral, Bedsonial and Rickettsial Diseases. Springfield, Charles C. Thomas, 1972.

Benenson, A. S. (ed.): Control of Communicable Diseases in Man. Washington, D.C., American Public Health Association, 1970.

Brown, H. W.: Basic Clinical Parasitology. New York, Appleton-Century-Crofts, 1969.

Brown, W. J., et al.: Syphilis and Other Venereal Diseases. Cambridge, Harvard University Press, 1970.

Brunner, L., et al.: Textbook of Medical-Surgical Nursing, 2nd ed. Philadelphia, J. B. Lippincott, 1970, pp. 891–945.

Conant, N. F., et al.: Manual of Clinical Mycology. Philadelphia, W. B. Saunders, 1971.

Cutting, W. C.: Handbook of Pharmacology. New York, Appleton-Century-Crofts, 1969, pp. 373–380.

Edams, E. B., et al.: Tetanus. Oxford, Blackwell Scientific Publications, 1969.

Emmons, C. W., et al.: Medical Mycology. Philadelphia, Lea and Febiger, 1970.

Gibson, G. L.: Infections in Hospitals. Baltimore, Williams and Wilkins, 1971.

Jawetz, E., et al.: Review of Medical Microbiology. Los Altos, Lange Medical Publications, 1970.

Johnston, D. F.: Essentials of Communicable Disease. St. Louis, C. V. Mosby, 1968.

King, A., and Nicol, C.: Venereal Disease. Philadelphia, F. A. Davis, 1969.

Maegraith, B. G., and Gilles, H. M. (eds.): Management and Treatment of Tropical Diseases. Oxford, Blackwell Scientific Publications, 1971.

Riemann, H. (ed.): Food-borne Infections and Intoxications. New York, Academic Press, 1969.

Schwartz, S. I.: Tropical Surgery. New York, McGraw-Hill, 1971.

Top, F. H., and Wehrle, P. F.: Communicable Infectious Diseases. St. Louis, C. V. Mosby, 1972.

U.S. Dept. of Health, Education and Welfare: Isolation Techniques for Use in Hospitals. Washington, D.C., U.S. Government Printing Office, 1970.

Articles

Altemeier, W. A., et al.: Prevention and treatment of gas gangrene. JAMA, *217*:806–813, Aug. 9, 1971.

Brashear, R. E., et al.: Trichinosis and respiratory-failure. Am. Rev. Resp. Dis., *104*:245–248, Aug. 1971.

Brooks, G. F., et al.: Tetanus toxoid immunization of adults: a continuing need. Ann. Intern. Med., *73*:603–606, Oct. 1970.

Canfield, C. J., et al.: Treatment of acute falciparum malaria from Vietnam with Trimethoprim and Sulfalene. Amer. J. Trop. Med. Hyg., *20*:524–526, July 1971.

Carruthers, M. M.: Diagnosis and management of flu. Amer. Fam. Phys., *2*:118–122, Nov. 1970.

Chen, W. J., et al.: Colon perforation in amebiasis. Arch. Surg., *103*:676–680, Dec. 1971.

Clinicopathologic Conference: The Medical complications of influenza. Amer. J. Med., *50*:105–112, Jan. 1971.

Counts, G. W., et al.: Shiga bacillus dysentery acquired in Nicaragua. Arch. Inter. Med., *128*:582–584, Oct. 1971.

Feigin, R. D., et al.: Treatment of penicillin-resistant staphylococcal infections with Clindamycin. Amer. J. Med. Sci., *261*:207–212, April 1971.

Foster, M. T., Jr.: Diagnosis and treatment of venereal disease. Postgrad. Med., *50*:67–73, July 1971.

Garner, J. S., and Kaiser, A. B.: How often is isolation needed? Amer. J. Nurs., *72*:733–737, April 1972.

Gould, S. E.: The story of trichinosis. Amer. J. Clin. Path., *55*:2–11, Jan. 1971.

Hart, M.: Gonorrhea in women. JAMA, *216*:1609–1611, June 1971.

Herban, N. L.: Nursing care of patients with tropical diseases. Nurs. Clin. N. Amer., 5:157–164, March 1970.

Holmes, K. K., et al.: Disseminated gonococcal infection. Ann. Intern. Med., 74:979–993, June 1971.

Kvale, P. A., et al.: Single oral dose Ampicillin-Probenecid treatment of gonorrhea in the male. JAMA, 215:1449–1453, March 1971.

Lentz, J.: The nurse's role in extending infection control to the community. Nurs. Clin. N. Amer., 5:165–174, March 1970.

Lenz, P. E.: Venereal disease. Women, the unwitting carriers of gonorrhea. Amer. J. Nurs., 71:716–719, April 1971.

Lindsay, M. I., Jr., et al.: Hong Kong influenza: clinical, microbiologic and pathologic features in 127 cases. JAMA, 214:1825–1832, Dec. 7, 1970.

————: Primary influenzal pneumonia. Postgrad. Med., 49:173–178, May 1971.

Martin, J. E., et al.: Comparative study of gonococcal susceptibility to penicillin in the United States, 1955-1969. J. Infect. Dis., 122:459–461, Nov. 1970.

Neal, R.: Pathogenesis of amoebiasis. Gut, 12:483–486, July 1971.

Parker, J. D., et al.: Treatment of chronic pulmonary histoplasmosis. New Eng. J. Med., 283:225–229, July 30, 1970.

Powell, S. J.: New developments in the therapy of amoebiasis. Gut, 11:967–969, Nov. 1970.

Prather, J. R., et al.: Actinomyocosis of the thorax. Ann. Thorac. Surg., 9:307–312, April 1970.

Reddy, P., et al.: Progressive disseminated histoplasmosis as seen in adults. Amer. J. Med., 48:629–636, May 1970.

Richards, T., et al.: Gentamicin treatment of staphylococcal infections. JAMA, 215:1297–3000, Feb. 22, 1971.

Sabin, A. B.: Control of infectious diseases. J. Infect. Dis., 121:91–94, Jan. 1970.

Schroeter, A. L., and Pazin, G. J.: Gonorrhea. Ann. Intern. Med., 72:553–559, April 1970.

Sodeman, W. A., Jr.: Amebiasis. Am. J. Dig. Dis., 16:51–60, Jan. 1970.

Sparling, P. F.: Diagnosis and treatment of syphilis. New Eng. J. Med., 284:642–653, March 1971.

Storlie, F.: Ann: A child with botulism poisoning. Nurs. Clin. N. Amer., 6:563–566, Sept. 1971.

Tong, M. J., et al.: Clinical and bacteriological evaluation of antibiotic treatment in shigellosis. JAMA, 214:1841–1844, Dec. 7, 1970.

Utz, J. P.: Symposium on treatment of the systemic mycoses. Mod. Treat., 7:509–615, May 1970.

Vanek, J., and Schwartz, M.: The gamut of histoplasmosis. Amer. J. Med., 50:89–104, Jan. 1972.

Walker, D. G.: Clinical manifestations and treatment of tetanus. J. Oral Surg., 27:826–827, Oct. 1969.

Webster, B. (ed.): Symposium on venereal diseases. Med. Clin. N. Amer., 56 (entire volume), Sept. 1972.

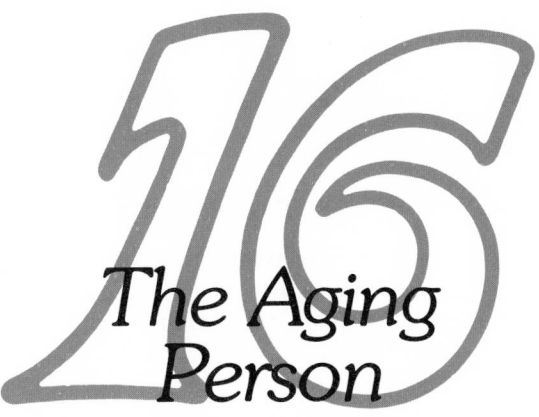

The Aging Person

Definitions

Gerontology is the study of older persons and the aging process.

Social gerontology is the study of the aging process and its impact upon the individual and his society.

Geriatrics is medical treatment of older persons.

BODILY CHANGES ASSOCIATED WITH AGING

General Principles

1. Aging begins at conception and proceeds at different rates in different individuals.
2. Aging proceeds at different rates in different systems in the same individual.
3. There is a reduction of reserve capacity due to actual loss of individual cells in various organs and tissues of the body.
4. So many changes come with aging that these changes cannot be termed abnormalities.

Changes in the Nervous System

1. Progessive loss of brain cells—nerve cell loss frequently is gradual and diffuse
2. Progressive atrophy of the convolutions (gyri) of the brain surface and consequently widening and deepening of the spaces (sulci) between the convolutions
3. Decrease in blood flow to the brain by 20% per unit of remaining brain cells
4. Increased reaction times and increased time in decision making
5. Associated psychological and motor impairment—impairment in short-term memory but not in long-term memory
6. Personality changes—appear to be related to blood supply to brain as well as changes in nervous system:
   a. Loss of interest; failure to accept new ideas
   b. Melancholia; pessimism

    c. Loss in intensity of emotional response; loss of adaptability
    d. Abnormal possessiveness
    e. Mental confusion (if patient has advanced senility)

Changes in Skin and Subcutaneous Tissues

1. Skin becomes inelastic and wrinkled (from changes in collagen and elastic fiber), wrinkled and atrophic (thinner).
    Fissuring may occur—from atrophy of dermal layer.
2. Focal pigmentary discolorations occur.
3. Ecchymoses appear—due to increased fragility of the dermal and subcutaneous vessels.
4. Sweating decreases.
5. Body unable to regulate temperature—in part due to loss of subcutaneous tissue.

Changes in the Skeletal System

1. Loss of muscle power—thinning of muscle fibers, loss of cross striations
2. Postural changes—from structural changes in ligaments, joints and bones. Ligaments calcify and ossify; joints stiffen from erosion of cartilaginous joint surfaces; and ossification and degenerative changes occur in synovium (lining of joint cavities)
3. Increase in curvature of spine—from atrophic changes of fibrocartilaginous discs which cushion the vertebrae
4. Bone changes—bones become porous and lighter and lose much of their density (osteoporosis, see p. 808)

Changes in the Special Senses

1. Vision—decrease in visual acuity, decreased accommodation to light, falling off of lateral vision, receding clarity
    Clinical problems include presbyopia (farsightedness), senile cataract, glaucoma
2. Hearing—loss of hearing ability, inability to hear higher pitches, increased difficulty in hearing normal ranges of sound
3. Voice—lower volume; increasing difficulty and slowing of speech (may be due to lesions involving motor nerves controlling muscles of speech, etc.)
4. Smell and taste—decrease in sense of smell and in number of taste buds

Changes in the Cardiovascular System

A. *Heart*

1. Decrease in effective heart function
2. Hypertrophy of the heart (from disease)—impedes facility of oxygen diffusion
3. Decreased cardiac output
4. Increase in peripheral resistance to blood flow and increased systolic blood pressure
5. Aged hearts exhibit more arrhythmias—leads to poor oxygenation of the heart

B. *Vascular*

1. Elongation of arteries (become tortuous and calcify)
2. Fibrosis and narrowing of inner lumen of arteries
3. Thickening of basement (supporting) membrane in vessels of all sizes

Changes in the Respiratory System

1. Decreased elasticity of lungs and chest wall—due to infiltration and deposition of collagen
2. Less oxygen diffusion—due to increase in collagen and scar tissue of lung and decreased blood flow to the lung
3. Decreased blood flow to lungs—contributes to arrhythmias
4. Decline in total lung capacity—producing decrease in function

Changes in the Gastrointestinal System

1. Diminishing volume of gastric acid
2. Decreasing peristalsis—from generalized weakness of muscle activity

Changes in the Urinary System

1. Decrease in kidney function and adaptability
2. Reduction of blood flow to kidneys—due to decreased cardiac output and increased peripheral resistance (from cholesterol deposits along the arteries)
3. Diminished filtration rate and tubular function
4. Structural changes in kidneys

Changes in the Endocrine Glands

1. Decrease in the effectiveness and interaction of hormones—exaggerated under stress
2. Decrease in glucose utilization
3. Decrease in adrenal activity—may affect older person's adaptation to stress
4. Deficit in anabolic steroids—may be responsible for loss of muscle power
5. Decreased basal metabolic rate
6. Decrease in body water—exhibited by decrease in body weight

Changes in the Reproductive System

1. Period of menopause for women
2. Sexual activity not necessarily impaired in men

Changes in Homeostasis

Homeostasis is the ability of body to restore equilibrium.
1. Decrease in functional capacity and decrease in functioning of coordinating systems within the body
    Progressively limited capacity to respond to stress
2. Diminution in functional reserve—person more vulnerable to disease, death more likely; increased time required for body to return to normal after illness

PSYCHOSOCIAL INFLUENCE OF AGING ON HEALTH

Psychosocial Aspects

Health is interrelated with psychosocial aspects of aging.
1. *Low self-esteem from many losses*
    a. Losses through death of spouse, children, other "significant persons."
    b. Loss of social roles and resources—affects status and prestige; person may withdraw and disengage himself from the mainstream of life.

    c. Socioeconomic losses—decreased income; inflation
        Affects quality of health care, self-esteem and position in society.
    d. Loss of work role—produces sense of uselessness; feelings of nonparticipation.
2. Social isolation and loneliness—can lead to mental and physical deterioration.
    Social participation is important to mental health.
3. Lack of resilience in recovery from illness and stress.
4. Lack of meaningful activity.
5. Youth worship by society—makes elderly feel inferior, inadequate and unattractive.
6. Decline in physical and mental capabilities—poor memory, loss of speed and agility.
7. Sensory disabilities—makes individual suspicious and distrustful of others.

Physical Disabilities Affecting Adaptation

1. Perceptual impairment
2. Hearing losses—lead to depression and suspiciousness
3. Lack of sexual desire and capacity
4. Loss of speed and psychomotor response
5. Subjective awareness of aging
6. Cultural devaluation
7. Slowing down of psychological processes

Adaptive Techniques Employed by the Aged

1. Disengagement—mutual withdrawal between individual and society; can produce chronic depression
2. Activity
3. Paranoid retreat
4. Integration—person accepts aging and ages gracefully

DISEASE ASPECTS OF AGING

Effects of Disease on Health

1. Manifestations of disease are modified by old age.
2. More than one disease may be present—over 40% of elderly have more than one illness.
3. Elderly respond more slowly and to a lesser degree to treatment.
4. There is less resistance to stress—one major illness lowers resistance and allows other illnesses to appear.
5. Illness tends to cluster around closing years of life with the very aged—chain types of reaction of one degenerative process leading to another and finally to death.

Physical Illness

1. Most common diseases are those of circulatory system and arteriosclerosis.
    Arterial disease causes cardiac, renal and neurologic problems.
2. Elderly are more vulnerable to acute infections of respiratory tract—increasing numbers have chronic lung disease.
3. Elderly are prone to gastrointestinal diseases; particularly functional diseases.
4. Incidence of cancer increases—may be of many years' duration.
5. Elderly have changes in arterial walls (arteriosclerosis), in joint spaces (arthritis) and in functioning of certain endocrine glands (diabetes).

Mental Illness

1. Older persons account for 25% of annual mental hospital admissions.
2. Underlying cause of mental illness in aged is frequently organic brain injury from strokes or vascular conditions—may produce major psychoses.
3. Patient may exhibit delusions, hallucinations and other signs of brain decompensation.
4. Most common emotional problem is *anxiety* (may be associated with depression).

MEDICAL AND NURSING MANAGEMENT OF THE AGED

Preventive Care and Health Maintenance

Objective: to maintain the health status and functioning ability of elderly people who are well.

1. Promote positive feelings about health of the aged.
2. Educate older person on ways to conserve his health.
3. Encourage periodic health appraisal and counseling to give attention to health before illness develops.
   a. Health assessment techniques utilize automated procedures and computer analysis and read-out results to obtain base-line health information.

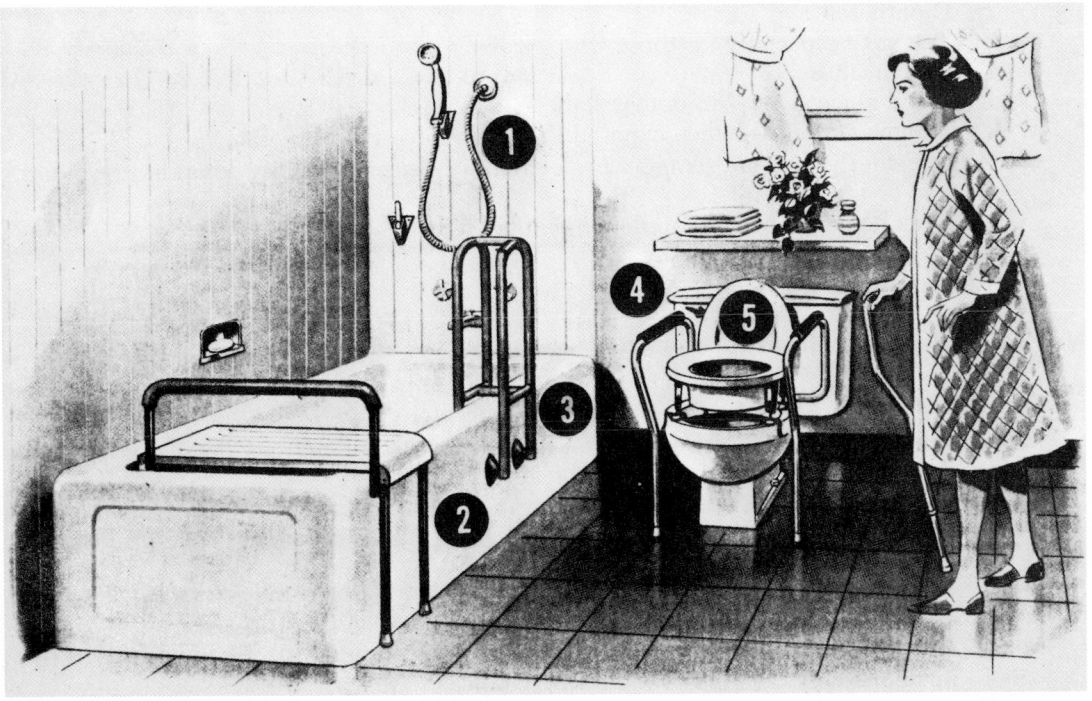

Figure 16-1. Aids to accident prevention in the bathroom. (1) Flexible-hose shower nozzle enables the person to be seated while showering, (2) tub seat; (3) grab-bar to help person step over the tub; (4) toilet equipped with arm rests to help retain balance and to aid in transfer to and from toilet; (5) raised toilet seat that is helpful to weak, elderly or arthritic person. (From the booklet, *Patient Care in the Home.* Courtesy, Lumex, Inc.)

b. Self-administered medical history is combined with certain physiological measurements to secure a health profile of the individual.
   (1) Collects a broad range of physiologic measurements and psychosocial data.
   (2) Helps in determining the state of wellness.
   (3) Aids in determining the probability of presence of one or more diseases.
   (4) Helps medical personnel to see *change*—provides patterns essential to early disease detection.
4. Promote accident prevention among the elderly and their families (Fig. 16-1).
   High incidence of falls due to age and pathological conditions, locomotor disabilities and environmental risks.
5. Schedule and coordinate restorative and therapeutic health services.
   a. Electrocardiogram—to show subtle heart abnormalities
   b. Chest x-ray—for tuberculosis, lung cancer, heart size, changes in large blood vessels and bony structure of chest
   c. Pulmonary function tests—to rule out chronic bronchitis and emphysema
   d. Tonometer test—to measure intraocular pressure for glaucoma
   e. Blood glucose test—to detect diabetes mellitus
   f. Papanicolaou smear—to detect cancer of cervix
6. Protect patient against infectious diseases with immunizations.
   a. Smallpox—every 5 to 10 years
   b. Diphtheria
   c. Tetanus (especially for those who garden)
   d. Poliomyelitis
   e. Blood glucose test—to detect diabetes mellitus
   f. Gamma globulin—when exposed to certain infectious diseases
7. Advise elderly to avoid temperature extremes (especially if individual has respiratory disease or arthritis).
   a. Keep home properly heated and ventilated.
   b. Wear appropriate clothing.
8. Ensure proper nutrition.

Nutritional Considerations for the Aged

1. Nutritional requirements of the elderly are similar to those of adults except that caloric intake should be reduced.
   a. Energy needs diminish with age—metabolic rate and activity decreases indicating that the caloric requirements of the aged are reduced.
   b. The caloric intake is adjusted on an individual basis to maintain normal weight.
   c. Protein requirements are not reduced but protein utilization may be decreased with age.
   d. Calcium intake should be as great as that of a younger person—high prevalence of osteoporosis in older person.
   e. Older persons usually have inadequate intake of calcium and ascorbic acid from inadequate use of milk, fruit and vegetables in the diet.
2. Nutritional deficiencies are frequently encountered in the aged.
   a. Vitamin C and vitamin K deficiency—ecchymoses from capillary fragility
   b. Vitamin A deficiency—fissuring of skin around mouth
   c. Vitamin B deficiency—glossitis, angular stomatitis
   d. Mineral deficiencies—demineralization of bone

3. Factors affecting nutritional habits of the elderly
   a. Food habits of a lifetime
   b. Social factors (eating alone)
   c. Food fads
   d. Poor dental health; ill-fitting dentures
   e. Shopping problems
   f. Reduced income
   g. Lack of motivation for meal planning and food preparation
   h. Decreased appeal of food—loss of taste buds; decreased sense of smell
4. Assistance programs
   Home delivered meals; "Meals on Wheels"

Nursing Approach to the "Confused" Elderly

1. Changes in mental status may be the first sign of illness in the elderly.
   a. Expect an underlying physical cause in any patient who has sudden changes in intellectual functioning.
   b. Confusion may develop from pneumonia, cardiac failure, coronary occlusion, strokes, dehydration, anemia, malignancy.
2. Aging is not synonymous with senility—senile dementia is a *degenerative* disease of the elderly.
3. A new environment may bring on senile behavior without physiological causes.
   a. Be optimistic in outlook over this turn of events; act on the assumption that this behavior is temporary.
   b. Accept the person as he is now, without judgment or criticism.
   c. Pay attention to what the patient is saying—often a person who is considered confused is only transiently so and much of what he is saying makes sense.
   d. Attempt to alleviate the patient's anxiety.
      (1) Try "laying on of hands"—many aged persons have no one to touch them.
      (2) Use warm baths, warm milk, back massage and understanding and compassion as therapeutic modalities.
   e. Call the person by name each time a contact is made.
   f. Show the person the nurse's name tag.
   g. Keep the patient oriented to time and place.
      Keep a calendar with easily seen numbers and a clock within his vision
   h. Schedule the patient's daily activities and adhere to the schedule to promote security.
   i. Arrange for visits from others to counteract isolation.
   j. Learn of former interests and talk about them.
   k. Keep a night-light on during the night.
   l. Remove unduly stressful stimuli.

Summary of the Principles Underlying the Nursing Management of the Elderly

1. Nursing care must be individualized, taking into consideration the patient's past experiences, needs and individual goals.
2. The patient should be an active participant in his own plan of care.
   a. Consult him for his preferences.
   b. Ask his opinions.
   c. Encourage him to make choices and decisions.

    d. Support him during his periods of anxiety.
    e. Urge him to remain active.
3. Nursing activities should be done *with* the patient rather than *for* him.
4. The individuality of the person should be encouraged.
    Preserve his identity and sense of control.
5. Necessary modifications and compromises imposed by the physiological limits of aging must be made in the medical and nursing management of the patient.
6. Realistic and attainable goals, understood by the aged individual, should be set to help him gain a sense of accomplishment and purpose.
    Communicate to the patient the planned goals of his care.
7. The elderly should be kept in the mainstream of life to prevent mental deterioration.
8. The nursing approach must communicate to the patient that he has value as an individual and status as a member of the family and society.
9. Utilize the potentialities of the patient.

BIBLIOGRAPHY

Books

Brunner, L., et al.: Textbook of Medical-Surgical Nursing, 2nd ed. Philadelphia, J. B. Lippincott, 1970, pp. 41–58.
Chinn, A. E. (ed.): Working With Older People: Clinical Aspects of Aging. Vol. IV. U.S. Department of Health, Education and Welfare, Washington, D.C. U.S. Government Printing Office, 1971.
Cowdry, E. V., and Steinberg, F. W.: The Care of the Geriatric Patient. St. Louis, C. V. Mosby, 1971.
Hoffman, A. M. (ed.): The Daily Needs and Interests of Older People. Springfield, Charles C Thomas, 1970.
Howell, T. H.: A Student's Guide to Geriatrics. Springfield, Charles C Thomas, 1970.
Jaeger, D., and Simmons, L. W.: The Aged Ill. New York, Appleton-Century-Crofts, 1970.
Koller, M. R.: Social Gerontology. New York, Random House, 1968.
Merkin, L.: The Old Age Story. New York, Vantage Press, Inc., 1971.
Poe, W. D.: The Old Person in Your Home. New York, Charles Scribner's Sons, 1969.
Rossman, I.: Clinical Geriatrics. Philadelphia, J. B. Lippincott, 1971.
Routh, T. A.: Choosing a Nursing Home. Springfield, Charles C Thomas, 1970.
Townsend, C.: The Nader Report. Old Age: The Last Segregation. New York, Grossman Publishers, 1971.
Working With Older People: The Practitioner and the Elderly. Vol. I. Washington, D.C., U.S. Government Printing Office, 1969.

Articles

Frenay, A. C., et al.: The climate of care for a geriatric patient. Amer. J. Nurs., 71:1747–1750, Oct. 1971.
Kamenetz, H.: Exercises for the elderly. Amer. J. Nurs., 72:1401, August 1972.
Knowles, L. N. (ed.): Symposium on putting geriatric nursing standards into practice. Nurs. Clin. N. Amer., 7:201–309, June 1972.
Murray, R. L.: Caring. Amer. J. Nurs., 72:1286–1287, July 1972.
Ornstein, S.: Objective—a national policy on aging. Amer. J. Nurs., 71:960–963, May 1971.
Rodstein, M.: Health problems of the aged. RN 35:39–43, August 1972.
Wilkiemeyer, D. S.: Affection: key to care for the elderly. Amer. J. Nurs., 72:2166–2168, Dec. 1972.

17 Nursing the Person with Cancer

GENERAL CONSIDERATIONS

Cancer's Warning Signals

C hange in bowel or bladder habits
A sore that does not heal
U nusual bleeding or discharge
T hickening or lump in breast or elsewhere
I ndigestion or difficulty in swallowing
O bvious change in wart or mole
N agging cough or hoarseness

Benign and Malignant Tumors

	BENIGN	MALIGNANT
Type of Cell	Adult	Young
Nature	Closely resembles parent tissue	Tends to be anaplastic (reverting to primitive cells)
Growth	Slow	Rapid, usually
Encapsulated	Often	Never
Effect on surrounding tissue	Never invades	Invades widely

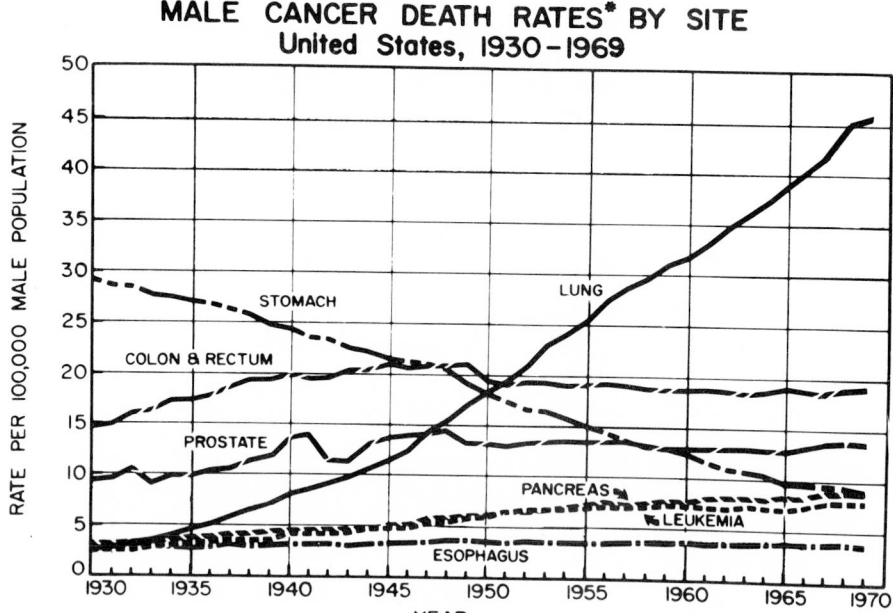

MALE CANCER DEATH RATES* BY SITE
United States, 1930-1969

*Rate for the male population standardized for age on the 1940 U.S. population.

Sources of Data: National Vital Statistics Division and
Bureau of the Census, United States.

RESEARCH DEPARTMENT
AMERICAN CANCER SOCIETY

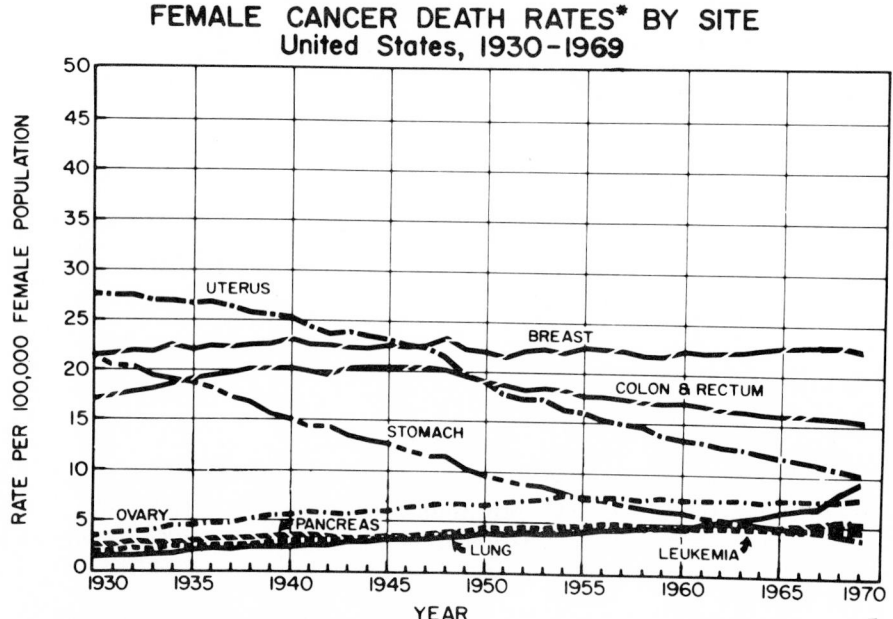

FEMALE CANCER DEATH RATES* BY SITE
United States, 1930-1969

*Rate for the female population standardized for age on the 1940 U.S. population.

Sources of Data: National Vital Statistics Division and
Bureau of the Census, United States.

RESEARCH DEPARTMENT
AMERICAN CANCER SOCIETY

	BENIGN	MALIGNANT
Localization	Remains at original site	Nonlocalized—forms secondary growths by metastasis
Recurrence after removal	Does not tend to recur	Tends to recur

Metastasis

Metastasis is the transfer of disease cells from one organ or part to another not directly connected.

1. *Extension and invasion*—because they are not encapsulated, it is easy for cancer cells to invade other tissues and extend themselves rapidly via lymphatic and blood circulatory systems; cancer may also recur in treated areas.
2. *Lymph*—secondary growths of tumor cells are often caught in the lymph filter, the lymph node.
3. *Blood*—by invasion, tumor cells enter the blood vessels and are carried to organs where the venous blood passes through a capillary bed.

Incidence

1. The annual death toll from malignancy in the U.S. is at least 350,000.
2. Cancer ranks second as the leading cause of death in the U.S.
3. About 1 million Americans are under medical care for cancer.
4. Cancer strikes at any age. It affects children as well as adults, but it strikes with increasing frequency with advancing age.
5. There will be about 650,000 new cancer cases this year (diagnosed for the first time).
6. No organ of the body is exempt. (See accompanying charts for cancer death rates by site.)

Treatment

1. Modalities of treatment include surgery, radiotherapy, radioactive substances including radioisotopes, and various drugs (pharmaceuticals and hormones). (See pp. 873–888.)
2. Method of treatment will depend upon the type of malignancy, stage, localization or spread, and the physician; a single method or combination of methods may be required.

Surgery

1. *Biopsy*—a piece of tissue is cut out surgically from the questionable area and sent to pathology laboratory for diagnostic verification.
2. *Preventive or prophylactic surgery*—removal of lesions which, if left in the body, are apt to develop into cancer. Example: polyps in rectum may lead to cancer of colon.
3. *Palliative surgery*—a type of surgery which attempts to relieve the complications of cancer, e.g., obstruction of the gastrointestinal tract, pain produced by tumor extension into surrounding nerves.

4. *Curative surgery*—the removal of the primary site of malignancy and any lymph nodes to which the neoplasm has extended. Such surgery in itself may be all that is required.

5. *Surgery combined with radiation or chemotherapy*—combinations of treatment required to halt the spread of a malignancy.

NOTE: Details of surgical treatment are given in the sections relating to specific disease entities.

CHEMOTHERAPY FOR CANCER

Value of Chemotherapy in Treating a Malignancy

1. As yet no drugs are available to cure most malignant tumors. Chemotherapy is used successfully in treating choriocarcinoma.

2. Cancer chemotherapy offers some relief to patients for whom surgery and irradiation are no longer beneficial.

3. Effects of chemotherapy:
   a. May produce a regression of the tumor or its metastasis.
   b. May reduce or slow the appearance of secondary growths.
   c. May relieve pain and other symptoms for a time.
   d. May improve quality of survival.

4. Chemotherapeutic agents are useful in treatment of lymphomas and leukemias, solid tumors of the breast and choriocarcinoma. Leads to remissions on occasion for many years.

5. Many chemotherapeutic agents have unpleasant systemic effects in addition to their effect on malignant tissue; therefore, it is imperative that these be recognized by the nurse.

Pharmacologic Action

1. These drugs are capable of destroying young, rapidly multiplying cells, such as malignant cells.

2. They interfere with manufacture of nucleic acids so that cellular growth and reproduction are inhibited.

3. Since many normal cells in the body also grow rapidly and have short life spans (e.g., bone marrow, gastrointestinal tract lining, hair follicles), many chemotherapeutic agents directly attack these normal cells. Herein lies the challenge.

Specific Agents Used in Cancer Chemotherapy (See Table 17-1)

A. *Polyfunctional Alkylating Agents* (cytotoxic or lethal to cell).
   Example: nitrogen mustard
   1. These agents destroy normal and tumor cells, particularly bone marrow cells.
   2. They act with deoxyribonucleic acid (DNA) in cell nucleus to hinder cell growth and division.
   3. Early toxic signs—nausea, vomiting, stomatitis and diarrhea.
   4. Later toxic manifestations—severe bone marrow depression with leukopenia, thrombocytopenia.

B. *Antimetabolites*—synthetic substances similar to those that nourish normal cells during growth and development.

    Examples: folic acid, methotrexate, 6-mercaptopurine, 5-fluorouracil

    1. Such drugs cannot be used by the cell; actually they deceive the cell.
    2. More suitable for prolonged constant administration.
    3. Toxic signs—nausea, vomiting, stomatitis, diarrhea.
    4. Major toxic manifestations—oral and digestive tract ulcerations, bone marrow depression with leukopenia, thrombocytopenia and bleeding.

C. *Steroid Compounds*

    Examples: Cortisone, estrogen therapy (androgen, estrogen, progestin) vs. ablative procedures (castration, hypophysectomy).

    1. Alters the endocrine environment, e.g., castration for prostatic cancer; androgen and estrogen therapy for breast cancer.
    2. Toxic signs—fluid retention, nausea, vomiting.
    3. Major toxic manifestations—masculinization or feminization (depending upon steroid), fluid retention, hypertension, increased susceptibility to infection.

D. *Major Drugs and Their Toxic Manifestations*

Drug	Toxic Manifestations
1. Vinca alkaloids	
Vinblastine	Nausea, vomiting, alopecia, bone marrow depression, areflexia, local irritation
Vincristine	Areflexia, peripheral neuritis, paralytic ileus, muscle weakness, bone marrow depression, alopecia, local irritation
2. Procarbazine	Nausea, vomiting, bone marrow depression, leukopenia, thrombocytopenia, central nervous system depression
3. Enzymes (L-asparaginase)	Nausea, vomiting, anorexia, somnolence, weight loss, lethargy, confusion, hypoproteinemia, hypolipidemia, azotemia, granulocytopenia, lymphopenia, thrombocytopenia
4. Antibiotics	
Dactinomycin	Erythema, ulceration of oral mucosa, local irritation
Mithramycin	Fever, nausea, vomiting, stomatitis, bleeding syndrome, drowsiness, hypocalcemia, bone marrow depression

Method of Administration

Drugs may be given orally, intravenously, intramuscularly or intra-arterially, depending upon the drug.

A. *Isolation-Perfusion*—administration of large doses of extremely toxic drugs to an isolated extremity, organ or region of the body (excluding systemic circulation). Usually such a dose cannot be tolerated by the entire body. By this means, short intensive recirculation of high doses of antineoplastic drugs is used.

TABLE 17-1. DRUGS USED AGAINST CANCER*

Common name	Other names	Acute Leukemia Granulocytic	Acute Leukemia Lymphocytic	Chronic Leukemia Granulocytic	Chronic Leukemia Lymphocytic	Adrenal cancer	Brain tumors	Breast cancer	Burkitt's lymphoma
ALKYLATING AGENTS:									
BCNU	1,3-Bis(2-chloroethyl)-1-nitrosourea						●		
Busulfan	Myleran			●					
CCNU							●		
Chlorambucil	Leukeran				●			●	
Cyclophosphamide	Endoxan, Cytoxan		●		●			●	●
Dibromomannitol	DBM, Myelobromal			●					
Nitrogen mustard	HN2, Mustargen, Mechlorethamine							●	
Phenylalanine mustard	L-Sarcolysin, Melphalan, Alkeran								
Pipobroman	Vercyte			●					
ThioTEPA	TSPA							●	
Triethylene melamine	TEM							●	
ANTIBIOTICS:									
Actinomycin D	Dactinomycin, Cosmegen, Meractinomycin								
Adriamycin		●	●						
Bleomycin									
Daunomycin	Rubidomycin, Daunorubicin	●	●						
Mithramycin	Mithracin								
Mitomycin C									
Streptozotocin									
ANTIMETABOLITES:									
6-azauridine triacetate	Azaribine								
Cytosine arabinoside	Ara-C, Cytarabine, Cytosar	●	●						
5-fluorouracil	5-FU							●	
6-mercaptopurine	6-MP, Purinethol	●	●	●					
Methotrexate	Amethopterin		●						
Thioguanine	TTG	●	●						
HORMONAL AGENTS:	Hormonal agents are known by a variety								
Adrenal cortical compounds:	of trade names.								
Cortisone			●					●	
Hydrocortisone			●					●	
Prednisolone			●					●	
Prednisone			●		●			●	
Androgens:									
Delta-1-testololactone								●	
Fluoxymesterone								●	
Testosterone propionate								●	
Estrogens:									
Diethylstilbestrol								●	
Ethinyl estradiol								●	
Other:									
ACTH			●						
Progesterone									
MISCELLANEOUS:									
Hydroxyurea	Hydrea			●					
Imidazole carboxamide	NSC-45388								
L-asparaginase	EC-2		●						
Methyl hydrazine derivative	MIH, Natulan, Procarbazine, Ibenzmethyzin, Matulane								
Methylglyoxal-bis-guanyl-hydrazone	Methyl-GAG	●							
o,p'-DDD	Mitotane					●			
MITOTIC INHIBITORS:									
TMCA	Trimethylcolchicinic acid	●						●	
Vinblastine sulfate	Velban								
Vincristine sulfate	Oncovin		●						

* Courtesy: National Institute of Health.

Choriocarcinoma	Colon cancer	Endometrial cancer	Ewing's sarcoma	Head & neck cancer	Hodgkin's disease	Lung cancer	Lymphosarcoma	Melanoma	Multiple myeloma	Mycosis fungoides	Neuroblastoma	Osteogenic sarcoma	Ovarian cancer	Pancreatic islet cell tumors	Polycythemia vera	Prostatic cancer	Reticulum cell sarcoma	Retinoblastoma	Rhabdomyosarcoma	Sarcomas (general)	Stomach cancer	Testicular cancer	Wilms' tumor
	•				•	•			•														
					•																		
					•		•						•				•					•	
			•		•	•	•		•		•		•				•						
					•	•	•						•				•						
								•	•			•											
														•									
					•		•						•					•					
					•		•						•					•					
•			•																	•		•	•
			•		•	•	•				•	•					•		•			•	
				•	•		•										•					•	
																						•	
												•									•		
														•									
•										•													
	•												•									•	
•																							
•				•																		•	
							•																
							•																
							•																
							•										•						
														•									
														•									
	•																						
								•															
								•															
					•																		
								•															
•					•		•																
			•		•		•				•						•			•			•

1. Areas
   a. Lower extremity—iliac, femoral, popliteal arteries and veins
   b. Pelvis—abdominal aorta, vena cava
2. Patient Preparation
   a. Weigh patient since drug dosage is calculated on basis of kilograms of body weight.
   b. Obtain blood, urine and x-ray studies.
   c. Explain to the patient the nature of the procedure and the reason for applying tourniquets.
3. Operative Procedure
   a. A totally occlusive tourniquet may be applied to an extremity in order to separate this area from systemic circulation.
   b. A pump oxygenator is used to circulate patient's blood in a closed system for the involved part of the body.
   c. Concentrated doses of the chemotherapeutic agent are injected.
   d. Length of time of perfusion depends on drug and extent and location of growth.
   e. Oxygenated blood is pumped into the artery, passed through the extremity involved by the tumor and out through the vein where the blood is reoxygenated and recirculated.
   f. For an abdominal or lower pelvic tumor, a laparotomy may be done.
      (1) Blood supply to the tumor area is blocked from systemic circulation by means of pneumatic tourniquets on the legs and special clamps on the inferior mesentery artery and vein.
      (2) Catheters are inserted into the major vessels near the tumor site.
      (3) The desired drug is injected into the artery; venous blood is conveyed to an oxygenator for oxygenation, and is then pumped back into arterial system.
      (4) Upon completion of treatment, fresh blood may be transfused if necessary, clamps and tourniquets are removed and the surgical wound is closed.

B. *Intra-arterial Infusion*—the introduction percutaneously of a catheter into a major artery under fluoroscopic guidance. This does not require major surgery and can be repeated at intervals. The continuous administration of the chemotherapeutic agent into the artery leading to the tumor may last for several days or several weeks.

1. Routes
   Brachial, axillary, carotid or femoral artery—determined by location of tumors
2. Uses and Advantages
   a. This method is used preferably when the tumor is completely encompassed by the vessels in question; to check this, fluoroscein may be injected into the catheter and the tumor observed under a special lamp for fluorescence.
   b. Arterial infusion acts on the tumor over a longer period of time than is possible with isolation perfusion.

D. *Adjunct Chemotherapy*—administration of a chemotherapeutic agent at the time of surgery to kill any tumor cells which may spill into the bloodstream when the tumor is manipulated.

E. *Combined Chemotherapy and Irradiation*—permits drug to enhance the effect of irradiation. This has been particularly effective in treating head and neck lesions.

Medical and Nursing Care of Patients Receiving Perfusion or Arterial Infusion

Before Special Treatment

1. The patient needs concerned care; these are procedures (perfusion and arterial infusion) which are tried because the disease is advanced but limited to an anatomic area.
2. Provide encouragement as well as enough description of the procedure to acquaint patient with the possible benefits as well as dangers.
3. Give emotional support since the effects of chemotherapy can cause depression because of the unpleasant side effects.

During Chemotherapy

1. Be familiar with the nature of the chemotherapeutic agent being used (toxic manifestations, etc.).
2. Observe arterial injection site to see that catheter is properly positioned. Hemorrhage, sepsis and tissue irritation are problems that also need to be guarded against.
3. Note any signs of malaise, nausea, vomiting, temperature elevation, changes in blood pressure and pulse.
4. Report input and output accurately.

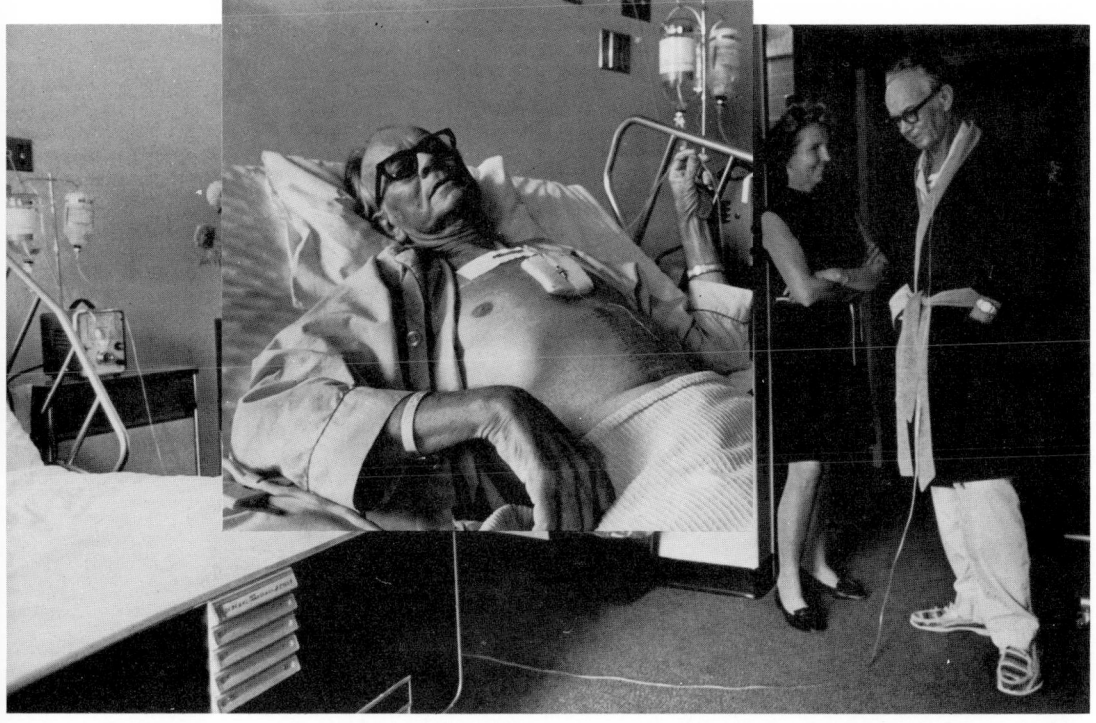

Figure 17-1. This patient is receiving regional chemotherapy via a catheter placed into the nutrient artery in the tumor region. Such medication can be received while he is ambulatory. Note tube leading to pump at left. When he goes home, he will use a portable pump. (From RN, Feb. 1972.)

5. If necessary, administer fluids intravenously for first 48 hours to maintain general hydration as well as dilution of post-treatment antineoplastic drugs.
6. Record local or systemic changes in detail, such as diarrhea or melena.
7. Observe skin tissue in local area for reaction—erythema, blistering, edema, petechiae.
8. Check mucous membranes for signs of tissue breakdown, hemorrhage or infection.
9. Turn patient frequently because of increased possibility of pressure area breakdown.

Management of Complications

A. *Blood Difficulties*
   1. Withdraw drugs if leukocyte or platelet counts fall to dangerous levels.
   2. If leukocyte count is below 1200, obtain a culture to assist in determining specific treatment.
   3. Practice reverse isolation when leukocyte count falls to low levels, or discharge the patient.
   4. Administer packed cells if anemia occurs.
   5. Give platelet transfusions if thrombocytopenia (deficiency of all the cell elements of the blood) is severe; steroids may also be used.

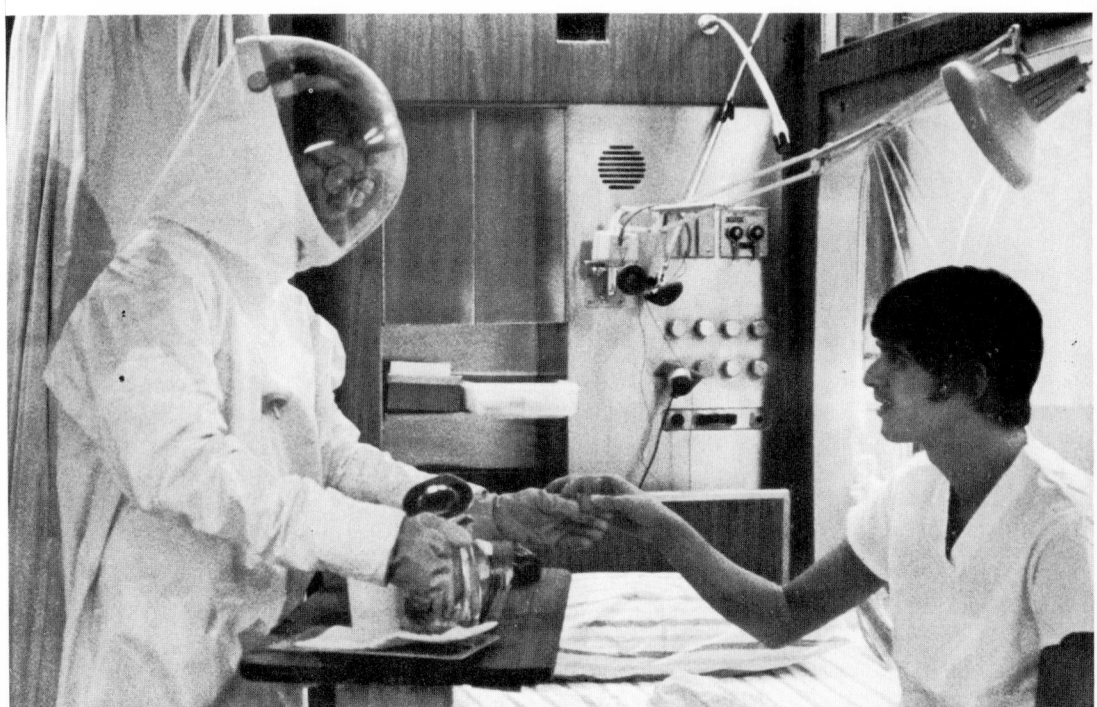

Figure 17-2. A nurse gives nursing care to the patient inside a germ-free unit. All materials in this unit are sterile, and vertical airflow (laminar) prevents cross-contamination from nurse to patient. The nurse wears a special outfit which is attached to a train allowing her to move about freely. (From RN, Feb. 1972.)

B. *Mucositis*
   1. Stop drug administration.
   2. Use hydrogen peroxide 1½ % as a mouthwash.
   3. Apply viscous Xylocaine jelly to mucous membrane as a topical anesthetic.
   4. See that patient avoids irritating foods and fluids, e.g., toast, citrus fruit juices.

C. *Alopecia (Loss of Hair)*
   1. Reassure patient that hair will grow back.
   2. Suggest a wig or hair piece if the hair loss is anticipated.

D. *Diarrhea*
   1. Withdraw drug if diarrhea is uncontrolled.
   2. Administer supplemental intravenous fluids to combat dehydration.
   3. Administer diphenoxylate hydrochloride (Lomotil).

E. *Nausea and Vomiting*
   1. Withdraw drug if not controlled.
   2. Administer supplemental intravenous fluids to combat dehydration.
   3. Give antiemetics: chlorpromazine (Thorazine), prochlorperazine (Compazine).
   4. Pass a nasogastric tube for hyperalimentation if anorexia is a problem.

F. *Infection*
   1. Administer antibiotics along with chemotherapeutic agents.
   2. Utilize "Life Island" where available to provide a protected environment. (Fig. 17-2).

Nursing Care of the Patient Receiving Chemotherapeutic Agents for Neoplastic Disease

1. Recognize signs of toxicity from the chemotherapeutic agent being administered.
   a. Note that signs vary from patient to patient.
   b. Utilize combative measures to offset minor disturbances.
   c. Anticipate that the patient will experience discomforts but avoid suggesting to the patient that they might occur since psychologically this might hasten their occurrence.
2. Be alert for manifestations of gastrointestinal tract disturbances.
   a. Observe for signs of discomfort.
   b. Symptoms—stomatitis, nausea and vomiting, diarrhea.
   c. Recognize that the patient's nutritional status may be jeopardized.
   d. Be cognizant of imbalance of fluids and electrolytes.
3. Note the manifestations of bone marrow depression.
   a. Check for reduction in number of leukocytes, erythrocytes and platelets.
   b. Observe for evidence of infection and bleeding tendencies.
   c. Guard against exposure to infection since patient's resistance is decreased.
4. Assess status of oral mucosa and utilize measures to minimize mucosal trauma.
   a. Initiate a program of administering oral care so that mouth does not become a breeding place for bacteria.
   b. Cleanse the mouth with nonabrasive soft materials.
   c. Apply a soothing coating such as glycerin and lemon swab.

5. Maintain adequate nutritional levels, recognizing that there may be nausea, vomiting, anorexia, stomatitis and oral mucositis.
    a. Regulate temperature of fluids and foods coming in contact with the oral mucosa; avoid temperature extremes—too hot or too cold.
    b. Modify chemical and mechanical factors in an effort to avoid tissue trauma of the mouth—use soft toothbrush and soothing dentifrices and mouthwash; avoid ill-fitting dentures.
    c. Avoid highly seasoned foods, particularly if patient ordinarily thrives on such foods.
    d. Discourage smoking and use of alcoholic beverages since these irritate the mucous membranes.
6. Attend to the psychosocial needs of the patient receiving chemotherapeutic agents.
    a. For hair loss, recognize that this change in physical appearance may result in antisocial behavior and depression.
    b. Recommend the wearing of a wig or attractive head scarves; hair pieces for men and women are fashionable.
    c. Utilize any and all measures that will tend to distract the patient from himself; provide diversional and recreational therapy.
    d. Provide rest periods that are conducive to rest—quiet, relaxing backrubs, soft music, comfortable surroundings.
    e. Be honest with the patient in all aspects of his therapy and condition. To promote self-sufficiency and self-esteem, allow him to be a participant in the planning of his care.
    f. Encourage the patient to stay on the therapeutic program.

RADIATION IN DIAGNOSIS AND THERAPY

Radiation is frequently used to diagnose and treat cancer.

Sources of Radiation

1. Naturally occurring radioactivity—radium, radon
2. Artificially produced radioactivity—radioisotopes
    a. Internal application

Gold	^{198}Au	Iodine	^{131}I
Phosphorus	^{32}P	Iridium	^{192}Ir
Cobalt	^{60}Co		

    b. External application

Cobalt teletherapy	^{60}Co
Cesium teletherapy	^{137}Cs

    c. X-ray machines

30–120 Kev	Van de Graaff (2 Mev)
250 Kev	Betatron (24 Mev)
Million Volt	

Definitions

1. *Nuclide*—any atomic entity capable of existing for a measurable lifetime, usually more than 10^{-9} seconds.
2. *Radionuclide* (radioactive nuclide)—one that disintegrates with the emission of particular or electromagnetic radiations.

3. *Radioactivity*—the disintegration of the atom which gives up energy in the form of rays or particles.

4. *Isotope*—an element whose nucleus contains a fixed number of protons but has a differing number of neutrons, thereby changing its weight.
   a. Optimal ratio between proton and neutrons is stable.
   b. By using nuclear reactors, it is possible to bombard a stable isotope with additional free neutrons.
   c. Most radioisotopes emit:
      (1) Particulate radiation—small fragments of the nucleus having mass and size (alpha and beta particles).
      (2) Electromagnetic radiations—rays that have no mass (x-rays).

5. *Radioactive Decay or Disintegration*
   a. The rate of decay varies from isotope to isotope.
   b. 'Half-life' or decay rate is the time required to reduce a particular radioactive substance by one-half of its atoms, thereby reducing it to half its initial activity. Example: Radium–225—half-life of over 1600 years.
   c. A radioisotope administered to a patient in unsealed form has a relatively short life and is essentially inactive after therapeutic use has been completed. Example: ^{131}Iodine—half-life about 8 days.
   d. Longer lasting isotopes are implanted temporarily in the patient in a sealed container, Example: ^{60}Co—half-life about 5 years.

6. *Units of Measurement (Activity)*
   a. Curie (c.)—basic unit to measure amount of activity in a radioactive sample
   b. Millicurie (mc.)—one thousandth of a curie
   c. Microcurie (μc.)—one millionth of a curie
   d. Picocurie (pc.)—one billionth of a curie

7. *Units to Measure Amount of Radiation Exposed to or Absorbed by a Substance.*
   a. Roentgen (r.)—a standard unit of exposure (usually applied to x-ray or gamma rays)
   b. Milliroentgen (mr.)—one thousandth of a roentgen
   c. Rad—a unit to measure absorbed dose
      (1 rad = amount of radiation required to deposit 100 ergs of energy per gram of irradiated material)
   d. Rem—a unit of measure of radiation-dose equivalent which relates to biological effectiveness (roentgen equivalent man)
      Standards have been established by the International Committee on Radiation Protection (I.C.R.P.) that the maximum permissible dose (M.P.D.) for radiation workers is 5 rems for persons over age 18.

Biological Aspects and Clinical Application

A. *Nature and Indications for Use*
   1. Individualized to produce effective ionization within a tumor while avoiding unnecessary irradiation of normal structures
   2. Low voltage—Kev (thousand electron volts)
      Super voltage—Mev (million electron volts)
   3. Tissues most likely to respond to radiation exposure—those originating from reticuloendothelial tissues (leukemia, lymphomas) and those from embryonal tissues (teratomas)
   4. Tissues least likely to respond—bone and muscle

B. *Factors Affecting the Benefit of Radiation Exposure vs. Risk of Tissue Damage*
   1. *Dose rate*—a prescribed dose causes less tissue destruction if given in small amounts over a long period of time rather than given all at once.
   2. *Area of Body Exposure*—the larger the area exposed, the greater the effect.
   3. *Cell susceptibility*
      Greater susceptibility—rapidly dividing cells with no specialized function (Example: lymphocytes and germ cells)
      Lesser susceptibility—nondividing cells and highly differentiated cells (Example: nerve or muscle cells)
   4. *Biological variability*—individual differences play a role in human susceptibility. Examples:
      a. Healthy person more responsive than malnourished individual.
      b. Skin is especially vulnerable to radiation injury.
      c. Bone marrow is very radiosensitive; therefore, such damage is potentially the most lethal.
      d. Radiation cataracts result from excessive eye exposure.
      e. Lung fibrosis occurs, following injudicious radiation of chest.

C. *Symptoms of Radiation Syndrome*
   Major portion of body exposed to large doses of irradiation (*over 100 rems*) in a short period of time
   1. Prodromal—nausea, vomiting, malaise
   2. Latent—symptoms subside
   3. Illness—general malaise, epilation (hair loss), hemorrhage (petechiae, nosebleed), pallor, diarrhea, inflammation of mouth and throat, leukopenia
   4. Recovery or death

D. *Symptoms of Radiation Syndrome*
   Low levels of radiation over a long period of time
   Examples:
   1. Radiologists may acquire leukemia
   2. Radium-containing luminizing paint (clock dial painters)—may develop sarcomas
   3. Gonad exposure to radiation—may affect progeny

E. *Roentgenologic Precautions During Radiography, Fluoroscopy or Radiotherapy*
   1. No one permitted in the room where the patient is undergoing x-ray therapy or roentgenography.
   2. Fluoroscopic equipment should not leak radiation.
   3. Fluoroscopic room attendants should be protected from scattered radiation by wearing lead aprons and, if necessary, lead-impregnated gloves.
   4. Appropriate lead shielding should be available to protect the patient's gonads during radiation exposure.

Nursing Support and Action in Radiation Therapy

A. *Physical and Psychological Preparation of the Patient.*
   1. Remove all opaque objects such as pins, buttons and hairpins, and replace clothing with a gown for body x-rays.
   2. Have patient remain perfectly still; maintain position with use of sandbags, etc. if required.

3. Tell patient that there will be no sensation or pain accompanying picture taking or penetration of x-rays.
4. Advise him that he will be alone in the room for the protection of the technician but that he will be in voice contact.
5. Determine from the physician what he has told the patient relative to radiotherapy, particularly if it is administered to the patient with advanced cancer.
6. If a series of treatments are to be given, include the patient in the planning phase.
7. Give special attention to diet and medications; administer antinauseants, analgesics, specifics for diarrhea, proctitis and cystitis.
8. Explain the need for routine blood counts.

B. *Skin Manifestations.*
   1. Inform the patient that some skin reaction can be expected but that it varies from patient to patient. Example: dry erythema, desquamation, moist erythema, healing, epilation, tanning, telangiectasis.
   2. Apply no lotions, ointments, cosmetics, etc. to the site of radiation unless prescribed by the physician; avoid talcum powder because it contains heavy metals which are irritating.
   3. Discourage vigorous rubbing, friction or scratching because it can destroy skin cells; apply a bland ointment (with vitamins A and D).
   4. Exert caution against irritation from friction, exposure to sunlight and extremes in temperature.
   5. Do not apply adhesive or scotch tape to the skin.

C. *Systemic Reactions.*
   Nausea, vomiting, fever, loss of appetite, malaise.
   1. Administer sedatives for greater comfort.
   2. Select fluids and foods that will not induce or aggravate nausea.
   3. Provide smaller frequent meals rather than 3 larger meals.
   4. Suggest time for rest and relaxation; avoid noise, confusion.
   5. Recognize that the patient needs encouragement and understanding.

RADIOISOTOPE THERAPY

Types of Radioisotope Therapy

A. *Teletherapy*—utilizing gamma rays from a radioactive source which is kept in a shielded unit placed at a distance from the patient.
   1. Radioisotope Cobalt-60 (^{60}Co) and Cesium-137 (^{137}Ce) deliver radiation similar to that produced by supervoltage x-ray apparatus.
   2. ^{60}Co therapy unit requires extra shielding because rays are being emitted constantly. Because gamma rays cannot be absorbed entirely, personnel are advised to spend minimum time in this room.
   3. *Advantages of ^{60}Co over conventional x-ray.*
      a. Skin problems are significantly reduced.
      b. Bone or cartilage involvement is lessened.
      c. Electronic circuits are not required.
   4. *Disadvantages of ^{60}Co.*
      a. Because it has a half-life of 5 years, it is necessary to replace the ^{60}Co.
      b. Radiation energy cannot be varied.
      c. Cost of room shielding is high.

B. *External Molds*—a packaged and screened container in which a radioisotope can be placed and applied directly to the skin surface.

    Examples:

    1. ^{60}Co can be applied in this manner to small areas such as in the treatment of carcinoma of the lip, larynx, ear, etc.

    2. ^{182}Ta (radioactive tantalum) can be applied in a flexible wire mold such as to the external surface of a retinoblastoma involving eyeball and optic nerve.

    3. ^{90}Sr (radioactive strontium) and ^{90}Y (yttrium) such as an external mold used for shallow irradiation of eye neoplasms.

C. *Intracavitary Isotope Therapy.*

    Examples:

    1. Liquid radioisotopes—^{198}Au (radioactive colloidal gold)
                       —^{20}Na (radioactive sodium)
                       —^{82}Br (radioactive bromine)
    used in the balloon of a catheter inside the bladder for internal bladder radiation of a few millimeters.

    2. Capsules containing ^{182}Ta (radioactive tantalum) may be packed in the body of the uterus, cervical canal or maxillary sinus.

D. *Interstitial Isotope Therapy*

    Examples:

    1. Radioactive needles, seeds, tubes or wires can be implanted directly into tumor tissue: Cobalt-60, Cesium-137, Gold-198, Radon-222, Tantalum-182, and Iodine-125.

    2. These may be temporary or permanent; they may be supplementary to surgery or to external beam irradiation.

    3. Radioactive solutions may be injected directly into the tumor or surrounding tissue. Colloidal solutions of radioactive colloidal gold (^{198}Au) is one of the most commonly used solutions.

E. *Internal Irradiation*

    Examples:

    1. Oral ingestion of solutions of radioiodine (^{131}I) are administered to patients with hyperthyroidism.

    2. Intravenous injection of sodium phosphate (^{32}P) is used in the treatment of myelogenous leukemia and polycythemia vera.

    Clinical Action

    In above instances, the target tissue has an affinity for the therapeutic agent; the isotope concentrates within the substance.

Nursing Management of Patients Receiving Radioisotopes

A. *Identification of the Patient as a Radiation Source*

    1. Have patient wear a wristband with a radioactive symbol.

    2. Identify the chart cover, doctor's and nurse's order sheets, and special radiation instruction sheet with the radioactive symbol.

    3. For patients receiving the most minute quantities of tracer radioisotopes, such identification (above) is not necessary.

    4. Personnel who may be exposed to penetrating radiation (x-ray or gamma rays) should wear film badges on front of the body.

B. *Radiation Instruction Sheet*
1. Type of radioactivity used
2. Time of insertion
3. Anticipated time of removal
4. Precautions to follow
5. Whom to notify when in doubt or in an emergency

C. *Factors Affecting the Amount of Radiation*
1. *Amount* of radioactivity present, 10mc., 20mc., 30mc., etc.
2. The *distance* of the nurse from the patient
   NOTE: The inverse square law applies: doubling the distance from a radiation source cuts intensity received to one-fourth.
3. Amount of *time* spent in actual contact with patient
4. Degree of *shielding* utilized
   Chosen according to type of radiation—alpha, beta, gamma (see Fig. 17-3).
5. Amount of *body area exposed* to radiation

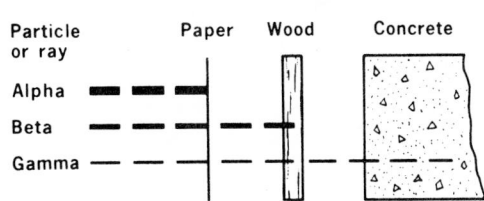

Figure 17-3. Relative penetration of alpha, beta and gamma radiation. (U.S. Atomic Energy Commission.)

NURSING ALERT: During the period of greatest radioactivity (24-72 hours), limit amount of time spent with the patient to that required for essential care. Require patient to remain in his bed or room during his course of treatment.

D. *Salient Nursing Measures in Caring for the Patient with Internal Radiation*
1. Be acquainted with the nomenclature describing disposition of radioisotopes.
   a. *Physical half-life*—a constant rate in which one-half of radioactivity is dissipated in a given time.
   b. *Biologic half-life*—the time it takes for a radioisotope to disappear from the body via normal metabolic processes.
   c. *Effective half-life*—a combination of physical half-life and biologic half-life.
2. Recognize that an isotope that is completely dispersed throughout the body (or a major portion of it) is less hazardous to an organ or tissue than another isotope concentrated by the body into a very localized area.
3. Recognize that an isotope that is excreted rapidly is less hazardous than radium which may be kept in the body for long periods.
4. Take appropriate measures associated with *sealed sources of radiation* implanted within a patient (sealed internal radiation).
   a. Follow directives on precaution sheet which is placed on chart of all patients receiving radiotherapy.
   b. Do not remain within 1 meter (3 feet) of the patient longer than required to give essential care.
   c. Know that the casing material absorbs all alpha radiation and most beta radiation, but that a hazard concerning gamma radiation may exist.
   d. Do not linger in giving patient care longer than necessary even though all precautions are followed.
   e. Be alert for implants which have become loosened when such are used in cavities that have access to the exterior, e.g., check the emesis basin following mouth care for a patient with an oral implant.

    f. Notify the radiologist of any implant that has moved out of position.

    g. Utilize long-handled forceps or tongs and handle at arm's length when picking up any accidentally dislodged radium needle, seeds, tubes, etc., that may appear on dressings, the bed or floor. *Never pick up a radioactive source with your hands.*

    h. Do not discard any dressings or linens unless sure that it does not contain a radioactive source.

    i. Wash hands with soap and water after caring for a patient who is being treated with a radioisotope. When wearing gloves, wash them with soap and water before removing them.
       NOTE: This is not necessary for sealed sources.

    j. Encourage patients who are ambulatory to remain in their own rooms.

    k. Upon discharge of a patient, it is a good policy for the radiologist to check the room with a radiograph or survey meter to be certain that all radioactive materials have been removed.

    l. Continue radiation precautions when a patient has a permanent implant until such time as the radiologist declares precautions unnecessary. (See p. 543 for nursing care of the patient receiving radium therapy.)

5. Take appropriate measures associated with *unsealed sources;* radioactivity may be (1) widely spread in the body, (2) localized, or (3) appear in any body tissue or fluid.

Examples:

1. *Radioactive iodine*
    a. Circulates in bloodstream, excreted by kidneys—urine and blood contain radioactivity.
    b. Can be secreted by sweat glands.
    c. May be found in vomitus of patient who recently took oral dose.

2. *Radioactive colloidal gold*
    a. May be noted in wound seepage as pink, red or purple stain following intracavitary injection.
    b. May be noted in small amounts in urine.

3. *Radioactive phosphorus solution*
    Be alert for contamination from excreta (urine and feces) and vomitus.

CARE OF THE PATIENT WITH ADVANCED CARCINOMA

Objectives of Nursing Management

A. *To halt the spread of the malignant growth.*

1. Prepare the patient for the prescribed modality of treatment: surgery, chemotherapy or radiation.
2. Assist with diagnostic evaluation in an attempt to determine precise location(s) of involvement or spread.
3. Control local and generalized infections.
4. Promote optimum nutritional, fluid and electrolyte levels by correcting deficiencies.
5. Provide the patient with psychosociological support.
    a. Listen to his concerns.
    b. Observe and support his reactions where appropriate.

    c. Explain the aspect of treatment that is pertinent at that time.

    d. Empathize with him and offer reassurance where appropriate.

  6. Assist with the prescribed forms of therapy.

B. *To encourage the patient to pursue purposeful or diversional activities as long as possible.*

  1. Invite him to participate socially, visit with other individuals, take walks, etc.

  2. Provide opportunities for communication and mind-occupying activities.

    Accept him as an individual with natural defense mechanisms; encourage him to talk about himself, his concerns, his understanding, his future—even the possibility of dying.

  3. Support the patient as he taps his spiritual resources.

  4. Understand his behavioral deviations, even when socially unacceptable; when the episode passes, assist him in restoring his self-esteem.

  5. Empathize with him in an effort to show concern and understanding.

  6. Include the patient's family in planning with him meaningful day-to-day activities.

C. *To promote comfort of the patient and relieve his pain.*

  1. Assist the patient in bathing and with personal hygiene; personal cleanliness is a comfort measure.

  2. Provide warmth when required; in cool seasons the debilitated patient is more sensitive to chilling.

  3. Assist him as required in moving, turning, getting out of bed, walking, etc., in an effort to promote maximum activity and minimum amount of pain.

  4. Evaluate objectively the nature of his pain, location, duration, quality and manner in which the patient tolerates or accepts his pain.

  5. Convey the impression that his pain is understood and that relief is forthcoming.

  6. Ascertain pain source—is it carcinoma-related? Is there some other physical source? Is it psychological?

  7. Administer medications as specifically required:

    a. Sedative and hypnotics—to induce and promote sleep

    b. Local anesthetics—for localized pain

    c. Ataractic drugs—for fear and apprehension

    d. Specific medications—for nausea and vomiting

    e. Muscle relaxant and antispasmodic drugs—to relieve tenseness

    f. Tranquilizers—to promote a sense of well-being

    g. Analgesics—for discomfort of pain

    h. Narcotics—for more intense pain

NURSING ALERT: Recognize that elderly debilitated patients have increased sensitivity: Avoid this cycle: a narcotic → drowsiness → less food and fluid → dehydration → nausea and vomiting → increased pain → more narcotic (and a resumption of the cycle).

---

  8. Prepare the patient for surgical pain-relieving interventions.

    a. Alcohol injections to block nerve pathways

    b. Localized radiotherapy

    c. Presacral neurectomy for visceral pain

    d. Cordotomy for intractable pain

    e. Neurosurgical nerve interruption

D. *To cope with the annoying and discomforting side effects of radiation therapy.*
   1. Radiation sickness
      a. Administer sedatives, antiemetics, and antihistamines as prescribed.
      b. Encourage adequate fluid intake.
      c. Tempt patient with small, frequent, high caloric, high protein feedings.
      d. Record his reactions.
   2. Skin reactions
      a. Observe skin for dryness, tautness, erythema, desquamation.
      b. Apply bland cream or oil to radiation site as directed.
      c. Cleanse skin gently with bland soaps (Neutrogena) and lukewarm water.
      d. Protect skin from sunlight, heat, trauma, constricting clothing.
      e. Note changes such as telangiectasis (small network of dilated arterioles).
      f. Offer medicated mouthwashes to sooth oral mucosa.
   3. Diarrhea
      a. Give antidiarrhea medications as prescribed.
      b. Avoid serving foods that aggravate the problem, such as stewed prunes.
      c. Provide suppositories as suggested.
      d. Keep diet restricted to low residue or bland foods.
   4. Blood cell depression
      a. Protect the patient from injury and infection.
      b. Observe for evidences of bleeding or infection and take measures to correct.

E. *To assist in overcoming bladder and bowel disturbances.*
   1. Bladder frequency or incontinence
      a. Keep an accurate input and output record.
      b. Establish a bladder control program (see p. 35).
      c. Maintain perineal cleanliness.
      d. Insert an indwelling catheter if other measures fail.
   2. Constipation
      a. Maintain an adequate fluid level.
      b. Omit constipating foods from diet—ensure adequate fruits and vegetables.
      c. Administer glycerin suppository or mild laxative as prescribed.

NURSING ALERT: Avoid giving enemas when patient has leukopenia or is taking drugs which irritate the intestinal tract (e.g., 5-fluorouracil).

F. *To maintain an intact skin and prevent tissue breakdown.*
   1. Offer regular back and body massages; these can stimulate poor circulation and promote relaxation as well.
   2. Ensure wrinkle-free, dry bedding which helps prevent skin breakdown in debilitated patients. Special mattress pads can be used.
   3. Control skin breakdown following radiation treatment as indicated on page 885.
   4. Maintain an exercise program utilizing range of motion activities.
   5. Control edema of extremities by elevating the part as well as supporting it.
   6. Initiate measure to prevent decubiti (see p. 20).

G. *To control odors which tend to emanate from the affected tissues.*
   1. Promote an esthetically comfortable environment.
   2. Encourage good personal hygiene.

3. Irrigate external wounds with saline and use mechanical cleansers as prescribed (half strength hydrogen peroxide, diluted antiseptic detergents, etc.).
4. Remove soiled dressings promptly and change all soiled linens frequently—wrap dressings in paper and place in covered container immediately.
5. Provide fresh circulating air—use aerosol deodorants when necessary.
6. Change packing or pads frequently, irrigate thoroughly any affected body cavities and shave where hair presents a problem—mouth, nasal area, vagina, rectum.
7. Prevent dressing changes at inopportune times—visiting hours, meal times, etc.

H. *To anticipate and control hemorrhage.*
1. Monitor vital signs to detect increase in pulse rate and respiration and decrease in blood pressure.
2. Apply pressure, if active bleeding occurs, at convenient pressure points between site and heart.
3. Employ emergency hemorrhage-control measures.
4. Note and record amount and nature of bleeding; notify physician.
5. Reassure and comfort patient.
6. Use packing if bleeding involves accessible cavity, e.g., rectum, vagina.
7. Administer platelet or whole-blood transfusion.
8. Prepare patient for cauterization and ligation if necessary.

I. *To assist patient as he strives for peace of mind in preparing for death.*

J. *To keep the patient at the optimum physical and psychological level of which he is capable.*
1. Provide a high caloric and high vitamin diet; cater to his personal food likes.
2. Offer between-meal feedings.
3. Change patient's environment if possible by encouraging him to walk and go outdoors.
4. Promote physical activities as much as possible; encourage rest periods.
5. Allow him to verbalize his feelings and thoughts; provide unhurried time to listen.
6. Maintain an optimistic atmosphere; limit the time plans to hour by hour, or day by day but not week by week, month by month or year by year.

PSYCHOSOCIAL SUPPORT OF THE DYING PATIENT

Reactions of the Patient to Dying*

A. *Stage of Denial*
1. Period of denial allows patient to mobilize his defenses.
2. Patient will exhibit withdrawal and avoidance of subject of death.
3. Usually a temporary defense to be replaced in time by partial acceptance.
4. Patient may talk of death and then change topic abruptly.
5. Patient may be in a temporary state of shock.

B. *Stage of Anger*
1. Denial may be replaced by anger, rage, envy and resentment.
2. Anger may be displaced and projected into environment.

* Adapted from Kübler-Ross, E.: On Death and Dying. New York, Macmillan, 1970.

     a. Anger frequently directed at hospital staff. (Avoid reacting personally to this anger.)

     b. Try to tolerate rational and irrational anger. Patient may experience considerable relief in expressing anger.

C. *Stage of Bargaining*

    Bargaining is an attempt to postpone the inevitable and to extend life.

D. *Stage of Depression*

   1. This is a stage in which the patient is preparing himself to accept the loss of everything and everyone he loves.

   2. Patient may be undergoing anticipatory grief to prepare himself for the final separation; may mourn the loss of meaningful people in his life.

     a. Allow the patient to express his sorrow—helps make the final acceptance easier.

     b. Sit with the patient.

     c. Use touch therapy if appropriate.

E. *Stage of Acceptance*

   1. Patient is neither depressed nor angry about his impending death; he bows to the sentence.

   2. May contemplate his demise with quiet acceptance and expectation—detachment may make death easier.

   3. During this stage patient may be almost void of feelings—his circle of interest diminishes.

   4. Patient will sleep and rest more—does not desire news or visitors from outside world.

   5. Patient may just wish someone to hold his hand—reassures him that he is not forgotten.

   6. Patient may reach the point where death comes as a relief.

   7. Family may require more support during this stage.

Supportive Attitudes and Actions to the Patient, Family and Health Team

Objectives: to allow the patient to live as fully as possible.

            to relieve the discomfort and distress.

            to be attuned to the special needs of the dying.

            to help the patient achieve death with dignity.

A. *Physical Support of the Dying Patient*

    See page 888.

B. *Emotional Support of the Dying Patient*

   1. Make sure the patient has continuing, personal and caring contacts—gives comfort and reassurance.

     a. Avoid changing personnel.

     b. Be willing to become involved with the patient—personal involvement is necessary if human interaction is supportive.

     c. Make sure the nursing approach reflects the mutuality of human interaction.

     d. Take *time* with the patient—gives him the feeling that he is being cared for.

     e. Do not withdraw from the presence of death.

   2. Give the patient an opportunity to talk about himself, his illness and his dying.

     a. Accept the patient as he is now.

     b. Be able to accept the patient's anger—whether overt anger or that expressed as depression.

      c. Encourage him to talk about changes made by his illness.

      d. Demonstrate interest in patient's total life style.

         (1) Learn what supports his ego and self-esteem.

         (2) Be accessible.

  3. Allow the patient to act out his feelings without judgment.

      a. Understand that the patient is increasingly overwhelmed by feelings of rage, anger, fear, guilt, futility, despondency and pain.

         (1) Understand the patient rather than judge him.

         (2) Demonstrate patience, tolerance and support.

      b. Allow the patient to keep his hold on *hope*—hope is therapeutic and will help maintain the patient through his suffering.

         (1) Maintain hope with the patient.

         (2) Avoid reinforcing hope after the patient has given up (stage of acceptance).

      c. Understand the patient's dread of being deserted.

  4. Be alert for behavioral changes—patient may be trying to communicate something. Anticipate that the patient's behavior will be altered by his deteriorating physical condition.

         (1) Withdrawal from customary interests

         (2) Impairment of self-esteem

  5. Encourage the patient to retain confidence in his health team.

      a. Emphasize to the patient that he and the health team are in the battle together—patient will not be as fearful of loneliness, rejection, deceit.

      b. Reassure him that everything possible will be done for him.

      c. Let the patient know that he is respected and understood; treat him as a fellow human being.

      d. Seek the opinions of the patient—bolsters his self-esteem.

      e. Encourage the patient to take some initiative in his care.

      f. Keep the room neat and confusion at a minimum.

  6. Help the patient who must undergo the "business" of dying.

      a. Settling of affairs, settling problems in human relationships, planning future for children, parent, spouse.

      b. Utilize services of chaplain, legal counselor, social worker, etc.

  7. Pay attention to the patient's day-to-day complaints.

      a. Recognize the wide variety of symptoms accompanying anxiety—palpitation, nausea, insomnia, diarrhea, irritability.

      b. Be aware of the symptoms of depression—fatigue, lethargy, disturbances of sleep and appetite, inability to concentrate, psychomotor retardation.

      c. Try to alleviate each symptom.

      d. Reassure the patient that his pain will be relieved—helps the patient to cope with his discomfort.

      e. Give appropriate drugs to help the dying patient face death, cope with his anxiety and depression and alter his sensitivity to pain (see p. 895).

      f. Help make each day as good a day as possible.

C. *Support of the Family of the Dying Patient*

    Anticipatory grief—mourning that occurs over an extended period of time before actual death:

             Bereavement starts when one realizes that loss is inevitable.

             Family experiences awareness of loss and depression.

Family may begin to make the physical and psychological adaptions to the consequences of death.

1. Understand that the family may be undergoing anticipatory mourning and is reacting to anticipated loss.
   a. Recognize that various family members behave differently while working out their anticipatory grief.
      (1) Avoid showing disapproval of the behavior of others—may produce feelings of shame, guilt and inadequacy.
      (2) Understand that family members may feel guilty when they are unable to demonstrate grief—there may be little or no feeling at actual time of death because family members have worked through their grief during the anticipatory period.
      (3) Family may withdraw emotional investment from the patient as they perceive he has no future.
   b. Be alert for untoward reactions to death—family member may need supportive therapy and counseling.
2. Accept the feelings and attitudes of the family—helps avoid mutual hostility and recriminations.
   Feelings include:
   (1) Fear and anxiety
   (2) Sorrow and grief
   (3) Overt or suppressed hostility interwoven with guilt feelings; self blame
   (4) Ambivalent feelings toward dying member
   (5) Overly protected attitude
   (6) Depersonalization
   (7) Projection of guilt to medical personnel
   (8) Submission or excessive courtesy—may mask hostility
3. Realize the problems faced by the family—anticipated separation of loved one, financial problems, disruption of family life, problems of communication.
4. Demonstrate concern for the family.
   a. Inform them of practical help—financial assistance, social worker, other supporting services of local helping agencies.
   b. Reassure family that they will not be left alone.
   c. Provide opportunity for family member to ventilate his conflicts—anger, depression, victimization by illness.

D. *Support of the Health Team*
   1. Examine one's own attitudes and ability to face terminal illness and death.
      a. Look at possessions and relationships in context of inevitability of death.
      b. Plan for disaster and death.
   2. Monitor one's own feelings.
      a. Accept the idea of denial, fear and guilt.
      b. Assess and correct one's own biases and fears.
      c. Watch emotional responses to challenges of incurable disease and "difficult" families.
   3. Do not withdraw from the presence of death.
      a. Face the reality of the dying patient.
      b. Become skilled and sensitive in the art of human interaction.

Psychotherapeutic Agents* for the Support of the Seriously Ill Patient

The use of drugs is indicated when:
  (1) there is decreasing ability to function (eat, sleep, care for hygienic needs, etc.),
  (2) duration of symptoms is abnormally long.

Objective: to assist the patient to maintain his daily activities

DRUG	NURSING IMPLICATIONS

Antianxiety Agents *Sedatives*
  Pentobarbital sodium (Nembutal)
  Secobarbital sodium (Seconal)
  Methyprylon (Noludar)
  Ethchlorvynol (Placidyl)
  Amobarbital (Amytal)
  Gluthethimide (Doriden)
  Phenobarbital
	1. Sedatives act as central nervous system depressants; given to relieve anxiety and induce sleep.
	2. Dosage varies with physiologic and psychologic state of patient.
	3. Evaluate patient for drowsiness, impaired judgment and performance, dizziness, drug habituation.

Tranquilizers
  Methotrimeprazine (Neozine, Veractil)
  Acetapromazine (Notensil)
  Chlorpromazine (Thorazine)
  Carisoprodol (Soma, Rela)
  Meprobamate (Equanil, Miltown)
  Chlordiazepoxide hydrochloride (Librium)
  Diazepam (Valium)
	1. Tranquilizers act in all parts of the brain; principally on the subcortical areas to produce mental relaxation and emotional calmness.
	2. Tranquilizers act at different subcortical levels, have different pharmacological properties and varying degrees of clinical usefulness.
	3. Synthetic tranquilizers cause dry mouth, visual problems, constipation and tachycardia.
	4. *Watch for postural hypotension and syncope,* drowsiness and delayed reflexes.

Antidepressant Agents
  Imipramine (Tofranil)
  Disipramine (Pertofran, Norpramin)
  Amitriptyline (Elavil)
  Nortriptyline (Aventyl)
  Protriptyline (Vivactil)
	1. Drug is started at a low dose and increased gradually until a maximum daily dose is reached (according to efficacy and side effects).
	2. Treatment may be continued for several months; then the drug is gradually withdrawn.
	3. Evaluate for weakness, drowsiness, or deepening of depression; patient may also demonstrate agitation, tremulousness, visual hallucinations and agitation.
	4. *Assess for postural hypotension;* dry mouth and constipation also occur.

Combinations

Antianxiety agents and antidepressants may be used in combination—to treat combination of symptoms (anxiety and depression).

* Reader is referred to a pharmacology textbook for a more complete listing.

BIBLIOGRAPHY

Books

Ackerman, L. V., and del Regato, J. A.: Cancer, 4th ed. St. Louis, C. V. Mosby, 1970.

Bouchard, R., and Owens, N. F.: Nursing Care of the Cancer Patient, 2nd ed. St. Louis, C. V. Mosby, 1972.

Browning, M. H., and Lewis, E. P. (eds.): The Dying Patient: A Nursing Perspective. New York, American Journal of Nursing Co., 1972.

Brunner, L. S., et al.: Textbook of Medical and Surgical Nursing, 2nd ed. Philadelphia, J. B. Lippincott, 1970, pp. 179–207.

Consumer Radiation Protection, FDA Papers, Washington, D.C., Food and Drug Administration, U.S. Department of Health, Education and Welfare, Oct. 1971.

Healy, J. E., Jr. (ed.): Ecology of the Cancer Patient. Washington, D.C., Interdisciplinary Communication Associates, Inc., 1970.

Kastenbaum, R., and Aisenberg, R. B.: The Psychology of Death. New York, Springer Publishing Co., 1972.

Kübler-Ross, E.: On Death and Dying. New York, Macmillan, 1970.

National Council on Radiation Protection and Measurements: MCRP Report No. 37: Precautions in the Management of Patients Who Have Received Therapeutic Amounts of Radionuclides, 1970.

Schoenberg, B., et al. (eds.): Loss and Grief: Psychological Management in Medical Practice. New York, Columbia University Press, 1970.

————: Psychosocial Aspects of Terminal Care. New York, Columbia University Press, 1972.

University of Rochester: Clinical Oncology, 3rd ed., American Cancer Society, 1970–71.

Winter, A. (ed.): The Moment of Death: A Symposium. Illinois, Charles C Thomas, 1969.

Articles

Barckley, V.: A visiting nurse specializes in cancer nursing. Amer. J. Nurs., 70:1680–1683, Aug. 1970.

Benoliel, J. Q.: Talking to patients about death. Nurs. Forum, 9:254–268, 1970.

Blewett, L. J.: To die at home. Amer. J. Nurs., 70:2602–2604, Dec. 1970.

Branson, H. K.: The terminal patient and his family. Bedside Nurse, 3:21–23, June 1970.

Craytor, J. K.: Talking with persons who have cancer. Amer. J. Nurs., 69:744–748, April 1969.

Dollinger, M. R.: How to use cancer chemo-therapy. Amer. Fam. Phys., 3:73–84, June 1971.

Francis, G. M.: Cancer: The emotional component. Amer. J. Nurs., 69:1677–1681, Aug. 1969.

Freckman, H. A.: Results in 169 patients with cancer of the head and neck treated by intra-arterial infusion therapy. Amer. J. Surg., 124:501–509, Oct. 1972.

Hilkemeyer, R.: Nursing care in radium therapy. Nurs. Clin. N. Amer., 2:83–95, March 1967.

Hoffman, E.: Don't give up on me. Amer. J. Nurs., 71:60–62, Jan. 1971.

Isler, C.: Radiation therapy II, The nurse and the patient. RN, 34:48–51, March 1971.

————: The cancer nurses. RN, 35:27–37, Feb. 1972.

Klagsbrun, S. C.: Communications in the treatment of cancer. Amer. J. Nurs., 71:944–948, May 1971.

Lee, J. A. H.: Prevention of cancer. Postgrad. Med., 51:84–88, Jan. 1972.

Leitch, W. H.: Review your knowledge of tumors. AORN J., 17:71–82, Feb. 1973.

Livingston, B. M., and Krakoff, I.: L-asparaginase. Amer. J. Nurs., 70:1910–1915, Sept. 1970.

Mervyn, F.: The plight of dying patients in hospitals. Amer. J. Nurs., 71:1988–1990, Oct. 1971.

Nichols, E. G.: Jeannette: no hope for cure. Nursing Forum, 11:95–113, 1972.

Prosnitz, L. R.: Radiation therapy I, Treatment for malignant disease, RN, 34:42–47, March 1971.

Ross, E. K.: What is it like to be dying? Amer. J. Nurs., 71:54–60, Jan. 1971.

Shepardson, J.: Team approach to the patient with cancer. Amer. J. Nurs., 72:488–491, March 1971.

Symposium on death and attitudes toward death. Geriatrics, 27:52–60, Aug. 1972.

Vernick, J. J.: Selected bibliography on death and dying. Washington, D.C., U.S. Government Printing Office, 1970.

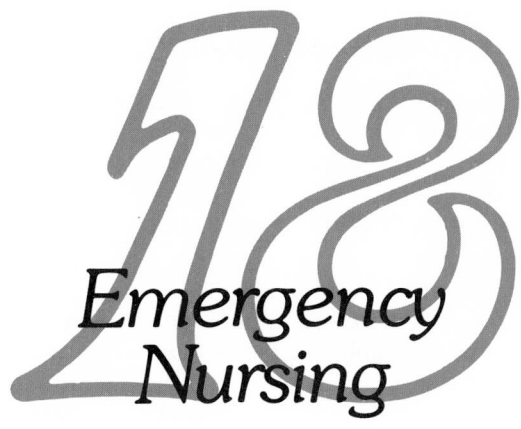

Emergency Nursing

EMERGENCY MANAGEMENT

Emergency medical care refers to the care given to patients with urgent and critical needs. The circumstances under which the care is given may or may not be optimal; whatever facilities are at hand are used in the most effective manner.

Principles of Emergency Management

Objectives: to preserve life.
  to restore the patient to useful living.
  to prevent deterioration before more definitive treatment can be given.

1. Maintain a patent airway, employing resuscitation measures if necessary.
2. Stop bleeding.
3. Prevent and treat shock.
4. Assess for chest injuries and airway obstruction (sucking chest wounds, tension pneumothorax, etc.).
5. Protect wounds with sterile dressings or with dressings that are as clean as possible.
6. Splint suspected fractures.
7. Start a chart of patient's vital signs; monitor blood pressure, pulse and respiration at frequent intervals.
8. Allay anxiety and keep patient as comfortable as possible.
9. Observe and re-evaluate patients at frequent intervals.
10. Carry out special procedures and assist with history and physical examination.

Psychological Management of Patients in Emergencies

1. Understand and accept the basic anxieties of the acutely traumatized patient.
   a. Be aware of the patient's fear of death, mutilation and isolation.
   b. Understand and support the patient's feelings concerning his loss of control (loss of emotional, physical and intellectual control).
2. Be prepared to handle all aspects of acute trauma; know what to expect and what to do—alleviates nurse's anxieties and increases patient's confidence.
3. Maintain and convey optimism and a concern for the welfare of the patient.
4. Caution the family not to be shocked or horrified by the patient's condition; encourage them to reassure the patient that they value him.
5. Accept the rights of the patient and family to have their own feelings.
6. Maintain a calm and reassuring manner—helps emotionally distressed patient or family to mobilize their own psychological resources.

EMERGENCY RESUSCITATION PROCEDURES

GUIDELINES: *Giving Mouth-to-mouth and Mouth-to-nose Resuscitation*

Artificial respiration is the maintenance of respiratory movements by artificial means.

Methods

1. Mouth-to-mouth resuscitation
2. Mouth-to-nose resuscitation

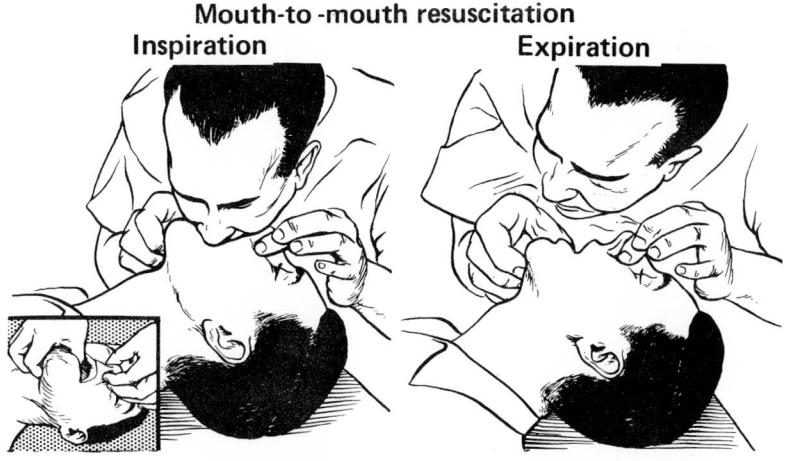

Mouth-to-mouth resuscitation

Inspiration   Expiration

Mouth-to-nose resuscitation

Inspiration   Expiration

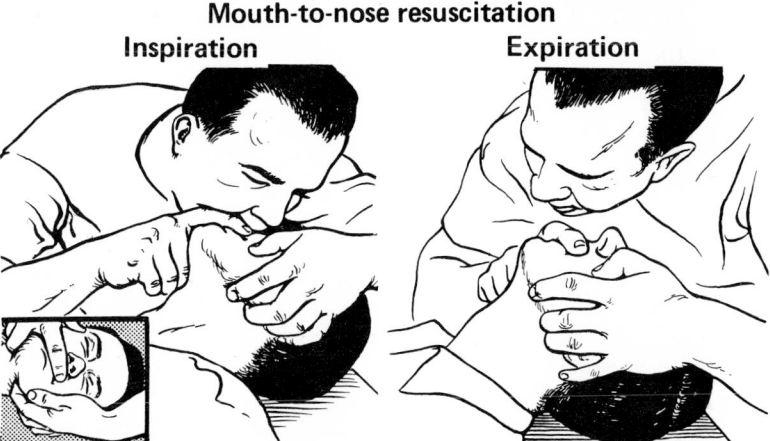

Figure 18-1. Technics for mouth-to-mouth and mouth-to-nose resuscitation. (Gordon, Archer S., *et al.*: Mouth-to-mouth versus manual artificial respiration for children and adults, J.A.M.A., *167:326, 1958.*)

Principle

1. The patient's lungs are directly inflated with air from the operator's mouth (Fig. 18-1).
2. These methods ensure pulmonary ventilation in an emergency situation when resuscitation equipment is not available.

Procedure

Nursing Action	*Rationale / Amplification*
1. Place palm of hand over patient's mouth and feel for air movement. If patient is not breathing start some form of pulmonary ventilation immediately.	

Nursing Action	Rationale/Amplification
2. Place the patient supine on a hard table or floor. Position yourself on the left side at the patient's head.	
3. Clear the mouth of mucus and foreign objects by wiping or suctioning.	3. The first requirement is that the airway be open. It may be necessary to place the patient on his abdomen to accomplish this.
4. Place one hand under the patient's neck and the other hand on the patient's forehead. Tilt the head back as far as possible.	4. Backward tilt of the head lifts the base of the tongue off the posterior pharyngeal wall, opens the air passage and permits inflation of the lungs.
5. For *mouth-to-mouth resuscitation,* pinch the nostrils closed. Blow forcefully into the patient's mouth with a smooth steady action until the patient's chest rises. The operator's mouth should be placed tightly over the patient's mouth.	5. In mouth-to-mouth resuscitation the nose must be held closed to seal the nasopharynx so that the air goes into the lungs. The rising chest indicates inflation of the lungs with operator's expired air.
6. For *mouth-to-nose resuscitation,* the mouth is held closed and the air is blown through the nose into the nasopharynx and lungs.	
7. After blowing, turn the head to the side and *watch* the patients' chest expand; *listen* to detect if air is leaving the lungs. (Blow, watch, listen.)	7. After the patient's lungs are inflated there is an unassisted expiration phase brought about by elastic recoil of the patient's chest and lungs.
8. The operator should take his next breath while listening to the sound of the patient exhaling.	8. If abdominal distention occurs, have an assistant apply pressure over the patient's epigastrium.
9. Reinflate the lungs as soon as the patient has exhaled.	
10. Continue the cycle at the rate of 12–20 inflations per minute.	10. The operator should take a breath about twice the volume of ordinary respiration. At every 20 cycles, he should take one deep breath for himself.

GUIDELINES: *Cardiac Arrest and Cardiopulmonary Resuscitation*

Cardiac arrest is the sudden and unexpected cessation of the heart endangering effective circulation.

Cardiopulmonary resuscitation is restoration of life or consciousness in an apparently dead person (Fig. 18-2).

Procedure

Nursing Action	Rationale/Amplification
Performance Phase	
1. Note the time as soon as cardiac arrest is determined. Summon help immediately (telephone).	1. Lack of effective circulation to the central nervous system of more than 4–6 minutes may result in irreversible changes.
2. Administer 1 or 2 sharp blows over the lower sternum.	2. Cardiac standstill may sometimes be terminated by a sharp blow, particularly if asystole is mechanism of arrest.
3. Carry out artificial ventilation and external cardiac massage *simultaneously.*	

Nursing Action

Artificial Ventilation

1. Clear airway of foreign material.
2. Hyperextend (tilt back) head and pull jaw forward.
3. Insert oropharyngeal tube if available.
4. Ventilate the patient. Inflate the patient's lungs by a forceful expiration of a full breath through a mouth-to-mouth airtight seal (see p. 900).
5. Provide 12 breaths per minute. (Utilize bag and mask if someone is available to operate it.)

External cardiac massage

1. Place patient on firm surface.

Rationale/Amplification

2. This tends to lift the tongue off the back wall of the pharynx and open the airway.

4. With each attempted inflation, the patient's chest should rise to a visible degree. Absence of chest expansion indicates airway obstruction. Keep the jaw pulled forward during ventilation to relieve obstruction.

External cardiac compression is necessary to circulate blood that has been oxygenated by artificial ventilation.

1. A firm surface supports the spine and allows the heart to be compressed between the spine and the sternum.

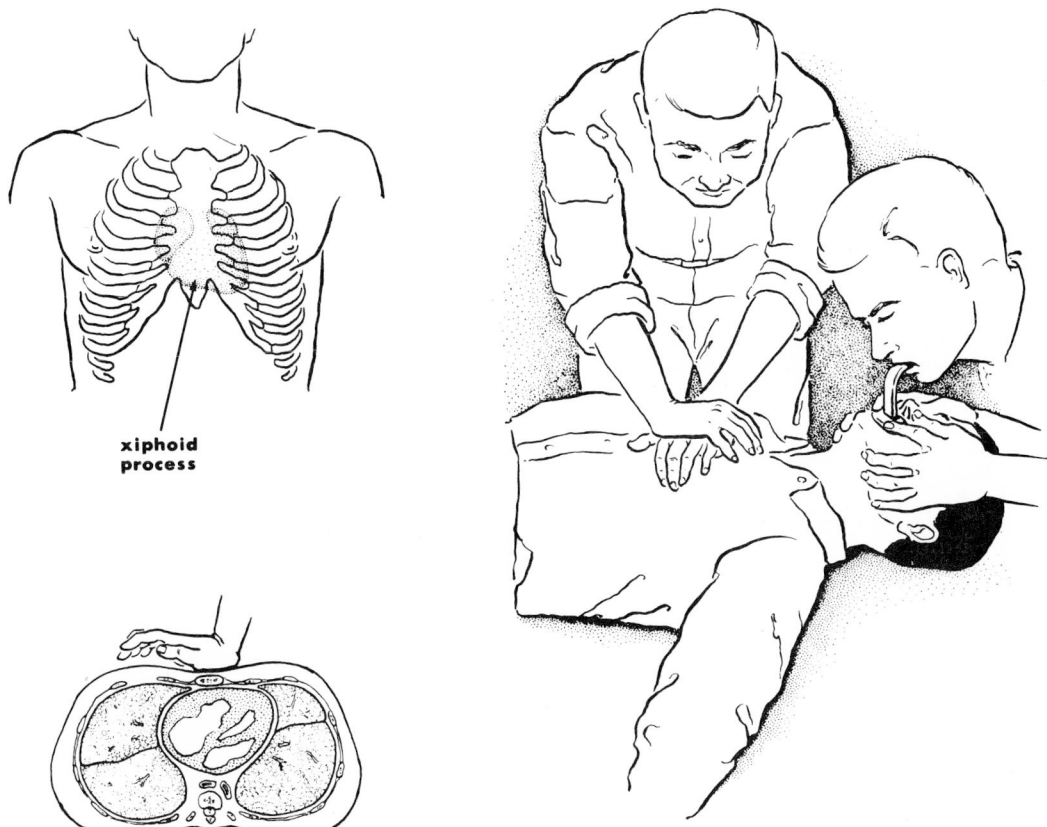

xiphoid process

Figure 18-2. Closed-chest cardiac massage.

Nursing Action	*Rationale / Amplification*
2. Place the heel of one hand on the lower half of the sternum and place the opposite hand on top of the first hand.	
3. Using the operator's weight, quickly and forcefully depress the lower sternum 7.5–10 cm. (1.5–2 inches) and then suddenly release the sternal pressure.	3. Each compression forces blood from the heart into the arterial system. Rapid sternal release facilitates filling of the right heart from the great veins and the left heart from the pulmonary veins.
4. Use 60–80 compressions per minute.	
5. Deliver 1 deep breath for each 5 cardiac compressions without interruption of the compression cycle.	5. If only 1 person is available alternate 30 seconds of external massage with 5 seconds of ventilation.
6. Palpate for carotid pulse and note size of pupils as an indication of response.	6. The presence of a palpable carotid pulse and constriction of pupils are evidence of effective circulation of oxygenated blood.

Follow-up Phase

See page 247 for drug therapy after resuscitation and during postresuscitation care.

ANAPHYLACTIC REACTION

Anaphylactic reaction is a generalized systemic and frequently fatal reaction occurring within minutes after administration of foreign sera or drugs.

Causes

Penicillin, sera, other antibiotics, bee and wasp stings or almost any repeatedly administered parenteral or oral therapeutic agent

Clinical Manifestations

1. Apprehension and flushing.
2. Itching or burning (Generalized itching over entire body indicates a general systemic reaction is developing).
3. Sneezing or coughing.
4. Hives on face and upper chest—appear within first few seconds after injection (With massive facial angiodema, expect that upper respiratory edema may occur).
5. *Respiratory difficulty*—tightness or pain in chest.
6. *Wheezing and shortness* of breath, hoarseness, respiratory stridor.
7. Cyanosis.
8. Pallor, imperceptible pulse—circulatory failure leading to coma and death.

Emergency Management

1. Establish vital functions.
   a. Employ resuscitative measures (especially for patient with stridor and progressive pulmonary edema).
   b. Ensure adequate airway; use positive pressure oxygen therapy.
   c. Use closed-chest cardiac massage or mouth-to-mouth resuscitation.

2. Give epinephrine hydrochloride (Adrenalin) I.M. or I.V. as directed.
   a. Dosage may be repeated in 5–10 minutes if patient does not respond.
   b. Apply tourniquet above injection site if anaphylactic reaction followed an injection—give epinephrine in opposite arm.
   c. Infiltrate injection site with 0.3 ml. of 1:1000 solution of epinephrine.
3. Give antihistamine drugs, e.g., diphenhydramine hydrochloride (Benadryl), I.M. or I.V. if patient requires adjunctive treatment.
4. Administer hydrocortisone I.V. if patient is having a prolonged reaction—helpful in preventing late relapses.
5. Give vasopressor agent (levarterenol) I.V. for extreme hypotension.
6. Give aminophylline, I.V. (250 mg. diluted in 10–20 ml. of normal saline) over a 10-minute period—for patients with severe bronchospasm and asthmatic symptoms.

Preventive Measures

1. Be aware of the danger of anaphylactic reactions.
2. Ask about patient's previous allergies to medications; if positive, do not give medication or injection.
3. Question patient before giving a foreign serum or other type of antigenic agent to determine if he has had it at some earlier time.
4. Question patient concerning previous allergic reactions to food or pollen.
5. Avoid giving drugs to patients with hay fever, asthma and other allergic disorders unless absolutely necessary.
6. Do skin testing before administering foreign serum.
7. If patient is being treated as an out-patient, keep him in office, hospital or clinic at least 30 minutes after injection of any agent.
8. Caution patients who are sensitive to insect bites to carry first-aid kits or kits equipped to treat insect stings.
9. Encourage allergic individual to wear identification tag.

HEMORRHAGE

Emergency Management

Objective: to maintain an adequate circulating blood volume.

1. Undress the patient (and drape adequately) so that a complete examination may be carried out.
2. Apply firm manual pressure over the wound or artery involved (Fig. 18-3). Unchecked arterial bleeding produces death.
3. Apply a firm pressure bandage. Do not constrict circulation.
4. Treat for hypovolemic shock (see p. 905).
5. Immobilize an injured extremity to control the blood loss—elevate the affected part.
6. Insert intravenous cannula to provide means of blood replacement.
   a. Withdraw blood sample for analysis, typing and cross-matching.
   b. Give replacement fluids including isotonic electrolyte solutions, plasma and blood (depending on clinical estimates of type and volume of fluids lost).
   c. Rate of infusion depends upon severity of blood loss and clinical evidence of hypovolemia.

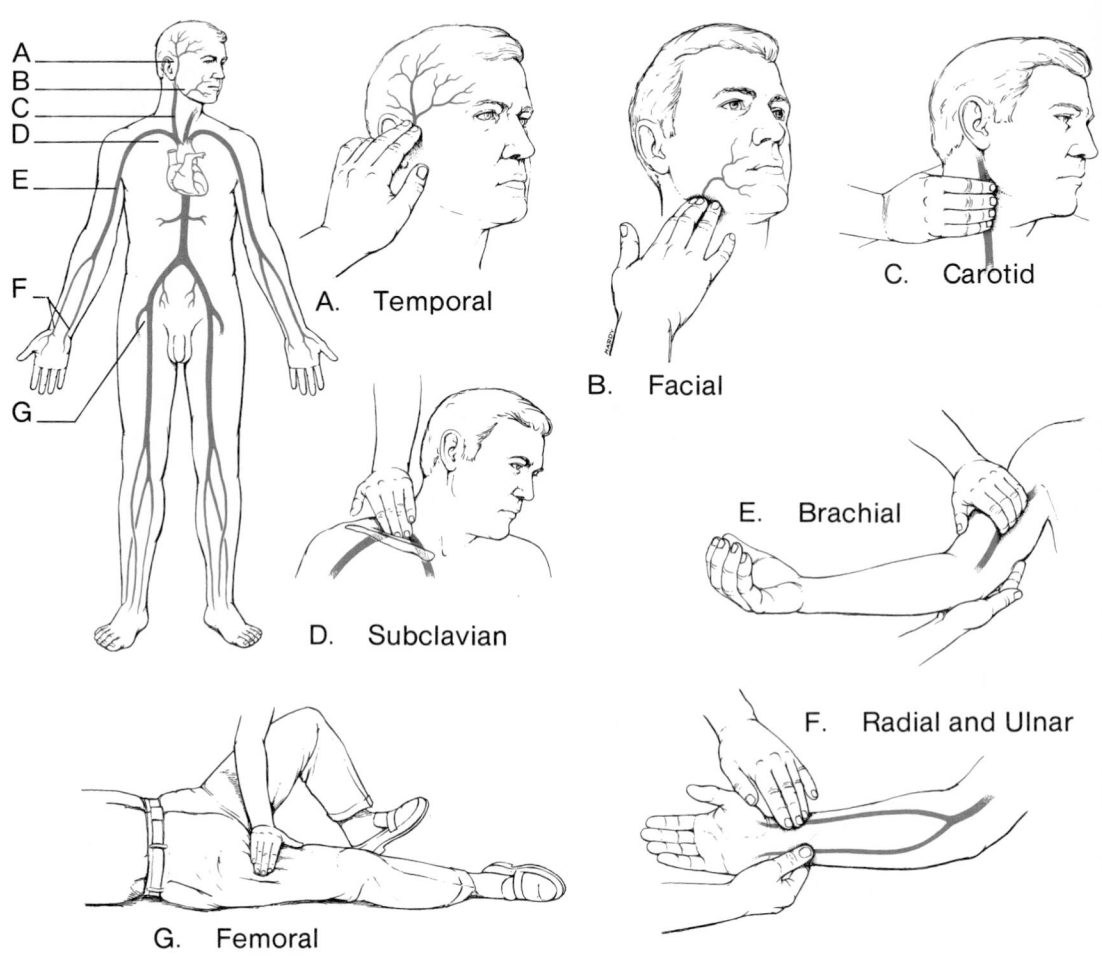

A. Temporal

B. Facial

C. Carotid

D. Subclavian

E. Brachial

F. Radial and Ulnar

G. Femoral

Figure 18-3. Pressure points for control of hemorrhage.

7. Give whole blood or plasma expanders at the rate of blood loss if the patient is hemorrhaging internally.

    Prepare patient immediately for surgical intervention.

8. Apply a tourniquet only as a last resort when the hemorrhage of an extremity cannot be controlled by any other method.

    a. Apply the tourniquet just above the wound.

    b. Apply it tightly enough to control arterial blood flow.

    c. Do not loosen tourniquet until facilities are available for surgical control.

    d. Tag the patient with a notation stating the location of the tourniquet and the time applied.

9. See page 81 for further discussion.

SHOCK

Shock is a state of profound prostration and hypotension resulting when blood flow is inadequate to sustain normal cell activity.

Clinical Manifestations

1. Decreasing arterial pressure (Systolic usually falls more rapidly than diastolic pressure.)
2. Tachycardia
3. Prostration; cold moist skin
4. Circumoral pallor
5. Alterations of mental status
6. Suppression of kidney function

Emergency Management

Objective: to restore tissue perfusion and reduce peripheral vasoconstriction.

1. Establish and maintain an airway.
   a. Clear the airway of mucus and foreign material.
   b. Administer oxygen.
   c. Start resuscitation procedures if necessary.
2. Control hemorrhage—hemorrhage will compound the shock state.
3. Establish an adequate venous return.
   a. Insert intravenous catheter or needle—2 catheters may be necessary in profound shock.
   b. Withdraw blood for specimens (blood pH, pO_2, pCO_2, and hematocrit) and for typing and cross-matching.
   c. Start intravenous infusion (5% dextrose in normal saline)—to restore circulation and to serve as an adjunct to whole blood.
   d. Use plasma volume expanders if indicated until blood can be obtained.
   e. Start blood transfusion as soon as available.
   f. Maintain the systolic blood pressure at 80–90 mm. Hg via fluid and blood volume replacement.
   g. Carry out serial hematocrit examinations if continued bleeding is suspected.
4. Insert a central venous catheter in or near right atrium (see page 241). (Continuing CVP reading gives direction and degree of change from baseline reading; also is vehicle for emergency fluid volume replacement.)
5. Insert a urinary catheter. Urinary volume indicates adequate kidney perfusion. (1 ml. of urine per kg. of body weight per hour is desirable.)
6. Give appropriate medication for patients with cardiogenic or septic shock if indicated.

7. Support the defense mechanisms of the body.
   a. Reassure and comfort the patient—sedative may be necessary for apprehension.
   b. Relieve pain by cautious use of narcotics or analgesics.
   c. Maintain the body temperature.
      (1) Too much heat produces vasodilatation which counteracts the body's compensatory mechanism of vasoconstriction and also increases fluid loss by perspiration.
      (2) A patient who is in septic shock should be kept cool, since high fever will increase cellular metabolic effects of shock.

8. Elevate the feet slightly to improve cerebral circulation. (This position is contra-indicated in patients with head injuries.)
9. Digitalize the patient prophylactically if signs of cardiac failure occur.
10. See page 78 for complete discussion of shock.

WOUNDS

Wounds vary from minor lacerations to severe crushing injuries. The aims of emergency treatment are to maintain the airway, stop bleeding, relieve shock and control infection.

Emergency Management

1. Stop the bleeding.
   a. Remove gross foreign material from the wound.
   b. Apply sterile pressure dressing.
   c. If extremity is involved, elevate.
   d. Apply tourniquet as low on extremity as possible *if hemorrhage is not controllable in other ways.*
      (1) Apply tourniquet tightly; do not loosen at intervals.
      (2) Remove tourniquet only when facilities for surgical control are available.
2. Relieve shock (see p. 905).
3. Prevent injuries to respiratory tract.
   a. Maintain adequate airway.
   b. Position patient on side or on back with head turned to side to allow drainage of pharyngeal secretions.
   c. Cover gaping chest wounds with an airtight dressing and adhesive.
4. Relieve pain—sedation should not exceed 10 mg. morphine.
5. Control infection.
   a. Keep wound covered.
   b. Give tetanus prophylaxis (see p. 825).
   c. Give antibiotic therapy.
6. Debride wounds.
   a. Open wound for inspection.
   b. Remove devitalized tissue and foreign bodies.
   c. Irrigate gently with saline.
   d. Pack loosely with dry gauze and cover with sterile dressing; immobilize part.

INTRA-ABDOMINAL INJURIES

Clinical Manifestations

1. Pain
2. Muscular rigidity
3. Tenderness or rebound tenderness
4. Diminished bowel sounds
5. Hypotension—shock

Emergency Management

1. Avoid moving the patient until initial assessment is done. (Movement may fragment a clot in a large vessel and produce massive hemorrhage.)
2. Evaluate for signs and symptoms of hemorrhage. (Hemorrhage frequently accompanies abdominal injury, especially if the liver has been traumatized.)

3. Control the bleeding and maintain blood volume until surgery can be performed.
   a. Provide compression of external bleeding wounds and occlusion of chest wounds.
   b. Insert indwelling intravenous catheter(s) for rapid fluid replacement to restore circulatory dynamics.
      Use upper extremity veins to avoid pumping fluids out through a wound in the inferior vena cava.
4. Cover protruding abdominal viscera with sterile saline dressings—prevents drying of viscera.
   a. Do not attempt to manipulate or replace protruding viscera—this maneuver enhances possibility of peritonitis and increases danger of additional trauma and shock.
   b. Flex the patient's knees. (The flexed position prevents further protrusion.)
   c. Withhold fluids. (Intake of oral fluid increases peristalsis, leading to further contamination by fecal matter.)
5. Insert indwelling urethral catheter—to determine presence of hematuria and to monitor urinary output.
6. Keep record of vital signs (blood pressure, pulse, respiration and temperature), hourly urinary output, central venous pressure and amount of fluid administered.
7. Carry out tetanus prophylaxis (see p. 825).
8. Give broad spectrum antibiotic (penicillin, streptomycin)—to prevent infection as bacterial contamination is a frequent complication.
9. Transport patient to operating room for exploratory laparotomy—to determine location of missiles (bullets), to debride wound, or to close injured abdominal viscera, etc.
   Keep patient on stretcher from time of arrival in emergency department until surgery.

CRUSH INJURIES

Crush injuries occur when a person is crushed beneath debris, run over or compressed by machinery.

Clinical Manifestations

1. Oligemic shock—due to extravasation of blood and plasma into injured tissues after compression has been released.
2. Paralysis of part, erythema and blistering of skin—damaged part (usually an extremity) becomes swollen, tense, hard.
3. Renal dysfunction—prolonged hypotension causes kidney damage and acute renal insufficiency.

Emergency Management

1. Control shock.
2. Observe carefully for acute renal insufficiency (see p. 472).
3. Splint major soft tissue injuries to control bleeding and pain.
4. Expose extremity to air to reduce tissue metabolism.
5. Incise fascia if blood supply is blocked to relieve pressure of extravasated fluid.
6. Apply pressure bandages as indicated.
7. Administer medication for pain and anxiety.

BURNS

Immediate Management

Stop burning process to prevent further tissue destruction.

1. Remove hot and burning clothing.
2. Cover with moist sheets—for patient with extensive thermal injuries.
3. Immerse small areas of burns in cold water for 10 minutes—inhibits capillary permeability thereby suppressing or preventing edema, blister formation and tissue destruction.
   a. Reimmerse part for additional 10 minutes if pain resumes.
   b. Immersions may be repeated for a period of 40 minutes.

Emergency Treatment of Specific Burns

A. *Chemical Burns*

1. Irrigate copiously with large quantities of running water (except those caused by phosphorus).
2. Cover with loosely applied clean cloth.

B. *Electrical Burns*

Electrical energy affects all tissues that it traverses.

1. Remove electrical source with a nonconductor.
2. Treat for coma, circulatory and respiratory collapse.
3. Determine points of entrance and exit of current—to ascertain the organs that may be damaged.
4. Debride entrance and exit wounds.
   a. Remove charred and devitalized skin.
   b. Use sutures to close wound if necessary.
5. Monitor for cardiac irregularities—death may ensue from ventricular fibrillation.
6. Watch for complications of myoglobinuria—large amounts of myoglobin pigment result from electrical muscle destruction.

C. *Acute Burns*

1. Establish adequate airway; maintain adequate oxygenation.
2. Prepare for tracheostomy for:
   a. Patients with deep burns of face, neck and respiratory tract; injuries from inhalation of gases
   b. Stridor and inadequate respiratory exchange
   c. Patient unable to handle tracheobronchial secretions
3. Replace fluids.
   a. Withdraw blood for typing, cross-matching and blood gas samples.
   b. Start intravenous fluids; use cut down in brachial vein for extensive burns.
   c. Replace blood volume deficit—use plasma volume expander until blood is available.
   d. Start fluid summary record.
4. Combat shock—from local blood vessel damage with increased capillary permeability and loss of fluid into injured tissues.
   a. Insert central venous pressure catheter (see p. 241).
   b. Assess patient for fractures, bleeding, head injuries, hemothorax, cardiac tamponade.
   c. Give definitive treatment for shock (see p. 905).

5. Remove eschar (decompression).
6. Insert indwelling catheter—to monitor hourly urinary output and to serve as a guide to adequacy of fluid replacement.
     0.5–1.5 ml./kg./hourly is considered adequate.
7. Give analgesic as indicated.
   a. Patients with extensive superficial burns will complain of pain.
   b. Pain of extensive burns may require no medication during shock phase.
8. Assist with evaluation of thermal injury—to assess extent of burns and their probable depth.
   Determine:
   a. Circumstances of accident
   b. Approximate duration of exposure to heat
   c. Age and previous health condition
   d. Time, place and mechanism of injury
   e. Mental status
9. Assist with systemic review of patient (physical).
10. Start a record of vital signs.
11. Initiate care of burn wound (see p. 606).
12. Give systemic (and topical) antibacterial drugs—for burn wound sepsis.
13. Administer tetanus immune globulin or toxoid—for tetanus prophylaxis.
14. Insert nasogastric tube—to allow evacuation of air from stomach and prevent gastric dilation; patient with extensive burn is likely to have decreased gastrointestinal motility.
15. Prepare to digitalize patient if decreased cardiac output becomes evident.
16. Secure laboratory tests as ordered.

HEAD INJURIES

Head injuries are classified as open or closed injuries. About 15 to 20% of all patients coming to emergency departments for treatment have some form of head trauma. (See page 722 for more complete discussion of treatment of head injuries.)

Emergency Management

1. Maintain the airway and exchange of air.
   a. Keep the patient prone (or semiprone) with head to one side after making certain there is no cervical spine injury. Prone position facilities drainage from the tracheobronchial tree and minimizes aspiration of nasopharyngeal and gastric secretions.
   b. Clear the respiratory passages via suctioning.
   c. Ensure adequate oxygenation and humidification. (Hypoxia of the brain, which leads to increased intracranial pressure, is the most frequent cause of death after head injury.)
   d. Assist with endotracheal intubation if patient is comatose.
   e. Utilize assisted ventilation if necessary. (The brain is very sensitive to lack of oxygen.)
2. Control hemorrhage and shock.
3. Determine base-line condition of the patient.
   a. Assess level of responsiveness (see p. 724).
   b. Determine presence of headache, double vision, nausea or vomiting.

      c. Evaluate pupil size and reaction to light.

      d. Measure blood pressure, pulse, respirations.

      e. Evaluate motion and strength of extremities.

      f. Assess for injuries to other organ systems.

4. Evaluate for changes in patient's condition. *(Change in level of responsiveness is most sensitive sign of improvement or deterioration.)*

5. Prepare for surgical intervention.

SPINAL CORD INJURY

Clinical Manifestations

1. Total sensory loss and motor paralysis below level of injury.
2. Priapism—persistent erection of penis.
3. Loss of bowel and bladder control; usually urinary retention and bladder distention.
4. Loss of sweating and vasomotor tone below level of cord lesion.
5. Marked reduction of blood pressure—from loss of peripheral and vascular resistance.

Emergency Management

1. Keep the patient on a flat hard stretcher or board.
    a. Do not move the spine; keep the back straight—flexion or extension can increase the cord injury.
    b. Move the patient on stretcher or transfer board.
       (1) Carry out x-ray procedures while patient is on board.
       (2) Transfer patient to Stryker frame after initial evaluation.

2. Evaluate and examine patient for level of spinal cord injury and associated injuries.
    a. Test for strength and motion of extremities.
       (1) Request patient to flex and extend elbows; squeeze fingers of examiner.
       (2) Request patient to move hips, knees, ankles, toes.
       (3) Observe pattern of respirations—intercostal muscle paralysis causes paradoxical movement of chest and abdomen.
       (4) Observe for priapism—a sign of spinal cord injury.
    b. Test for sensory impairment—prick the skin with a pin.
    c. Test the biceps, triceps, quadriceps and achilles reflexes.
    d. Evaluate vital signs.
    e. Look for the presence of associated injuries.

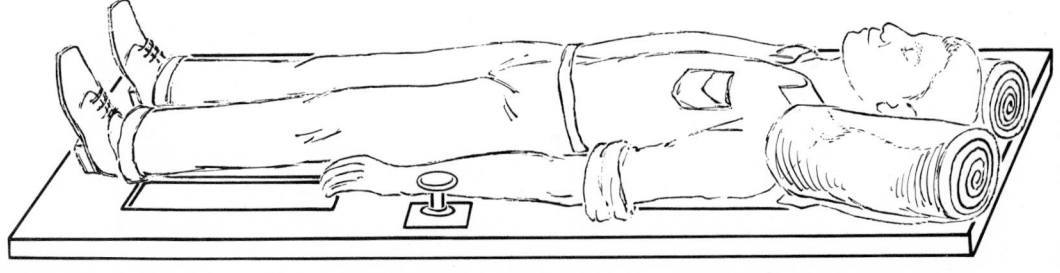

Figure 18-4. When transporting patient with a cervical injury of spine, assign someone to stabilize the patient's head. (From Amer. J. Orthoped. 9 (2) 36-37, Feb. 1967.)

3. Evaluate the patient's respiratory exchange.
   Prepare for tracheostomy if level of cord transection is high.
4. Introduce nasogastric tube—to prevent and treat adynamic ileus, gastric and intestinal distention.
5. Catheterize the patient—patient with spinal cord injury cannot empty his bladder.
6. Start intravenous infusion.
7. Prepare patient for skeletal traction (Crutchfield tongs) if he has a cervical spinal cord injury (see p. 757).
   a. Shave patient's head.
   b. Tongs are applied at the vertex, parallel to coronal suture and directly above mastoid process.

CHEST INJURIES

Injuries to the chest are dire emergencies and are potentially life-threatening because of disturbances to cardiorespiratory physiology. See page 171 for more complete discussion of chest injuries.

Emergency Management (Fig. 18-5)

Objective: to restore normal cardiorespiratory function as rapidly as possible.

A. *Airway Assessment*
   1. Undress patient completely to evaluate patient's respiratory pattern and to look for other injuries; multiple injuries frequently occur with chest injuries.
   2. Assess for signs of obstruction, sternal retraction, stridor, wheezing and cyanosis.
   3. Determine if patient is ventilating properly; auscultate both sides of thorax.

B. *Sucking wounds*—air passing through hole in the chest wall causing collapse of lungs and mediastinal shift. There is an audible passage of air during inspiration and expiration.
   1. Instruct the patient to exhale.
   2. Cover the wound with petrolatum gauze and a pressure bandage applied by circumferential strapping—prevents further shifting of mediastinum and allows for airtight closure of wound; petrolatum gauze dressing helps seal the leak.
   3. Assess respiratory status and assure adequate airway and ventilatory function.
   4. Treat the patient symptomatically until surgical closure of the chest wall wound can be carried out.

C. *Flail chest*—loss of stability of chest wall with subsequent respiratory impairment. This is usually the result of multiple rib fractures.
   1. Immobilize the flail portion of the chest by stabilizing it with the hands and then applying a pressure dressing with adhesive strapping.
   2. Prepare for tracheostomy or endotracheal intubation plus mechanical ventilation—to expand the lungs and give adequate oxygenation.
   3. Place patient on his injured side with compression by padding (folded blanket, sandbag).
   4. Prepare for operative internal fixation of fracture segments.

D. *Hemothorax*—accumulation of fluid and clotted blood in the pleural cavity.
   1. Drain the hemothorax with chest tube and suction (see p. 150).
   2. Prepare patient for emergency thoracotomy if necessary.

EMERGENCY MANAGEMENT OF PATIENT WITH CHEST INJURIES

Objective: Restore normal cardiopulmonary function as rapidly as possible

Assess Patient to Determine Psychological Status

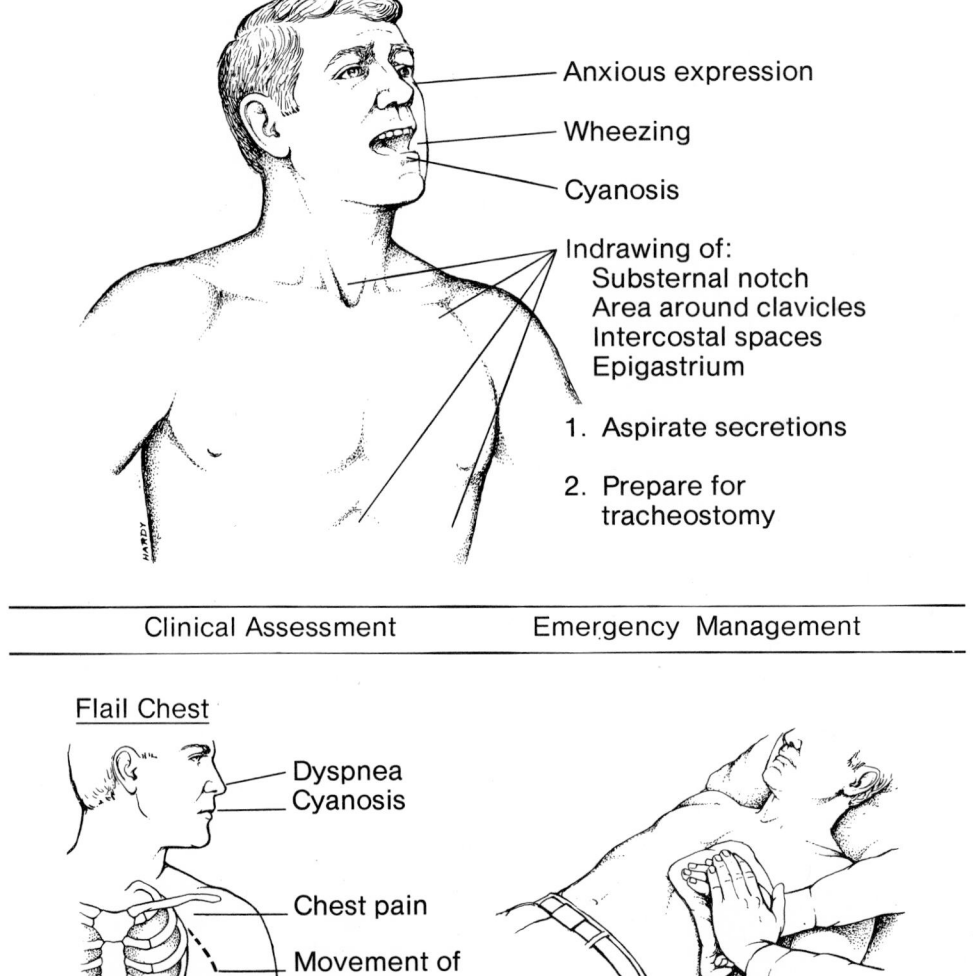

Anxious expression

Wheezing

Cyanosis

Indrawing of:
 Substernal notch
 Area around clavicles
 Intercostal spaces
 Epigastrium

1. Aspirate secretions

2. Prepare for
   tracheostomy

Clinical Assessment	Emergency Management

Flail Chest

Dyspnea
Cyanosis

Chest pain

Movement of
involved chest
wall

Stabilize flail segments with hands.
Apply a pressure dressing.
Place patient on affected side.

Figure 18-5. Emergency management of patients with chest injuries.

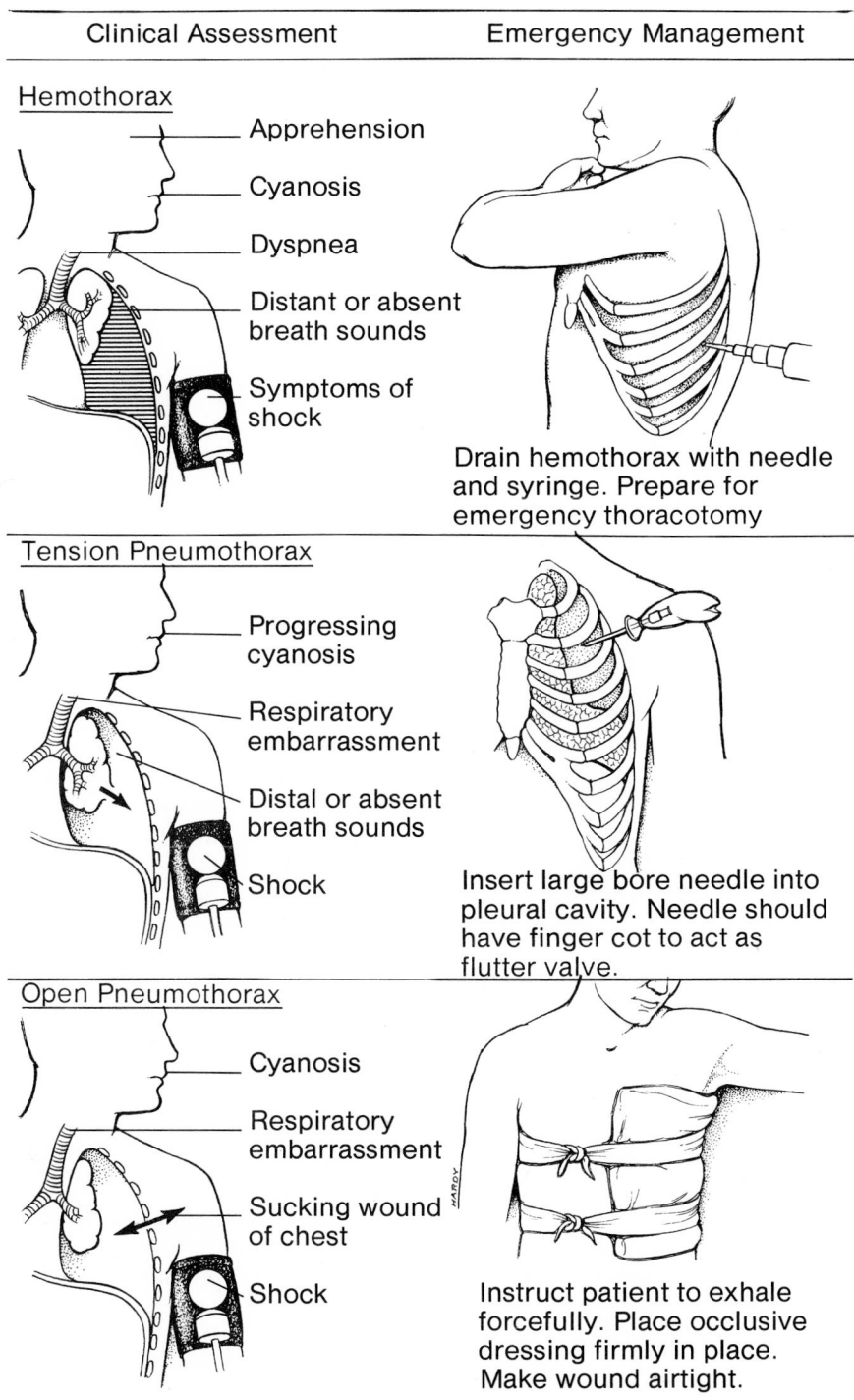

Clinical Assessment	Emergency Management

Hemothorax

Apprehension

Cyanosis

Dyspnea

Distant or absent breath sounds

Symptoms of shock

Drain hemothorax with needle and syringe. Prepare for emergency thoracotomy

Tension Pneumothorax

Progressing cyanosis

Respiratory embarrassment

Distal or absent breath sounds

Shock

Insert large bore needle into pleural cavity. Needle should have finger cot to act as flutter valve.

Open Pneumothorax

Cyanosis

Respiratory embarrassment

Sucking wound of chest

Shock

Instruct patient to exhale forcefully. Place occlusive dressing firmly in place. Make wound airtight.

E. *Tension pneumothorax*—air in the pleural cavity producing displacement of the mediastinum to the uninvolved side with resultant severe cardiorespiratory embarrassment.
   1. Insert large bore needle (No. 16 or 18) into pleural cavity.
   2. Attach incised finger cot to hub of needle to act as a flutter valve.

F. *Cardiac tamponade*—compression of heart resulting from accumulation of fluid within the pericardial sac (see p. 243).

EYE INJURIES

Basic Assumption

   1. Do no harm.
   2. Suspect a penetrating ocular injury with every eye wound until it is proved otherwise.

Emergency Management

A. *Corneal abrasion*—injury to the cornea which goes no deeper than the epithelium.
   1. Instill 0.5% tetracaine (Pontocaine) solution—to relieve pain and facilitate eye examination.
   2. Stain the cornea with sterile fluorescein—to detect existence of an abrasion and its extent.
   3. Apply a pressure bandage, firmly but gently, over eye—to prevent movement of the eyelid and resultant irritation of abraded corneal area.
   4. Give oral analgesic as necessary—abrasions of the cornea are painful.
   5. Advise patient to rest his eyes for 24 hours for greater comfort.
   6. Instruct patient to return to ophthalmologist the following day for dressing change and inspection of eye for evidence of infection or ulcer formation.

B. *Contusion*—blackeye; hemorrhage into the orbit from trauma; hyphema (hemorrhage into anterior chamber of eye).
   1. Contusions usually clear slowly and without treatment.
      a. Apply cold compresses intermittently for first 24 hours to control pain and swelling.
      b. Apply warm compresses (after 24 hours) intermittently.
   2. Place patient on bedrest with both eyes bandaged if intraocular hemorrhage occurs.

C. *Foreign bodies lodged in cornea*—treatment by ophthalmologist or emergency department physician.
   1. Instill sterile anesthetic into the conjunctival sac—to facilitate examination.
   2. Ophthalmologist will remove superficial particles with a moist cotton-tipped applicator.
   3. Instill antibiotic ointment (Neomycin, Neosporin) in conjunctival sac—to prevent bacterial contamination.
   4. Apply eye patch and reinforce instruction to return to ophthalmologist the following day to determine if healing is under way.

D. *Penetrating injuries to the eye*—lacerations or intraocular foreign bodies.
   1. Cover eye with sterile dressing and call ophthalmologist.
   2. Apply eye patch lightly—pressure of pad may cause further penetration.

E. *Burns of the eye*—cause drying of the cornea with resulting chronic conjunctivitis and corneal ulceration.
    1. *Thermal burns* (associated with face or body burns).
        a. Call ophthalmologist.
        b. Thermal burns are treated as burns of skin structures.
    2. *Chemical burns*—may be either acid or alkali in nature. Both cause intense pain and inflammation.
        a. *Irrigate eye with copious amounts of water*—holding the patient's eye directly under running water with lids retracted by gauze flats is the best way to irrigate the eye when immediate irrigation is required.
            (1) Irrigate for at least 5 minutes.
            (2) Repeat irrigation every 15–20 minutes until patient is seen by ophthalmologist.
        b. Instill 2 drops of 5% tetracaine (Pontocaine) to control severe pain (upon order).

FRACTURES

A *fracture* is a break in the continuity of the bone.

Emergency Management

    1. Give immediate attention to the patient's general condition.
        a. Evaluate for respiratory difficulties—from edema due to facial and neck injuries, accumulation of secretions in respiratory tract, etc.
            (1) Examine chest for evidences of sucking chest wounds, pneumothorax, flail chest, etc.
            (2) Prepare for tracheal intubation or emergency tracheostomy.
        b. Control hemorrhage.
            (1) Control venous bleeding by direct pressure.
            (2) Apply digital pressure over artery nearest to bleeding area.
            (3) Suspect internal hemorrhage (pleural, pericardial or abdominal) in the event of continuing shock and in the presence of injuries to chest and abdomen.
        c. Treat for shock—usually the result of blood loss in patients with fractures.
            (1) Assess for falling blood pressure, cold and clammy skin and rapid thready pulse.
            (2) Keep in mind that a large amount of blood loss may accompany a fracture of the femur.
            (3) Maintain the blood pressure with intravenous infusions, plasma or plasma expanders.
            (4) Give blood transfusion(s) as soon as blood is available.
            (5) Administer oxygen—cardiopulmonary embarrassment produces decreased oxygen supply to the tissues and circulatory collapse.
        d. Look for evidence of head, chest and other injuries—patients with multiple fractures may have other serious injuries.
    2. Inspect the fractured part(s).
        a. Cut away clothing if necessary.
        b. Observe the entire body using a methodical head-to-toe system—inspect for lacerations, swelling and deformities.
        c. Look for *angulation* (bending), *shortening* and *rotation*.

      d. Assess for coolness, blanching, decreased sensation and motor function, diminished or absent pulses—indicate injury to the blood supply.
      e. Check peripheral pulses.
      f. Handle the part gently and as little as possible.
   3. Apply the splint before the patient is moved.
      a. Immobilize the joint above and below the fracture—to prevent further soft tissue injury from the motion of the fracture fragments.
      b. Extend the splints well beyond the joints adjacent to the fracture.
      c. Use the patient's clothing for padding (tie, shirt) if nothing else is available.
      d. Use newspapers, magazines, pillows, tree limbs and boards for splints if necessary. (Specialized splints, traction are used in the hospital.)
      e. Splint joints in functional positions.
   4. Investigate any complaint of pain or pressure.
   5. Transport the patient carefully and gently.
   6. See page 785 for more complete discussion of treatment of fractures of specific sites.

Emergency Splinting and Transporting

A. *Skull*
   1. Elevate the head slightly.
   2. Transport with the head to one side to promote drainage of mucus, blood and vomitus if there is no spinal cord injury.

B. *Jaw*
   1. Hold jaw up and in by tying with bandage (if there is no spinal cord injury).
   2. Transport patient in a sitting position with head slightly forward.

C. *Cervical Spine*
   1. Hold the patient's head, keeping it in line with the body.
   2. Slide the patient on a rigid surface *flat on his back, face up.*
   3. Move the entire body as a unit. Avoid twisting, turning or pulling of the spine.
   4. Immobilize the head on each side with padded stones, bricks, sandbags, etc.
   5. Assign someone to keep head immobilized while patient is being transported.

D. *Lumbar Spine*
   1. Straighten patient carefully and place him on a rigid surface.
   2. If a rigid surface is not available, transport him face down on a blanket using at least 4 persons.

E. *Pelvis*
   1. Turn the patient carefully on his back.
   2. Place padding between the legs and splint them together to prevent unnecessary motion.
   3. Immobilize the pelvis by binding a folded blanket around the pelvis.
   4. Transport on a stretcher.

F. *Shoulder, Arm and Elbow*
   1. Place elbow at right angle and apply sling.
   2. Bind arm and sling to body with a circular bandage or binder.

G. *Forearm, Wrist, Hand*

Immobilize with newspaper splint (or other suitable splinting apparatus) and place in sling.

H. *Hip*

1. Splint from axilla to ankle with board, or bind legs together.
2. Use a Thomas splint if available.
3. Transport on a stretcher.

I. *Lower extremity*

1. Apply steady even traction and splint fracture from hip to ankle.
2. Transport on stretcher.

J. *Ankle*

1. Wrap pillow around ankle and leg.
2. Transport on stretcher.

MULTIPLE INJURIES

Underlying Considerations

1. The *evidence* of gross trauma may be slight or completely absent.
2. Any injury interfering with vital physiologic function which is an immediate threat to life takes priority for immediate treatment (obstructed airway, hemorrhage).
3. The patient should be completely undressed and a rapid physical examination carried out as quickly as possible.

Emergency Management

Objectives: determine the extent of injuries.
establish priorities of treatment.

1. Carry out a rapid physical examination to determine if patient is breathing, bleeding or in shock; determine the status of his responsiveness and if he has severe wounds or fracture deformities.
2. Establish an open airway.
   a. Apply suction to clear the trachea and bronchial tree.
   b. Hold hand above patient's nose to determine adequacy of ventilation.
   c. Prepare for endotracheal intubation if necessary (p. 104).
   d. Suspect serious intrathoracic injuries if respiratory distress continues after adequate airway has been established.
      (1) *Flail chest* (p. 173).
         (a) Provide endotracheal intubation with IPP ventilation to provide for expansion of lungs, ventilation and prevention of atelectasis or pneumonia.
         (b) Stabilize chest wall with hands, pressure dressing and subsequent fixation of rib fractures.
         (c) Introduce 18 gauge needle into 2nd interspace of midclavicular line for emergency treatment (p. 912, Fig. 18-5).
         (d) Prepare for subsequent chest drainage.
         (e) Give supplemental oxygen.

(2) *Sucking wound of chest* (p. 172).
Cover wound with sterile dressing.
(3) *Hemothorax* (p. 172).
(a) Insert chest tubes (No. 28 French) connected to a water-sealed bottle.
(b) Prepare for emergency thoracotomy if operative control of bleeding is necessary.
(4) *Cardiac tamponade*
(a) Watch for falling blood pressure, rising venous pressure, quiet heart, narrowing pulse pressure.
(b) Prepare for needle pericardiocentesis (p. 244).
(5) *Tracheal or bronchial rupture*—produces pneumomediastinum or pneumothorax (p. 172).
Assess for cardiac embarrassment, subcutaneous emphysema of neck.
3. Control hemorrhage.
   a. Apply pressure over bleeding points if hemorrhage is overt (see p. 904).
   b. Expect significant blood loss in patient with fracture of shaft of femur, with multiple fractures or with major pelvic trauma.
   c. Prepare for immediate surgical intervention if patient is bleeding internally.
4. Prevent and treat hypovolemic shock.
   a. Insert I.V. needle or catheter; draw blood for laboratory analysis as directed (fasting blood sugar, electrolytes, type, cross matching, etc.).
   b. Introduce catheter into right antecubital space for central venous pressure readings as required (see p. 241).
   c. Start I.V. infusions in both upper extremities (if necessary) with large bore needles or catheters; assist with venous cut down as directed.
   d. Give balanced saline solution in sufficient quantity to maintain blood pressure until blood is available.
   e. Give saline solution rapidly enough to keep central venous pressure reading at 5–15 cm. of water.
   f. Prepare for immediate surgical intervention if patient does not respond to fluids or blood. Inability to restore blood pressure and circulatory volume in patient usually indicates hemorrhage.
5. Splint fractures to prevent further trauma to soft tissues and blood vessels and relieve pain; note presence or absence of pulses in fractured extremities.
6. Assess for head and neck injuries (p. 722).
   Make definite statements concerning base-line neurologic status of patient regarding his level of responsiveness, size and reactivity of pupils, motor power, reflexes.
7. Assess patient for gastrointestinal injuries.
   a. Examine patient repeatedly for abdominal pain, muscular rigidity, tenderness, rebound tenderness, diminished bowel sounds, hypotension and shock.
   b. Prepare for laparotomy if patient shows continuing signs of unlocalized hemorrhage and deterioration.
   c. Assist with insertion of nasogastric tube if upper gastrointestinal bleeding is suspected.
8. Insert an indwelling catheter to determine possible injury to urinary system and to monitor hourly urinary output.
   Assess for hematuria and oliguria.
9. Evaluate patient for other injuries and institute appropriate treatment.
10. Carry out continuing observation of patient; make repeated physical examinations.

POISONING

Poison is any substance which when ingested, inhaled, absorbed, applied to the skin or developed within the body, in relatively small amounts, produces injury to the body by its chemical action. (See page 1383 for prevention of poisoning.)

Swallowed Poisons

General Nursing Management

1. Maintain the airway.
   a. Administer oxygen for respiratory depression (respirations below 10), unconsciousness, cyanosis, shock.
   b. Give artificial respiration if respiration is depressed.
2. Treat shock with the administration of whole blood.
3. Support the patient having convulsions (p. 731)—many poisons excite the central nervous system or else the patient convulses from oxygen deprivation.
   a. Give intravenous pentobarbital (or other anticonvulsant) until specific therapy can be instituted.
   b. Give positive pressure respiration if oxygen is necessary.
4. Give analgesics for pain—severe pain causes vasomotor collapse and reflex inhibition of normal physiologic functions.
5. Watch for fluid imbalance and acidosis.
6. Reduce elevated temperature by tepid sponges (see p. 726).
7. Give specific therapy. Administer special chemical antidotes or specific pharmacological antagonists [naloxone hydrochloride (Narcan)] as early as possible.
8. Give constant nursing surveillance and attention to the patient in coma (see p. 728) —coma from poisoning results from interference with brain cell function or metabolism.

Corrosive Poisons

A. *Clinical Manifestations*
   1. Severe pain; burning sensation in mouth and throat
   2. Vomiting
   3. Destruction of oral mucosa
   4. Drooling in children; painful swallowing or inability to swallow

B. *Types of Corrosive Poisons*
   1. Acid and acid-like corrosives; sodium acid sulfate (toilet bowl cleaners), acetic acid (glacial), sulfuric acid, nitric acid, oxalic acid, hydrofluoric acid (rust removers), iodine, silver nitrate.
   2. Alkali corrosives—most common are sodium hydroxide (lye; drain cleaners), dishwasher detergents, sodium carbonate (washing soda), ammonia water, sodium hypochlorite (household bleach).

C. *Emergency Management*

   If the patient can swallow after ingestion of a *corrosive poison,* the following substances and amounts may be given:

    a. For acids: milk, water or milk of magnesia (1 tablespoon to 1 cup of water)

    b. For alkalies: milk, water, any fruit juice or dilute vinegar (1–2 cups for patients aged 1–5, or up to 1 quart for individuals 5 years old or older)

NOTE: A hospital with a 24-hour emergency department can qualify as a poison control center and receive U.S.P.H. service card service and statistical support.

Noncorrosive Poisons

Emergency Management

1. *Remove poison from patient's stomach immediately by inducing vomiting.*

NURSING ALERT: Do not induce vomiting if victim has consumed a strong acid, alkali or other corrosive or hydrocarbon solvent. Do not induce vomiting if patient is in a coma, is unconscious or having convulsions.

---

    a. Give 3–4 glassfuls of milk or water to drink to dilute poison.

    b. Induce vomiting by giving syrup of ipecac or inserting the index finger or blunt end of a spoon at the back of the patient's throat.

    c. Do not take more than 5 minutes to induce emesis.

2. Carry out gastric lavage procedure (p. 923) to remove any unabsorbed poison. This procedure is *not* done if corrosives or hydrocarbon solvents have been ingested. (Example: turpentine, varsol, gasoline, kerosine, liquid wax, etc.)

3. Instruct family to bring unused poison to hospital for identification.

4. Know the poison control center in the area; call the center if unknown toxic agent has been taken or if it is necessary to identify an antidote for a known toxic agent.

Inhaled Poisons

Emergency Management

1. Carry patient to fresh air immediately.

2. Open all doors and windows.

3. Loosen all tight clothing.

4. Apply artificial respiration (by direct inflation of the patient's lungs) if breathing has stopped or is irregular (see p. 898).

5. Prevent chilling. (Wrap patient in blankets.)

6. Keep patient as quiet as possible.

7. Do not give alcohol in any form.

Carbon Monoxide Poisoning

May occur as an industrial or household accident or as an attempted suicide.

A. *Basic Understandings*

1. The effect of carbon monoxide is to render the hemoglobin useless as an oxygen-carrying chemical, because it unites so firmly with the pigment in place of oxygen. As a result, tissue anoxia occurs.

2. A concentration of carbon monoxide as low as 0.03% is potentially dangerous.

B. *Clinical Manifestations*

    Headache, lassitude, drowsiness, coma

    Cherry red skin color

C. *Emergency Management*

1. Give 100% oxygen by mask until blood carboxyhemoglobin is reduced and respiration is normal.
2. Give artificial respiration (see p. 898).
3. Maintain the blood pressure and body warmth.
4. Administer 50 ml. of 50% glucose (or give mannitol)—to reduce cerebral edema.
5. Observe patient constantly—psychoses, spastic paralysis, visual disturbances may persist following resuscitation; these may be symptoms of permanent central nervous system damage.

Skin Contamination Poisons

Emergency Management

1. Drench skin with water (shower, hose, faucet).
2. Apply stream of water on skin while removing clothing.
3. Cleanse skin thoroughly with water; rapidity in washing is most important in reducing extent of injury.

Injected Poisons

Snake Bites

Emergency Management

Objective: to remove as much venom as possible and retard the spread of venom; venom may be neurotoxic or hemotoxic.

1. Make patient lie down as soon as possible; prepare for immediate transportation to the hospital.
2. Do not give alcohol in any form.
3. Apply tourniquet above the injection site.
   a. The pulse in vessels below the tourniquet should not disappear, nor should the tourniquet produce a throbbing sensation.
   b. Loosen the tourniquet for 1 minute every 15 minutes.
4. Make linear incisions through the fang marks.
5. Apply suction to venom.
6. Apply icepacks to the site of bite—slows absorption of venom and relieves pain of bite.
7. Carry patient to physician or hospital: DO NOT LET HIM WALK!

Stinging Insects

(Bee, hornet, wasp, yellow jacket)

NURSING ALERT: Patient may have extreme sensitivity to hymenoptera venom (bees, hornets, wasps, yellow jackets). This constitutes an acute emergency—death may occur within 1 hour.

A. *Clinical Manifestations*

Anaphylactic shock

Severe fall of blood pressure	Itching
Difficult breathing	Bronchial constriction
Edema of face, lips	

B. *Emergency Management*

1. Give epinephrine hydrochloride (Adrenalin) as directed.
2. See page 902 for treatment of anaphylactic shock.
3. Patients known to be sensitive to hymenoptera venom should carry an emergency kit with tourniquet, epinephrine (with syringe and needles) an aerosol inhalator containing epinephrine, and oral antihistamine tablets.

Food Poisoning

Food poisoning is a sudden, explosive illness that occurs after ingestion of food or drink that contains bacteria (or their products), chemicals and poisonous plants or animals.

Emergency Management

1. Induce vomiting.
   a. Have patient drink warm water; stimulate back of pharynx with finger or blunt end of spoon to induce vomiting.
   b. Save vomitus for possible laboratory analysis.
2. Monitor vital signs on a continuing basis.
   a. Assess respiration, blood pressure, sensorium, central venous pressure, muscular activity.
   b. Weigh patient.
3. Determine source and type of food poisoning.
   a. Bring suspected food to medical facility for identification.
   b. Determine:
      (1) How soon after eating did the symptoms occur? Immediate onset suggests chemical, plant or animal poisoning.
      (2) What was eaten in the previous meal? Did the food have any unusual odor or taste?—Most foods causing bacterial poisoning do not have unusual odor or taste.
      (3) Did vomiting occur? What was the appearance of the vomitus?
      (4) Did diarrhea occur?—Usually absent with botulism, shell-fish or other fish poisoning.
      (5) Are any neurologic symptoms present?—Occur in botulism (p. 833), chemical plant and animal poisoning.
      (6) Does the patient have fever?—Seen in salmonella, favism (ingestion of fava beans) and some fish poisoning.
      (7) What is the patient's appearance?
4. Support the respiratory system—deaths from respiratory paralysis occur with botulism, some insecticides, fish poisoning, etc.
   a. Insert oropharyngeal airway or endotracheal tube.
   b. Prepare for tracheostomy if necessary.

5. Maintain fluid and electrolyte balance—severe vomiting produces alkalosis and severe diarrhea produces acidosis; large amounts of electrolytes and water lost by vomiting and diarrhea.
   a. Watch for oligemic shock—from severe fluid and electrolyte losses.
   b. Assess for apathy, rapid pulse, fever, oliguria, anuria, hypotension, delirium.
   c. Carry out blood electrolyte studies—sodium, potassium, chloride, arterial blood gas determinations, pH, carbon dioxide.
6. Correct and control hypoglycemia.
7. Control the nausea.
   a. Give sips of weak tea, carbonated drinks, tap water for mild nausea.
   b. Give rectal suppositories (anti-emetics, sodium phenobarbital) if patient cannot tolerate fluids or medications by mouth.
   c. Give clear liquids 12–24 hours after nausea and vomiting subside.
   d. Graduate to a low residue bland diet.
8. Control the diarrhea—diarrhea may be desirable to rid body of ingested toxins.
   a. Give atropine, meperidine or codeine as ordered.
   b. Apply warm compresses and moist mild heat to abdomen—for comfort.
   c. Give antidiarrheal agents as ordered (kaolin, bismuth subcarbonate, aluminum oxide gels)—to adsorb and bind toxins.

GUIDELINES: *Assisting with Gastric Lavage*

Gastric lavage involves passing a large tube into the stomach to wash out the stomach.

Purpose

To remove unabsorbed poison after poison ingestion (may be done anytime within 3 hours after ingestion of poison; up to 10 hours with salicylate ingestion).

> NURSING ALERT: Gastric lavage is dangerous after ingestion of strong corrosive agents (lye, ammonia, mineral acids).

Equipment

Stomach tubes: No. 20 (0.5 cm.) and No. 30 (1.5 cm.)
Large irrigating syringe with adapter
Large funnel (plastic) with adapter to fit stomach tube
Water-soluble lubricant
Tap water or appropriate antidote (milk, saline solution, sodium bicarbonate solution, fruit juice, activated charcoal)
Bucket for aspirate
Suction machine
Mouth gag; endotracheal tubes with inflatable cuffs
Containers for specimens

Procedure

Nursing Action	Rationale/Amplification
Preparatory Phase	
1. Give patient a glass of water to drink if he is conscious.	1. This delays absorption of poison.
2. Remove dentures.	
3. Apply appropriate restraint for a child (see pp. 1073-1076).	
4. Lubricate tube with water-soluble lubricant.	
Performance Phase	
1. Measure the distance between the bridge of the nose and the xiphoid process. Mark with indelible pencil or tape.	
2. If the patient is comatose he is intubated with a cuffed endotracheal tube.	2. A cuffed endotracheal tube prevents aspiration of gastric contents.
3. Place the patient in a supine Trendelenburg position. *Have standby suction available.*	3. This position prevents fluid from running into the trachea and keeps reflux vomitus from being aspirated.
4. Pass the tube via the nasal route while keeping the head in a neutral position. Pass the tube to adhesive marking (about 50 cm. or 20 inches).	4. When this marking is level with the mouth, the stomach should have been entered. If tube enters the larynx instead of esophagus the patient will experience coughing and dyspnea.
5. Submerge free end of tube below water level at moment of patient's exhalation.	5. If tube has inadvertently entered the lungs, bubbling of water will occur with each exhalation.
6. Aspirate stomach with syringe attached to the tube before instilling water or antidote. Save the specimen.	6. Aspiration is carried out to remove the stomach contents.
7. Remove syringe. Attach funnel to the stomach tube or use 50-ml. syringe to put water in gastric tube.	7. Overfilling may cause regurgitation and aspiration or force stomach contents through the pylorus.
8. Elevate funnel above patient's head and pour 120–500 ml. of water or antidote into funnel. Avoid overfilling stomach.	8. If the syringe method is used, the turbulence from the pressure of the syringe will force the fluid to mix with the stomach contents, helping to wash all the mucosal surface.
9. Lower the funnel and siphon gastric contents into bucket.	
10. Save samples of first 2 washings.	10. Keep first washings isolated from other washings for possible analysis.
11. Repeat lavage (washing) procedure for 10–15 times or until returns are clear. (1–2 liters).	
12. At completion of lavage: a. Stomach may be left empty. b. Antidote may be instilled in tube (a demulcent) and allowed to remain in stomach. c. Cathartic (saline) may be put down tube.	
13. Pinch off tube during removal or maintain suction while tube is being withdrawn.	13. Pinching off the tube prevents aspiration and initiation of gag reflex. Keeping the patient's head lower than his body also gives this protection.

Nursing Action	**Rationale/Amplification**

Follow-up Phase

1. Give patient a carthartic if ordered.

2. Have the patient under close observation for 24 hours.
3. Record the poison ingested (if known) and the condition of patient after lavage.
4. Check blood salicylate level 6 hours after aspirin ingestion to determine maximum blood level.

1. If the poison has no corrosive action on the bowel a cathartic may be given to remove unabsorbed material from the intestines. Mineral oil may help absorb petroleum distillates.
2. Latent symptoms may develop.

4. Aspirin is the most common accidental overdose.

HEAT STROKE

Heat stroke is a medical emergency caused by the failure of the heat-regulating mechanisms of the body.

Clinical Manifestations

Headache and visual disturbances
Dizziness and nausea
Hot, flushed dry skin
Weak, rapid and irregular pulse

Sudden loss of consciousness
High fever
Cessation of sweating
Muscle cramping

Emergency Management

Objective: to reduce high temperature as rapidly as possible.

1. Reduce the body temperature to 39°C. (102.2°F.) rectally as rapidly as possible.
   a. Place the patient in a cool environment.
   b. Remove patient's clothing.
   c. Sponge patient liberally with water at room temperature—or
   d. Place patient in a tub of cool water—or
   e. Apply hypothermia blanket.
   f. Give chilled saline enemas—if temperature does not come down.
   g. Place electric fan so that it blows on patient—air movement increases evaporation.
2. Massage body and extremities—to maintain circulation.
3. Administer oxygen under positive pressure by face mask if cyanosis is present.
4. Start intravenous infusion of hypotonic multiple electrolyte solution; give slowly because of danger of pulmonary edema.
5. Give antipyretic and chlorpromazine (I.V.) as directed.
6. Give supportive care for convulsions (see p. 731).
7. Measure urinary output—acute tubular necrosis is a complication of heat stroke.
8. Advise patient to avoid immediate re-exposure to high heat (after his condition has stabilized). Patient may remain hypersensitive to high heat for considerable length of time.

COLD INJURIES

Local *cold injuries* include cold sensitivity, chilblains, frost bite, immersion foot and trench foot.

Clinical Manifestations

First degree—hyperemia, edema, skin peeling, slight swelling, redness, mild cyanosis
Second degree—redness and slight swelling, vesicles, black eschars (sloughing)
Third degree—vesicles, edema, black, hard dry eschar, shrivelling toes
Fourth degree—destruction of entire area involved; gangrene

Emergency Management

Objective: to restore circulation to the part and to relieve vasospasm.
1. Do not allow patient to walk if lower extremities are involved.
2. Remove all constrictive clothing.
3. Rewarm extremity rapidly by immersing it in water at 40.6°C. (105°F.) for several minutes.
4. Expose extremity to air at room temperature after rapid rewarming.
5. Administer analgesic for pain.
6. Give tetanus prophylaxis (human tetanus immune globulin or toxoid) (see p. 825) if ulceration has occurred.
7. Place patient on bedrest—to prevent him from walking on thawed toes which will cause tissue destruction and to assess extent of tissue damage over a period of time.
   a. Elevate the affected part(s).
   b. Avoid pressure or friction on extremity.
8. Give prophylactic antibiotic therapy.
9. Instruct patient to avoid subsequent exposure to cold.

DRUG ABUSE

Narcotics

Examples

Heroin (most frequently involved)
Opium
Morphine, codeine, synthetic narcotics (methadone)

Clinical Manifestations

Acute Intoxication

1. Pinpoint pupils
2. Decreased vital signs
3. Coma
4. Fresh needle marks along course of superficial veins
5. Thrombophlebitis
6. Healed skin abscesses

Emergency Management

1. Support vital functions. Use mechanical artificial ventilation.
2. Give naloxone hydrochloride (Narcan) or levallorphan tartrate (Lorfan)—antinarcotics which reverse effect of heroin toxicity.

3. Send urine for analysis—opiates can be detected in urine.
4. Gastric lavage may be necessary to obtain sample of drug for analysis.
5. Hemodialysis is indicated for severe drug intoxication.

Heroin Withdrawal Syndrome

A. *Clinical Manifestations*
1. Lethargy, yawning
2. Perspiration, lacrimation, runny nose
3. Dilated pupils, which react poorly to light
4. Gooseflesh, muscular aches
5. Twitching, anorexia, nausea, vomiting
6. Chills and fever

B. *Emergency Management*
1. Give methadone (Dolophine) daily 10–20 mg. orally to a total of 40–60 mg. Dosage is then reduced if patient is receiving treatment in an appropriate methadone center. Substitution therapy should be given in a hospital setting.
2. Give intravenous fluids—patient may be dehydrated from vomiting; may progress to toxic delirium.
3. Assess for concomitant medical problems (hepatitis, pneumonia, severe diarrhea).
4. Place patient in protective environment under proper medical supervision.

Barbiturates

Examples

Pentobarbital (Nembutal)
Secobarbital (Seconal)
Amobarbital (Amytal)

Clinical Manifestations

1. Flushed face
2. Decreased pulse rate
3. Increasing nystagmus
4. Decreasing tendon reflexes
5. Decreasing mental alertness
6. Difficulty in speaking
7. Poor motor coordination
8. Mental confusion

Emergency Management

1. Maintain airway and stimulate depressed respiration.
2. Support cardiovascular and respiratory functions.
3. Prepare patient for dialysis as directed.

Withdrawal Syndrome

A. *Clinical Manifestations*
1. Shakiness, anxiety, muscular irritability
2. Orthostatic hypotension, tachycardia
3. Grand mal convulsions, hyperpyrexia
4. Possible death

NURSING ALERT: Symptoms of barbiturate withdrawal are serious because abrupt withdrawal from the drug may be life-threatening.

B. *Emergency Management*
1. Maintain airway and stimulate depressed respiration.
2. Administer pentobarbital according to level of patient's tolerance.
3. Carry out gastric lavage to evacuate stomach.
4. Give oxygen, antibiotics, intravenous fluids as required.
5. Gradually reduce dosage of barbiturates.
6. Watch for excessive agitation, confusion and convulsions.

Salicylate Poisoning
(Aspirin)

Clinical Manifestations

1. Hyperpnea
2. Disturbed acid-base balance
3. Tinnitus and vertigo
4. Mental aberrations
5. Hyperventilation
6. Convulsions, coma

Emergency Management

1. Treat respiratory depression.
2. Give water, milk or activated charcoal—to delay absorption of ingested poison.
3. Carry out gastric lavage—will remove significant amounts of salicylates up to 10 hours. (Give Ipecac as directed.)
4. Support patient with intravenous infusions to correct electrolyte imbalance and maintain hydration.
5. Give blood transfusion if blood pressure is low.
6. Give sodium bicarbonate or sodium lactate parenterally in severe poisoning.
7. Prepare for peritoneal dialysis (p. 476) or hemodialysis for patients with severe intoxication.
8. Give vitamin K for bleeding—salicylates lower plasma prothrombin by interfering with vitamin K utilization in the liver.

Amphetamine-type Drugs

Examples

Amphetamine (Benzedrine)
Dextroamphetamine (Dexedrine)
Methamphetamine (Desoxyn, Methedrine)

Clinical Manifestations

1. Aggressive type of behavior
2. Irritability, insomnia
3. Hyperactivity, stereotyped activities
4. Dilated pupils
5. Increase in pulse and blood pressure
6. Paranoid suspiciousness
7. High temperature
8. Convulsions, coma, death

Emergency Management

1. Try to communicate with patient.
2. Use specific drug therapy to calm patient.

   a. Chlorpromazine (Thorazine)—Assess patient carefully as chlorpromazine may lower convulsive threshold.
   b. Barbiturates for insomnia.
3. Place patient in protective environment—observe for suicidal attempts.

Hallucinogens or Psychedelic-type Drugs

Examples

LSD, Mescaline,
Cannabis (marihuana)
Psilocybin

Clinical Manifestations

1. Marked anxiety bordering on panic
2. Confusion, incoherence
3. Hallucinations
4. Hazardous behavior
5. Flashback—recurrence of LSD-like state; may occur weeks or months after drug was taken

Emergency Management

1. Try to communicate with patient—use "vocal anesthesia" to reassure him.
2. Reassure patient that he will be cared for—isolation may intensify his isolation and panic.
3. Instruct patient to keep his eyes open—reduces intensity of reaction.
4. Sedate the patient if his hyperactivity cannot be controlled.
5. Watch patient closely—his behavior may become hazardous.
6. Place patient in a protected environment under proper medical supervision.

Nonbarbiturate Sedatives

Examples

Glutethimide (Doriden)
Methyprylon (Noludar)
Ethchlorvynol (Placidyl)

Ethinamate (Valmid)
Meprobamate (Miltown, Equinal)
Chlordiazepoxide (Librium)
Diazepam (Valium)

Clinical Manifestations

1. Decreasing mental alertness
2. Confusion
3. Slurred speech
4. Ataxia
5. Coma, possible death

Emergency Management

1. Watch for sudden apnea and laryngeal spasm (especially in patients habituated to Doriden).
2. Insert endotracheal tube as a precaution.
3. Utilize assisted ventilation.
4. Give vasopressor agents as indicated.
5. Use hemodialysis therapy if needed.

ALCOHOLISM
Acute Alcoholism

Clinical Manifestations

Drowsiness, incoordination, slurring of speech
  or
Belligerency, grandiosity
Odor of alcohol on breath
Blood alcohol concentrations:
  Mild intoxication—blood alcohol 0.05–0.15%; 0.5–1.5 mg./ml.
  Moderate intoxication—blood alcohol 0.15–0.3%; 1.5–3 mg./ml.
  Severe intoxication—blood alcohol 0.3–0.5%; 3–5 mg./ml.

Emergency Management

1. Allow the drowsy patient to "sleep off" state of alcoholic intoxication.
   a. Observe for symptoms of respiratory depression.
   b. Protect the airway.
2. Sedate the belligerent, noisy patient—chlordiazepoxide (Librium), chlorpromazine (Thorazine).
3. Examine patient for injuries and organic disease.
   a. Look for symptoms of head injury.
   b. Evaluate for pneumonia—common in alcoholics.
   c. Assess the neurologic status of the patient.
4. Hospitalize if necessary.

Delirium Tremens (Alcoholic Hallucinosis)

Delirium tremens is a toxic state that follows a prolonged bout of steady drinking or diminution or withdrawal of alcoholic intake.

Clinical Manifestations

1. Anxiety; uncontrollable fear
2. Tremulousness, irritability, agitation, insomnia
3. Talkativeness; preoccupation
4. Visual, tactile and auditory hallucinations
5. Autonomic overactivity—tachycardia, profuse perspiration
6. Loss of pride in personal appearance

NURSING ALERT: Delirium Tremens is a serious complication and poses a threat to the life of the alcoholic patient.

Emergency Management

Objective: to give proper sedation to enable patient to rest and recover without the danger of injury or exhaustion.

1. Take the blood pressure as the patient's subsequent medication may depend on his blood pressure reading.
2. Sedate the patient.
   a. Give chlordiazepoxide (Librium) 100 mg. I.M. then 50 mg. every 30 minutes until agitation ceases.

The dosage may be adjusted according to the patient's blood pressure response.

  b. Chlorpromazine (Thorazine) 100 mg. is also used occasionally.

3. Place the patient in a private room where he can be observed closely.

  a. Keep room lighted—to reduce incidence of visual hallucinations.

  b. Observe patient closely—patient may become homicidal or suicidal in response to his hallucinations if he is having alcoholic hallucinosis.

  c. Have someone stay with the patient as much as possible—presence of another person has a reassuring and quieting effect.

4. Maintain hydration via oral or intravenous routes.

5. Give supplemental vitamin therapy and a high protein diet.

6. Administer diphenylhydantoin (Dilantin) or other analeptics as prescribed to prevent or control alcoholic convulsions.

7. Assess respiratory hepatic and cardiovascular status of patient—cirrhosis, pneumonia and cardiac failure are complications of delirium tremens.

PSYCHIATRIC EMERGENCY

Psychiatric emergency is a sudden serious disturbance of behavior, affect or thought which makes the patient unable to cope with his life situation and interpersonal relationships.

Behavioral Manifestations

A. *Overactive*

1. Disturbed, uncooperative, paranoid behavior
2. Anxiety and panic-like state
3. Assaultive and destructive impulses and behavior (patient may be noisy or disturbed from acute alcohol or drug intoxication)

B. *Underactive*

1. Depression
2. Fearfulness
3. Slowing of responses
4. Sad facial expression

C. *Suicidal*

Emergency Management

A. *Overactive*

1. Determine (from family, ambulance driver, etc.) if patient has had past mental illness, hospitalizations, injuries or serious illnesses, uses alcohol or drugs or has experienced crises in interpersonal relationships or intrapsychic conflicts.

2. Try to gain control of the situation.

  a. Approach the patient with a calm, confident and firm manner—this attitude is therapeutic and will help calm the patient.

  b. Be interested in and listen to the patient—encourage him to talk of his thoughts and *feelings*.

  c. Offer appropriate explanations. Tell the truth.

3. Sedate the patient with chlorpromazine (Thorazine) 100 mg. I.M. if he is assaultive or continues to be hyperactive.

4. Use restraints only as a last resort.

5. Admit to psychiatric unit or arrange for psychiatric out-patient treatment.

B. *Underactive*
   1. Listen to the patient in a calm unhurried manner—offer follow-up services.
   2. Give antidepressants with antianxiety agents—amitriptyline (Elavil) or nortriptyline (Aventyl).
   3. Attempt to find out if patient has thought about or attempted suicide.
   4. Anticipate that the patient may be suicidal.
   5. Notify relatives about a seriously depressed patient.
   6. Refer patient to hospital psychiatric unit.

C. *Suicidal*
   1. Treat the emergency condition brought about by the suicide attempt.
      a. Maintain airway.
      b. Treat for shock.
      c. Carry out gastric lavage, hemodialysis, etc.
   2. Prevent further self injury—a patient who has made a suicidal gesture may do so again.
   3. Admit to intensive care unit or psychiatric unit.

SUSPECTED RAPE

Rape is assaultive sexual attack on any unwilling victim.
Statutory rape is carnal knowledge of any girl below a legally set age (16 to 18 in most states) with or without her consent.

Emergency Management
   1. Respect the privacy and sensitivity of the patient. Be kind and supportive.
   2. Observe objectively and record accurately the findings concerning the events of the alleged act. Get the history in the patient's words only if the patient has not already talked to police officers.
      a. Date and time of alleged act
      b. Events of attack
      c. Description of emotional status of patient
   3. Secure written permission from patient (or parent or guardian if patient is a minor) for examination and taking of photographs if necessary.
      a. Record general appearance of patient—evidence of bruises, lacerations, secretions, torn and bloody clothing.
         (1) Help patient undress. Drape properly.
         (2) Save clothing, label appropriately and turn over to proper law enforcement authorities.
      b. Assist with vaginal examination.
         (1) Use water-moistened vaginal speculum for examination; do not use lubricant.
         (2) Children with genital injuries may be examined and injury repaired under general anesthesia.
   4. Assist with securing laboratory specimens.
      a. Swab from vaginal pool:
         (1) Acid phosphatase
         (2) Blood group antigen of semen
         (3) Precipitin tests against human sperm and blood
      b. Secure wet mount of material from fornix—examined immediately for motile sperm.

   c. Obtain smears from vulva.
   d. Obtain culture from cervix for *Neisseria gonorrhoeae;* place in Thayer-Martin
      Medium (see p. 836).
5. Give prophylactic treatment against gonorrhea and syphilis.
   a. Gonorrhea—4.8 million units penicillin G; repeat in 3 days (see p. 835).
   b. Syphilis—2.4 million units of penicillin; 1 dose only.
6. Give diethylstilbestrol to prevent pregnancy.
   a. Give medication to women of child-bearing age.
   b. Dosage—25 mg. twice daily starting immediately and daily thereafter for 5 days.
   c. A cleansing douche may be offered patient if she desires.
7. Support the patient psychologically. Provide follow-up emotional support as indicated.

EMERGENCY DRUGS

Table 18-1 lists the drugs frequently used in emergency situations. Included are their actions, indications and contraindications.

DISASTERS

Disaster is a catastrophe which may be either natural in origin or man-made. If man-made, it may be produced accidentally or by design, such as by a hostile enemy act.

Emergency Management

1. Provide first aid, including but not limited to artificial respiration emergency treatment of open chest wounds; relief of pain; treatment of shock and the preparation of casualties for movement.
2. Control hemorrhage.
3. Attain and maintain patent airway, and intratracheal catheterization, to include emergency tracheostomy.
4. Provide proper and adequate cleansing and treatment of wounds.
5. Bandage wounds and splint fractures.
6. Administer anesthetics under medical supervision.
7. Assist in surgical procedures.
8. Insert nasogastric tubes (lavage or gavage) as directed.
9. Administer whole blood and intravenous solutions, as directed.
10. Administer parenteral medications, as directed.
11. Catheterize males and females.
12. Administer immunizing agents, as directed.
13. Manage the psychologically disturbed.
14. Manage normal deliveries.
15. Operate treatment and aid stations in reception areas and in communities where physicians are inadequate in number, to diagnose and treat minor illnesses and injuries, institute life-saving measures and refer more serious cases to physicians.*

Sorting of Casualties

1. Sorting is done by the most responsible and able person of the medical team.
2. Initial evaluation is done rapidly to detect threats to life and evaluate the patient's general condition.

* Adapted from Summary Report on National Emergency Care, American Medical Association.

TABLE 18-1. EMERGENCY DRUGS*

Drug	Preparations and Dosages	Actions	Indications	Contraindications and Cautions
Aminophylline	0.25–0.5 gm. as 2.5% solution slowly I.V.; or 0.5 gm. as rectal suppository.	Bronchial dilator, myocardial stimulator, coronary vasodilator (?), diuretic.	Pulmonary edema, bronchial or cardiac asthma, Cheyne-Stokes respirations, status anginosus (?).	
Amobarbital sodium (Amytal Sodium)	0.25–0.5 gm. (3¾–7½ gr.) powder in ampules; make up as fresh 10% solution. Give slowly I.V. or I.M. or 0.13 gm. (2 gr.) rectal suppositories.	Hypnotic, sedative, anticonvulsant.	Convulsions, status epilepticus, excitement, hysterical reactions, mania.	Delirium, respiratory distress, hepatic insufficiency.
Atropine sulfate	0.3–0.6 mg. (1/200–1/100 gr.) orally or subcutaneously.	Parasympathetic depressant.	Colicky pain, nausea; methacholine, organic $PO_4^{\equiv}$, mushroom poisoning; carotid sinus syncope, Stokes-Adams syncope.	Glaucoma, drug sensitivity.
Calcium gluconate	5–10 ml. of 10% solution I.V.	Reduces CNS irritability due to Ca^{++} deficiency.	Hypocalcemic tetany (due to nephritis, hypoparathyroidism, alkalosis, hyperventilation); intense pruritus, spider bites, poisoning.	
Deslanoside injection (Cedilanid-D)	6 ml. (1.2 mg.) I.M. or I.V. followed by 2 ml. (0.4 mg.) I.M. or I.V. every 3–5 hours until effect is obtained.	Increases myocardial efficiency; slows AV conduction.	Acute congestive failure, atrial flutter or fibrillation with rapid rate, long-standing atrial paroxysmal tachycardia.	Relatively contraindicated in acute myocarditis, acute myocardial infarction, ventricular tachycardias, and in incomplete heart block, unless failure occurs. Question patient regarding recent digitalis therapy.
Dextrose	50% solution, 10–50 ml. for I.V. use.	Dehydrating agent; elevates blood sugar.	Symptoms secondary to increased intracranial pressure (tumor, cerebral edema); hypoglycemia due to insulin; hyperinsulinism.	

TABLE 18-1. (Continued)

	Dosage	Classification/Action	Indications	Remarks
Dimercaprol injection (BAL)	10% solution in oil, 3 mg./kg./dose. Give I.M. 1st and 2nd day: 1 injection q. 4 h. day and night. 3rd day: 1 injection q. 6 h. for 4 doses. 4th day on: 1 injection b.i.d. for 10 days or until recovery is complete.		Arsenic, mercury, gold, antimony, bismuth poisoning.	Lead, iron, cadmium poisoning.
Epinephrine	0.1–0.5 ml. of 1:1000 solution subcutaneously, I.M., or I.V.	Sympathomimetic	Ventricular standstill, bronchial asthma, angioneurotic edema, anaphylactic shock.	Advanced hypertensive vascular disease, advanced cerebral arteriosclerosis, serious organic heart disease; during inhalation anesthesia.
Hydrocortisone sodium succinate	100–200 mg. in 1–10 ml. fluid I.M. q. 6 h. p.r.n., or in 500–1000 ml. fluid I.V. p.r.n.	Replacement, anti-inflammatory	Acute adrenocortical insufficiency, addisonian crisis, exfoliative dermatitis.	
Magnesium sulfate	0.5–1 ml. of 50% solution I.V.	CNS depressant; supplies Mg^{++} ion.	Tetany, eclamptic convulsions, uremic convulsions.	A syringe of 10% calcium gluconate should be available in case respiratory failure results.
Morphine sulfate	8–32 mg. (⅛–½ gr.) subcutaneously, I.M., or I.V.	Narcotic (analgesic and hypnotic).	Severe pain due to various causes; pulmonary edema, severe diarrhea.	Head injury, morphine sensitivity, bronchial asthma, undiagnosed surgical abdominal disease, hepatic insufficiency, hypothyroidism.
Nalorphine hydrochloride (Nalline)	5–10 mg. I.V. Repeat in 15 minutes and then in 1–2 hours. Maximum total dose: 40 mg.	Reverse effects of narcotics.	Opiate (morphine, etc.), meperidine, and methadone poisoning or overdosage.	Not effective against hypnotics and sedatives (barbiturates, paraldehyde, chloral hydrate, etc.).
Chlorpromazine (Thorazine)	50–100 mg. orally or I.M. every 2–3 hours p.r.n.	Tranquilizer	Acute alcoholism syndromes, psychiatric excitement, vomiting, and to supplement narcotics in control of severe pain.	In comatose states due to CNS depressants (alcohol, barbiturates, or opiates), do not give more than 50 mg.
"Universal antidote"	2 parts powdered charcoal; 1 part magnesium oxide. Give 1 tsp (heaping) in warm water and repeat as necessary.		Many ingested poisons.	Should not be used as a substitute for removal of poisons or administration of specific antidote.

* From Chattom, M. J, Margen, S., and Brainerd, H.: Handbook of Medical Treatment. Los Altos, California, Lange Medical Publications, 1970.

Classification for Priority in Treatment

1. *Minimal treatment*—patients who can be returned to active duty immediately.
2. *Immediate treatment*—patients for whom the available expedient procedures will save life or limb.
3. *Delayed treatment*—patients, who, after emergency treatment, will incur little increased risk by having surgery withheld temporarily.
4. *Expectant treatment*—critically injured patients who will be given treatment if time and facilities are available.

Priorities of Treatment

The following is a priority schedule which serves as a guide to establish the flow of casualties from the disaster area through the First Aid Station to Forward Treatment Center and Hospital.

A. *First Priority* (individuals needing immediate attention to save life)
1. Any wound interfering with airway or causing airway obstruction. (This includes sucking chest wounds, tension pneumothorax and maxillofacial wounds in which asphyxia is present or an impending threat.
2. Any wound requiring immediate pressure.
3. Shock due to major hemorrhage, to wounds of any organ system, fractures, etc. (some of these conditions may be so urgent that immediate life-saving measures will be required by the person doing the sorting.)

B. *Second Priority* (individuals needing early surgery)
1. Visceral injuries, including perforations of the gastrointestinal tract; wounds of the biliary and pancreatic system; wounds of the genitourinary tract; and thoracic wounds without asphyxia.
2. Vascular injuries requiring repair. All injuries which require the use of a tourniquet fall into this group.
3. Closed cerebral injuries with increasing loss of consciousness.

C. *Third Priority* (patients who require surgery but can tolerate a delay)
1. Spinal injuries in which decompression is required.
2. Soft-tissue wounds in which debridement is necessary, but in which muscle damage is less than major.
3. Lesser fractures and dislocations.
4. Injuries of the eyes.
5. Maxillofacial injuries without asphyxia.

Identification of Casualties

1. Identification is done by an emergency medical tag.
2. Place the tag directly on the body, preferably the wrist; do not attach to clothing as it may be lost.
3. Tags are written out by a clerk who accompanies the sorting officer; clerk completes admission records, clinical records and emergency tags.
4. Following abbreviations are used on the tag:
   H—severe hemorrhage
   L—litter case
   T—tourniquet case (add time of application)
   X—person who is definitely dead

BIBLIOGRAPHY

Books

Birch, C. A.: Emergencies in Medical Practice. Edinburgh and London. Churchill Livingstone, 1971.

Bridges, P. K.: Psychiatric Emergencies. Springfield, Charles C Thomas, 1971.

Brunner, L., et al.: Textbook of Medical-Surgical Nursing, 2nd ed. Philadelphia, J. B. Lippincott, 1970, pp. 946–968.

Cole, W. H., and Puestow, C. B.: Emergency Care. New York, Appleton-Century-Crofts, 1972.

Committee on Injuries. American Academy of Orthopaedic Surgeons: Emergency Care and Transportation of the Sick and Injured. Menasha, Wisconsin, George Banta Co., 1971.

Dreisbach, R. H.: Handbook of Poisoning. Los Altos, Lange Medical Publications, 1971.

Eckert, C. (ed.): Emergency Room Care. Boston, Little, Brown and Co., 1971.

Flint, T., and Caine, H.: Emergency Treatment and Management. Philadelphia, W. B. Saunders, 1970.

Gardiner-Hill, H. (ed.): Compendium of Emergencies. New York, Appleton-Century-Crofts, 1971.

Gurdjian, E. S., et al.: Impact Injury and Crash Protection. Springfield, Charles C Thomas, 1970.

Grant, H., and Murray, R.: Emergency Care. Washington, D.C., Robert T. Brady Co., 1971.

Henderson, J.: Emergency Medical Guide. New York, McGraw-Hill, 1969.

Lowenfels, A. B.: The Alcoholic Patient in Surgery. Baltimore, Williams and Wilkins, 1971.

Mitchell, A. R. K.: Psychological Medicine in Family Practice. Baltimore, Williams and Wilkins, 1971, pp. 3–10.

McNichol, R.: The Treatment of Delirium Tremens and Related States. Springfield, Charles C Thomas, 1970.

Naclerio, E. A.: Chest Injuries. New York, Grune and Stratton, 1971.

Pridgen, J. E., et al.: Penetrating Wounds of the Abdomen. Springfield, Charles C Thomas, 1970.

Raney, R. B., et al.: Shands' Handbook of Orthopaedic Surgery. St. Louis, C. V. Mosby, 1971.

Riehl, C. L.: Emergency Nursing. Peoria, Charles A. Bennett Co., Inc., 1970.

Sharpe, J. C., and Marx, F. W.: Management of Medical Emergencies. New York, McGraw-Hill, 1969.

Articles

Craven, R. F.: Anaphylactic shock. Amer. J. Nurs., 72:718–721, April 1972.

Dimijian, G. G., et al.: Evaluation and treatment of the suspected drug user in the emergency room. Arch. Intern. Med., 125:162–170, Jan. 1970.

Fink, M., et al.: Narcotic antagonists; another approach to addiction therapy. Amer. J. Nurs., 71:1359–1363, July 1971.

Foreman, N. J., et al.: Drug crisis intervention. Amer. J. Nurs., 71:1736–1739, Sept. 1971.

Gallaher, H. L., et al.: The occupational health nurse and the patient with trauma. Nurs. Clin. N. Amer., 5:609–619, Dec. 1970.

Hayman, C. R., et al.: Sexual assault on women and girls. Amer. J. Obstet. Gynecol., 109:480–486, Feb. 1, 1971.

Kline, N. S., and Davis, J. M.: Psychotropic drugs. Amer. J. Nurs., 73:54–62, Jan. 1973.

Lee, J. M.: Emotional reactions to trauma. Nurs. Clin. N. Amer., 5:577–587, Dec. 1970.

Lister, J.: Nursing intervention in anaphylactic shock. Amer. J. Nurs., 72:720–721, April 1972.

Madding, G. F., and Kennedy, P. A.: Symposium on nonpenetrating thoracoabdominal injuries. Surg. Clin. N. Amer., 52, June 1972 (entire vol.).

Massey, J. B., et al.: Management of sexually assaulted females. Obstet. Gynecol., 38:29–36, July 1971.

Phillipson, R.: Emergency treatment of drug abusers. Medical Annals of D.C., 40:436–438, July 1971.

Wagner, M. M.: Assessment of patients with multiple injuries. Amer. J. Nurs., 72:1822–1827, Oct. 1972.

Weinstock, F. J.: Emergency treatment of eye injuries. Amer. J. Nurs., 71:1928–1931, Oct. 1971.

PART II

Maternity Nursing

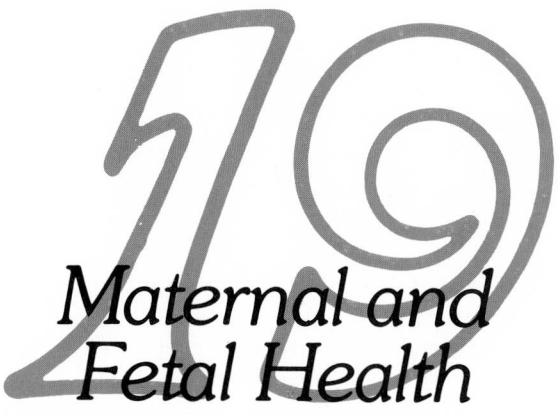

Maternal and Fetal Health

INTRODUCTION TO MATERNITY NURSING

Maternity nursing is the care and related activities relevant to maternity patients and their infants during all phases of the child-bearing experience.

Current Problems Affecting Maternal and Infant Morbidity and Mortality

1. Poor distribution or lack of care among disadvantaged low-income families living in urban industrial areas, rural areas and ghetto areas
2. Shortage of professional personnel—physicians, nurses, midwives, social workers
3. Nutritional problems among the disadvantaged and adolescent mothers
4. Increased incidence of prematurity, congenital defects and birth injuries in the newborn

THE EXPECTANT MOTHER
Nomenclature for Gravida and Parity

Gravidity

1. *Gravida*—a pregnant woman
2. *Primigravida*—a woman pregnant for the first time
3. *Multigravida*—a woman who has been pregnant several times

Parity

1. *Para*—alludes to past pregnancies that have reached viability.
2. *Parity*—refers to number of past pregnancies that have gone to viability and have been delivered regardless of the number of children involved (NOTE: The birth of triplets increases the parity by 1).
3. *Primipara*—a woman who has delivered 1 pregnancy where the child has reached viability without regard to the child's being alive or dead at the time of birth.
4. *Multipara*—a woman who has had 2 or more pregnancies terminated at the stage when the children were viable.

Gravida and Para

1. A woman pregnant for the first time is a primigravida and is described as Gravida 1, Para 0
2. If she aborts before viability, she remains Gravida 1, Para 0.
3. If she delivers a fetus which has reached viability she becomes a Primipara regardless of whether the child is alive or dead; Gravida 1, Para 1.
4. During a second pregnancy she is Gravida 2, Para 1.
5. A patient with 2 abortions and no viable children is Gravida 2, Para 0.

Manifestations of Pregnancy

Presumptive Signs and Symptoms

1. Cessation of menses—pregnancy is indicated if more than 10 days have elapsed since the missed period.
2. Breast changes
   a. Breasts enlarge and become tender. Veins in breast become increasingly visible.
   b. Nipples increase in size and pigmentation.
   c. Colostrum, a thin milky fluid, may be expressed after the first few months.
   d. Montgomery glands, small elevations among the areolar, may appear.
3. Vaginal and vulval color changes (Chadwick's sign)—a bluish discoloration and congestion.
4. Abdominal striae (striae gravidarum)—sometimes appear on the breasts and thighs as a result of increased pigmentation of the skin.
5. Nausea and vomiting (morning sickness)—may occur at any time of day and usually lasts a few hours.
6. Quickening (sensations of movement in the abdomen)—occurs between 16th and 19th week after the last menses.

7. Frequency of urination
   a. Caused by the pressure of an expanding uterus on the bladder.
   b. Disappears when the uterus rises out of the pelvis.
   c. Reappears when the fetal head engages in the pelvis at the end of pregnancy.
8. Fatigue

Probable Signs and Symptoms

1. Enlargement of abdomen—near the end of the 3rd month the uterus can be felt through the abdominal wall.
2. Changes in shape, size and consistency of the uterus.
   a. A soft, cushion-like consistency in early pregnancy nourishes and protects the implanted ovum.
   b. Uterine thickness gradually decreases as the stretching of later pregnancy occurs.
3. Changes in cervix
   a. Softening may not occur until much later in pregnancy.
      (1) Goodell's sign—softening of the cervix.
      (2) Hegar's sign—softening of the lower uterine segment.
   b. In certain pathologic conditions the cervix may remain firm.
4. Intermittent contractions of the uterus (Braxton Hicks sign)—painless, palpable contractions occurring at irregular intervals.
5. Ballottement—a sinking and rebounding of the fetus in its surrounding amniotic fluid as a response to a sudden tap on the uterus (occurs in 4th or 5th month of pregnancy).
6. Outlining of the fetus through the abdomen—abdominal palpation in the 2nd half of pregnancy.
7. Positive hormonal tests for pregnancy (test reactions produced by gonadotropin in maternal plasma and urine).

Positive Signs and Symptoms

1. Fetal heartbeat (separate and distinct from that of the mother)—usually heard between 20th and 22nd week of gestation.
2. Perception of fetal movements by the examiner.
3. X-ray visualization of the fetus (after the 4th month).
4. Sonographic examination.

Maternal Physiology During Pregnancy

Duration of Pregnancy

280 days or 40 weeks, 9 calendar months, 10 lunar months, counting from the 1st day of the last menstrual period.

General Alterations in Function

1. Changes become recognizable shortly after first missed period.
2. Pregnancy imposes a stress on the maternal organism, particularly upon the vascular circulation.
3. Many changes represent the response of the body to additional metabolic demands.
4. Physical and functional alterations involve all the body systems.

Changes in Reproductive Tract

1. Uterus
   a. Uterus increases in size: 7–35 cm. in length; 60–1200 gm. at term—hypertrophy of muscle cells becomes 5–10 times normal.
   b. By 2nd month, uterus triples in size and weight—may cause shift in position and exaggerated antiflexion, retrocession or retroversion.
   c. By 3rd month, uterus occupies pelvic cavity; may be felt suprapubically—myometrium 2–3 cm. in thickness.
   d. By 4th month, uterus becomes an abdominal organ—fundus has reached the level of the umbilicus.
   e. By 36–38 weeks, fundal portion has reached the ensiform process.
   f. Last 3–4 weeks, uterus recedes slightly—due to descent into pelvis. Walls of uterus become thinner (1–2 cm.).
   g. Changes in contractibility occur—during 1st trimester regular painless contractions occur (Braxton-Hicks contractions)—result of combination of muscle stretch, increased actinomycin in the muscle cells and changes in estrogen, progesterone and electrolyte levels.
   h. Blood flow remains fairly constant
      (1) 10–15 ml./100 gm./minute.
      (2) Total flow, 500–700 ml./minute at term.
2. Cervix
   a. Pronounced softening and cyanosis—due to increased vascularity, edema and hypertrophy and hyperplasia of the cervical glands.
   b. Common erosions of cervix—represents an extension of proliferating endocervical glands and columnar endocervical epithelium due to increased estrogen production.
3. Ovaries
   a. Ovulation ceases during pregnancy and maturation of new follicles is suspended. One large corpus luteum remains on 1 ovary.
   b. Ovarian veins increase in caliber from 0.9–2.6 cm. at term.
4. Vagina
   a. Chadwick's sign noted—characteristic violet color due to increased vascularity and hyperemia.
   b. Vaginal walls prepare for labor: mucosa increases in thickness, connective tissue loosens and small muscle cells hypertrophy.
   c. Vaginal secretions increase with pH of 3.5–6—due to increased production of lactic acid from glycogen in the vaginal epithelium by *Lactobacillus acidophilus.* (Acid pH probably aids in keeping vagina relatively free of pathogenic bacteria.)

Changes in the Abdominal Wall

Striae gravidarum often develop—reddish, slightly depressed streaks in the skin of abdomen, breast and thighs. (Become glistening silvery line after pregnancy).

Breast Changes

1. Are tender and tingly in early weeks of pregnancy.
2. Increase in size by 2nd month leading to hypertrophy of mammary alveoli.
3. Nipples become larger, more deeply pigmented and more erectile early in pregnancy.
4. Colostrum may be expressed by 2nd trimester.

5. Areola become broader and more deeply pigmented. The depth of pigmentation varies with the individual's complexion.
6. Scattered through the areola are a number of small elevations (glands of Montgomery) which are hypertrophic sebaceous glands.

Metabolic Changes

1. Are numerous and intensive—response to rapidly growing fetus and placenta.
2. Weight gain averages 9.1 kg. (20 lbs.).
   a. Fetus, 3.4 kg. (7½ lbs.).
   b. Placenta, 0.454 kg. (1 lb.).
   c. Amniotic fluid, 0.91 kg. (2 lbs.).
   d. Hypertrophy of uterus, 0.91 kg. (2 lbs.).
   e. Breasts, 0.91 kg. (2 lbs.).
   f. Increase in blood volume, 1.60 kg. (3½ lbs.).
   g. Water retention and fat and protein deposition, 1.7 kg. (4 lbs.).
3. Water metabolism
   a. Increased water retention (fetus, placenta, amniotic fluid) comprises 3.5 liters; uterus, maternal blood volume and breast tissue comprise 3.5 liters, producing intracapillary hydrostatic pressure which favors filtration from the vascular bed and increased capillary permeability.
   b. Increased sodium retention.
4. Protein metabolism
   a. Fetus, uterus and maternal blood are rich in protein rather than fat or carbohydrates.
   b. At term fetus and placenta weigh about 4 kg. and contain 500 gm. of protein.
   c. Approximately 500 gm. more of protein are added to maternal blood in form of hemoglobin and plasma proteins.
5. Carbohydrate and insulin metabolism
   a. Diabetes mellitus is aggravated by pregnancy.
   b. Clinical diabetes appears in some women only during pregnancy. Normal pregnancy level of plasma insulin is higher, and destruction of insulin more rapid; thus secretion of insulin during pregnancy is increased.
6. Fat metabolism
   Plasma lipids increase during latter half of pregnancy. (Reasons are not known.)
7. Iron metabolism
   a. Iron requirements increase—often exceed amounts available.
   b. Total volume of circulating red blood cells increases by about 450 ml. during pregnancy, resulting in increased need of nearly 500 mg. of iron (6–7 mg.)/day.
   c. Supplemental iron is valuable during latter half of pregnancy and for several weeks after pregnancy.

Changes in Cardiovascular System

1. Heart
   a. Diaphragm is progressively elevated during pregnancy; heart is displaced to the left and upward with apex moved laterally.
   b. Pulmonic systolic and apical systolic murmurs are common—created by lowered blood viscosity and displacement causing torsion in the great vessels.
2. Circulation
   a. Cardiac volume increases by 10%—causes slight hypertrophy of the heart.
   b. Red cell volume increases but lags behind the plasma volume—may lead to reduced hematocrit and hemoglobin concentration.

    c. Femoral venous pressure increases—due to retardation of blood flow from lower extremities as a result of pressure of enlarged uterus on pelvic vein and inferior vena cava.

    d. In the supine position, the large uterus of pregnancy compresses the venous system, thereby slowing cardiac filling and decreasing cardiac output.

    e. Resting pulse rate increases 10 beats per minute—due to increased blood volume and cardiac output.

3. Hematologic changes

    a. Leukocyte count is elevated to values ranging between 6000–12,000/cu. mm. during pregnancy and rising to 25,000 or more during labor—cause unknown but probably represents the reappearance in the circulation of leukocytes previously shunted out of active circulation.

    b. Fibrinogen levels increase 50%—influence of estrogen and progesterone.

Changes in Urinary Tract

1. Dilation of ureters and renal pelvis begins early in pregnancy—due to effect of progesterone.

2. Dilation later in pregnancy—mechanical pressure is greater on right side above the pelvic brim.

3. Glomerular filtration increases early in pregnancy and persists almost to term—due to pressure on the inferior vena cava and iliac veins.

4. Renal plasma flow increases early in pregnancy, decreases to prepregnant range during 3rd trimester—may be due to effect of antidiuretic hormone, upright position or vena cava congestion.

5. Glucosuria is evident—due to increase in glomerular filtration without increase in tubular reabsorptive capacity for filtered glucose.

Changes in Gastrointestinal Tract

1. Generalized softening of gingiva occurs—associated with bleeding or irritation.

2. Stomach and intestines are displaced upward and laterally by enlarging uterus.

3. Liver is displaced backwards, upward and to the right—hepatic blood flow remains unaltered and various liver function tests are within normal lines.

4. Alkaline phosphatase activity doubles during normal pregnancy—due to placental enzymes and maternal estrogen level.

5. Tone and motility of gastrointestinal tract decreases, leading to prolongation of gastric emptiness and relaxation of pyloric sphincter—due to large amount of progesterone produced by placenta.

Changes in Respiratory Tract

1. Hyperventilation occurs—increase in respiratory rate, tidal volume and minute volume, probably due to increased consumption of oxygen and production of carbon dioxide by products of conception.

2. Diaphragm is elevated during pregnancy—chiefly by the enlarging uterus.

3. Thoracic cage expands through flaring of the ribs—result of increased mobility of rib attachments.

Changes in Endocrine System

1. Pituitary enlarges slightly.

2. Thyroid is moderately enlarged due to hyperplasia of glandular tissue and increased vascularity.

a. Basal metabolic rate increases progressively during normal pregnancy to as high as 25%—due to metabolic activity of fetus.

b. Level of protein-bound iodine and thyroxin rises sharply and is maintained until after delivery—due to increased circulatory estrogen.

3. Adrenal secretions considerably increased—amounts of aldosterone increase as early as 15th week—due to augmented renin, renin-substrate and angiotensin.

Changes in Integumentary System

1. Pigmentary changes occur from melanocyte-stimulating hormone which is elevated from the 2nd month of pregnancy until term.
2. Chloasma gravidarum (pigmentation of circumscribed areas of the skin during pregnancy) occurs.

Changes in Musculoskeletal System

1. The increasing mobility of sacroiliac, sacrococcygeal and pelvic joints during pregnancy is result of hormonal (progesterone) changes.
2. This mobility contributes to alteration of maternal posture and to back pain.

Nursing and Obstetrical Support During the Antepartal Period

Antepartal care is the medical and nursing supervision of the pregnant woman during the course of gestation until the onset of labor.

Purposes

1. To ensure optimum health for both mother and infant.
2. To prevent complications or accidents during childbirth.
3. To educate the mother-to-be in self-care and infant care.
4. To provide medical, sociological and psychological support as necessary.

Categories of Antepartum Care

1. Monitoring the physical well being and progress of pregnancy.
2. Educating the mother in healthful living, especially during the period of pregnancy.

Physical Examination

A. *Initial Examination*

1. Weight
   a. The average woman may gain up to 9.1 kg. (20 lbs.) during a normal gestation period.
   b. A woman whose prepregnant weight was subnormal may safely gain more, and conversely the overweight woman will be encouraged to gain less.
   c. Marked weight gain or loss is a significant symptom and requires further follow-up.
2. Blood pressure
   Any rise in systolic or diastolic blood pressure is cause for concern (see Toxemias, p. 1007).
3. Urinalysis
   a. Urine is tested for sugar and albumin at each visit.
   b. Glucose threshold is normally lowered in pregnant women. (*The urine specimen should be taken before breakfast to avoid false-positive reports of glucose*).

TABLE 19-1. DELIVERY PREDICTION DATES

Date of delivery (2) (3) (4) can be predicted when one of three dates (1) are known:

Example:

(1) Date of first day of last menstruation → (4)
(1) Date of first day life is felt for a primipara → (2)
(1) Date of first day life is felt for a multipara → (3)

(1) Jan. 1 —Date of first day of last menstruation → (4) Oct. 8
(1) Jan. 1 —Date of first day life is felt for a primipara → (2) June 4
(1) Jan. 1 —Date of first day life is felt for a multipara → (3) June 18

	1	2	3	4	5	6	7	8	9	10	11	12	13	14	15	16	17	18	19	20	21	22	23	24	25	26	27	28	29	30	31
Jan. (1)	1	2	3	4	5	6	7	8	9	10	11	12	13	14	15	16	17	18	19	20	21	22	23	24	25	26	27	28	29	30	31
June→July (2)	4	5	6	7	8	9	10	11	12	13	14	15	16	17	18	19	20	21	22	23	24	25	26	27	28	29	30	1	2	3	4
June→July (3)	18	19	20	21	22	23	24	25	26	27	28	29	30	1	2	3	4	5	6	7	8	9	10	11	12	13	14	15	16	17	18
Oct.→Nov. (4)	8	9	10	11	12	13	14	15	16	17	18	19	20	21	22	23	24	25	26	27	28	29	30	31	1	2	3	4	5	6	7
Feb. (1)	1	2	3	4	5	6	7	8	9	10	11	12	13	14	15	16	17	18	19	20	21	22	23	24	25	26	27	28			
July→Aug. (2)	5	6	7	8	9	10	11	12	13	14	15	16	17	18	19	20	21	22	23	24	25	26	27	28	29	30	31	1			
July→Aug. (3)	19	20	21	22	23	24	25	26	27	28	29	30	31	1	2	3	4	5	6	7	8	9	10	11	12	13	14	15			
Nov.→Dec. (4)	8	9	10	11	12	13	14	15	16	17	18	19	20	21	22	23	24	25	26	27	28	29	30	1	2	3	4	5			
March (1)	1	2	3	4	5	6	7	8	9	10	11	12	13	14	15	16	17	18	19	20	21	22	23	24	25	26	27	28	29	30	31
Aug.→Sept. (2)	2	3	4	5	6	7	8	9	10	11	12	13	14	15	16	17	18	19	20	21	22	23	24	25	26	27	28	29	30	31	1
Aug.→Sept. (3)	16	17	18	19	20	21	22	23	24	25	26	27	28	29	30	31	1	2	3	4	5	6	7	8	9	10	11	12	13	14	15
Dec.→Jan. (4)	6	7	8	9	10	11	12	13	14	15	16	17	18	19	20	21	22	23	24	25	26	27	28	29	30	31	1	2	3	4	5
April (1)	1	2	3	4	5	6	7	8	9	10	11	12	13	14	15	16	17	18	19	20	21	22	23	24	25	26	27	28	29	30	
Sept.→Oct. (2)	2	3	4	5	6	7	8	9	10	11	12	13	14	15	16	17	18	19	20	21	22	23	24	25	26	27	28	29	30	1	
Sept.→Oct. (3)	16	17	18	19	20	21	22	23	24	25	26	27	28	29	30	1	2	3	4	5	6	7	8	9	10	11	12	13	14	15	
Jan.→Feb. (4)	6	7	8	9	10	11	12	13	14	15	16	17	18	19	20	21	22	23	24	25	26	27	28	29	30	31	1	2	3	4	
May (1)	1	2	3	4	5	6	7	8	9	10	11	12	13	14	15	16	17	18	19	20	21	22	23	24	25	26	27	28	29	30	31
Oct.→Nov. (2)	2	3	4	5	6	7	8	9	10	11	12	13	14	15	16	17	18	19	20	21	22	23	24	25	26	27	28	29	30	31	1
Oct.→Nov. (3)	16	17	18	19	20	21	22	23	24	25	26	27	28	29	30	31	1	2	3	4	5	6	7	8	9	10	11	12	13	14	15
Feb.→March (4)	5	6	7	8	9	10	11	12	13	14	15	16	17	18	19	20	21	22	23	24	25	26	27	28	1	2	3	4	5	6	7
June (1)	1	2	3	4	5	6	7	8	9	10	11	12	13	14	15	16	17	18	19	20	21	22	23	24	25	26	27	28	29	30	
Nov.→Dec. (2)	2	3	4	5	6	7	8	9	10	11	12	13	14	15	16	17	18	19	20	21	22	23	24	25	26	27	28	29	30	1	
Nov.→Dec. (3)	16	17	18	19	20	21	22	23	24	25	26	27	28	29	30	1	2	3	4	5	6	7	8	9	10	11	12	13	14	15	
March→April (4)	8	9	10	11	12	13	14	15	16	17	18	19	20	21	22	23	24	25	26	27	28	29	30	31	1	2	3	4	5	6	
July (1)	1	2	3	4	5	6	7	8	9	10	11	12	13	14	15	16	17	18	19	20	21	22	23	24	25	26	27	28	29	30	31
Dec.→Jan. (2)	2	3	4	5	6	7	8	9	10	11	12	13	14	15	16	17	18	19	20	21	22	23	24	25	26	27	28	29	30	31	1
Dec.→Jan. (3)	16	17	18	19	20	21	22	23	24	25	26	27	28	29	30	31	1	2	3	4	5	6	7	8	9	10	11	12	13	14	15
April→May (4)	7	8	9	10	11	12	13	14	15	16	17	18	19	20	21	22	23	24	25	26	27	28	29	30	1	2	3	4	5	6	7
Aug. (1)	1	2	3	4	5	6	7	8	9	10	11	12	13	14	15	16	17	18	19	20	21	22	23	24	25	26	27	28	29	30	31
Jan.→Feb. (2)	2	3	4	5	6	7	8	9	10	11	12	13	14	15	16	17	18	19	20	21	22	23	24	25	26	27	28	29	30	31	1
Jan.→Feb. (3)	16	17	18	19	20	21	22	23	24	25	26	27	28	29	30	31	1	2	3	4	5	6	7	8	9	10	11	12	13	14	15
May→June (4)	8	9	10	11	12	13	14	15	16	17	18	19	20	21	22	23	24	25	26	27	28	29	30	31	1	2	3	4	5	6	7
Sept. (1)	1	2	3	4	5	6	7	8	9	10	11	12	13	14	15	16	17	18	19	20	21	22	23	24	25	26	27	28	29	30	
Feb.→March (2)	2	3	4	5	6	7	8	9	10	11	12	13	14	15	16	17	18	19	20	21	22	23	24	25	26	27	28	1	2	3	
Feb.→March (3)	16	17	18	19	20	21	22	23	24	25	26	27	28	1	2	3	4	5	6	7	8	9	10	11	12	13	14	15	16	17	
June→July (4)	8	9	10	11	12	13	14	15	16	17	18	19	20	21	22	23	24	25	26	27	28	29	30	1	2	3	4	5	6	7	
Oct. (1)	1	2	3	4	5	6	7	8	9	10	11	12	13	14	15	16	17	18	19	20	21	22	23	24	25	26	27	28	29	30	31
March→April (2)	4	5	6	7	8	9	10	11	12	13	14	15	16	17	18	19	20	21	22	23	24	25	26	27	28	29	30	31	1	2	3
March→April (3)	18	19	20	21	22	23	24	25	26	27	28	29	30	31	1	2	3	4	5	6	7	8	9	10	11	12	13	14	15	16	17
July→Aug. (4)	8	9	10	11	12	13	14	15	16	17	18	19	20	21	22	23	24	25	26	27	28	29	30	31	1	2	3	4	5	6	7
Nov. (1)	1	2	3	4	5	6	7	8	9	10	11	12	13	14	15	16	17	18	19	20	21	22	23	24	25	26	27	28	29	30	
April→May (2)	4	5	6	7	8	9	10	11	12	13	14	15	16	17	18	19	20	21	22	23	24	25	26	27	28	29	30	1	2	3	
April→May (3)	18	19	20	21	22	23	24	25	26	27	28	29	30	1	2	3	4	5	6	7	8	9	10	11	12	13	14	15	16	17	
Aug.→Sept. (4)	8	9	10	11	12	13	14	15	16	17	18	19	20	21	22	23	24	25	26	27	28	29	30	31	1	2	3	4	5	6	
Dec. (1)	1	2	3	4	5	6	7	8	9	10	11	12	13	14	15	16	17	18	19	20	21	22	23	24	25	26	27	28	29	30	31
May→June (2)	4	5	6	7	8	9	10	11	12	13	14	15	16	17	18	19	20	21	22	23	24	25	26	27	28	29	30	31	1	2	3
May→June (3)	18	19	20	21	22	23	24	25	26	27	28	29	30	31	1	2	3	4	5	6	7	8	9	10	11	12	13	14	15	16	17
Sept.→Oct. (4)	7	8	9	10	11	12	13	14	15	16	17	18	19	20	21	22	23	24	25	26	27	28	29	30	1	2	3	4	5	6	7

    c. Any sign of albumin in the urine should be reported immediately as it is considered a serious sign of toxemia.

4. Blood evaluation

    Includes complete blood count, blood typing and cross-matching.

5. Patient history

    a. Family history—presence of inheritable diseases, difficult births, abortions, etc.

    b. Personal medical history—usual childhood diseases, major illnesses, surgery, previous pregnancies, etc.

    c. Personal history of the present pregnancy—date of last menstrual period (LMP), symptoms, and estimated date of birth.

        Expected date of confinement (EDC) is calculated by counting back 3 calendar months from the 1st day of the last menstrual period and adding 7 days. (For specific delivery prediction dates, see Table 19-1.)

6. Pelvic examination

    The patient should be asked to empty her bladder before the procedure and should be properly draped to prevent unnecessary exposure (see p. 524).

    a. Palpation and auscultation of the abdomen—size and position of the fetus can be ascertained as well as the fetal heart rate.

    b. Estimation of pelvic measurement—to anticipate difficult delivery in the case of cephalopelvic disproportion (see p. 960).

    c. Vaginal examination to:

        (1) Rule out abnormalities of the birth canal

        (2) Obtain further pelvic measurement

        (3) Secure a Papanicolaou smear for the detection of abnormal cells

B. *Subsequent Visits*

    1. All of the above physical signs are monitored except the vaginal examination, which is done only occasionally to check the progress of the pregnancy.

    2. These visits are also used for teaching purposes, an integral part of antepartum care.

Teaching the Maternity Patient Principles of Hygiene

A. *Rest and Relaxation*—aimed at the prevention of fatigue

    1. Symptoms of fatigue

        a. Irritability   c. Tendency to worry

        b. Apprehension   d. Restlessness

    2. Prevention of fatigue

        a. Adequate sleep at night

        b. Supplemental naps in morning and afternoon, or both if possible

        c. Household chores performed from the most comfortable position, preferably with expectant mother sitting with feet elevated, as when ironing, sewing or performing some aspects of cooking

B. *Exercise*—in moderation and individualized according to:

    1. Age and physical condition

    2. Customary amount of exercise (Exercise is never continued to the point of fatigue.)

    3. Stage of pregnancy

C. *Employment*—in moderation and individualized so as to:
  1. Avoid fatigue
  2. Prevent accidents to which the pregnant woman is especially vulnerable because of changes in center of gravity
  3. Reduce environmental hazards, both physical and chemical
  4. Avoid any job requiring manual labor, delicate balance or inverted living hours.

D. *Traveling*—usually not contraindicated during pregnancy
  1. Long-distance traveling should be punctuated with frequent rest periods (10–15 minutes every 2 hours).
  2. The obstetrician's advice should be enlisted before any traveling is undertaken.

E. *Skin Care*
  1. Daily bath
     a. Stimulates and refreshes
     b. Favors elimination of waste products through skin
  2. Sponge baths or showers—if sense of balance is affected

F. *Breast Care and Preparation for Breast Feeding*
  1. A well-fitting supporting brassiere
     a. Relieves discomfort of pendulous breasts
     b. Prevents sagging after childbirth
  2. Daily washing with clean washcloth and warm water
     The use of soap, alcohol and other commercial products should be discussed with the obstetrician as these materials can cause drying of the nipples.
  3. Drying nipple with rough towel in final trimester—to help toughen the nipples for breast feeding
  4. Nipple creams or lanolin applied to each nipple—to help minimize irritations from colostrum and to prevent drying

G. *Clothing*
  1. Nonrestrictive
  2. Attractive style and fit
  3. Abdominal support in later pregnancy— to prevent fatigue
  4. Comfortable shoes that assist in maintaining balance

H. *Bowel Habits*
  1. Tendency to constipation increased because of:
     a. Reduced activity
     b. Pressure of expanding uterus
  2. Treatment
     a. Ample fluids
     b. Fruits, vegetables
     c. Rest
     d. Glycerin suppositories or mild laxatives

I. *Vaginal Douches*
   Should only be taken if prescribed by obstetrician. (See p. 535 for douche procedure.)

J. *Sexual Intercourse*
   Individualized, but the following points may be noted:
  1. Sexual desire may be unpredictable in the woman during early pregnancy.
  2. If there is danger of abortion or premature labor, coitus is avoided.

3. During last few weeks before term, some obstetricians advise abstaining from sexual activity.
4. The male-superior position is avoided as the pregnancy progresses.

K. *Smoking*
   1. Causes peripheral vasoconstriction affecting heart rate, blood pressure and cardiac output.
   2. Small birth weights have been associated with the incidence of smoking in pregnant women.

Teaching the Maternity Patient About Nutrition

A. *Diet*
   1. Significant relationship found between maternal nutrition and well-being of infant, especially concerning protein intake.
   2. Energy requirements—change during course of pregnancy; caloric intake regulated accordingly.
   3. Meals—should be individually balanced and consumed on a regular consistent schedule.
   4. Best index of nutritional needs—is the condition of the patient, her body weight and pregravid status of nutrition.
   5. Total weight gain—8.2-10 kg. (18-22 lbs.) (1.4 kg. or 3 pounds first 4 months, with subsequent average gain of 0.36 kg. or 0.8 pounds per week).
   6. Caloric intake—sufficient to maintain calculated ideal body weight with additional 200 calories per day during last 5 months of gestation.
   7. Protein intake—needs should be met easily with additional 10 gm. to maintain level of 0.9 gm./kg. of ideal body weight provided that at least two-thirds of total nitrogen component is of animal origin.
   8. Fat intake—should constitute approximately 25% of total calories.
   9. Carbohydrate intake—consists predominantly of complex polysaccharides.
   10. Sodium intake—2.5-5 gm. daily intake allowed unless contraindicated by water retention.
   11. Vitamins
       a. During pregnancy and lactation, vitamin needs increase.
       b. Best sources found in natural foods.
       c. Supplements usually recommended by most physicians.
          (1) Vitamin A
              (a) Essential for maintenance of body resistance to infection.
              (b) Sources—whole milk, dairy products containing butterfat, eggs, green leafy or yellow vegetables and liver.
          (2) Vitamin B complex
              (a) Fetus depletes mother's reserves.
              (b) Sources—milk, eggs, lean meat, whole grains or enriched bread and cereals, riboflavin and nicotinic acid found in meat, milk, eggs and green vegetables.
          (3) Vitamin C
              (a) Water-soluble vitamin, not stored—daily intake required.
              (b) Sources—fresh citrus fruits, berries and green leafy vegetables are excellent sources—preferably taken raw as cooking destroys one-half vitamin content.

      (4) Vitamin D

        (a) Relationship of calcium and phosphorus metabolism important.

        (b) Sources—liver, eggs, fortified milk and fish (400 I.U. recommended).

12. Iron—indicated for all pregnant women especially for those with a history of anemia multiple births or frequent pregnancies.

    a. Hemoglobin below the following rates indicates iron deficiency:

        11 gm./100 ml. in 1st trimester

        10.5 gm./100 ml. in 2nd trimester

        10 gm./100 ml. in 3rd trimester

    b. Iron is needed to maintain satisfactory hemoglobin concentration during pregnancy and to compensate for blood loss during delivery.

    c. Frequency of complicated deliveries and postpartal hemorrhage requires a reserve supply of iron.

    d. Adequate reserves of iron together with protein and other essential nutrients are conducive to rapid recovery and ability to breast feed.

    e. Oral preparation of 100 mg. of iron daily is usually effective.

        (1) During 3rd trimester, absorption increased 3-fold.

        (2) Ferrous gluconate, 1 gm. daily, recommended.

    f. Long-lasting, sustained-release preparations are useful for patients with impaired absorption.

NURSING ALERT: Parenteral administration of large doses of iron is frequently accompanied by adverse reactions and should be reserved for patients who have extremely low levels and are close to term. A large intake of milk may interfere with iron absorption.

---

13. Folic acid—may be necessary for patients with macrocytic patterns, refractory anemia or hemoglobinopathy (3 mg. daily given with vitamin B_{12}).

14. Calcium—may be advocated for some patients with repeated pregnancy or leg cramps. Supplementation unnecessary if daily intake is 1.3–1.8 gm.

15. Magnesium, copper, potassium and iodine—assured intake in balanced diet.

B. *Foods to be eaten daily*

    1. Milk—1 quart of whole milk (or 1 quart of skimmed milk if weight control desired).

      a. Skimmed powdered milk may be used as a substitute for or supplement to liquid milk (1–2 tablespoons to 1 glass of liquid).

      b. 1 oz. of cheddar cheese may substitute for 1 glass of milk.

    2. Eggs—at least 1 daily (5 weekly if animal fats are restricted).

    3. Meat—6 to 8 oz. lean meat (beef, veal, lamb, chicken, turkey or fish—2 servings). Organ meats substituted 2 times weekly.

    4. Fat—2 tablespoons butter, margarine or vegetable oil.

    5. Bread and cereal—2 slices of whole grain or enriched bread plus ½ cup enriched or cooked whole grain cereal.

    6. Vegetables

      a. Potato—1 medium or ¾ cups cooked rice, noodles, spaghetti or macaroni substituted 2 times weekly.

      b. 1 cup dark green or deep yellow vegetables.

      c. 1 cup of another vegetable, raw or cooked, or ½ cup of peas, beans, corn or lentils.

7. Fruit
   a. Citrus fruit—2 oranges or 1 grapefruit or 8 oz. of orange juice or tomato juice.
   b. 1 fresh fruit or ½ cup cooked unsweetened fruit or 4–5 prunes or 5–6 dried apricots may be substituted.
8. Desserts—1 serving simple pudding made with milk, eggs or fruit, if desired.
9. Water—4 glasses minimum requirement unless specifically restricted.

Discomforts of Pregnancy

Frequency of Urination

1. Cause—pressure of enlarging uterus on bladder.
2. Course—usually subsides spontaneously by the 2nd or 3rd month when the uterus rises into the abdominal cavity only to return in the last weeks of pregnancy when the vertex drops into the pelvic cavity (engagement).

Morning Sickness

Nausea sometimes accompanied by mild vomiting—usually occurs in morning but may occur at any time of day.
1. Possible causes
   a. Changes in hormonal balance
   b. Emotional upset
   c. Sluggish peristalsis
2. Duration (4–12 weeks)
3. Aim of treatment—to prevent exaggeration of symptoms (see hyperemesis gravidarum, p. 1011).
4. Treatment
   Instruct patient as follows:
   a. Before breakfast:
      (1) Eat dry toast or a cracker one-half hour before rising.
      (2) Drink hot tea, clear coffee or hot milk.
      (3) Remain in bed and rest one-half hour before rising.
   b. Eat simple light foods 5–6 times a day rather than 3 full meals.
   c. Avoid foods that are difficult to digest.

Heartburn

1. Causes
   a. May occur anytime during pregnancy as a result of diminished gastric motility causing reflux of stomach contents into the esophagus with resulting irritation.
   b. Nervous tension and emotional disturbances contribute to heartburn.
2. Treatment
   Instruct patient as follows:
   a. Avoid fatty and fried foods.
   b. Take antacid medications.

NURSING ALERT: Soda bicarbonate should not be used as it promotes retention of fluid.

Flatulence

1. Cause—gas-forming bacterial action in the intestines.
2. Treatment
   Instruct patient as follows:
   a. Chew food thoroughly.
   b. Avoid gas-forming foods (fried foods, beans, corn).

Constipation

1. Cause—impaired intestinal peristalsis from the pressure of gravid uterus.
2. Treatment
   Instruct patient as follows:
   a. Take adequate fluids.
   b. Establish regular patterns of elimination.
   c. Eat an appropriate diet (fruits, vegetables, coarse bread).
   d. Take laxatives only when prescribed by obstetrician.

Backache

1. Cause
   a. Postural adjustments of pregnancy.
   b. Relaxation of sacroiliac joints in late pregnancy.
2. Treatment
   Instruct patient as follows:
   a. Maintain good posture, avoid fatigue, use good body mechanics.
   b. Wear appropriate clothing.
      (1) Flat, wide-based shoes.
      (2) Supporting maternity girdle.

Respiratory Discomfort

1. Cause—pressure of enlarged uterus on diaphragm
2. Treatment
   a. Spontaneous relief occurs with "lightening" (sensation of decreased abdominal distention caused by descent of uterus into pelvis) or with the birth of the baby
   b. Provide relief by semi-Fowler's position arranged with pillows.
   NOTE: The possibility of heart disease may need to be ruled out.

Varicose Veins

1. May affect the lower extremities, vulva and pelvis (Fig. 19-1).
2. Causes
   a. Heredity
   b. Pressure of gravid uterus on the great veins of the pelvis
   c. Prolonged standing
   d. Constrictive clothing
3. Treatment
   Instruct patient as follows:
   a. Avoid restrictive clothing.
   b. Elevate legs and hips on pillows above the level of the heart.
   c. Wear elastic stockings or bandages (support hose).
   d. Take frequent rest periods.

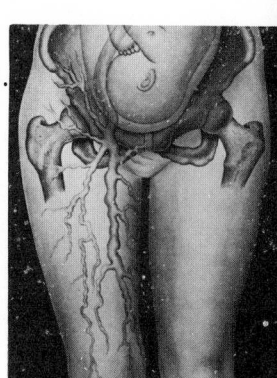

Figure 19-1. Varicose veins due to gravid uterus. (Courtesy Jobst Co.)

Hemorrhoids

1. Causes
   a. Pressure of gravid uterus interfering with venous circulation
   b. Aggravated by constipation.
2. Treatment
   Instruct patient as follows:
   a. Prevent and treat constipation.
   b. Replace protruding internal hemorrhoids using lubricated finger.
   c. Apply cold compresses with or without witch hazel or Epsom salts.
   d. Use suppositories, if prescribed.

Leg Cramps

1. Causes
   a. Increased pressure from gravid uterus
   b. Fatigue
   c. Chilling
   d. Muscle tenseness
   e. Excessive amounts of phosphorus
   f. Inadequate dietary calcium
2. Treatment
   Instruct patient as follows:
   a. Provide for frequent rest periods with feet elevated.
   b. Assure adequate intake of calcium (diet, medication or both).
   c. Wear comfortable, warm clothing.
   d. *Push the toes upward while applying pressure to the knee to flatten the affected extremity to provide immediate relief.*

Edema of the Lower Extremities

1. Most common in hot weather.

NURSING ALERT: Edema is one of the early signs of toxemia (see p. 1008).

2. Treatment
   Instruct the patient as follows:
   a. Take frequent rest periods.
   b. Elevate legs.
   c. Provide abdominal support.

Vaginal Discharge

1. Increased vaginal discharge is normal in pregnancy. Generally a perineal pad is all that is needed.
2. Excessive or green, yellow, foul-smelling or irritating vaginal discharge may be caused by any of the following:
   a. Venereal disease
   b. Trichomonas vaginalis
   c. Moniliasis
3. Treatment
   According to the cause (see p. 532).

THE FETUS

Fetal Development

1st Lunar Month

1. *Length* 0.75–1 cm. (0.3–0.4 inch)
2. Trophoblasts imbed in decidua.
3. Chorionic villa form.
4. Foundations formed for nervous system, genitourinary system, skin, bones and lungs.
5. Buds of arms and legs begin to form.
6. Rudiments of eyes, ears and nose appear.

4 weeks

2nd Lunar Month

1. *Length* 2.5 cm. (1 inch)
   Weight 4 gm.
2. Fetus is markedly bent.
3. Head is disproportionately large due to brain development.
4. Sex differentiation begins.
5. Centers of bone begin to ossify.

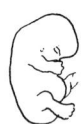

8 weeks

3rd Lunar Month

1. *Length* 7–9 cm. (2.8–3.6 inches)
   Weight 5.20 gm.
2. Fingers and toes are distinct.
3. Placenta is complete.
4. Fetal circulation is complete.

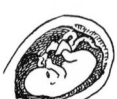

3 months

4th Lunar Month

1. *Length* 10–17 cm. (4–6.7 inches)
   Weight 55–120 gm. (1.9–4.2 oz.)
2. Sex is differentiated.
3. Rudimentary kidneys secrete urine.
4. Heart beat is present.
5. Nasal septum and palate close.

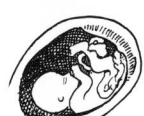

4th month

5th Lunar Month

1. *Length* 30 cm. (12 inches)
   Weight 280–300 gm. (9.9–10.6 oz.)
2. Lanugo covers entire body.
3. Fetal movements are felt by mother.
4. Heart sounds are perceptible with fetoscope.

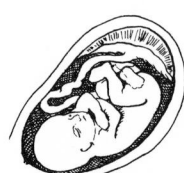

5th month

6th Lunar Month

1. *Length* 28–34 cm. (11.2–13.4 inches)
   Weight 650 gm. (1.4 lb.)
2. Skin appears wrinkled.
3. Vernix caseosa appears.
4. Eyebrows and fingernails develop.

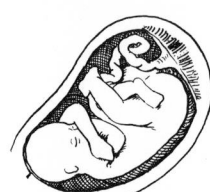

6th month

7th Lunar Month

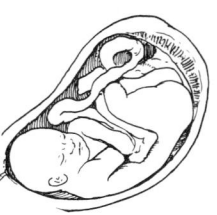

1. *Length* 35–38 cm. (13.8–15 inches)
   Weight 1200 gm. (2.6 lb.)
2. Skin is red.
3. Pupillary membrane disappears from eyes.
4. If born, infant cries, breathes but usually expires.

7th month

8th Lunar Month

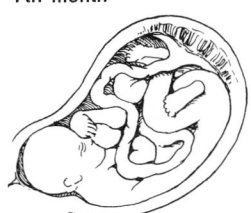

1. *Length* 38–43 cm. (15–17 inches)
   Weight 2000 gm. (3.5–4.2 lb.)
2. Fetus is viable.
3. Eyelids open.
4. Fingerprints are set.
5. Vigorous fetal movement occurs.

8th month

9th Lunar Month

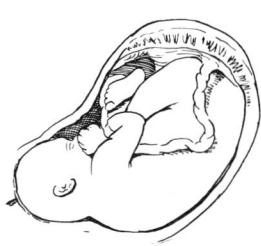

1. *Length* 42–49 cm. (16.5–19.3 inches)
   Weight 1700–2600 gm. (3.7–5.7 lb.)
2. Face and body has loose wrinkled appearance due to subcutaneous fat deposit.
3. Lanugo disappears.
4. Amniotic fluid decreases somewhat.

10th Lunar Month

9th month

1. *Length* 48–52 cm. (18.9–20.5 inches)
   Weight 3000–3600 gm. (6.6–7.9 lb.)
2. Skin is smooth.
3. Eyes are uniformly slate-colored.
4. Bones of skull are ossified and nearly together at sutures.

The Fetal Head

The *fetal head* (Fig. 19-2), from obstetrical standpoint is the most important part of the fetus because (1) it is the largest part of the baby, (2) it is the least compressible and (3) it is the most frequently presenting part.

Base of the Skull

1. Characteristics of Bones
   a. Large
   b. Ossified
   c. Firmly united
   d. Not compressible
2. Function is to protect vital centers on the brain stem.

Vault of the Skull (the cranium)

1. Composed of:
   a. Occipital bone posteriorly
   b. 2 parietal bones on the sides
   c. 2 temporal bones anteriorly
   d. 2 frontal bones anteriorly
2. The cranium is thin, poorly ossified and easily compressible; permits overlapping known as *molding*.

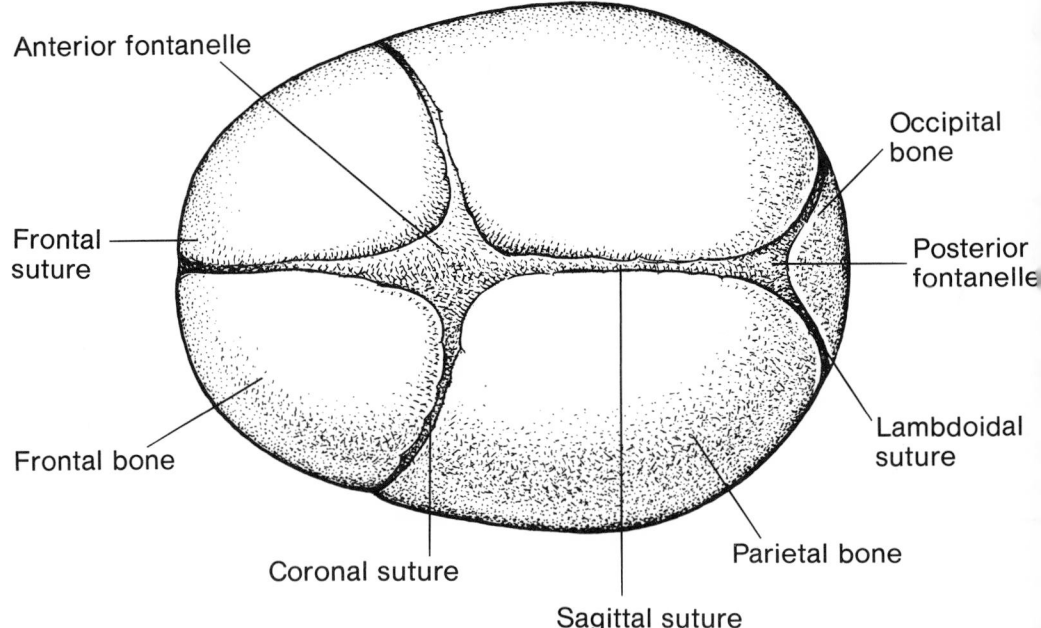

Figure 19-2. Fetal skull.

Sutures of the Skull

1. Aids in molding process and in identifying the position of fetal head during labor.
2. Sagittal suture—lies between the parietal bones.
3. Lambdoidal suture—lies between the occipital and 2 parietal bones.
4. Coronal suture—extends transversely from the anterior fontanelle; lies between the parietal and frontal bones.
5. Frontal suture—is between the 2 frontal bones and is an anterior continuation of the sagittal suture.

Fontanelles

1. Membrane space where the sutures intersect.
2. Anterior fontanelle—junction of the sagittal, frontal and coronal sutures (3 × 2 cm.)—*closes by 18 months of age.*
3. Posterior fontanelle—located where the sagittal suture meets the lambdoidal (smaller than anterior)—*closes at 6–8 weeks of age.*

Changes in Fetal Circulation*

Structure	Before Birth	After Birth
Umbilical vein	Brings arterial blood to liver and heart	Obliterated, becomes the round ligament of liver
Umbilical arteries	Brings arteriovenous blood to the placenta	Obliterated, becomes vesical ligament on anterior abdominal wall

* Adapted from Williams, J. F.: Anatomy and Physiology. Philadelphia, W. B. Saunders.

Structure	Before Birth	After Birth
Ductus venosus	Shunts arterial blood into inferior vena cava	Obliterated, becomes ligamentum venosum
Ductus arteriosus	Shunts arterial and some venous blood from the pulmonary artery to the aorta	Obliterated, becomes ligamentum arteriosum
Foramen ovale	Connects right and left atria	Usually obliterated
Lungs	Contain no air and very little blood	Filled with air and well supplied with blood
Pulmonary arteries	Bring little blood to lungs	Bring much blood to lungs
Aorta	Receives blood from both ventricles	Receives blood from left ventricle only
Inferior vena cava	Brings venous blood from body and arterial blood from placenta	Brings venous blood only to right atrium

GUIDELINES: *Assisting with an Amniocentesis*

Amniocentesis is the transabdominal aspiration of amniotic fluid.

Purposes

1. Cytogenetic evaluation
   a. To detect trisomy 21 (Mongolism).
   b. To establish the fetal sex (important when sex-linked disorders such as hemophilia are anticipated).
2. Amniotic fluid studies
   a. To determine ABO blood groups and amounts of Rh factor sensitization.
   b. To assess fetal maturity.
   c. To identify homozygous biochemical defects (inborn errors of metabolism) in fetuses of known heterozygous parents.
   d. To determine through biochemical analysis of cells if any fatal fetal disorders exist such as Tay-Sachs disease or galactosemia.

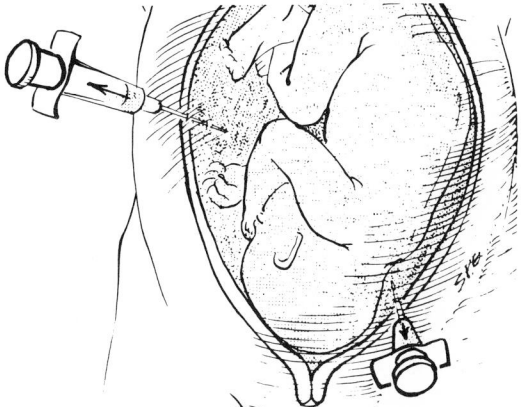

Figure 19-3. Technique of amniocentesis indicating the direction of the needle in relation to the fetal position, to avoid fetal injury. (From Fitzpatrick, E., et al.: Maternity Nursing, 12th ed. Philadelphia, J. B. Lippincott, 1971.)

Equipment

> Sterile amniocentesis tray
>> Draping towels
>> Skin antiseptic
>> 25 gauge needle on 3-ml. syringe for local skin injection
>> Vial of local anesthetic (Xylocaine)
>> 22-gauge spinal needle 12.5 cm. (5 inches) in length, with stylet in place
>> 10-ml. syringe
>> Test tube
> Sterile surgical gloves

Procedure

Nursing Action	Rationale/Amplification
Preparatory Phase	
1. Identify patient's concerns and if necessary provide additional explanation of procedure.	1. Patient may consider procedure hazardous to self or fetus.
2. Assist patient to undress and put on patient gown.	2. Procedure will be done in delivery or operating room.
3. Have patient void.	3. To prevent injury to bladder.
4. Transfer the patient to delivery or operating room.	4. Procedure is performed under sterile conditions.
Performance Phase	
1. The physician determines fetal position by palpation. (X-ray location is sometimes done.)	1. Fetal position must be determined to prevent inadvertent fetal injury.
2. He localizes the placenta through ultrasound.	2. This is a feasible technique after 13 weeks gestation. Puncture of fetal placental vessels could cause exsanguination and contamination of the fluid by blood, making specimen useless for chemical or cytogenic analysis.
3. Carry out surgical skin preparation.	3. Since the needle will be inserted through the skin into the amniotic cavity, asepsis is carried out to prevent infection.
4. Drape patient's abdomen using sterile technique.	4. Same as above.
5. Local anesthesia is infiltrated in the site.	5. The site is determined by the position of the fetus and placenta.
6. The 12.5-cm. (5-inch), 22-gauge spinal needle with stylet in place is introduced into the amniotic cavity.	
7. The stylet is removed and the 10 ml. syringe attached; 2–10 ml. of fluid is slowly withdrawn and placed in test tube.	7. The fluid obtained is sent to the lab or shipped to a center equipped for the analysis; 2–4 weeks are required for cellular growth.
8. The needle is withdrawn and a small dressing applied.	

Follow-up Phase

1. Be aware of complications (fetal or maternal hemorrhage, premature labor, infection).
2. Assess patient for fainting, pain, nausea or onset of contractions.
3. Return patient to dressing room and outpatient clinic.

FETOPELVIC RELATIONSHIPS
The Obstetrical Pelvis

Pelvic Bones and Joints

A. *Bones*

The pelvis is composed of 5 bones.
1. 2 innominate bones
2. Sacrum
3. Coccyx

B. *Joints*

The bones articulate through 4 joints.
1. 2 sacroiliac joints—link the sacrum to the iliac part of the innominate bones.
2. Symphysis pubis—joins the 2 pubic bones.
3. Sacrococcygeal joint—attaches the sacrum to the coccyx.

C. *True and False Pelvis*

1. *False pelvis*—lies above the linea terminalis. Its obstetrical function is to support the enlarged uterus during pregnancy.
2. *True pelvis* lies below the pelvic brim or linea terminalis and is the bony canal through which the infant must pass. It is divided into 3 parts (Fig. 19-4).
   a. The inlet
   b. The pelvic cavity
   c. The pelvic outlet

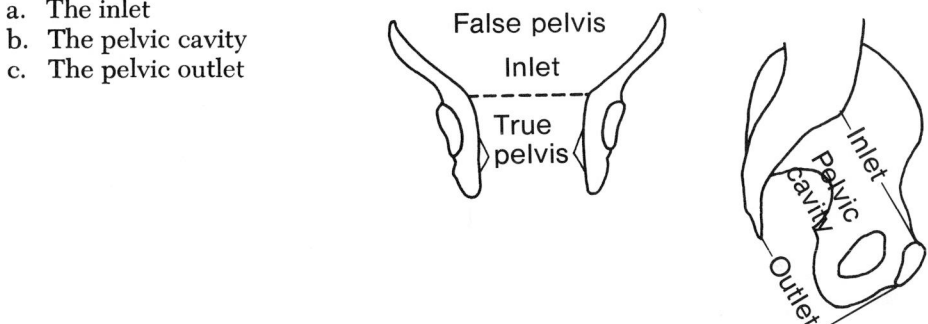

Figure 19-4. The true pelvis.

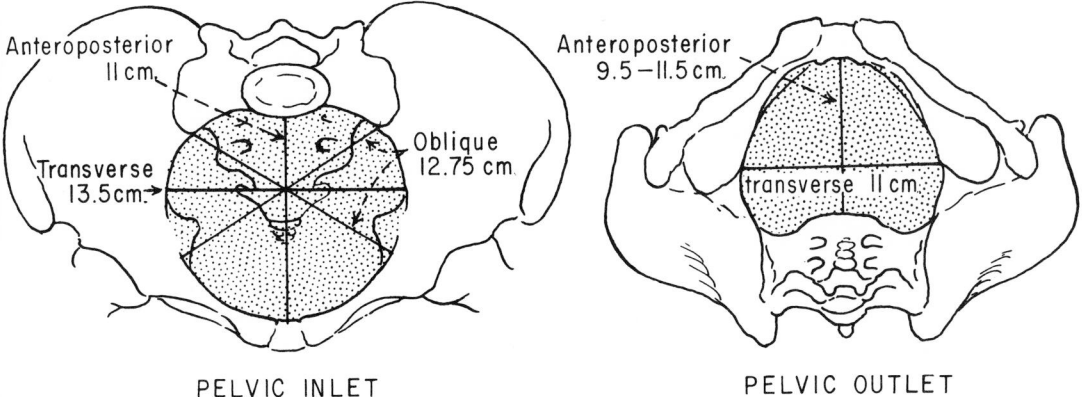

PELVIC INLET

PELVIC OUTLET

Figure 19-5. The pelvic inlet.

The Normal Female Pelvic Inlet and Planes

A. *Diameters of Female Pelvis*

Four diameters traverse the female pelvis (Fig. 19-5):
1. The anteroposterior diameter
   a. Extends from the middle of the promontory of the sacrum to the upper margin of the symphysis pubis.
   b. Is the most important diameter because it is the point of departure in estimating the size of the pelvis. *It is the true conjugate and measures 11 cm. or more.*
2. The transverse diameter
   a. Constructed at right angles to the true conjugate.
   b. Represents the greatest distance between the linea terminalis on either side and measures 13.5 cm.
3. Two oblique diameters
   a. Each extends from one of the sacroiliac synchondroses to the iliopectineal eminence on the opposite side of the pelvis.
   b. The oblique diameters measure 12.75 cm.

Classification of the Pelvis

Name based on structure of the inlet (Fig. 19-6).
1. Gynecoid   3. Anthropoid
2. Android   4. Platypelloid

Presentations and Position of Fetus

General Terms

1. *Lie*—the relationship of the long axis of the fetus to the long axis of the mother. The 2 lies are longitudinal or transverse.
2. *Presentation*—the part of the fetus which lies over the inlet; may be vertex (Fig. 19-7A), face (Fig. 19-7B), breech (Fig. 19-7C) or shoulder.

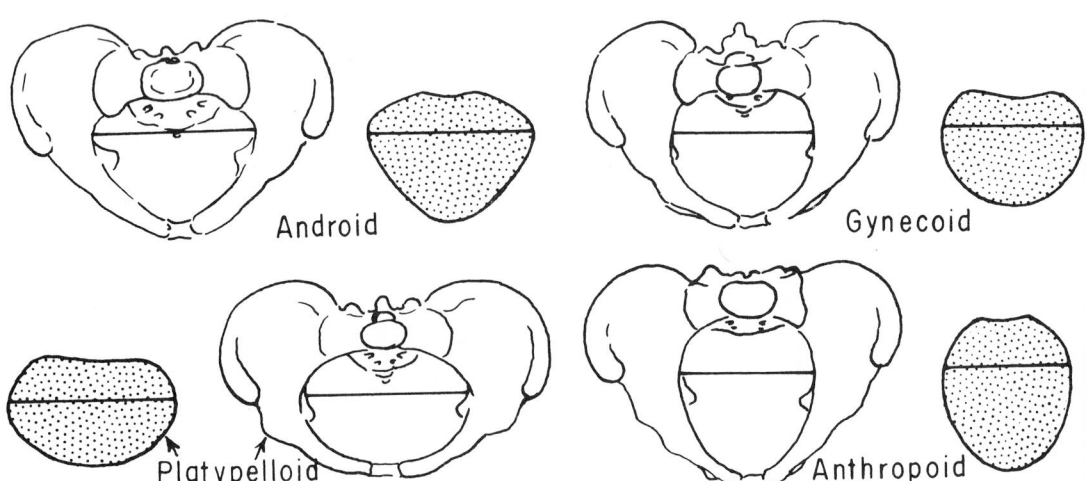

Android   Gynecoid

Platypelloid   Anthropoid

Figure 19-6. The four types of female pelvis.

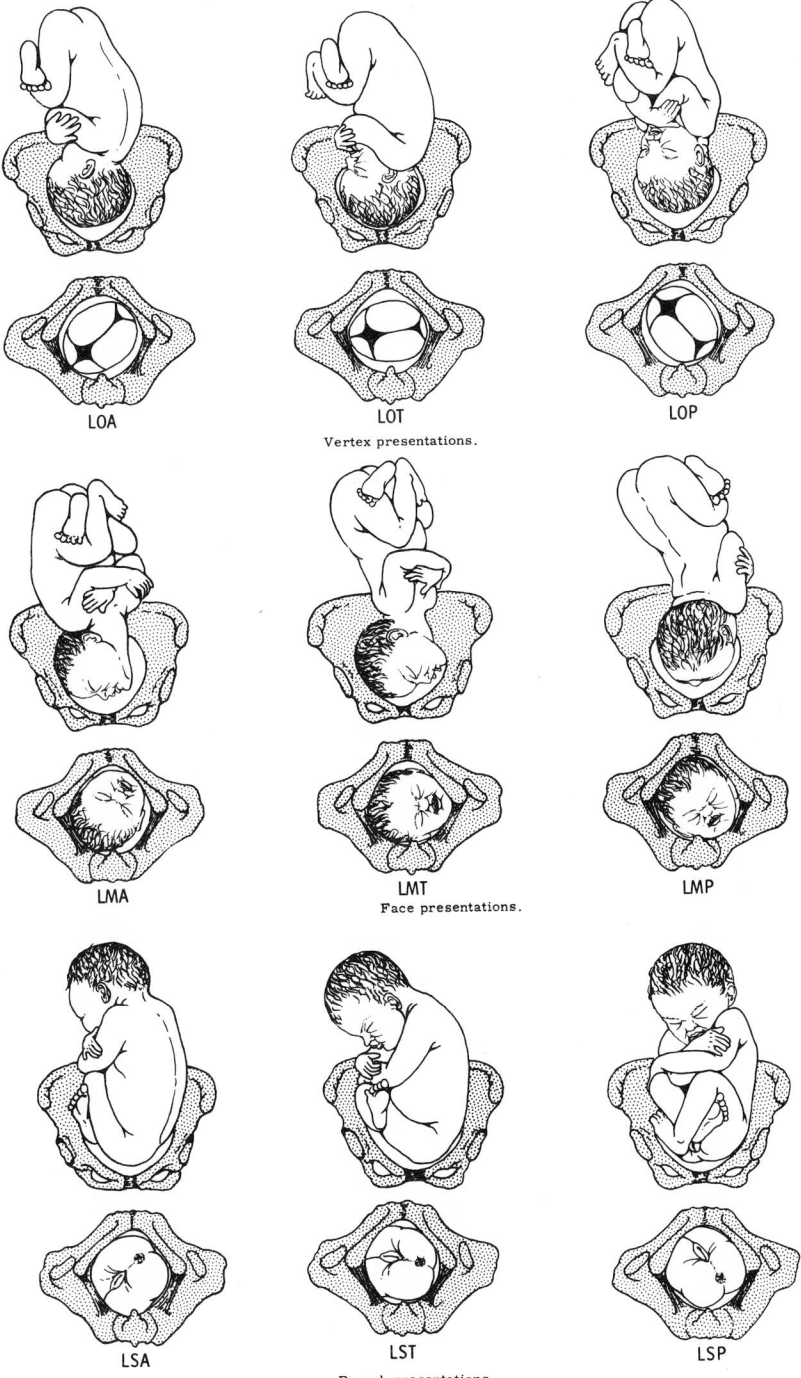

LOA LOT LOP

Vertex presentations.

LMA LMT LMP

Face presentations.

LSA LST LSP

Breech presentations.

Figure 19-7. Fetal presentations. (From Benson, R.C.: Handbook of Obstetrics and Gynecology. Los Altos, California, Lange Medical Publications, 1971.)

3. *Presenting part*—the part of the fetus that lies over the internal os of the cervix.
4. *Attitude*—the relation of the fetal parts to each other; basic attitudes are flexion and extension.
5. *Position*—the relationships of the denominator to the front, back or sides of the maternal pelvis.

Terms Describing Position

1. *Denominator*—an arbitrarily chosen spot on the presenting part of the fetus.
2. *Right or left*—depending on which side of the maternal pelvis the denominator is in
3. *Anterior, posterior or transverse*—according to whether the denominator is in the front, the back or at the side of the pelvis.

BIBLIOGRAPHY

Books

Benson, R. C.: Handbook of Obstetrics and Gynecology. Los Altos, Lange Medical Publications, 1971.
Danforth, D. N.: Textbook of Obstetrics and Gynecology. New York, Harper and Row, 1971.
Fitzpatrick, E., et al.: Maternity Nursing. Philadelphia, J. B. Lippincott, 1971.
Greenhill, J. P.: Obstetrics. Philadelphia, W. B. Saunders, 1965.
————: The Miracle of Life. Chicago, Chicago Year Book Medical Publishers, Inc., 1971.
Hellman, L. M., and Pritchard, J. A.: Williams Obstetrics. New York, Appleton-Century-Crofts, 1971.
Hungerford, M. J.: Childbirth Education. Springfield, Charles C Thomas, 1972.
Odell, W. D., and Moyer, D. L.: Physiology of Reproduction. St. Louis, C. V. Mosby, 1971.
Page, E. W., et al.: Human Reproduction. Philadelphia, W. B. Saunders, 1972.
Reid, D. E., et al.: Principles and Management of Human Reproduction. Philadelphia, W. B. Saunders, 1972.
Taylor, E. S.: Beck's Obstetrical Practice. Baltimore, Williams and Wilkins, 1971.

Articles

Cole, W.: The right to be well-borne. Today's Health, *49*:42–44, Jan. 1971.
Cominos, H.: Teaching infant care to adopting parents. Nurs. Outlook, *19*:421, June 1971.
Conant, L.: What helps mothers to speak out? Amer. J. Nurs., *69*:2650–2653, Dec. 1969.
Daniels, A.: Reaching unwed adolescent mothers. Amer. J. Nurs., *69*:332–335, Feb. 1969.
Edwards, J.: Notes to a maternity clinician. RN, *34*:46–48, Nov. 1971.
Fort, A. T.: Adequate prenatal nutrition. Obstet., Gynecol., *37*:286–288, Feb. 1971.
Hommel, F.: Natural childbirth: nurses in private practice as monitrices. Amer. J. Nurs., *69*:1446–1450, July 1969.
Hunscher, H. A., and Tompkins, W.: The influence of maternal nutrition on the immediate and long-term outcome of pregnancy. Clin. Obstet. Gynecol., *13*:130–144, March 1970.
Obrig, A.: "A nurse-midwife in practice." Amer. J. Nurs., *71*:953–957, May 1971.
Rubin, R.: Cognitive style in pregnancy. Amer. J. Nurs., *70*:502–508, March 1970.
Ulin, P.: Changing techniques in psychoprophylactic preparation for childbirth. Amer. J. Nurs., *68*:2586–2591, Dec. 1968.
Wonnell, E.: The education of expectant fathers for childbirth. Nurs. Clin. N. Amer., *6*:591–601, Dec. 1971.
Yeaworth, R. C.: Maternity nursing—challenge or routine? Nurs. Clin. N. Amer., *6*:247–252, June 1971.

Obstetrical and Nursing Management During Labor and Delivery

20

THE LABOR PROCESS

Phenomena Preliminary to the Onset of Labor

1. Lightening (the settling of the fetus in the lower uterine segment) occurs 2–3 weeks before term in the primigravida and later or during labor in the multigravida.
   a. Respiration becomes easier as fetus falls away from the diaphragm.
   b. Lordosis is increased as the fetus enters the pelvis and falls more forward.
   c. Frequency of urination due to pressure on the bladder occurs.
2. Vaginal secretions increase.
3. Some weight is lost—from excretion of body fluid and loss of appetite.
4. Mucous plug is discharged from cervix—is a protective mechanism which forms by 7th month.
5. Bloody show appears—effacement or thinning of cervix causes capillary bleeding.
6. Cervix becomes soft and effaced (thinned).
7. Backache becomes persistent.
8. False labor pains occur with variable frequency; myometrium becomes irritable.

Stages of Labor

1. First stage of labor or stage of cervical dilatation begins with first true labor contractions and ends with complete dilatation of the cervix.
2. Second stage of labor or stage of expulsion begins with complete dilatation and ends with the birth of the baby.
3. Third stage of labor or the placental stage begins with delivery of the baby and ends with the delivery of the placenta.
4. Fourth stage lasts from the delivery of the placenta until the postpartum condition of the patient has become stabilized.

Signs of True Labor

1. Uterine contractions occur at regular intervals. They occur every 20–30 minutes at the beginning; later they appear closer together and increase in duration and intensity.
2. Uterine contractions are painful and hard.
3. Pain is felt in both back and front of abdomen.
4. Dilatation and effacement of the cervix is accomplished.
5. Presenting part descends.
6. Fetal head is fixed between contractions.
7. Bulging or rupture of the membranes at the cervix may occur.
8. Moderate sedation will not stop contractions.

False Labor

1. Due to inefficient contractions of the uterus or painful spasms of the intestines, bladder and abdominal wall muscles.
2. Appears a few days to a week before term.
3. May be brought on by digestive upset.
4. Contractions are irregular and short and felt more in front.
5. May be slight uterine contractions which are not hard and do not bring about dilatation and effacement.
6. May be stopped by sedation.

Mechanisms of Labor

1. *Descent*—includes engagement of head; continues through labor.
2. *Flexion*—resistance to descent causes head to flex so that the chin approaches the chest, reducing the presenting diameter by 1.5 cm.
3. *Internal rotation*—takes place in 2nd stage of labor. Head enters pelvis in transverse diameter of the inlet—occiput is at 3 o'clock and rotates 90 degrees to arrive under the pubic symphysis. The sequence is L.O.T. (left occipital transverse) to L.O.A. (left occipital anterior) to O.A. (occipital anterior). The shoulders are flexed 45 degrees in the left oblique.
4. *Extension*—birth is by extension. Back of neck pivots under the pubis with the vertex, bregma, forehead, face and chin born over the perineum.
5. *Restitution*—when the head has been delivered the neck twists and the head turns back 45 degrees to the left, resuming the normal relationship with the shoulders—O.A. (occipital anterior) to L.O.A. (left occipital anterior).
6. *External rotation*—the shoulders now rotate 45 degrees to the left to bring their bisacromial diameter into the anteroposterior diameter of the pelvis. The head follows the shoulder and rotates another 45 degrees to the left—L.O.A. (left occipital anterior) to L.O.T. (left occipital transverse). (See Fig. 20-1.)

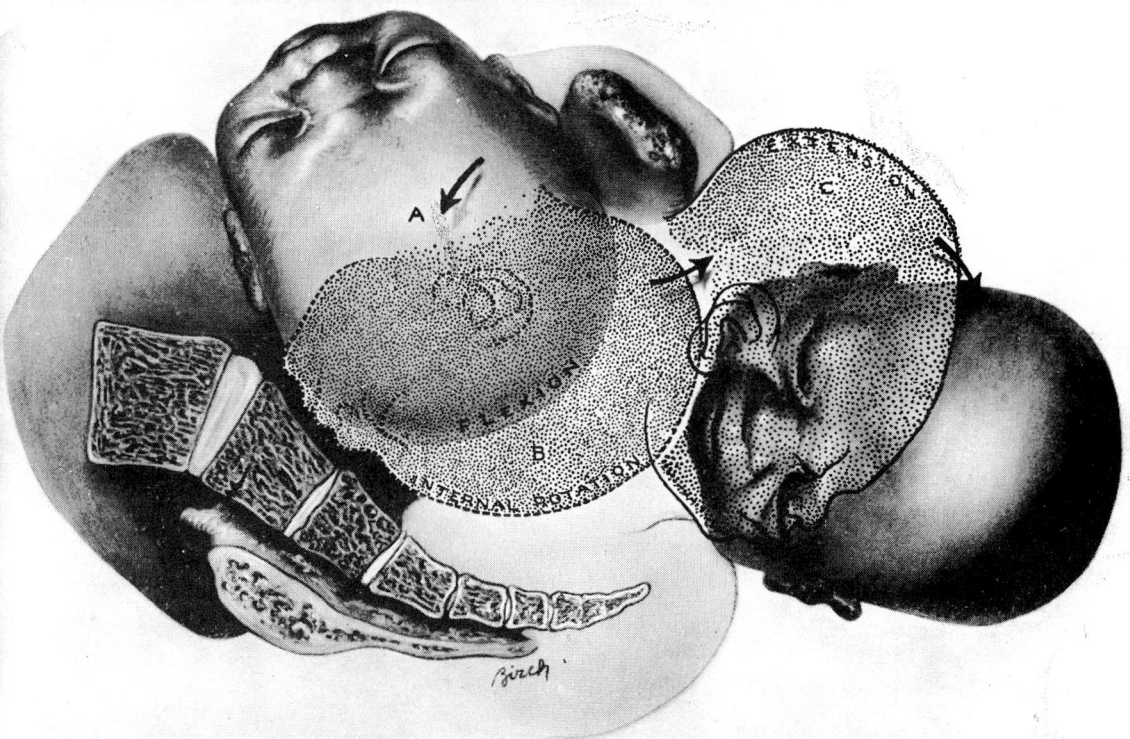

Figure 20-1. L.O.A. Positional changes of head in passing through birth canal. (From Fitzpatrick, E., et al.: Maternity Nursing, 12th ed. Philadelphia, J. B. Lippincott, 1971.)

EXAMINATION OF THE PATIENT DURING LABOR

Abdominal Palpation or Leopold Maneuvers

A. *First Maneuver*

Examiner grasps the lower uterine segment between the thumb and fingers of 1 hand to feel the presenting part. The head is at the inlet or in the pelvis in 90% of cases.

B. *Second Maneuver*

Hands are placed on the sides of the abdomen to identify the location of the back and small parts.

C. *Third Maneuver*

Hands are moved up the sides of the uterus, and the fundus is palpated. In most cases the breech is felt and is softer, more irregular, less globular and not as mobile as the head.

D. *Fourth Maneuver*

Examiner turns and faces the patient's feet. Gently the fingers are moved down the sides of the uterus. The cephalic prominence is felt on the side where there is greater resistance to the descent of the fingers into the pelvis. In addition it is noted whether the head is free and floating or fixed and engaged.

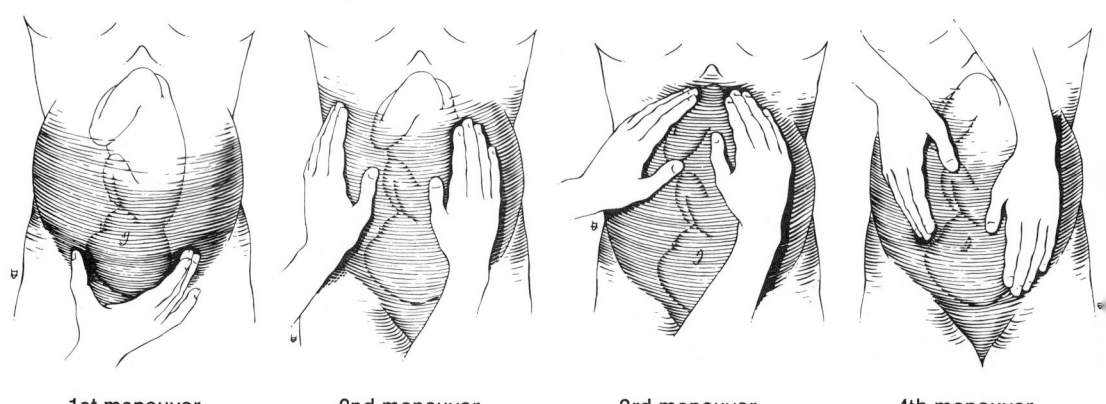

1st maneuver   2nd maneuver   3rd maneuver   4th maneuver

Vaginal Examination (Fig. 20-2)

1. Vaginal examination is preferable to rectal examination in several ways:
    a. Is more accurate in determining:
        (1) Condition and dilatation of the cervix
        (2) Station and position of the presenting part
        (3) Relationship of the fetus to the pelvis

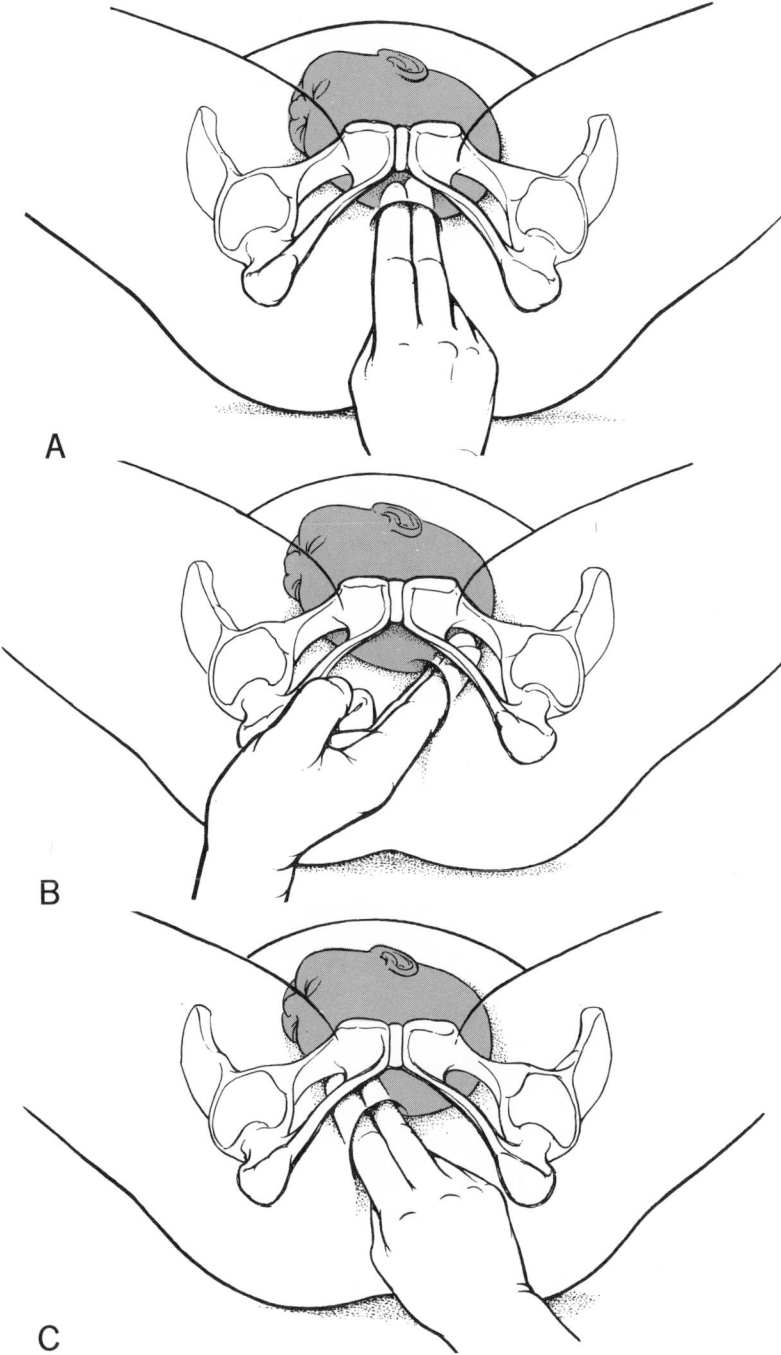

Figure 20-2. Vaginal Examination. *A.* Determining the station and palpating the sagittal suture. *B.* Identifying the posterior fontanelle. *C.* Identifying the anterior fontanelle.

    b. Takes less time since it requires less manipulation.

    c. Causes less pain.

    d. Abnormal presentation diagnosed earlier.

    e. Accidents or complications identified.

       (1) Prolapse of the umbilical cord

       (2) Placenta previae

2. Examination carried out as follows:

    a. Gently and carefully

    b. Under aseptic conditions

    c. With patient in the lithotomy position

3. After palpation, cervix determined as being:

    a. Soft or hard

    b. Effaced and thin or thick and long

    c. Easily dilatable or resistant

    d. Closed or open (dilated)

4. Presentation

    a. Breech, cephalic (head) or shoulder

    b. Caput succedaneum (edema occurring in and under fetal scalp) present (small or large)

    c. Station identified

5. Position

    a. Cephalic presentation (identification of the sagittal suture and its direction)

    b. Location of posterior fontanelle

6. Membranes

    a. Intact

    b. Ruptured

       (1) Drainage of fluid

       (2) Passage of meconium

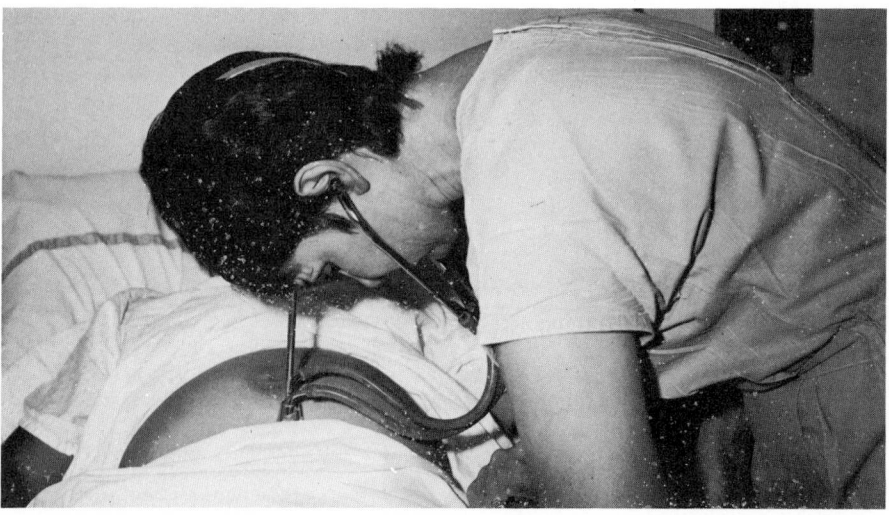

Figure 20-3. Auscultation of the fetal heart beat using the fetoscope.

Auscultation with Fetoscope

1. Fetal heart beat can be monitored with a fetoscope (Fig. 20-3).
2. Location of the fetal heart beat may be used to aid in identifying the presentation and position of the fetus.

Assessment of Fetal Position and Descent

Engagement—has taken place when the widest diameter of the presenting part has passed through the inlet (Fig. 20-4C). In cephalic presentations this diameter is the biparietal diameter of the head.

Floating—the presenting part is entirely out of the pelvis and is freely movable above the pelvic inlet (Fig. 20-4A).

Dipping—the presenting part has passed through the plane of the inlet but engagement has not occurred (Fig. 20-4B).

A. *Engagement*
1. The presence or absence of engagement is determined by abdominal and vaginal or rectal examination.

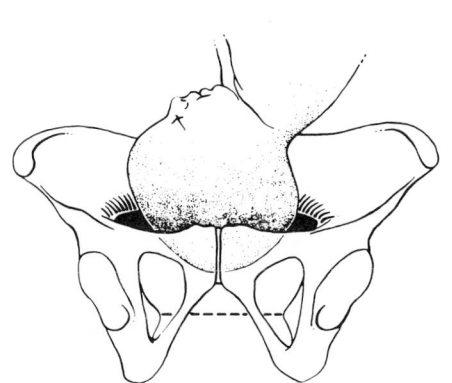

Dipping.

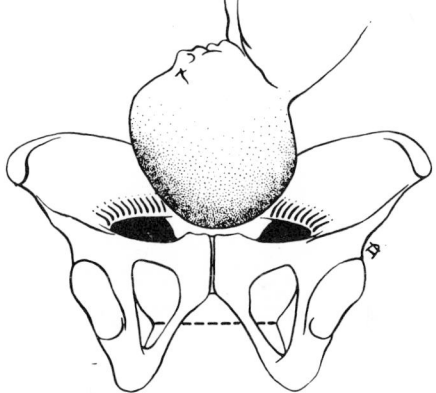

Floating.

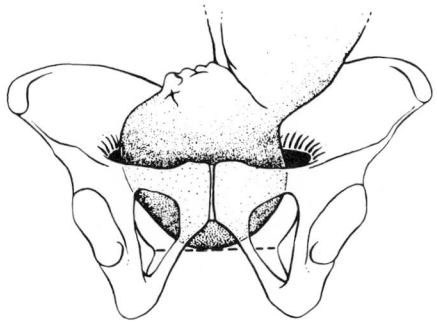

Engagement.

Figure 20-4. Dipping, floating and engagement. (From Oxhorn, H., and Foote, W. R.: Human Labor and Birth. New York, Appleton-Century-Crofts, 1968.)

The location of the presenting part in relation to the level of the ischial spines is designated *station,* and indicates the degree of advancement of the presenting part through the pelvis.

Stations are expressed in centimeters above (*minus*) or below (*plus*) the level of the ischial spines (*zero*). The presenting part is usually engaged when it reaches the level of the ischial spines.

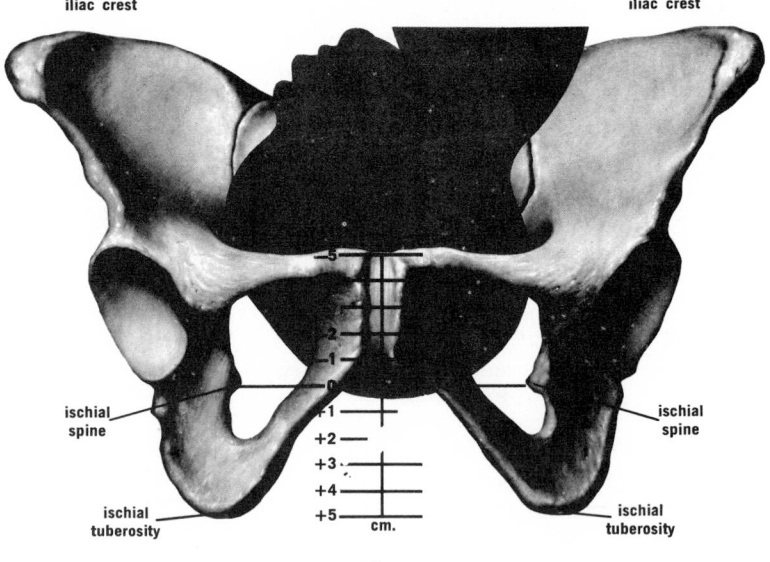

Figure 20-5. Stations of presenting part. (Courtesy, Ross Laboratories.)

    2. In primigravidas, engagement usually takes place 2–3 weeks before term.
          (Lack of engagement in primiparas calls for investigation to rule out disproportion, abnormal position or some condition blocking the birth canal.)
    3. In multigravidas, engagement occurs any time before or after onset of labor.

B. *Station* (Fig. 20–5)
    1. The relationship of the presenting part to an imaginary line drawn between the ischial spines.
    2. The location of the buttocks in breech presentations or the bony skull in cephalic presentations at the level of the spines indicates that the station is zero.
    3. Above the spines the station is —1, —2 and so forth.
    4. At the spine the station is —5 at the inlet.
    5. Below the spines it is +1, +2 and so forth.

MANAGEMENT OF THE PATIENT DURING LABOR AND DELIVERY

Admitting the Patient to the Unit

    1. Establish positive relationships by greeting and reassuring the patient and by providing supportive nursing care.
    2. Assist the patient to undress and get into bed.
    3. Provide for safekeeping of personal belongings.
    4. Listen to fetal heart tones to identify location, rate, and character. *Detection of fetal distress may require that the clinical management of the patient be adjusted.*
    5. Assess and evaluate the following by means of vaginal examination (p. 967).
        a. Cervical dilatation
        b. Status of membranes
        c. Presentation, position and station of the fetus

6. Accept husband's presence or absence.
7. Ascertain patient's desires concerning the management of her labor and delivery, such as natural childbirth, type of analgesia and anesthesia.
8. Obtain pertinent information from the patient or from records previously submitted by the obstetrician.
   a. Expected date of delivery (May indicate complications of pre- or postmaturity of the fetus.)
   b. Parity and character of previous labors
   c. Time when contractions began; their frequency, duration and intensity
   d. If membranes are ruptured, at what time and general characteristics
   e. Food and fluid intake during the 6 hours prior to admission (Digestion is inhibited during labor which leads to danger of aspiration during delivery when inhalation anesthesia is used.)
   f. Rh-factor, blood type, hemoglobin and hematocrit (obtained from obstetrician's records)
   g. Contact lenses, dentures or removable bridges—removed if the patient has general inhalation anesthesia
9. Record blood pressure and report any elevations of systolic over 140 mm. Hg or diastolic over 80 mm. Hg or any unusual reading in relation to the stage of labor.
10. Measure pulse and respiration rate and temperature.
    a. Anxiety and exertion may cause increased pulse and respiration rate but temperature will remain normal.
    b. Elevated temperature suggests maternal infection—isolation techniques may be indicated and the infant placed in the observation nursery.
11. Carry out perineal preparations.
    a. Shaving the vulva and perineal areas promotes cleanliness and reduces possibilities of postpartum infection.
    b. Vaginal opening will be more easily visible.
12. Obtain urine specimen only if specifically ordered. It is difficult to obtain an uncontaminated voided specimen if membranes have ruptured or if show is present.
13. Administer enema (soapsuds or Fleet).
    Emptying the lower large intestine has following effects:
    (1) Increases space available for passage of the fetus.
    (2) Decreases fecal contamination of the field during delivery.
    (3) Usually increases frequency and intensity of uterine contractions.

> NURSING ALERT: An enema is contraindicated when vaginal bleeding, premature labor or abnormal fetal presentation or position is present.

First Stage of Labor

A. *Characteristics of Labor During First or Dilating Stage*
1. Cervix dilates to 3–4 cm.
2. Uterine contractions occur regularly 5–10 minutes apart and are of short duration (20 seconds).
3. Patient usually experiences low back pain and abdominal discomfort with contractions.
4. Patient may feel anticipation, excitement, relief or apprehension.
5. Patient usually appears alert and talkative; however, if patient is unprepared and improperly informed, she may be fearful and withdrawn.

B. *Nursing Management During Latent Phase of First Stage*
  1. Provide diversion.
     a. Encourage patient to time contractions.
     b. Provide reading materials.
     c. Teach breathing techniques to be used in active phase.
     d. Involve husband in activities if he is present.
     e. Permit patient to listen to fetal heart tones.
  2. Provide explanations of nursing activities.
  3. Share information of patient's progress following examinations.
  4. Continue constant nursing surveillance.
     a. Major concern of most patients is being left alone and unattended.
     b. Identify any deviations from the normal status of both mother and fetus.
  5. Continue to monitor fetal heart tones every 30 minutes.
  6. Evaluate vital signs every 2 hours; blood pressure every hour and more often if indicated.
  7. Encourage patient to void every 3 hours—a full bladder will inhibit contractions and interfere with descent of fetus.

C. *Characteristics of Labor During the Active Phase of the First Stage of Labor*
  1. Cervical dilation from 4–8 cm.
  2. Labor becomes active—contractions occur at 2- to 5-minute intervals with greater intensity and duration of 30–40 seconds.
  3. When cervical dilation reaches 6 cm. there is noticeable change in character of labor and patient reaction.
  4. If membranes are intact, rupture usually occurs spontaneously.

NURSING ALERT: Monitor fetal heart tones following amniotomy or spontaneous rupture of membranes; flow of fluid may cause prolapse of cord.

---

  5. Patient becomes serious, pays little attention to external stimuli and is concerned with progress of labor.
  6. Patient may feel unable to cope with contractions and begins to lose control.

D. *Nursing Management During Active Phase*
  1. Ascertain patient progress by vaginal examination.
  2. Monitor fetal heart tones every 5 minutes.
  3. Observe contractions for frequency, intensity and duration.
  4. Assist patient with controlled abdominal breathing to reduce tension and prevent hyperventilation.
  5. Encourage patient to assume Sims' position whenever possible.
     a. Favors anterior rotation of the fetal head.
     b. Prevents continual pressure of the gravid uterus on the inferior vena cava.
     c. Promotes relaxation between contractions.
  6. Provide comfort measures.
     a. Provide sacral hand pressure and backrest.
     b. Change damp or soiled linen.
     c. Assist with mouth care.
     d. Give partial sponge bath.
     e. Continue to provide encouragement and information in accordance with the patient needs.

7. Administer I.V. fluids as prescribed.
   a. Dehydration leads to acidosis—fetus may be born with respiratory acidosis.
   b. Electrolyte imbalance may occur.
   c. Drugs can be given more effectively if complications occur.
8. Administer analgesia as prescribed. Check dosage according to: (a) weight of patient, (b) status of labor, (c) size and gestation of fetus.
9. Assist anesthesiologist in administering regional anesthesia (caudal or lumbar epidural block).
   a. For even distribution of agent, supine position is necessary following placement of catheter.
   b. Since Carbocaine or Xylocaine are vasodilators, the blood pressure may drop rapidly.
   c. Pressure of the gravid uterus in the supine position affects blood flow of the large vessels—also predisposes to hypotension.
   d. Monitor blood pressure constantly until stabilized,
      (1) Adjust patient's position as indicated.
      (2) Elevate lower extremities to increase blood flow to vital centers.
      (3) Oxygen, 5 liters by mask, may be used.

Transitional Stage of Labor

A. *Characteristics of the Transitional Stage*
   1. Dilation progresses from 8 cm. to full dilatation.
   2. Average time is 40 minutes and 20 contractions in primigravidas; 20 minutes and 10 contractions with multigravidas.
   3. Bloody show increases as more capillary vessels in the cervix rupture.
   4. Nausea and vomiting may occur due to reflex action as the cervix stretches and retracts over the fetal head.
   5. Patient experiences feelings of rectal pressure.
   6. Patient may have partial amnesia between contractions; if narcotics and scopolamine have been given, she may be restless and may cry with contractions.

B. *Nursing Management During the Transitional Stage*
   1. Assist with controlled chest (costal) breathing as contractions occur.
   2. Discourage patient from bearing down until cervical dilatation is complete.
   3. Encourage rest between contractions to conserve energy.
   4. If epidural analgesia is being used, continue to monitor blood pressure and renew agent if hospital policy permits; if not, notify anesthesiologist when more medication is needed.
   5. Continue to monitor fetal heart tones.
   6. Observe for onset of second stage.

Second Stage of Labor

A. *Characteristics of Second Stage or Expulsive Stage of Labor*
   1. Usually lasts from 2–60 minutes; average of 20 contractions for the primigravida, 10 contractions for the multigravida.
   2. Reflex bearing down of the abdominal wall occurs with contractions due to pressure of the presenting part against the pelvic floor.
   3. Vaginal discharge increases.

4. Perineal muscles stretch and central portion of perineum thins.
5. There is marked distention of anus.
6. Perineal bulge increases with each contraction.
7. Fetal head descends with each contraction and recedes slightly between contractions.
8. The introitus becomes an anteroposterior slit, then an oval, and finally a circular opening with exposure of the fetal head (caput).
9. An episiotomy (perineal incision) may be done at this time to prevent laceration (see Fig. 20-6).
10. The head continues to advance and recede with contractions until the largest diameter of the head (crown) is forced through the vulva.
11. The head is born by process of extension, and the forehead, nose, mouth and chin appear over the perineum (Fig. 20-1).
12. Mucus and fluid are removed from the face, and the oropharynx is suctioned before infant gasps and aspirates with first breath.
13. Restitution occurs as the head rotates back to the original position.
14. External rotation takes place as the shoulders move from the oblique to the anteroposterior diameter of the pelvis.
15. The anterior shoulder emerges under the symphysis pubis.
16. Head is raised so that the posterior shoulder can be born over the perineum.
17. When the head and shoulders are delivered, the rest of the body slips out easily, usually with a gush of amniotic fluid.
18. Umbilical cord is clamped and cut usually after pulsation has ceased.
19. Infant is (a) placed in heated resuscitator on sterile drape to avoid contamination of doctor's gloves or (b) received by nurse with sterile receiving blanket.
20. Placental separation occurs usually within 5 minutes.
21. Pressure upon the fundus expresses the placenta.

B. *Nursing Management During the Second Stage*
1. Transfer multigravida to the delivery room; primigravidas usually remain in the labor room until caput is observed.
2. Provide direction to the patient to accomplish effective pushing.
3. Provide encouragement with each effort.
4. Monitor fetal heart tones following each contraction and pushing effort; transient fetal bradycardia is not unusual at this stage due to pressure exerted upon the fetal head or compression of the cord.

NURSING ALERT: Fetal bradycardia is pathologic if (1) the recovery period is delayed beyond 20 seconds (2) it is preceded by period of acceleration, 160 beats or more per minute or (3) meconium is observed in the amniotic fluid.

5. Transfer primigravida to delivery room.
6. Carry out activities designated to the circulating nurse.
   a. Assist the patient onto the delivery table and place in lithotomy position.
   b. Provide hand grips and wrist restraints; explain purpose if patient is awake.
   c. Wait for instructions before adjusting position if inhalation anesthesia is to be given.
   d. Simultaneously elevate both of the patient's legs in stirrups to avoid backache, injury or ligament strain. Adjust stirrups to leg length and provide padding to prevent pressure upon the popliteal veins.

 e. Cleanse vulva and perineal area.

 f. Uncover sterile table and check infant resuscitator. Attach sterile suction catheter and oxygen mask.

 g. Check infant weight scale for correct balance.

 h. Prepare silver nitrate ampule and sterile water for newborn eye care.

 i. Assist physician to drape patient, utilizing correct aseptic technique.

 j. Adjust instrument table and provide additional materials as requested by the obstetrician.

 k. Observe delivery of the infant and complete written records of birth.

 l. Administer oxytocics as requested.

NATURAL CHILDBIRTH

Natural childbirth is a normal or natural process in which an infant is delivered without medical analgesia or anesthesia. The mother is prepared for this type of delivery through prenatal training.

Underlying Principles

 (As advocated by Grantly Dick-Read and Herbert Thoms)

1. Fear stimulates the sympathetic nervous system and causes the circular muscles of the cervix to contract.
2. The longitudinal muscles of the uterus have to act against increased cervical resistance, causing tension and pain.
3. Tension and pain aggravate fear which produces a vicious cycle of tension, pain and fear.
4. Minor degree of pain, magnified by fear, becomes unbearable.

Objectives of Prenatal Training

A. *To provide the patient with an opportunity to acquire understanding of birth processes and to gain self-confidence.*

1. Explain processes of fetal development and childbirth.
2. Describe methods available to relieve pain.
3. Teach exercises that strengthen certain muscles and relax others.
4. Teach breathing techniques that will enable the patient to relax in first stage of labor and work effectively with muscles used in the delivery.
5. Stress improvement of physical health and emotional stability.

B. *To eliminate fear.*

1. Never tell patient that labor and delivery will be painless; indicate that analgesia and anesthesia are available if needed or desired.
2. Assure patient that she will be given empathetic understanding and support during labor by her husband, the nurse and the physician.

Psychoprophylactic Childbirth

Psychoprophylactic childbirth is another version of natural childbirth with rationale based on Pavlov's concept of pain perception and his theory of conditioned reflexes (the substitution of favorable conditioned reflexes for unfavorable ones). The *Lamaze method* is an example of this technique.

Underlying Principles

Programs teaching this method of childbirth are based on the neurophysiology of cortical excitement and conditional response.

1. The mother is taught to replace responses of restlessness and fear and the loss of control with more useful activity. High level of activity can excite the cerebral cortex efficiently to inhibit other stimuli, such as pain in labor.
2. Mother-to-be is taught exercises which strengthen the abdominal muscles and relax the perineum.
3. Breathing techniques to help the process of labor are practiced.
4. Mother is conditioned to respond with respiratory activity and disassociation or relaxation of the uninvolved muscles, while controlling her perception of the stimuli associated with labor.
5. One method of control is by normal breathing while the patient silently mouths the words to a song and simultaneously taps the rhythm with her fingers.

Similarity Between Psychoprophylactic and Natural Childbirth Theories

1. Fear enhances the perception of pain but may diminish or disappear when the patient understands the physiology of labor.
2. Since psychic tension enhances perception of pain, relaxation is achieved more easily in a calm agreeable atmosphere with supportive contacts.
3. Muscular relaxation and a specific type of breathing diminish or abolish the pains of labor.

Breathing Techniques for Childbirth

During First Stage of Labor

1. A complete breath is taken once at the beginning of a contraction and once again when the contraction is completed.
2. At the peak of each contraction breathing should be quiet and shallow.
3. The technique for complete breathing involves 3 steps:
   a. Breathing in as deeply as possible.
   b. Hissing or blowing the air out slowly.
   c. Allowing the whole body to go limp (relaxation phase).

During Second Stage of Labor

Pushing breath should augment uterine contractions and aid in the delivery of the baby.

1. Mother breathes in as deeply and quickly as possible.
2. She holds her breath. (This fixes the diaphragm and allows more effective downward pressure on the uterus.)
3. She takes catch-breaths as needed. Catch-breaths are taken whenever breath can no longer be held comfortably.
4. She pushes as if straining at defecation. (Pushing is not necessary during practice sessions.)
5. *Panting* may be necessary in the middle of a contraction during the second stage of labor. Panting physically prevents pushing although it does not decrease the desire to push.

OPERATIVE OBSTETRICS

Operative obstetrics refers to a number of special procedures (episiotomy, forceps delivery, cesarean section, induction of labor) which the physician may use to assist the mother in labor and delivery.

Episiotomy

An *episiotomy* is an incision of the perineum during delivery to facilitate the birth of the baby.

Types of Episiotomies

1. Median—incision is made in the middle toward the rectum (Fig. 20-6).
2. Mediolateral—incision is begun in the middle and directed laterally and downward away from the rectum. A mediolateral episiotomy reduces incidents of third-degree laceration (extends through skin, mucous membrane, perineal body and the rectal sphincter).

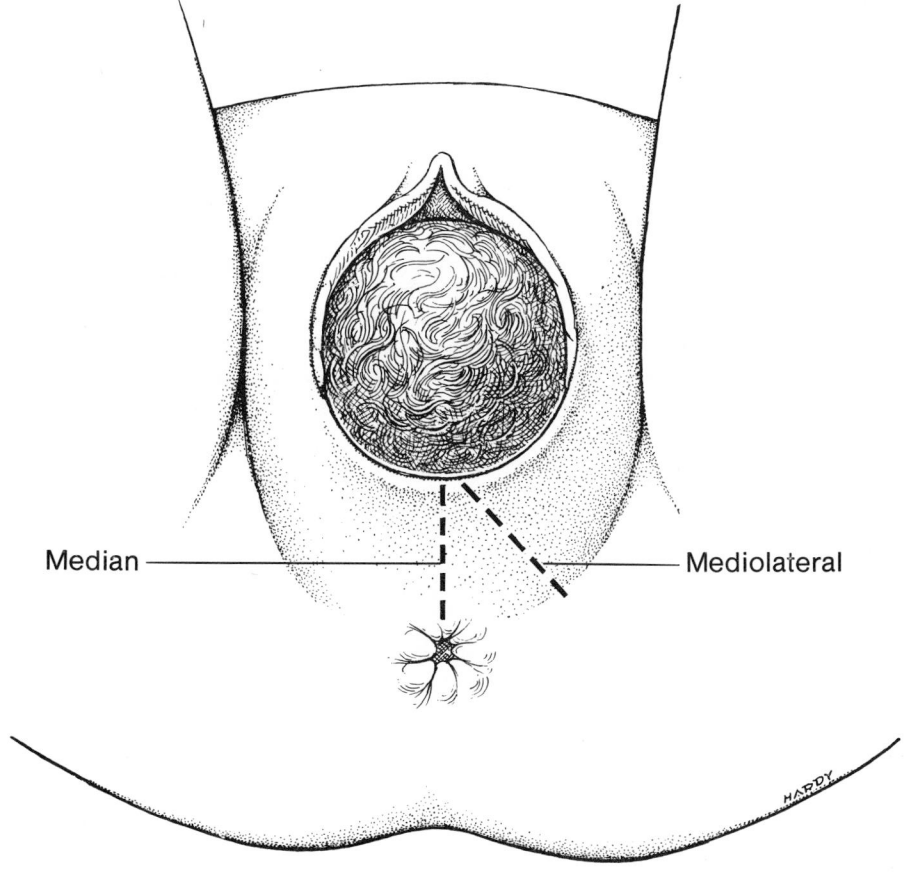

Figure 20-6. Types of episiotomies.

Purposes

1. To substitute a straight surgical incision for the laceration that otherwise frequently occurs.
2. To enable laceration to be repaired more easily and to heal better.
3. To spare the infant's head from prolonged pressure and pushing against the rigid perineum which may result in brain damage especially with the premature infant.
4. To shorten the second stage of labor.

Nursing Management

1. Assess the healing processes; inspect for signs of infection or pain.
2. Provide analgesics for pain relief (Darvon or codeine) or apply ice bag *early* to reduce edema and allay discomfort.
3. Evaluate degree of pain; *excessive pain may be a signal of vulval, paravaginal or ischiorectal hematoma or abscess.*
4. Return patient to the operating room for ligature of bleeding vessels if hematoma is identified.
5. Provide antibiotic therapy for infection and incision and drainage of abscess.

Forceps Delivery

Obstetric forceps is an instrument, consisting of 2 crossing blades, designed to extract the fetus by means of traction and rotation.

Types of Forceps Deliveries

1. *Low forceps operation*—forceps are applied after the head has reached the perineal floor with the sagittal suture in the anteroposterior diameter of the outlet.
2. *Midforceps operation*—forceps are applied before the criteria for low forceps are met but after engagement has taken place.
3. *High forceps operation*—forceps are applied before engagement has taken place (only used in modern obstetrics in very rare circumstances).

Prerequisites for Application of Forceps

1. Pelvis should be adequate with no disproportion.
2. Fetal head must be engaged—preferably deeply engaged.
3. Cervix must be completely dilated.
4. Accurate diagnosis of position and station must be made (see pp. 969–970).
5. Membranes must be ruptured.
6. Some form of anesthesia should be used.
7. Rectum and bladder should be empty.

Indications

1. Fetal distress as identified by:
   a. Irregular fetal heart rate
   b. Bradycardia under 100 beats per minute
   c. Rapid fetal heart rate more than 160 beats per minute
   d. Passage of meconium in cephalic presentation
   e. Prolapse of the cord

2. Maternal conditions
   a. Maternal exhaustion
   b. Maternal disease (cardiac or pulmonary disease, hemorrhage, intrapartal infection)
   c. Failure of progress in the second stage due to poor uterine contractions, rigid perineum
   d. Failure of fetal head to rotate

Complications

1. Maternal complications
   a. Lacerations of the vagina and cervix, predisposing to hemorrhage and infection
   b. Rupture of the uterus
   c. Injury to bladder or rectum
2. Fetal complications
   a. Cephalhematoma
   b. Brain damage and intracranial hemorrhage
   c. Skull fracture
   d. Facial paralysis
   e. Cord compression

Nursing Management

1. Carry out surveillance during the postpartum period for signs and symptoms of complications.
2. Assess the newborn for indications of injury.
3. Provide explanation to parents if bruising is apparent.

Cesarean Section

Cesarean section is removal of the infant from the uterus through an incision made in the abdominal wall and the uterus.

Indications

1. Cephalopelvic disproportion
2. Uterine dysfunction, inertia, inability of cervix to dilate, lack of progress
3. Neoplasm obstructing birth canal or pelvis
4. Malposition and malpresentation
5. Previous uterine surgery (cesarean section, myomectomy, hysterotomy) or cervical surgery
6. Complete or partial placenta previa
7. Certain cases of premature separation of the placenta
8. Certain cases of toxemia of pregnancy
9. Maternal diabetes
10. Certain cases of elderly primigravida (35–40 years old)
11. Prolapse of the umbilical cord
12. Fetal distress
13. Post-term pregnancy
14. Failed forceps

Types of Cesarean Section

A. *Low Segment Cesarean Section* (operation of choice)—incision made transversely in lower segment of uterus.
  1. Incision is made in thinnest portion so that blood loss is minimal and uterus is easier to open.
  2. Lower segment is area of least uterine activity.
  3. Postoperative convalescence is more comfortable.
  4. Possibility of later rupture is lessened.
  5. Peritoneal flap is brought over uterine incision, preventing lochia from entering peritoneal cavity.
  6. There is less incidence of postoperative adhesions and danger of intestinal obstruction.

B. *Classical Cesarean Section*—vertical incision is made directly into the wall of the body of the uterus.
  1. Bleeding is profuse and more scar tissue will form.
  2. Useful when bladder and lower segment involved in extensive adhesions.
  3. Selected when anterior placenta previa exists.
  4. Useful when fetus is in a transverse lie.

C. *Extraperitoneal Cesarean Section*—the tissue around the bladder is dissected, providing access to lower uterine segment without entering into the peritoneal cavity.
  1. Devised to prevent peritonitis.
  2. Availability of blood and antibiotics has reduced use of this method.

D. *Cesarean Section and Hysterectomy (Porro's operation)*—cesarean section followed by removal of the uterus.

  Indications:
  1. Hemorrhage from uterine atony after conservative therapy fails
  2. Uncontrollable hemorrhage from placenta previa and abruptio placenta
  3. Placenta accreta (abnormal attachment of placenta to uterine endometrium)
  4. Rupture of the uterus, not repairable
  5. Gross multiple fibromyomata
  6. Certain cases of cancer of the cervix or ovary

Nursing Management

A. *Preoperative Care*
  1. Carry out physical examination.
  2. Request routine laboratory studies, including type and cross-matching of blood.
  3. Monitor fetal heart tones.
  4. Shave abdomen and perineal area.
  5. Insert a retention catheter.
  6. Administer prescribed preoperative atropine. (Narcotic drugs are avoided.)
  7. Start I.V. infusion with 19-gauge needle and double hook-up so that blood may be administered quickly if necessary.
  8. Prepare oxytocic drugs to be added to the infusion following delivery of the infant.
  9. Notify pediatrician or pediatric resident of surgery to provide initial care and resuscitation of infant.

B. *Postoperative Care*
1. Provide postoperative care similar to that following abdominal surgery.
2. Observe for hemorrhage
    a. Inspect perineal pads and abdominal dressings.
    b. Assess vital signs frequently.
3. Administer oxytocics as prescribed.
4. Check fundus frequently for firmness.
5. Continue I.V. fluids for 24 hours.
6. Check drainage from indwelling catheter.
7. Provide medication for relief of pain.
8. Encourage patient to turn from side to side, to breathe deeply and to cough.
9. Assist with ambulation during first postoperative day.

Induction of Labor

Induction of labor means to bring about labor by amniotomy (surgical rupture of fetal membranes) or administration of oxytocin.

Indications

1. Maternal Condition
    a. Toxemia of pregnancy when medical therapy has been unsuccessful
    b. Uncontrollable antepartal bleeding in late pregnancy (premature separation of the marginal placenta previa)
    c. Premature spontaneous rupture of membranes (Infant should be delivered within 24 hours.)
    d. History of rapid labors
    e. Patients living far from hospital
2. Fetal Condition
    a. Maternal diabetes (pregnancy terminated about 37 weeks)
    b. Rh incompatibility with rising titer
    c. Excessive size of fetus or postmaturity

Prerequisites for Successful Induction

1. Normal cephalopelvic relationship
2. Single fetus with vertex engaged
3. Stage of pregnancy—the closer to term the easier the induction
4. Fetal maturity—chance of survival before 32 weeks is reduced
5. Cervix amenable to induction—effaced or partially effaced and dilated 1–2 cm.

Nursing Management

A. *For Induction by Oxytocin*
1. Prepare infusion of 1000 ml. 5% glucose with 10 units of Pitocin added.
2. Regulate number of drops per minute prescribed by physician—usually started slowly (4–5 drops per minute), increased gradually to 20.
3. Check rate of flow frequently; patient's movement may change rate of flow.
4. Observe uterine contractions—*keep hand on fundus to time beginning and termination of contractions.*

5. Turn off infusion if there are any abnormalities in contractions or fetal heart tones or if attending physician leaves labor suite.

B. *For Artificial Rupture of Membranes*

> NURSING ALERT: Artificial rupture of membranes is usually done to enhance labor begun by oxytocin rather than to initiate labor. The membranes serve as a barrier against bacterial invasion and delivery should be accomplished as soon as possible after membranes have been artificially ruptured.

1. Explain procedures to patient.
2. Carry out antiseptic preparation of vulva.
3. Carry out vaginal examination.
4. Insert amniohook or allis clamp or orangewood stick to rupture membranes.
5. Allow as much fluid as possible to escape.
6. Note quality of fluid (normal, amber, clear).
7. *Check fetal heart tones immediately as there is an increased possibility of cord prolapse.*

OBSTETRICAL ANALGESIA AND ANESTHESIA

Obstetrical Analgesia

Method	Comment	Precautions
Natural childbirth (Read, Lamaze methods)	Requires patient preparation and psychologic support, controlled breathing, voluntary muscle relaxation.	Requires commitment of patient and husband and support of obstetric staff
Hypnosis		Requires specially trained obstetrician, a willing patient, considerable prenatal training
Narcotics (Demerol most frequently used)	Given I.M. or I.V. in 50–100 mg. doses (smaller doses given I.V.)	Must be withheld until active labor starts Not to be administered when delivery imminent lest depression of infant occur
Tranquilizers (ataractics)	May be used in combination with narcotics Reduced dose of narcotic required Allays anxiety Has antinauseant effect	
Barbiturates	Given in combination with analgesic Produces sedation and hypnosis.	Produces excitement when given alone Depresses infant for many hours after birth Caution must be exercised when there is maternal liver or renal impairment

Method	Comment	Precautions
Scopolamine	Depresses parasympathetic nervous system Produces amnesia	Must be given with narcotics or will produce excitation, delirium, hallucinations
Trichlorethylene (Trilene)	Usually is self-administered by cannister and face mask	Should not be given with another form of inhalation anesthesia for delivery Cardiac arrhythmias may occur Administration should be carried out by anesthesia service or by physician or nurse

General Anesthesia

Halothane	Produces good uterine relaxation quickly Useful for intrauterine manipulations such as version and extraction Postpartum hemorrhage is a problem	
Methoxyflurane (Penthrane)	Contraindicated in patients with a history of liver disease Slow-acting Rarely used in obstetrics	
Thiopental (Pentothal sodium)	For rapid induction of anesthesia for vaginal deliveries and cesarean sections Fetal depression is a problem Maternal laryngospasm may lead to fetal and maternal hypoxia	

Regional Analgesia and Anesthesia

See Table 20-1.

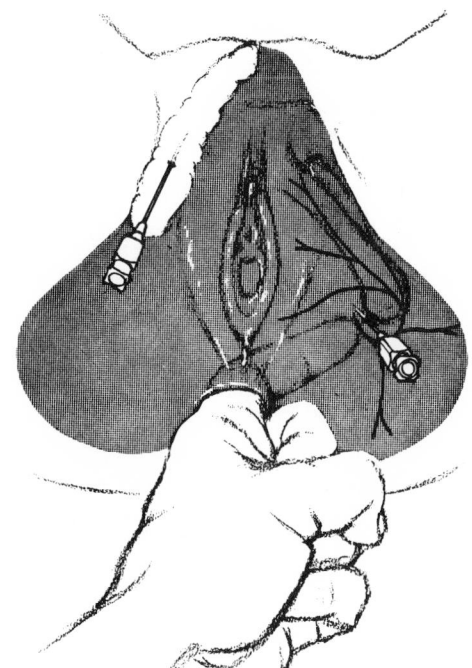

Figure 20-7. The pudendal block is used for perineal anesthesia in uncomplicated obstetrical procedures. The pudendal nerve lies medial to the ischial tuberosity, and the physician inserts his index finger into the rectum to guide the needle point to the tuberosity.

The other part of the block is done to anesthetize the iliohypogastric, ilioinguinal and genitocrural nerves which innervate the skin over the mons pubis and the labia. (From Nealon, T. F.: Fundamental Skills in Surgery. Philadelphia, W. B. Saunders, 1971.)

TABLE 20-1. REGIONAL ANALGESIA AND ANESTHESIA

Type	Method	Advantages	Disadvantages
Paracervical block	Transvaginal injection of a local anesthetic into the tissue on either side of the cervix Lasts 45 to 60 minutes	1. Started in the 1st stage of labor 2. Useful in a rapidly progressing labor 3. Causes cervix to dilate more rapidly	1. May cause transient fetal bradycardia 2. Danger of direct injection into maternal circulation or fetal tissue 3. Constant fetal heart monitoring required
Caudal	Blocking of nerves in the peridural space at the sacral hiatus Can be given as single or continuous injection	1. Provides analgesia in the 1st and 2nd stages of labor and anesthesia for delivery 2. Patient is awake 3. Has little effect on fetus 4. Better than narcotics for patients with metabolic diseases, lung or heart disease and some patients with toxemia	1. Specially trained anesthesiologist is needed 2. Produces hypotension (agents are vasodilators) 3. May prolong labor in primigravida 4. Higher incidence of forceps deliveries if unassisted with pushing 5. May prolong labor if administered too early 6. Sacral hiatus may be difficult to locate 7. Inadvertent puncture of dura mater into subarachnoid space — with large needle causing severe postanesthesia headache 8. Difficult to keep site clear
Local infiltration	Regional anesthesia produced by local infiltration of the nerves of the perineum	1. Simple to administer 2. Does not affect fetus 3. Toxic effects minimal	1. No value for analgesia during labor 2. Takes time for infiltration and for agent to take effect 3. Useful for perineal repair with natural childbirth

TABLE 20-1. REGIONAL ANALGESIA AND ANESTHESIA (Continued)

Type	Method	Advantages	Disadvantages
Lumbar epidural	Extradural analgesia produced by injection of a local anesthetic into the epidural space in the lumbar region Can be given in single or continuous injection	1. Provides analgesia in the 1st and 2nd stages and anesthesia for delivery 2. Patient is awake and cooperative 3. No effect on fetus unless hypotension occurs 4. Useful when general anesthesia is contraindicated and when patient has diabetes, cardiovascular disease, pulmonary, renal and hepatic disease or is in premature labor	1. Risk of dural puncture greater than in caudal 2. May cause hypotension 3. Requires expert administration by anesthesiologist 4. Patient requires assistance in pushing 5. Greater incidence of uterine atony following delivery 6. May prolong labor 7. Higher incidence of forceps delivery if patient unable to push effectively
Subarachnoid block (spinal anesthesia, saddle block) 1. Low spinal (saddle block) limited to the sacral segment 2. Midspinal analgesia extends to 10th thoracic dermatoma 3. High spinal analgesia to T5 or T6 used for cesarean section	Form of regional anesthesia produced by injection of a local anesthetic solution into the cerebrospinal fluid in the spinal canal	1. Relative simplicity of procedure 2. Is rapid and certain and has lasting action 3. Low failure rate 4. Low incidence of side effects when properly performed	1. Frequency and degree of hypotension higher than with either caudal or epidural block 2. Postspinal headache 3. Anesthesia from a single injection is of short duration (used primarily for delivery)
Pudendal block (Fig. 20-7)	Form of regional anesthesia produced by blocking the pudendal nerve with a local anesthetic agent	1. Simple and safe method of securing perineal analgesia for normal deliveries 2. Does not depress infant	1. Short duration, may be done in patient's room 30 minutes before delivery (may need to be repeated) 2. May fail to produce adequate pain relief 3. Patient must be cooperative

[985]

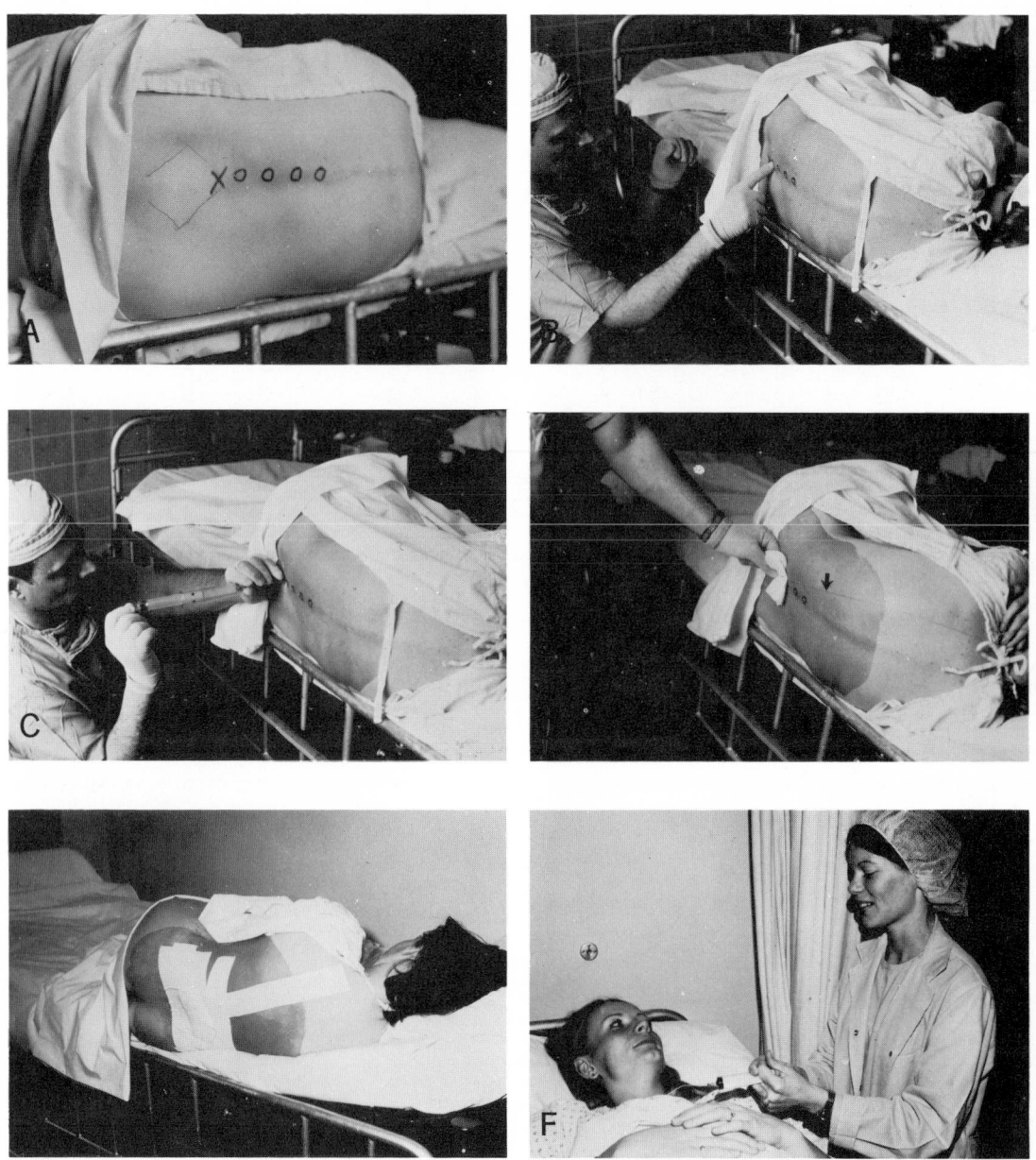

Figure 20-8. Epidural block. *A.* The X marks the L$_{4-5}$ interspace where epidural needle is to be inserted. *B.* The anesthesiologist is pointing to the needle puncture site. *C.* He uses the loss of resistance test to identify the epidural space. *D.* The epidural catheter has been threaded into the needle and is in position (arrow). The needle is removed and the catheter is folded over a sponge to prevent kinking. *E.* The catheter is taped in place so it will not become dislodged. *F.* The delivery room nurse is giving a maintenance dose. (Photographs, courtesy of John O'Connor, M.D.)

GUIDELINES: *Assisting with a Continuous Lumbar Epidural Block*

Continuous lumbar epidural block is a form of analgesia achieved by blocking the nerves in the epidural space (Fig. 20-8).

Purpose

To provide pain relief during labor and delivery.

Equipment

Sterile surgical gloves
Vials of Xylocaine 1 and 2% and Carbocaine 1.5%
Adhesive tape 4 cm. (1½ inches) width
Vinyl plastic epidural catheter in sterile package
Antiseptic solution for skin preparation
Sterile epidural tray containing
2 medicine glasses (1 for antiseptic solution and 1 for anesthetic agent)
10-ml. glass syringe
3-ml. glass syringe with 1½-inch 25-gauge needle
No. 17 Touhy spinal needle with stylet in place
Draping towels
Sponge forceps with sponges for applying antiseptic solution for the skin preparation

Procedure

Nursing Action	Rationale/Amplification
Preparatory Phase	
1. Provide explanation of procedure to the patient.	1. Cooperation by the patient is essential. She must not move while the needle and catheter are being positioned.
2. Have the patient void.	2. It is difficult, if not impossible, to void after the anesthesia has taken effect.
3. Take blood pressure.	3. Anesthetic agent usually causes some degree of hypotension. (Anesthesiologist should be aware of blood pressure levels before proceeding.)
4. Assist the patient to lie on the left side with shoulders parallel, head flexed toward chest and knees drawn upward.	4. The spinal column should not be too convex or the epidural space will be reduced and the dura stretched, making it more susceptible to puncture.
5. Open the outer covering of the surgical gloves and the epidural tray.	
Performance Phase (by the anesthesiologist)	
1. Put on surgical gloves and open inner sterile covering. (Assistant fills the medicine glasses with anesthetic agent and antiseptic solution for skin preparation.)	1. Aseptic technique is required since needle is injected through the skin into the epidural space.
2. Skin is cleansed with solution and area draped as for a spinal puncture (see p. 720).	
3. Skin, interspinous ligament and the ligamentum flavum are infiltrated with the same anesthetic solution used for the continuous block.	

Nursing Action	*Rationale/Amplification*
4. The Touhy needle is introduced into the 3rd, 4th or 5th lumbar interspace.	4. The largest epidural spaces are found in the lumbar area.
5. Position of the needle in the epidural space is tested.	5. When an attempt is made to inject air into the ligamentum flavum, the plunger of the syringe rebounds, when air is injected into the epidural space, the plunger falls into space.
6. When the needle is properly placed and no spinal fluid is aspirated, the plastic catheter is introduced through the needle into the epidural space.	6. The passage of the catheter often elicits a neurologic response in the leg or hip as the tip of the catheter touches a nerve in the space.
7. A test dose of 5–8 ml. of anesthetic agent is given.	7. If catheter has been placed inadvertently in subarachnoid space, a spinal rather than epidural anesthesia will result. The patient will have difficulty moving her legs.
8. Larger doses (8–12 ml.) of the anesthetic agent are given as indicated by the patient's response.	8. Amount of agent is determined by process of labor and need for pain relief.

Follow-up Phase

1. The catheter is held in place by adhesive tape, and the patient is turned on her back.	
2. The blood pressure is monitored continuously until stabilized. Systolic should not be allowed to fall below 100 mm. Hg.	2. The agent is a vasodilator—some degree of hypotension usually occurs. The fall of pressure can be corrected easily by turning patient on her side so that the gravid uterus falls away from large vessels. Elevation of legs will also aid circulation.

EMERGENCY DELIVERY BY THE NURSE

Immediate Needs of Mother and Baby

1. Baby must breathe.
2. Mother needs reassurance.

Essentials of Care until Physician Arrives

1. Using a clean or sterile towel, exert gentle pressure against the head of the fetus to control its progress.
   a. Prevents undue stretching of the perineum.
   b. Prevents sudden expulsion through the vulva with subsequent infant and maternal complications.
2. Encourage mother to pant at this time to prevent bearing down.
3. If membranes have not ruptured by the time the head is delivered, they must be removed immediately by tearing them at the nape of the infant's neck.
4. Holding the baby's head in both hands, gently exert downward pressure toward the floor, thereby slipping the anterior shoulder under the symphysis pubis (Fig. 20-9).
5. If the cord is looped around the baby's neck, gently slip it over the head. If the cord is too tight to permit this, it must be clamped in 2 places and cut between the clamps before the rest of the body is delivered.
6. Support the infant's body and head as it is born.

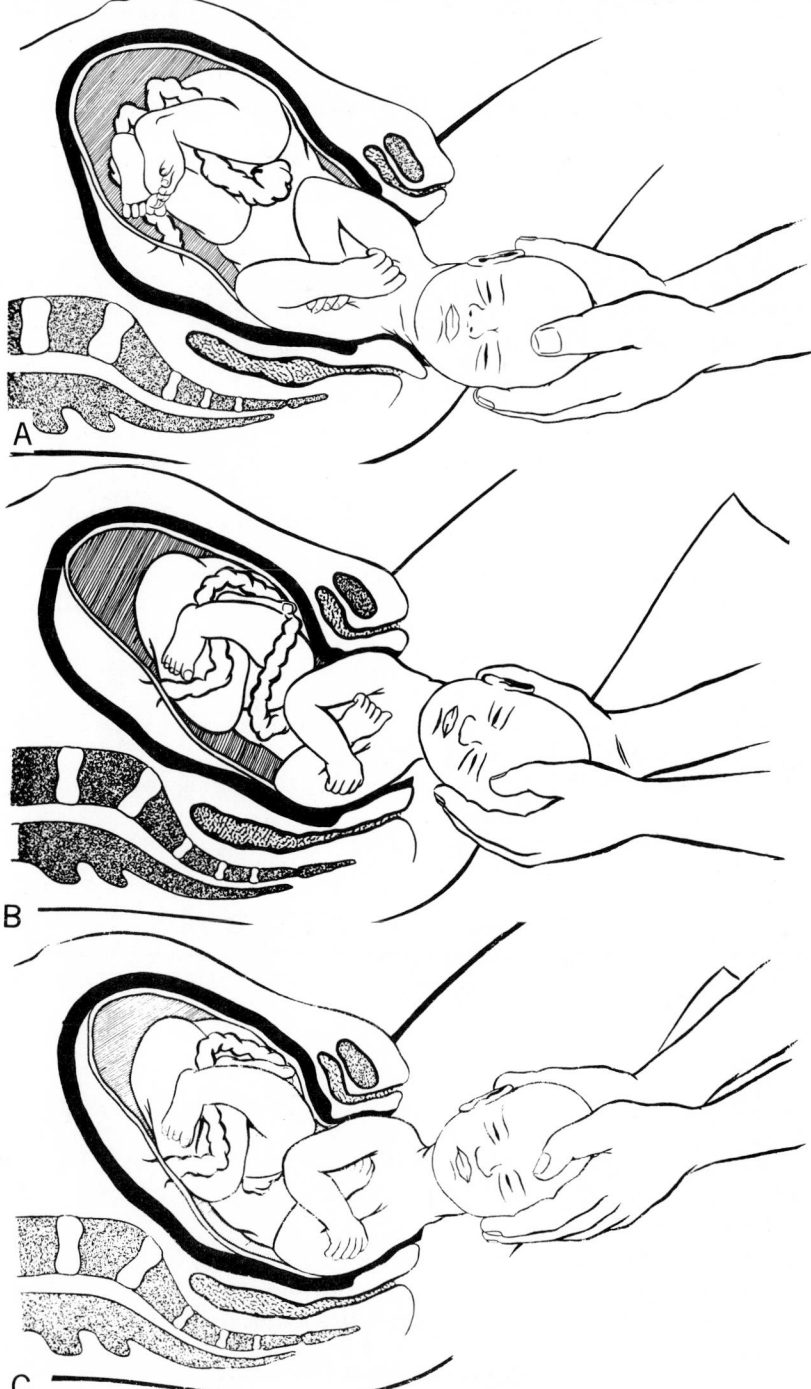

Figure 20-9. Emergency delivery by the nurse. *A.* Controlling the head during delivery. *B.* Delivering the upper shoulder. *C.* Delivering lower shoulder while maintaining support of the head. (From Emergency Birth in Disaster. U.S. Army Film and Equipment Exchange.)

7. Pick baby up gently by feet, with head down to prevent aspiration of fluid. Drainage of mucus is stimulated when the infant cries; gentle rubbing of the back may stimulate breathing.
8. Encourage mother.
9. After baby cries, place him gently on mother's abdomen where she can see him. This serves 2 purposes:
    a. Reassures mother.
    b. Weight over the uterus will help uterus contract.
10. Avoid touching perineal area so as not to cause infection.
11. Avoid pulling on cord which might break and cause hemorrhage.
12. Watch for signs of placental separation.
13. When placenta is delivered, do the following:
    a. Clamp cord with surgical clamp when cord stops pulsating. If clamp is not available, tie off cord with any suitable material several inches from the infant's abdomen.
    b. Do not cut cord; the physician will cut it later under more stable conditions.
    c. Wrap the baby and placenta in a blanket.
14. Check fundal contractions; massage if indicated. *Putting the baby to breast may help the uterus to contract.*
15. Give mother fluids.
16. Encourage mother to move; if she is not in bed or in a place where she can lie down, she may move to a more suitable environment.
17. Do not leave mother alone until help arrives. Mother should never be alone during the first hour and a half after delivery.
18. Instruct mother so that she may care for herself and her newborn.
19. Explain why cord has not been cut.
20. Keep accurate record of delivery.

COMPLICATIONS OF LABOR

Dystocia

Dystocia or difficult labor may be due to either mechanical or functional factors or to a combination of both.

Mechanical Dystocia

1. *Maternal Causes*
    a. Contracted pelvis
    b. Obstructive tumors (ovarian or uterine fibromyoma)
2. *Fetal Causes*
    a. Failure of the vertex to rotate as in occiput posterior or occiput transverse
    b. Malpresentations (shoulder, brow, face or breech)
    c. Malformation of the fetus (as in hydrocephalus) or excessive size of the infant

Functional Dystocia (Uterine Dysfunction or Inertia)

Conditions in which uterine contractions are deviating from the normal.
1. *Types of Uterine Inertia*
    a. Primary inertia—occurring at onset of labor
    b. Secondary inertia—occurs later; prolongation of the active phase of labor

2. *Contributing Conditions*
   a. Uterine abnormalities (such as double uterus)
   b. Minor degrees of pelvic contraction and fetal malposition
   c. Overdistention of the uterus, associated with multiple pregnancy, polyhydramnios
   d. Postmaturity or delayed labor
   e. Grande multiparity
   f. Excessive cervical rigidity as with the older primigravida
   g. Excessive or too early administration of analgesic drugs
   h. Unknown causes
3. *Complications of Uterine Dysfunction*
   a. Fetal injury and death
   b. Maternal exhaustion and dehydration if labor is too prolonged
   c. Intrauterine infection
   d. Deleterious effect on future childbearing

Treatment and Nursing Management

A. *For Mechanical Dystocia*
   1. Re-evaluate pelvis with X-ray pelvimetry.
   2. Prepare for cesarean section if vaginal delivery appears to be hazardous to either mother or infant.
   3. Plan nursing intervention if occiput posterior is identified.
      a. Relieve back pain as much as possible by sacral pressure, back rubs, frequent change of position from side to side (may also assist fetal head to rotate).
      b. Observe the character and frequency of contractions and monitor fetal heart rate constantly and critically.
      c. Assess the amount of discomfort the mother is experiencing and her general condition.
      d. Prevent dehydration during the lengthened labor by starting I.V. fluids.
      e. Rotate fetal head manually or by forceps when cervical dilation is complete.
   4. Plan obstetrical and nursing intervention if breech presentation is identified.
      a. Provide explanation and appropriate reassurance.
      b. Identify type of breech presentation:
         (1) Complete breech—when feet and legs are flexed on the thighs and the thighs flexed on the abdomen so that the buttocks and feet present.
         (2) Footling—when one or both feet present through the cervix.
         (3) Frank breech—when legs are extended and lie against the abdomen and the chest, with the feet meeting the shoulders; the buttocks present.
      c. Provide comfort measures.
         (1) Labor is generally longer since the soft buttocks do not aid in cervical dilation as well as vertex presentation.
         (2) Analgesia may be limited so as not to interfere with the mother's ability to push effectively.
         (3) Amniotomy is not done until breech is well engaged as there is greater danger of prolapse of the cord with footling.
      d. Assist with delivery.
         (1) Breech cases may be delivered spontaneously with strong contractions, particularly in multiparae.

(2) More aid is indicated (manual extraction of the head or application of Piper forceps to the aftercoming head) in the majority of patients, especially in primigravidae.

(3) Cesarean section is a better approach than difficult extraction.

e. Assess newborn's condition.

1 breech in every 15 succumbs as the result of delivery due to tentorial tears and subsequent intracranial hemorrhage, lesions of the spinal cord and extrusion of the medulla into the foramen magnum.

f. Assess condition of the mother and observe for postpartum bleeding; lacerations of birth canal are more frequent.

B. *For Functional Dystocia*

1. *Hypertonic uterine dysfunction*—muscle of the uterus is in a state of greater than normal tension, so that contractions are ineffective for accomplishing dilatation.

a. Provide rest with aid of sedation. (Morphine, 16 mg., usually stops contractions.)

b. Provide fluids to maintain hydration and electrolyte balance.

c. Observe for normal contractions when patient awakens.

2. *Hypotonic uterine dysfunction*—tone or tension of the uterine muscle is defective or inadequate—usually occurs during the active phase of labor.

a. Confirm diagnosis with x-ray pelvimetry and sterile vaginal examination to ascertain:

(1) Accurate pelvic measurement

(2) Abnormalities of presentation and position

(3) State of cervical dilation

(4) Level of presenting part

b. Prepare for cesarean section if indicated.

c. Provide comfort measures to promote relaxation if cesarean section not indicated.

d. Provide explanations and continue supportive care.

e. Administer enema to stimulate contractions.

f. Perform amniotomy—rupture of membranes often stimulates contractions (see p. 982).

g. Start I.V. fluids to prevent dehydration.

h. Administer intravenous infusion of oxytocin or give subcutaneously.

(1) Pitocin I.V. (5 units) in 500 ml. of 5% dextrose in water or 10 units pitocin in 1000 ml. of 5% dextrose in water.

(2) Pitocin (0.5 minims) subcutaneously PRN every 20–30 minutes up to 3–5 times.

(3) Spartocin sulfate (75–150 mg.) I.M., up to a total and not to exceed 600 mg., I.M.

i. Provide continuous surveillance.

(1) Observe contractions for character and frequency. If contractions last more than 60–70 seconds, adjust infusion. (Tetonic contractions may cause premature separation of the placenta or rupture of the uterus.)

(2) Observe I.V. drip; be certain infusion is running at prescribed drops per minute.

(3) Report any maternal or fetal aberrations immediately.

(4) Record observations and nursing activities.

Precipitate Labor

Precipitate labor is a labor which lasts 2 hours or less and possibly includes precipitate delivery (sudden and unexpected delivery without professional attendance).

Predisposing Factors

1. Multiparity
2. Large pelvis
3. Lax and unresistant soft tissue
4. Tumultuous contractions
5. Small baby in good position
6. Induction of labor by rupture of membranes and oxytocin infusion

Complications

1. Impaired blood flow may have hypoxic effect on fetus. (May be an etiologic factor in cerebral palsy.)
2. Rapid transit of fetus through bony pelvis may produce cerebral trauma.
3. Delivery may be unattended and baby may not receive the benefit of immediate resuscitation.
4. Maternal birth canal may be lacerated.
5. Uterus may rupture.

Treatment and Nursing Management

1. Obtain obstetrical history. Patients with previous rapid labor may be candidates for elective induction of labor and control of labor.
2. Provide constant surveillance.
3. If contractions become excessively strong, anesthesia is given to decrease strength of contractions.
4. Administer oxygen by mask to aid fetus.

Uterine Rupture

Uterine rupture is a spontaneous or traumatic rupture of the uterus.

Causes

1. Excessive strain on the myometrium
2. Rupture of the scar from a previous cesarean section or hysterotomy
3. Prolonged or obstructed labor
4. Faulty presentation
5. Forced delivery of fetus with abnormalities, e.g., hydrocephalus
6. Ill-advised podalic version
7. Application of forceps and extraction before cervical os has completely dilated
8. Injudicious use of oxytocin
9. Excessive manual pressure applied to the fundus during delivery

Clinical Manifestations

1. Complete rupture
   a. Sudden sharp abdominal pain during contractions
   b. Abdominal tenderness

    c. Cessation of contractions
    d. Bleeding into the abdominal cavity and sometimes into the vagina
    e. Fetus easily palpated; fetal heart tones cease
    f. Signs of shock—rapid weak pulse, cold clammy skin, pale color, flaring of nostrils with air hunger
  2. Incomplete rupture—develops over a period of a few hours
    a. Abdominal pain during contractions
    b. Contractions continue but cervix fails to dilate
    c. Slight vaginal bleeding
    d. Rising pulse rate and skin pallor
    e. Loss of fetal heart tones

Treatment and Nursing Management

  1. Fetal prognosis is grave, fetus often dies of asphyxia prior to delivery or suffers permanent damage from effects of hypoxia.
  2. Maternal prognosis is guarded, especially in uterine rupture of traumatic origin (5–10% mortality rate).
  3. Treatment begins with prevention of spontaneous rupture:
    a. Accurate evaluation of maternal pelvis
    b. Identification of fetal position
    c. Avoidance of prolonged labor
    d. Judicious use of pitocin
    e. Cesarean section for subsequent deliveries
  4. Prepare for immediate hysterectomy after rupture.
    a. Obtain complete hemostasis at earliest possible moment.
    b. Ensure adequate amount of blood by 1 or 2 venous cutdowns.
    c. Ligation of the hypogastric arteries may be considered preliminary to hysterectomy.
    d. Administer antibiotics to combat peritonitis.

Amniotic Fluid Embolism

Amniotic fluid embolism is the escape of amniotic fluid containing debris such as meconium, lanugo and vernex caseosa into the maternal circulation, usually resulting in deposition of fluid or debris in the pulmonary arterioles (rare but usually fatal).

Clinical Manifestations

  1. Sudden dyspnea   4. Profound shock due to:
  2. Cyanosis   a. Anaphylaxis causing vascular collapse
  3. Pulmonary edema   b. Uterine bleeding with development of hypofibrinogenemia

Treatment and Nursing Management

  1. Treatment initially directed to relief of respiratory difficulties.
  2. Administer oxygen therapy and provide assisted ventilation (see pp. 125 and 137).
  3. Start fresh whole blood transfusion immediately.
  4. Give I.V. administration of fibrinogen.

5. Administer heparin to control intravascular coagulation, especially in the pulmonary circulation.
6. Prepare for immediate sterile vaginal examination. If cervix is dilated, forceps delivery may salvage fetus and reduce maternal respiratory difficulty.

Prolapsed Umbilical Cord

Prolapsed umbilical cord—descent of the cord following rupture of the membranes.

Causes

1. Rupture of membranes when the presenting part is not engaged in the pelvis.
2. More common in shoulder and foot presentations.
3. Prematurity—small fetus allows more space around presenting part.
4. Hydramnios—causes greater amount of fluid with more force when membranes rupture.

Clinical Manifestations

1. Cord may be seen protruding from vagina.
2. Fetal distress occurs following rupture of membranes.
3. Cord can be palpated in the vaginal canal or cervix.

Treatment and Nursing Management

1. Place mother in deep Trendelenburg position.
2. Administer oxygen (5 liters) by mask.
3. Place sterile gloved hand in vagina and push head upward relieving compression on the cord.
4. Prepare for immediate vaginal delivery if cervix is dilated.
5. Prepare for immediate cesarean section if cervix is incompletely dilated.
   General anesthesia administered to prevent uterine contractions while preparation for cesarean section is being made.

Inverted Uterus

Inverted uterus—uterus inverted or turned inside out usually during the delivery of the placenta.

Causes

1. Excessive traction on the cord when the placenta is firmly attached to the uterine wall
2. Markedly lax or thin uterine walls
3. Fundal pressure when the uterus is relaxed
4. May occur spontaneously

Clinical Manifestations

1. Shock with faintness, severe uterine pain and hemorrhage
2. Mild symptoms observed with incomplete version in the later postpartum period

Treatment and Nursing Management

1. Uterus is manually replaced while the patient is under anesthesia.
2. Treatment for shock.
3. Uterus may need to be replaced surgically.

Postpartum Hemorrhage

Postpartum hemorrhage involves a loss of 500 ml. or more of blood which occurs most frequently in the first hour following delivery.

Causes (in order of frequency)

1. Uterine atony—relaxation of the uterus secondary to:
   a. Multiple pregnancy—causes overdistention of uterus and a larger placental site
   b. Polyhydramnios
   c. High parity
   d. Prolonged labor with maternal exhaustion
   e. Deep anesthesia
   f. Fibromyomata—prevents uterus from contracting
2. Laceration of the vagina, cervix or perineum secondary to:
   a. Forceps delivery, especially rotation forceps
   b. Large infant
   c. Multiple pregnancy
   d. Unsutured vessel in the episiotomy site
3. Retained placental fragments secondary to:
   a. Manual removal of the placenta
   b. Abruptio placenta
   c. Placenta previa

Clinical Manifestations

1. Effects of hemorrhage depend on maternal blood volume and degree of anemia previous to delivery.
2. Bleeding from lacerations is bright red and usually occurs with a firm fundus.
3. Moderate blood loss often not reflected by depression of blood pressure or pulse.
4. Blood loss usually occurs by constant seepage rather than in a sudden massive hemorrhage episode.
5. Excessive blood loss indicated by pallor, restlessness, dyspnea, thready pulse, lowered blood pressure, chills and air hunger.
6. Soft uterus that is difficult to palpate indicates uterine atony.

Treatment and Nursing Management

A. *For Uterine Atony*
   1. Massage the uterus firmly.

NURSING ALERT: Overmassage of the uterus will contribute to muscle fatigue and cause further relaxation and increased bleeding.

---

2. Administer oxytocins as prescribed.
3. Start I.V. fluids to increase blood volume.
4. Replace blood loss by transfusion.
5. Examine uterine cavity for blood clots or placental fragments which would keep the uterus from contracting.

B. *For Lacerations*
1. Return patient to delivery room for inspection and repair.
2. Administer I.V. fluids and blood transfusion if necessary.

C. *For Retained Placental Fragments*
1. Symptoms usually occur late after the patient has been discharged from the hospital.
2. Patient is returned to the hospital for dilatation of the cervix and curettage of the uterus.

Fetal Distress

Fetal distress is fetal compromise leading to a stressful, harmful and potentially lethal fetal environment, requiring relief or rescue of the fetus.

Causes

1. Maternal complications
   a. Diabetes mellitus
   b. Heart disease
   c. Toxemias of pregnancy
   d. Hemorrhagic conditions
   e. Infection, hypotension
   f. Prolonged or abnormal labor
2. Uteroplacental circulatory insufficiency
   a. Cord compression
   b. Prolapse of cord
   c. Fetal hypoxia
3. Rh or ABO incompatibility
4. Prematurity
5. Congenital malformations

Manifestations

(in order of clinical significance)
1. Fetal heart rate (FHR) changes:
   a. Type II fetal bradycardia (late deceleration) begins at or after the peak of the contraction and continues 20–30 seconds or more after the cessation of the contraction.

      NOTE: Type I fetal bradycardia, probably due to vagal nerve stimulation by head compression, occurs simultaneously with the force of the contraction. This is much less ominous.

   b. Persistent fetal tachycardia (160 beats/minute)
   c. Persistent fetal bradycardia (120 beats/minute)
   d. Persistent irregularity
2. Passage of meconium into the amniotic fluid from the fetal gastrointestinal tract in late pregnancy as a response to stress.
3. Fetal hyperactivity—hyperreflexia caused by carbon dioxide retention with stimulation of the respiratory center.

Diagnostic Evaluation

A. *FHR monitoring*

Methods	Uses
1. Auscultation (stethoscope monitoring)	Most useful when FHR is counted throughout and just after a contraction
2. Phonocardiography (Microphone amplification of FH sounds)	Requires accurate placement of microphone Also amplifies maternal sounds
3. Doppler probe (Ultrasound flow probe)	Requires frequent repositioning Detects difficult-to-hear FH tones Useful in localizing the placenta Detects maternal pulse as well
4. Direct FHR monitor (corometric fetal monitor) (direct application of electrode to fetus)	Cervix must be dilated and membranes ruptured Often combined with intrauterine pressure recording Useful in determining accurate FHR and patterns of change Unaffected by maternal or fetal changes of position
5. Indirect monitor (cardiotocograph) (FHR and contractions obtained from transducers placed on patient's abdomen)	Easily connected by nurse Requires no internal examination or manipulation No rupture of membranes or cervical dilation is necessary Major disadvantage—necessity of frequent repositioning of the sensor since changes in both maternal and fetal positions cause discontinuity in the recordings

B. *Amniotic Fluid Studies*

To test for:

    a. Meconium (in fetal distress)
    b. Desquamated fetal skin cells and creatinine (as indices of fetal maturity)
    c. Bilirubin (if hemolytic disease is suspected)

	Clinical Considerations
1. Amniocentesis (transabdominal aspiration of amniotic fluid)	Color of fluid is evaluated Risk of inadvertent rupture of membranes Requires aseptic technique Accurate fetal position and placental location must be determined
2. Amnioscopy (visualization of the membranes with an endoscope without rupturing the membranes)	Color of fluid is evaluated Cervix must be dilated Risk of inadvertent rupture of membranes Occasionally no fluid is visualized

C. *Maternal Estriol Studies*

Index to placental and fetal well-being (precursor of estriol formed in fetal adrenals, metabolized by the placenta and excreted by the maternal kidneys; value for 24 hours excretion increases with the progression of pregnancy)

1. Urinary estriol
   (24-hr. urine collection)　　　Maternal kidney function must be normal
2. Blood estriol
   (blood samples taken
   same time each day)　　　Not dependent on maternal kidney function

D. *Fetal Blood Sampling*

Membranes must have ruptured and vertex must be in the pelvis (Fig. 20-10). Fetal compromise causes the following changes:

1. pH—decreased (normal 7.30–7.40)
   　　　(below 7.20, fetus may be suffering
   　　　from severe asphyxia)
2. pCO_2—increased
3. pO_2—decreased

E. *Estimation of Fetal Maturity*

1. Ultrasonography
2. X-ray for evaluation of fetal bone formation. (At 35–36 weeks gestation the distal femoral epiphyses are formed in most infants.)
3. Estriol, pregnanediol and human placental lactogen (HPL) all rise during pregnancy
4. Amniotic fluid analysis
   a. Creatinine rises with fetal maturity (must compare to maternal value)
   b. Fetal cells—percentage increases with maturity
   c. Lecithin—sphingomyeline ratio increases with maturity

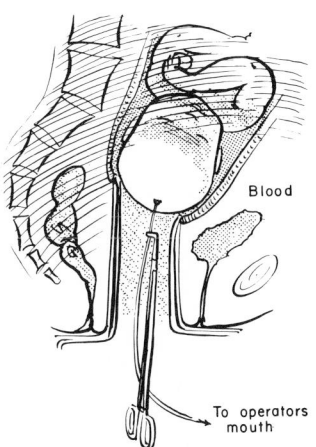

Figure 20-10. Technique of obtaining blood samples from the fetal scalp during labor.

Treatment and Nursing Management

1. Change maternal position from supine to left lateral to relieve pressure on cord and maternal hypotension. If improvement in heart tones does not immediately occur, further measures are necessary.
2. Administer oxygen (6–7 liters/minute) by mask as an aid to fetal hypoxia.
3. Start I.V. fluids if maternal hypotension is severe.
4. Prepare for immediate delivery by cesarean section if vaginal delivery is not imminent and fetal distress is persistent in spite of above measures.

BIBLIOGRAPHY

Books

Benson, R. C.: Handbook of Obstetrics and Gynecology. Los Altos, Lange Medical Publications, 1971.

Bonica, J. L.: Principles and Practice of Obstetric Analgesia and Anesthesia. Philadelphia, F. A. Davis, 1969.

Danforth, D. N.: Textbook of Obstetrics and Gynecology. New York, Harper and Row, 1971.

Fitzpatrick, E., et al.: Maternity Nursing. Philadelphia, J. B. Lippincott, 1971.

Greenhill, J. P.: Obstetrics. Philadelphia, W. B. Saunders, 1965.

Hellman, L. M., and Pritchard, J. A.: William's Obstetrics. New York, Appleton-Century-Crofts, 1971.

Hungerford, M. J.: Childbirth Education. Springfield, Charles C Thomas, 1972.

Oxhorn, H., and Foote, W. R.: Human Labor and Birth. New York, Appleton-Century-Crofts, 1968.

Page, E. W., et al.: Human Reproduction. Philadelphia, W. B. Saunders, 1972.

Reid, D. E., et al.: Principles and Management of Human Reproduction. Philadelphia, W. B. Saunders, 1972.

Shnider, S. M.: Obstetrical Anesthesia. Baltimore, Williams and Wilkins, 1970.

Taylor, E. S.: Beck's Obstetrical Practice. Baltimore, Williams and Wilkins, 1971.

Articles

Barber, H. R. K., et al.: Augmented labor. Obstet. Gynecol., 39:933–941, June 1972.

Case, L.: Ultrasound monitoring of mother and fetus. Amer. J. Nurs., 72:725–727, April 1972.

Chan, W. H., et al.: Intrapartum fetal monitoring. Obstet. Gynecol., 41:7–13, Jan. 1973.

Estey, G.: Natural childbirth: word from a mother. Amer. J. Nurs., 69:1451–1454, July 1969.

Greiss, F. C., and Pritchard, J. A.: Obstetrical anesthesia. Amer. J. Nurs., 71:67–69, Jan. 1971.

Hoff, F.: Natural childbirth: how any nurse can help. Amer, J. Nurs., 69:1451–1454, July 1969.

Hutchinson, S.: Anxiety, ecstasy, and the nurse's role. RN, 34:35–39, Nov. 1971.

Lasater, C.: Electronic monitoring of mother and fetus. Amer. J. Nurs., 72:728–730, April 1972.

Laros, R. K., et al.: Amniotomy during the active phase of labor. Obstet. Gynecol., 39:702-704, May 1972.

Paul, R. H., and Hon, E. H.: Clinical fetal monitoring. Obstet. Gynecol., 37:779–784, May 1971.

Reed, B., et al.: Management of the infant during labor, delivery and in the immediate neo-natal period. Nurs. Clin. N. Amer., 6:3–14, March 1971.

Rice, G. T.: Recognition and treatment of intrapartal fetal distress. J. Obstet., Gynecol., Neonatal Nurs., 2:15, Aug. 1972.

Roberts, J.: Suctioning the newborn. Amer. J. Nurs., 73:63–65, Jan. 1973.

Sasmor, J. L., et al.: The childbirth team during labor. Amer. J. Nurs., 73:444–447, March 1973.

Smith, B. A., et al.: The transition phase of labor. Amer. J. Nurs., 73:448–450, March 1973.

Williams, B. L., and Richards S. F.: Fetal monitoring during labor. Amer. J. Nurs., 70:2384–2388, Nov. 1970.

Obstetrical and Nursing Support of the Mother and Newborn During the Postpartal Period

POSTPARTUM CARE

Immediate Postpartum Care

The first hour after delivery of placenta ("fourth stage of labor") is a critical period during which postpartum hemorrhage is most likely to occur.
1. Check fundus frequently and massage gently if not firm.
2. Inspect perineum frequently for visible signs of bleeding.
3. Evaluate vital signs at frequent intervals as determined by mother's condition.
4. Avoid leaving mother alone at this time since changes in condition can occur precipitously.

Subsequent Postpartum Care

A. *For Postpartum Bleeding.*
1. Check firmness of the fundus at regular intervals.
2. Inspect the perineum regularly for frank bleeding.
    a. Note color, amount and odor of the lochia (perineal discharge).
    b. Count the number of perineal pads that are saturated in each 8-hour period.
3. Assess vital signs at least once daily and more frequently if indicated.

B. *For Comfort and Healing*
1. Provide perineal care.
    a. Pour warm water gently over the perineum while cleansing the labia, always from front to back.
    b. It is not necessary to separate the labia for this procedure as this may introduce infection.
    c. Wash the anal region separately.

2. Sitz baths are frequently used to promote perineal hygiene.
3. Teach the mother to handle the perineal pad from the outside so the fingers do not come in contact with the side that will touch the perineum.
4. Give perineal heat lamp, 20 minutes, 2-3 times a day to promote healing.
5. Use anesthetic sprays or ointment to alleviate perineal discomfort.
6. Some patients feel that foam rubber rings offer some relief.

C. *Ambulation*
   1. Normally patients are out of bed within the first 24 hours after childbirth.
   2. The mother should be assisted in her first effort out of bed to prevent accidents caused by weakness.

D. *Diet*
   1. After the first postpartum hour, the mother may eat or drink as desired providing she is not nauseated.
   2. The diet of a lactating mother should be increased somewhat in protein and calories.

E. *Voiding*
   1. The patient should be encouraged to void within 8 hours after delivery.
   2. Catheterize the patient if she is unable to void and the bladder is distended.
   3. Evaluate urinary output.

F. *Breast Care*
   1. Observe nipples for fissures daily.
   2. Wash nipples at least once a day to remove dried and seeping colostrum.
   3. Give the following care to nursing mothers.
      a. Cleanse nipples with warm water before each feeding; soap may be drying to the nipples.
      b. Lotion or ointment may help to prevent cracks or drying and may be applied after the baby's feedings.
   4. Treat breast engorgement as follows:
      a. A well-fitting supportive brassiere or breast binder should be worn night and day.
      b. Hot packs 15–20 minutes before nursing may be helpful
      c. For removal of milk
         (1) Oxytocin encourages the "let down" reflex.
         (2) Express milk manually or with breast pump.

G. *Suppression of Lactation*
   1. Administer hormones as prescribed; estrogen, progesterone or testosterone may be administered alone or in combination. (A single I.M. injection may be given or oral hormones prescribed.)
   2. Apply ice bags to breasts.
   3. Offer mild analgesic agent as needed.
   4. Advise the patient to wear a supporting brassiere.
   5. Avoid pumping the breasts.

H. *Menstruation*
   1. For non-nursing mothers, menstrual flow usually returns within 6–8 weeks.
   2. For nursing mothers, menstruation does not usually recur until after the child is weaned from the breast.

I. *Follow-up Examination*
   A routine examination is usual within 3–6 weeks postpartum.
   1. General physical condition is evaluated.

2. Vital signs are checked.
3. Urine is examined for sugar and protein.
4. Muscle tone is checked, particularly that of the abdominal wall.
5. Pelvic examination conducted.
6. Counselling and information regarding birth control methods are provided as indicated or requested.

GUIDELINES: *Teaching the Mother Breast Feeding Procedure*

Procedure

Teaching Points	*Rationale/Amplification*
1. Wash hands before breast feeding.	1. Protects infant and breast from infection.
2. Prepare to nurse shortly after birth and at least every 4 hours.	2. Prevents engorgement and helps bring in milk supply quickly.
3. Nurse infant at night feeding.	3. Regular feeding (every 4 hours) establishes nursing pattern.

Position of Mother

1. Lie on left side with pillow under head. Position left arm above head—or	1. The mother should be relaxed and comfortable.
2. Use a chair with a back support. Place pillow on lap to hold infant.	2. The infant's head should be higher than his abdomen to prevent regurgitation.

Nursing Technique

1. With the right hand, press darkened area around nipple into infant's mouth.	1. This maneuver is necessary for adequate suction.
2. If breast is full and firm, use 1 finger to press breast away from infant's nose.	2. Prevents obstruction of airway; infant breathes mainly through his nose.
3. Use both breasts at each feeding; 5 minutes on each breast, then increase nursing time to 10 minutes.	
4. At each feeding alternate the breast that is used first. Pin a safety pin to the bra as a reminder of which breast to start with at the next feeding.	4. The infant will empty the first breast; nursing at the second breast will increase milk production.
5. Break the suction by putting a finger into the corner of infant's mouth.	5. Pulling the nipple abruptly away from the infant will result in sore nipples.
6. "Burp" infant midway through the feeding. Pat gently on the back or hold in upright position.	6. Helps infant to release air bubbles in stomach.
7. Uterine cramps may occur.	7. Nursing stimulates release of oxytocin hormone, causing uterine contractions.

Other Considerations for Mother

1. Drink water for two. Continue eating a balanced nutritional diet. (May require 1000 more calories and an additional 8–10 gm. of protein daily.)	1. Necessary for adequate milk production.
2. Get adequate rest.	
3. Avoid emotional stress and do not become discouraged.	3. It takes time to establish a good nursing routine.
4. Avoid taking medications and drugs unless approved by the physician.	4. Cold or allergy medication will limit fluid output. Birth control medication may suppress milk production.

POSTPARTUM COMPLICATIONS
Puerperal Infection

Puerperal infection is a postpartum infection of the genital tract, usually of the endometrium, that may remain localized or may extend to various parts of the body.

Causes

Bacterial organisms either introduced from external sources or normally present in the generative tract.

Predisposing Factors

1. Prolonged labor
2. Postpartum hemorrhage
3. Premature rupture of membranes
4. Urinary tract infections
5. Intrauterine manipulation
6. Anemia
7. Retention of placental fragments

Clinical Manifestations

Symptoms depend on site and degree of extension.
1. Sustained fever of 38°C. (100.4 F.) or higher
2. Pain
3. Profuse foul-smelling vaginal discharge, sometimes frothy
4. Burning on urination
5. Secondary abscesses elsewhere in the body
6. Thrombophlebitis, caused by extension of infection along veins
7. Pyemia

Complications

1. Pulmonary embolism
2. Peritonitis
3. Pelvic cellulitis

Preventive Measures

1. Prompt treatment of anemia
2. Well-balanced diet
3. Avoidance of coitus in late pregnancy
4. Strict asepsis during labor and delivery
5. Sterile perineal pads changed every 4 hours
6. Separation of infected from noninfected patients

Treatment and Nursing Management

1. Antibiotic therapy
2. Warm sitz baths, warm compresses or heat lamp
3. Drainage—established when possible (Fowler's position is helpful.)
4. Maintenance of fluid and electrolyte balances

Mastitis

Mastitis is inflammation of the breasts.

Etiology

Usually due to *Staphylococcus aureus* derived from the nursing infant's nose and throat.

Clinical Manifestations

Usually appear in 3rd or 4th week of puerperium.

1. Marked breast engorgement
2. Chills
3. Elevated temperature
4. Increased pulse rate
5. Hardness and reddening of breasts
6. Pain in breasts

Preventive Measures

1. Nursery routine
   a. Careful handscrubbing between handling of infants
   b. Prompt isolation of any infant who appears to be developing an infection
   c. Exclusion from the nursery of all personnel with infections
2. Proper care of maternal breasts
   a. Washing nipples before and after nursing
   b. Prompt attention to fissures and cracks in nipples

Treatment

Antibiotic therapy

NURSING CARE OF THE NEWBORN INFANT

Objective

To support the infant in adjusting to extrauterine life.

Physical Care

1. Maintain patent airway.
   a. Place in modified Trendelenburg position to drain mucus while suctioning.
   b. Aspirate mucus from mouth and pharynx with suction catheter.
   c. Turn to side Trendelenburg position to promote drainage from mouth and to prevent aspiration.

> NURSING ALERT: Gentle manipulation and careful suctioning are required or stimuli may produce laryngeal spasm or cause pharyngeal edema.

2. Maintain or improve body temperature.
   a. Remove excess vernix, mucus and fluid and dry the infant.
   b. Wrap infant in heated blankets and expose only to obtain birth weight.
   c. Keep infant in heated resuscitator until transferred to heated crib in nursery.
3. Provide proper cord care.
   a. Asepsis is used to prevent cord infection—sterile clamp and scissors used.
   b. Cord is clamped 2.5 cm. (1 inch) from skin. The cord clamp is left on longer in babies of Rh negative mothers for possible transfusion purposes.
   c. Check cord for presence of 3 vessels—abnormal vessels indicate possibility of other birth defects.

Observations

1. Evaluate infant's condition by Apgar scoring system taken at 1 and 5 minutes after birth. The infant is evaluated in 5 different areas listed in rank of importance.
2. Interpretation
   a. Apgar score of 7–10 indicates the infant's condition is good. No special procedures are necessary.

b. Score of 4–6 means the infant is in fair condition, may have moderate central nervous system depression, some muscle flaccidity, cyanosis and poor respiratory effort. Air passage must be cleaned and oxygen given.

c. Score of 0–3 indicates extremely poor condition. Resuscitation required immediately.

APGAR SCORING CHART

Sign	0	1	2
Heart rate	absent	slow (less than 100)	over 100
Respiratory effort	absent	slow, irregular	good, crying
Muscle tone	flaccid	some flexion of extremities	active motion
Reflex irritability	no response	cry	vigorous cry
Color	blue, pale	body pink, extremities blue	completely pink

Care of the Eyes

Instill prophylactic agent as protection against ophthalmia neonatorum (gonorrheal conjunctivitis). Is mandatory in all states.

a. Silver nitrate 1%, 1–2 drops in the conjunctival sac. After diffusion, flush gently with sterile distilled water.

b. Penicillin ophthalmic ointment or drops instilled in conjuctival sac.

Identification

1. Before taking infant to nursery apply bracelet or anklet with mother's name, hospital number, infant's sex and time and date of birth.
2. Apply bracelet with same information to mother's wrist.
3. Infant and mother wear identification bands during the hospital stay and should be discharged with the identification bands still in place (not to be removed).

BIBLIOGRAPHY

Books

Benson, R. C.: Handbook of Obstetrics and Gynecology. Los Altos, Lange Medical Publications, 1971.

Danforth, D. N.: Textbook of Obstetrics and Gynecology. New York, Harper and Row, 1971.

Fitzpatrick, E., et al.: Maternity Nursing. Philadelphia, J. B. Lippincott, 1971.

Greenhill, J. P.: Obstetrics. Philadelphia, W. B. Saunders, 1965.

Hellman, L. M., and Pritchard, J. A.: William's Obstetrics. New York, Appleton-Century-Crofts, 1971.

Page, E. W., et al.: Human Reproduction. Philadelphia, W. B. Saunders, 1972.

Reid, D. E., et al.: Principles and Management of Human Reproduction. Philadelphia, W. B. Saunders, 1972.

Taylor, E. S.: Beck's Obstetrical Practice. Baltimore, Williams and Wilkins, 1971.

Articles

Beck, W. W.: Prevention of the postpartum spinal headache. Amer. J. Obstet. Gynecol., *115*:345–356, Feb. 1973.

Strachan, M.: International cooperation in family planning. Nurs. Outlook, *19*:103, Feb. 1971.

Yunek, M. J.: Postpartum care is more than a routine. Nurs. Outlook, *17*:50–52, Jan. 1969.

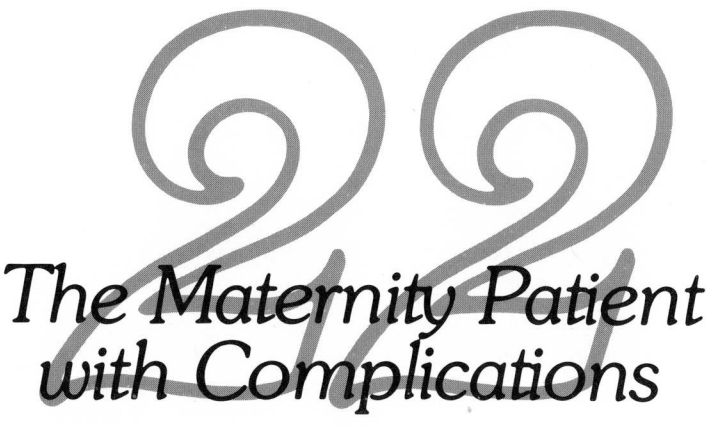

The Maternity Patient with Complications

TOXEMIAS OF PREGNANCY

Toxemias of pregnancy are disorders specific to pregnancy, encountered during the last trimester or early puerperium and characterized by generalized vasospasm, excessive retention of sodium and water and renal lesions.

Types of Toxemia

A. *Mild preeclampsia*—hypertension, proteinuria or edema appearing after the 24th week of gestation.

1. Systolic blood pressure of 140 mm. Hg or a rise of 30 mm. Hg or more above usual level

2. Diastolic pressure of 90 mm. Hg or more or a rise of 20 mm. Hg above the usual level

3. Proteinuria—observed in 2 or more successive days

4. Persistent edema

B. *Severe preeclampsia*—increased clinical signs and symptoms.
   1. Systolic blood pressure of 160 mm. Hg or more
   2. Diastolic pressure of 110 mm. Hg or more on 2 separate occasions with the patient at rest
   3. Proteinuria of 5 gm. or more in 24 hours
   4. Oliguria of 400 ml. or less per 24 hours
   5. Cerebral or visual disturbances

C. *Eclampsia*—convulsions or coma (usually both) associated with hypertension, proteinuria or edema.

D. *Chronic hypertensive vascular disease*
   1. Process not peculiar to pregnancy.
      Manifestations may exist before 24th week of pregnancy and persist indefinitely after delivery.
   3. Blood pressure usually exceeds 140/90.
   4. Usually develops into superimposed preeclampsia.

Incidence
   1. Hypertension in pregnancy occurs in 5% of all pregnancies in the U.S.
   2. Is currently the second leading cause of maternal mortality in U.S.

Predisposing Factors
   1. Age and gravida—predilection for the younger primigravida and for those with multiple gestation.
   2. Diet—high carbohydrate, high salt, and low protein—influenced by socioeconomic status, race and cultural patterns, geographic location and psychologic state of patient.

Etiology
   1. Unknown.
   2. Current research suggests:
      a. Decreased uterine and placental blood flow—result of vascular spasm caused by hormonal influence.
      b. Overstimulated adrenal cortex due to hypertrophic anterior pituitary and placental function. This activity decreases with reduction of oxygen tension caused by the uterine ischemia observed with overdistention of the uterus (twins, hydramnios), increased tension on abdominal walls (primigravida) or constricted blood vessels (pre-existing hypertension).

Clinical Manifestations
   1. Weight gain—first indication, over 0.45 kg. (1 lb.) per week as early as the 20th week.
   2. Ankle edema, digital swelling, periorbital edema, then pretibial fluid collection.
   3. Optic fundi—reveal segmental or generalized arteriolar spasms.
   4. Hypertension—140/90 or increase of 30 mm. systolic or 15 mm. diastolic.
   5. Proteinuria—may develop into oliguria.
   6. Cerebral and neurological involvement—frontal headache, vertigo, tinnitus, visual disturbance, drowsiness, hyperreflexia, apprehension, excitability, nausea and vomiting.

NURSING ALERT: Feelings of thoracic pressure or epigastric pain due to liver pathology may herald onset of convulsions or coma.

7. Poor prognostic signs
   a. Increasing number of convulsions
   b. Prolonged time between first convulsion and delivery
   c. Persistence of coma, high fever, pulse rate 120 or over, cyanosis and hemoglobinuria
8. Fatal outcome due to:
   a. Pulmonary edema
   b. Cardiac failure
   c. Massive cerebral hemorrhage
   d. Pneumonitis
   e. Renal failure

Objectives of Treatment

A. *To provide for frequent periods of observation and assessment during the antepartal period and attempt to prevent the development of severe preeclampsia or eclampsia.*
   1. Create an awareness of the importance of limited caloric and salt intake. (Any tendency toward hypertensive disease is enhanced by unlimited food intake.)
   2. Institute salt-poor diet upon first indication of eclampsia or hypertensive disease—less than 3 gm. per day is recommended but is difficult to achieve on an out-patient basis.
   3. Encourage bedrest—provides decrease in blood pressure and increase in filtration rate and decrease in proteinuria.
   4. Evaluate blood pressure readings and report any sudden or persistent elevations.
   5. Test urine weekly—examine for proteinuria.

B. *To provide medical management for further control of signs and symptoms.*
   1. Diuretics—limited effect of dietary regimen in achieving sodium reduction.
      a. Meralluride, acetazolamide and chlorothiazide are safe and efficient if used intermittently (see p. 278).
      b. Potassium supplements are usually given.

NURSING ALERT: Occasionally a "low sodium" syndrome may result from the combination of strict low sodium diet and effective diuretic therapy, indicated by nitrogen retention, oliguria and vascular collapse.

   2. Barbiturates and analgesics—provide sedation by depressing central nervous system.
   3. Antihypertensive agents:
      a. Hydralazine (Apresoline)—provides both adrenalytic and sympatholytic action, increasing blood flow through kidneys.
      b. Rauwolfia derivatives (central nervous system depressant and tranquilizer)—suppresses sympathetic branch of the autonomic nervous system.
   4. Assist the patient to accept the therapeutic plan. Provide understanding support and encourage the patient to verbalize concerns.

C. *To provide care and therapy for the patient with severe preeclampsia or eclampsia so as to prevent maternal and fetal pathology.*
   Provide hospitalization and therapy to treat severe hypertension, marked edema and advanced proteinuria.

1. Heavy sedation—depresses central nervous system to reduce irritability.
2. Morphine sulphate 15 mg. I.M. every 4–6 hours. Magnesium sulphate I.V., 10 gm. initially then 5 gm. every 6 hours. (Also increases cerebral blood flow and provides antihypertensive action.)

NURSING ALERT: Repeat doses of magnesium sulphate only if (1) deep tendon reflexes are present, (2) respirations are above 12 per minute and (3) urine output is at least 100 ml. per 6 hours. Calcium Gluconate 10% I.V. must be available to counteract magnesium toxicity.

---

3. Anticonvulsants—diphenylhydantoin (Dilantin) 100 mg. I.M. every 4–6 hours.
   a. Requires several days to become effective but has little sedation effect on fetus.
   b. Used after sedation is achieved.
4. Diuretics –meralluride (Mercuhydrin) 2 ml. I.M.
   a. Produces rapid diuresis.
   b. Use with caution—toxic reactions may occur.
5. Hypotensive drugs with more radical action:
   a. Protoveratrines (Veralba) 2 mg. in 200 ml. of 5% dextrose solution I.V.
      (1) Controls hypertensive crisis.
      (2) Used with caution—produces bradycardia.
   b. Ephedrine 25 mg. or atropine 0.4 mg. on hand for I.V. administration to counteract severe hypotension or bradycardia.
   c. Hydralazine (Apresoline) 20 mg. and Cryptenamine Tannates (Unitensen) 5 mg. in 500 ml. of 5% dextrose solution I.V. drip—slower acting agent.
6. Digitalis—indicated by signs and symptoms of cardiac failure (see p. 275).
7. Broad spectrum antibiotics—prophylactic measure to prevent pneumonitis.
8. I.V. fluids—given slowly to provide adequate hydration.
9. Indwelling catheter—ascertain exact renal output for comparison with fluid intake.
10. Oxygen—(administered by nasal catheter or mask at 6 liters per minute)—increases oxygen supply to the fetus.
11. Nasopharyngeal suctioning—prevents aspiration.
12. Tracheostomy—may be necessary to facilitate respiration (extreme measure).

Nursing Management

1. Provide constant nursing surveillance.
2. Provide quiet, restful environment—prevent stimuli that could provoke convulsions.
3. Monitor patient's physical condition—observe vital signs and fetal heart tones.
4. Assess patient's response to medication.
5. Provide safety measures—be prepared for sudden convulsive episodes.
   a. Have side rails in place.
   b. Alert personnel to watch for signal light.
   c. Have rolled washcloth to place between teeth (used more realistically than padded tongue blade).
   d. I.V. sedation or inhalation anesthesia constitutes current management for convulsions. (See p. 731 for nursing management of patient with convulsions.)
6. Have emergency equipment and medications in the room ready for immediate use.

Treatment During Labor and Delivery

Management based on assessment of the disease and viability of the fetus.

1. If fetus is thought to be viable and if the disease is not controllable, induction or cesarean section is usually recommended.
2. Delays may result in fetal death.

HYPEREMESIS GRAVIDARUM

Hyperemesis gravidarum is exaggerated nausea and vomiting during pregnancy.

Incidence

Fewer than 1 in 300 pregnancies (becoming more rare due to lessened fear of pregnancy and early correction of ordinary nausea and vomiting).

Predisposing Factors

1. Hormonal changes of pregnancy—chorionic gonadotropin levels are high during the first trimester.
2. Emotional factors—uncontrollable vomiting more common in neurotic women.
3. Psychopathology—vomiting may symbolize subconscious rejection of the pregnancy.

Clinical Manifestations

1. Weight loss—due to anorexia.
2. Alkalosis—due to loss of hydrochloric acid.
3. Acidosis—from starvation.
4. Hypokalemia—due to electrolyte imbalance.
5. Increased pulse rate—due to anemia.
6. Increased blood concentration—due to dehydration.
7. Oliguria—due to dehydration.

Treatment and Nursing Management

A. *Initial Step*

Rule out other diseases—gastroenteritis, hepatitis, cholecystitis, peptic ulcer or brain tumor present similar signs and symptoms.

B. *Management of Mild Disease*

1. Provide understanding support; often the only therapy required is discussion of the patient's concerns.
2. Prevent morning nausea by instructing the patient to:
   a. Eat 2 or 3 crackers and remain in bed 15 minutes after awakening. (Dry carbohydrates have an effective antiemetic action.)
   b. One-half hour after rising eat a small dry breakfast.
3. Give prochlorperazine (Compazine) 10 mg. on awakening and 10 mg. every 6–8 hours (acts as an antiemetic).

C. *Management of Moderately Severe Disease*

(When nausea and vomiting extend throughout the 24 hours without remission, or if the patient has a weight loss of more than 4.5 kg. or 10 pounds.)

1. Restrict solid food and give orange or lemon juice over cracked ice—supplies fluid and vitamin C and is acceptable to the patient.
2. Provide for bedrest (at home if facilities are adequate or patient may need to be hospitalized).
3. Administer compazine suppositories—have antiemetic and sedative action.
4. Provide 6 small dry meals per day—give only if nausea and vomiting have subsided.
5. Provide fluids—offer hot fluids or very cold fluids.
6. Decrease sedation and allow patient activity.

D. *Management of Severe Disease*—vomiting very severe

1. Provide hospitalization in quiet private room and permit no visitors including husband—prevents stimuli.
2. Restrict the patient's activity by complete bedrest—conserves energy.
3. Repeat laboratory evaluation of patient's electrolyte and chemical balance. Tests of carbon dioxide, chlorides and total proteins, as well as diacetic acid and acetone in the urine, are done. (They aid in replacement therapy and indicate the patient's condition.)
4. Allow nothing by mouth for 24 hours—provide parenteral fluids 1500 ml. of 5% glucose followed by 1000 ml. of 5% glucose in saline.
5. Give B complex factor with vitamin C in I.V. fluids—prevents avitaminosis.
6. Give promazine hydrochloride (Sparine) in I.V. fluid, and Compazine 10 mg. I.M. t.i.d.—provides sedation and antiemetic action.

NURSING ALERT: Antiemetic and antihistaminic agents may have teratogenic effects during early pregnancy (proven with laboratory animals).

---

7. Allow oral feedings when patient no longer experiences nausea.
8. Arrange for psychiatric interview—indicated if patient does not improve with therapeutic regimen.
9. Consider therapeutic abortion—recommended if following conditions occur:
   a. Jaundice
   b. Delirium
   c. Rising pulse rate to 130
   d. Fever of 38.3°C. (101°F.) despite adequate hydration
   e. Retinal hemorrhage

HEMORRHAGIC DISORDERS
Ectopic Pregnancy

In an *ectopic pregnancy*, gestation is located outside the uterine cavity. Although the majority of ectopic pregnancies are tubal implantations, other types include cervical, abdominal or ovarian implantations.

Contributing Causes

1. Salpingitis
2. Pelvic inflammatory disease
3. Endometriosis
4. Infantile tubes or imperfect development
5. Spasm of the tubes with muscular insufficiency

RECOGNIZING AN ECTOPIC PREGNANCY

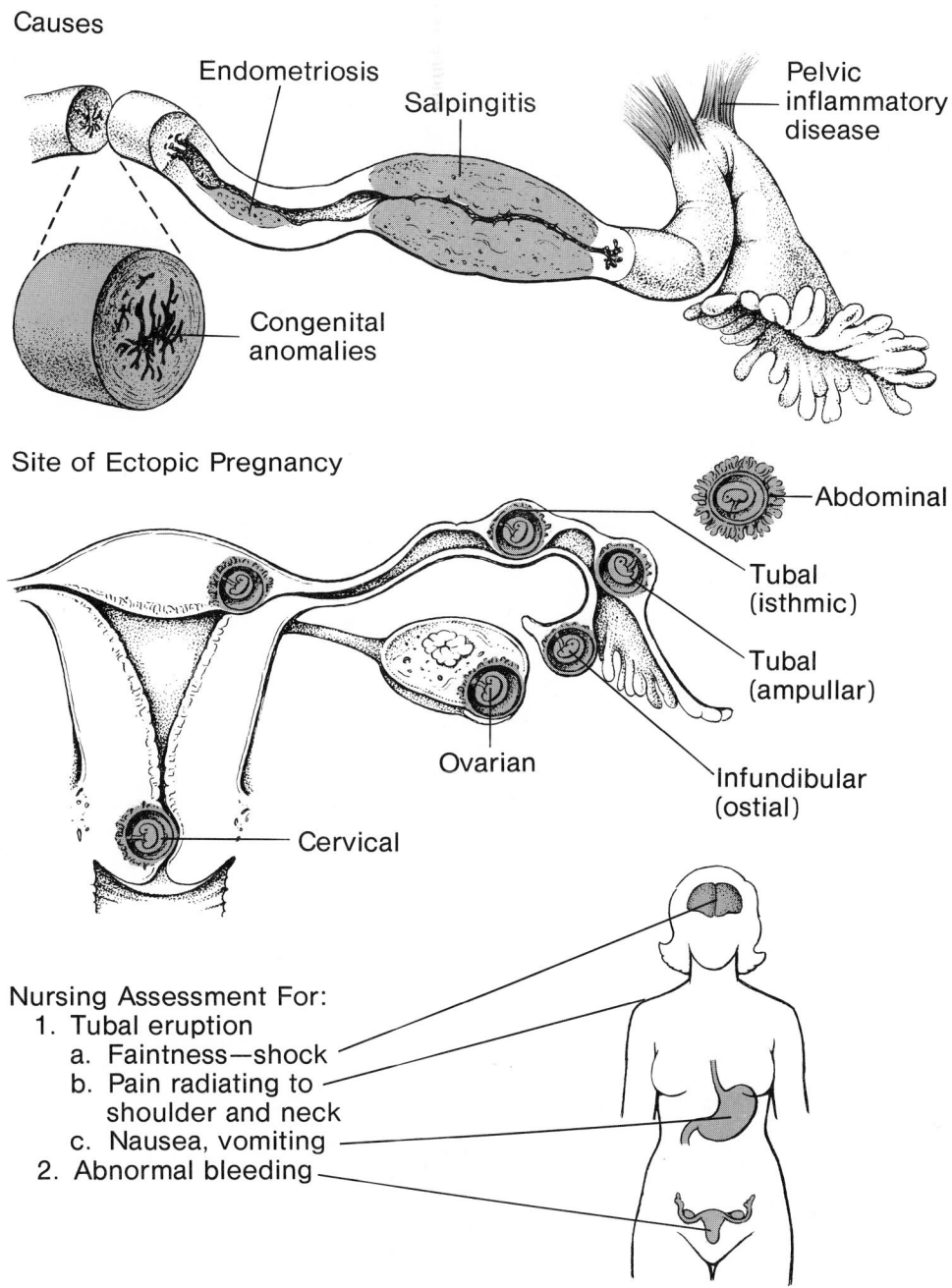

Causes

Endometriosis

Salpingitis

Pelvic inflammatory disease

Congenital anomalies

Site of Ectopic Pregnancy

Abdominal

Tubal (isthmic)

Tubal (ampullar)

Ovarian

Infundibular (ostial)

Cervical

Nursing Assessment For:
1. Tubal eruption
    a. Faintness—shock
    b. Pain radiating to shoulder and neck
    c. Nausea, vomiting
2. Abnormal bleeding

Figure 22-1. Ectopic pregnancy.

Clinical Manifestations

1. Vary with the site of implantation and usually occur after tubal rupture
2. Early signs and symptoms
   a. Abnormal menstrual period
   b. Symptoms of early pregnancy
   c. Dull pain on affected side
3. Signs and symptoms of tubal rupture
   a. Pain; sudden, severe and unilateral—later generalized and radiating to shoulder and neck due to diaphragmatic irritation
   b. Nausea, vomiting, faintness
   c. Shock manifested by pallor with slight cyanosis around the lips, yawning, rapid weak pulse
   d. Normal or low temperature—fever important in distinguishing ruptured tubal pregnancy from acute salpingitis
   e. Leukocyte count—normal if rupture is old or if only leakage is occurring, but after sudden hemorrhage usually exceeds 15,000
   f. Tenderness over abdomen upon palpation
   g. Pelvic mass—posterior or lateral to uterus
   h. Cervical pain during vaginal examination and motion of the cervix
   i. Distention of the posterior fornix with blood in the cul-de-sac

Treatment and Nursing Management

Objective: to establish the diagnosis without delay and to initiate immediate surgical intervention.

1. Provide constant nursing surveillance—note any changes in patient's condition.
2. Monitor vital signs—assess for indications of impending shock.
3. Start I.V. fluids with 19-gauge needle—in preparation for administration of blood.
4. Observe for vaginal bleeding—may indicate a uterine abortion rather than ectopic pregnancy.
5. Give narcotics or analgesic agents as prescribed—shock may be due to pain rather than blood loss.
6. Request hematology reports—CBC, type and cross-matching (blood replacement often necessary).
7. Offer intelligent support and provide explanation of nursing activities—reduces fear and anxiety.
8. Prepare patient for vaginal examination or surgery—to establish or confirm diagnosis and to institute surgical correction.
   a. Culdocentesis—aspiration of fluid from the cul-de-sac of Douglas. Presence of bloody fluid indicates intraperitoneal bleeding.
   b. Culdoscopy—visualization of the pelvic organs through the punctured posterior fornix.
   c. Colpotomy—incision through the posterior fornix to remove the tube. (If the tube is observed to be ruptured, the incision is closed and a laparotomy and salpingectomy are performed.)
9. Provide postoperative care—this is the same as for the patient having abdominal laparotomy.

Placenta Previa

Placenta previa is the development of the placenta in the lower uterine segment, partially or completely covering the internal cervical os.

Incidence

1. Common cause of bleeding during the last trimester.
2. Occurs once in every 200 deliveries.
3. 3 out of 4 women with placenta previa are multigravidas.

Contributing Causes

1. Largely unknown, although multiparity and advancing age favor occurrence.
2. Unfavorable decidua in upper uterine segment (fibroid tumors, old cesarean section scars).

Clinical Manifestations

Hemorrhage—first and most constant symptom
a. *Painless* causeless bleeding—not accompanied by uterine contraction.
b. Occurs most frequently in 8th month—dilation of the internal os causes tearing of placental attachments.

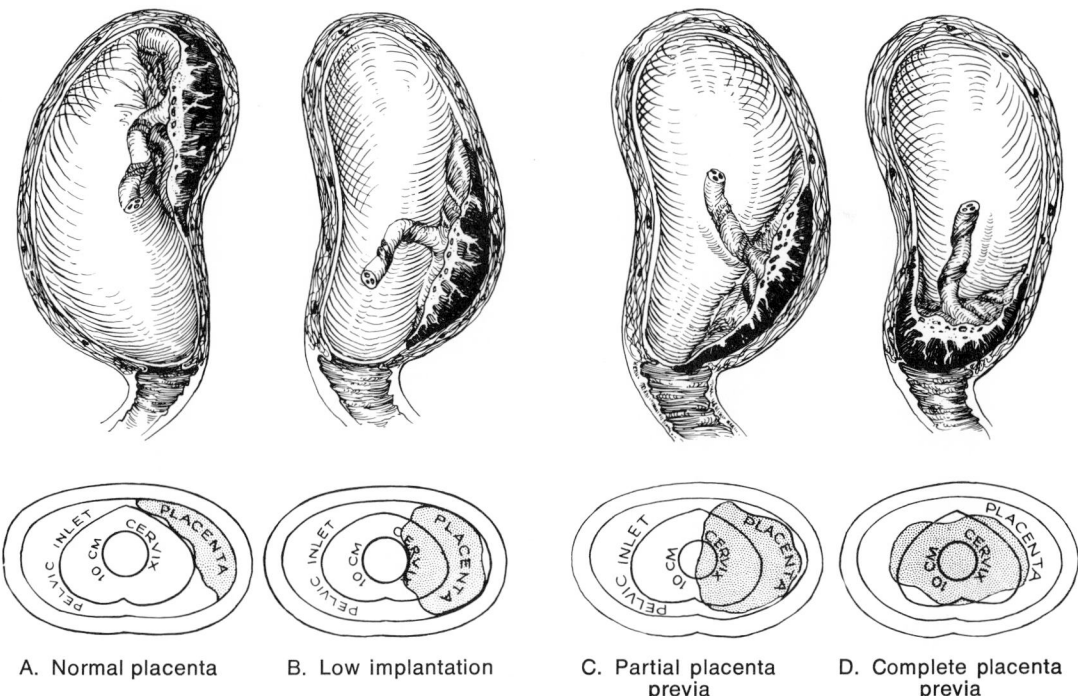

A. Normal placenta   B. Low implantation   C. Partial placenta previa   D. Complete placenta previa

Figure 22-2. Placenta previa. (From Benson, R. C.: Handbook of Obstetrics and Gynecology. Los Altos, California, Lange Medical Publications, 1971.)

    c. Each succeeding hemorrhage is greater—further dilation is taking place.

    d. Constant seepage of blood-stained serum—indicates a large clot is forming in lower uterine segment.

    e. Partial placenta previa may not cause bleeding until labor begins or until complete dilation has occurred.

    f. Bleeding occurs earlier and is more profuse with total placenta previa.

Treatment and Nursing Management

1. Provide constant nursing surveillance during critical phase.
   a. Provide hospitalization—delivery is recommended except when bleeding is slight and the fetus is not viable.
   b. Prepare for blood replacement—obtain hemoglobin and hematocrit, type and cross-matching of blood.
   c. Prepare patient for pelvic examination. (For 8th month pregnancy, examination must be done in operating room prepared for emergency cesarean section since this maneuver may induce profuse hemorrhage.)
   d. Differentiate between total and partial placenta previa if fetus is immature and delay in delivery is advisable.
      (1) Ultrasonography—simplest most precise and least hazardous procedure.
      (2) Radiology—soft tissue x-ray—least accurate.
      (3) Radioactive isotope scan—localization of placenta by noting area of maximal count.
      (4) Amniography—contrast material injected into amniotic sac.
      (5) Angiography—injection of contrast material into maternal femoral artery.
   e. Reduce patient fear and anxieties—explain nursing activities and x-ray procedure.
2. Provide for rest and diversional activities—if fetus is immature and hemorrhage moderate, the patient is managed with supportive therapy and bedrest.
3. Prepare patient for vaginal delivery—if pregnancy is near term, the cervix favorable and partial placenta identified, labor is induced by amniotomy.
4. Provide constant nursing surveillance during labor.
   a. Correct anemia—be prepared for further blood loss.
   b. Start I.V. fluids—avoid dehydration and hypoglycemia during labor.
   c. Assess vaginal bleeding—cesarean section may be indicated.
   d. Assess progress of labor—malposition of fetus and slow descent common with placenta previa.
   e. Monitor fetal heart tones—use of cardiotocograph monitor or corometric fetal monitor indicated for more accurate fetal assessment.
   f. Provide continuing observation during 3rd and 4th stages of labor and delivery—lower uterine segment may be atonic leaving open venous sinuses. Oxytocins given and uterine packing placed.
   g. Provide meticulous attention to antiseptic and aseptic precautions—hemorrhage predisposes to postpartal infection; placental site slower to heal than with normal implantation.

Abruptio Placenta

Abruptio placenta is premature separation of the placenta.

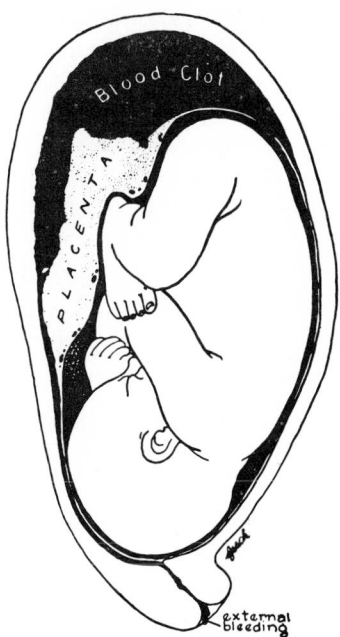

Predisposing Factors

1. Toxemias of pregnancy
2. Trauma (severe coughing, blow on abdomen, coitus)
3. Delivery of twins—placenta of 2nd fetus disturbed
4. Traction on placenta by a short cord during labor contractions
5. Sudden rupture of the membranes, especially with hydramnios
6. Injudicious use of Pitocin during labor with resulting hard and long contractions

Altered Physiology

Separation of the placenta is always accompanied by hemorrhage, either concealed or external.
  a. Concealed hemorrhage usually occurs during pregnancy—placental separation occurs centrally with large amount of blood stored under the placenta.
  b. External hemorrhage usually occurs during labor —blood flows outward from the edge of the placenta under the membranes through the cervix.

Figure 22-3. Abruptio placenta with large blood clot between placenta and uterine wall. (From Fitzpatrick, E., et al.: Maternity Nursing, 12th ed. Philadelphia, J. B. Lippincott, 1971.)

Clinical Manifestations

1. Hemorrhage, slight or profuse—blood escapes under the decidua basalis.
2. Shock—often out of proportion with blood loss manifested by hypotension, rapid pulse, dyspnea, pallor, syncope.
3. Pain, usually sudden and severe—produced by accumulation of blood behind the placenta and infiltration into the myometrium.
4. Rigidity and tenderness of uterus—myometrium becomes board-like (Couvelaire uterus).
5. Uterine contractions—begin spontaneously due to uterine irritability.
6. Excessive fetal movement with onset of severe pain—indicates fetal distress from anoxia.
7. Loss of fetal heart tone—indicating fetal death.

Objectives of Treatment and Nursing Management

A. *To control hemorrhage and overcome shock.*
  1. Monitor blood pressure, pulse, respiration and fetal heart tones—indicates impending shock and assesses fetal condition.
  2. Assess external blood loss and compare with vital signs—indications of internal hemorrhage.

3. Administer I.V. fluids or whole blood—replacement therapy imperative to prevent irreversible shock.
4. Determine plasma fibrinogen levels frequently—entry of thromboplastin into the circulation from the uterus and placenta causes small fibrin clots in the capillaries and consumes fibrinogen, leaving the patient with nonclotting blood.

> NURSING ALERT: Human fibrinogen (Cohn Fraction I) has been responsible for transmitting hepatitis more frequently than other blood components.

B. *To relieve the patient's pain and anxiety.*
   1. Give analgesic medications with caution—central nervous system depressant may intensify shock symptoms.
   2. Provide intelligent explanation of activities.

C. *To accomplish delivery of infant as promptly as possible.*
   1. Prepare patient for amniotomy and vaginal delivery (treatment of choice)—cervix is dilated, bleeding moderate and shock minimal.
   2. Prepare patient for cesarean section—immediate delivery desirable for best chance of fetal survival and for control of hemorrhage.

D. *To prevent postpartal complications.*
   1. Provide nursing surveillance during the puerperium—early detection of complications.
   2. Monitor vital signs and uterine muscle tone—traumatized myometrium may cause uterine atony necessitating hysterectomy.
   3. Be alert for indications of postpartum infections—blood loss and shock greatly reduce resistance to infections.
   4. Observe urinary output for oliguria or hematuria—renal failure may result from acute tubular necrosis or bilateral cortical necrosis.

HYDATIDIFORM MOLE

Hydatidiform mole is a developmental anomaly of the placenta resulting in the conversion of the chorionic villi into a mass of clear vesicles. It is the most common lesion anteceding choriocarcinoma, a malignant tumor of the trophoblast with a tendency to rapid and widespread metastasis.

Incidence
1. Occurs in 1 of every 2000 pregnancies.
2. Relatively high frequency in women over 45.

Clinical Manifestations
1. Enlargement of the uterus out of proportion to the duration of pregnancy.
2. Continuous or intermittent brownish bloody discharge about the 12th week of pregnancy.
3. Signs and symptoms of preeclampsia, proteinuria, hypertension or edema earlier in pregnancy than usual.

Diagnostic Evaluation

1. Absence of fetal parts on palpation or by x-ray.
2. High chorionic gonadotropin level in serum 100 days or more after last menstrual period.
3. Care must be taken in differential diagnosis to rule out multiple pregnancy.

Objectives of Treatment and Nursing Management

A. *To prepare patient for immediate abortion or evacuation of the mole.*
   1. Administer oxytocic agents—stimulates uterine contractions.
   2. Evaluate blood loss—have ample blood for transfusion; hemorrhage may be severe.
   3. Prepare patient for surgery—abortion of mole is either completed or followed by D & C or suction curettage (deferred for several days until uterus is firmer to prevent perforation).
   4. Prepare patient for hysterotomy or hysterectomy—if the mole is not passed spontaneously, surgical intervention is indicated.
   5. Request microscopic examination of curetted tissue—identification of residual or proliferative trophoblastic tissue.

B. *To provide follow-up for detection of malignant change.*
   1. Measure chorionic gonadotropin levels—levels become negative within a week after normal pregnancy; extend to 50–60 days following a hydatidiform mole.
   2. Assess chorionic gonadotropin titer—if titer is rising, D & C is performed and tissue examined.
   3. Give chemotherapy if malignant cells are found—Methotrexate is usually drug of choice.
   4. Assess for indication of impending perforation of the uterus by the tumor—hysterectomy recommended.

MEDICAL COMPLICATIONS OF PREGNANCY
Cardiac Involvement

The most common form of heart disease in pregnancy is *rheumatic heart disease* (90% of patients). The other 10% is divided among the arteriosclerotic, hypertensive and congenital types.

Normal Cardiopulmonary Symptoms During Pregnancy

1. Shortness of breath on effort—due to increased ventilation rate and elevated diaphragm.
2. Tachycardia and palpitations at rest or on mild exertion—heart rate increases gradually reaching a peak 1–2 months before term; average increase 15 beats per minute.
3. Cardiac enlargement—increased plasma volume 30–50% greater during 25th and 35th week, causing increased pulmonary blood flow.
4. Edema of lower extremities—disproportionate increase in venous pressure in the lower extremities as compared with upper extremities, predisposing to dependent edema, varicosities and hemorrhoids.
5. Functional heart murmurs—due to overactive heart, increased blood velocity and anemia.

Pathological Cardiopulmonary Signs and Symptoms

1. Dyspnea, increasing at rest or with mild exertion.
2. Diastolic murmur at the heart apex—indicative of mitral stenosis.
3. Tachycardia, increasing with activity.
4. Cough, hemoptysis and rales at the lung bases—indicates development of pulmonary edema and congestive heart failure.

Treatment and Nursing Management

A. *General Considerations*
   1. Obtain history and physical examination—to establish functional classification and determine prognosis and diagnosis of specific heart lesions.
   2. Provide constant observation throughout pregnancy—note evidence of increasing pulmonary, arterial and venous pressure and venous congestion particularly from 20th to 30th week.
   3. Prevent venous congestion and fluid retention or provide therapy if they occur.
   4. Prevent precipitating causes of heart failure such as infection, nutritional deficiencies, physical stress and anemia; if any of these occur, treat immediately.

NURSING ALERT: A serious anemia (hemoglobin, 8 gm./100 ml. or less) may produce all of the signs simulating congestive heart failure, especially if a functional heart murmur is present.

B. *Specific Aspects of Management*
   1. Limit patient's activities.
      Instruct the patient as follows:
      a. Obtain adequate rest—10 hours sleep at night and frequent rest periods during the day and ½ hour after each meal.
      b. Secure housekeeping help—arrange with social worker if necessary.
      c. Avoid crowds—in social functions or shopping areas to avoid infection.
      d. Avoid stress.
      e. Should any signs of decompensation appear, notify physician and remain in bed.
   2. Set down diet guidelines for patient.
      a. Prevent excessive weight gain with lower caloric intake—excessive weight increases load on heart and predisposes to hypertension, toxemia, venous stasis, edema and dyspnea.
      b. Prevent excessive fluid retention by restricting salt intake—retention of water and electrolytes, which occurs in normal pregnancy due to adrenocortical hormone changes, is exaggerated in cardiac patients.

C. *Medical Management*
   1. Diuretic therapy—to increase the excretion of sodium, chlorides and water to counteract the predisposition to congestive failure.
   2. Antibiotics—to control infection which is often a precipitating cause of pulmonary edema; antibiotics are often used as a prophylactic measure.
   3. Digitalis—to exert a depressant action on the A-V conduction system and slow ventricular rate in atrial fibrillation and other arrhythmias (see p. 276).
   4. Oxygen therapy—to facilitate breathing.

Physiologic Changes in the Heart and Circulation During Labor and Delivery

1. Oxygen consumption is greatly increased during periods of uterine contractions with parallel acceleration of pulse and respiratory rate.
2. Cardiac output increases 20% during each contraction.
3. Blood pressure rises; there are increases in both systolic and diastolic pressures, usually at the peak of uterine contraction.
4. Venous pressure is usually elevated during labor and 24 hours postpartum—increased venous return is associated with muscular exercise of labor and closure of the A-V placental shunt.
5. Heart rate increases during early seconds of a uterine contraction then slows as the contraction continues due to reduction of placental blood flow; during delivery there is a persistent tachycardia.

Management During Labor and Delivery

1. Provide hospitalization for most cardiac patients for several days (or even weeks, if necessary) before "due date"—to evaluate signs and symptoms of cardiac decompensation.
2. Perform cesarean section only when absolutely necessary—to avoid hazards:
   a. Risk of infection
   b. Longer need of anesthesia
   c. Greater blood loss
   d. Higher incidence of postoperative thromboembolic complications
3. Insure constant nursing surveillance to:
   a. Provide support and encouragement, allay anxiety and evaluate progress of labor.
   b. Take and record vital signs and fetal heart rate.
   c. Observe for evidence of obstetrical or cardiac complications.
   d. Assist the respiratory effort of the patient by placing her in semi-Fowler's position.
   e. Apply elastic stockings to help prevent venous congestion in the lower extremities.
4. *Analgesia*—to relieve pain and apprehension, avoid hypotension and maintain good oxygenation (essentially the same as for the noncardiac patient).
   a. Early labor
      Barbiturate therapy—to control restlessness.

> NURSING ALERT: These agents are slowly metabolized by the fetus and may cause central nervous system depression in the newborn.

   b. Advanced labor
      (1) Meperidine or morphine I.M.—use with caution since it depresses respiratory and vasomotor centers and may cause anoxia.
      (2) Meperidine given I.V. may cause vomiting and create unwanted stress.
      (3) Scopolamine (widely used in obstetrics to produce amnesia) is contraindicated for the cardiac patient because it causes restlessness and undesired physical activity.
5. *Anesthesia*
   a. Inhalation anesthesia with high level of oxygen is considered safe for short duration.

b. Regional anesthesia, especially epidural or caudal, is a superior alternative which provides excellent anesthesia while eliminating the need for barbiturates and narcotics during labor. Note that occasionally hypotension may occur.

This can be corrected by:

(1) Positioning patient on her side.

(2) Elevating her legs.

(3) Administering oxygen and vasopressor drugs, if necessary.

Management During the Postpartum Period

Continue observation and assessment.

1. Evaluate blood loss—excessive blood loss or hypotension may cause shock.
   a. Massage uterine fundus.
   b. Record vital signs.
   c. Administer oxytocic drugs.
2. Administer fluids slowly by mouth or intravenously—to replace fluid loss.
3. Provide narcotics and sedation as prescribed—to relieve pain and provide comfort following episiotomy and trauma to tissues.

NURSING ALERT: Patient may show no signs of difficulty during 1st and 2nd stages of labor, BUT may collapse following delivery because of the sudden decrease of intra-abdominal pressure with consequent engorgement of vessels.

The Diabetic and Prediabetic Pregnant Patient

Diabetes Mellitus is a chronic hereditary disease characterized by hyperglycemia (abnormally high level of blood sugar) due to a relative insufficiency or lack of insulin which leads to abnormalities in the metabolism of carbohydrates, protein and fat.

Predisposing Factors

1. Heredity factor—recessive trait
2. Obesity—increased demand on the secretory activity of the beta cells of the islands of Langerhans in the pancreas
3. Stress—emotional and physical (e.g., infections, trauma, surgery, pregnancy)

Mortality

1. Maternal mortality
   a. More than 50% before insulin therapy
   b. Currently comparable to nondiabetic
2. Infant mortality
   a. 40–50% before insulin therapy
   b. Currently 15–20% in mothers with pre-existing diabetes
   c. High rates of spontaneous abortion, extrauterine and neonatal deaths and congenital abnormalities
   d. Figures lower but still substantial for mothers with diabetes diagnosed for the first time during pregnancy

Metabolism Changes During Normal Pregnancy

1. Lowered glucose tolerance—alteration in metabolic rate and increased secretion of adrenocortical and pituitary hormones.
2. Decreased glucose utilization—insulin antagonists produced by the fetus.
3. Loss of reactivity to insulin—insulin tolerance tests performed throughout pregnancy show a significant reduction in effectiveness because of insulin degradation influenced by the placenta as it increases in size.
4. Hypoglycemic patients return to normal levels during pregnancy—islands of Langerhans increase in size and number during pregnancy.

Altered Physiology

1. Insulin requirements usually increase during the 1st trimester, remain stable during the 2nd and increase considerably during the 3rd—due to increased basal metabolic rate.
2. Increased tendency to ketosis and acidosis—nausea and vomiting during 1st trimester and diminished CO_2-combining power of the blood.
3. Spontaneous abortion—vascular complications affect placental circulation.
4. Diabetic nephropathy and retinopathy may develop or be aggravated during pregnancy—arteriosclerotic changes.
5. Hydramnios—(excessive accumulation of amniotic fluid)—mechanism unknown.
6. Rapid fetal growth with acceleration of skeletal development, excessive deposition of fat and water retention because of:
   a. Excessive supply of glucose from maternal hyperglycemia
   b. Increased production of growth hormone from maternal pituitary
   c. Increased secretion of insulin from fetal pancreas
   d. Increased action of adrenocortical hormones which favor passage of glucose from mother to fetus
7. High fetal and neonatal death rate because of:
   a. Ketoacidosis—a single episode can cause fetal death—due to electrolytic imbalance with severe circulatory alteration
   b. Hyaline membrane disease—combination of prematurity and water retention
   c. Birth injuries—cephalopelvic disproportion

Objectives of Treatment and Nursing Management

A. *To identify and diagnose the prediabetic or diabetic patient as early as possible.*

1. Obtain complete history.
   a. Signs and symptoms of diabetes (see p. 638)
   b. Diabetes within family
   c. Previous unexplained stillbirths
   d. Large babies weighing over 9 pounds (4000 gm.)
   e. Habitual spontaneous abortions
   f. Delivery of infants with multiple congenital anomalies
   g. Presence of hydramnios
   h. Excessive obesity
2. Carry out thorough physical examination.
   a. Determine patient's medical and obstetrical status.
   b. Assess patient's individual needs and plan management with her.

B. *To provide best possible outcome for mother and newborn by rigid control of the diabetes.*
  1. Observe and examine patient frequently—patient should be seen every week alternately by the internist and obstetrician; pediatrician also must be aware of patient's progress.
     a. Provide continuing education of the patient regarding diet, medications, signs and symptoms of diabetes and its complications.
     b. Keep record of weight and blood pressure.
     c. Examine ocular fundus.
     d. Observe for signs of edema or hydramnios.
     e. Assess if diet or medication is controlling disease; adjust as necessary.
  2. Laboratory tests
     a. Urinalysis for sugar and albumin at each visit—indicates effectiveness of medication or diet and renal function.
     b. Frequent glucose tolerance test—normal test may become abnormal as pregnancy progresses.
     c. Monthly hemoglobin determination—increased need for iron same as for non-diabetic patient.

NURSING ALERT: Tes-tape and Diastix are specific for glucose and should be used for urine testing in preference to Benedict's solution or Clinitest tablets which give a positive reaction for sugar in such benign melliturias as pentosuria, fructosuria and lactosuria late in pregnancy and during lactation.

Management of Delivery

  1. Pregnancy is terminated 2–4 weeks before term—major concern is fetal size and viability determined by abdominal palpation, x-ray and fetal heart tones; earlier delivery is recommended if there is evidence of the following:
     a. Excessive fetal size
     b. Toxemias with history of fetal deaths before 36th week
     c. Diabetes difficult to control
  2. Pediatrician should be notified of patient's status—to plan management of newborn.
  3. Patient hospitalized several days before delivery—to prepare for delivery; long-lasting insulin changed to regular, and fractional urinalysis begun to prevent hypoglycemic reactions while patient is in labor or undergoing cesarean section.
  4. Patients being treated with oral agents are maintained on medication until day of delivery; medication resumed if necessary postdelivery.
  5. Labor induced by stripping of membranes, amniotomy and I.V. Pitocin drip.
  6. Patient is given nothing by mouth and administered continuous I.V. 10% glucose covered by regular insulin.
  7. Cesarean section indicated if induction of labor fails.
  8. Patient maintained on regular insulin until able to eat, then returned to long-lasting insulin; dosage usually decreases in the postpartum period.

INFECTIONS DURING PREGNANCY

There are numerous types of infections which the mother can contract during pregnancy. The implications of many of these infections in terms of maternal effects, fetal effects and nursing management are presented in Table 22-1.

TABLE 22-1. EFFECTS OF INFECTIONS DURING PREGNANCY

Disease	Maternal Effects	Fetal Effects	Management
Scarlet fever	High fever Puerperal infection	Abortion	Isolation Penicillin
Erysipelas	Puerperal infection Septicemia	Fetal infection Fetal death	Isolation Penicillin or erythromycin
Typhoid fever	High fever	Abortion Premature labor	Isolation Chloramphenicol Antityphoid vaccine
Urinary tract infections	Fever with chills Hematuria Pyuria Dysuria Pain	No effects from maternal infection Large doses of antibiotics in late pregnancy may cause kernicterus in newborn	Sulfonamides Furadantin Ampicillin Tetracycline
Syphilis	Increased resistance with pregnancy Primary and secondary lesions May be asymptomatic	Infection of fetus occurs from 3 months to day of delivery Untreated—premature stillbirth 20% surviving newborns have congenital syphilis	Procaine penicillin G, 2.4 million units In late syphilis, 6 million–9 million units I.M. in divided doses
Gonorrhea	Infection of genitourinary tract Closure of fallopian tubes May be asymptomatic during pregnancy	Ophthalmia neonatorum acquired during birth	Preventive—silver nitrate 1% eye drops at birth

Rubella	Fever and rash	If infected during first 8 weeks:
		    Congenital cataracts
		    Heart anomalies
		    Deafness
		    Central nervous system damage
			12 ml. of rubella convalescent gamma globulin, I.M., for exposure

Cytomegalovirus disease	Asymptomatic	Hydrocephaly Microphthalmia, Seizures Encephalitis Hepatosplenomegaly Hematologic changes Microcephaly Blindness	No effective treatment
Herpes simplex	Gingivostomatitis Vulvovaginitis	May be lethal to fetus Skin eruptions on newborn Septicemia with respiratory and circulatory failure	Cesarean section if maternal vaginal canal infected

TABLE 22-1. EFFECTS OF INFECTIONS DURING PREGNANCY (Continued)

Disease	Maternal Effects	Fetal Effects	Management
Coxsackie virus	Minor illness	Fatal to fetus—myocarditis Encephalomyelitis	No effective treatment
Mumps	Parotitis	Abortion Premature labor Congenital defects Fetal death	Intradermal mumps skin test used to determine immunity If susceptible, convalescent gamma globulin given
Measles (rubeola)	Rash and fever	Abortion Premature labor If late in pregnancy, infant born with infection in same stage as mother	Gamma globulin if exposed
Smallpox	Skin lesions Fever	Abortion Premature labor Born with disease	If vaccination indicated (exposure to smallpox), Vaccinia Immune Globulin is given with the vaccine (particularly in primary vaccine cases)
Poliomyelitis	More susceptible during pregnancy Labor proceeds normally even in presence of paralysis	Abortion Infant may develop poliomyelitis or be completely normal	Both inactivated vaccine (Salk) and attenuated live vaccine (Sabin) are safe for immunization during pregnancy Antibodies may be transmitted from mother to fetus
Influenza	Prognosis excellent in uncomplicated influenza, serious if pneumonia develops	Abortion Premature labor	Vaccination with specific immune serum
Toxoplasmosis	Asymptomatic	Abortion Death Chorioretinitis Mental retardation Cerebral calcification Anomalies of head size Convulsions	No effective treatment Diagnosis verified rising antibody titer
Malaria	Fever and chills	Abortion May involve placenta extensively	Commonly used anti-malarial drugs
Common cold	More susceptible during pregnancy Becomes serious if hemolytic streptococci infect upper respiratory system	Not known	Symptomatic

TERMINATION OF A PREGNANCY
Abortion

Abortion is termination of pregnancy at any time before the fetus has attained viability (20 weeks gestation or fetal weight of 400 gm.).

Incidence

1. Frequent complication of pregnancy.
2. 1 pregnancy in every 10 terminates in spontaneous abortion.

Predisposing Factors

1. Faulty germ plasm—imperfect ova or sperm cells.
2. Decrease in production of progesterone—insufficient progesterone leads to increased uterine sensitivity and contractions causing expulsion of the ovum or embryo.
3. Incompetent cervix—mechanical defect in the cervix causing dilatation and effacement in early pregnancy.
4. Acute infections—cause fetal death by:
   a. Transmission of bacterial toxins from mother to fetus
   b. Passage of microorganisms from mother to fetus
   c. High temperature, which stimulates uterine contractions
   d. Excessive carbon dioxide in blood (as associated with respiratory infections)

Types of Abortion

1. Threatened abortion
2. Inevitable abortion
3. Habitual abortion
4. Incomplete abortion
5. Missed abortion

	Classification	Clinical Manifestations	Management
1.	Threatened	Vaginal bleeding or spotting Mild cramps Cervix closed or slightly dilated Symptoms subside or develop into an inevitable abortion	Vaginal examination Pregnanediol test if progesterone low Bedrest Pad count
2.	Inevitable	Bleeding more profuse Cervix dilated Painful uterine contractions	Embryo delivered followed by D & C
3.	Habitual abortion	Spontaneous abortion occurs in successive pregnancies (3 or more)	Hysterogram to rule out uterine abnormalities, infections Surgical constriction of the cervix if incompetent cervix D & C
4.	Incomplete abortion	Fetus usually expelled Placenta and membranes retained	D & C
5.	Missed abortion	Fetus dies in utero and is retained Maceration occurs No symptoms of abortion but malaise, anorexia and headache are common	D & C and oxytocin contraindicated Intra-amniotic injection of saline usually successful in expulsion of retained material

> NURSING ALERT: Serious hemorrhage from alteration in the blood clotting mechanism may occur with prolonged retention of a dead fetus. Fibrinogen concentrations should be measured weekly. If concentrations are reduced to 150 mg./100 ml. of blood, the uterus should be emptied; fibrinogen and whole blood may need to be administered.

Nursing Management

1. Provide constant nursing surveillance.
   a. Measure and record vital signs—to determine presence of shock.
   b. Assess amount of blood loss—perineal pad count.
   c. Save all tissue and clots—for examination by pathologist for presence of decidua or embryo.
2. Relieve the patient's pain and anxiety—uterine contractions may be as severe as those experienced during childbirth.
   a. Give analgesic medication within prescribed limit.
   b. Monitor the blood pressure, pulse and respiratory rate before administering or repeating narcotics—narcotics are central nervous system depressants and may contribute to development of shock.
   c. Offer intelligent reassurance—avoid statement that would imply a favorable outcome for the fetus even with threatened abortion—prognosis very uncertain.
3. Be alert for developing complications.
   a. Assess for signs of shock from excessive blood loss.
      (1) Reduced blood pressure   (4) Restlessness
      (2) Rapid weak pulse   (5) Apathy
      (3) Cool moist skin
   b. Provide emergency measures to combat shock
      (1) Elevate patient's legs.
      (2) Notify physician.
      (3) Start I.V. fluids with 19 gauge needle.
   c. Prepare patient for surgical completion of the abortion—patient will continue to bleed or hemorrhage until uterus is emptied and able to contract.
   d. Observe patient postoperatively for infection—hemorrhage lowers resistance to infection, and retained blood clots or tissue provides excellent bacterial media.
   e. Prepare patient for artificial termination of the pregnancy by intra-amniotic instillation of hypertonic solution.

GUIDELINES: *Saline Infusion Into the Amniotic Cavity*

Saline infusion is replacement of the amniotic fluid with a hypertonic saline solution which chemically stops fetal and placental function thereby initiating labor.

Purpose

Interruption of pregnancy after 12 weeks gestation

Equipment

A receptacle for the amniotic fluid
200 ml. of a 20% solution of sodium chloride

Skin disinfectant
Sterile infusion tray
    Sterile draping towel
    Medicine glass for saline solution
    50-ml. syringe for removal of amniotic fluid and injection of the saline solution
    20-ml. syringe, a 25 gauge 3.8-cm. (1½-inch) needle and a 20 gauge 3.8-cm. (1½-inch) needle for anesthetizing the anterior abdominal wall
    10-cm. (4-inch), 14-gauge spinal needle with stylet
    A No. 5 teflon catheter, 1 meter (approximately 36 inches) long with 3 holes at the top
    Vial of local anesthetic agent
    Sterile surgical gown and gloves

Procedure

Nursing Action	Rationale/Amplification
Preparatory Phase	
1. Obtain history and assist with general physical examination.	1. Problems elicited may indicate referral to an appropriate specialist or decision to perform procedure in hospital rather than office or clinic.
2. Discuss present pregnancy.	2. Identifying patient's feelings toward abortion is important. Further counselling may be indicated.
3. Have patient void.	3. To avoid injury to the bladder.
4. Assist patient to disrobe, put on examining gown and assume supine position.	
5. Expose the abdomen and wash with antiseptic solution.	5. Since the needle will be inserted through the skin into the amniotic cavity, asepsis is carried out to prevent infection.
Performance Phase	
The physician does the following:	
1. A skin wheal is made with the 25-gauge needle.	1. The site chosen for injection is usually the mid-uterus.
2. A 20-gauge 3.8-cm. (1½-inch) needle is used to anesthetize the other layers of the anterior abdominal wall.	
3. For actual amniocentesis, a 10-cm. (4-inch) No. 14 gauge spinal needle with stylet is placed at the site of analgesia and firmly inserted through the abdominal wall into the uterus.	3. A loss of resistance may be felt when the needle enters the amniotic cavity. The needle will be inserted to a depth of 7.6 cm. (3 inches) before fluid is reached.
4. Stylet is removed and amniotic fluid returns through the needle.	
5. The No. 5 teflon catheter is threaded slightly beyond the needle top, and the needle is withdrawn.	
6. Approximately 150 ml. of amniotic fluid is withdrawn through the catheter.	

Nursing Action	**Rationale/Amplification**
7. 200 ml. of 20% solution of sodium chloride is injected through the catheter.	7. The first 20–30 ml. of solution is injected slowly and patient is observed for any unusual symptoms such as pain at the site of injection, feeling of warmth, thirst, headache, numbness which indicate that the catheter is no longer in the amniotic space and adjustments must be made.
8. 1 million units of aqueous penicillin are instilled through the catheter.	8. This is a prophylactic measure to prevent intrauterine infection.
9. The catheter is withdrawn and a small dressing applied.	

Follow-up Phase

The patient is discharged with the following instructions:

1. Drink at least 2 liters (quarts) of water during the afternoon the procedure is performed.	1. To combat hypernatremia and to promote diuresis.
2. When contractions become uncomfortable, return to the clinic or hospital for completion of abortion.	2. Labor contractions should begin within 12 to 24 hours.
3. If fever develops or bleeding commences, call physician and plan to return to hospital.	3. Fever may be caused by chorioamnionitis, or by chemical necrosis of tissue. Tetracycline or ampicillin may be prescribed. Bleeding is usually due to partial placenta separation.

BIBLIOGRAPHY

Books

Benson, R. C.: Handbook of Obstetrics and Gynecology. Los Altos, Lange Medical Publications, 1971.

Danforth, D. N.: Textbook of Obstetrics and Gynecology. New York, Harper and Row, 1971.

Fitzpatrick, E., et. al.: Maternity Nursing. Philadelphia, J. B. Lippincott, 1971.

Greenhill, J. P.: Obstetrics. Philadelphia, W. B. Saunders, 1965.

Haynes, D. M.: Medical Complications During Pregnancy. New York, McGraw-Hill Book Co., 1969.

Hellman, L. M., and Pritchard, J. A.: William's Obstetrics. New York, Appleton-Century-Crofts, 1971.

Page, E. W., et al.: Human Reproduction. Philadelphia, W. B. Saunders, 1972.

Reid, D. E., et al.: Principles and Management of Human Reproduction. Philadelphia, W. B. Saunders, 1972.

Rovinsky, J., and Guttmacher, A. F.: Medical, Surgical and Gynecologic Complications of Pregnancy. Baltimore, Williams and Wilkins, 1965.

Taylor, E. S.: Beck's Obstetrical Practice. Baltimore, Williams and Wilkins, 1971.

Articles

Charles, D., and MacAulay, M.: Use of antibiotics in obstetric practice. Clin. Obstet. and Gynecol., *13*:255–271, June 1970.

Cronenwett, L. R., and Choyce, J. M.: Saline abortion. Amer. J. Nurs., *71*:1754–1757, Sept. 1971.

Daly, M.: The unwanted pregnancy. Clin. Obstet. and Gynecol., *13*:713–726, Sept. 1970.

Davis, L., and Grace, H.: Anticipatory counseling of unwed pregnant adolescents. Nurs. Clin. N. Amer., *6*:581–590, Dec. 1971.

Edwards, J.: When the baby is stillborn. RN, *34*:44, Nov. 1971.

Gause, R. W.: Multiple pregnancies: diagnosis, delivery and problems of development. J. Obstet., Gynecol., and Neonatal Nurs., *1*:22–26, Sept.–Oct. 1972.

Goldman, A.: Learning abortion care. Nurs. Outlook, *19*:350–352, May 1971.

Goodheart, B.: A second look at the German measles vaccine. Today's Health, *49*:46–47, March 1971.

Heisseman, G. S., and Lee, J. H.: Bacteriuria in pregnancy. Obstet. and Gynecol., *41*:22–26, Jan. 1973.

Hershey, N.: Abortion and sterilization: status of the law in mid-1970. Amer. J. Nurs., *70*:1926–1927, Sept. 1970.

Kass, E. H.: Pregnancy, pyelonephritis and prematurity. Clin. Obstet. and Gynecol., *13*:239–254, June 1970.

Lucas, M., et al.: Recurrent abortions and chromosome abnormalities. J. Obstet. and Gynecol. of the British Commonwealth, *79*:1119–1127, Dec. 1972.

Malo-Juvera, P.: Preparing students for abortion care. Nurs. Outlook, *19*:347–349, June 1971.

Milio, A., and Adamsons, K.: Fetal blood sampling. Amer. J. Nurs., *68*:2149–2152, Oct. 1968.

Nitowsky, H. M.: Prenatal diagnosis of genetic abnormality. Amer. J. Nurs., *71*:1551–1557, Aug. 1971.

Penza, J., and Rankin, J.: Infectious vaginopathies in pregnancy. Clin. Obstet. and Gynecol., *13*: 223–238, June 1970.

Ruoss, C. F., and Bourne, G. L.: Toxoplasmosis in pregnancy. J. Obstet. and Gynecol. of the British Commonwealth, *79*:1115–1118, Dec. 1972.

Schaefer, G.: Legal abortions in New York State: medical, nursing, social aspects. Clin. Obstet. and Gynecol., *14*, March 1971. (Entire volume.)

Schulman, H., et al.: Outpatient saline abortion. Obstet. and Gynecol., *37*:521–526, April 1971.

Seetz, S. D.: When the baby isn't normal. RN, *34*:40–43, Nov. 1971.

Siegler, A.: A review of tubal sterilization. J. Obstet., Gynecol. and Neonatal Nurs., *1*:23, Aug. 1972.

Wentz, A. C., et al.: Methodology in premature pregnancy termination. Obstet. and Gynecol. Survey, *28*:2–19, Jan. 1973.

White, C. A., and Koontz, F. P.: B-hemolytic streptococcus infections in postpartum patients. Obstet. and Gynecol., *41*:29–32, Jan. 1973.

PART III

Pediatric Nursing

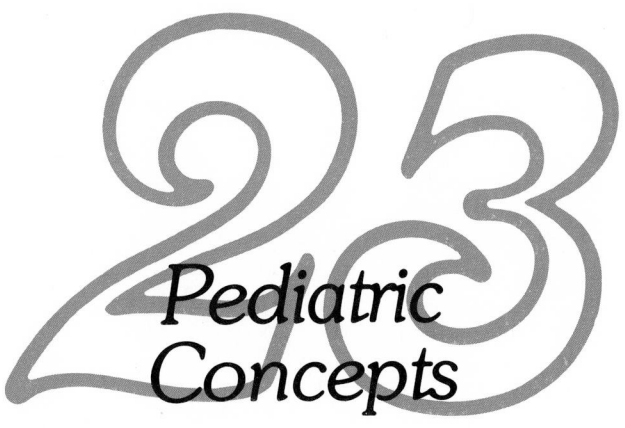

Pediatric Concepts

GROWTH AND DEVELOPMENT

Reflexes of the Newborn

1. *Pupillary reflexes*—ipsilateral constriction to light.
2. *Rooting*—when corner of mouth is touched and object is moved toward cheek, infant will turn head toward object and open mouth.
3. *Palmer grasp*—pressure on palm of hand will elicit grasp.
4. *Plantar grasp*—pressure on sole of foot behind toes will cause flexion of toes.
5. *Tonic neck reflex*—sudden jolt will cause head to turn to one side with leg and arm on that side extended, while the extremities on the other side flex.
6. *Neck righting*—when head is turned to one side, the shoulder and trunk will turn to that side, followed by the pelvis.
7. *Moro reflex*—response to sudden loud noise causing body to stiffen and arms to go up and out then forward and toward each other. Thumb and index finger will assume c-shape.

GROWTH AND DEVELOPMENT

Age	Physical Growth	Behavior Patterns	Related Nursing Actions
Birth–4 weeks (1 month)		*Motor Development* Visual fixation—stares at windows and ceiling Eyes follow bright moving objects Lies awake on back with head averted *Socialization and Vocalization* Mews and makes throaty noises Intently interested in human face	*Play Stimulation* Use human face—smile and talk Dangle bright and moving object in field of vision (mobile) Hold, touch, caress, fondle Rock, pat, change position Play soft music-clock or have infant listen to ticking clock *Parental Guidance* Keep infant near Allow him to sleep Play with him when awake Hold him during feeding
8 weeks (2 months)		*Motor Development* If bell is sounded near him, he will stop activity and listen Eyes follow better, vertically and horizontally Crossed extensor reflex disappears *Socialization and Vocalization* Social smile Eyes follow person more intently	*Play Stimulation* (8–12 weeks) Hang wind chimes near infant Hang bright colored pictures on wall (yellow and red-colored stripes) Use cradle gym and infant seat Use rattles Hold infant and walk around room Allow freedom of kicking with clothes on *Parental Guidance* Talk to him and smile, get excited when he coos Place infant seat where he cannot fall off or tip over Put in prone position in bed or on floor

Age	Motor Development / Socialization and Vocalization	Play Stimulation / Parental Guidance
12 weeks (3 months)	**Motor Development** When prone, he will rest on forearms and keep head midline Discovers and stares at hands Positive supporting reflex disappears 3–4 months, stepping reflex disappears Landau reflex appears **Socialization and Vocalization** Smiles more readily Babbles and coos	**Play Stimulation (4–6 months)** Mirror play Soft squeeze toys in vivid colors of varying texture Enjoys splashing in bath Still enjoys holding and playing with rattles Enjoys old fashioned clothes pins **Parental Guidance** Be certain button eyes, etc. cannot be pulled off Hold rattle for him and let him reach and grasp it When in high chair, strap in Let him play with food Move mobile out of reach—he may grab it and cause injury
16 weeks (4 months)	**Motor Development** Eyes focus on small objects; may pick up dangling ring Likes being propped up Holds head up More interested in environment Hand comes to meet rattle Listens—turns head to familiar sound Stepping reflex disappears Rooting reflex disappears **Socialization and Vocalization** Laughs and chuckles socially Demands social attention by fussing Recognizes mother	
26 weeks (7 months)	**Motor Development** Momentary sitting and hand support Bounces and bears some weight when held in standing position Reaches for objects Transfers and mouths objects in one hand Discovers feet 5–6 months, tonic neck reflex disappears 6–7 months, palmar grasp disappears	**Play Stimulation (6–9 months)** Bounce chair Large nesting toys (round rather than square) Likes to drop and retrieve things Likes metal cups and wooden spoons and things to bang with Loves crumpled paper Enjoys squeeze toys in bath

GROWTH AND DEVELOPMENT (Continued)

Age	Physical Growth	Behavior Patterns	Related Nursing Actions
26 weeks (7 months) (*cont.*)		Inspects objects, localizes sound	Likes peek-a-boo, bye-bye and pat-a-cake
		Likes to sit in high chair	
		Drops and picks up objects	
		Displays exploratory behavior with food	
			Parental Guidance
		Socialization and Vocalization	Will play as long as you can
		Discriminates strangers	Tie toys to chair with short string
		Crows and squeals	Let play with extra spoon at feeding
		Starts to say "ma, da"	Give soft finger foods
		Self-play is self-contained	Since infant puts everything in mouth, use safety precautions. Keep small items away from him; he could choke on them
			Show excitement at his achievement
40 weeks (10 months)	9–12 months, plantar reflex disappears	*Motor Development*	*Play Stimulation (10–15 months)*
	9–12 months, neck-righting reflex disappears	Sits without support	Learns by imitation
		Recovers balance	Likes new objects (blocks)
		Manipulates objects with hands	Likes freedom of creeping and walking, but closeness of family is important
		Creeps	
		Pulls self upright at crib rails	Good toys: milk carton, bean bag for tossing, fabric books, things to move around, fill up, empty out, pile up and knock down toys
		Uses index finger and thumb to hold objects	
		Rings a bell	
		Can feed himself cracker and can hold bottle	
		Can control lips around cup	
		Doesn't like supine position	
			Parental Guidance
		Socialization and Vocalization	Do things with him
		Claps hands on request	Protect him from dangerous objects—cover electrical outlets, block stairs, move breakable objects from tables
		Responds to own name	
		Very aware of social environment	
		Imitates gestures, facial expressions and sounds	Use plastic bottle
		Smiles at image in mirror	

10–15 months	12–18 months, Babinski sign disappears 12–24 months, Landau reflex disappears	*Motor Development* Walks alone Builds tower of 2 blocks Puts ball in box Uses spoon Can release objects at will Can dress in simple garments Has regular bowel movements *Socialization and Vocalization* Uses jargon Points to indicate wants Loves give-and-take game Shares fear, anger, affection, jealousy, anxiety and sympathy Responds to music Enjoys being center of attention and will repeat laughed-at activities	*Play Stimulation* Pull toys and push toys Selects a favorite toy Likes teddy bears, dolls, pots and pans, cloth picture books with colorful large pictures, telephone, musical top, nested blocks
15–18 months	Anterior fontanelle closes Big muscles become well developed Fine-muscle coordination begins to develop Abdomen protrudes	*Motor* Walks and runs with a stiff gait and wide stance Falls less frequently Climbs stairs with help Stoops to pick up toys Mimics household chores, like dusting Places one block on top of another Holds a cup with both hands Throws a ball *Social* Develops new awareness of strangers Wants to explore everything in his reach Finds security in a blanket, favorite toy or thumb sucking	*Parental Guidance* Begin to teach tooth brushing to establish good dental habits Safety teaching—child gets into everything within his reach. Place medications in safe, locked place. Create a safe environment for child

GROWTH AND DEVELOPMENT (Continued)

Age	Physical Growth	Behavior Patterns	Related Nursing Actions
15–18 months (*cont.*)		*Vocalization* Has vocabulary of 10 words which have meanings Uses phrases	
18 months–2 years	Landau reflex disappears	*Motor* Walks up and down stairs Opens doors, turns knobs Has steady gait Drinks well with 1 hand Uses spoon without spilling (may prefer fingers) Kicks a ball in front of him without support Builds a tower of 4–6 blocks Scribbles *Social* Uses word "mine" constantly Has fear of parents leaving *Vocalization* Has 200–300 words in his vocabulary Begins to use short sentences *Mental* Obeys simple commands Does not know right from wrong	*Play Stimulation* Parallel play—although he enjoys having other children around him Very short attention span Toys (same as for 15–18 months) *Parental Guidance* Has need for peer companionship although his immaturity is evidenced by his inability to share and take turns A decrease in appetite normally occurs at this stage Toilet training should be started (each child follows his own pattern) Begin to have child eat his meals with the family Begin to read to child—likes storybooks with large pictures
2–3 years		*Motor* Throws objects overhand Pedals tricycle Walks backward Washes and dries hands Begins to use scissors Can string large beads Can undress himself Feeds himself well Tries to dance	*Play Stimulation* Plays simple games with other children

Social

Negativism grows out of child's sense of developing independence—says no to every command

Ritualism—important to toddler for his security (follows certain pattern, especially at bedtime)

Temper tantrums—may result from toddler's frustration in wanting to do everything himself

Vocalization

Talks in short sentences

Uses plurals

May attempt to sing simple songs

Has vocabulary of 900 words

Mental

Begins to understand what it means to take turns

Can repeat 3 numbers

Develops interest in colors

Parental Guidance

From 2–3 years the child develops a seeming maturity—do not expect more of him than he is able to do

First visit to the dentist to have teeth checked

Be aware that negativistic and ritualistic behavior is normal

Be consistent in discipline

Control temper tantrums

Begin to teach traffic safety

Supervise outdoor play

3—4 years

Grows relatively slowly during preschool years

Gains less than 2.3 kg. (5 pounds) per year

Grows 5–6.25 cm. (2–2½ inches) a year

Motor

Dresses himself with supervision

Climbs and jumps well

Buttons buttons

Can lace his shoes

Social

Can tolerate separation from mother for a few minutes without anxiety

Exaggerates, boasts and tattles on others

Talks with imaginary companion —usually of same age and sex

Vocalization

Has vocabulary of 900 words

Play Stimulation

Plays with other children, so they interact

Toys and games: record player, nursery rhymes, housekeeping toys, transportation toys (tricycle, trucks, cars, wagon), blocks, hammer and peg bench, floor trains, blackboard and chalk, easel and brushes, clay, crayon and finger paints, outside toys (sandbox, swing, small slide), books (short stories, action stories), drum

GROWTH AND DEVELOPMENT (Continued)

Age	Physical Growth	Behavior Patterns	Related Nursing Actions
3–4 years (*cont.*)		*Mental* Knows first and last name Understands what to do when told Identifies longer of 2 lines Is less negativistic Can be given simple explanation as to cause and effect	*Parental Guidance* Give small errands to do around the house (putting silverware on table, drying a dish) Expand child's world with trips to the zoo; go to supermarket, out to lunch, etc.
4–5 years	Gains less than 2.3 kg. (5 pounds) Grows 5–6.25 cm. (2–2½ inches)	*Motor* Hops 2 or more times Dresses without supervision Has good motor control—climbs and jumps well Walks up stairs without grasping handrail Walks backwards	*Play Stimulation* Likes to jump rope, skip, etc. Prefers group play and cooperates in projects
		Vocalization Has a vocabulary of 1500 words	*Parental Guidance* No longer takes an afternoon nap Prepare for kindergarten Loves to have parents tell him stories Provide opportunities for group play; have his friends over for lunch and an afternoon of playing
		Mental Knows primary colors Can count to 10 Can copy a triangle Has high power of imagination Questioning at a peak	
		Social May have an imaginary companion Has a sense of order (likes to finish what he has started) Is obedient and reliable Is protective toward younger children Begins to develop an elementary conscience with some influence in governing his behavior Has increased self-confidence	

5–6 years

Since child grows proportionally more than he gains weight, he appears taller and slimmer

Lordosis has disappeared

Motor
Begins to ride 2-wheel bicycle
Runs skillfully and plays games at the same time
Can use hammer and hit nail on head
Can wash himself without wetting clothes

Social
Likely to do what is expected of him
Begins to take more responsibility for his actions

Vocalization
Vocabulary of 2100 words
Talks constantly
Repeats a sentence of 10 syllables or more

Mental
Can form some letters correctly
Copies a triangle
Can name 4 colors—usually red, yellow, green, blue
Interested in meaning of relatives —aunts and uncles
Asks meaning of words
Asks searching questions
Can identify penny, nickel and dime
Knows names of days of week and recognizes that a week is a unit of time

Play Stimulation
Plays with other children and is less likely to inflict injury on other child
Plays house and begins to imitate firemen and teachers
Bicycle

Parental Guidance
Begins kindergarten. Keep in touch with teacher

GROWTH AND DEVELOPMENT (Continued)

Age	Physical Growth	Behavior Patterns	Related Nursing Actions
6–7 years	Growth spurt begins Gains approximately 1.82–3.18 kg. (4–7 pounds) per year Begins to lose baby teeth Acquires first molars at about 7 years	*Motor* Is very active, impulsive Likes to bathe self Dresses self with help *Social* Plays well alone Enjoys group play with small groups Considers ideas of teachers as important Begins to accept authority outside of home Uses telephone *Mental* Has vocabulary of about 2500 words Knows comparative value of coins Begins to learn to read Knows number combinations to 10 Knows right from left Knows morning from afternoon	*Play Stimulation* Painting, coloring, pasting, drawing Imaginary dramatic play Girls—"dress-up", school Boys—firemen, soldiers, etc. Table games Dolls Airplanes, cars, trucks, etc. Collections of various items
7–8 years	Gains approximately 1.36–2.27 kg. (3–5 pounds) per year Eyes become fully developed	*Motor* Less impulsive and boisterous in activities Nervous habits such as nail biting are common Capable of fine hand movements Improved muscular skills—ball throwing, etc. *Social* Competition is important Aware of differences between his home and others Wants to be like friends	*Play Stimulation* Enjoys games which develop physical and mental skills More realism in play Radio, T.V., records Magic tricks Paper dolls Books Table games and card games Paper mache *Parental Guidance* Frequently has "quiet days," periods of shyness which should be

tolerated as part of growing up and deciding who he is. May be subject to nightmares which require reassurance and understanding

Mental
Counts by 1, 2, 5, 10's
Tells time
Knows what month it is
Curious about sex differences
Grasps basic ideas of addition and subtraction
Knows days of week

8–9 years

Has 10–11 permanent teeth
Arms grow longer in proportion to body
Onset of secondary sex characteristics appear in some females (ranges from 8–14 years)
Breast bud formation
Breasts enlarge, hips widen
Early development of pubic hair

Motor
Has coordination of fine muscles
Bathes self without help
Engages in active play

Social
More self-assured in environment
Likes group projects, clubs
Not quite ready for team play
Selective in choice of friends
Recognizes property rights
Modesty is increased
Demonstrates a sense of humor
Needs help accepting defeat in games

Mental
Interested in history (Indians, etc.)
Knows day of month, year
Interested in distant places
Makes change for small amounts of money

Play Stimulation
Detailed drawings
Comics and funny papers
Clay, play-dough
Cooking sets for girls
Erector sets for boys
Cards, marbles, checkers
Dramatics
Sports
Books—geography, adventure

Parental Guidance
Needs to be considered important by adults—can be given small household responsibilities
Sex-conscious. Should be able to discuss his questions at home rather than with his friends. Requires simple, honest answers to questions
Common problems include: teasing, quarreling, nail-biting, enuresis, whining, poor manners, swearing. These are usually fleeting phases and should not be handled negatively. The causes for such behavior should be investigated and dealt with constructively

Lippincott Manual of Nursing Practice

GROWTH AND DEVELOPMENT (Continued)

Age	Physical Growth	Behavior Patterns	Related Nursing Actions
9–10 years	Growth in height decreases Hand-eye coordination is developed	*Motor* Constantly on the go Cares for his own physical needs completely Uses tools fairly well Uses both hands independently *Social* Play is more varied Likes to have secrets Sex differences in play Antagonism often develops between sexes More interested in family life *Mental* Less interested in fantasy Grasps easy multiplication and division Interested in how things are made Knows seasons, rhymes	*Play Stimulation* Books Musical instruments T.V., records Clubs and "organizations" Practical projects—simple sewing, ceramics, models Art—tissue paper, modeling *Parental Guidance* Lying and stealing are more serious problems. Again, the causes must be determined. (Usually these are attempts to gain recognition or remedy inadequacies) Harsh and severe punishment should be avoided Understanding is important
10–11 years	Weight gain often intensified Onset of major secondary sex characteristics appear in some males (ranges from 10–15 years) Early development of testes, scrotum Physique changes as fat and muscle are added Further enlargement of testes, scrotum, penis	*Motor* Very active Marked differences in motor skills according to sex Works hard to perfect physical skills *Social* Companionship becomes more important than play Enjoys team work Occasional privacy is important	*Play Stimulation* Experiments Gangs and club houses Weaving (pot-holders) Jewelry T.V. Leather Group singing *Parental Guidance* Encourage participation in organized clubs, youth groups

Mental
Continue sex education and preparation for adolescent body changes

Mental
Has more ability to plan ahead
Able to discuss problems
Sees others ideas and opinions
Has growing capacity for thought and conceptual organization
Sees physical qualities as constant despite changes in size, shape, weight, volume

11–12 years

Females may begin menstruation (develop axillary hair)
12-year molars erupt

Motor
Females can no longer compete on equal terms with males in the area of physical strength

Social
Club membership is important
Enjoys team games
Participates in community and school affairs
Sexes tend to remain segregated
Likes to be alone occasionally

Mental
Able to understand human reproduction
Can be critical of own work
Comprehends world of possibility and abstraction
Interested in world affairs

Play Stimulation
Likes to do jobs, run errands
Ceramic projects
Copper and metal work
Knitting, crocheting
Records
Link belts

Parental Guidance
Democratic guidance is essential as child works through a conflict between dependence (on his parents) and independence. Needs realistic limits set
Needs help channeling energy in proper direction—work and sports
Requires adequate explanation of body changes. Special understanding required for the child who lags in physical development

GROWTH AND DEVELOPMENT (Continued)

Age	Physical Growth	Behavior Patterns	Related Nursing Actions
Early adolescence	Further development of secondary sex characteristics	*Motor*	*Play Stimulation*
		Often awkward, uncoordinated; has poor posture	*Girls*
	Males	Tires easily	Social functions
	Growth of pubic and facial hair		Romantic T.V. shows and movies
	Height spurt accelerates	*Social*	Make-up
	Shoulders broaden	Increased interest in the opposite sex	Cooking, sewing
	Voice changes	Peer group extremely important	Art, poetry
	Axillary hair develops	Emancipation from the family begins—may become hostile toward parents	*Boys*
	Production of spermatozoa, nocturnal emissions	Strong bonds of friendship between 1–2 close peers	Sports
			Mechanical and electrical devices
	Females		Part-time employment
	Axillary and pubic hair becomes coarser, darker	*Mental*	*Parental Guidance*
	Further development of breasts	Concerned with morality, ethics, religion and social customs	Requires reassurance and help in accepting his changing body image—make the most of his positive qualities
	Menarche occurs if it has not already done so	Great variation in academic interest and ability	Gentle encouragement and guidance regarding dating—avoid strong pressures in either direction
	Sebaceous glands in face, back and chest become more active		Understanding of his conflicts as he attempts to deal with social, moral and intellectual issues is important
			Limits are still necessary for the adolescent's security; avoid threats
			Provide opportunities to earn their own money, and allow some financial independence
			Encourage independence, but allow child to lean on parents for support when frightened or unable to attain his aspirations

Late adolescence

Completion of sexual development

Males (13–18 years)
Genital size and pubic hair are adult in appearance
Hair present on side of face
Structural growth near completion
Physique that of mature male

Females (13–18 years)
Breasts and pubic hair are adult in appearance
Height may increase from 5–10 cm. (2–4 inches) after menarche

Capable of reproduction
Wisdom teeth erupt

Motor
More energy as growth spurt tapers
Muscular ability and coordination increase

Social
More mature, interdependent relationship with parents
Romantic love affairs which form the basis for more mature relationships preceding marriage
Able to balance responsibility and pleasure
Loosened grasp of peer group

Mental
Has an identity concern about himself and the kind of person he will become

Play Stimulation
Working for altruistic causes
Sports
Reading
T.V.
Music—records

Parental Guidance
Provide assistance in selection of and preparation for a vocation
Provide safety education—especially regarding driving
Provide assistance to develop good attitudes toward health—smoking, drinking, drugs, nutrition, etc.
Parents themselves may require assistance facing the loss of their dependent child
Assistance with solving problems of late adolescence, early adulthood

8. *Positive-supporting reflex*—when held in an erect position, baby will stiffen lower extremities and support his weight.

9. *Stepping reflex*—when infant is held in an erect position and then moved forward while tilted to one side, stepping action will be elicited on the other side.

10. *Babinski's sign*—scratching sole of foot causes great toe to flex and toes to fan.

11. *Crossed extensor reflex*—when one leg is extended and the knee is held straight, while the sole of foot is stimulated, the opposite leg will flex.

12. *Landau's sign*—when baby is suspended horizontally with head depressed against trunk and neck flexed, legs will flex and be drawn up to trunk.

13. Other characteristics of the newborn:

Cries	Makes discriminating sounds
Sucks	Sleeps for long intervals
Has extremely sensitive skin	Has little head control (head lag)

Infant to Adolescent

See tables on pages 1034–1047.

ESSENTIAL ELEMENTS OF PEDIATRIC NURSING

1. Parents must be closely involved with the child's hospitalization and the plan for his care. Parent participation is to be encouraged.

2. Nursing care should allow the child dependency thereby helping him to develop confidence and trust in the situation and at the same time assisting him to develop independency.

3. Nursing histories should be taken when child is admitted to the hospital. Questions should be asked to obtain information related to the following:
   a. Family situation
   b. Toilet habits
   c. Food preferences
   d. Home routines
   e. Schooling
   f. Experiences with illness
   g. Preparation for hospitalization

4. Explanation of the treatment plan and preparation for special tests, procedures and surgery are essential. These should be appropriate to:
   a. The child's age
   b. His level of comprehension

5. Play is a natural part of nursing care. It is important for the child's physical, emotional and social development.

6. Nursing care should relate illness to the child's personality, individual reaction and previous experiences. Recognition must be given to:
   a. What the child comes from
   b. What he is returning to
   c. What he is experiencing during his hospitalization

7. The ultimate goal in pediatric nursing is directed toward:
   a. Reduction of stress
   b. Increase in the child's feeling of well being

8. Nursing care is successful when its outcome is therapeutic and encompasses growth.

THE HOSPITALIZED CHILD
General Principles of Care

Emotional and Social Needs

1. The child has the same emotional and social needs during hospitalization as he does at home. He needs a chance to develop the following:
   a. Motor skills
   b. Social skills
   c. Language skills
   d. Psychological strengths
      (1) A sense of autonomy
      (2) Ego strength
      (3) A sense of identity
   e. Patterns of behavior

2. The hospitalized child has special needs—to deal with the many new problems that confront him:
   a. Separation from home and all that such a separation implies
   b. Problems concerning the illness itself
   c. Hospital rules and regulations
   d. Surgery
   e. Death

Impact of Age and Stage of Development on Hospitalized Child

The reactions and concerns of the hospitalized child are greatly influenced by his age and stage of growth and development.

A. *Infants and Toddlers*
   1. Concerns
      Separation anxiety—strong need to provide for continuity of care and affection
   2. Reactions
      a. May experience stages of protest, denial and despair
      b. Protest
         (1) Has urgent desire to find his mother.
         (2) Expects that she will answer his cries.
         (3) Frequently cries, shakes the crib, etc.
         (4) Rejects attention of nurses.
      c. Despair
         (1) Feels increasingly hopeless of finding his mother.
         (2) Becomes apathetic.
         (3) May cry monotonously or intermittently.
      d. Denial
         (1) Represses all feelings for his mother.
         (2) Does not cry when she leaves.
         (3) May seem more attached to nurses.
         (4) Finds little satisfaction in relationships with people.
   3. Tools for nursing intervention
      a. Rooming-in
      b. Promoting parent substitutes
      c. Explanations to parents regarding their child's reactions
      d. Diversional play
      e. Consistency in nursing personnel and approach to care

B. *Preschool Child*
  1. Concerns
      a. Separation anxiety continues.
      b. Is concerned about his body image and medical manipulations that may affect his body.
  2. Reactions
      a. Prone to develop fantasies associated with his illness and treatment.
          Need exists to help the child distinguish between reality and fantasy.
  3. Tools for nursing intervention
      a. Play
      b. Verbalization
      c. Allowing temporary regression
      d. Liberalized visiting hours
      e. Parent participation
      f. Consistency in nursing personnel and approach to care

C. *School-age Child*
  1. Concerns
      a. Has questions regarding his body and illness.
      b. Has additional concerns of helplessness, passivity and defenselessness.
  2. Reactions
      a. Tends to be phobic (normal tendency).
          (1) Fears include fear of:
              (a) Dark
              (b) Doctors
              (c) Hospitals
          (2) Unrealistic fears are commonly attached to needles, x-ray procedures, blood tests, etc.
      b. Frequently views hospitalization as a punishment for his misdeeds. Holds himself responsible for his illness.
  3. Tools for nursing intervention:
      a. Honesty in all explanations
      b. Play—especially in group situations
      c. Sharing in ward management
          (1) Pencil sharpening
          (2) Bed making
          (3) Errands, etc.
      d. Learning
          (1) Continuation of formal education
          (2) Informal education
              (a) How to use a microscope
              (b) How to apply a bandage, etc.

D. *Adolescent*
  1. Concerns
      a. Interference with his struggle for independence and emancipation from his parents.
      b. Illness is a major threat to his ego.
          Image is created which is different from his treasured self-image.
      c. Very threatened by helplessness.
      d. May see illness as a punishment for feelings not mastered or for breaking rules imposed by his parents or physician.
  2. Reactions
      a. Denial
      b. Withdrawal
      c. Disappointment
      d. Anger and hostility

3. Tools for nursing intervention
   a. Introduce the adolescent to the hospital staff and regular routines soon after admission.
   b. Provide opportunities for asking questions.
      (1) Answers must be honest.
      (2) Questions related to prognosis and therapeutic plan should be answered by one trusted person in whom he can confide.
   c. Allow independence in caring for his personal needs whenever feasible. Support the patient's active involvement in finding solutions to his problem.
   d. Provide privacy.
   e. Permit patient socialization and continuation of peer relationships with outside friends.
   f. Serve meals which reflect adolescent food preferences.
   g. Allow freedom in clothing.
   h. Encourage continuation of education.

Family Centered Care (Parent Participation)

Family centered care provides an opportunity for the family to care for the hospitalized child under nursing supervision.

Benefits for Parents and Child
1. Continued close family interactions during stress
2. Absence of separation anxiety
3. Greater sense of security for the child
4. Opportunity for family to fulfill their needs to care for their child physically and emotionally
5. Comfort for the family provided by other families
6. Greater absorption of staff teaching by the family
7. Lessening of guilty feeling parents have after a short visit

Benefits for Child
Family centered care can be of most benefit to the child while he is placed in this strange, frightening environment.
1. Healthy mother-child relationships can be maintained by helping to keep the child in touch with his family.
2. Reactions of protest, denial and despair are decreased or nonexistent.
   a. There is little inconsolable crying.
   b. Sleep is more relaxed.
3. The hospital experience can become but one event in the child's life.
4. Posthospital reactions are diminished.
5. The child receives a great sense of security from his parents.

Atmosphere
Family centered care units should present a relaxed, comfortable atmosphere.
1. Do not require parents to stay, but allow them to stay if they desire.
   a. Some mothers may be too anxious or guilty to participate.
   b. Outside responsibilities may prohibit parents staying.

2. Provide physical comfort for participating parents.
   a. Folding chair or bed in child's room.
   b. Comfortable lounge or waiting room.
   c. Eating facilities.
3. Encourage parent(s) to take frequent breaks from attending to the child.
   a. Provides rest for the parent.
   b. Helps child learn parent(s) will return and not abandon him.

Parent Needs in Family Centered Care

1. When parents are active participants in their child's care, they too have certain needs because they are concerned about their ill child.
   a. They want to care for their child like they would do at home.
   b. They are interested in working with the staff and learning from the staff how they can help their child.
   c. They like to keep busy and have something to do. This lessens their feeling of helplessness.
2. If parents know what is expected of them and what they can expect of the staff, many problems can be avoided. It helps parents feel more comfortable.
   a. What can parents do for their child?—bathe, play, feed.
   b. What activities will the nurse do in caring for the child?—give medications, assist with procedures.
   c. Parent should allow child to become involved with peers on the unit.
   d. Nursing and medical observations and care will be continued with or without the parents (mother) present.
   e. Parents are to take care of their own needs and not ask for personal services.

Parental Teaching

1. Parents have many methods of coping with their child's illness, i.e., denial, hope, anger, repeatedly asking same questions of everyone, doing everything for the child, being over-protective, etc. When parents are active in caring for their child, the nurse has an excellent opportunity to assess mother's (parents') state. This can be valuable.
   a. Spotting problems in parent-child relationships.
   b. Observing parents' attitudes, skills and techniques and the child's behavior and response to them.
   c. Helping to assess what teaching needs to be done.
   d. Evaluating the degree of participation of parent in physical and emotional care of the child.
   e. Helping parents not feel guilty because they cannot stay.
   f. Helping father establish or maintain his role of supporting mother and child, of keeping things going at home and of relieving mother in the hospital.
2. Families can offer a great deal of support to one another. Many times they have similar problems.
   a. Allow families to gather in groups—informal or formally planned group meetings.
   b. Formal group meetings usually provide a professional mental health team composed of social worker, psychiatrist, physician and nurse, as needed.

Nurse's Role

1. Staff must realize that parents are not time savers for nurses when they are participating in their child's care. The parents are not there to relieve the nurse of her routines and care.

   Additional nursing time is necessary to answer questions, orient parents to the unit, teach child care and comfort parents.

2. Family centered care places a great deal of responsibility on the nurse and offers an opportunity to administer total patient care to the child and his family. The nurse should begin to establish a positive working relationship with the parents and child upon admission.
   a. Parent teaching
      (1) Prepare parents to meet the child's needs during hospitalization.
      (2) Provide health teaching.
      (3) Offer anticipatory guidance.
   b. Interpret and reinforce what physician has told parents. Answer questions thoroughly and honestly as knowledge permits.
   c. Help to maintain healthy mother-child relationship. (Mother should not be threatened by the nurse.)
   d. Be perceptive of parents' physical and emotional needs and limitations.
      (1) Do not allow parents to become fatigued.
      (2) Allow parents to leave, take a break.
   e. Interpret medical procedures and diagnostic tests.
   f. Help parents adapt to this situation, increase their knowledge and develop their own feeling of value by coping with this illness.
   g. Supplement the family in the common goal of the child's welfare.
   h. Demonstrate understanding and acceptance of the parents and their feelings.

PREVENTIVE PEDIATRICS

Dental Care

Primary Teeth

1. Eruption
   a. 2 lower incisors—appear by 6–7 months
   b. 4 upper incisors—appear by 9 months
   c. 2 lower incisors—appear by 1 year
   d. 4 first molars—appear by 14 months
   e. 4 cuspids—appear by 18 months
   f. 4 second molars—appear by 2–2½ years
2. Importance of Primary Teeth and Dental Care for Primary Teeth
   a. By age 3, child should be examined by dentist when all primary teeth have erupted.
   b. When decayed primary teeth are neglected they endanger the child's health and may cause abscesses, fever and excessive pain. The infected teeth may damage the permanent tooth that is forming within the jaw. A child with advanced tooth decay finds it difficult to chew some foods that are essential to a well-balanced diet.

c. Primary teeth act as a guide for the proper positioning of permanent teeth. Each primary tooth is holding the space for a permanent tooth that will replace it. If a primary tooth is lost permanently, there will be a loss of space. This usually results in crowding of permanent teeth, ultimately requiring orthodontic work when a child is older.

d. Primary teeth serve as a stimulus for growth of the jaws, aid in the development of speech and serve a cosmetic function. Some young people become very self-conscious when they lose a tooth in the front of their mouth and realize that they look different. Indirectly, a child's speech may be affected if self-consciousness about his loss of teeth prevents him from opening his mouth for proper talking. Ability to use the teeth for pronunciation is acquired entirely with the aid of the primary teeth. Early loss of front teeth may lead to difficulty in pronouncing "s", "f", "l", "z", and "th". Even after the permanent teeth erupt, difficulty in pronouncing "s", "z", and "th" may persist to the point of requiring speech correction.

Permanent Teeth

1. Eruption
   a. 4 "6-year molars"—appear 6–7 years
   b. From this point onward, until 12–13 years of age, the primary teeth loosen, one by one, and each is replaced by a permanent tooth
   c. 4 additional molars appear at 12–13 years
   d. 4 molars ("wisdom teeth") appear at 17–21 years
2. Importance of Early Dental Care
   Care of teeth during infancy and childhood is necessary in order to:
   a. Promote proper development of the teeth
   b. Prevent dental caries

Nursing Management

1. Take advantage of incidental opportunities to teach children and their parents information that will promote dental health.
   Provide a well-balanced diet that is necessary for tooth development.
2. Provide supplemental fluoride if the local drinking water supply does not contain fluoride.
3. Maintain child's general health.
4. Encourage parents to arrange a dental visit when child is 3 years old and to continue to see the dentist on a regular basis.
5. Teach child good brushing habits.
6. Practice measures that will aid in avoiding cavities.
   a. Do not let child take bottle to bed with him; if child does take a bottle, put plain water in the bottle.
   b. Brush teeth after every meal and at bedtime.
   c. Reduce the amounts of sugar and sweets eaten by the child.
   d. Beware of foods that contain large amounts of sugar:

   Bubble and chewing gum
   Colas
   Peanut butter and jelly on white bread
   Candies, cookies, cakes
   Malted and sweet chocolate drinks
   Synthetic orange juice (artificially sweetened)
   White bread and raisin bread
   Sugar coated cereals

e. For the above foods substitute the following:

Sugarless gum

Diet colas

Cold cuts, cheese and hamburgers

Popcorn or potato chips

Skim milk

Orange juice

Peanuts

Whole wheat bread

Unsugared cereal

Immunization

Recommended Immunization Schedule

Age	Immunization
2–3 months	DPT[1], Trivalent OPV[2], or Type 1 OPV
3–4 months	DPT, Trivalent OPV, or Type 3 OPV
4–5 months	DPT, Trivalent OPV, or Type 2 OPV
9–11 months	Tuberculin test
12 months	Measles vaccine (live, attenuated)
15–18 months	DPT, Trivalent OPV, rubella vaccine (live attenuated)
2 years	Tuberculin test
3 years	DPT, Tuberculin test
4–5 years	Tuberculin test
6 years	TD[3], Tuberculin test, Trivalent OPV
7, 8, 9 and 10 years	Tuberculin test
12–16 years	TD, Tuberculin test

[1] DPT—Diphtheria and tetanus toxoids, and pertussis vaccine combined.

[2] OPV—Oral polio vaccine. If Trivalent OPV is used, interval should be 6 weeks longer.

[3] TD—Tetanus and diphtheria toxoids, adult type, for those over 6 years of age in contrast to DT (diphtheria and tetanus) containing a larger amount of diphtheria antigen.

General Considerations

1. Immunizations may be started at any age.
2. Immune response is limited in a proportion of young infants, and the recommended booster doses are designed to ensure and maintain immunity.
3. *Pertussis*
   a. Protection of infants against pertussis should start early.
   b. In newborn infants, the best protection against pertussis is avoidance of household contacts by adequate immunization of older siblings.
4. *DPT, OPV and measles immunizations*
   Some authorities recommend that these immunizations should always be given singly and never in combination.
5. *Tuberculin tests*
   a. Frequency of repeated tests dependent on:
      (1) Risk of exposure of children.
      (2) Prevalence of tuberculosis in the population group.
   b. In high risk situations, intervals between routine testing should not exceed 6 months.
   c. Under normal conditions where risk of exposure to active tuberculosis is remote, yearly testing should be adequate.
6. *Smallpox vaccination*
   a. No longer recommended in U.S.
   b. Where indicated (i.e., traveling), initial smallpox vaccine may be given at any time between 12–24 months of age (after age 12, every 3–10 years).

7. *Rubella vaccine*
   a. Live vaccine is recommended for boys and girls between the age of 1 year and puberty.
   b. Children in kindergarten should be given priority because they are the major source of virus dissemination.
   c. A history of rubella illness is not reliable enough to exclude children from immunization.
8. *Tetanus toxoid booster*
   After age 12, booster should be given every 10 years as TD.
9. *Mumps vaccine*
   All preadolescent or older males who have not experienced mumps should be immunized.

Nursing Management

1. Teach parents the importance of routine immunizations and tuberculin testing.
2. Refer parents whose children have not been immunized to either a pediatrician or health center where they may receive routine immunization and tuberculin testing.
3. Stress the importance of routine immunizations to the parents who have a chronically ill child and believe that immunizations would be harmful to him.
4. Be aware that immunizations are not given at a time when a child has signs of an acute illness.
5. Be aware that an interrupted primary series of immunizations need not be started again, but simply continued.
6. Inform parents that child may experience a low grade fever, irritability and soreness at the site of the injection following immunizations.

Safety

Principles of Safety

1. The child's developmental stage influences the types of accidents that are likely to occur.
   Potential accident situations may be foreseen by parents who have knowledge of their own child's typical patterns of growth and development.
2. Children are naturally curious, impulsive and impatient. The young child needs to touch, feel and investigate.
   a. Patient, adult supervision will enable the child to learn what he wants to know within the limits of safety for his stage of growth and development.
   b. Young children should never be left alone at home.
3. Children copy the behavior of their parents and absorb parental attitudes.
   Parents and other adults should be certain that their ways of doing things are safe.
4. Children become less careful and less willing to listen to warnings and observe routine safety precautions when they are tired or hungry.

General Areas of Adult Safety Responsibility

A. *Motor Vehicle*
   1. All automobiles should be maintained in good mechanical condition.
   2. Seat belts should be worn at all times.
   3. Driver should look carefully in front of and in back of the car before accelerating.

B. *Sports and Recreation*
   1. Keep equipment in good condition and proper working order.
   2. Wear appropriate clothing for the activity.
   3. Do not attempt activities beyond one's physical endurance.
   4. Keep firearms and ammunition locked up.

C. *Electrical and Mechanical Equipment*
   1. Only underwriter-approved devices should be installed; they should be inspected periodically.
   2. Dry hands before touching appliances.
      Keep radios, fans, portable heaters and hair dryers out of the bathroom.
   3. Disconnect appliances after use or before attempting minor repairs.
   4. Keep garden equipment and machinery in a restricted area.
      Teach proper use of the equipment as soon as the child is old enough.

D. *Prevention of Falls*
   1. Keep stairs well lighted and free from clutter.
   2. Provide sturdy railings.
   3. Anchor small rugs securely.
   4. Use rubber mats in the bathtub and shower.
   5. Use only sturdy ladders for climbing.

E. *Poisonings and Ingestions*
   1. Do not mix bleaches with ammonia, vinegar and other household cleaners.
   2. See section on ingested poisons, page 919.

F. *Fire*
   1. Maintain an adequate fire escape plan.
      Teach the child escape routes as soon as he is old enough.
   2. Keep a pressure-type hand fire extinguisher on each floor.
      Instruct all family members who are old enough in its use.
   3. Fit fireplaces with snug fireplace screens.
   4. Store gasoline and other flammable fluids in tightly covered containers that are clearly labeled and away from heat and sparks.
   5. Dispose of paint and oil soaked cloths quickly.

G. *Emergency Precautions*
   1. Record emergency phone numbers in an obvious and easily accessible place.
   2. Keep a well-stocked first-aid kit immediately available for emergencies.
   3. Instruct all family members who are old enough in principles of first aid.
      a. Responsible adults should enroll in first-aid courses offered by the Red Cross, adult education programs, etc.
      b. Be aware of first-aid procedures for:

Burns	Cuts, scrapes and punctures
Electric shock	Drowning
Poisoning	Fractures
Bites and stings	

   4. Know the location of gas, water and electrical switches and how to turn them off in an emergency.

H. *Miscellaneous*
   1. Take advantage of preventive health care.
      a. Obtain recommended immunizations.
      b. Have regular physical examinations.
   2. Seek immediate treatment of all diseases and health problems.
   3. Balance periods of work, rest and exercise in daily living.

Specific Safety Concerns Related to Child's Stage of Growth and Development

A. *Infants*

   Newborn babies are helpless and need absolute protection. When they begin to move about they need close supervision.
   1. They may wiggle, roll and shift position.
      a. The sides of the crib should be kept up at all times.
      b. The bars of the crib should be spaced so that the infant can't catch his head between them.
      c. The crib should not be placed near a radiator or heating unit.
      d. The crib should be away from windows with venetian blinds as the infant may become fatally entangled in a dangling cord.
      e. Babies should not be left unattended on anything from which they might fall.
         Infant seats should not be left on tables, beds, or other furniture.
      f. Infants should be strapped carefully in feeding chairs, infant seats, etc.
         A means should be provided to prevent the child from slipping down and being strangled by his waist strap.
      g. Well-constructed car seats should be used for traveling.
         (1) The car seat should carry the recommendation of the American Safety Belt Council.
         (2) The infant's seat belt should be secure around him.
   2. They may start to suck on toys, crib slats and other objects.
      a. Paints containing lead should not be used on toys, furniture or any other objects that the child is likely to put into his mouth.
      b. Stuffed toys should be checked carefully to be certain that eyes, etc., cannot be pulled off and eaten by the child.
      c. Small objects should not be left within the reach of the infant.
   3. They are helpless in water for the next several years.
      a. The temperature of the bath water should be checked carefully to avoid scalding.
      b. The child should never be left unattended in the bathtub for any reason.
   4. They are frequently victims of rats in highly populated metropolitan areas.
      a. The rats should be exterminated before the baby is discharged from the hospital.
      b. Infant beds should be high above the floor.
   5. They must be carried from one place to another.
      The adult who carries the infant should avoid walking on slippery floors or where toys or other small objects have been scattered.

B. *Toddlers*

   Toddlers are adventurous and are anxious to explore everything around them. Although they sometimes seem very mature and independent, they still require close adult supervision.
   1. They want to roam all over the house.
      a. Gates should be used at the head and foot of stairways to prevent falls.

    b. Fireplaces should be screened.

    c. Radiators should be enclosed or covered.

2. They poke and probe with their index finger.

    a. Sharp objects such as scissors, nail files, etc. should be kept out of reach.

    b. Bureau drawers and cabinets with anything potentially dangerous in them should be locked.

    c. Unused light sockets should be taped or capped.

    d. Electric fans or heaters should be out of reach.

    e. Electrical cords should be kept in good repair.

3. They are curious about many things, especially those things higher than their eye level.

    a. They should be lifted occasionally to satisfy their curiosity.

    b. Furniture should be balanced to prevent the child from pulling it over on himself.

    c. Hot, scalding foods should be kept out of the reach of children.

    d. All handles of pots and pans should be turned to the back of the stove.

    e. Tablecloths should not hang over the edge of the table.

    f. A small child should never be left alone in the kitchen. Hot ovens, toasters, coffee pots, irons, etc., pose a special threat to small children.

4. They put almost anything into their mouths.

    a. Medicines, lye, and household cleaning products should be locked up out of the reach of children.

    b. Pins, buttons, needles, etc., should be put away.

    c. Unbreakable toys that have no small removable parts should be used.

    d. The child should be closely supervised if he plays with a balloon. Aspiration of rubber from broken balloons can be fatal.

    e. Foods such as popcorn, peanuts and carrot sticks should not be offered to toddlers because of the danger of aspiration.

5. They climb onto things.

    a. Toddlers should be protected from falls.

      (1) Windows should have guards on them.

      (2) Screens should be firm and securely fastened.

    b. Car doors should be locked.

    c. Special equipment for climbing (small wooden grates, etc.) should be provided, and climbing should be done under adult supervision.

6. They like to play outside and in water.

    a. The toddler must have close supervision while playing outside.

    b. His play yard should be fenced.

    c. Ponds, pools, wells, etc., should be fenced or covered.

    d. The child should never be left alone in a wading pool.

    e. Caution should be used in allowing the toddler to play with older children. He may easily be injured by bats, hard balls, bicycles and rough play.

C. *Preschool Children*

Preschool children are very active and inquisitive. They begin to develop increased self-control, but still have an immature understanding of danger.

1. They can reach doorknobs and are anxious to explore the world beyond.

    a. Doors that open to potential danger should be locked.

    b. Bathroom doors should have locks which can be opened from the outside to prevent the child from locking himself in the room.

2. They enjoy taking things apart, putting them together again and experimenting with their use.
   a. Dangerous items such as knives, electrical equipment, etc., should be put away.
   b. Matches, lighters, etc., should be kept well out of the child's reach.
3. They are nimble on their feet and usually in a hurry.
   a. The child should not be allowed to walk or run while eating a lollipop.
   b. Stairs should have strong railings. They should be clear of objects or defective coverings on which a child can trip.
   c. Stairs and floors should not be highly waxed.
   d. Area rugs should be fixed.
4. They often enjoy cooperative play with others.
   a. Toy trucks or wagons should be strong enough to bear their weight as well as their playmates.
   b. They should be taught to ride tricycles on the sidewalk and to watch for cars in driveways.
   c. They should be cautioned not to run after the ball if it rolls into the street or driveway.
   d. Clothes should allow the child freedom of action and shoes should be suitable for running and climbing.
   e. The play area should be checked for such hazards as old refrigerators, deep holes, construction, broken glass and trash heaps.
   f. Swings and other equipment should be properly installed and maintained.
5. They are proud to run simple errands.
   They should not be asked to do anything hazardous such as crossing the street or carrying a knife or glass container.
6. They can take verbal direction and their attention span is lengthening. They can be instructed in the following areas.
   a. Personal safety
      (1) To identify information such as their name, address and telephone number.
      (2) To identify firemen, policemen, and other safety officials.
      (3) Not to accept gifts or rides from strangers.
   b. Home safety
      (1) The reasons for various safety measures such as keeping the floor clear of their toys, etc.
      (2) The safe way to use tools.
      (3) Kitchen safety.
      (4) The danger of matches, open flames, hot objects, and gas and electric equipment.
   c. Recreational safety
      Swimming instructions
   d. Motor-vehicle and pedestrian safety
      (1) Safety rules and the dangers of traffic.
      (2) Obedience to the rules.

D. *School-age Children*

School-age children are usually fairly independent. They still need discipline and rules but they also need to know *why* precautions are necessary and what the consequences are for failing to follow the rules.

1. They are anxious to make things and participate in household activities.
   a. They should be taught the proper use and storage of equipment.
      (1) Saws
      (2) Nails and hammer
      (3) Kitchen implements
      (4) Sewing machines
      (5) Gas and electric appliances
   b. They should be taught to wear protective devices over their eyes when doing anything potentially dangerous to their vision.
2. They enjoy holding and attending parties, carnivals, etc.
   Party costumes and equipment should be checked to be certain that they are flameproof.
3. They enjoy sports and outdoor play.
   a. Their whereabouts should be known at all times.
   b. The play areas should be inspected for broken glass, rusty nails, etc.
   c. They should be instructed regarding the dangers of playing in sand pits, old refrigerators, excavations, rickety shacks and deserted buildings.
   d. They must learn the rules of the sports that they play. They should have the proper equipment and keep it in good working condition.
   e. Ice skating and other water sports should always be closely supervised.
4. Areas for teaching:
   a. The rules of cycling safety should be emphasized.
      A child with a bicycle must learn the rules of the road as well as respect for the traffic officers and their directions.
   b. Pedestrian safety rules should also be stressed as motor accidents are the most common cause of accidental injury in this age group.
   c. Swimming instruction should be continued.
   d. The older child should be taught respect for fire, its uses and dangers.

E. *Adolescents*

Adolescents are increasingly independent. They should be able to build on their past experiences and accept responsibility for their own safety. Limits must still be set and direction given by adults because adolescents lack emotional maturity.
1. They may obtain driving licenses.
   a. They should learn to maintain their automobile in good mechanical condition.
   b. Seat belts should be worn at all times.
   c. They must be aware of traffic regulations and the penalty for not obeying them.
   d. They should be encouraged to participate in driver education and safety programs at school.
   e. Proper clothes should be worn while riding on motorcycles, motor scooters or motor-bikes. A safety helmet is essential.
2. They enjoy competing in competitive sports.
   Safeguards should be taken to prevent physical trauma when they want to do something beyond their physical endurance.
3. Their values and habits are greatly influenced by their peer groups and cliques.
   a. Parents should be aware of their child's activities.
   b. Constructive group activities should be encouraged.
   c. Formal instructions should be continued in the areas of sex education, drug and alcohol abuse and smoking.
      Open discussions with responsible adults should be encouraged.
4. Older adolescents are capable of assuming some responsibility for family safety measures.

a. They should be included in safety planning.
b. Their opinions and suggestions should be considered.
c. Specific areas of responsibility may be delegated to them.

LABORATORY VALUES: NORMAL RANGES IN CHILDREN

Urine

pH:	5–7
Specific gravity	
Infant	1.002–1.006
Child	1.005–1.018
Glucose	trace
Reducing substance	negative
Protein	less than 100 mg./24 hrs.
Sodium	43–211 mEq./L.
Potassium	26–125 mEq./L.
Chlorides	170–250 mEq./L.
Nitrogen	85–500 mg./24 hrs.
Creatinine	
Newborn	10–15.5 mg./kg./24 hrs.
2–3 years	12 mg./kg./24 hrs.
6–12 years	6.4–21.9 mg./kg./24 hrs.
RBC	<1,000,000 ⎫
WBC	<1,000,000 ⎬ Addis Count/12 hrs.
Casts	<10,000 ⎭

Blood Chemistries

Enzymes

Amylase	90–300 mg./100 ml.
	70–200 Somogyi units
	6–33 Close Street units
Alkaline phosphatase	
1–3 months	4.4–14.0 BLB units
	7.3–226 mU./ml.
2–12 years	2.8–9 BLB units
	46.5–111.2 mU./ml.
Adolescent	3.4–15.5 BLB units
	57–258 mU./ml.
SGPT	
Infant	27–54 mU./ml.
Child	1–30 mU./ml.
SGOT	
Infant	0–54 mU./ml.
Child	1–25 mU./ml.
Acid phosphatase	
Newborn	0.62–0.99 BLB units
	10.4–16.4 mU./ml.
2–13 years	0.52–0.78 BLB units
	8.6–13.0 mU./ml.

Nitrogen Constituents

Urea nitrogen	5–20 mg./100 ml.
Creatinine	2–6 mg./100 ml.
Ammonia	
Newborn	90–150 mg./100 ml.
Child	40–80 mg./100 ml.

Proteins

Total proteins (plasma)	
Birth	0.6–10 gm./100 ml.
1–4 years	6.5–7.3 gm./100 ml.
5–12 years	6.8–7.8 gm./100 ml.
over 12 years	7.16 gm./100 ml.
Total protein (serum)	6.5–7.5 gm./100 ml.

Carbohydrates and Pigments

Fasting glucose	55–110 mg./100 ml.
Total bilirubin	
Premature at 24 hrs.	1.0–6.0 mg./100 ml.
Premature at 48 hrs.	6.0–8.0 mg./100 ml.
Premature at 3–5 days	10–15.0 mg./100 ml.
Full term at 24 hrs.	2.0–6.0 mg./100 ml.
Full term at 48 hrs.	6.0–7.0 mg./100 ml.
Full term at 3–5 days	4.0–12.0 mg./100 ml.
After newborn period	less than 0.8 mg./100 ml.

Acid-Base Constituents (Electrolytes and Blood Gases)

Sodium	134–151 mEq./L.
Potassium	
0–10 days	up to 7 mEq./L.
After 10 days	3.2–6 mEq./L.
Chlorides	94–108 mEq./L.
Phosphorus	
1st year	4.2–8.5 mg./100 ml.
1–12 years	4.5–6.5 mg./100 ml.
pH	7.35–7.45
pO_2	80–100 mm.Hg
pCO_2	35–45 mm.Hg
CO_2	20–25 mm./L.
CO_2 combining power	19–30 mEq./L.
Calcium	
Neonate	8–11 mg./100 ml.
	4.5–5.5 mEq./L.
Child	9.0–12 mg./100 ml.
	5.0–6.0 mEq./L.

Hematology

Age	% Gm. Hg.	% Hct.	Platelets/cu. mm. (in thousands)	WBC/cu. mm.	% Reticulocytes
Birth	16–22	53–73	350.0	15–18	2.5–6.5
3 months	11.4–12.2	36–38	260.0	5–18	0.7–3.0
6 months	11.8–12	35–40	250.0	6–16	0.7–2.3
1 year	11.2–12.2	35–40	250.0	6–15	0.6–1.7
2–8 years	11.5–13.1	35.5–43	250.0	7–13	0.5–1.5
8–12 years	12–14.1	37–46	250.0	5–12	0.5–1.0

Age	RBC/cu. mm. (in millions)	% Polymorphonuclear Leukocytes	Eosinophils Basophils	Lymphocytes	Monocytes
Birth	5.1	45–85	3	30	12
3 months	4.3	30–50	3	55	7
6 months	4.6	30–50	3	51	6
1 year	4.7	30–50	2	53	5
2–8 years	4.8	35–55	2	40–50	8
8–12 years	5.1	60	2	30	8

Cerebrospinal Fluid

Initial pressure
  Newborn — 50–90 mm. CSF
  Infant — 40–150 mm.
  Child — 70–200 mm.
Specific gravity — 1.005–1.009
pH (at 38° C.) — 7.33–7.42
Cell count
  Newborn — up to 25 WBC (8 average), up to 650 RBC/mm.
  1–12 months — up to 10 cells/cu. mm.
  1–4 years — up to 8 cells/cu. mm.
  5–13 years — 0–5 cells/cu. mm.
Calcium — 4.5–5.5 mg./100 ml.
Chlorides — 120–125 mEq./L.
Glucose
  Infant — 40–80 mg./100 ml.
  6–10 months — 71–90 mg./100 ml.
  over 10 years — 50–80 mg./100 ml.
Protein
  Newborn — 40–120 mg./100 ml.
  over 1 month — 20–70 mg./100 ml.
LDH
  0–10 days — 2.3–84 mU./ml.
  over 10 days — 6.3–30 mU./ml.

BIBLIOGRAPHY

Books

Ausubel, D. P., and Sullivan, E. V.: Theory and Problems of Child Development, 2nd ed. New York, Grune and Stratton, 1970.
Blake, F. G.: The Child, His Parents and The Nurse. Philadelphia, J. B. Lippincott, 1954.
Blake, F. G., et al.: Nursing Care of Children, 8th ed. Philadelphia, J. B. Lippincott, 1970.
Children are Different. Ross Laboratories, Columbus, Ohio, 1971.
Hammer, S. L., and Eddy, J.: Nursing Care of the Adolescent. New York, Springer Publishing Company, 1966.
Hardgrove, C. B., and Dawson, R. B.: Parents and Children in the Hospital. Boston, Little, Brown and Co., 1972.
The Harriet Lane Handbook: A Manual for Pediatric House Officers. Johns Hopkins Hospital. Chicago, Year Book Medical Publishers, Inc., 1969.
Hellmuth, J. (ed.): Exceptional Infant. New York, Brunner-Mazel, 1967.
Hughes, J. G.: Synopsis of Pediatrics. St. Louis, C. V. Mosby, 1971.
James, J. A.: Renal Disease in Children. St. Louis, C. V. Mosby, 1972.
Marlow, D.: Textbook of Pediatric Nursing. Philadelphia, W. B. Saunders, 1973.
Nelson, W. E.: Textbook of Pediatrics. Philadelphia, W. B. Saunders, 1969.
Petrillo, M.: The Emotional Care of Hospitalized Children. Philadelphia, J. B. Lippincott, 1972.
Petrillo, M., and Sanger, S.: Emotional Care of the Hospitalized Child. Philadelphia, J. B. Lippincott, 1972.
Plank, E. N.: Working With Children in Hospitals. Chicago, The Press of Case Western Reserve University, 1971.
Standards of Child Health Care, 2nd ed. Evanston, Illinois, American Academy of Pediatrics, 1972.
Stone, L., and Church, J.: Childhood and Adolescence, 2nd ed. New York, Random House, 1968.
Vernon, D., et al.: The Psychological Responses of Children to Hospitalization and Illness: A Review of the Literature. Springfield, Illinois, Charles C Thomas, 1965.
Whipple, D. V.: Dynamics of Development: Euthenic Pediatrics. New York, McGraw-Hill, 1966.

Articles

Colella, R. F.: Dental care. Ped. Clin. N. Amer., *15*:325, 1968.
Condon, M., and Peters, C.: Family participation unit. Amer. J. Nurs., *68*:504–8, March 1968.
Davis, V.: Through the bars of a crib. Amer. J. Nurs., *71* (No. 9), 1752–1753, Sept. 1971.
Francis, B. J.: Current concepts in immunization. Amer. J. Nurs., *73*:646–649, April 1973.
Petrillo, M.: Preventing hospital trauma in pediatric patients. Amer. J. Nurs., *68*:1469–1473, July 1968.
Schowalter, J. E., and Lord, R. D.: The hospitalized adolescent. Children, *18*:127–132, July-August 1971.
Scofield, C.: Parents in the hospital. Nurs. Clin. N. Amer., *4*:59–67, March 1969.
Selected Papers from the Sixth Annual Conference, American Association for Child Care in Hospitals. "Needs of Children in the Hospital." May 19–22, 1971. Cleveland, American Association for Child Care in Hospitals, 1972.
Selected articles: Symposium on family-centered care in a pediatric setting. Nurs. Clin. N. Amer., *7* (No. 1):1–94, March 1972.
Smith, M.: Ego support for the child patient. Amer. J. Nurs., *63* (No. 10):90–95, October 1963.
Stokes, J.: Pediatric immunization and the new academy schedule. Hosp. Prac., *7*:127, 1972.

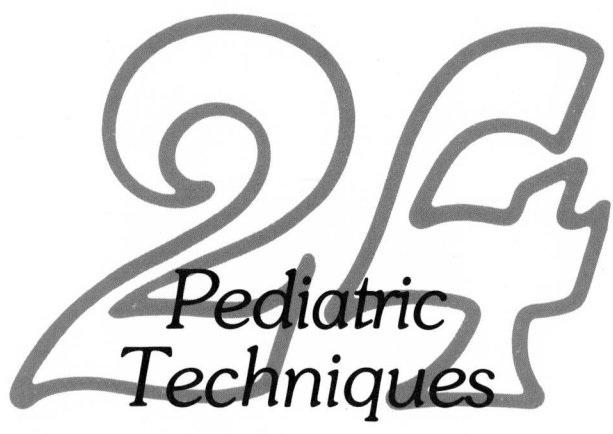

Pediatric Techniques

MEASURING VITAL SIGNS IN CHILDREN

Normal Vital Sign Ranges in Children

Pulse or Heart Rate

Age	Range	Average
0–24 hrs	70–170/minute	120/minute
1–7 days	100–180/minute	140/minute
1 month	110–188/minute	160/minute
1 month–1 year	80–180/minute	120–130/minute
2 years	80–140/minute	110/minute
4 years	80–120/minute	100/minute
6 years	70–115/minute	100/minute
10 years	70–110/minute	90/minute
12–14 years	60–110/minute	85–90/minute
14–18 years	50–95/minute	70–75/minute

Respiration Rate

Age	Range
Birth	30–60/minute
1 month–1 year	26–34/minute
2 years	20–30/minute
2–6 years	20–30/minute
6–10 years	18–26/minute
10–18 years	15–24/minute

Temperature

Oral 36.4–37.2°C. (97.6–99°F.)
Rectal 37.0–37.8°C. (98.6–100°F.)
Axillary 35.9–36.7°C. (96.6–98°F.)

Blood Pressure

Age	Systolic	Diastolic
Birth	40	—
1 month	80	—
4 years	85	60
5 years	87	60
6 years	90	60
8 years	95	62
10 years	100	65
11 years	105	65
13 years	110	67
15 years	115	72
16 years	118	75

Temperature

1. Normal body temperature represents a balance between the body heat produced and body heat lost.
2. Rectal temperature is indicated when the following conditions exist:
   a. Child is under 5 years of age (varies with the child).
   b. Child has seizures.

     c. Child exhibits poor muscle control and therefore may bite the thermometer.

     d. Child has had oral surgery.

     e. Child has difficulty breathing.

     f. Child is receiving oxygen.

  3. Rectal temperature is contraindicated in the following instances:

     a. Following rectal surgery

     b. Diarrhea

  4. Never leave the child alone when taking his temperature.

  5. For security, safety and accuracy keep one hand on the thermometer when it is in place.

  6. Record and report an elevated or subnormal temperature.

Pulse

  1. Take apical rate on an infant.

     a. Place stethoscope between left nipple and sternum.

     b. Take heart rate for 1 full minute.

  2. With an older child, the pulse rate may be obtained at the radial, temple or neck locations. (The pulse may be taken for 30 seconds and multiplied by 2.)

  3. Take pulse rate prior to taking temperature because child may cry when temperature is taken, thereby increasing the pulse rate and making it more difficult to hear the apical rate.

  4. Record accurately the following:

     a. Activity of child at time pulse is taken   c. Quality of pulse

       (1) Sleeping   d. Rate

       (2) Crying

     b. Regularity or irregularity of rate

  5. Record and report immediately any changes in pulse characteristics.

Respirations

  1. Count respirations on an infant for 1 full minute.

     Observe chest movements as well as abdominal movements.

  2. Respirations may be counted for 30 seconds and multiplied by 2 in the older child.

  3. Obtain respiratory rate prior to taking temperature since child may cry when temperature is taken.

  4. Note and record accurately the following:

     a. Rate and character of respirations   d. Any signs of respiratory distress

     b. Activity of the child during observation   (1) Retractions

     c. Color of patient   (2) Nasal flaring

  5. Record and report immediately any change in respirations.

Blood Pressure

Generally, the technique for taking the blood pressure of a child is the same as for the adult. The following principles are important to observe when dealing with the pediatric patient.

  1. The cuff must cover two-thirds of the length of the upper arm or leg. Even small variations in cuff size may produce significant inaccuracies in blood pressure readings.

     a. A cuff that is too narrow will produce an apparent increase in blood pressure.

b. A cuff that is too wide will produce an apparent decrease in blood pressure.

c. A flexible blood pressure cuff that can be folded to the correct size is frequently easier and more effective for the nurse to use than choosing among several assorted premeasured cuffs.

2. If the child is excited, uncomfortable or distrusts the person taking the blood pressure, the systolic pressure may rise as much as 50 mm. Hg above the usual level.

   a. The blood pressure should be taken when the child is at rest and in a consistent position.

   b. The procedure should be explained to the child before it is done.
      (1) He should know that it will not hurt.
      (2) He should be allowed to handle the equipment, pump the cuff, etc.
      (3) It may be necessary for the child to use the equipment on his parents, the nurse or a doll in order for him to overcome his fears or understand its use.

3. It is very difficult to obtain an accurate blood pressure reading in infants. The following methods may be used.

   a. Auscultatory method
      (1) Can frequently be obtained if the stethoscope head is small enough.
      (2) This is the method of choice whenever possible.

   b. Palpatory method
      (1) The cuff is inflated to about 200 mm. Hg.
      (2) The reading is taken when the pulse distal to the cuff becomes palpable in the course of deflation.
      (3) The reading lies between the systolic and diastolic pressures obtained by the auscultatory method.

   c. Flush method
      (1) The infant should be quiet and in the supine position.
      (2) A blood pressure cuff is applied to the wrist or ankle.
      (3) The extremity is compressed by firm wrapping so that blood is pressed from the area distal to the cuff.
      (4) The cuff is inflated to about 200 mm. Hg and the wrapping is removed.
      (5) The pressure in the cuff is slowly deflated.
      (6) The reading is taken at the point at which blood re-enters the hand or foot causing a sudden flushing.
      (7) This method also has the disadvantage of providing only an approximate mean pressure.

Principles Related to Pediatric Blood Pressure Values

1. The blood pressure varies with the age of the child and is closely related to his height and weight.

   a. There is a gradual rise in systolic blood pressure during growth.

   b. Diastolic blood pressure rises only slightly between the ages of 6–18 years.

   c. Significant increases in blood pressure occur during adolescence with many temporary variations.

2. Variability of blood pressure among children of approximately the same age and body build is normal.

3. The pressure in the legs with the cuff technique is ordinarily 20 mm. Hg higher than in the arms.

ADMINISTERING MEDICATIONS TO CHILDREN

Purpose

To safely administer medications to the child as prescribed by the physician.

Important Considerations

1. The nurse's manner of approach should indicate that she firmly expects the child to take the medication. This manner often convinces the child of the necessity of the procedure.
2. Explanation about the medication should appeal to the child's level of understanding (i.e., color, comparison to something familiar).
3. The nurse must mask her own feelings regarding the medication.
4. Always be truthful when the child asks, "Does it taste bad?" or "Will it hurt?" Respond by saying, "The medicine does not taste good, but I will give you some juice as soon as you swallow it", or "It will hurt for just a minute, like a mosquito bite."
5. It is often necessary to mix distasteful medications or crushed pills with a small amount of coke or cherry syrup, honey or applesauce.
6. Never threaten a child with an injection if he refuses an oral medication.
7. Medications should not be mixed with large quantities of food or any food that is taken regularly (i.e., milk).
8. Medications should not be given at mealtime unless specifically ordered.

Calculating the Pediatric Dosage

It is not the nurse's responsibility to decide upon the dosage of a drug.
1. Know what factors determine the amount of drug ordered.
2. Be alert to an order that would be inappropriate for a child.
3. Consult drug literature for recommended dosage per kg. (or lb.) of body weight— is the most accurate method of calculating appropriate drug dosage for child. (Dosages recommended according to age groups are not satisfactory since a child may be much smaller or larger than the average child in his age group.)

Clark's Rule

The following rule may be used as an estimate of the pediatric dosage based on the child's weight in respect to the adult dose of the drug.

$$\frac{\text{Child's Weight in Pounds}}{150} \times \text{Adult Dose} = \text{Approximate Dose for Child}$$

Identifying the Patient

Always check a child's identification bracelet before administering a medication.

Oral Medications

A. *Infants*
1. Draw up medication in a plastic dropper or disposable syringe.
2. Elevate infant's head and shoulders: depress chin with thumb to open mouth.
3. Place dropper or syringe on the middle of the tongue and slowly drop the medication on the tongue.
4. Release thumb and allow child to swallow.

B. *Toddlers*
   1. Draw up medication in syringe or medicine cup.
   2. Elevate the child's head and shoulders.
   3. Squeeze cup and put the cup to the child's lips, or place the syringe (without the needle) in the child's mouth and slowly expel the medicine.
   4. Allow child time to swallow.
   5. A child may be able to hold the medicine cup and take the medicine himself.

C. *School-age children*
   1. When a child is old enough to take medicine in pill or capsule form, he should be taught to place the pill near the back of his tongue and immediately swallow fluid such as water or fruit juice. If the swallowing of the fluid is emphasized, the child will no longer think about the pill.
   2. Always praise a child after he has taken his medication.

Intramuscular Injections (Fig. 24-1)

A. *Infants*
   1. Site selection
      Lateral and anterior aspect of the thigh
   2. Administration
      a. Place the child in a secure position to prevent movement of the extremity.
      b. Do not use a needle longer than 2.5 cm.

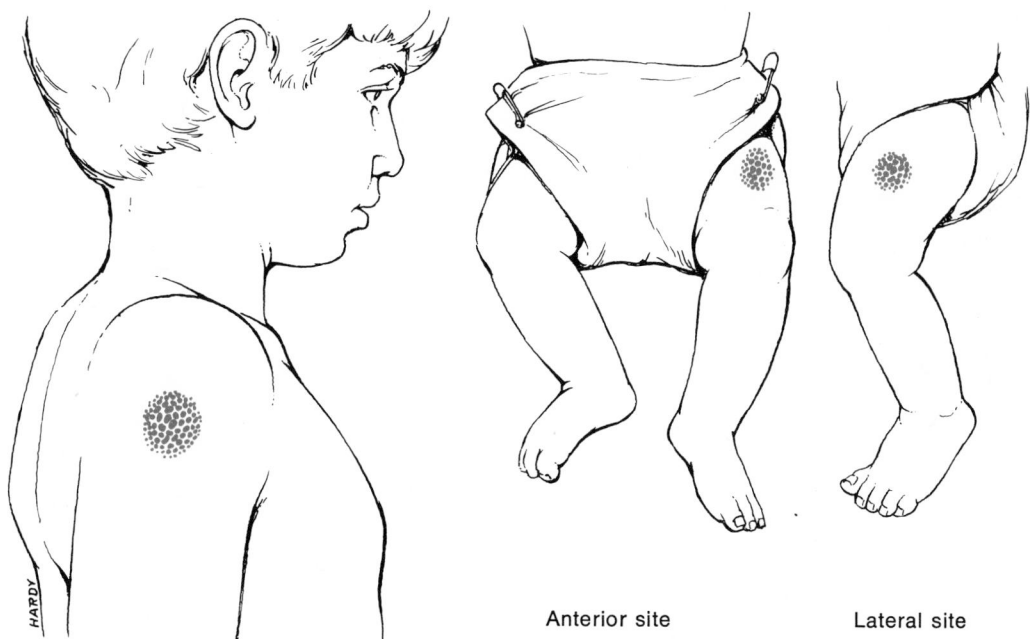

Anterior site   Lateral site

Arm for older child   Leg for small infants

Figure 24-1. Sites for I.M. injections.

     c. Use upper outer quadrant of the thigh.

     d. Insert needle at a 45-degree angle in a direction downward toward the knee.

     e. Hold and cuddle the infant following the injection.

B. *Toddlers and School-age Children*

  1. Site selection

    a. *Dorsogluteal*—upper outer quadrant

      (1) Gluteal muscles do not develop until child begins to walk; they should be used only when child has been walking for one year or more.

      (2) Upper outer quadrant of the young child's buttock is smaller in diameter than an adult's; thus accuracy in determining the area comprising the upper outer quadrant is essential.

      (3) Administration

        (a) Do not use a needle longer than 2.5 cm.

        (b) Position the child in a prone position.

        (c) Place thumb on the trochanter.

        (d) Place middle finger on the iliac crest.

        (e) Let index finger drop at a point midway between the thumb and middle finger to the upper outer quadrant of the buttock.

        (f) Insert needle perpendicular to the surface on which the child is lying, not perpendicular to the skin.

    b. *Ventrogluteal*

      (1) This site provides a dense muscle mass which is relatively free of the danger of injuring the nervous and vascular systems.

      (2) The disadvantage is that the injection site is visible to the child.

      (3) Administration

        (a) Place child on his back.

        (b) Place index finger on the anterosuperior spine.

        (c) With the middle finger moving dorsally, locate the iliac crest; drop finger below the crest. The triangle formed by the iliac crest, index finger and middle finger is the injection site.

    c. *Deltoid*

      (1) May be used for older, larger children.

      (2) Determine injection site as with an adult.

    d. *Lateral and anterior aspect of the thigh*

      (1) Do not use a needle longer than 2.5 cm.

      (2) Use the upper outer quadrant of the thigh.

      (3) Insert needle at a 45-degree angle in a direction downward toward the knee.

  2. Nursing support

    a. Explain to the child where you are going to give him the injection (site) and why he must receive the injection.

    b. Allow the child to express his fears.

    c. Carry out procedure quickly and gently.

    d. Always secure the assistance of a second nurse to help immobilize the child and divert his attention.

    e. Praise the child for his behavior after the injection.

    f. Utilize play opportunities to help him master his feelings about injections.

PROTECTIVE MEASURES TO LIMIT MOVEMENT
(Restraints)

Protective measures to limit movement are mechanisms for restraining children (Fig. 24-2).

Purpose

1. To maintain the child's safety and protect him from injury.
2. To facilitate examination and minimize the child's discomfort during special tests, procedures and specimen collections.

Underlying Principles

1. Protective devices should be used only when necessary and never as a substitute for careful observation of the child.
2. The reason for using the protective device should be explained to the child and his parents to prevent misinterpretation and to ensure their cooperation with the procedure.
3. Any protective device should be checked frequently to make sure that it is effective. It should be removed periodically to prevent skin irritation or circulation impairment.
4. Protective devices should always be applied in a manner which maintains proper body alignment and ensures the child's comfort.
5. Any protective device which requires attachment to the child's bed should be secured to the bed springs or frame, *never* the mattress or side rails. This allows the side rails to be adjusted without removing the restraint or injuring the child's extremity.
6. Any knots which are required, should be tied in a manner which permits their quick release. This is a safety precaution.

Mummy Device

The mummy device involves securing a sheet or blanket around the child's body in such a way that his arms are held to his sides and his leg movement is restricted (Fig. 24-2).

A. *Purpose*

To restrain infants and small children during treatments and examinations involving the head and neck.

B. *Equipment*

Small sheet or blanket
Several large safety pins

C. *Nursing Action*
1. Place the blanket or sheet flat on the bed.
2. Fold over one corner of the blanket.
3. Place the child on the blanket with his neck at the edge of the fold.
4. Pull the right side of the blanket firmly over the child's right shoulder.
5. Tuck the remainder of the right side of the blanket under the left side of the child's body.
6. Repeat the procedure with the left side of the blanket.
7. Pin the blanket in place.

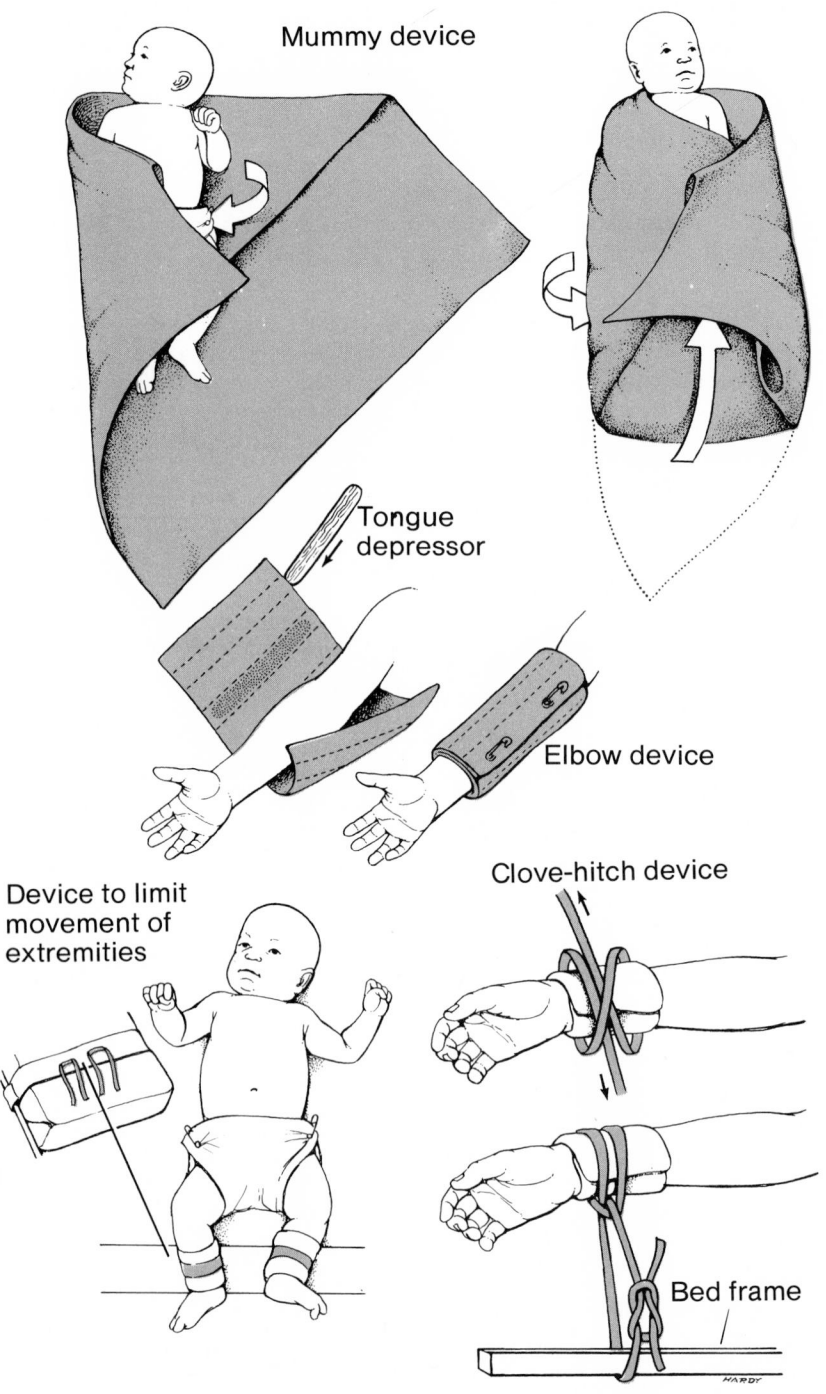

Figure 24-2. Restraints.

D. *Special Precautions*

Make certain that the child's extremities are in a comfortable position during this procedure.

Jacket Device

The *jacket device* is a piece of material which fits the child as a jacket or halter. Long tapes are attached to the sides of the jacket.

A. *Purpose*

To keep the child in his wheelchair, highchair or crib.

B. *Nursing Action*

1. Put the jacket on the child with the opening in the back.
2. Tie the strings securely.
3. Position the child in his highchair, wheelchair or crib.
4. Secure the long tapes appropriately:
   a. Under the arm supports of a chair.
   b. Around the back of the wheelchair or highchair.
   c. To the springs or frame of the crib.

C. *Special Precautions*

The child in a crib must be observed frequently to make certain that he does not entangle himself in the long tapes of the jacket device.

Belt Device

The *belt device* is exactly like the jacket method of restraining, except that the material fits the child like a wide belt and buckles in the back.

Elbow Device

The *elbow device* consists of a piece of material into which tongue depressors have been inserted at regular intervals (Fig. 24-2). It is especially useful for infants receiving scalp-vein infusion, those with eczema or cleft lip repair and children having eye surgery.

A. *Purpose*

To prevent flexion of the elbow.

B. *Equipment*

Elbow cuff
Tongue depressors
Safety pins, tapes or string

C. *Nursing Action*

1. Insert tongue depressors into the appropriate places in the elbow cuff.
2. Place the child's arm in the center of the elbow cuff.
3. Wrap the cuff around the child's arm.
4. Secure the cuff with pins, tapes or string.

D. *Special Precautions*
1. The tongue depressors should be cut to about 10 cm. (4 inches) in length if the elbow cuff is to be used for an infant—is most comfortable for infant.
2. Additional security may be provided by dressing the child in a long-sleeved shirt prior to the application of the elbow cuff. The ends of the shirt can then be turned back over the cuff and pinned securely.

Devices to Limit Movement of the Extremities

There are many different kinds of devices to limit motion of one or more extremities. One commercial variety consists of a piece of material with tapes on both ends to be secured on the frame of the crib. The material also has 2 small flaps sewn to it for securing the ankles or wrists of the child (Fig. 24-2).

A. *Purpose*
To restrain infants and young children for such procedures as intravenous therapy and urine collections.

B. *Equipment*
Extremity restraint of appropriate size for the child (small, medium or large)
Several safety pins
Cotton wadding covered with gauze

C. *Nursing Action*
1. Secure the device to the crib frame.
2. Pad the extremities to be used with cotton wadding covered with gauze or other suitable material.
3. Pin the small flaps securely around the child's ankles or wrists.
4. Adjust the device by pinning a tuck in the center of the material if it is too large.

D. *Special Precautions*
The infant's fingers or toes should be observed frequently for coldness or discoloration and the skin under the device checked for signs of irritation.

Clove-hitch Device

The clove-hitch device is a mechanism for restraining an extremity by tying gauze strips or a diaper in a certain manner (Fig. 24-2).

A. *Equipment*
Cotton wadding covered with gauze
Gauze bandage or diapers cut in lengths of 137 cm. (1½ yards)

B. *Nursing Action*
1. Pad the extremity to be restrained with the cotton wadding covered with gauze or other suitable material.
2. Spread out the gauze strip or diaper on the bed.
3. Make a figure-8 loop in the center of the gauze strip or diaper (Fig. 24-2).
4. Place the child's wrist or ankle in the loop of the device.
5. Pull the ends of the device to the desired tightness.
6. Tie the ends to the crib springs or frame.
7. Check the device to make certain that it does not tighten when both ends are pulled taut or slip over the child's hand or foot.

FEEDING AND NUTRITION

GUIDELINES: *Breast Feeding the Ill or Hospitalized Infant* *

Breast feeding is suckling of an infant at the mother's breast to provide him with nourishment.

Purposes

1. To provide psychological and emotional satisfaction for the infant and the mother.
2. To feed the infant a natural and ideal food that will supply him with adequate nutrition.
3. To always have milk available, at the right temperature.
4. To prevent chance of gastrointestinal disturbances and development of allergies.
5. To provide a physical closeness of baby to mother during feeding.

Equipment

Clear water
Cotton balls

Procedure

Nursing Action	Rationale/Amplification
Preparatory Phase	
1. When an infant who is nursing is hospitalized, it is nurse's responsibility to encourage the mother to continue breast feeding if the infant's condition does not contraindicate it. Explain to the mother that: a. Supplemental artificial formula can be given to the infant if she is not available or b. She can pump her breasts and bring in her milk to be given to the infant via bottle when she is not available.	1. Some mothers have very strong feelings about wanting to nurse their baby. It gives them an emotional satisfaction that is vitally important to the mother-child relationship. The nurse must help to foster this relationship as much as she can.
2. When nursing is to be done in the hospital pediatric setting, the physical setting may need to be altered somewhat. Provide the mother and infant with a relatively quiet area that is as private as possible and free from interruption.	2. This will provide the mother and infant with an opportunity to continue to develop their relationship during the crisis of illness and hospitalization.
3. Provide the mother with a comfortable armchair or pillow so that she can assume a comfortable position during the feeding. A footstool should also be available so she can support her feet and the infant.	3. Proper and comfortable position of the mother will enable her to hold the baby correctly and support him while he is at the breast.
4. The infant should be awake and dry before the feeding is started.	4. If the infant is comfortable he will settle down and feed better.
5. Dress the infant appropriately so that he is not too warm or too cool during the feeding. The infant should also be hungry.	5. If he is too warm, he may fall asleep after the first few sucks of milk. A sleepy baby will not nurse well. If he is too cool, he may be fussy and restless.
6. Have mother wash her hands. Then she should wash her nipples with clear water and cotton balls.	6. Washing the nipples will remove any old milk that may have leaked and dried on them, providing a good media for bacteria to grow and cause gastrointestinal disturbance in the infant.

* See p. 1003 for breast feeding the newborn.

Nursing Action	**Rationale/Amplification**
7. Position the baby at breast. Put him in a semi-sitting position with his face close to the breast supported by one arm and hand. A pillow may be used under the baby to support him. The breast may need to be supported by mother's other hand.	7. Proper positioning will provide the infant with comfort and security and make it easier for him to suck and swallow. This makes the nipple more easily accessible to the infant's mouth and prevents obstruction of nasal breathing.

Performance Phase

1. When the feeding is to start, let the breast touch the infant's cheek. Do not hold his cheek and try to help him find the nipple.	1. The rooting reflex will take over and the infant will turn his head toward the breast with his mouth open. If his cheek is touched with a hand, he will become confused, perhaps turning toward the hand.
2. The infant's lips should be out over the areola and not just around the nipple before he begins to suck.	2. Since the nipple is so small, suction cannot be achieved merely by grasping it. The areola must be in the infant's mouth in order to establish suction and make the suck effective.
3. Note the presence or absence of the "let-down" reflex during the nursing period.	3. Milk flowing from the other breast during nursing is quite normal. It is not usually present when the mother is worried.
4. The length of feeding time may vary from 5–20 minutes. Let the infant nurse until he is satisfied.	4. When the infant is satisfied and has nursed well, he will be relaxed and usually falls asleep. He will stop sucking.
5. Instruct the mother to bubble the baby during and at the end of the feeding.	5. When the infant is sucking he swallows some air. Bubbling will help prevent abdominal distention and discomfort as well as regurgitation.
6. One or both breasts may be used at each feeding. It doesn't matter as long as (a) baby is satisfied at the end of the feeding and (b) one breast is completely emptied at the feeding.	6. Regular and complete emptying of the breast is the only stimulation for the production and secretion of milk.
7. Once the infant has stopped sucking, he likes to cling to the breast. To break this suction, instruct mother to put her finger to the corner of the baby's mouth and gently pull.	7. Pulling will not hurt mother or infant.

Follow-up Phase

1. When the infant has finished feeding, change his diaper if it is wet or soiled.	1. To provide comfort for a restful sleep and to prevent diaper rash.
2. Position infant on his right side or on his abdomen in his bed.	2. This facilitates emptying of the stomach and decreases the possibility of regurgitation.
3. Note if baby appears satisfied or still seems to be hungry.	3. Mother may not have enough milk to satisfy the baby. Supplemental formula may be necessary.
4. Chart descriptively and accurately: a. How baby fed b. How baby went to breast c. Satiety or hunger after feeding d. Breast or breasts used; which breast was emptied and which breast was nursed from thereafter.	d. If both breasts were used, the second breast is not usually emptied and should be used first at the next feeding.

GUIDELINES: *Artificial or Nipple Feeding*

Artificial or nipple feeding is a method of supplying nutrition to the infant by oral feedings, using a bottle and nipple set-up.

Purposes

1. To provide the baby adequate fluid and caloric intake for appropriate growth.
2. To supplement breast feeding with formula or water.
3. To provide additional fluid intake between feedings.

Equipment

Sterile nipple and bottle
Sterile formula or feeding fluid

Procedure

Nursing Action	Rationale/Amplification
Preparatory Phase	
1. Baby should be awake and hungry. Change wet or soiled diaper.	1. A sleepy baby will not feed well. A dry diaper will provide comfort so the baby will settle down and eat more easily.
2. Check formula for correct type and amount.	2. To prevent error.
3. Sit in a comfortable chair. Cradle baby with one hand and arm, while supporting baby against your body or lap.	3. Proper position will provide the baby with comfort and security and will make it easier for him to suck and swallow.
Performance Phase	
1. Let the baby root for the nipple by touching the corner of his mouth with the nipple. When he opens his mouth, insert the nipple.	1. Place the nipple on top of the tongue and far enough in his mouth so suction can be created when he sucks.
2. Hold the bottle at an angle to completely fill the nipple with fluid.	2. This prevents the baby from sucking and swallowing excessive amounts of air.
3. NEVER prop the bottle or leave the baby unattended during feeding.	3. This is unsafe. Should vomiting occur, aspiration is more likely.
4. The bottle should be handled so as not to contaminate the nipple or fluid.	4. Contamination will increase the chances of gastrointestinal disturbances.
5. Baby's feeding time will vary from 10–25 minutes.	5. The length of time will depend upon the age of the baby and how vigorously he sucks.
6. Bubble the baby at least once during the feeding and at the end of feeding.	6. Most babies swallow some air during feeding.
a. Place the baby in sitting position in nurse's lap, tilt him slightly forward and gently rub or pat his back.	These positions aid in expulsion of air thus preventing abdominal distention, discomfort and regurgitation.
b. Place baby in prone position on nurse's shoulder and gently pat or rub his back.	
c. Place baby in prone position on nurse's lap and gently rub or pat his back.	
7. Take nipple out of mouth periodically.	7. To allow baby to rest and to let air into the bottle so the nipple does not collapse.

Nursing Action	**Rationale/Amplification**

Follow-up Phase

1. After final bubbling, change wet or soiled diaper and place baby in crib on stomach or right side.

2. Check baby in a few minutes. If he is restless, pick him up and bubble him. Note if any spitting-up has occurred.

3. Accurate and descriptive charting:
   a. What was fed and amount
   b. How feeding was tolerated
   c. Any regurgitation or emesis, amount and material
   d. Length of time of feeding
   e. How baby sucked and took the feeding

1. This position aids in emptying the stomach and prevents regurgitation.

2. Some babies relieve themselves of air when in the crib and also bring up small amounts of formula at the same time.

NOTE: When feeding a premature infant, the same principles apply. The premature infant, however, will tire more easily and fall asleep. Allow him frequent rest periods and use a soft nipple so less energy is needed to suck. To stimulate this infant to suck, the nurse can brush the infant's cheek with finger, place thumb or finger under infant's chin or move the nipple back and forth in his mouth. Feeding time should not exceed 45 minutes.

GUIDELINES: *Gavage Feeding*

Gavage feeding is a means of providing food via a catheter passed through the nares or mouth, past the pharynx, down the esophagus and into the stomach, slightly beyond the cardiac sphincter.

Purposes

1. To provide a method of feeding or receiving medications that requires minimal patient effort when the infant is unable to suck or swallow.
2. To provide a route that allows adequate caloric or fluid intake.
3. To prevent fatigue or cyanosis which is apt to occur from nipple feeding.
4. To provide a safe method of feeding a limp and listless patient.

Equipment

Sterile rubber or plastic catheter, rounded-tip, size 5–10	Stethoscope
Clear, calibrated reservoir for feeding fluid	Water for lubrication
Syringe	Tape
	Feeding fluid

Procedure

Nursing Action	**Rationale/Amplification**

Preparatory Phase

1. Position patient on his side or back with his neck hyperflexed. A mummy restraint may be necessary to help maintain this position.

2. Measure feeding catheter and mark with tape.
   a. *Premature infant and neonate:* measure from bridge of nose to just beyond the tip of sternum.
   b. *Older child:* measure from tip of nose past the ear, to the tip of sternum.

1. This position allows for easy passage of the catheter, facilitates observation and helps avoid obstruction of the airway.

2. Premeasuring the catheter provides a guideline as to how far to insert catheter. Chilling catheter will stiffen it and facilitate insertion.

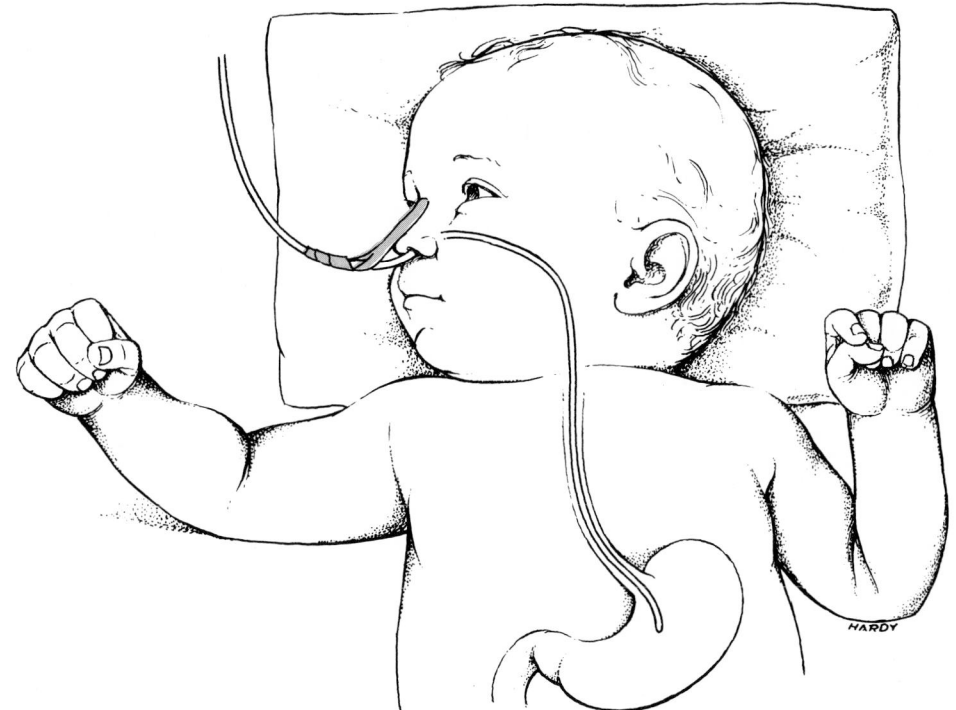

Gavage tube in place in stomach

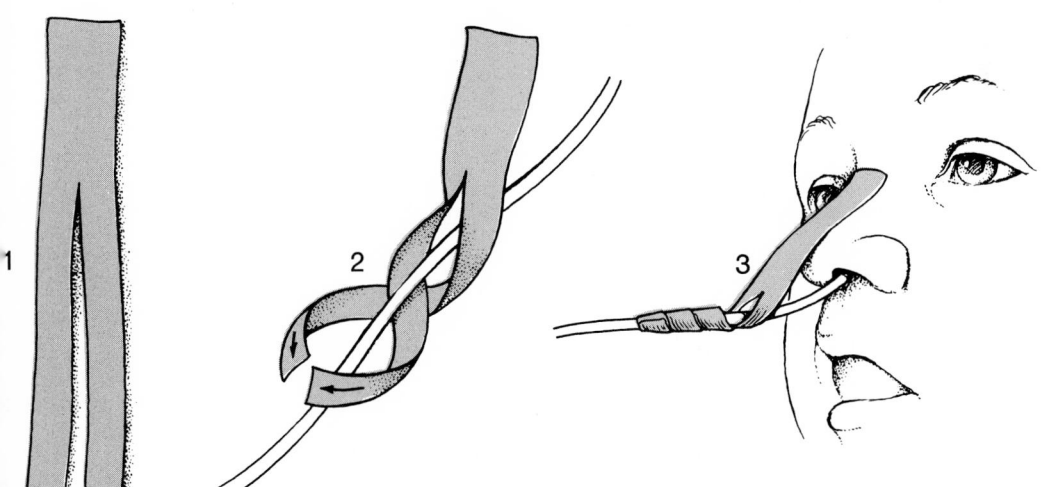

Steps in preparing adhesive tape to retain gavage tube

Figure 24-3. Gavage feeding.

Nursing Action	**Rationale/Amplification**

Performance Phase

1. Lubricate catheter with water.

1. Do not use oil because of danger of aspiration.

2. Stabilize patient's head with one hand; use the other hand to insert catheter.
   a. *Insertion through nares:* slip the catheter into nostril and direct toward the occiput in a horizontal plane.
   b. *Insertion through the mouth:* pass the catheter through the mouth toward the back of the throat.

   a. This direction will follow the nares passageway into the pharynx. Do not direct the catheter upward.

3. If patient swallows, passage of the catheter may be synchronized with the swallowing.

3. Swallowing motions will cause esophageal peristalsis, thus opening the cardiac sphincter and facilitating passage of the catheter.

4. If there is no swallowing, insert the catheter smoothly and quickly.

4. Because of cardiac sphincter spasm, resistance may be met at this point. Pause a few seconds, then proceed.

5. In the infant, especially, observe for vagal stimulation, i.e., bradycardia (slow heart rate) and apnea.

5. The vagus nerve pathway lies from the medulla through the neck and thorax to the abdomen. Above the stomach, the left and right branches unite to form the esophageal plexus. Stimulation of these nerve branches with the catheter will directly affect the cardiac and pulmonary plexus.

6. Once the catheter has been inserted to the premeasured length, tape the catheter to the patient's face (Fig. 24-3).

6. This prevents movement of catheter from the premeasured, pre-established correct position.

7. Test for correct position of the catheter in the stomach:
   a. Inject 0.5–1 ml. air into the catheter and stomach. At the same time listen to the typical growling stomach sound with a stethoscope placed over the epigastric region.
   b. Aspirate small amount of stomach content.

   a. Aspirate injected air from the stomach to prevent abdominal distention.

   b. Failure to obtain aspirant does not indicate improper placement as there may not be any stomach content or the catheter may not be in contact with the fluid.

   c. Avoid inserting catheter into infant's trachea. (An infant's anatomy makes it relatively difficult to enter the trachea.)

   c. If improper placement occurs and the catheter enters the trachea, the patient may cough, fight and become cyanotic. Remove the catheter immediately and allow the patient to rest before attempting intubation again.

8. The feeding position should be supine with head and chest slightly elevated. Attach reservoir to catheter and fill with feeding fluid.

8. This position allows the flow of fluid to be aided by gravity.

9. The flow of the feeding fluid should be slow. Do not apply pressure. Elevate reservoir 15–20 cm. (6–8 inches) above the patient's head.

9. The rate of flow is controlled by the size of the feeding catheter: the smaller the size, the slower the flow. If the reservoir is too high, the pressure of the fluid itself affects the rate of flow.

Nursing Action	**Rationale/Amplification**
10. Food taken too rapidly will interfere with peristalsis, causing abdominal distention and regurgitation.	10. The presence of food in the stomach stimulates peristalsis and causes the digestive process to begin.
11. Feeding time should take approximately as long as a corresponding amount given by nipple.	
12. When the feeding is completed, the catheter may be irrigated with clear water. Before the fluid reaches the end of the catheter, clamp it off and withdraw it quickly.	12. Clamp the catheter before air enters the stomach causing abdominal distention. Clamping also prevents fluid from dripping from the catheter into the pharynx, causing patient to gag and aspirate.

NOTE: Intermittent gavage feeding is often preferred to indwelling gavage feeding. An indwelling catheter may coil and knot, perforate the stomach, and cause nasal airway obstruction, ulceration, irritation to the mucous membranes, and epistaxis. However, if intermittent intubation is not tolerated well and the indwelling method is used, the catheter should be changed every 48–72 hours. (Alternate sides of the nares.) Constant alertness to the above problems should be stressed.

Follow-up Phase

1. Burp or bubble patient.	1. Adequate expulsion of air swallowed or ingested during feeding will decrease abdominal distention and allow for better tolerance of the feeding.
2. Place patient on right side or on abdomen.	2. To minimize regurgitation and aspiration.
3. Observe condition after feeding; bradycardia and apnea may still occur.	3. Because of vagal stimulation as mentioned above.
4. Note any vomiting or abdominal distention.	4. Due to overfeeding or too rapid feeding.
5. Note infant's activity.	5. Fatigue or peaceful sleep.
6. Accurately describe and chart procedure, including time of feeding, type of gavage feeding, type and amount of feeding fluid given, the amount retained or vomited, how patient tolerated feeding and activity following feeding.	

GUIDELINES: *Feeding via Hyperalimentation*

Hyperalimentation is a method of providing complete nutrition entirely by the intravenous route. It involves the infusion of a solution of protein hydrolysate, glucose, electrolytes, minerals and vitamins at a constant rate through an indwelling catheter placed in the superior vena cava (Fig. 24-4). The procedure has been used successfully in patients with intestinal obstruction requiring multiple surgical procedures, in infants and young children with chronic diarrhea and malabsorption syndromes, and in small premature infants.

Purpose

To sustain life and promote growth in patients whose gastrointestinal function is deranged to such an extent that adequate oral intake is prevented for an extended period of time.

DAILY CALORIC RECOMMENDATIONS*

Age	Recommended Allowance	
Infant		
0–2 months	115–120 cal/kg./24 hrs.	
2–6 months	110 cal/kg./24 hrs.	
6–12 months	100 cal/kg./24 hrs.	
Toddler		
1–2 years	1000 cal	
2–3 years	1250 cal	
Pre-schooler		
3–4 years	1400 cal	
4–6 years	1600 cal	
School-age Child		
6–8 years	2000–2100 cal	
8–10 years	2100–2200 cal	
10–12 years	*Boys*	*Girls*
	2500 cal	2250 cal
Adolescent		
12–14 years	2700 cal	2300 cal
14–16 years	3000 cal	2300–2400 cal
14–16 years	3000 cal	2300 cal

* Based on recommendations from the Food and Nutrition Board, National Academy of Science, National Research Council and the American Academy of Pediatrics, Committee on Hospital Care, "Care of Children in Hospitals" 1971.

Equipment

Silastic catheter of appropriate size
Hyperalimentation solution
Millipore intravenous filter
Constant infusion pump
All of the equipment listed in the procedure for intravenous therapy by cutdown method

Procedure

Nursing activities for all phases of the administration of hyperalimentation solution are the same as those specified in the procedure for intravenous fluid therapy with the following additions:

Nursing Action	Rationale/Amplification
Preparatory Phase	
1. Mix the components of the hyperalimentation solution under strict aseptic conditions. Culture each bottle to assure the adequacy of the technique.	1. It is essential to prevent microbial contamination of the infusate in order to protect the child from septicemia.
2. Place a millipore filter in the intravenous line.	2. The filter is a final attempt to remove any bacteria or fungi from the solution.

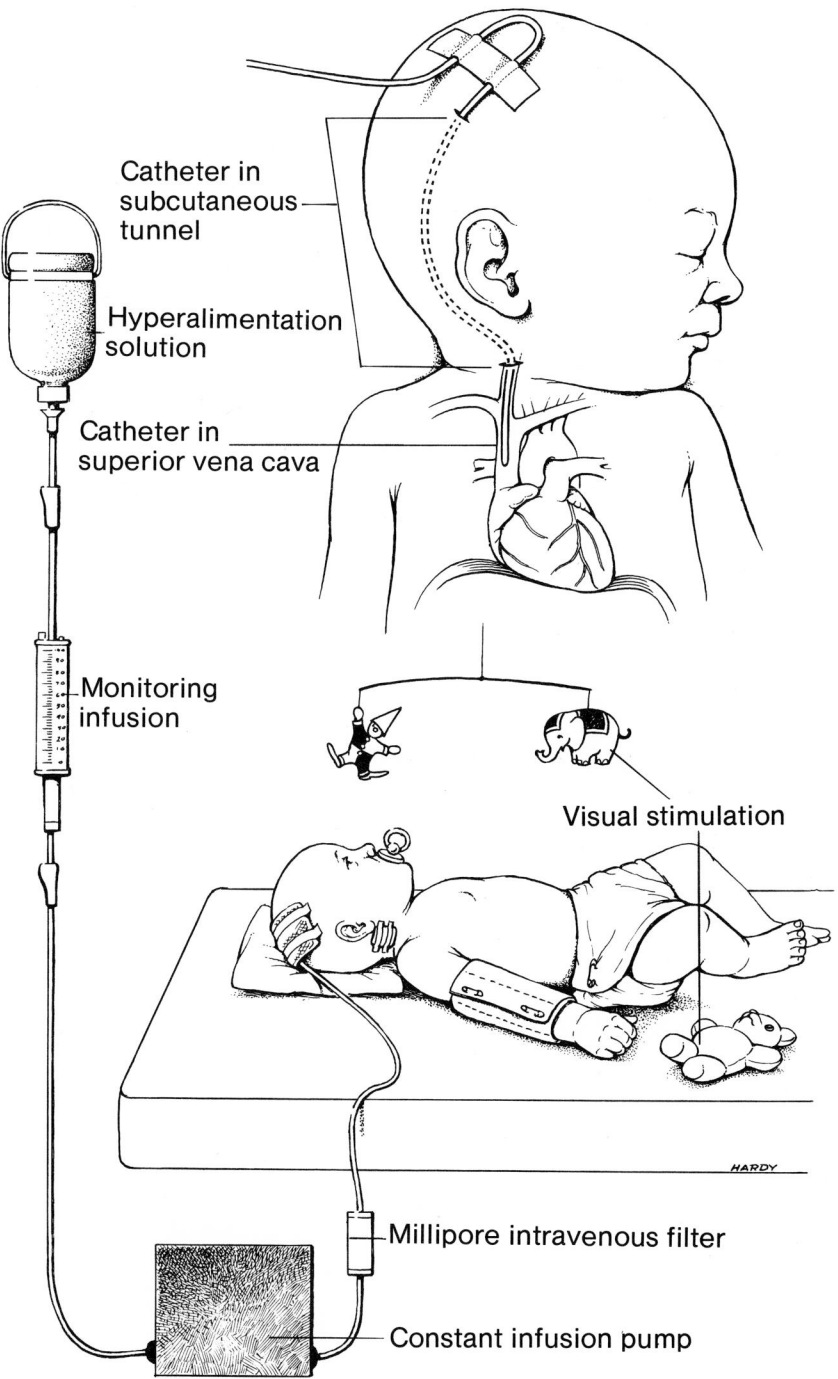

Catheter in
subcutaneous
tunnel

Hyperalimentation
solution

Catheter in
superior vena cava

Monitoring
infusion

Visual stimulation

Millipore intravenous filter

Constant infusion pump

Figure 24-4. Hyperalimentation.

Nursing Action	**Rationale/Amplification**

Performance Phase

1. The hyperalimentation catheter should be inserted under sterile operating room conditions.

1. Violation of aseptic techniques at the time of insertion can result in overwhelming septicemia and death.

Follow-up Phase

1. Do not use the catheter for the administration of medications or for blood sampling.
2. Make certain that the solution is infused continuously and at a constant rate.
   a. Use a constant-infusion pump if one is available.
   b. Never slow or increase the drip to make up for an excess or deficit without consulting the physician.

1. This increases the risk of infections and the possibility of dislodging the catheter.
2. Continuous infusion is necessary to prevent such metabolic complications as osmotic diuresis, hypoglycemia and pulmonary edema.

3. Change the entire length of the intravenous tubing from the bottle to the catheter, including the filter, at least every other day.
   a. Use sterile gloves for this procedure.
   b. Culture the filter each time it is changed.

3. This is another attempt to prevent contamination and reduce the possibility that the child will develop infection.

   b. It is possible to detect microbial contamination prior to the development of clinical signs, by culturing the filter.

4. Change the dressing around the catheter at least 3 times each week using strict aseptic technique.
   a. Remove the dressing carefully.
   b. Cleanse the skin with alcohol and paint it with an iodine preparation.
   c. Apply a prescribed antibiotic ointment.
   d. Apply benzoin to the area where tape will be applied.

   e. Apply sterile dressings.
5. Monitor the child's weight daily. Weigh at the same time each day and on the same scales.
6. Provide the infant with a pacifier.

4. This reduces the possibility of infection at the catheter site.

   a. Extreme care is necessary to avoid dislodging the catheter.

   d. Even nonirritating tape may produce damage to the underlying skin with prolonged use.

5. Weight gain is one of the most reliable indications of a positive response to therapy.
6. It is especially important to meet the sucking needs of the infant as hyperalimentation therapy may be necessary for several weeks or months.

7. Observe for signs of complications resulting from therapy.
   a. Complications related to the catheter:
      (1) Septicemia
      (2) Thrombosis of a major blood vessel
      (3) Plugging or dislodging of the catheter
      (4) Local skin infection
      (5) Cardiac arrhythmia
   b. Metabolic Complications
      (1) Persistent glucosuria
      (2) Dehydration
      (3) Postinfusion hypoglycemia
      (4) Acidosis
      (5) Amino acid imbalance

   a. Three-fourths of the major complications of therapy are of this variety. Sepsis accounts for more than half of these problems.

   b. Careful clinical and chemical monitoring especially during the initial period of hyperalimentation can greatly reduce the incidence of these types of complications.

GUIDELINES: *Intravenous Fluid Therapy*

Intravenous therapy refers to the infusion of fluids directly into the venous system. This may be accomplished through the use of a needle or by venous cutdown and insertion of a small catheter directly into the vein (Fig. 24-5).

Purpose

To restore and maintain the child's fluid and electrolyte balance and body homeostasis when his oral intake is inadequate to serve this purpose.

Equipment

A. *Needle Method*

I.V. solution
   The kind of solution is specified by the physician.
   For small children, 250-ml. bottles should be used for purposes of safety.
I.V. pole
I.V. administration set
   The set should include a closed reservoir with a minidropper to ensure that the child will not receive an excessive amount of fluid in a brief period of time.
Syringe, 10 ml.—filled with approximately 6 ml. of normal saline
Scalp-vein or short No. 21–24 gauge needle
   The size of the needle depends on the age and size of the child and the type of fluid to be administered.
Alcohol sponges
Small tourniquet
Adhesive tape, 1.2 cm. (½ inch), 2.5 cm. (1 inch), 5 cm. (2 inches)
Padded armboard
Dry sponges
Gauze bandage for securing the extremity to the armboard
Restraining devices—bath blanket, extremity restraint, covered sandbags
   The type of restraint depends on the child's age, his level of cooperation and the kind of I.V. to be started.
Safety razor (if scalp vein is to be used)

B. *Cutdown Method*

I.V. solution
I.V. pole
I.V. administration set
Alcohol sponges
Adhesive tape, 1.2 cm. (½ inch), 2.5 cm. (1 inch), 5 cm. (2 inches)
Padded armboard
Dry sponges
Gauze bandage
Cutdown tray
   The tray should include the following equipment: medicine cups, treatment towels, wound towel, syringe, No. 1–25 gauge 1.5-cm. (⅝-inch) needle. No. 1–20 gauge 2.5-cm. (1-inch) needle, knife handle and No. 15 blade, forceps, scissors, gauze sponges, 4–0 black silk suture, needle holder.

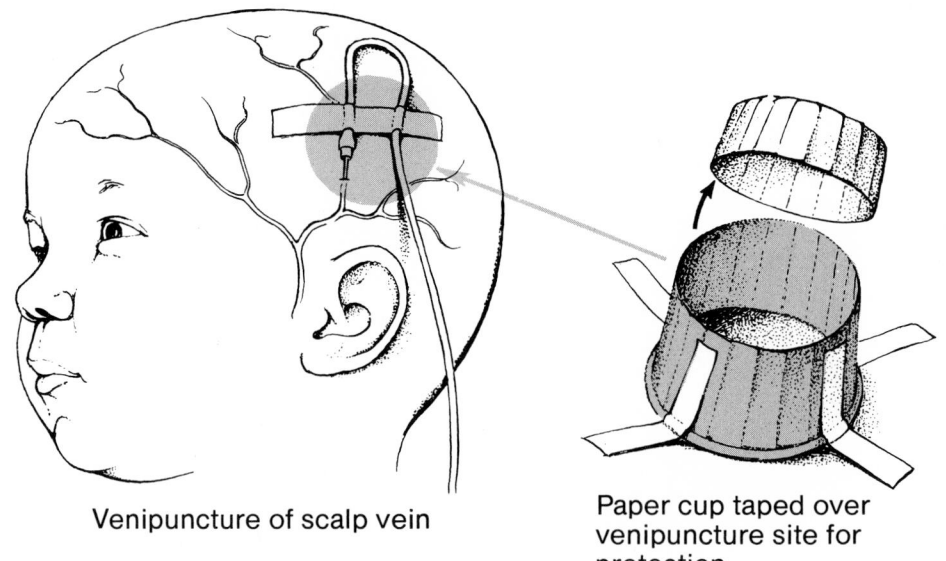

Venipuncture of scalp vein

Paper cup taped over
venipuncture site for
protection

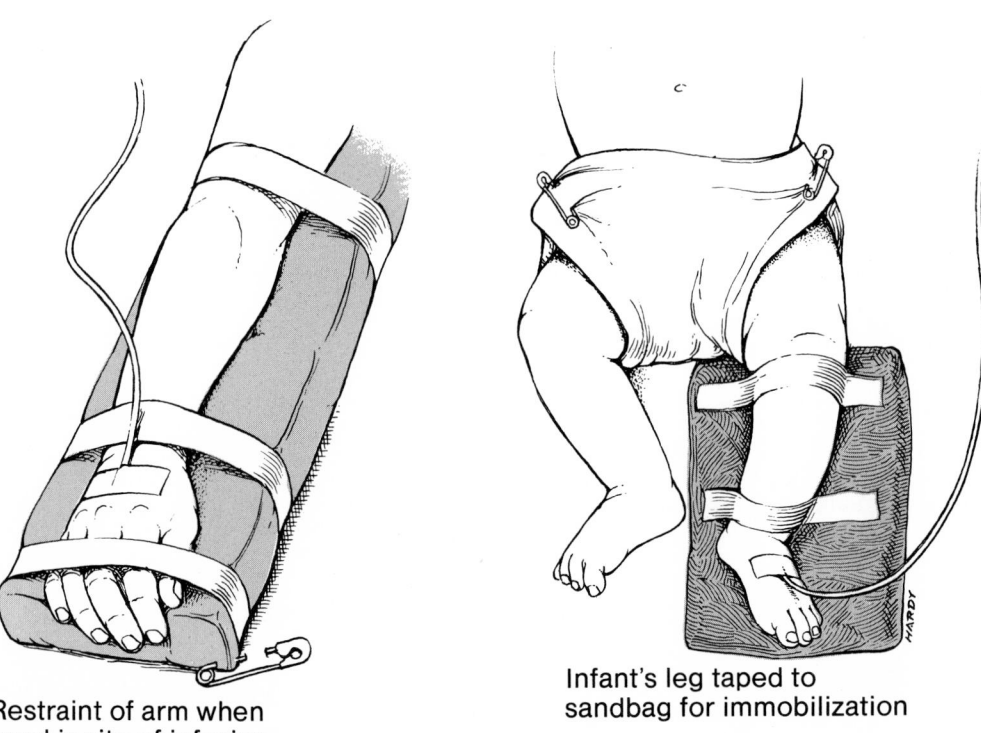

Restraint of arm when
hand is site of infusion

Infant's leg taped to
sandbag for immobilization

Figure 24-5. I.V. fluid therapy.

Assorted sizes of polyethylene tubing and luer stubs
5–0 black silk suture with a straight eye needle
1–2% procaine
Normal saline
Tourniquet
Sterile gloves
Restraining devices

Procedure

Nursing Action	**Rationale/Amplification**

Preparatory Phase

1. Check the I.V. fluid for sediment or contaminant by holding the bottle up to the light.

1. Contaminant is most easily identified with the bottle in this position. If sediment is observed, the solution should be discarded.

2. Connect the bottle to the infusion administration set. Use aseptic technique.
3. Hang the bottle from the I.V. pole and allow the fluid to fill the tubing. Make sure that there are no air bubbles present.
4. Shut off the fluid flow and keep the end of the tubing sterile until ready to connect it to the needle.
5. Promote the cooperation of the child.
   a. *Infant:* Provide with a pacifier.
   b. *Older child:* Explain the procedure and its purpose.

5. The procedure will be least traumatic for the child if he is able to cooperate and is not frightened or resistant.

6. Transport the child to the treatment room.

6. Since this is a relatively traumatic procedure for the child, it should not be done in his room or in front of other children on the ward.

7. Position the child so that he is comfortable.
8. Restrain the child as necessary.
   a. *Infant or young child:* Restraints may include mummy wrapping, jacket or elbow restraints or small sandbags.
   b. *Older child:* The extremity to be used should be comfortably restrained on the armboard. Free extremities may also require light restraints to remind the child not to move.

8. Protective devices may be necessary to prevent the child from dislodging the I.V. needle. The type and size of such devices should be appropriate for the child's age and the position of the I.V.

Performance Phase

1. Assist the physician as necessary. This may involve holding the child, cutting tape, regulating fluid flow, etc.
2. Check the restraints at intervals and adjust them as necessary.

2. The restraints may become loose after a period of time and must be secured to ensure the child's safety. They may also become too tight and require loosening to maintain adequate circulation.

3. Comfort and reassure the child.

3. The procedure is usually disturbing for the child. This should be acknowledged. If crying and upset, the child should be reassured that his behavior is acceptable.

Nursing Action   **Rationale/Amplification**

4. Regulate the I.V. flow at the designated rate.
5. Record:
      Type of solution being used
      Reading on the bottle or reservoir
      Rate of flow
      Time that the infusion began
      Name of the physician who started the I.V.
      Site of administration
      Reaction of the child to the procedure
6. Return the child to his room.

Follow-up Phase

1. Check the child at least hourly.   1. The child must be observed frequently to
   a. Note the location of the I.V.   make certain that the I.V. is not infiltrating and
   b. Note the color of the skin at the needle   is functioning properly. Report any swelling,
      point.   discoloration or leakage.
   c. Check for swelling of the skin at the needle
      point.
      (1) If in a hand or foot, compare with the
          opposite extremity.
      (2) If in the head, look at the face to deter-
          mine asymmetry.
   d. Feel the area around the I.V. site for spon-
      giness or leakage.
   e. Check for blood return into the tube when
      the flow of fluid is stopped.
   f. Make certain that the child is adequately
      restrained.
2. Observe closely for complications.   2. Complications associated with the administra-
   a. *Local reactions:*   tion of intravenous fluids to infants and chil-
      (1) Compromised circulation   dren are very serious and may have fatal con-
      (2) Pressure sores   sequences. Any signs of complications must
      (3) Thrombophlebitis   be reported immediately.
   b. Dehydration or overhydration
      (1) Maintain an accurate record of intake
          and output.
          (a) Total the intake and output every
              8 hours.
          (b) Describe carefully the amount
              and consistency of all stools and
              vomiting.
          (c) Collect all urine and weigh dia-
              pers if more accurate measure-
              ment of the child's output is
              necessary.
      (2) Weigh the child at regular intervals,   (2) An increase or decrease of 5% within
          using the same scales each time.   a relatively brief period of time is usu-
          (a) Record the amount of clothes the   ally significant and should be reported.
              child is wearing, etc.
      (3) Report:
          (a) Decreased skin turgor

Nursing Action	Rationale/Amplification

Nursing Action

    (b) Marked increase or decrease in urination
    (c) Fever
    (d) Sunken or bulging fontanelles in an infant
    (e) Sudden change in weight or vital signs
    (f) Diarrhea
    (g) Weakness, apathy or lethargy

3. Record essential information.
  a. Reading on the bottle or reservoir
  b. Amount of fluid absorbed in the hour
  c. Total amount of fluid absorbed
  d. Total amount of fluid intended to have been absorbed
  e. Rate of flow
  f. Apparent condition of the child

4. Regulate the rate of flow as necessary by any of the following methods:
  a. Raising the height of the bottle
  b. Adjusting the flow regulator
  c. Adjusting the position of the extremity

5. Irrigate the I.V. as necessary.
  a. Gather equipment:
    (1) Syringe with 1–3 ml. of normal saline
    (2) Several alcohol wipes
  b. Clamp off the I.V. solution.
  c. Disconnect the I.V. tubing at the needle insertion site.
  d. Remove the needle from the syringe.
  e. Connect the syringe to the tubing at the needle insertion site.
  f. Slowly inject the normal saline.

  g. Disconnect the syringe and reconnect the I.V. tubing to the needle insertion site.
  h. Unclamp the I.V. and regulate the flow of the solution.
  i. Check frequently to make certain that the I.V. is functioning properly.

6. Change the I.V. bottle and tubing every 24 hours.

7. Disconnect the I.V. when ordered or if it is obviously infiltrated.
  a. Gather equipment.
    (1) Scissors
    (2) 4 x 4 gauze square
    (3) Bandaid
  b. Explain the procedure to the child, depending on his age.

Rationale/Amplification

5. Irrigation may be required to dislodge small clots in the needle or to maintain the infusion rate of a sluggish I.V.

  f. Great force of injector should be avoided as this may cause the vein to rupture or the needle to become dislodged from the vein.

6. The I.V. set-up should be changed daily to maintain sterility and prevent contamination of the I.V. fluid during I.V. therapy.

Nursing Action	Rationale/Amplification

c. Clamp off the flow of the I.V. fluid.
d. Determine the location of the needle.
e. Loosen the tape around the needle, holding the needle firmly in position so that it does not slip out.
f. Hold the 4 x 4 lightly over the insertion site and remove the needle quickly and carefully.
g. Apply pressure to the site immediately and hold until bleeding stops.
h. Apply bandaid.

    h. The bandaid should not be applied until all bleeding has stopped to minimize the possibility of prolonged or unnoticed bleeding.

i. Remove the tape and armboard from the extremity.
j. Comfort the child as required.
k. Note the fluid level on the bottle or reservoir and complete recordings.
l. Record that the I.V. was discontinued.

SPECIAL PEDIATRIC CONSIDERATIONS

The Child Undergoing Surgery

Preoperative Care

1. Provide emotional preparation and preoperative teaching appropriate for age—helps establish good nurse-parent-patient relationship.
    a. Orient patient and family to the unit, room, location of operating room and recovery room and introduce to some of the personnel.
    b. Answer questions honestly.
        Explain at appropriate time what is going to be done.
    c. Provide opportunity for child and parents to work out concerns and feelings (play, talk).
2. Assist in physical preparation of patient for surgery.
    a. Assist with necessary laboratory studies.
    b. See that patient has nothing by mouth (NPO).
        Explain what NPO means to child and parents.
    c. Assist with fever reduction.
        (1) Fever will result from some surgical diseases, i.e., intestinal obstruction.
        (2) Fever increases risk of anesthesia and need for fluid and calories.
    d. Administer appropriate medications as ordered.
        Sedatives and drugs to dry the secretions are often given on the unit.
    e. Establish good hydration.
        Parenteral therapy may be necessary to hydrate the child, especially if he is NPO, vomiting or febrile.
3. Support parents in this time of crisis.
    a. May be an emotionally distressing experience.
    b. Parents may have feelings of fear or guilt.

Postoperative Care

A. *Immediate*
1. Maintain a patent airway and prevent aspiration.
    a. Position child on his side or abdomen to allow secretions to drain and prevent tongue from obstructing pharynx.
    b. Suction any secretions present.
2. Make frequent observations of general condition and vital signs.
    a. Take vital signs every 15 minutes until child is awake and his condition stable.
    b. Note respiratory rate and quality, pulse rate and quality, blood pressure, skin color.
    c. Watch for signs of shock.
        (1) All children have signs of pallor, coldness, increased pulse and irregular respirations.
        (2) Older children have decreased blood pressure and perspiration.
    d. Change in vital signs may indicate airway obstruction, hemorrhage or atelectasis.
    e. Restlessness may indicate pain or hypoxia.
        Medication for pain is not usually given until anesthesia has worn off.
    f. Check dressings for drainage or constriction and pressure.
3. See that all drainage tubes are connected and functioning properly.
        Gastric decompression relieves abdominal distention and decreases the possibility of respiratory embarrassment.
4. Monitor parenteral fluids as ordered. (See p. 1090.)
5. Be physically near the child as he awakens to offer soothing words and a gentle touch.

B. *After Recovery from Anesthesia*
    After undergoing simple surgery and receiving a small amount of anesthesia, the child may be ready to play and eat in a few hours. More complicated and extensive surgery debilitates the child for a longer period of time.
1. Continue to make frequent and astute observations in regard to behavior, vital signs, dressings or operative site and special apparatus (I.V., chest tubes, oxygen).
    a. Note signs of dehydration.
        (1) Dry skin and membranes   (3) Poor skin turgor
        (2) Sunken eyes   (4) Sunken fontanelle in infant
    b. Record any passage of flatus or stool.
2. Record accurately intake and output.
    a. Parenteral fluids and oral intake.
    b. Drainage from gastric tubes or chest tubes, colostomy, wound, and urinary output.
        Dressing may need to be weighed for more accurate estimate of output.
    c. Parenteral fluid is evaluated and ordered by considering output and intake.
        Parenteral fluid is usually maintained until child is taking adequate oral fluids.
3. Advance diet as tolerated, according to child's age and the physician orders.
    a. First feedings are usually clear fluids; if tolerated, advance slowly to full diet for age.
        Note any vomiting or abdominal distention.
    b. Since anorexia may occur, offer child what he likes in small amounts and in an attractive manner.

4. Prevent infection.
   a. Keep child away from other children or personnel with respiratory or other infections.
   b. Change the child's position every 2–3 hours.
        Prop infants with a blanket roll.
   c. Encourage patient to cough and breathe deeply.
        Let infant cry for short periods of time.
   d. Keep operative site clean.
        (1) Change dressing as needed.
        (2) Keep diaper away from wound.
5. Provide good general hygiene.
   a. Good skin care will increase circulation and prevent pressure sores.
   b. Provide proper rest and sleep periods.
   c. Allow child exercise and movement out of bed when he feels better.
        Advance gradually.
   d. Allow diversional activity at intervals appropriate for age.
6. Offer the child measures of comfort.
   a. See that child is warm and changes position as needed.
   b. Provide mouth care.
   c. Allow child to have and hold favorite toy or object.
   d. Anticipate his needs.
   e. Holding and rocking the infant or young child may be comforting.
7. Provide emotional support and psychological security.
   a. Encourage child to talk about his operation.
   b. Allow child to play out his feelings.
   c. Return often to see and talk to the child.
   d. Reassure him that things are going well.
8. Continue to offer support to the parents.
   a. Help to maintain healthy family relationships. (Encourage parents to care for their child.)
   b. Encourage parents to talk about their concerns.
   c. Begin early to prepare for discharge.
        (1) Teach any special procedures to be continued at home.
        (2) Arrange for community nurse referral.
        (3) Determine limits of activity for the child.
        (4) Make follow-up appointments.
        (5) Anticipate reactions of the child as a result of the hospitalization.

GUIDELINES: Oxygen Therapy for Children

Indications for Use of Oxygen

(In order of sequence)
1. Shallow breathing
2. Flaring of nostrils
3. Restlessness
4. Tachycardia
5. Elevation of blood pressure followed by decrease in blood pressure
6. Cyanosis
7. Bradycardia
8. Gasping, irregular respirations

Underlying Considerations

1. Cyanosis can be observed clinically in the child with a blood oxygen saturation of 75–80% or less.
2. Relief of cyanosis alone is not an adequate parameter to measure the effect of oxygen. It is necessary also to monitor the tension of the arterial blood.
3. If oxygen needs are not met, coma and death will ensue.
4. Retrolental fibroplasia may occur in preterm infants when high arterial oxygen saturations are maintained in the retinal vessels for a prolonged time. Thus it is imperative that this situation be avoided. (However, when hypoventilation and hypoxia exist, oxygen administration is vital and is extremely important in managing the infant.)

Complications of Oxygen Therapy

1. Nausea
2. Dyspnea
3. Substernal distress
4. Carbon dioxide narcosis
   a. Stimuli to spontaneous respiration is removed.
   b. Delirium may result.
5. Retrolental fibroplasia

Purpose

To provide a sufficient concentration of oxygen to the alveoli so that the tension and saturation of oxygen can be maintained in the circulating blood.

Procedure

Nursing Action	Rationale/Amplification

Preparatory Phase

(For most forms of oxygen therapy)

1. Explain the procedure to the child and allow him to feel the equipment and the oxygen flowing through the tube, mask, etc.
2. Suction the nose and mouth to clear airway.
3. See that the oxygen is delivered via a humidified source.

4. Turn on oxygen supply slightly higher than required and then adjust to desired rate.

1. The child will be reassured if he understands the procedure and knows what to expect.

2. The delivery of oxygen requires a clear airway.
3. Oxygen is a dry gas and requires the addition of moisture to prevent drying of the tracheo-bronchial tree and thickening and consolidation of secretions.

Performance Phase

NASAL CATHETER

1. Fit catheter into child's nose and secure elastic head grip.
2. Observe the child's response to the oxygen:
   a. Decreased restlessness
   b. Decreased respiratory distress
   c. Improvement of color
   d. Changes in vital signs

1. Infants and small children rarely tolerate oxygen via nasal catheter.

MASK OXYGEN

1. Choose an appropriate size mask that covers the mouth and nose but not the eyes.

Nursing Action	*Rationale/Amplification*
2. Place the mask over the child's mouth and nose so that it fits securely. Secure the mask with an elastic head grip.	2. Make sure that the mask is adjusted properly over the mouth and nose. Do not allow the oxygen to blow in child's eyes.
3. Remove the oxygen mask at hourly intervals and wash the face and apply a cream to area where mask hits the face.	3. Makes the patient feel more comfortable.

4. Observe the child's response to the oxygen:
  a. Decreasing restlessness
  b. Decreasing respiratory distress
  c. Improvement of color
  d. Changes in vital signs	

OXYGEN TENT

1. Set up oxygen tent.	1. An ideal way to administer oxygen to a small child—allows child free movement within tent where a high oxygen concentration can be maintained.
2. A concentration of 50–60% oxygen can be produced at 3–4 liters/minute.	2. Concentration of oxygen within the tent depends on the efficiency of the tent and the rate of flow of oxygen.
3. Temperature should be maintained at 17.8–21.1°C. (64–70°F.).	
4. Place child in comfortable position inside the tent.	4. Provide nursing care through the sleeves or pockets in the tent.
5. Observe the child's response to oxygen.	

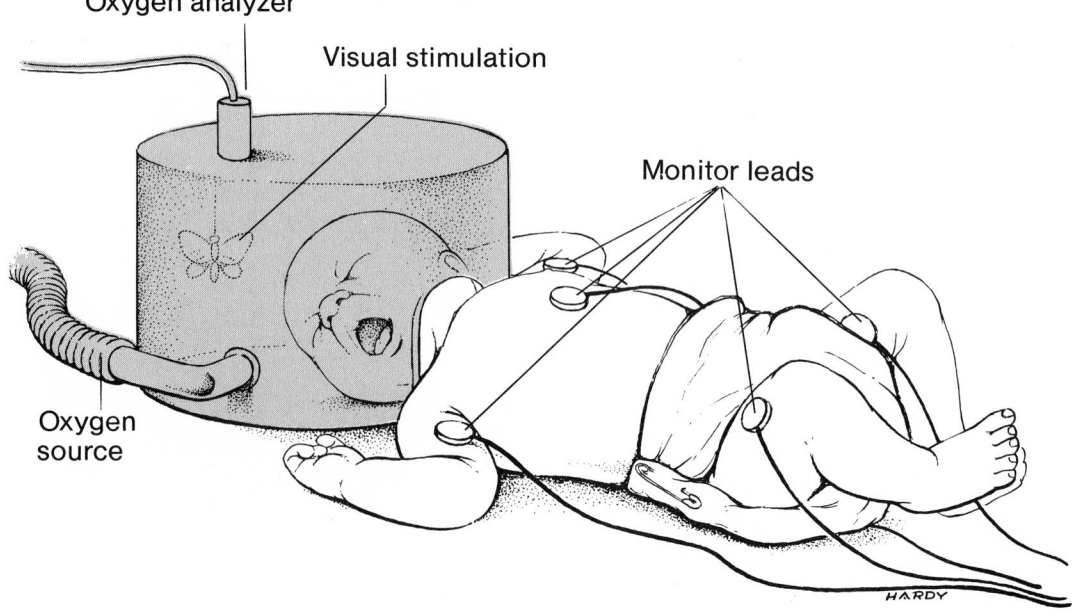

Figure 24-6. Oxygen hood.

Nursing Action	**Rationale/Amplification**
CROUPETTE (Oxygen tent equipped with a humidification system) See procedure under oxygen tent	Cover the child with a cotton blanket to prevent chilling.
INCUBATOR WITH OXYGEN 1. A humidified oxygen supply is administered via a heated incubator. 2. Keep sleeves of incubator closed to prevent loss of oxygen.	2. When incubator or sleeves are opened, supply supplemental oxygen with oxygen mask to face and nose.
HEAD HOOD (Doghouse Frame) 1. A humidified oxygen supply is administered via a plastic container which fits over the head. Oxygen is concentrated around the infant's head (Fig. 24-6). (May be used in an incubator or with a warming unit.) 2. Observe infant's response to oxygen.	1. Prevent any air leaks in the area where hood fits around infant's neck. Area should be sealed with a small piece of surgical dressing (4 x 4 gauze square).

GENERAL PROCEDURES
1. Provide a method for measuring oxygen concentrations:
  a. Measure concentration only when the oxygen environment is closed.
  b. Record oxygen concentrations.
2. When child is being weaned from oxygen observe closely for:
  a. Pulse elevation.
  b. Respiratory distress with increased respirations and retractions.
  c. Cyanosis.
3. First reduce liter flow gradually; observe response; if tolerated, gradually continue to reduce liter flow until child is completely weaned.
	1. Oxygen concentration should be measured once each hour when child is receiving oxygen via incubator, hood, tent or croupette.
	
	3. Child should be weaned from oxygen gradually.

Follow-up Phase
1. Continually monitor the child's response.
2. Remove and clean equipment as indicated.

Cardiopulmonary Resuscitation

Cardiopulmonary resuscitation involves measures instituted to provide effective ventilation and circulation when the patient's respiration and heart have ceased to function.

Causes

1. Anesthesia
2. Trauma
3. Chemicals and drugs
4. Anoxia or prolonged hypoxia
5. Electrolyte imbalance
6. Hypothermia
7. Cardiac arrhythmia

Underlying Considerations

A. *Cardiac arrest*

1. Due to either asystole or ventricular fibrillation which immediately interrupts the oxygen supply to the brain.
2. Within 2–4 minutes, the cells have used up the small amount of oxygen lying stagnant in the vascular bed—irreversible brain damage and cell death will occur unless circulation is restored.

B. *Respiratory arrest*

1. Although the cardiac action may maintain circulation, the oxygen reserves to the vital centers are rapidly depleted.
2. Produces hypoxia and finally anoxia with resultant cardiac asystole.

C. *Emergency preparation*

1. Every hospital should have a well-defined and organized plan to be carried out in the event of cardiac or respiratory arrest.
2. Emergency carts should be placed in strategic locations in the hospital and checked daily to assure that all equipment is available.

Equipment

Emergency Cart—assembled and ready for use
    Positive pressure breathing bag with nonrebreathing valve
    Masks (premature infant, infant, child, adult sizes)
    Endotracheal tubes (complete sterile set with connectors)
    Oropharyngeal airways (Guedel size 0,1,2,3,4)
    Laryngeal handle and blades of various sizes
    Extra light and bulbs for laryngoscope
    Portable suction equipment and sterile catheters of various sizes
Portable oxygen supply (oxygen gauge and tubing)
Drugs

Sodium bicarbonate	Dextrose
Epinephrine	Pentobarbitol
Isoproterenol	Saline (for dilution)
Calcium chloride	
Syringes of various sizes	Alcohol swabs
Needles of various sizes	Tongue blades
Intracardiac needle	Sterile 4 x 4 gauze sponges
Scalp-vein infusion sets of various sizes	Sterile hemostat
Intravenous solutions and infusion sets	Sterile scissors

Emergency Procedure

A. *Cardiac Massage*

1. *Newborn and Premature Infant*

a. Place the thumb on the lower sternum with the finger extended behind the infant's back.

    In infants and children the location of the sternum is determined as in the adult.

b. Bring thumb and fingers together *gently* but forcibly at the rate of 80–100 compressions per minute.

Technique for closed
chest heart massage
in the small infant

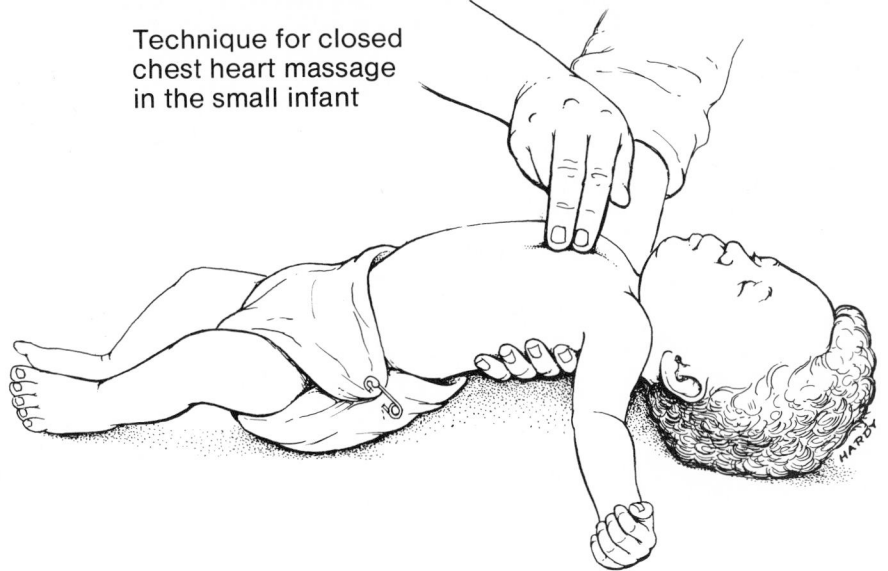

In the young child, the
heel of the hand is placed
over the lower sternum

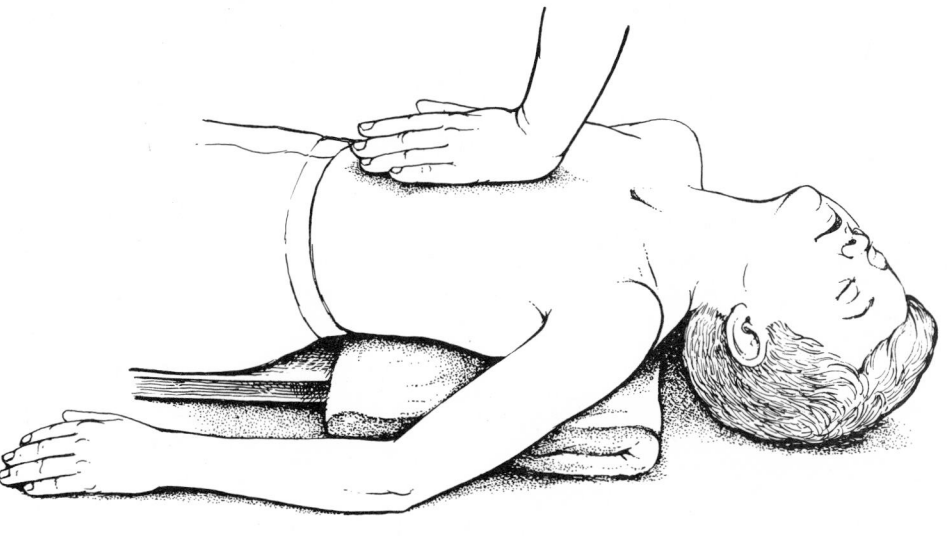

In older children
and adults, both
hands are used

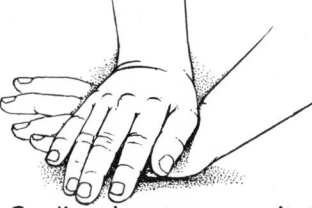

Figure 24-7. Cardiopulmonary resuscitation.

(1) The amount of pressure applied to infant and children is much less than the adult since the size of the thorax is less and the structure much more flexible.

(2) The criterion of good technique is a palpable femoral or carotid pulse.

2. *Infants* (Fig. 24-7)
   a. Place infant on flat firm surface.
   b. Place the index and middle finger of one hand on the lower sternum and gently but forcibly apply pressure at the rate of 80–100 compressions per minute.

3. *Small Children* (Fig. 24-7)
   a. Place child on a flat, firm surface—a firm, flat surface allows compression against a solid surface rather than a yielding surface which would absorb too much of the energy of a downward stroke.
   b. Place the heel of one hand on the middle and lower third of the sternum parallel with the long axis of the body.
      (1) Pressure should be applied to the lower half of the sternum only and not to the ribs on either side.
      (2) Only the heel not the palms and fingers should be in contact with the chest wall.
      (3) Rapid compression of the lower sternum is accomplished for systole and equally rapid release of pressure is necessary to allow for diastolic filling.
      (4) The criterion of good technique is a palpable femoral or carotid pulse.
   c. With the arm in a vertical position, elbow straight, apply rhythmic pressure downward. Depress the sternum 1.2–2.5 cm. (½–1 inch).
   d. The thrust should be rapid and held for approximately 0.4 second, and then instantly released so the chest wall can recoil.
   e. The compression should be repeated 60–80 times per minute or faster.

4. *Older Children and Adolescents*
   a. Place the child on a flat surface or place a board under the thorax.
   b. Place the heel of one hand on the lower half of the sternum parallel with the long axis of the body.
   c. The heel of the second hand is placed over the first.
   d. Place yourself above the child so that you will be able to use your own weight on his body in the application of pressure.
   e. With the arms in a vertical position, elbows straight, apply rhythmic pressure downward. The downward thrust on the sternum goes directly posterior toward the vertebral column. Depress the sternum 2.5–5 cm. (1–2 inches) (depending on whether the patient is a child or adolescent).
   f. The thrust is rapid and should be held for approximately 0.4 second and then instantly released so that the chest wall can recoil. The compression should be repeated 60 times per minute or faster.

B. *Mouth-to-mouth Breathing*

   1. *Premature Infants, Newborns, Infants*
      a. Clear mouth of mucus or vomitus with finger or suction.
      b. Hyperextend neck with towel or diaper roll.
      c. Place mouth over infant's mouth and nose.
      d. Gently blow air from cheeks and observe for chest expansion.
      e. Remove mouth from infant's mouth and nose.

      f. Replace mouth over infant's mouth and nose and gently blow air from cheeks and observe for chest expansion.

      g. Repeat 40 times per minute.

      h. Observe for abdominal distension. If this occurs, place hand on abdomen and gently apply pressure to force air out. Do this between breaths.

  2. *Older Children and Adolescents*

      a. Clear mouth of mucus or vomitus with finger or suction—the airway must be patent in order to ventilate successfully.

      b. Hyperextend head with a towel roll.

      c. Clamp the nostrils with fingers.

      d. Take a deep breath.

      e. Press mouth firmly against the child's mouth and force air into the lungs until chest expansion is observed.

      f. Release mouth from child's mouth and release nostrils.

      g. Replace mouth over child's mouth and clamp nostrils with fingers and force air into lungs until expansion is observed.

      h. Release mouth.

      i. Repeat 15–20 times a minute.

      j. The criteria for adequate ventilation are chest expansion and breath sounds and improvement in nailbed and skin color.

C. *Hand Resuscitators*

  1. Remove secretions from mouth and throat and move mandible forward.

  2. Hyperextend the neck with one hand or a diaper roll.

  3. Hold the mask snugly over the mouth and nose, holding the chin forward and the neck in extension. An appropriate size mask must be used in order to obtain an adequate seal.

  4. Squeeze the bag, noting inflation of the lungs by chest expansion.

  5. Release the bag, which will expand spontaneously. The child will exhale and the chest will fall.

  6. Repeat 20–40 times a minute (depending on size of the child).

Nursing Management

A. *Emergency Phase*

  1. Recognize cardiac and respiratory arrest.

  2. Call for help and note time.

  3. If alone:

      a. First ventilate the child's lungs rapidly 2–3 times and then proceed with external cardiac compression at the rate of 60–80 per minute.

      b. After each series of 15 cardiac compressions, reventilate the lungs rapidly 2–3 times. Then proceed with external cardiac compression at the rate of 60–80 per minute.

      c. Continue repeating this cycle until additional help arrives.

  4. When help arrives:

      One operator performs mouth-to-mouth resuscitation or institutes bag breathing. Other operator performs cardiac massage.

  5. Administer medication as ordered and record.

  6. Assist with intubation and other definitive measures.

B. *After Emergency*
  1. Attend to needs of the child.
  2. See that the family members have been notified and are being cared for by other personnel.
  3. Record all events.
  4. Restock emergency cart.

GUIDELINES: *Assisting with Exchange Transfusion*

Exchange transfusion is replacement of circulating blood by withdrawing blood and injecting donor's blood in equal amounts.

Purposes

  1. To prevent accumulation of bilirubin in the blood above a dangerous level.
  2. To prevent kernicterus.
  3. To prevent accumulation of other by-products of hemolysis from hemolytic disease, i.e., ABO incompatibility.

Equipment

Fresh donor blood
Monitoring equipment
Disposable exchange transfusion set containing:
  Sterile stopcock with extension tubing
  Extra extension tubing
  Umbilical catheters sizes 5 and 8, French
  2 20-ml. syringes
  1 5-ml. syringe and No. 23-gauge needle
  Waste-blood container
  Blood administration set
  Gauze sponges

Transfusion record
Cleansing solution
Means of heating infant
Means of heating blood
Calcium gluconate in 5-ml. syringe
50% glucose solution in 10-ml. syringe
Sodium bicarbonate in 10-ml. syringe
Sterile drapes
Sterile gown and gloves for physician
Cap and mask for physician

Procedure

Nursing Action	Rationale/Amplification
Preparatory Phase	
1. Place infant under heat lamps or radiant heating unit.	1. Chilling of the infant during the procedure can result in apnea and increased caloric need and oxygen consumption which can be exhausting to a baby with already limited amount of energy.
2. If the infant has not been NPO for 3–4 hours it may be necessary to empty stomach content via stomach tube.	2. To prevent aspiration should vomiting occur during the procedure.
3. Attach electronic monitoring device to infant if available. Otherwise place stethoscope over apex of heart.	3. Apnea, bradycardia and cardiac arrest are complications of an exchange transfusion. Close monitoring will allow for immediate observation of signs of trouble.
4. Place infant on his back. Restrain all 4 extremities.	4. This will prevent the infant from moving and inadvertently pulling out the exchange catheter.

Nursing Action	**Rationale/Amplification**
5. Have resuscitative equipment ready for immediate use: oxygen supply, mask, breathing bag, suction, sodium bicarbonate, and 50% glucose solution.	5. Should the infant develop bradycardia, hypoglycemia or cyanosis during procedure, these items will be necessary for immediate and supportive treatment.
6. Check donor blood for type, age and other identifying data.	6. To eliminate any errors. Heparinized fresh blood is desirable because it eliminates the hazards of ACD blood, i.e., acid blood and increased potassium.
7. Assist the physician in setting up blood and exchange equipment. Blood should be run through a coil of tubing through a water bath at 38° C. (100° F.).	7. Hypothermia, increased blood viscosity and ventricular fibrillation can result from administering cold blood.

EXCHANGE TRANSFUSION RECORD

HOSPITAL NO. _____

NAME OF BABY: Johnson, Clarence David

NAME OF MOTHER: Marsha Johnson

BIRTH WEIGHT: 7-4 ½

BLOOD GROUP: O pos

TIME COMMENCING EXCHANGE: 3:45 PM

TIME FINISHING EXCHANGE: 4:17 PM

DATE OF DELIVERY: 8-28-72

TIME: 4:10 AM

APGAR SCORE AT DELIVERY: 8 at 1 min.; 9 at 5 min.

INITIAL HEMOGLOBIN: 42

BILIRUBIN: 16.3

POST-EXCHANGE BILIRUBIN: 11.8

AGE OF BABY IN HOURS: 30

TIME	OUT Amount	OUT Total	IN Amount	IN Total	PULSE	RESPIRATION	VENOUS PRESSURE	MEDICATION	COMMENTS
3:45	20	20	20	20					
3:48	20	40	20	40					
3:51	20	60	20	60					
3:55	20	80	20	80					
3:58	20	100	20	100	150	48		Ca 1ml	
4:02	20	120	20	120					
4:06	20	140	20	140					
4:10	20	160	20	160					
4:13	20	180	20	180					
4:17	20	200	20	200	160	56			

Nursing Action	**Rationale/Amplification**

Performance Phase

1. The infant's skin is cleansed with antiseptic solution. Sterile drapes are applied by the physician who is gowned and gloved. Strict attention should be paid to maintaining aseptic technique.

2. Once the umbilical catheter is in place in the umbilical vein, the venous pressure is measured and the exchange will begin. (Preferred site is the umbilical artery; jugular or femoral vessels may be used.)

3. Note and record the time the exchange started. Record each successive withdrawal and infusion of blood in exact amount and time. Report to the physician when each 100 ml. of blood is exchanged. (See Record Chart, p. 1103.)

4. After each 100 ml. of blood is exchanged, calcium gluconate is injected. Monitor cardiac rate very carefully during the injection.

5. Constant monitoring of the cardiac rate is imperative. Also note respirations, skin color and color of withdrawn blood.

1. To prevent infection or sepsis. A foreign body introduced into the blood vessel is always a potential for infection due to an infected cord stump or contaminated equipment.

2. Record the venous pressure. This will be maintained at about 10–12 cm. by equal volume exchanges. An increase in pressure during the procedure is an indication to stop and assess the infant.

3. Blood is exchanged slowly in amounts of 5–20 ml., depending upon the infant's size and condition. The total amount exchanged is about 170 ml. of blood/kilogram of body weight (80 ml./pound). About 75–85% of the infant's total blood volume is exchanged.

4. Calcium decreases the irritability and irregularity of the heart. Too rapid an injection will cause bradycardia.

5. Observation and monitoring will allow immediate treatment if untoward signs appear. Bradycardia may occur at any time during the procedure due to a low pH of donor blood or old blood.

Follow-up Phase

1. When transfusion is completed, umbilical catheter may be:
   a. Left in place with an I.V. plug or intravenous infusion or
   b. Removed.

1. If catheter is left in place, it is usually done for future exchange transfusions, easy withdrawal of blood for blood studies, administration of intravenous fluids and medications. Keep infant restrained. If catheter is removed, apply small pressure dressing and observe for any bleeding.

2. Finish charting by recording accurately:
   a. Time transfusion was completed
   b. Total amount blood withdrawn and infused
   c. Any changes in vital signs
   d. Medications administered during exchange
   e. Infant's color and current vital signs
   f. Catheter removed or left indwelling
   g. How infant tolerated the procedure
   h. Any blood samples taken before or after exchange

3. Observe infant closely following the procedure: respirations, pulse (heart rate), temperature, evidence of lethargy or jitteriness, increasing jaundice, pigmentation of urine, cyanosis, edema, or convulsions. Report any of these signs immediately.

3. The complications of an exchange transfusion can be: heart failure, hypocalcemia, hypoglycemia, sepsis, acidosis, shock.
   Change infant's position frequently but handle gently and minimally following procedure.

SPECIMEN COLLECTION

GUIDELINES: Assisting with Blood Collection

Blood collection from a venous puncture in the extremity of an infant or young child is the same as for an adult with the following exceptions or additions.

Equipment

No. 23–19 gauge short needle or scalp-vein needle
Smaller volume or micro blood-collecting tubes
Smaller tourniquet (rubber band may be used)

Procedure

Nursing Action	Rationale/Amplification

Preparatory Phase

1. Immobilize the child by placing him in a mummy restraint if necessary (see p. 1073).

2. Position the patient.
   a. *Femoral venipuncture:* place patient on his back with legs in frog-like position. Nurse places her hands on patient's knees. (See position for bladder puncture p. 1107).
   b. *External jugular venipuncture:* place patient in mummy restraint and lower his head over the side of the bed or table. Stabilize his head.

1. Infants and young children squirm. Immobilizing them allows easier access to the venipuncture site. It also helps keep infant warm.

2. These positions allow for optimum visualization and stabilization of the patient.

Performance Phase

1. After the specimen is collected and needle is removed, apply pressure to the site with a dry gauze for 3–5 minutes.
   a. Jugular venipuncture: while applying pressure to the site, place the patient in an upright sitting position.

2. When the bleeding has been stopped, soothe and comfort the child before leaving him.

1. Both the femoral and jugular veins are large vessels. Since respiratory pressure is great, bleeding, oozing and hematoma formation may result. External pressure prevents this from happening.

2. Crying and thrashing about may initiate bleeding.

Follow-up Phase

1. Check patient frequently for an hour after procedure for oozing, bleeding or evidence of a hematoma.

2. Record carefully and accurately:
   a. Site of venipuncture
   b. How patient tolerated procedure
   c. Bleeding stopped or continued and for how long
   d. What test the specimen was collected for

1. Reapply pressure and report if oozing continues.

GUIDELINES: *Collecting Urine Specimen from the Infant and Young Child*

Urine collection is a safe method of collecting urine for a specified purpose.

Purposes

1. To check urine for presence of sugar, acetone, bacteria and other urinary products.
2. To aid in diagnosis.
3. To determine the condition of the patient.
4. To determine effectiveness of therapy.

Equipment

Collecting device—plastic, disposable urine bag or collector
Cleansing agent
Wiping material 4 x 4's or cotton balls
Clean or sterile water
Containers for solutions
Specimen container

Procedure

Nursing Action	Rationale/Amplification
Preparatory Phase	
1. Position patient so that genitalia are exposed by placing him on his back with legs in frog-like position. Assistance may be needed to hold the legs of the young child in proper position.	1. Proper positioning will facilitate cleansing and allow for proper placement of collection device.
Performance Phase	
1. Cleanse genital area.	1. This method of cleansing the female will prevent contamination of the genitalia from the anus, and will prevent contamination of the urine specimen obtained.
a. *Female:* using cotton balls, dip into cleansing agent, wipe labia majora from top to bottom (clitoris to anus) only once with each cotton ball. Repeat this once more. Wipe again with clear water. Then spread labia apart with one hand, while wiping the labia minora in the same manner with other hand. Wipe area dry.	During the cleansing, be gentle to avoid any injury or possible stimulation of urination.
b. *Male:* wipe tip of penis in circular motion down towards the scrotum. Be certain to retract foreskin, if present. Wipe first with cleansing agent 2–3 times, then clear water. Dry the area.	
2. Apply collecting bag firmly so that the opening is exposed to receive urine.	2. If collecting bag is properly and securely placed, the procedure will not have to be repeated.
3. Diaper patient and leave him comfortable.	
4. Check the patient frequently (30–60 minutes) to see if he has voided. When patient has voided, remove bag gently. Clean area and rediaper patient.	4. The adhesive on the collecting bag may tend to be sticky. Careful removal of the bag will prevent skin injury on and around genitalia. Also avoid spilling urine out of the bag during removal.

Nursing Action	**Rationale / Amplification**

Follow-up Phase

1. Pour specimen into proper collecting container. Send specimen to the laboratory within 30 minutes.

1. Prompt delivery of specimen to the laboratory will prevent growth of organisms in an uncontrolled environment and distortion of the test results.

2. Accurately chart and describe the following in the nurses' notes:
   a. Time specimen collection was started and ended
   b. Amount of urine voided
   c. Color of urine (cloudy, clear, any sediment)
   d. Type of test to be done
   e. Condition of skin of perineal area

GUIDELINES: *Assisting with a Percutaneous Bladder Puncture*

A percutaneous bladder puncture is an aseptic method of entering the bladder in the suprapubic location with a needle to obtain a urine specimen.

Purposes

1. To obtain urine in an aseptic manner for culture.
2. To aid in diagnostic work-up.
3. To determine condition of the patient and aid in treatment.

Equipment

Skin cleansing solution
Sterile 4 x 4's
Sterile gloves
Sterile needle, No. 21 gauge, 3.7 cm.
   (1½ inches) long

Sterile syringe, 20-ml.
Sterile specimen container
Bandaid

Procedure

Nursing Action	**Rationale / Amplification**

Preparatory Phase

1. Check diaper for wetness. If patient has just voided, report this to the physician or report last voiding time.

1. In order to perform a successful bladder puncture, there must be enough urine in the bladder to distend the bladder up above the pubic symphysis thus making it accessible.

2. Position patient on his back on the examining table. His head should be toward nurse, his feet toward the physician. Spread his legs apart in a frog-like position. Place hands on his knees and thumbs along his side at the hip level.

2. This position allows the nurse to stabilize the patient. It also gives a full view of the patient, making it easier to observe him, talk to him and soothe him.

3. Ensure that the skin over the puncture site is cleansed in an antiseptic manner.

3. To prevent infection from being introduced into the bladder by inserting the needle through unclean skin, thereby contaminating the specimen.

Nursing Action	Rationale/Amplification

Performance Phase

1. While the procedure is being performed, note the condition of the patient and any signs of distress.
Comfort him by talking to him and smiling at him.

2. When urine has been obtained or the procedure is discontinued and the needle is removed, apply pressure over the puncture site with a 4 x 4 and fingers.

3. Apply a Bandaid if necessary. Rediaper patient. Hold and comfort patient for a few minutes.

Follow-up Phase

1. Check patient periodically for 1 hour after procedure to see that bleeding or oozing has not occurred.

2. Note time of first voiding after procedure. Note color of urine (it may be pink). Bloody urine should be reported to the physician.

3. Accurately describe and chart the procedure including:
   a. Time of procedure
   b. Whether or not a specimen was obtained
   c. How the patient tolerated the procedure
   d. Description and amount of urine obtained
   e. Patient's condition and activity following the procedure

1. Report any changes in color or respiration rate or other signs.
Soothing the patient will help him to relax so that he will not move about so much. Crying increases the muscle tone of the lower abdomen making it more difficult to insert the needle.

2. This prevents any bleeding from occurring either internally or externally. Pressure should be maintained about 3 minutes or until oozing ceases and coagulation has taken place.

3. Holding the patient will help to restore and maintain a good nurse-patient relationship and will help the patient relax after a frightening and painful procedure.

1. This is not likely if pressure was applied properly after procedure and patient was left quiet.

2. It is important to note any changes in voiding pattern following the procedure, since it might indicate injury. The first voided urine may be bloody due to a small amount of local capillary bleeding at the time of the procedure.

GUIDELINES: *Collecting a Stool Specimen*

Stool collection is a method of obtaining stool specimen from the patient.

Purposes

1. To check stool for presence of specific material, i.e., blood, ova and parasites or bacteria.
2. To aid in diagnosis.
3. To determine condition or status of the patient.
4. To determine effectiveness of therapy.

Equipment

Diaper
Cellophane or plastic liner (used when stool is loose or watery)

Tongue blade
Specimen container

NOTE: Collecting a stool specimen from an older child who is toilet trained is the same as collecting such a specimen from an adult.

Procedure

Nursing Action	**Rationale / Amplification**
Preparatory Phase	
1. If a specimen is needed from a patient whose stools are loose or watery enough to be absorbed in the diaper, line the diaper with a piece of cellophane or plastic. Place this liner between the diaper and the skin. Then diaper patient and place him in a position with his head slightly elevated. If stools are soft or formed, simply diaper patient.	1. The liner and position will allow the loose stool specimen to collect in the liner and not be absorbed by the diaper.
Performance Phase	
1. Check patient frequently to see if stooling has occurred.	1. A fresh specimen should be obtained so test results will not be distorted by time-lapse. This will also decrease the chance of the stool becoming contaminated with urine and will prevent skin irritation from the stool.
2. Remove soiled diaper from patient. Clean perineal area, apply clean diaper, and leave patient comfortable.	
3. Remove small amount of stool from diaper with the tongue blade and place it in the specimen container.	
4. Send labeled specimen to the laboratory promptly.	4. Prompt delivery to the lab will prevent changes from taking place in the specimen that could alter the test results.
Follow-up Phase	
1. Accurately describe and chart the following: a. Time specimen was collected b. Color, amount and consistency of stool (Note any foul smell.) c. Type of specimen collected d. Nature of test for which the specimen was collected. e. Condition of the skin	

GUIDELINES: *Assisting with a Spinal Tap—Lumbar Puncture*

A *spinal tap* in an infant or young child is based on the same principles and is essentially the same as for an adult with the following exceptions.

Equipment

No. 21–20 gauge, 3.7-cm. (1½-inch) long spinal needle

Procedure

Nursing Action	Rationale/Amplification
Preparatory Phase	
1. Position the patient.	1. In either position the patient may squirm. Hold him securely to prevent him from moving and causing injury to himself or causing the spinal needle to be inserted too far, resulting in a traumatic tap.
a. *Side position* (similar to the adult): wrap the lower extremities in a sheet, if an older child; place the patient on his side facing the nurse; flex knees and neck by placing one hand on his shoulders and head and the other hand on buttocks and upper thigh.	
b. *Sitting position:* this position is primarily used with small infants. Place patient in sitting position; extend legs and arms in front of the patient; flex his neck so chin is almost resting on his chest; back is rounded by placing thumbs on his shoulders and hands along side of his hips.	

> NURSING ALERT: Observe for signs of respiratory distress. Because the trachea in the infant is so soft, it can kink very easily when the neck is flexed. If this happens and the airway is obstructed, the infant will stop breathing. This is an emergency situation.

Follow-up Phase

1. It is not usually necessary to keep the infant or young child flat in bed following the procedure unless there are contraindications to his being up and the physician has ordered that he be kept in bed.

TRACTION

Traction refers to the extension of an injured extremity in the direction and position which will promote healing and optimal functioning. It is accomplished by the use of weights which pull a part in the desired direction in the presence of countertraction.

Purpose

1. To maintain the approximation of fractured segments of a bone until union occurs.
2. To prevent resulting deformities in the presence of injury or inflammation.
   a. Fractures
   b. Arthritis
   c. Trauma
3. To correct existing deformities.
   a. Congenital dislocation of the hip
   b. Flexion contractures of the knees

Types of Traction

1. *Skeletal traction*—exerted against the bone via any of the following mechanisms:
   a. A pin driven into the bone.
   b. A device such as Crutchfield tongs.
   c. A wire passed through a hole drilled in the bone.
2. *Skin traction*
   Applied to the skin of the affected part of the body.

GUIDELINES: *Assisting the Child in Bryant's Traction*

Bryant's traction involves a bilateral vertical extension of the child's legs. It is used commonly in small children with fractured femurs. It is more effective than Buck's extension used for adults because children cannot provide sufficient countertraction with the weight of their bodies against the *horizontal* pull of the weights. In Bryant's traction the child's weight serves as countertraction to the *vertical* pull of the weights (Fig. 24-8).

Equipment

Moleskin
Adhesive tape
Ace bandage
Jacket restraint

Square wooden block
Ropes, weights, pulleys
Traction bars

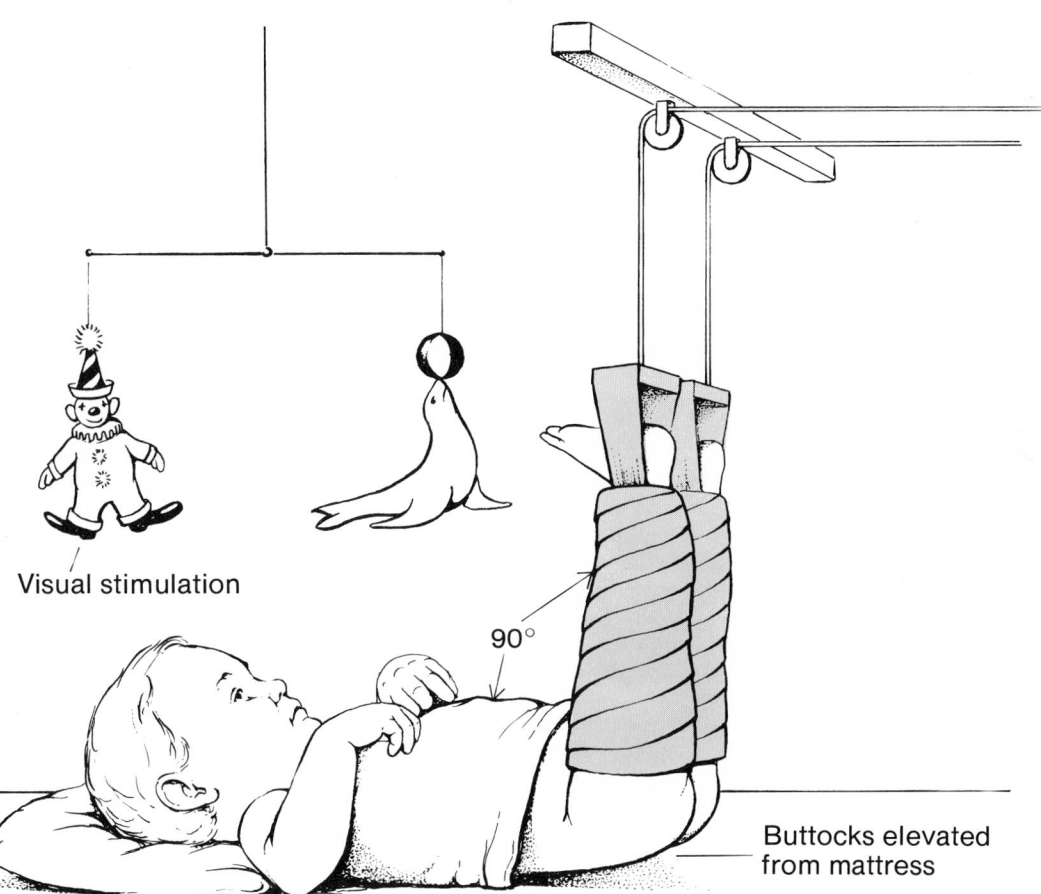

Visual stimulation

90°

Buttocks elevated
from mattress

HARDY

Figure 24-8. Bryant's traction.

Procedure

Nursing Action	*Rationale/Amplification*

Preparatory Phase

1. Gather equipment.

2. Explain the procedure to the child and his parents.

3. Shave the legs if hair is present and paint the skin with tincture of benzoin.

4. Pad bony prominences (ankles) with cotton padding.
5. Cut the moleskin into strips of appropriate length.

1. The amount of weight to be used will be prescribed by the physician.
2. If the traction is to be effective, it is essential that the parents understand the procedure and cooperate while the child is in traction.
3. This allows the adhesive to grasp the skin more firmly. Benzoin also disinfects the skin, allays itching and prevents skin breakdown under the tape.
4. The skin must be protected from injury.

5. The moleskin should extend above the knee on each side of the leg and under the foot.

Performance Phase

1. Assist the physician in applying the traction so that:
   a. The legs are extended at right angles to the body.
   b. The hips are elevated slightly from the bed.
   c. The buttocks are elevated and clear of the bed.
2. Apply a jacket restraint.

3. Record:
   a. Time of the procedure
   b. Position of the child at the end of the procedure
   c. Reaction of the child to the procedure

1. This position is essential in order to achieve the desired results.

2. It is important to keep the child flat in the bed and prevent him from turning from side to side.

Follow-up Phase

1. Maintain even, constant traction:
   a. Do not add or remove weights.
   b. Allow the weights to hang free at all times. Do not allow them to touch the floor or bed.
   c. Be certain that the ropes are in the wheel grooves of the pulleys.
   d. Keep the weights out of the child's reach.
   e. Wrap knotted areas of the ropes with adhesive tape to prevent slipping.
   f. Do not elevate the head or foot of the bed without consulting the physician.
   g. Do not allow the child to turn or move about in the bed.
2. Check the circulation to the toes at frequent intervals.

3. Provide skin care:
   a. Wash and dry all exposed areas thoroughly.

1. Traction must be kept constant in order to achieve the desired results. Any change in the amount of weights or countertraction affects the entire traction system.

2. Cyanosis, tingling, coldness or loss of sensation are indications that local circulation may be impaired.
3. Immobilized children readily develop areas of decubiti unless meticulous skin care is provided.

Nursing Action	**Rationale/Amplification**
b. Rub the child's back and buttocks frequently and apply cornstarch.	b. Cornstarch absorbs moisture and prevents maceration of the skin.
c. Keep the linen clean, dry and free from wrinkles and crumbs.	
4. Plan for short periods of muscle exercise every day.	4. Disuse of muscles can result in atrophy and deformities.
a. Encourage the child to move and exercise his unaffected extremities. Provide diversional therapy which requires the use of these muscles.	
b. Assist him to exercise his toes.	
5. Have the child breathe deeply at intervals. Provide him with soap bubbles to make this more fun.	5. Prolonged periods of immobilization may cause the child to develop hypostatic pneumonia.
6. Provide a diet high in roughage and fluid intake.	6. Lack of exercise may result in the child becoming constipated.

7. Record:
   a. Color, temperature and appearance of toes
   b. Skin condition
   c. Evidence of local edema
   d. Body alignment
   e. Functioning of traction ropes, weights, and pulleys	

8. Do not allow the weights to hang directly over the child's body.	8. This is a safety precaution.
9. Provide daily diversion and encourage the child's family to visit frequently.	9. Enforced bedrest makes the time pass very slowly and can be very traumatic for a small child.

GUIDELINES: *Assisting the Child in Split-Russell Traction*

Split-Russell traction is a type of skin traction used for children with injuries to the lower extremities.

Purposes

1. To aid in reducing muscle spasm around the hip or knee.
2. To immobilize the hip or knee.
3. To correct a deformity of the hip or knee.

Equipment

Appropriate size bed for the child
Bradford frame if the child is small
Additional equipment is the same as for the adult

Procedure

Nursing activities for the child in split-Russell traction are the same as for the adult. In addition, the following points should be considered.

Nursing Action	**Rationale/Amplification**
Application of Ace Bandages	
1. Wrap bandages from the ankle to the thigh on patients under 18 months of age.	1. The length of the leg from the knee to the foot is usually not long enough to maintain traction.
2. Wrap bandages from the ankle to the knee on patients over 18 months of age.	2. This length in an older child is sufficient to maintain traction.
Countertraction	
1. Use a Bradford frame for patients whose weight is not sufficient to provide effective countertraction.	1. Usually children who are 4 years of age or younger.
Diversion	
1. Suspend toys over the child's head so he can reach them. (Punching bag can help child relieve hostility.)	1-4. Since the child will be immobilized for a long period of time, he needs to have diversions appropriate for his age.
2. Provide continuing education for the school-age child.	
3. Encourage projects that will allow child a feeling of accomplishment: painting, puzzles, knitting, ceramics.	
4. Patients who are immobilized in traction or casts should be grouped together.	

GUIDELINES: *Assisting the Child in Cervical Traction*

Cervical traction is used for children with spinal fractures to provide immobilization in a position of hyperextension which causes least pressure on the spinal cord. Cervical traction may be applied directly to the skull bone by a device such as the Crutchfield tong, or indirectly by using a head halter.

Equipment

Equipment is the same as for the adult.

Procedure

Nursing activities for the child in cervical traction are essentially the same as for the adult. The following points are important to observe when maintaining the traction.

Nursing Action	**Rationale/Amplification**
1. Check the position of the head halter frequently:	1. It is important to prevent continuous pressure and rubbing on these areas in order to avoid skin breakdown.
a. The halter should not press on the ears.	
b. The rope should not rest against the skin.	
c. The chin piece should not press on the throat.	
2. Keep the position of the bed flat and avoid lifting the child's head or flexing his neck.	2. Raising the head increases countertraction which may be undesirable.
3. Keep the child flat on his back.	
a. A Stryker frame may be useful if the child must be maintained in this position for a long period of time.	a. A Stryker frame makes it easier to turn the child.

4. Diversion
   a. Position an adjustable mirror at the head of the bed so that the child can see around the room.
   b. Encourage companionship:
      (1) Place the child in a room with other children his age.
      (2) Allow liberal visiting by parents, older siblings and friends.
   c. Place colorful objects, cards, pictures, etc. within sight of the child.
   d. Utilize audiovisual stimulation—records, radio, television, etc.
   e. Provide for continuing education for the child of school age.

GUIDELINES: *Assisting the Child in a Bradford Frame*

A *Bradford frame* is a piece of equipment which facilitates the nursing of young children who must be immobilized for extensive periods of time. It is frequently used for young infants with meningoceles, children in hip–spica casts and children with extensive burns.

Purposes

1. To ensure correct positioning.
2. To facilitate the collection of urine and stools.
3. To protect the child from injury.

Equipment

Frame of appropriate size for the child
2 pieces of canvas of appropriate size to cover the head and foot of the frame
Plastic sheeting
2 crib sheets or draw sheets
Bedboard
Linen for the bed
Plastic draw sheet
Heavy blocks for supporting the frame
Material such as canvas strips for attaching the frame to the bed
Protective device to limit the child's movement

Procedure

Nursing Action	Rationale/Amplification
Preparatory Phase	
1. Select frame according to the size of the child.	1. Frame should be approximately 15 cm. (6 inches) longer and 5 cm. (2 inches) wider than the patient.
2. Cover the head and foot areas with canvas.	
a. Leave an open area between the head and foot sections for the drainage of urine and feces.	a. Make sure that the size of the opening is adequate for the size of the child.
b. Stretch the canvas tightly over the frame.	b. If the canvas is not tight, it will stretch.
3. Cover the top and bottom sections of the canvas with heavy plastic sheeting.	3. This protects the canvas from becoming soiled.
4. Place a small sheet tightly over each section of the frame.	
Performance Phase	
1. Place a bedboard on the mattress.	1. A firm base is required for proper use of the frame.

Nursing Action	**Rationale/Amplification**
2. Place 2 draw sheets on the bed, one at each end.	2. The entire bed will not require changing when only one part is soiled.
3. Place a plastic draw sheet under the center opening of the frame.	3. This is the area most likely to become soiled by urine or feces.
4. Place blocks on the bed. Place the frame on the blocks.	4. The position of the blocks and frame will be ordered by the physician. The blocks should always be placed under the child's shoulders, never directly under his head if the head of the frame is to be elevated.
5. Secure the frame to the bed at the head and foot.	5. This is a safety precaution to prevent slipping.
6. Place the bedpan below the center opening.	
a. Plastic sheeting may be draped over the top and bottom edges of the opening of the frame.	a. This permits urine and feces to drain into the bedpan if the child is incontinent.
b. Place diapers over the plastic.	b. This prevents irritation of the skin.
7. Place the child on the frame.	
a. Maintain his position by use of a jacket restraint. (See procedure for protective measures to limit movement.)	
8. Place pillows at the sides of the frame to support the child's arms.	8. It is important to maintain proper body alignment.

Follow-up Phase

1. Check frequently:	1. These are principles of safety. (See procedure for protective devices to limit movement.)
a. Position of the frame on the blocks.	
b. Security of all knots and materials which are used to fasten the frame to the bed.	
c. Position of the child on the frame.	
2. Provide meticulous general hygiene:	2. See procedure for Bryant's traction and for congenital dislocation of the hip.
a. Empty the bedpan frequently.	
b. Check the linen for soiling by urine or feces and change it if necessary.	
c. Cleanse the buttocks after each bowel movement and apply lotion or cornstarch.	
d. Bathe daily and provide skin care frequently.	
3. Provide for the prevention of contractures, muscle wasting and the development of hypostatic pneumonia.	3. See procedure for Bryant's traction.
4. Provide diversion.	4. See procedures for split-Russell traction and congenital dislocation of the hip.
a. Move the child's bed from room to room for a change of scenery or out into the hall so that he can watch unit activities.	
5. Reconstruct the child's frame as necessary.	
a. The child can usually be placed on a firm bed or stretcher while his frame is being changed.	a. Special care must be taken to ensure correct body alignment during this procedure.
b. If a second frame is available, this can be prepared and placed on another bed. The child can then be easily transferred from one frame to another.	

CASTS

Nursing Considerations

Nursing activities related to the application and care of casts are essentially the same in pediatrics as for adults. The following points of consideration are important.

1. The child is usually more troubled by immobilization than the adult. A special attempt should be made to ensure that his activities are as normal as possible and that full use is made of his unaffected joints and muscles.
2. The younger child may not be able to understand why the cast is necessary. He may attempt to remove it, put pieces of toys or food under it, etc.
   a. An attempt should be made to allow the child to work through his questions and feelings via play (i.e., give him a doll with a cast).
   b. Close supervision is necessary to prevent the child from destroying the cast or injuring himself.
3. There is a danger of soiling a long-leg or hip-spica cast with feces or urine. (The area of the cast near the buttocks and genitalia should be protected with waterproof material.)
4. See section on the nursing care of the child with congenital dislocation of the hip (pp. 1374–1376).

BIBLIOGRAPHY

Books

Abbott Laboratories. Intravenous Hyperalimentation, Intravenous Therapy In-Service Training Series. Clinical Seminar Number 8. Illinois, 1969.
Blake, F., et al.: Nursing Care of Children. Philadelphia, J. B. Lippincott, 1970.
Leifer, G.: Principles and Techniques in Pediatric Nursing. Philadelphia, W. B. Saunders, 1972.
Marlow, D. R.: Textbook of Pediatric Nursing. Philadelphia, W. B. Saunders, 1973.
Silver, H. K., et al.: Handbook of Pediatrics. Los Altos, California, Lange Medical Publications, 1969.
Zimmerbook: Traction Handbook. Zimmer Manufacturing Company, Warsaw, Indiana.

Articles

Barnes, L. A.: Fluid and electrolyte problems. Ped. Clin. N. Amer., 11:789–1103, 1964.
Brandt, P. A., et al.: I.M. injections in children. Amer J. Nurs., 72:1402–1406, Aug. 1972.
Chinn, P. L.: Infant gavage feeding. Amer. J. Nurs., 71:1964–1967, Oct. 1971.
Heid, W. C., et al.: Intravenous alimentation in pediatric patients. J. Ped., 80 (No. 3):351–372, 1972.
Humphrey, N. M., Wright, P., and Swanson, A.: Parental hyperalimentation for children. Amer. J. Nurs., 72:286–288, Feb. 1972.
Lane, P.: A mother's confession—Home care of a toddler in a spica cast: What it is really like. Amer. J. Nurs., 71:2142–2143, Nov. 1971.
Sinclair, J. C., et al.: Supportive management of the sick neonate. Ped. Clin. N. Amer., 17:881–890, 1970.
Wiley, L.: Hyperalimentation, its help and risk. Nursing '72, 2:26–32, April 1972.
Wilmore, D. W., et al.: Growth and development of an infant receiving all nutrients exclusively by vein. J.A.M.A., 203:860, 1968.

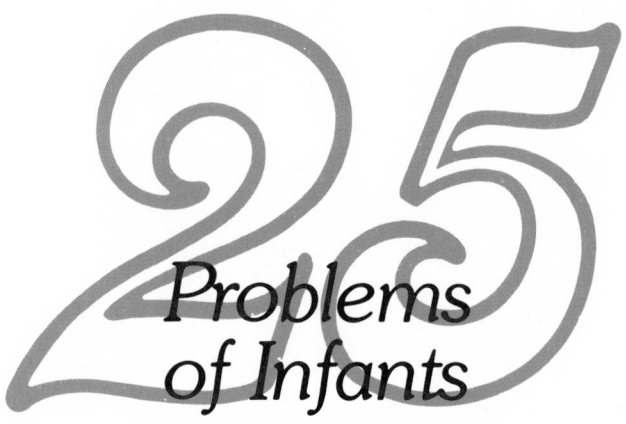

Problems of Infants

MANAGEMENT OF THE PREMATURE INFANT

The *premature infant* is a viable infant born before 38 weeks gestation.

Etiology

1. Not known in many cases
2. Maternal factors associated with prematurity:
   a. Chronic poor nutrition
   b. Diabetes
   c. Multiple births
   d. Chronic disease
      (1) Heart disease
      (2) Kidney disease
      (3) Infection
   e. Complications of pregnancy
      (1) Toxemia
      (2) Bleeding
      (3) Placenta previa or abruptio placenta
      (4) Incompetent cervix
      (5) Premature rupture of membranes
      (6) Polyhydramnios
3. Fetal factors associated with prematurity
   a. Chromosomal abnormalities
   b. Anatomic abnormalities
      (1) Tracheoesophageal atresia or fistula
      (2) Intestinal obstruction
   c. Fetoplacental unit dysfunction

Altered Physiology

The premature infant is generally immature with poorly developed systems that sustain life.

1. Respiratory system is susceptible to difficulty.
   a. Alveoli begin to form at 22 weeks gestation (weight, 1000 gm. or 2 pounds 6 ounces); therefore, lungs are poorly developed.

    b. Respiratory muscles are poorly developed.

    c. Chest wall lacks stability.

    d. Thoracic cage is flexible.

    e. Respiratory center is poorly developed and not as sensitive to decreased oxygen.

    f. Breathing may be dyspneic and irregular with periods of apnea and cyanosis.

    g. Infant is prone to atelectasis, respiratory distress syndrome and hyaline membrane disease.

    h. Gag and cough reflexes are poor; thus, aspiration is a problem.

2. Digestive system is immature.

    a. Stomach is small—vomiting more likely to occur.

    b. Decreased tolerance and impaired ability to absorb fat.

3. Thermal stability is poor.

    a. Has very little subcutaneous fat; thus, there is no heat storage.

    b. Cannot shiver.

    c. There is a large surface area in comparison to weight.

    d. Cannot perspire because has few sweat glands.

    e. Usually less active.

4. Renal function is immature.

    a. Difficulty in excreting sodium and calcium; therefore, water is retained and edema results.

    b. Cannot concentrate urine well, thus when vomiting or diarrhea occur, dehydration is likely to follow.

    c. Has difficulty in excreting acid, so acidosis becomes a possibility.

5. Nervous system is immature.

    a. Slow to respond to stimulation.

    b. Suck, swallow and gag reflexes are poor, making feeding and aspiration a problem.

    c. Cough reflex is weak or absent.

    d. Centers that control respirations, temperature and other vital functions are poorly developed.

6. Infant is susceptible to infection.

    a. White blood cells are adequate, but they do not mobilize to attack.

    b. Because gamma globulin level is lower, there is less resistance to disease.

    c. Poor ability to localize infection; therefore, greater chance of generalized sepsis.

7. Liver function is immature.

    a. Inability to handle and conjugate bilirubin.

    b. Does not store or release sugar well; thus, a tendency for hypoglycemia.

    c. There is a steady decrease in hemoglobin after birth and in the production of blood; therefore, anemia may occur.

    d. Does not make or store vitamin K.

8. Retina of the eyes are immature.

    Oxygen given beyond the point of infant need will cause retinal arteries to constrict, resulting in anoxic damage. The retinae detach from the surface of posterior chambers and a fibrous mass forms, resulting in an inability to receive visual stimulation. This is *retrolental fibroplasia.*

9. Tendency toward hemorrhage is increased.

    a. Blood prothrombin level is low.

    b. Increased fragility of capillary walls.

    c. Intracranial hemorrhage is very likely.

Clinical Manifestations

1. Physical appearance
   Hair—lanugo, fluffy
   Poor ear cartilage
   Skin—very thin; capillaries are visible
     (may be red and wrinkled)
   Lack of subcutaneous fat
   Sole of foot is smooth
     (36 weeks gestation—
     ⅓ of foot is creased)
     (38 weeks gestation—
     ⅔ of foot is creased)
   Breast buds 5 mm.
     (36 weeks gestation—none)
     (38 weeks gestation—3 mm.)

   Testes—undescended
   Labia majora—undeveloped
   Rugae of scrotum—very fine
   Fingernails—softer
   Abdomen—relatively large
   Thorax—relatively small
   Head—appears disproportionately large
   Facies resembles "an old man"
   Muscle tone poor—reflexes weak

2. Generally, maturation and growth rate increase after birth

Diagnostic Evaluation

Neurologic Assessment

   Maturation of the nervous system goes on at its own pace and is not increased by birth. The value of a neurologic evaluation increases after 48 hours of life. This examination is used primarily to estimate the infant's gestational age.

A. *Evaluation of muscle tone*
   1. Posture normally assumed by the infant is a supine position.
   2. The extensor tone usually predominates earlier than flexor tone.
   3. Posture—at 24 weeks gestation, infant rolls over on his side when placed supine.
   4. Recoil
      a. The liveliness with which extremity returns to original position after passive stretching and relaxing.
      b. Helpful in determining gestational age between 37–40 weeks.
   5. Mobility
      As gestational age advances, spontaneous movements range from extensive and generalized to localized and brief.
   6. Heel-to-ear movement.
      a. The degree of resistance met when attempt is made to approximate an extended leg to the ear.
      b. At 34 weeks gestational age—begins to be difficult.
         At 37 weeks gestational age—meets great resistance.
   7. Scarf sign
      a. The degree of head turning toward acromion when the examiner carries one of infant's hands across chest to opposite shoulder.
      b. At 36–40 weeks gestational age, there is great resistance.
   8. Neck muscle tone
      a. In sitting position, the ease with which the chin is raised away from the chest.
      b. At 34 weeks gestational age—movement is fairly good.
         At 36 weeks gestational age—movement is good.

B. *Evaluation of reflexes and reactions* (see p. 1033 normal newborn reflexes)
   1. Moro reflex
       Fully developed at 28 weeks gestation.
   2. Grasp reflex
       a. 24 weeks gestational age—is feeble.
       b. 28 weeks gestational age—is fair.
       c. 32 weeks gestational age—arm becomes involved.
       d. 36 weeks gestational age—there is arm flexion at elbow and shoulder becomes involved.
   3. Rooting
       a. Accomplished 24–28 weeks gestational age when neck is slightly elevated.
       b. Well developed at 32 weeks gestational age.
   4. Sucking
       a. Present to some degree at 24 weeks gestational age.
       b. At 32 weeks gestational age, it is strong.
       c. At 34 weeks gestational age, it is synchronized with swallowing.
   5. Pupillary response
       Usually present after 30 weeks gestational age.
   6. Stepping
       a. Just present at 34 weeks gestational age.
       b. Fairly well-developed; infant using tip toes at 37 weeks gestational age.
       c. Good at 37 weeks gestational age.
   7. Crossed extensor
       a. Evaluated in 3 phases of (1) withdrawal, (2) extension and (3) adduction.
       b. At 24 weeks gestation—all are absent, but at 28 weeks gestation there is slight withdrawal.
       c. At 32–34 weeks gestational age—good withdrawal.
       d. At 37 weeks gestational age—withdrawal and extension.
       e. At 41 weeks gestational age—withdrawal, extension and adduction are seen.
   8. Cry
       a. At 24 weeks gestation—cry is weak.
       b. At 28 weeks gestation—cry is brief and high-pitched.
       c. At 32 weeks gestation—cry is good.
   9. Tonic neck reflex and neck righting
       May be seen as early as 32 weeks gestational age.

Complications in Premature Infants

   1. Hyaline membrane disease
       (respiratory distress syndrome)
   2. Aspiration
   3. Infection
   4. Hypoglycemia
   5. Hypocalcemia
   6. Patent ductus arteriosus

Nursing Objectives

ADMISSION TO THE NURSERY

A. *To observe for any gross abnormalities as in the case of a full-term infant on admission, and to pay special attention to respirations, heart rate, muscle tone and activity.*
   1. Respirations above 40/minute over a period of time may be indicative of respiratory difficulty.

      a. Expiratory grunting, retractions or nasal flaring should be reported immediately.

      b. Cyanosis (other than acrocyanosis—coldness and cyanosis of hands and feet) should be watched for along with other signs of respiratory distress.

  2. Increased (above 120/minute) or irregular heart rate may indicate cardiac or circulatory difficulties.

  3. Muscle tone and activity can be a good guide to degree of prematurity.

B. *To maintain a patent airway.*

  1. Have oxygen, suction and resuscitative equipment readily available.

  2. Suction mouth and pharynx if mucus is present—to prevent aspiration.
"Preemies" often have an excess amount of mucus as well as poor cough, swallow and gag reflexes.

  3. Position infant in incubator to allow for easy drainage of mucus from his mouth.

      a. Very small "preemie"—place on side.

      b. Larger "preemies"—place on abdomen.

      c. Head may be tilted down—this may be contraindicated because of increased intracranial pressure or increased respiratory distress due to liver pushing against diaphragm decreasing lung expansion.

  4. Administer emergency oxygen to just barely relieve cyanosis.

C. *To stabilize infant's temperature.*

  1. Obtain weight and temperature quickly and place infant in warm environment (incubator); then let him rest.
Incubator temperature should be between 30–32.2°C. (85–90°F.) usually with humidity.

  2. Omit bath until infant's temperature is stabilized.

D. *To ensure that prophylactic measures have been administered against ophthalmia neonatorum and that vitamin K₁ has been administered.*
Since the "preemie" is frequently taken from the delivery room as soon as possible after birth, prophylactic measures may have been omitted.

E. *To be aware of early complications that may arise as a result of complications of the pregnancy, labor or delivery.*

  1. Maternal medication

      a. Drugs pass quickly from mother's blood, across the placenta into the infant's blood.

      b. Infant may be drowsy and have slowed respirations.

      c. Because of poor development, respiratory difficulty may occur.

  2. Blood incompatibility of mother and infant.

      a. "Preemie" is more susceptible to jaundice, even without incompatibilities.

      b. Observe closely for early signs of jaundice (see p. 1127, hyperbilirubinemia).

  3. Maternal conditions that may predispose to infant problems.

      a. Infection or illness

      b. Diabetes

      c. Drugs

  4. Hypoglycemia

      a. "Preemie" has low blood sugar 24–36 hours after birth.

      b. Low blood sugar is less than 20 mg./100 ml.

      c. Symptoms are nonspecific.

        (1) Jitteriness   (4) Lethargy

        (2) Sweating   (5) Convulsions

        (3) Tachypnea or apnea   (6) Cyanosis

      d. Try to maintain blood sugar at 30–40 mg./100 ml.

      e. Predisposing factors of hypoglycemia:

        (1) Infant of a diabetic mother   (4) Intrauterine malnutrition

        (2) Erythroblastosis fetalis   (5) Developmental defects

        (3) Sepsis

      f. Treatment is to increase blood sugar intake by intravenous or oral feedings. If given too rapidly, it will stimulate insulin production.

   5. Hypocalcemia

      a. Low blood calcium is reached the first day of life.

      b. Try to maintain serum calcium above 8 mg./100 ml.

      c. Symptoms are nondescript.

        (1) Twitching   (4) Hypotonia

        (2) Convulsions   (5) Abdominal distention with ileus

        (3) Lethargy

      d. Predisposing factors of hypocalcemia

        (1) Hypoglycemia   (3) Low infant Apgar rating

        (2) Previous maternal abortion   (4) Hyaline membrane disease

      e. Treatment is to give calcium intravenously or orally.

        Intravenous calcium given too rapidly will cause bradycardia.

THE FIRST 24–48 HOURS OF LIFE

    This period after birth is the most critical time for the premature infant.

A. *To be constantly aware of the infant's condition and to make frequent observations.*

   1. This poorly developed, immature infant is prone to sudden changes in condition.

   2. Early recognition of symptoms is the most valuable contribution the nurse can make in caring for and saving the "preemie's" life.

   3. Note bleeding from the umbilical cord.

      a. Should bleeding occur, apply pressure.

      b. Estimate amount of bleeding and record.

      c. Notify the physician immediately—replacement transfusion may be necessary.

   4. Note first voiding.

      a. This may occur up to 36 hours after birth.

      b. Note amount, color and frequency of voidings.

      c. Lack of voiding may indicate renal system anomalies.

   5. Note stools

      a. Note when first stool occurred and its characteristics.

      b. Abdominal distention and lack of stool may indicate intestinal obstruction or other intestinal tract anomalies.

   6. Note activity and behavior.

      a. Note amount of lethargy or activity or need for stimulation.

      b. Look for sucking movement, hand-to-mouth maneuver. This can help to determine oral feeding initiation.

      c. Note quality of cry.

7. Observe for a tense and bulging fontanelle.
   a. Full fontanelle may indicate hydrocephalus or intracranial hemorrhage.
   b. Be alert to twitching and seizures.
8. Note color of skin.
   a. Cyanosis
      (1) Circulatory or cardiac difficulties may be present.
      (2) Respiratory effort may be ineffective.
   b. Jaundice
      (1) May indicate infection.
      (2) Erythroblastosis fetalis is another possible difficulty.

B. *To maintain respirations.*
   1. Immediate emergency support may be necessary since respiratory system is poorly developed and ability to control respirations is often barely sufficient.
   2. Have available resuscitative equipment, oxygen and suction apparatus.
      a. Mucus may not be handled well because of poor gag, cough, and swallowing reflexes.
         (1) Clearing the airway is of major importance.
         (2) A rubber ear bulb syringe is often all that is necessary for clearing the mouth.
         (3) Frequent suctioning of the pharynx may not be necessary.
   3. Position infant so mucus and secretions can drain easily from mouth (see above).
   4. Use only the percent of oxygen necessary to relieve cyanosis or maintain color.
      a. Oxygen is used with moisture to prevent mucous membranes from drying and becoming irritated.
      b. Monitor oxygen with analyzer every hour to ensure consistency in percentage used.
   5. Note any changes in respiratory effort.
      a. Note quality and rate particularly.
      b. Hyaline membrane disease or respiratory distress syndrome occurs during the first 24–48 hours of life. Observe for and report immediately any signs and symptoms of respiratory difficulty.
         (1) Increased respiratory rate   (4) Cyanosis
             (usually above 60/minute)   (5) Expiratory grunting
         (2) Thoracic retractions   (6) Developing exhaustion
         (3) Nasal flaring   (7) Periods of apnea

C. *To conserve the infant's energy while providing necessary care.*
   1. Be organized in caring for the infant.
      Collect all equipment before starting care, do what needs to be done, and then let the infant rest.
   2. Premature infants tire very easily.
      Any activity increases oxygen need, thus increasing respiratory rate, taxing already limited energy.

D. *To provide and maintain thermal stability of the "preemie."*
   1. An incubator or warming bed is usually used.
      a. This allows for better observation of the undressed infant.
      b. Temperature control is made easier.
      c. When using an incubator:
         (1) Minimize entrance activities.
         (2) Keep portholes tight around arm when entering.

2. The "preemie's" skin temperature should be maintained at 36–36.5°C. (96.8–97.8°F.).
   a. Environmental temperature should be between 30–32.2°C. (85–90°F.). Smaller premature infants may need a temperature around 32.2°C. (90°F.); larger premature infants, around 30°C. (85°F.).
   b. When infant's temperature is maintained at this level, his oxygen consumption and caloric usage is at a minimum.
   c. Avoid constant changing of temperature control dials on incubator.
   d. Check the incubator temperature each time the infant's temperature is taken for use as a point of reference.
   Temperature control centers are poorly developed in the premature infant and his temperature is easily influenced by his environment.

E. *To prevent infection of this very susceptible premature infant.*
   1. Practice scrupulous hand washing.
   2. Use gown and mask technique as prescribed by hospital.
   3. Minimize infant's contact with unsterile equipment.
   4. Any nurse or other personnel with any kind of infection should not enter the nursery.

F. *To offer support to the parents of the premature infant during this crucial period.*
   1. Most parents, particularly mothers, are physically and emotionally unprepared for the early arrival of their baby.
   2. Allow parents to see their infant and touch him if this is feasible.
   3. Listen to parents talk and express their concerns. Encourage them, but do not give them false hope.

THE GROWING OR OLDER PREMATURE INFANT

After the first few days have passed without any complications the premature infant is very busy growing. During this time, however, it must be remembered that other complications can occur. The areas of concern mentioned above are still important, along with the following:

A. *To be constantly alert to signs and symptoms of complications.*
   1. Aspiration
      a. The growing "preemie" may still have poor reacting gag and cough reflexes.
      b. The "preemie" will show signs of respiratory distress.
         Suction mouth and pharynx immediately and get medical assistance.
   2. Infection or sepsis
      a. Infant becomes less active, lethargic and sleepy and will not suck or eat well.
      b. Temperature may be subnormal or elevated.
      c. Skin may be mottled or jaundiced.
   3. Latent acidosis of prematurity
      a. Infant begins to feed poorly and takes longer to eat. He is also sleepy and needs stimulation to keep awake.
      b. There will be no weight gain.
   4. Neonatal tetany (see hypocalcemia, p. 1123)
      a. Onset is between 5–10 days.
      b. Formula with a low phosphorus content is used in treatment.
         (1) Regular infant formula has a high phosphorus content.
         (2) Immature kidneys cannot handle the high phosphorus load that results when calcium is low in the infant.

B. *To provide and maintain adequate nutrition to allow for growth and development.*
   1. The premature infant has a small stomach but a great need for calories.
      a. Small, frequent feedings are offered.
      b. High calorie formula may be given, but may cause edema.
         (1) Kidneys are immature and cannot handle the high protein load in the formula.
         (2) Infant has difficulty in excreting acid so he may become acidotic.
      c. Overfeeding can increase the risk of vomiting.
            Vomiting can lead to dehydration, loss of hydrochloric acid and alkalosis.
      d. Tilt mattress to elevate head, shoulders and chest after feeding to decrease chance of vomiting.
      e. Bubble infant frequently during feeding.
   2. Allow the infant to rest prior to feeding.
         The "preemie" tires easily from procedures and will eat better if rested.
   3. Feed appropriately for individual patient.
      a. Gavage is indicated for very small "preemie" who does not demonstrate good sucking or synchronized sucking and swallowing.
      b. Dropper or nipple feeding is indicated for a vigorous "preemie" with good suck, gag and swallowing reflexes.
      c. Gastrostomy may be indicated for "preemie" who has no gag reflex.

C. *To meet the psychological needs of the "preemie" who is an individual in his own right.*
   1. At first, even though handling is minimal, the nurse should talk to and caress the infant while performing procedures.
      a. Stroking and gentle handling will provide necessary sensory stimulation.
      b. A soft musical sound may also be comforting.
   2. Once the "preemie" is able to leave the incubator, even for short periods of time, he should be held for feedings.
      a. While holding him, stroke him and talk to him.
      b. Keep him warmly wrapped—this will also give him a feeling of security.
   3. If the infant is restless in his incubator, he may be calmed by propping him against a blanket or diaper roll.
         The freedom of movement, restrained only by the mattress, cannot offer much security to the infant.
   4. Encourage parents to touch, fondle, caress and talk to their baby whenever they visit.

D. *To foster healthy family relationships with the premature baby.*
   1. Encourage parents to make frequent visits to the nursery so they can become familiar with all aspects of care of their infant.
      a. When they visit, explain the equipment and procedures that may be foreign to them.
      b. Help them to feel comfortable and confident in handling their infant.
      c. Parents may lose interest in the infant if the hospitalization is long.
            If parents cannot visit daily, encourage them to call.
   2. The support and help given to parents during hospitalization will make home care easier.
      a. Teach mother how to care for her infant.
      b. The small size of the infant often is the thing that frightens parents the most.
   3. Initiate community nurse referral if parents seem anxious about caring for their baby at home.
         If this "preemie" is the first baby, this may be particularly helpful to the mother.

4. Encourage parents to talk about their feelings or fears concerning their infant and how they will care for him.
   a. By listening, the nurse can gain some insight as to what to talk about or teach the parents.
   b. Parents' feelings can frequently interfere with appropriate home care.
   c. Parents often treat the "preemie" like he is fragile and more prone to illness.
   d. Parents worry about how to feed and protect the infant.
5. Help the family prepare for the time when their new baby will arrive home.
   Because of the early, unexpected arrival of the infant, things such as clothing, bed and bottles may not be ready.

Parental (Family) Teaching

1. Help the family to understand that caring for the premature at home should not be any different from caring for a full-term infant.
   a. Special treatment may lead to behavior problems later.
   b. At first a little extra caution should be practiced.
      (1) Keep room temperature fairly constant—about 22.2°C. (72°F.).
      (2) Sponge-bathe infant instead of bathing in tub and keep him warm during procedure.
      (3) Feed him the recommended amount of formula to be certain he receives the necessary calories for continual growth.
      (4) Keep him away from crowds and people who have colds.
2. Spend enough time with the mother teaching her how to feed and care for her infant.
   Show her how, then watch her and help her improve and gain confidence.
      (1) Infant needs gentle, firm handling.
      (2) He needs to be mothered and kept comfortable with minimal tensions.
      (3) A soothing voice can be comforting.
      (4) Sucking provides a pleasant experience.
3. Stress the importance of medical follow-up for the baby after discharge from the hospital.
   Anemia and failure to thrive are common long-term side effects of prematurity.
4. Help mother understand the importance of good, early prenatal care for subsequent pregnancies.
   Once a woman has had one premature infant, this classifies her as high-risk for another premature delivery with future pregnancies.

JAUNDICE IN THE NEWBORN
(Hyperbilirubinemia)

Hyperbilirubinemia (jaundice) in the newborn is an accumulation of serum bilirubin above normal levels.

Etiology

1. The red blood cell is destroyed.
   a. When the RBC is destroyed, hemoglobin is released.
   b. Hemoglobin eventually breaks down into indirect or unconjugated bilirubin. (This bilirubin is fat-soluble.)
   c. Indirect bilirubin attaches to albumin in the plasma.
      Indirect bilirubin is also in the tissues in a state of equilibrium with that in the plasma.

2. Serum indirect bilirubin is transported to the liver where it is:
   a. Acted upon by enzymes, one being glucuronyl transferase.
   b. The result is direct or conjugated bilirubin. (This is water-soluble.)
3. From the liver, direct bilirubin is excreted in bile, to the intestines and out of the body in stool.
4. Newborn serum bilirubin stays around 3–7 mg./100 ml. of blood. This level varies depending upon age or physical condition of the newborn.

Altered Physiology

A. *Physiologic jaundice*
1. Normal newborn's hemoglobin ranges from 16–20 mg./100 ml. of blood.
2. Peak serum bilirubin levels of 12 mg./100 ml. of blood in the full-term infant and 15 mg./100 ml. of blood in the premature in physiologic jaundice.
3. The first few days of life there is slightly more rapid red blood cell hemolysis.
      Each gram of hemoglobin breakdown forms 35 mg. of bilirubin.
4. This hemolysis combined with an immature liver results in an increase of serum indirect bilirubin—jaundice may be seen.

B. *Erythroblastosis fetalis*
1. Immune hemolysis or Rh/ABO blood group incompatibility
      Mother's and infant's blood are different.
            Rh factor
            Different ABO blood groups
2. Mother produces antibodies against the antigen of baby's blood. Fetal cells frequently cross placenta.
3. Antibodies of mother's blood are present in baby's blood at birth.
   a. Therefore there is hemolysis of infant's red blood cells.
   b. Hemolysis leads to rising level of indirect bilirubin.

C. *Other Considerations*
1. Rapid increase in indirect bilirubin due to hemolysis.
   a. Some bilirubin might not bind to albumin. (This cannot be measured.)
   b. Free indirect bilirubin is very toxic. (Causes brain damage—kernicterus.)
2. Other causes of hyperbilirubinemia:
   a. Sepsis   d. Decreased liver metabolism
   b. Enclosed hemorrhage of the newborn   e. Intestinal obstruction
   c. Red blood cell enzyme defects

Clinical Manifestations

1. Onset
   a. Onset in physiologic jaundice—occurs 3–5 days after birth
   b. Onset in erythroblastosis—may be within 24 hours after birth
2. Major symptoms
   a. Skin appears light to bright yellow   c. Lethargy
   b. Sclera appear yellow before skin does   d. Dark amber and concentrated urine
3. Minor symptoms
   a. Poor feeding
   b. Dark stools

4. Complications—kernicterus
   a. Kernicterus (brain damage) occurs when there is yellow staining of the brain tissue from the deposits of indirect bilirubin.
   b. Early signs of kernicterus:
      (1) Refusal or vomiting of feedings
      (2) Hypotonia
      (3) High-pitched cry
      (4) Decrease of normal reflexes, i.e., Moro reflex, sucking reflex
   c. Later signs of kernicterus:
      (1) Opisthotonus
      (2) Apnea
      (3) Cyanosis
      (4) Convulsions

Diagnostic Evaluation

1. All infants who have clinical signs of hyperbilirubinemia should be given the following work-up:
   a. Total bilirubin levels—indirect and direct
   b. Peripheral smear—for evidence of red blood cell immaturity or abnormality
   c. Reticulocyte count—to determine rate of hemolysis
   d. Coomb's test—to check for Rh or ABO group incompatibility between mother and baby
   e. Blood typing of mother and infant
   f. Total serum protein—to measure binding capacity
2. If serum indirect bilirubin is rising or has reached the level of 15–20 mg./100 ml. of blood, exchange transfusion is considered.
3. Measuring the bilirubin-albumin binding capacity of the plasma can be valuable in determining the risk of kernicterus and the need for an exchange transfusion. This test defines the upper limits to which serum bilirubin is allowed to rise when an exchange transfusion is done.
   a. $\dfrac{\text{Total bilirubin}}{\text{Total serum protein}}$ = 1. if less than 3.7—no danger of kernicterus
      2. if greater than 3.7—treatment by exchange transfusion is indicated.
   b. Total serum protein $\times$ 3.7 = level of bilirubin at which to do exchange transfusion
4. The level of bilirubin at which the infant is at risk for brain damage depends upon the degree of prematurity, presence of acidosis, hypoxia, or drugs which bind albumin. (20 mg. of bilirubin/100 ml. of blood is not necessarily the upper limit of bilirubin as formerly thought.)

Nursing Objectives

A. *To observe infant's skin for appearance of or increase in icterus or yellowish coloring.*
   1. Make observations in daylight, sunlight or white fluorescent light.
   2. Blanch the skin during the observation to clear away capillary coloration.
B. *To be aware of the age of the infant. Know if mother's and baby's blood are incompatible.*
   1. Between age 3–5 days, physiologic jaundice can be expected to occur, if it is going to occur.
   2. If mother's and baby's blood types are incompatible, signs of jaundice may occur at about 24 hours of age and should be watched for.

C. *To note any changes in urine pigmentation and frequency.*

> Careful notation of frequency, amount and color of urine should be made so changes will be noticed immediately.

D. *To maintain adequate fluid intake.*
  1. Be aware of feeding history and amount of fluid taken.
  2. If infant is a slow eater, feed small amounts frequently.
  3. The amount of fluid intake determines amount of hydration and in turn determines excretion of bilirubin.
  4. If infant is receiving intravenous fluid, keep an accurate hourly record of fluid intake. Do not allow intake to fall behind ordered rate. Observe I.V. site for infiltration so I.V. can be discontinued and restarted immediately.

E. *To be alert to any behavior changes.*

> Note particularly: increasing lethargy, change in sucking activity or quality or vomiting.

F. *To be alert to signs of kernicterus.*

> Observe for signs of: decreased muscle tone, no sucking, no hand grasp, or regurgitation of feedings where not previously observed. In time infant becomes opisthotonic and irritable.

G. *To administer the treatment of phototherapy safely and properly should it be ordered.*
  1. 200–400 footcandles of fluorescent light directly to the exposed skin of the infant reduces tissue bilirubin which in turn reduces serum bilirubin by (a) photo-oxidizing tissue bilirubin to biliverdin, to secondary yellow pigments, to colorless, nontoxic compounds and (b) tissue-serum bilirubin equilibrium, or as the bilirubin decreases in the tissue, bilirubin is pulled from the serum into the tissue to maintain this equilibrium.
  2. The physician will determine the length of time the infant is to be under the lights based on serum bilirubin levels and clinical condition of the infant.
  3. Nursing care peculiar to phototherapy includes:
     a. Having infant completely undressed so entire skin surface is exposed to light.
     b. Keeping infant's eyes covered to protect them from the constant exposure to high intensity of light which may cause retinal injury. Do not apply pressure when the eyes are covered as this may cause corneal ulceration.
     c. Develop a systematic schedule of turning infant so all surfaces are exposed.
     d. Be aware of side effects of the light:
        (1) Lethargy
        (2) Loose green stools
        (3) Possible temperature change
        (4) Skin changes such as a rash due to capillary dilatation
        (5) Continual erection of penis—turn infant on abdomen for short periods of time and this will cease.
     e. Note sleeping and eating patterns. The feeding schedule may need to be adjusted to the infant's pattern for better feeding.
     f. Develop a schedule for changing light bulbs. The effectiveness of the wave length decreases after 200 hours of use; thus the bulbs should be changed at that time. A record of hours of use will be helpful.

H. *To assist in the treatment of exchange transfusion (see p. 1102).*

I. *To foster a healthy family-child relationship.*

1. Encourage parents to visit infant as much as possible during hospitalization.
2. Allow parents to fondle, care for and hold and feed infant as much as possible or as his condition permits.
3. Initiate a community nursing referral if parents are particularly anxious about caring for infant at home after discharge.

Parental Teaching

1. Help family to understand what is wrong with their baby. Explain in simple terms what the doctor has already told them. Allow them to ask questions about the baby and treatment.
2. If the baby has erythroblastosis fetalis, help parents understand the importance of prenatal care and monitoring should another pregnancy occur.
3. Stress the importance of close follow-up of the baby after hospital discharge. Anemia is a common long-term side effect of red blood cell hemolysis and exchange transfusion. The baby's hemoglobin level should be monitored for some time after illness so appropriate treatment can be initiated if necessary.

SEPTICEMIA NEONATORUM
(Sepsis)

Septicemia Neonatorum (sepsis) is a generalized infection which may occur in the newborn and is characterized by the proliferation of bacteria in the bloodstream.

Etiology

1. The distribution of etiologic agents vary from year to year and from institution to institution.
2. Gram negative organisms:
    E. coli
    Klebsiella (enterobacteriaceae)
    Pseudomonas
    Proteus
    Salmonella
    H. influenzae
3. Gram positive organisms:
    Staphylococcus aureus
    Staphylococcus epidermidis
    Beta hemolytic streptococci
    (usually Group B)
    Streptococcus faecalis
    D. pneumoniae
4. Sepsis occurs most frequently in the first month of life.

Altered Physiology

1. Infection may gain access into the amnionic sac either prior to or after rupture of the membranes; the fetus may aspirate some of this infected fluid.
2. Bacteria may enter the fetal circulation following invasion of the decidua from the amnionic cavity.

3. After birth, bacteria may enter the infant's circulation by a variety of routes. Infection may originate in the skin, umbilical stump, or mucous membranes of the eyes, nose, pharynx, ear, respiratory, gastrointestinal and renal tracts.

4. It is difficult to identify the site of the initial invasion because there may be a minimal local inflammatory response.

5. The organism causing sepsis can be acquired originally from many sources:
    a. Mother's vaginal tract
    b. Nursery personnel
    c. Other infants (airborne spread)
    d. Contaminated medications applied to the infant's skin, mucous membrane or umbilical cord
    e. Oxygen and humidification equipment
    f. Soap dispensers

Clinical Manifestations

1. The early symptoms of sepsis are usually vague and subtle. The infant is often described as being "lethargic" and not doing well.
    The symptoms often include:
    a. Reluctance to feed or refusal to feed
    b. Lack of vigor, lethargy, decreased activity and loss of muscle tone
    c. Loss of weight

2. More specific symptoms soon develop and include any of the following:
    a. Pallor, cyanosis or apneic attacks
    b. Hypothermia or hyperthermia
        (Frequent adjustment of incubator is required after period of initial stabilization.)
    c. Convulsions
    d. Bulging fontanelles
    e. Anemia
    f. Jaundice (of sudden onset)
    g. Hepatomegaly
    h. Splenomegaly
    i. Abdominal distention
    j. Vomiting and diarrhea

Diagnostic Evaluation

1. Cultures to detect specific organism
    a. Spinal fluid culture
    b. Blood cultures
    c. Urine cultures
    d. Umbilical stump cultures
    e. Skin lesions culture
    f. Mouth and throat culture

2. CBC—may be normal or may show varying degrees of anemia, leukocytosis or leukopenia

3. Platelet count—may be decreased

4. Blood glucose—may be low, elevated or normal

5. Chest X-ray—may demonstrate pulmonary infection

Complications

1. Meningitis—very common complication
2. Pyarthrosis
3. Shock

Treatment

1. Antimicrobial therapy, based on the identified organism; when the specific organism is not identified the antimicrobial therapy is based on the more common causative agents and their anticipated antimicrobial susceptibilities.
2. Supportive therapy.

Nursing Objectives

A. *To practice measures which will prevent the transmission of infection in the nursery.*
1. Practice careful handwashing technique and serve as a model of good technique.
2. Personnel with infection should avoid contact with infants.
   a. Seek medical care for infection. (Cultures should be done.)
   b. Remain out of the nursery.
   c. Wear a mask when it is necessary to enter the nursery.
3. Teach parents and other persons entering the nursery proper handwashing and gown technique.
4. Maintain sterile technique when procedures demanding this technique are performed.
5. Promote general cleanliness of the nursery environment.

B. *To observe infants for the vague symptoms which appear early in the course of sepsis.*
1. Observe for the following:
   a. Lethargy, decreased activity and loss of muscle tone
   b. Poor feeding or refusal to feed
   c. Loss of weight
2. Be consistent in planning for the care of infants to provide a means whereby these early symptoms may be detected.
   a. Accurate charting of the infant's previous behavior
   b. Assigning the same nurse to care for an infant on successive days
3. Report to the physician the symptoms observed.

C. *To observe for episodes of apnea and initiate measures to stimulate respiration.*
1. Observe the infant closely for apnea or have the infant placed on a respiratory monitor.
2. Stimulate infant when apnea does occur.
   a. Slap feet and provide more vigorous stimulation if necessary.
   b. Apply hand pulmonator or mouth-to-mouth resuscitation when spontaneous respiration does not occur within 15 to 30 seconds.
3. Report frequent periods of apnea to physician.
4. Record length of apneic episode and response to stimulation.

D. *To observe the infant for convulsions which may occur with sepsis.*
1. Immediately report to the physician any twitching or convulsive activity.
   a. Remain with infant.
   b. Suction mouth and nose if infant has secretions or vomitus in his mouth.
   c. Turn head to side.
   d. Protect infant from banging against side of isolette or incubator.
   e. Provide oxygen if cyanosis or respiratory distress occurs.
   f. Administer any medication prescribed to control the convulsions.
2. Record the length of and the type of convulsion, the parts of the body involved, the infant's general appearance before and following the convulsion, and response to any therapy given.

E. *To provide for the nutritional needs of the infant in order to provide for his caloric needs.*
  1. During the acute phase of the illness the infant may not be able to take or tolerate feedings.
    a. Monitor the administration of intravenous fluids.
    b. Provide for the sucking needs of the infant by providing him with a pacifier.
    c. Gavage feedings may be given to the infant.
  2. Initiate oral feedings of formula as soon as the infant's condition improves.
    a. Begin by offering small feedings and observe following responses:
       Vomiting
       Abdominal distention
       Infant's interest in feeding and ability to suck
       How the infant tires with feeding
    b. Daily feedings may be supplemented with gavage feedings.
    c. Gradually increase amount of feeding.
    d. Resume regular feeding schedule based on infant's ability to tolerate feeding.
  3. Hold the infant for feedings as soon as his condition warrants it.

F. *To provide measures to maintain the infant's temperature within normal range.*
  1. Take infant's temperature at hourly intervals.
  2. Adjust the incubator temperature to maintain infant's temperature between 36–37°C. (97–98°F.).
  3. When infant is placed in an open crib, maintain temperature and cover the infant appropriately.
  4. Report hypothermia or hyperthermia to the physician.

G. *To administer the prescribed antibiotic therapy to control the infection.*
  1. Administer the prescribed medications.
    a. Be aware of the action and side effects of the specific medications.
    b. Be aware of the route of excretion.
    c. Be aware of drug incompatibilities.
  2. Observe the infant's apparent response to therapy.
    a. Note child's activity, feeding behavior and weight.
    b. Observe for the development of new symptoms.

H. *To provide for the emotional needs of the infant.*
  1. Place bright colorful objects in the crib or isolette.
  2. Talk gently and quietly while caring for the infant.
  3. Touch and gently stroke the infant.
  4. Encourage the parents to visit and allow them to hold the infant as soon as possible.

I. *To involve the parents in the infant's care in the hospital and prepare them for the infant's discharge.*
  1. Encourage parents to visit the infant.
    a. Allow them to hold and feed the baby.
    b. Answer questions they may have regarding the infant's progress and care.
    c. Provide them with an opportunity to explain their concerns.
  2. Discuss symptoms of complications which may occur and should be watched for following discharge.
  3. Give specific instruction regarding medications to be given at home.

BIBLIOGRAPHY

Books

Babson, S. G., and Benson, R. C.: Management of High-risk Pregnancy and Intensive Care of the Neonate. St. Louis, C. V. Mosby, 1971.
Black, J.: Neonatal Emergencies and Other Problems. New York, Appleton-Century-Crofts, 1972.
Ingalls, A. J., and Salerno, M. C.: Maternal and Child Health. St. Louis, C. V. Mosby, 1971.
Latham, H. C., and Heckel, R. V.: Pediatric Nursing. St. Louis, C. V. Mosby, 1972.
Nelson, W. E.: Textbook of Pediatrics. Philadelphia, W. B. Saunders, 1969.
Oski, F. A., and Naiman, J. L.: Hematologic Problems in the Newborn. Philadelphia, W. B. Saunders, 1972.
Pierog, S. H., and Ferrara, A.: Approach to the Medical Care of the Sick Newborn. St. Louis, C. V. Mosby, 1971.

Articles

Hasselmeyer, E. G., and Hon., E. H.: Effects of gavage feeding of premature infants upon cardio-respiratory patterns. Military Med., *136*:252–257, March 1971.
Plight of the premature and Counseling parents of preemies. Nursing 71, *1*:5–9, Dec. 1971.
James, L. S.: Symposium on the newborn. Ped. Clin. N. Amer., *13*: Aug. 1966.

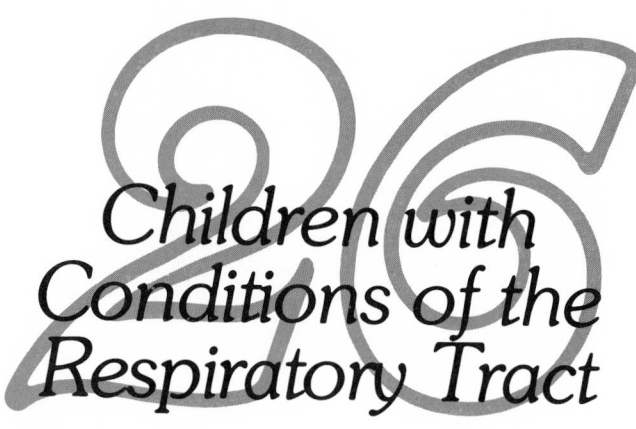

Children with Conditions of the Respiratory Tract

"STREP THROAT"

"Strep throat" is severe pharyngitis caused by the streptococcus organism.

Etiology

Beta hemolytic streptococcus—group A strains

Altered Physiology

Pharynx involvement—cellulitis of throat

Clinical Manifestations

1. Onset is generally acute:
   a. High fever
   b. Headache
   c. Vomiting

2. After 12–24 hours:
   a. Sore throat, varying degree of severity
   b. Dryness of throat
   c. Cervical lymphadenopathy
   d. White tongue coating gives way to strawberry-red tongue

Diagnostic Evaluation

Throat culture
a. Reveals beta hemolytic streptococcus A.
b. Drug sensitivity of organism is determined.

Complications

Peritonsillar abscess, pneumonia, otitis media, meningitis, acute glomerulonephritis or rheumatic fever.

Nursing Objectives

A. *To isolate patient from other patients since the mode of transmission is by direct or indirect contact with nasopharyngeal secretions.* (Period of communicability varies.)
Personnel in contact with patient should:
1. Practice good handwashing techniques.
2. Use disposable dishes whenever possible.
3. Use precautions with soiled tissues.

B. *To anticipate physical, emotional and psychological needs of the isolated child, who is usually on bedrest.*
1. Make frequent visits with the child—stop and talk or comfort him.
2. Provide the child with some sort of call system.
3. Provide child with some diversional activities appropriate for age.
4. Have fluids available for him to drink.

C. *To establish and maintain adequate nutritional and fluid intake.*
1. Offer fluids frequently that the child likes.
2. Allow the child to eat what he feels like eating until he feels better.

D. *To administer antibiotics to which the organism is sensitive as ordered by the physician.*
1. Analgesics may be ordered also.
Give medication if child seems uncomfortable or restless.
2. Warm saline throat irrigations may be soothing.
a. Used primarily in older child.
b. Encourage child to participate in treatment.
3. Hot or cold compress applications to cervical nodes may be comforting. (Many children find them irritating, however.)
4. Mouth care will help moisten dry mucous membranes.
5. Increased humidity will help loosen secretions when there is upper respiratory tract infection.

Parental Teaching

1. Help parents understand the importance of follow-up medical care and urine examinations after acute infection has subsided.
Rheumatic fever, a complication of this type of streptococcal infection, can be diagnosed early by careful observation. (See p. 1186 rheumatic fever.)
2. Impress upon parents the need for immediate medical attention should symptoms of illness occur.

TONSILLECTOMY AND ADENOIDECTOMY

Tonsillectomy and adenoidectomy is the surgical removal of the adenoid and tonsil structures, part of the lymphoid tissue that circles the pharynx. (The function of the tonsils and adenoids is to serve as a first line of defense against respiratory infection.)

Etiology

1. Acute or chronic infection of tonsils and adenoids
2. Hypertrophy produces obstruction to:
   a. Breathing
   b. Swallowing
   c. Eustachian tube

Clinical Manifestations

1. Indications for tonsillectomy
   a. Recurrent or persistent sore throat
   b. Persistent hyperemia of anterior pillars
   c. Enlargement of cervical nodes
   d. Peritonsillar abscess or retrotonsillar abscess
   e. Suppurative cervical adenitis with tonsil focus
   f. Small contracted tonsil or hypertrophy
2. Indications for adenoidectomy
   a. Chronic otitis media; impaired hearing
   b. Mouth breathing
   c. Persistent rhinitis
   d. Alterations of voice
   e. Persistent cough
   f. Hypertrophied adenoids

Diagnostic Evaluation

Since bleeding is a likely complication of surgery to this highly vascular area, pre-operative blood studies are completed.
   a. Clotting time
   b. Smear for platelets
   c. Prothrombin time
   d. Partial prothrombin time

Nursing Objectives

PREOPERATIVE CARE

A. *To assess upon admission the psychological preparation of the child for hospitalization and surgery.*
   1. The child should know why he has been admitted to the hospital and what will happen to him.
   2. When parents have not told the child about hospitalization, it may be because they cannot.
      a. They do not know what will happen.
      b. They do not know how to tell the child because of their own anxieties.
      c. They do not understand the importance of telling the child the truth in order to perpetuate the child's trust in the parents.
   3. Help parents in preparing the child by talking at first in general terms about hospitalization.
   4. Child may have preconceived ideas from parents and peers about what to expect. (These may pose as a threat to the child.)
      a. Expose child to other children on the unit, especially those who have had and are recovering from surgery.
      b. Correct any misunderstandings the child may have.
   5. The pre-school child is very vulnerable to psychological trauma as a result of this experience.
      a. Tell the child the truth.
      b. Include parents when helping the child.

B. *To take nursing history from parents at the time of admission to obtain any pertinent information that would contraindicate surgery.*
   1. Infection
      a. When was last recent infection?
      b. Has child been exposed to any contagious diseases?
   2. Safety
      a. Does the child have any loose teeth?
      b. Are there any bleeding tendencies in child or family?

C. *To maintain adequate hydration prior to surgery since blood loss may be extensive during surgery.*
   1. Encourage the child to drink fluids the night before surgery.
   2. Child usually is N.P.O. a few hours prior to surgery.

D. *To prepare the child specifically (appropriate for age) for what to expect postoperatively.*
   1. Where he will wake up.
   2. Sore throat, emesis of blood, position
   3. Ice collar, medications
   4. Fluid regimen

E. *To encourage mother to stay with her young child the day and night of surgery or at least before surgery and when the child returns to his room and is waking up.*
   Prepare the mother as to what to expect when she sees the child postoperatively.
      a. Vomiting
      b. Color
      c. Crying, angry or frightened

F. *To know if the child has a history of chronic infection or rheumatic fever so antibiotics may be given pre- and postoperatively.*

POSTOPERATIVE CARE

A. *To administer good postoperative care based on general principles and to observe for usual postoperative complications (see p. 1093).*

B. *To assist the child in maintaining a patent airway, by draining secretions and preventing aspiration of vomitus.*
   1. Place child prone or semiprone before he becomes alert.
   2. Allow the child to assume position of comfort when he is alert. (Mother may hold child.)
   3. Child may vomit old blood initially.

C. *To observe the child constantly until he is awake, and then frequently thereafter; monitor vital signs and be alert to signs of hemorrhage.*
   1. Indications of hemorrhage (the most frequent complication)
      a. Increasing rapid pulse
      b. Frequent swallowing
      c. Pallor
      d. Restlessness
      e. Clearing of throat and vomiting of blood
      f. Continuous slight oozing of blood over a number of hours postoperatively
   2. Have emergency equipment readily available.
      a. Suction equipment
      b. Packing material

D. *To offer measures of comfort to the child.*
   1. Cool liquids offer some relief from sore throat, as well as prevent dehydration and temperature elevation.
      a. Give ice chips 1–2 hours after awakening.
      b. Advance clear liquids cautiously until vomiting has ceased.
      c. Offer cool, synthetic fruit juices and milk at first as they are best tolerated.
   2. Ice collar to neck may provide some comfort. (Remove ice collar if child becomes restless.)
   3. Give analgesic, especially to older child.
   4. Rinse mouth with cool water or alkaline solution.

E. *To provide opportunity for child to have as much rest as possible.*
   1. Encourage mother to be with the child when he awakens as he is usually frightened. (Mother's presence can be very comforting.)
   2. When mother must leave, reassure child she will return.
   3. Keep child in bed in a quiet room.

Parental Teaching

1. Explain and write instructions as to the care of the child at home after discharge (usually the day after surgery).
   a. Diet should still consist of large amounts of fluids as well as soft, cool non-irritating foods. (Supply list of suggestions.)
   b. Bedrest should be maintained for a couple of days, then daily rest periods for about a week.
   c. If signs and symptoms of impending trouble occur, the physician should be called immediately.
      (1) Earache accompanied by fever
      (2) Any bleeding, often indicated only by frequent swallowing
   d. How to give any medications the physician may order.
   e. The telephone number of the physician or emergency room if trouble occurs.
2. Discuss with the mother (parents) what results they can expect from the surgery.
   a. Decreased number of sore throats
   b. Improvement in obstructive symptoms
   c. Decreased incidence of cervical lymphadenitis
   d. Improvement in nutritional status
3. Guide parents in helping child make the hospital experience a positive one once he has returned home.
   a. Talk about what happened.
   b. Let child play out his feelings.

ASTHMA

Asthma is a form of reversible airway obstruction involving both lung fields, with paroxysmal attacks of dyspnea accompanied by wheezing.

Classification of Asthma

1. *Acute attack*—sporadic in nature, with varying intervals of freedom from difficulty and with precipitating factors often readily defined.

2. *Latent asthma*—no outward signs or symptoms of asthma, but there is some shortness of breath on occasion, transitory wheezing on strenuous exercise, and wheezy rales heard during deep inspiration.
3. *Intractable asthma*—persistent wheezing requiring regular, daily medication, for either the control of symptoms or the ability to function.
4. *Status asthmaticus*—severe attack in which the patient deteriorates in spite of adequate treatment with sympathomimetic drugs.

Etiology

The stimuli responsible for attacks of asthma are as follows:
1. Antigen-antibody reaction
2. Infection
3. Physical factors
   a. Cold
   b. Meteorological factors (i.e., humidity, sudden changes in temperature and barometric pressure)
4. Irritants
   a. Dust
   b. Chemicals
   c. Air pollutants (i.e., nitric oxide, sulfur dioxide, carbon monoxide, particulate matter)
5. Psychic or emotional factors
6. Exercise

Incidence

1. The incidence of asthma in infancy is rare but increases in children 3 years and older.
2. Childhood asthma may cease at puberty.

Altered Physiology

1. The turbinates warm and moisten all air which passes into the lung.
2. Inspired air contains particulate matter which is removed by the blanket of mucus present in the tracheobronchial tree. This mucus is kept moistened by inspired moist air.
3. The blanket of mucus is moved constantly upward by the propelling action of the cilia, and if mucus becomes thickened or inspissated it cannot be moved.
4. An increased local deposition and concentration of allergens occurs.
5. This produces intrabronchial accumulation and stagnation of mucus which is the primary cause of the respiratory embarrassment.
6. Chemical mediators in asthma:
   a. Primarily involved are histamine and SRS-A. SRS-A appears after histamine release, and persists for a longer period. It is not inhibited by the action of the antihistamines.
   b. These materials are primarily responsible for changes in the blood vessels and mucus membrane in the bronchi and bronchioles, as well as for the initiation of bronchospasm.

Clinical Manifestations

1. The onset of an asthmatic attack may be gradual with nasal congestion, sneezing and a watery nasal discharge present before the attack.
2. Attacks may occur suddenly, often at night, when the child awakens with the following symptoms.
   a. Wheezing which occurs primarily with expiration
   b. Anxiety and apprehension
   c. Diaphoresis
   d. Uncontrollable cough

3. With treatment the attack may be controlled. The asthmatic attack may progress, however, and the child will develop the following symptoms.
   a. Increasing dyspnea
   b. Thick, tenacious mucus
   c. Coarse and fine musical rales
   d. Flaring of the alae nasi
   e. Use of accessory muscles
      for respiration
   f. Cyanosis
   g. Hypercapnia
   h. Increased heart and respiratory rates
   i. Abdominal pain from severe coughing
   j. Vomiting
   k. Extreme anxiety and apprehension

Diagnostic Evaluation

1. Eosinophilia in peripheral blood, nasal secretions and sputum
2. Polymorphonuclear leukocytosis in the presence of infection
3. Pulmonary function studies—diminished maximal breathing capacity, tidal volume and timed vital capaicty

Complications

1. Bronchiectasis
2. Emphysema
3. Cor pulmonale

Treatment

1. Removal of the suspected allergen
2. Desensitization in order to build up child's resistance to his allergens
3. Drug therapy to control symptoms

Nursing Objectives

A. *To become informed regarding the child's symptomatology and the medical plan of care.*
   1. Make a base-line nursing assessment of the child's condition in order to determine the severity of the attack and the degree of respiratory distress.
      a. Observe the child's breathing pattern:
         (1) Determine whether the expiratory phase of respiration is increased.
         (2) Determine whether the child is wheezing. (In severe attacks wheezing is audible at a distance from the child.)
         (3) Determine whether the child is using accessory muscles for breathing.
      b. Listen to the child's chest with a stethoscope to determine whether rales are present and to determine whether all areas of the lung fields are being aerated.
      c. Assess the child's level of anxiety and apprehension.
      d. Observe for flaring of the alae nasi.
      e. Observe the child for the development of cyanosis, utilizing adequate light.
   2. Determine the heart and respiratory rates; record and report to the physician any significant change.
   3. Discuss with the physician the plan of medical care.

B. *To provide measures to relieve the respiratory distress the child is experiencing.*
   1. Position the child in high Fowler's position to allow maximum lung expansion.
      a. Raise the head of the bed to achieve high Fowler's position.
      b. Place an overbed table padded with a pillow in front of the child and have him extend his arms over the table—this provides a comfortable position and allows maximum utilization of accessory muscles for breathing.

2. Administer oxygen when signs of air hunger are present.
   a. Do not wait for the appearance of cyanosis before administering oxygen.
   b. Oxygen must be administered with caution since the child with severe respiratory distress may be dependent upon his low pO_2 to stimulate spontaneous respiration. In the face of a rising pCO_2 and a potential CO_2 narcosis, the administration of oxygen may remove the last stimulus to spontaneous respirations.
3. Explain to the child the purpose of the oxygen equipment before oxygen is administered and allow the child to feel and touch the equipment.

C. *To relieve the anxiety and apprehension which results from the respiratory embarrassment.*
   1. Place the child in a quiet, clean room, where he can be closely observed.
   2. Provide the child with maximum reassurance.
      a. Allow parents to remain with the child.
         (1) Keep the parents informed as to the child's progress—what is being done and why—in order to relieve their apprehension. Parental anxiety is readily transmitted to the child.
         (2) Talk calmly and quietly to the child.
         (3) Assure the child that you will not leave him alone.
         (4) Allow the child to have his favorite security object.
   3. Organize care so as to avoid disturbing the child any more than necessary.
   4. When the child falls asleep, allow him to continue to sleep and do not disturb him unless absolutely necessary.
   5. Evaluate the need for sedation.

D. *To provide adequate hydration in order to liquefy bronchial secretions and maintain electrolyte balance.* (Dehydration occurs secondary to decreased fluid intake, excessive perspiration, increased respiration and infection.)
   1. Observe for signs of dehydration.
      a. Lack of skin turgor
      b. Lack of tears
      c. Dry parched lips
      d. Depressed fontanelle
      e. Decreased urinary output—high specific gravity; concentrated appearance.
   2. Maintain parenteral fluid administration.
   3. Encourage oral fluid intake.
      a. Determine child's fluid preferences.
      b. Offer small sips of fluid frequently.
      c. Avoid iced fluids which may provoke bronchospasm.
      d. Avoid carbonated beverages when wheezing.
   4. Allow the child to return to a regular diet as soon as possible.

E. *To be aware of the action and side effects of drugs used in the treatment of asthma.*
   1. *Epinephrine*—relaxes bronchial smooth muscle and constricts bronchial mucosal vessels, thereby reducing congestion and edema.
      a. The smallest dose affording relief should be used.
      b. Side effects—insomnia, headache, nervousness, palpitations, precordial pain, nausea, sweating, urinary retention. (May potentiate aminophylline toxicity.)
   2. *Ephedrine*—relaxes bronchial smooth muscle and constricts bronchial mucosal vessels, thereby reducing congestion and edema.

      a. Has the advantage of prolonged action and oral administration.

      b. Side effects—as for epinephrine.

   3. *Aminophylline*—bronchodilator

      a. Toxic reaction may occur but is more likely to occur with prolonged overdose.

      b. Side effects—irritability, excitement, continued dehydration, vomiting, hematemesis, albuminuria, stupor, convulsions, coma, death.

      c. Occasionally cyanosis and syncope may appear after only a small amount of the prescribed dose—this is considered an idiosyncracy and the drug should be discontinued.

   4. *Expectorants*—given as an adjunct to hydration; thins secretions and helps the child to cough productively.

   5. *Corticosteroids*—anti-inflammatory agents.

      a. Produces beneficial effects only after several hours.

      b. Used when other drugs fail to bring beneficial relief from an asthmatic attack.

      c. Side effects—Use for mild attacks may lead to suppression of adrenal activity. Prolonged use may lead to growth retardation and steroid dependency.

   6. While drugs are being administered intravenously:

      a. Monitor carefully the rate of administration.

      b. Observe closely the patient's reactions.

      c. Report side effects promptly to the physician.

F. *To encourage the child and his parents to practice measures which will help to maintain optimal health.*

   1. Promote a well-balanced diet.

   2. Avoid fatigue and chilling.

   3. Attempt to keep child emotionally calm and at ease.

   4. Provide regular medical follow-up.

G. *To teach the child and involve the parents in the teaching of proper breathing habits.* (The exercises strengthen the diaphram so that breathing will become much better and the total lung capacity increased.)

   1. Instruct the child to clear his nasal passages before beginning exercises.

   2. Each exercise should start with a short gentle inspiration through the nose, followed by a prolonged expiration through the mouth.

   3. During inspiration, the upper portion of the thorax should be kept immobilized.

   4. During expiration, abdominal muscles should be pulled in.

   5. On no account should the child take a deep inspiration during the exercise, but instead he should see how long he can continue the expiration.

      Exercise I—Abdominal Breathing

         1. Lie on back with knees drawn up, body relaxed and hands resting on upper abdomen.

         2. Exhale slowly, gently sink the chest and then upper abdomen until retracted at end of expiration (through mouth).

         3. Relax upper abdomen (bulges forward) while taking brief inspiration through nose (chest is not raised).

         Repeat 8–16 times; rest 1 minute; repeat.

      Exercise II—Side Expansion Breathing

         1. Sit relaxed in a chair and place palms of hands on each side of lower ribs.

2. Exhale slowly through mouth, contracting upper part of thorax, then lower ribs, then compress palms against ribs. (This expels air from base of lungs.)
3. Inhale, expanding lower ribs against slight pressure from hands. Repeat 8–16 times; rest 1 minute; repeat.

Excise III—Forward Bending
1. Sit with feet apart, arms relaxed at sides.
2. Exhale slowly, drop head forward and downward to knees, while retracting abdominal muscles.
3. Raise trunk slowly while inhaling and expand upper abdomen.
4. Exhale quickly, sinking chest and abdomen, but remain erect.
5. Inhale, expanding upper abdomen.

Exercise IV—Elbow Arching
(This exercise is performed between breathing exercises.)
1. Sit leaning slightly forward, back straight, fingers on shoulders.
2. Move elbows in circles forward, upward, backward and downward. Repeat 4–8 times; rest; repeat.

General Instructions
Perform exercises:
1. In the morning before breakfast when child is feeling fresh
2. At night, before getting into bed to clear the lungs before sleep, and
3. At the first sign of an impending attack to prevent asthma from developing.

NOTE: Many patients can abort their attacks entirely by doing simple exercises gently. Should child become short of breath or wheeze slightly, take single dose of whatever medication relieved him before beginning the exercises. Exercise may occasionally produce wheezing or coughing at the end of exercise. It may distress the child, but with perseverance the mucus in the bronchial tubes becomes loosened and the patient may be able to cough it up with consequent relief of attack.

H. *Assist the parents to develop a realistic attitude toward the child's illness.*
1. Try to treat the child as a completely normal child who only needs a few additional restrictions imposed because of his illness.
2. Allow child the same duties and rights as other children in family.
3. Try to explain why he must watch out for certain things and why restrictions are there. Give explanations instead of orders and show him confidence and respect.
4. Avoid overprotection and unnecessary surveillance.
5. Teach child to gradually manage for himself rather than being dependent on parents.
6. If child is too much engrossed with his illness, he can be diverted with kindly scolding, friendly minimizing of his ailments or with other interests, so that he forgets his troubles as much as possible.
7. Do not talk about child's illness any more than necessary—no secrecy or whispering.
8. Inform friends and relatives of problems so that the necessary consideration is given him (i.e., teacher).
9. Create an atmosphere at home that is not full of nervousness or unrest—but not artificially calm.

10. Prepare child for approaching events (if bursts of emotions have an effect on his illness).

11. Teach child special skills. Let him develop special hobbies and interests that can be combined with his illness. Accomplishments that develop respect and admiration in peers are particularly desirable and aid in building self-confidence and a feeling of security.

12. Both parents and child feel greater assurance if they are aware of how you should treat special expression and stages of disease. Have special instructions and medications on hand.

13. If child takes medications for his allergy or specific symptoms, administer in an everyday manner without making any fuss.

14. Child needs security, self-confidence and love. (Don't force these on the child.) Exaggeration is never beneficial.

I. *To teach the child and his parents protective measures which will encourage environmental control and help to avoid the offending allergen.*

1. Keep child's bedroom as free from dust as possible.
   a. Keep in bedroom only the furniture which is absolutely necessary.
   b. Remove upholstered furniture, draperies, carpets, pictures, books, toys and unnecessary dust-collecting objects.
   c. Use washable curtains and cotton or synthetic rugs.
   d. Use cotton or synthetic blankets and washable bedspreads (not chenille or tufted types).
   e. Do not use insect or other sprays in the bedroom.
   f. Do not store outer clothing or household articles in bedroom closets.
   g. Enclose mattresses, box-springs and pillows in dust-proof covers (unless they are synthetic).
   h. Blankets and clothing that have been stored should be thoroughly aired before use.

2. Avoid irritating odors such as paint, tobacco smoke, insect powders, pine oils and jellies and irritating cooking odors.

3. If possible, use an exhaust fan in the kitchen to remove cooking odors.

4. Remove all overstuffed furniture and rugs.

5. Avoid sitting and playing on overstuffed furniture and down pillows.

6. Avoid carbonated drinks, such as ginger ale and colas (especially when wheezing).

7. Avoid any physical exertion that causes wheezing or excessive shortness of breath.

8. Avoid using irritating salves on chest or in nose.

9. Avoid dusty and musty places (basements, storerooms, etc.).

10. Avoid felt rug pads because of animal hair content.

11. Purchase foam furniture and foam rubber pads if possible when refurnishing the home.

12. If home is heated by a circulating hot-air system, shut it off in the bedroom (use electric heater if necessary). A central air filter in the furnace is desirable; clean or replace it frequently.

13. Take only drugs prescribed by the physician.

14. Report for treatment as directed by physician.

BRONCHIOLITIS

Bronchiolitis is an infection of the bronchioles. In children it occurs in infants under the age of 1 year. Bronchiolitis involves an inflammatory reaction resulting in an attack of dyspnea, cough, expiratory wheezing and sternal retractions, which may progress to respiratory and cardiac failure.

Etiology

The etiology of bronchiolitis is associated with infection by the RS virus (respiratory syncytial virus) or the para-influenza viruses.

Incidence

The infection occurs most frequently in the winter and spring months, and often appears in epidemic numbers.

Altered Physiology

1. The virus produces generalized inflammation of the respiratory mucosa.
2. The inflammation may be confined to the upper respiratory passages or may spread downward through the respiratory tree and into the alveoli.
3. Swelling of the cells of the bronchi, together with the production of viscous mucus leads to partial or complete blockage of the smaller passageways.
4. Air becomes trapped behind the partially obstructed radicles, since it can be pulled in during inspiration but cannot be expelled because the narrowed passages collapse during expiration.
5. When obstruction is complete, the air is absorbed and areas of atelectasis or consolidation distal to the point of obstruction may occur.

Clinical Manifestations

1. Expiratory wheezing
2. Dyspnea
3. Cough
4. Lethargy
5. Cyanosis
6. Sternal retractions
7. Fever

Diagnostic Evaluation

Viral studies—may isolate the RS virus or para-influenza viruses

Complications

1. Pneumonia
2. Right-heart failure
3. Electrolyte imbalance
4. Respiratory failure

Nursing Management

1. Determine the severity of the respiratory distress that the child is experiencing.
    a. Make an initial nursing assessment.
        (1) Observe the respiratory rate and pattern.
            (a) Count the respirations for 1 full minute.
            (b) Observe for retractions and note severity and location.
            (c) Listen to the chest with a stethoscope to determine if rales are present and to evaluate the breath sounds.
        (2) Observe the child's color and note the presence of cyanosis.

(3) Observe for nasal flaring.

(4) Evaluate the child's degree of restlessness and apprehension.

(5) Note any wheezing, stridor or hoarseness.

   b. Record these observations on the nursing record.

2. Provide a warm, humidified environment enriched with oxygen in order to combat anoxia and liquefy secretions.

   a. Place child in a croupette. (See section on oxygen therapy, pp. 1094–1097.)

   b. Observe the child's response to this environment.

3. Provide the child with adequate hydration.

   a. Maintain the administration of intravenous fluids at the prescribed rate.

   b. When the child is in severe respiratory distress he is given nothing by mouth because of the danger of aspiration.

   c. Offer the child small sips of a clear fluid when the respiratory status improves.

     (1) Note any vomiting or abdominal distention following the oral fluid.

     (2) As the child begins to take more fluid by mouth, notify physician so that intravenous fluid rate may be adjusted in order to prevent fluid overload.

   d. Record child's intake and output.

     (1) Measure urinary output and record.

     (2) Check specific gravity.

4. Provide the child with both physical and psychological rest.

   a. Disturb the child as little as possible by organizing nursing care.

   b. The presence of the child's parents will alleviate some of his apprehensions.

   c. Provide opportunities for quiet play as the child's condition improves.

5. Provide good skin care while the child is confined to bed. Turn child frequently.

6. Provide measures to improve ventilation of affected portion of the lung.

   a. Move position frequently.

   b. Provide postural drainage if prescribed.

7. Provide for adequate nutrition to meet the growth and development needs of the child.

   a. Determine the child's food preferences.

   b. Offer the child small meals.

8. Administer appropriate antibiotic therapy.

   a. Observe for drug sensitivity.

   b. Observe child's response to therapy.

EPIGLOTTITIS AND LARYNGOTRACHEITIS
(Croup)

Croup is a general term used to describe inflammatory laryngeal disease. Croup is divided into 2 separate entities: (1) epiglottitis and (2) laryngotracheitis.

Epiglottitis

Epiglottitis is a life-threatening disease involving the false cords, aryepiglottic fold and the epiglottis.

Etiology

1. Epiglottitis occurs in children of all ages but is most severe in the young infant.

2. The most frequent bacterial agents causing epiglottitis include

   a. Hemophilus influenza   c. *Staphylococcus aureus*

   b. Pneumococci   d. Beta hemolytic streptococci

Altered Physiology

1. Inflammation and edema occur as a result of bacterial invasion of the false cords, the aryepiglottic fold and the epiglottis.
2. The mucous membranes of the glottis and epiglottis appear red and swollen, with thick superficial secretions.
3. This inflammation and edema either partially or totally obstructs the airway and may ultimately produce asphyxia.

Clinical Manifestations

After an upper respiratory infection of 1 or 2 days, the child develops progressively severe respiratory distress.
1. Severe inspiratory stridor with marked retraction in the supraclavicular and intercostal spaces
2. Hoarseness
3. Fever 39–40°C. (102–104°F.)
4. Apprehension, restlessness and anxiety
5. Cyanosis

Clinical Evaluation

1. Blood gases
   a. Increased pCO_2
   b. Decreased pO_2
2. Leukocytosis

Treatment

Objective: to maintain a patent airway.
1. Provide a warm, humidified environment.
2. Give oxygen.
3. Institute endotracheal intubation or tracheostomy in the case of rapidly increasing obstruction.

Complications

Airway obstruction

Nursing Management

1. Determine the severity of the respiratory distress that the child is experiencing.
   a. Make an initial nursing assessment.
      (1) Observe the respiratory rate and pattern.
         (a) Count the respirations for 1 full minute.
         (b) Observe for retractions and note severity and location.
         (c) Listen to the chest with a stethoscope to determine if rales are present and to evaluate the breath sounds.
      (2) Observe the child's color and note the presence of cyanosis.
      (3) Observe for nasal flaring.
      (4) Evaluate the child's degree of restlessness and apprehension.
      (5) Note any wheezing, stridor or hoarseness.
   b. Record these observations on the nursing record.

2. Provide a cool, humidified environment enriched with oxygen in order to combat anoxia and liquefy secretions.
    a. Place child in a croupette (see p. 1097).
    b. Observe the child's response to this environment.
3. Provide the child with adequate hydration.
    a. Maintain the administration of intravenous fluids at the prescribed rate.
    b. When the child is in severe respiratory distress he is given nothing by mouth because of the danger of aspiration.
    c. When the respiratory status improves, offer the child small sips of a clear fluid.
        (1) Note any vomiting or abdominal distention following the oral fluid.
        (2) As the child begins to take more fluid by mouth, notify physician so that intravenous fluid rate may be adjusted in order to prevent fluid overload.
    d. Record child's intake and output.
        (1) Measure urinary output and record.
        (2) Check specific gravity.
4. Have in readiness equipment for intubation and tracheostomy which may be necessitated by severe respiratory distress.
    a. If tracheostomy is performed observe the site for infection and bleeding.
    b. Provide the child with a great deal of security to alleviate his fear of the tracheostomy.
        (1) Place the child where he can be vigilantly observed, and where he can see nursing personnel.
        (2) Apply protective devices to prevent child from disturbing the tube (see p. 1073).
        (3) Assist the child in communicating his needs, and try to anticipate his needs.
        (4) Give the older child a bell to ring when he needs attention.
        (5) Explain to the child that the tracheostomy is only temporary.
    c. Maintain patency of the tracheostomy and observe for danger signals.
        (1) Restlessness   (4) Pallor
        (2) Fatigue   (5) Tachycardia
        (3) Cyanosis   (6) Noisy breathing
5. Administer drugs as prescribed.
        The child should not be sedated since restlessness is a good indicator of respiratory distress.
6. Prepare the parents for the child's discharge.
    a. Teach care of the tracheostomy if the child goes home with the tube in place.
    b. Provide them with the necessary equipment for care at home.
    c. Make a community nursing referral if indicated.

Laryngotracheitis

Laryngotracheitis is an inflammatory disease involving the vocal cords, subglottic tissue and the trachea.

Etiology

Laryngotracheitis is due to the following viral agents:
    1. Influenza   4. Adenoviruses
    2. Para-influenza virus   5. Respiratory syncytial viruses
    3. Echo viruses

Altered Physiology

1. Viral inflammation is primarily subglottal and produces an obstructing fibrinous exudate on the tracheal wall.
2. The airway may be partially or totally obstructed, ultimately resulting in asphyxia.

Clinical Manifestations

After an upper respiratory infection of 1 or 2 days, the child develops more severe respiratory difficulty.

1. Inspiratory stridor with suprasternal and intercostal retractions on inspiration
2. Hoarseness
3. Fever 38–39°C. (100–102°F.)
4. Apprehension, restlessness and anxiety
5. Cyanosis

Diagnostic Evaluation

1. Blood gases
   a. Increased pCO_2
   b. Decreased pO_2
2. Leukocytosis

Treatment

Treatment and Nursing Management
Same as for epiglottitis, page 1148.

IDIOPATHIC RESPIRATORY DISTRESS SYNDROME
(Hyaline Membrane Disease)

Idiopathic Respiratory Distress Syndrome is a syndrome of newborn infants characterized by a progressive and frequently fatal respiratory disorder which is the result of a hyaline type membrane in the lungs.

Etiology

The exact etiology of idiopathic respiratory distress syndrome is not clearly defined. The following theories have been proposed:

1. Alteration in the fibrinolytic enzyme system in the lungs or blood. A principal component of membrane is fibrin which is derived from fetal pulmonary tissues. Hyaline membrane would then result from an excessive outpouring of fluid from the terminal respiratory segments, either transudate from congested capillaries, or secretion from mucus-forming glands, or both. It is not known what is responsible for this.
2. Alteration or absence of pulmonary surfactant, producing a high surface tension at the alveolar surface. A high surface tension would produce decreased lung compliance, atelectasis and an increase in the work of breathing. Ventilation would decrease as the infant tired and as asphyxia developed which would produce pulmonary vasoconstriction. Blood would bypass the lung via the patent ductus arteriosus and foramen ovale and produce still more pulmonary vasoconstriction and further diminish pulmonary blood flow. Ischemia that results would interfere with lung metabolism and limit the production of surfactant.

3. Another theory is that the primary problem is pulmonary hypoperfusion rather than surfactant deficiency. Intrauterine asphyxia increases pulmonary vascular resistance and causes shunting of blood returning to the heart through the foramen ovale and patent ductus arteriosus away from the lung. Pulmonary ischemia would damage the alveolar lining cells that produce surfactant.

Incidence

Idiopathic respiratory distress syndrome occurs most frequently in:
1. Premature infants (primarily weighing between 1000–1500 gm.)
2. Infants of diabetic mothers
3. Infants delivered by cesarean section
4. Infants of mothers who have experienced intrauterine vaginal bleeding.

Altered Physiology

1. Altered physiology is based on the above theories.
2. The membrane occurs on the walls of the bronchioles, the alveoli and alveolar ducts, thus interfering with gaseous exchange and causing hypoxia, cyanosis and respiratory distress.

Clinical Manifestations

Symptoms are usually observed immediately after birth
1. Expiratory grunting or whining (when infant is not crying)
2. Sternal and substernal retractions
3. Nasal flaring
4. Tachypnea
5. Hypothermia
6. Cyanosis in room air (Infants with severe disease may be cyanotic even when given oxygen.)
7. Decreased breath sounds and fine rales (occasionally)—on auscultation of chest
8. Hypotension
9. Edema of hands and feet
10. Bowel sounds absent early in the illness
11. Urine output decreased
12. As the disease progresses:
    a. Seesaw retractions become marked.
    b. Peripheral edema increases.
    c. Muscle tone decreases.
    d. Cyanosis increases.
       (1) Body temperature drops.
       (2) Short periods of apnea occur.
       (3) Bradycardia may occur.
    e. Asphyxia becomes more severe.
       Apneic episodes develop.
       Changes in distribution of blood throughout body resulting in pale gray skin color.

Diagnostic Evaluation

A. Laboratory tests
   1. pCO_2—elevated.
   2. pO_2—low.
   3. Blood pH—low due to metabolic acidosis.
   4. Potassium—elevated.
   5. Calcium—low.

B. Chest x-ray—demonstrates a diffuse, fine granularity on an air bronchogram

C. Pulmonary function studies—demonstrate stiff, small lungs with a reduced effective pulmonary blood flow

Treatment

1. Early recognition is imperative so that treatment may be instituted immediately.
2. Transportation to a facility providing specialized care is desirable when possible.
3. The objectives of treatment include supportive measures.
    a. Maintenance of oxygenation
    b. Maintenance of respiration with ventilatory support if necessary
    c. Maintenance of body temperature
    d. Maintenance of fluid and electrolyte balance
    e. Maintenance of nutrition
4. No specific therapy is known.

Complications

1. Complications related to respiratory therapy:
    a. Pneumothorax
    b. Pneumonia
    c. Tracheal stenosis
2. Brain damage usually does not result if the infant survives.

Nursing Objectives

A. *To check the birth history for pertinent information to assist in determining the intensity of observation and care that the infant may require.*

1. The Apgar score 1 minute after birth and 5 minutes after birth (see p. 1006)
2. The type of resuscitation required
3. Any treatment or medication administered
4. Any medication or anesthesia the mother received during labor

B. *To make a generalized nursing assessment of the infant's condition immediately upon admission.*

1. Determine the degree of respiratory distress.
    a. Observe the type of retraction present.
        (1) Determine the type of retraction present.
        (2) Determine the degree and severity of retracting.
    b. Count the respiratory rate for 1 full minute.
        (1) Observe and determine if respirations are regular or irregular.
        (2) Observe to determine if the infant experiences any periods of apnea.
            (a) Note length of apnea.
            (b) Note what type of stimulation initiated breathing.
        (3) Note the infant's activity at the time respirations are recorded (e.g., crying, sleeping).
    c. Listen for expiratory grunting or whining sounds from the infant when he is not crying.
    d. Observe for nasal flaring.
    e. Observe for cyanosis.
        (1) Note location of cyanosis.
        (2) Note if cyanosis improves with oxygen administration.

      f. Listen to the chest with a stethoscope.
         (1) Note diminished breath sounds and location.
         (2) Note the presence of rales.
  2. Determine the infant's cardiac rate and rhythm.
      a. Count the apical pulse for 1 full minute.
      b. Note any irregularity in the heart rate.
  3. Observe the infant's general activity.
      a. Determine if the infant is lethargic or listless.
      b. Determine if the infant is active and responds to stimuli.
      c. Determine if the infant cries.
  4. Observe the infant's skin color.
      a. Note cyanosis as to degree and location.
      b. Note evidence of jaundice.
      c. Note skin mottling.
      d. Note paleness or grayness.
  5. Observe the general appearance of the infant's body.
      a. Note edema and location (face, hands, feet, etc.).
      b. Note any other abnormal appearance of body.
  6. Check infant's body temperature.
  7. Listen to abdomen with a stethoscope to determine if bowel sounds are present. Note any stool passed and observe and record type of stool.
  8. Note any urinary output.
      a. Apply urine collector to obtain sample of urine.
      b. Observe color of urine.
      c. Check specific gravity of urine.
      d. Record amount of urine.

C. *To provide measures to relieve respiratory distress.*
  1. Have emergency equipment readily available for use in the event of cardiac or respiratory arrest.
  2. Provide measures for monitoring ECG and respiratory rate.
  3. Place the infant in an oxygen-rich environment.
      a. Incubator with oxygen at prescribed concentration.
      b. Plastic hood with oxygen at prescribed concentration.
      c. Plastic hood with oxygen at prescribed concentration in warming unit.
      d. Measure oxygen concentration every hour and record.
  4. Observe the infant's response to oxygen.
      a. Observe for improvement in color, respiratory rate and pattern and nasal flaring.
      b. Note response by improvement in pH, pO_2, and pCO_2 (arterial).
  5. Observe closely for apnea.
      a. Stimulate infant if apnea occurs.
      b. If unable to produce spontaneous respiration with stimulation within 15–30 seconds:
         (1) Call for help.
         (2) Clear airway.
         (3) Hyperextend head.
         (4) Apply hand resuscitator attached to an oxygen supply, or apply mouth-to-mouth resuscitation (see pp. 1100–1101).

(5) Intubation may be necessary:
  (a) Obtain heart rate during intubation by physician.
  (b) Initiate cardiac massage if severe bradycardia or asystole occurs.
  (c) Listen to breath sounds once intubated.
  (d) Attach infant to appropriate ventilator
      Secure endotracheal tube.
      Suction tube to maintain patency.
  (e) Continue to monitor vital signs.
  c. Record events.

D. *To maintain the method used for the administration of intravenous fluids necessary to meet the metabolic demands of the infant.*
  1. Monitor flow.
  2. Observe site for infiltration or infection.
  3. If umbilical-artery catheter is in place, observe for bleeding.
  4. Record the amount of blood drawn for laboratory analysis (small infants can become anemic from having large amounts of blood removed for samples).
  5. Prepare and administer prescribed medications.

E. *To maintain the infant's body temperature between 36.5–37°C. (97 and 98°F.).*
  1. Adjust incubator accordingly.
  2. Prevent frequent opening of incubator.

F. *To disturb the infant as little as possible.*
  Attempt to accomplish as many things as possible during any single interruption.

NOTE: The premature infant with respiratory difficulty should continue to be observed very closely and his therapy adjusted as his condition changes. When his condition stabilizes, then resume care as for premature infant (see p. 1118).

BRONCHOPNEUMONIA

Bronchopneumonia is an inflammation of the lungs. The term includes 2 types of pneumonia: disseminated lobar pneumonia, and interstitial pneumonia.
  1. *Disseminated lobar pneumonia* involves scattered lobules in 1 or more lobes of the lungs.
  2. *Interstitial pneumonia* is a diffuse bronchiolitis in 1 or more lobes of the lungs.

Etiology

Bronchopneumonia may be caused by a bacteria or a virus.
  1. Bacterial agents include:
    a. Pneumococcus
    b. Streptococcus (Group A)
    c. Staphylacoccus
    d. Gram negative organisms
       Hemophilus influenza
       Klebsiella pneumoniae
       Pseudomonas

  2. Viral agents:
    a. Para-influenzal virus
    b. Adenoviruses

Altered Physiology

1. The physiologic alterations may occur in scattered lobules (lobar pneumonia) or in the entire lobe (interstitial pneumonia).
2. Blood serum and cells pour into alveoli.
3. Alveoli become congested with red blood cells and fibrinous exudate. Affected areas cannot be aerated properly.

Clinical Manifestations

1. The initial symptoms are usually vague:
   a. Poor feeding or refusal to feed
   b. Listlessness
   c. Gastrointestinal symptoms
      (1) Vomiting
      (2) Diarrhea
   d. Pallor or cyanosis
2. Fever (infants may be hypothermic)
3. Tachypnea and tachycardia
4. Progressive respiratory distress
5. Pulmonary rales

Diagnostic Evaluation

1. Nose and throat cultures
2. Blood cultures
3. Chest x-ray will demonstrate infiltrate

Treatment

1. Oxygen therapy is employed to relieve respiratory distress.
2. Antibiotics
3. Supportive care

Nursing Management

1. Determine the severity of the respiratory distress that the child is experiencing.
   a. Make an initial nursing assessment.
      (1) Observe the respiratory rate and pattern.
         (a) Count the respirations for 1 full minute.
         (b) Observe for retractions and note severity and location.
         (c) Listen to the chest with a stethoscope to determine if rales are present and to evaluate the breath sounds.
      (2) Observe the child's color and note the presence of cyanosis.
      (3) Observe for nasal flaring.
      (4) Evaluate the child's degree of restlessness and apprehension.
      (5) Note any wheezing, stridor or hoarseness.
   b. Record these observations on the nursing record.
2. Provide a warm, humidified environment enriched with oxygen in order to combat anoxia and liquefy secretions.
   a. Place child in a croupette (see p. 1097).
   b. Observe the child's response to this environment.
3. Provide the child with adequate hydration.
   a. Maintain the administration of intravenous fluids at the prescribed rate.
   b. When the child is in severe respiratory distress he is given nothing by mouth because of the danger of aspiration.

    c. When the respiratory status improves, offer the child small sips of a clear fluid.

       (1) Note any vomiting or abdominal distention following oral fluid intake.

       (2) As the child begins to take more fluid by mouth, notify physician so that intravenous fluid rate may be adjusted in order to prevent fluid overload.

    d. Record child's intake and output.

       (1) Measure urinary output and record.

       (2) Check specific gravity.

4. Provide the child with both physical and psychological rest.

    a. Disturb the child as little as possible by organizing nursing care.

    b. The presence of the child's parents will alleviate some of his apprehension.

    c. Provide opportunities for quiet play as the child's condition improves.

5. Provide good skin care while the child is confined to bed. Turn child frequently.

6. Provide measures to improve ventilation of affected portion of the lung.

    a. Change position frequently.

    b. Provide postural drainage if prescribed.

7. Provide for adequate nutrition to meet the child's growth and development needs.

    a. Determine the child's food preferences.

    b. Offer the child small meals.

8. Administer appropriate antibiotic therapy.

    a. Observe for drug sensitivity.

    b. Observe child's response to therapy.

9. Observe closely for the development of complications of pneumonia.

    a. Tension pneumothorax

       (1) Abrupt onset of chest pain

       (2) Dyspnea

       (3) Cyanosis

    b. If child develops these symptoms, notify physician immediately.

BIBLIOGRAPHY

Books

Avery, M. E.: The Lung and its Disorder in the Newborn Infant, 2nd ed. Philadelphia, W. B. Saunders, 1968.

Barnett, H. L. (ed.): Pediatrics, 15th ed. New York, Appleton-Century-Crofts, 1972.

Black, J.: Neonatal Emergencies and Other Problems. New York, Appleton-Century-Crofts, 1972.

Blake, F. G., et al.: Nursing Care of Children, 8th ed. Philadelphia, J. B. Lippincott, 1970.

Facts About Asthma For Parents. Evansville, Indiana, Mead Johnson and Company, 1970.

Fontana, V. J.: Practical Management of the Allergic Child. New York, Appleton-Century-Crofts, 1969.

Green, M., and Haggerty, R. (eds.): Ambulatory Pediatrics. Philadelphia, W. B. Saunders, 1968.

Gustafson, S. R., and Coursin, D. B.: The Pediatric Patient—1966. Philadelphia, J. B. Lippincott, 1966.

Ingalls, A. J., and Salerno, M. C.: Maternal and Child Health Nursing. St. Louis, C. V. Mosby, 1971.

Kendig, E. L. (ed.): Pulmonary Disorders (Vol. I of Disorders of the Respiratory Tract in Children). Philadelphia, W. B. Saunders, 1972.

Korones, S. B.: High Risk Newborn Infants: The Basis for Intensive Nursing Care. St. Louis, C. V. Mosby, 1972.

Latham, H. C., and Heckel, R. V.: Pediatric Nursing. St. Louis, C. V. Mosby, 1972.

Marlow, D.: Textbook of Pediatric Nursing. Philadelphia, W. B. Saunders, 1973.

Moore, M.: The Newborn and The Nurse. Philadelphia, W. B. Saunders, 1972.
Nelson, W. E.: Textbook of Pediatrics. Philadelphia, W. B. Saunders, 1969.
Petrillo, M.: The Emotional Care of Hospitalized Children. Philadelphia, J. B. Lippincott, 1972.
Raffensperger, J. G., and Primrose, R. B. (eds.): Pediatric Surgery for Nurses. Boston, Little, Brown and Company, 1968.
Tuft, L., and Mueller, H. L.: Allergy in Children. Philadelphia, W. B. Saunders, 1970.

Articles

Balog, T. G.: A mother's reaction to diagnosis of congenital anomalies in her child. Maternal-Child Nurs. J., *1*:143–156, Summer 1972.
Barber, T. K.: The handicapped adolescent. Dent. Clin. N. Amer., *13*:313–328, April 1969.
Bigos, D.: The role of the nurse on the cleft palate team. Unpublished paper for Masters degree, Boston University, 1970.
Canby, J. B., and Redd, H. J.: Tracheotomy in the management of severe bronchiolitis. Pediatrics, *36*:406, 1965.
Clifford, E., et al.: Psychological findings in the adulthood of 98 cleft lip-palate children. Plastic Reconstruc. Surg., *50*:234–237, Sept. 1972.
DiMaggio, G.: The child with asthma. Nurs. Clin. N. Amer., *3*:453–461, Sept. 1968.
Massler, M.: Teen-age cardiology. Dent. Clin. N. Amer., *13*:405–424, April 1969.
Reeves, K. R.: Acute epiglottitis—pediatric emergency. Amer. J. Nurs., *71*:1539, 1971.
Richards, W., and Siegel, S. C.: Status asthmaticus. Ped. Clin. N. Amer., *16*:1, 1969.
Rudolph, J., et al.: Clinical diagnosis of respiratory difficulty in the newborn. Ped. Clin. N. Amer., *13*:669, 1966.
Weatcroft, M. G., and Sumter, S. A.: An effective program of oral hygiene the dentist can teach adolescents. Dent. Clin. N. Amer., *13*:375–386, April 1969.
Wright, F. H., and Beem, M. O.: Diagnosis and treatment: management of acute viral bronchiolitis in infancy. Pediatrics, *35*:334, 1965.

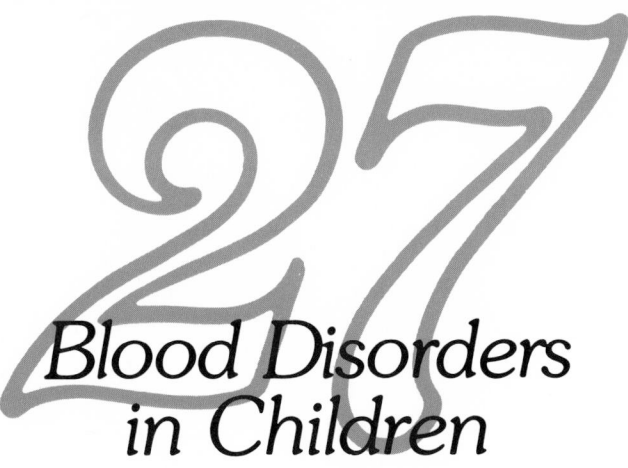

Blood Disorders in Children

ANEMIA

Anemia refers to a deficit of red blood cells or hemoglobin in the blood. It is the most frequent hematologic disorder encountered in children.

Etiology
1. Blood loss
2. Inadequate rate of blood formation
   a. Poor hemoglobin synthesis
      (1) Prematurity
      (2) Iron deficiency
   b. Infection
      (1) Chronic respiratory infection
      (2) Nephritis

   c. Delayed red cell maturation
      Megaloblastic anemia
   d. Drugs
   e. Poisons
   f. Invasion of bone marrow
      (1) Leukemia
      (2) Tumors

3. Increased blood destruction
   a. Antibody reactions
      Transfusion reaction
   b. Drugs

   c. Poisons
   d. Hereditary disease
      Sickle cell anemia

Clinical Manifestations
1. Condition may be acute or chronic
2. Early symptoms
   a. Listlessness
   b. Fatigability
3. Late symptoms
   a. Pallor
   b. Weakness
   c. Tachycardia
   d. Palpitations

4. Eventual symptoms
   a. Mental and physical sluggishness
   b. Cardiac enlargement
   c. Inability to carry out the usual childhood activities
5. Prognosis
   a. Varies with the type of anemia
   b. Death may result because of cardiac failure

1159

Altered Physiology

A. *General Considerations*

1. Red cells and hemoglobin are normally formed at the same rate at which they are destroyed.
2. Whenever formation of red cells or hemoglobin is decreased or their destruction is increased, anemia results.
3. The ability of the red blood cell to carry hemoglobin is decreased.
4. The ability of hemoglobin to oxygenate the tissues and remove carbon dioxide for excretion by the lungs is also decreased.
5. Less hemoglobin is available to act as a buffer in regulating the pH of the blood.

B. *Specific Anemias*

1. Iron Deficiency Anemia (Hypochromic Anemia)
   a. Most of the newborn's iron is contained in his circulating hemoglobin.
   b. The newborn's hemoglobin concentration decreases during the first 2–3 months of life.
      Considerable iron is reclaimed and stored.
   c. A diet inadequate in iron (less than 0.8–1.5 mg. of iron per day) results in decreased hemoglobin formation.
   d. Pallor of erythrocytes (hypochromia) results when hemoglobin is not synthesized.
   e. Hypochromia is accompanied by a decrease in the size of the red blood cell.
2. Megaloblastic Anemias
   a. Folic acid and vitamin B_{12} are necessary for the synthesis of nucleoproteins which are essential for the maturation of red blood cells.
   b. Deficiencies of folic acid or vitamin B_{12} or disturbances in their normal metabolism interfere with the synthesis of nucleoproteins.
   c. Red blood cells are immature and larger than normal at every stage of their development.
   d. The number of circulating red blood cells is decreased.
   e. Each red blood cell may carry a normal amount of hemoglobin.
3. Hypoplastic Anemias
   The bone marrow is unable to manufacture new red blood cells and hemoglobin at a rate necessary to maintain a normal concentration of these substances in the circulating blood.
4. Aplastic Anemia
   a. Formation of red blood cells stops altogether.
   b. There is usually an associated defective synthesis of other elements in the blood such as platelets and white blood cells.
5. Anemia of Infection
   a. Life span of the red blood cell is moderately decreased.
   b. The ability of the bone marrow to produce red blood cells is significantly decreased. (This is the principal factor in determining the degree of anemia.)
6. Hemolytic Anemias
   a. The red blood cells are destroyed at abnormally high rates.
   b. The activity of the bone marrow increases to compensate for the shortened survival time of the red blood cells.
   c. Products of red cell breakdown increase with hemolysis.

    d. Jaundice results when the liver is unable to clear the blood of the pigment resulting from the breakdown of hemoglobin from destroyed red cells.

    e. Bone marrow hypertrophies and occupies a larger than normal share of the inner structure of bones.

  7. Sickle Cell Anemia (See p. 1164.)

Nursing Objectives

A. *To build up resistance to infection.*

  1. See that child maintains good general body hygiene.

  2. Provide a diet high in vitamins, calories and iron.

    a. Be aware of the child's food preferences and plan his diet accordingly.

    b. Offer small amounts of food at frequent intervals.

    c. Provide food supplements and vitamins when necessary.

  3. Ensure adequate rest.

    a. Plan nursing care to allow for lengthy periods when the child is not disturbed by hospital routines, procedures, treatments, etc.

    b. Observe for early signs of fatigue such as irritability, hyperactivity, etc.

    c. Encourage sedentary rather than active projects.

  4. Avoid exposure to other children with colds, infections, etc.

B. *To administer blood and maintain the transfusion.*

  1. The procedure is similar to the administration of I.V. fluids. (See pp. 1087 and 1088.)

  2. Take special precautions.

    a. The patient's name, physician's name, hospital number and blood type must correspond with the information on the blood container from the blood bank.

    b. The rate of flow should be carefully regulated to prevent circulatory overload, especially in those children receiving multiple transfusions.

    c. The same blood should not be left running over a long period of time (usually over 4 hours).

  3. Observe the child for signs of transfusion reaction.

    a. Reaction usually occurs within 15–20 minutes from the start of the transfusion.

    b. Signs and symptoms:

      (1) Restlessness

      (2) Irritability

      (3) Chills

      (4) Elevation of temperature

      (5) Sudden changes in pulse and respiration

      (6) Rash or change in the color of the skin

      (7) Changes in the appearance or quantity of urine output

      (8) Hemorrhagic phenomena

C. *To minimize the child's anxieties and ensure his cooperation during hospitalization.*

  1. Allow the child to handle equipment used for tests and procedures (tourniquets, syringes, etc.).

  2. Explain all procedures and the treatment plan to the child in a way that he can understand.

  3. Allow the older child to look through a microscope at a blood smear.

  4. Permit the child to cleanse the area for a venipuncture or finger stick.

Nursing Management of Specific Anemias

A. *Iron Deficiency Anemia*

    1. Administer iron as ordered by the physician.

        a. Oral iron preparations

            (1) Administer between meals.

                Milk products and cereals inhibit the absorption of iron.

            (2) Administer with a dropper or straw.

                Staining of the teeth may be caused by iron.

            (3) Observe for side effects.

                (a) Gastric distress

                (b) Colic pain

                (c) Diarrhea

            (4) Caution the mother that iron medication causes the child's stools to be dark green or black.

        b. Intramuscular iron preparations

            (1) Dosage

                (a) Calculated by the physician

                (b) Depends on the child's weight and hemoglobin level

            (2) Special precautions

                (a) Should be injected into a large muscle, preferably the buttock.

                (b) Injection sites should be recorded and rotated.

                (c) The injection site should not be massaged.

                    Any pressure on the site may force the medication out of the muscle into the subcutaneous tissue.

                    Walking will help absorption.

                (d) Parenteral iron should be administered with discretion and only to those children whose anemia is not amenable to oral iron therapy.

                (e) Parenteral iron is contraindicated in children sensitive to the preparation or in anemias other than iron-deficiency anemia.

            (3) Technique of administration

                (a) Use a separate needle to withdraw the medication from the ampule and for injection.

                (b) Use a needle which is 5 cm. (2 inches) long.

                    Medication must be injected deeply into the muscle to avoid staining the tissue.

                (c) Allow 0.5 ml. of air in the syringe before injecting.

                (d) Retract the skin over the muscle laterally before inserting the needle.

                (e) Insert the needle and withdraw the plunger to check against entry into a blood vessel.

                (f) Inject the medication and the 0.5 ml. of air following the injection—to clear the needle and prevent leakage of the medication along the injection track when the needle is withdrawn.

                (g) Wait 10 seconds after injection before removing the needle.

            (4) Observe for side effects.

                (a) Local

                    Pain at the injection site

                    Skin discoloration

                    Local inflammation with lymphadenopathy

(b) Systemic toxicity (occurs within 10 minutes of injection)
Headache
Muscle and joint pain
Nausea and vomiting
Sweating
Tachycardia
Bronchospasm with dyspnea
Circulatory collapse, hypotension and dizziness
  2. Feed slowly and at frequent intervals.
  3. Do not allow the child to drink excessive quantities of milk.
  4. Offer a diet high in vegetables and meats.
  5. Provide vitamin supplements if necessary.
Vitamin C may enhance the absorption of iron.
  6. Parental education is especially important regarding:
     a. Administration of iron
     b. Child's need for iron-rich food
  7. Investigate social and economic problems which may contribute to the child's disease
Complete a referral to a community health nurse if it appears that the mother will need support in dealing with the child's chronic disease.

B. *Anemia of Infection*
  1. Provide supportive care relative to the underlying disease.
  2. Administer antibiotics as directed by the physician.

C. *Megaloblastic Anemias*
Administer folic acid or vitamin B_{12} as directed by the physician.
  1. Folic acid (pteroylmonoglutamic acid)
     a. Dosage—must be determined by trial for each patient.
     b. Route
        (1) Oral route is preferred.
        (2) May be administered deep subcutaneously or intramuscularly if malabsorption is suspected.
     c. Toxic effects—none.
  2. Vitamin B_{12} (cyanocobalamine)
     a. Dosage—regulated by individual trial for each patient.
     b. Route
        (1) Intramuscular or subcutaneous injection is preferred.
        (2) May be administered orally. (This method is very expensive.)
     c. Side effects—none.
     d. Points of emphasis
        Regular administration of the medication is essential. Patients may be tempted to miss injections because they are not in distress before the injection or do not feel significantly better after it.

Patient or Parental Teaching

  1. Discuss general hygiene measures, including adequate rest, diet, sunshine, fresh air.
  2. Encourage regular medical and dental evaluations.
  3. Explain that infection may be prevented by dressing the child according to the weather and keeping him away from persons with colds, sore throats and other infections.
  4. Teach parents how to administer medication.

SICKLE CELL DISEASE

Sickle cell anemia is a severe, chronic hemolytic anemia occurring in persons homozygous for the sickle gene. The clinical course is characterized by episodes of pain due to the occlusion of small blood vessels by sickled red cells. Persons heterozygous for the sickle gene are said to possess sickle cell trait which is associated with a benign clinical course.

Etiology

1. Genetically determined, inherited disease
2. Each person inherits 1 gene from each parent which governs the synthesis of hemoglobin (See Table 27-1)

TABLE 27-1. TRANSMISSION OF SICKLE CELL DISEASE

Genotype of Parents	Probability of Abnormal Hemoglobin in Offspring		
	Normal	Trait	Disease
1 parent with trait	50%	50%	0
Both parents with trait	25%	50%	25%
1 parent with trait, 1 parent with disease	0	50%	50%
Both parents with disease	0	0	100%

Incidence

1. More prevalent in the black race than the white race
2. Approximately 10% of black Americans have sickle cell trait
3. Approximately 1 out of every 400 black Americans has sickle cell anemia

Clinical Manifestations

A. *Symptoms*
1. Children are rarely symptomatic until late in the first year of life.
2. Clinical manifestations are sporadic.
   a. Child may be asymptomatic for several months.
   b. Periods of crisis occur at variable intervals.
   c. Precipitating factors of crisis include:
      (1) Dehydration   (4) Strenuous physical exertion
      (2) Infection   (5) Extreme fatigue
      (3) Trauma
3. Signs of crisis
   a. Loss of appetite   d. Pain in abdomen, legs or arms
   b. Paleness   e. Swelling of joints
   c. Weakness   f. Jaundice

B. *Thrombocytic Crisis*
1. Small blood vessels are occluded by the sickle-shaped cells causing distal ischemia and infarction.
2. Extremities
   a. Bony destruction
   b. Periosteal reaction
   c. Ulcers
3. Spleen
      Abdominal pain
4. Cerebral occlusion
   a. Strokes
   b. Hemiplegia
   c. Blindness
5. Pulmonary infarction

C. *Sequestrian Crisis*
   1. Large amounts of blood become pooled in the liver and spleen
   2. Spleen becomes massively enlarged
   3. Signs of circulatory collapse develop rapidly
   4. Frequent cause of death in infant with sickle cell disease

D. *Aplastic Crisis:*
   Bone marrow ceases production of red blood cells

E. *Chronic Symptoms*
   1. Jaundice
   2. Gallstones
   3. Progressive impairment of kidney function
   4. Fibrotic spleen
   5. High susceptibility to salmonella osteomyelitis and pneumococcal septicemia
   6. Delayed puberty
   7. Decreased life span

F. *Prognosis*
   1. Depends on severity of the disease
   2. No known cure
      Recent attention has been given to the possible, beneficial effects of intravenous infusion of large doses of urea for sickle cell crisis, but this treatment is still experimental and may be dangerous in children.
   3. Decreased life span
      Death occurs frequently before age 20

Altered Physiology

   1. Each hemoglobin molecule consists of 4 molecules of heme folded into 1 molecule of globin.
   2. Each globin molecule consists of 2 alpha chains and 2 beta chains.
   3. The amino acid sequence on the beta chain is altered in sickle cell hemoglobin.
      Valine is substituted for glutamic acid in the 6th position.
   4. Sickle cell hemoglobin aggregates into elongated crystals under conditions of low oxygen concentration.
   5. This distorts the membrane of the red blood cell causing it to assume a crescent or sickle shape.
   6. Sickled red cells are fragile and are rapidly destroyed in the circulation.
   7. Anemia results when the rate of destruction of red cells is greater than the rate of production.

Diagnostic Evaluation

   1. Stained blood smear
      a. Done by finger stick.
      b. Sickle cells are viewed under the microscope on a stained smear of blood.
      c. Cells are seen only in persons with sickle cell anemia (not sickle cell trait).
   2. Sickle cell prep
      a. Done by finger stick.
      b. Oxygen is removed from a drop of blood.

    c. The blood is observed under the microscope for the presence of sickle-shaped cells.

    d. Does not distinguish between persons with sickle cell trait and disease.

  3. Sickledex

    a. Done by finger stick.

    b. A small amount of blood is placed in a solution containing a chemical reducing agent.

    c. The presence of sickle hemoglobin is indicated if the solution turns cloudy.

    d. Also does not distinguish between persons with sickle cell trait and disease.

  4. Hemoglobin electrophoresis

    a. Requires venipuncture.

    b. Hemoglobin is subjected to an electric current which separates the various types and determines the amounts present.

    c. A person is diagnosed as having sickle cell trait if 2 types of hemoglobin are demonstrated in approximately equal amounts.

       A person is diagnosed as having sickle cell anemia if the majority of his hemoglobin is sickle hemoglobin.

Preventive Measures

1. Every black child admitted to the hospital should be tested for sickle cell anemia.
2. Parents at risk should be counseled regarding the genetic aspects of sickle cell anemia.
3. All siblings of any child who is admitted to the hospital with sickle cell anemia should be tested for the disease.

Nursing Objectives

A. *To alleviate the child's pain during a crisis.*

    Provide increased fluid intake to dilute the blood and reverse the agglutination of sickled cells within the small blood vessels.

    a. Maintain intravenous therapy if indicated. (See procedure for the administration of intravenous fluids, p. 1088.)

    b. Increase the amount and frequency of liquid intake.

       Offer fruit juice, water, milk, etc.

    c. Record the child's intake and output accurately. (Total his intake and ouput every 8 hours.)

B. *To provide emotional support to the child and his parents.*

  1. Encourage parents to talk about their child, his disease and how they feel about it.

    a. Accept negative feelings.

    b. Counsel parents concerning ways to recognize and alleviate their child's apprehension.

    c. Provide factual information so that parents are prepared to answer their child's questions.

       Make certain that parents understand the difference between sickle cell trait and sickle cell anemia.

  2. Alleviate the child's anxieties concerning his illness.

    a. Role playing and play activities are useful in identifying his fears.

    b. Explain what is happening to him in a way that he can understand.

3. Stress the positive aspects of his disease.
   a. Sickle cell disease does not affect intelligence.
   b. Between periods of crisis the child can usually participate in peer group activities with the exception of some strenuous sports.
4. Encourage quiet activities in which the child can excel—art painting, leather work, metal and woodworking, chess, etc.
5. Plan for the child to continue his education.
   a. Encourage parents to bring school work to the child during a lengthy hospitalization.
   b. Refer the child to a home teacher if necessary.

C. *To make certain that the child receives coordinated and continuous care.*

   Send a nursing care summary to a community health nurse or school nurse who will work with the child after he is discharged from the hospital.

Patient or Parental Teaching

1. Offer factual information concerning the disease so that:
   a. Conditions leading to crisis can be avoided.
   b. Medical attention is obtained as soon as symptoms or severe complications appear.
2. Discuss the genetic implications of sickle cell disease early so that the child, when he is old enough, can avail himself of counseling concerning marriage and family planning.

HEMOPHILIA

Hemophilia is an inherited, congenital blood dyscrasia which is characterized by a disturbance of blood clotting factors. It appears in males but is transmitted by females.

Etiology

1. Hereditary
2. Sex-linked, recessive trait
   a. Caused by a gene carried on the X chromosome, one of the sex chromosomes.
   b. Transmitted by asymptomatic females who carry the hemophilic gene on 1 of their X chromosomes.
   c. Appears only in males who have the hemophilic gene on their only X chromosome.
   d. Affected males may carry a latent form of the disease to female offspring.
3. Spontaneous mutations may cause the condition when the family history is negative for the disease.

Clinical Manifestations

A. *General Considerations*

1. Seldom diagnosed in infancy unless excessive bleeding is observed from the umbilical cord or after circumcision.
2. Usually diagnosed after the child becomes active.
3. Varies in severity:
   a. Most cases are mild.
   b. Degree of severity tends to be constant within a given family.

B. *Clinical Signs and Symptoms*
  1. Easily bruised
  2. Prolonged bleeding from the mucous membranes of the nose and mouth or from lacerations
  3. Intramuscular hematomas result from minor trauma
  4. Hemorrhages into the elbows, knees and ankles (hemarthrosis)
      a. Causes pain, swelling, limitation of movement
      b. Repeated hemorrhages may produce degenerative changes with osteoporosis and muscle atrophy
  5. Spontaneous hematuria
  6. Intracranial hemorrhage (rare)

C. *Prognosis*
  1. Uncertain
  2. Cycles may occur with periods of little bleeding followed by periods of severe bleeding
  3. Death may result from intracranial hemorrhage or from exsanguination following any serious hemorrhage.

Diagnostic Evaluation
  1. Routine bleeding and clotting tests—often normal
  2. Partial thromboplastin time, (PTT)—prolonged
  3. Prothrombin consumption—decreased
  4. Thromboplastin generation—decreased

Altered Physiology
  1. Hemophilia is not a single disease entity.
  2. May result from the absence or malfunction of any one of the blood clotting factors from the plasma.
  3. These blood clotting factors are necessary for the formation of prothrombin activator which acts as a catalyst in the conversion of prothrombin to thrombin.
      a. The rate of formation of thrombin from prothrombin is almost directly proportional to the amount of prothrombin activator available.
      b. The rapidity of the clotting process is proportional to the amount of thrombin formed.
  4. The most common types of hemophilia and the clotting factors involved are:

Type of Hemophilia	Clotting Factor
Hemophilia A, (Classic Hemophilia)	Factor VIII, (Antihemophilic globulin)
Hemophilia B, (Christmas Disease)	Factor IX, (Plasma thromboplastin component)
Hemophilia C	Factor XI, (Plasma thromboplastin antecedent)

Nursing Objectives
A. *To provide emergency care for bleeding wounds.*
  1. Cleanse wound thoroughly.
  2. Immobilize the affected part.
  3. Apply local measures for control of bleeding.
      a. Apply pressure on the area.
      b. Place fibrin foam or absorbable gelatin foam in the wound.

4. Administer blood or concentrated plasma containing the necessary factor. (See procedure for the administration of intravenous fluid and for blood transfusion, p. 1088.)
5. Keep the child quiet during treatment.
    a. Remain calm.
    b. Sedate the child if necessary.
6. Take special precautions.
    a. Suturing should be avoided if possible.
    b. Cauterization is always contraindicated.

B. *To provide supportive care for the child with hemarthroses.*
    1. Control bleeding.
        a. Immobilize the joint in a position of slight flexion.
        b. Elevate the affected part.
        c. Apply ice packs.
        d. Administer blood or plasma as directed by the physician.
    2. Alleviate pain.
        a. Administer sedatives or narcotics as ordered by the physician.
        b. Avoid excessive manipulation of the child.
        c. Use a bed cradle to keep the weight of the bedcovers off the affected part.
    3. Prevent further bleeding.
        a. Continue immobilization of the joint. (A bivalve plaster cast may be necessary.)
        b. Maintain the child on bedrest. (Careful handling of the child is essential.)
    4. Prevent permanent deformities and crippling.
        a. Begin gentle passive exercise and massage of the joint after the bleeding has been controlled for at least 48 hours.
        b. Refer the child for physical therapy on an out-patient basis if this is indicated by:
            (1) Presence of persistent deformity.
            (2) Need to use orthopedic devices such as crutches, braces, etc.

C. *To prevent hemorrhage during nursing procedures.*
    1. Temperature taking
        Insert the thermometer very gently.
    2. Injections
        a. Administer medications orally whenever possible.
        b. Choose intramuscular injection sites carefully and rotate them.
        c. Inject the medication slowly.
        d. Apply pressure to the area for 5 minutes.

D. *To provide emotional support to the child and his family.*
    1. Permit the child to participate in as many normal activities as possible within the realm of safety.
    2. Allow the child to handle equipment used in his care.
        Use play to help the young child adjust to his illness by "transfusing" his teddy bear, etc.
    3. Encourage the child's continuing education despite long periods of hospitalization and absence from school.
        a. Have parents bring assignments from the child's teacher.
        b. Refer to a home teacher if indicated.
        c. Investigate the possibility of a school-to-home telephone service.

4. Counsel the parents concerning:
   a. Financial problems caused by repeated hospitalizations and transfusions.
   b. Feelings of guilt at having given birth to the child or resentment of having to care for him.
   c. Practical considerations for caring for the child. (See Patient or Parent Teaching, below.)
   d. Refer the parents to a social worker or psychiatrist if indicated.
5. Introduce the child and his family to other hemophiliac families.
   a. Information concerning the location of parent groups may be obtained from the National Hemophilia Foundation, 25 West 39th St., New York 10018.
   b. Approximately 50 specialized hemophilia centers have been established in the United States.
6. Convey confidence to the patient and his family; they often are fearful of the diagnosis and need support.

Patient or Parent Teaching

1. Protecting the child from trauma
   a. Select toys which are soft and without rough edges.
   b. Pad the sides of cribs, playpens, etc.
   c. Offer food and liquids in plastic containers to avoid laceration.
   d. Guard against child falling when he is learning how to stand and walk.
      (1) Remove potential sources of injury from furniture.
      (2) Pad child's knees and buttocks.
      (3) Use a helmet for the child's head.
   e. Supervise play closely.
   f. Inform the child's teacher, school nurse, other adults and playmates of his condition so that his activities will be appropriately restricted.
   g. Have the child wear a medic-alert bracelet.
2. Emergency treatment for hemorrhage
   a. Immobilize the part.
         This may be done with splints or an elastic compression bandage. (These materials should be immediately available in the home.)
   b. Apply ice packs.
         Parents should keep 2 or 3 plastic bags of ice immediately available in the freezer.
   c. Transport the child to his physician or to the nearest hospital.
3. Regular medical and dental supervision
      Preventive dental care is important and hospitalization is often necessary for extensive dental work and extractions.
4. Diet
      Diet is important to avoid overweight which places additional strain on the child's weight-bearing joints and predisposes him to hemarthrosis.
5. Information concerning the disease itself
      The child should be helped to understand the exact nature of his illness as early as possible.
         Special attention should be given to the signs of hemorrhage, and the child should be told of the need to report even the slightest bleeding to an adult immediately.

6. Preventing emotional crippling by overprotection—this can be more disabling than the effects of the disease itself.
   a. Promote the sense of independence and self-care within the patient's limitations.
   b. Encourage healthful activity and reasonably aggressive pursuits—helps patient to cope with anxiety-driven behavior.
      Reinforce self-judgment of child or teenager in selection of physical activities.
   c. Help parents understand the importance of vocational guidance for their child—emphasis given to occupations using intellect or skills rather than physical effort.
7. Genetic counseling and family planning services should be offered to the family.

BIBLIOGRAPHY

Books

Blake, F., et al.: Nursing Care of Children. Philadelphia, J. B. Lippincott, 1970.
Guyton, A. C.: Textbook of Medical Physiology, 4th ed. Philadelphia, W. B. Saunders, 1971.
Katz, A. H.: Hemophilia: A Study in Hope and Reality. Springfield, Illinois, Charles C Thomas, 1970.
Marlow, D. R.: Textbook of Pediatric Nursing. Philadelphia, W. B. Saunders, 1973.
Nelson, W.: Textbook of Pediatrics. Philadelphia, W. B. Saunders, 1969.

Articles

Brinkhous, K. M.: Changing prospects for children with hemophilia. Children, *17* (No. 6): 222–228, November–December 1970.
Coleman, A., and Alpert, J. (eds.): Poisoning in children. Ped. Clin. N. Amer., *71* (No. 3): August 1970.
Davio, E.: Nursing management of the youngster with a coagulation disorder. J. Prac. Nurs., *21*:33–35, March 1971.
Deutsch, P., and Deutsch, R.: One man's fight against hemophilia. Readers Digest, August 1967.
Duckett, C. L.: Caring for children with sickle cell anemia. Children, *18*:227–231, November–December 1971.
Foster, S.: Sickle cell anemia: closing the gap between theory and therapy. Amer. J. Nurs., *71*: 1952–1956, October 1971.
Goldy, F. B., and Datz, A. H.: Social adaptation in hemophilia. Children, *10*:189–193, September–October 1963.
Pearson, H. A.: Progress in early diagnosis of sickle cell disease. Children, *18*:222–226, November–December 1971.
Pochedly, C.: Sickle cell anemia: recognition and management. Amer. J. Nurs., *71*:1948–1951, October 1971.

Children with Cardiovascular Disorders

CONGENITAL HEART DISEASE

Congenital heart disease is a structural malformation of the heart or great vessels, present at birth.

Etiology

1. Exact cause is unknown
2. Results from abnormal embryonic development or the persistence of fetal structure beyond the time of normal involution
3. Possible causes
   a. Fetal and maternal infection occurring during first trimester
   b. Teratogenic effects of drugs and radiation
   c. Maternal dietary deficiencies
4. Hereditary in some cases
5. Frequently associated with other congenital defects

Types of Congenital Heart Disease (Table 28-1)

1. Patent ductus arteriosus
2. Atrial septal defect
3. Ventricular septal defect
4. Coarctation of the aorta
5. Complete transposition of the great vessels
6. Tetralogy of Fallot

Patent Ductus Arteriosus

Patent ductus arteriosus is the persistence of a fetal connection (ductus arteriosus) between the pulmonary artery and the aorta.

Altered Physiology

1. During fetal life, the ductus arteriosus allows most of the right ventricular blood to bypass the nonfunctioning lungs by directing blood from the pulmonary artery to the aorta.
2. After birth, with the initiation of respiration, the ductus arteriosus is no longer necessary. It should functionally close within several hours after birth and anatomically close within several weeks after birth.
   a. The smooth muscle in the wall of the ductus arteriosus contracts to obliterate the lumen.
   b. Within several weeks after birth, degenerative changes occur in the ductus arteriosus and it becomes a cord of fibrous connective tissue (ligamentum arteriosum).
3. When the ductus arteriosus remains patent, oxygenated blood from the higher pressure systemic circuit (aorta) flows to the lower pressure pulmonary circuit (pulmonary artery) through the patent ductus arteriosus.

Clinical Manifestations

1. Small patent ductus arteriosus—usually asymptomatic
2. Large patent ductus arteriosus—may develop symptoms in very early infancy
   a. Slow weight gain
   b. Feeding difficulties
   c. Frequent respiratory infections
   d. Pale, delicate looking, scrawny appearance
   e. Congestive heart failure may develop

Diagnostic Evaluation

1. "Machinery-like" murmur
2. Chest x-ray—may be normal; may demonstrate cardiomegaly, large aortic knob, increased pulmonary vascularity and prominence of the left atrium and left ventricle
3. Electrocardiogram—may be normal; may demonstrate left ventricular hypertrophy
4. Cardiac catheterization
5. Angiocardiography

Complications

1. Congestive heart failure
2. Infectious endocarditis

Treatment

Surgical division of the patent ductus arteriosus
a. In early infancy if congestive heart failure develops and cannot be controlled
b. Electively by 2 to 3 years of age

Table 28-1. Congenital Heart Abnormalities*

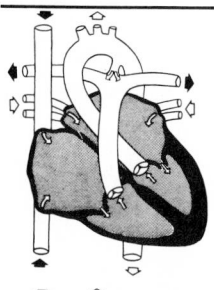

Patent Ductus Arteriosus

The patent ductus arteriosus is a vascular connection that, during fetal life, short circuits the pulmonary vascular bed and directs blood from the pulmonary artery to the aorta. Functional closure of the ductus normally occurs soon after birth. If the ductus remains patent after birth, the direction of blood flow in the ductus is reversed by the higher pressure in the aorta.

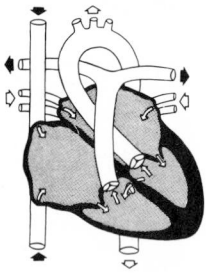

Ventricular Septal Defects

A ventricular septal defect is an abnormal opening between the right and left ventricle. Ventricular septal defects vary in size and may occur in either the membranous or muscular portion of the ventricular septum. Due to higher pressure in the left ventricle, a shunting of blood from the left to right ventricle occurs during systole. If pulmonary vascular resistance produces pulmonary hypertension, the shunt of blood is then reversed from the right to the left ventricle, with cyanosis resulting.

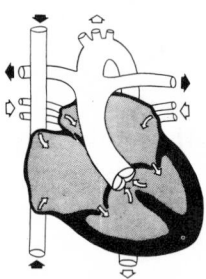

Truncus Arteriosus

Truncus arteriosus is a retention of the embryologic bulbar trunk. It results from the failure of normal septation and division of this trunk into an aorta and pulmonary artery. This single arterial trunk overrides the ventricles and receives blood from them through a ventricular septal defect. The entire pulmonary and systemic circulation is supplied from this common arterial trunk.

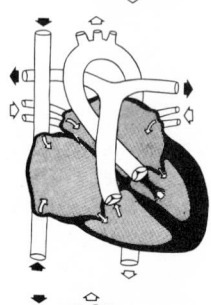

Subaortic Stenosis

In many instances, the stenosis is valvular with thickening and fusion of the cusps. Subaortic stenosis is caused by a fibrous ring below the aortic valve in the outflow tract of the left ventricle. At times, both valvular and subaortic stenosis exist in combination. The obstruction presents an increased work load for the normal output of the left ventricular blood and results in left ventricular enlargement.

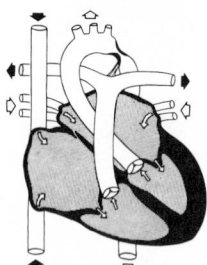

Coarctation of the Aorta

Coarctation of the aorta is characterized by a narrowed aortic lumen. It exists as a preductal or postductal obstruction, depending on the position of the obstruction in relation to the ductus arteriosus. Coarctations exist with great variation in anatomical features. The lesion produces an obstruction to the flow of blood through the aorta causing an increased left ventricular pressure and work load.

* Courtesy, Ross Laboratories.

Tetralogy of Fallot

Tetralogy of Fallot is characterized by the combination of 4 defects: (1) pulmonary stenosis, (2) ventricular septal defect, (3) overriding aorta, (4) hypertrophy of right ventricle. It is the most common defect causing cyanosis in patients surviving beyond 2 years of age. The severity of symptoms depends on the degree of pulmonary stenosis, the size of the ventricular septal defect and the degree to which the aorta overrides the septal defect.

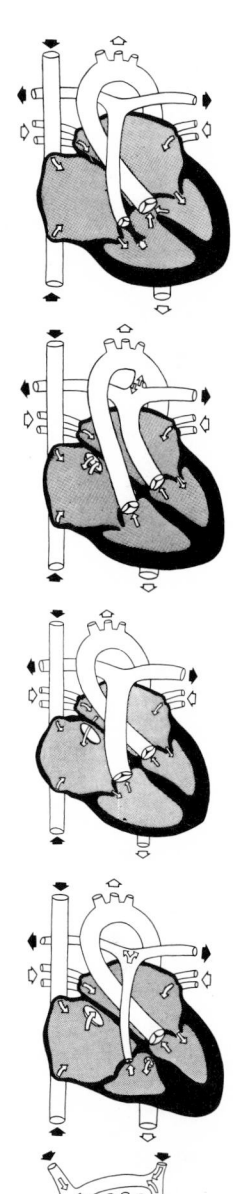

Complete Transposition of Great Vessels

This anomaly is an embryologic defect caused by a straight division of the bulbar trunk without normal spiraling. As a result, the aorta originates from the right ventricle, and the pulmonary artery from the left ventricle. An abnormal communication between the 2 circulations must be present to sustain life.

Atrial Septal Defects

An atrial septal defect is an abnormal opening between the right and left atria. Basically, 3 types of abnormalities result from incorrect development of the atrial septum. An incompetent foramen ovale is the most common defect. The high ostium secundum defect results from abnormal development of the septum secundum. Improper development of the septum primum produces a basal opening known as an ostium primum defect, frequently involving the atrioventricular valves. In general, left to right shunting of blood occurs in all atrial septal defects.

Tricuspid Atresia

Tricuspid valvular atresia is characterized by a small right ventricle, large left ventricle and usually a diminished pulmonary circulation. Blood from the right atrium passes through an atrial septal defect into the left atrium, mixes with oxygenated blood returning from the lungs, flows into the left ventricle and is propelled into the systemic circulation. The lungs may receive blood through 1 of 3 routes: (1) a small ventricular septal defect, (2) patent ductus arteriosus, (3) bronchial vessels.

Anomalous Venous Return

Oxygenated blood returning from the lungs is carried abnormally to the right heart by one or more pulmonary veins emptying directly, or indirectly through venous channels, into the right atrium. Partial anomalous return of the pulmonary veins to the right atrium functions the same as an atrial septal defect. In complete anomalous return of the pulmonary veins, an interatrial communication is necessary for survival.

Atrial Septal Defect

Atrial septal defect is an abnormal opening in the septum between the left atrium and the right atrium.

1. *Ostium secundum type*—located high in the atrial septum and may exist as one large opening or several small openings.
2. *Ostium primum type*—large gap at the base of the atrial septum frequently associated with deformities of the mitral and tricuspid valves and/or a small, high ventricular septal defect.

Altered Physiology

1. The pressure in the left atrium is greater than the pressure in the right atrium and promotes the flow of oxygenated blood from the left atrium to the right atrium.
2. The oxygenated blood that flows through the defect enters the right atrium and mixes with the systemic venous blood returning to the lung. The blood flow through the shunt recirculates through the lung, thus increasing the total blood flow through the lung.
3. If the pulmonary resistance is great, this may increase right atrial pressure, thus causing a reversal of the shunt, with unoxygenated blood flowing from the right atrium to the left atrium. (This situation will produce cyanosis.)

Clinical Manifestations

1. Ostium secundum type—generally asymptomatic even when this defect is large
2. Ostium primum type—generally asymptomatic, although the following may occur:
   a. Slow weight gain
   b. Fatigability
   c. Dyspnea with exertion
   d. Frequent respiratory infections

Diagnostic Evaluation

1. Murmur—not loud, systolic, medium-pitched ejection type
2. Chest x-ray—prominent main pulmonary artery, right atrial and right ventricular enlargement
3. Electrocardiogram—may demonstrate right atrial enlargement
4. Cardiac catheterization
5. Angiocardiography

Complications

Infectious endocarditis (rare)

Treatment

Surgical closure with cardiopulmonary bypass by suture or patch

Ventricular Septal Defect

Ventricular septal defect is an abnormal opening in the septum between the right and left ventricles. It may vary in size from very small defects (Roger defect) to very large defects, and may occur in either the membranous or muscular portion of the ventricular septum.

Altered Physiology

1. The pressure in the left ventricle is greater than the pressure in the right ventricle and promotes the flow of oxygenated blood from the left ventricle to the right ventricle.
2. The oxygenated blood that flows through the defect mixes with the blood returning from the right atrium. The blood flow through the shunt recirculates through the lung, thus increasing the total blood flow through the lung.
3. If the pulmonary resistance is great this may increase right ventricular pressure thus causing a reversal of the shunt with unoxygenated blood flowing from the right ventricle to the left ventricle. (This situation will produce cyanosis.)

Clinical Manifestations

1. Small ventricular septal defects—usually asymptomatic
2. Large ventricular septal defects—may develop symptoms as early as 1 to 2 months of age
   a. Slow weight gain
   b. Feeding difficulties
   c. Pale, delicate looking, scrawny appearance
   d. Frequent respiratory infections
   e. Congestive heart failure develops frequently

Diagnostic Evaluation

1. Murmur—loud, harsh systolic murmur over left lower sternum
2. Chest x-ray—cardiomegaly, biventricular and left atrial enlargement and increased pulmonary vascular markings
3. Electrocardiogram—left ventricular hypertrophy, may have right ventricular hypertrophy
4. Cardiac catheterization
5. Angiocardiography

Complications

1. Infectious endocarditis
2. Congestive heart failure

Treatment

1. Medical management of congestive heart failure if this occurs in infancy
2. If congestive heart failure is intractable to medical management a pulmonary artery banding procedure may be done to produce a significant obstruction to the pulmonary outflow tract and thus reduce the amount of blood flowing to the lungs.
3. Surgical closure with cardiopulmonary bypass (by suture or patch)

Coarctation of the Aorta

Coarctation of the aorta is a narrowing or constriction of the descending aorta in the vicinity of the ductus arteriosus.

1. *Preductal type*—the coarctation is located proximal to the ductus arteriosus (usually associated with other cardiac defects and the ductus arteriosus is widely patent).
2. *Postductal type*—the coarctation is located distal to the ductus arteriosus (usually not associated with other defects).

Altered Physiology

1. The narrowing of the aorta obstructs blood flow through the constricted segment of the aorta, thus increasing left ventricular pressure and work load.
2. Collateral vessels develop, arising chiefly from the branches of the subclavian and intercostal arteries, bypassing the coarcted segment of the aorta and supplying circulation to the lower extremities.

Clinical Manifestations

1. Usually asymptomatic in childhood—growth and development is normal
   a. Occasional fatigue
   b. Headache
   c. Nose bleeds
   d. Leg cramps
2. Severe coarctation—may develop congestive heart failure early in infancy
3. Absent or greatly reduced femoral pulsations
4. Hypertension in upper extremities and diminished blood pressure in lower extremities

Complications

1. Cerebral hemorrhage
2. Rupture of the aorta
3. Infectious endocarditis

Treatment

1. Infants—vigorous management of congestive heart failure and surgery only when congestive heart failure is intractable
2. Surgery—resection of the coarcted segment and an end-to-end anastomosis (done prior to pubertal growth spurt)

Complete Transposition of the Great Vessels

Complete transposition of the great vessels occurs when the pulmonary artery originates posteriorly from the left ventricle and the aorta originates anteriorly from the right ventricle.

Altered Physiology

1. This defect results in 2 separate circulations; the right heart manages the systemic circulation and the left heart manages the pulmonary circulation.
2. In order for life to be sustained, there must be an accompanying defect which provides for the mixing of oxygenated and unoxygenated blood between the 2 circulations.
3. The mixing of oxygenated and unoxygenated blood occurs through one or more of the following shunts:
   a. Atrial septal defect
   b. Ventricular septal defect
   c. Patent ductus arteriosus
   d. Propatent foramen ovale

Clinical Manifestations

1. Severe cyanosis, usually developing shortly after birth (day of birth to a week)
2. Shallow rapid respirations and fatigability
3. Slow weight gain
4. Clubbing of the fingers and toes
5. Congestive heart failure may develop

Diagnostic Evaluation

1. Murmurs—may be absent in infancy; may be murmur of an associated defect
2. Chest x-ray—cardiomegaly usually develops within 2 weeks; heart shape is described as "an egg on its side"; increased pulmonary vascularity; left atrial enlargement
3. Electrocardiogram—right axis deviation, right atrial hypertrophy, right ventricular hypertrophy
4. Laboratory tests
   a. Polycythemia
   b. Increased hemoglobin and hematocrit
5. Cardiac catheterization
6. Angiocardiography

Complications

1. Congestive heart failure
2. Infectious endocarditis
3. Brain abscess
4. Cerebral vascular accident (due to thrombosis or severe hypoxia)

Treatment

Objective: to improve oxygenation of arterial blood.
1. Palliative procedures
   a. Rashkind procedure—the creation of an atrial septal defect with a balloon catheter during cardiac catheterization
   b. Blalock-Hanlon procedure—surgical creation of an atrial septal defect
2. Complete correction
   Mustard procedure—with cardiopulmonary bypass, the atrial septum is removed, and a pericardial graft is sutured into the atrium in such a way that the pulmonary venous blood is directed toward the right ventricle and the systemic venous blood toward the left ventricle. (Usually done at 2½–4 years before pulmonary vascular disease develops.)

Tetralogy of Fallot

Tetralogy of Fallot consists of 4 abnormalities: (1) right ventricular-outflow stenosis or atresia, (2) ventricular septal defect, (3) overriding of the aorta (the aorta straddles the ventricular septal defect, and (4) right ventricular hypertrophy.

Altered Physiology

1. Obstruction of the blood flow from the right ventricle to the pulmonary circulation is caused by obstruction at the pulmonary valve level or the infundibular area of the right ventricle below the pulmonary valve.

2. Unoxygenated blood is shunted from the right ventricle through the ventricular septal defect directly into the aorta.
3. The right ventricle is hypertrophied due to high right ventricular pressure.

Clinical Manifestations

1. The clinical manifestations are highly variable and depend on the degree of right ventricular-outflow obstruction.
2. Cyanosis
   a. Initially, the shunt though the ventricular septal defect is mainly from left to right. Many infants with this defect are not cyanotic at birth, but they develop cyanosis as they grow and as the stenosis becomes relatively more severe.
   b. Cyanosis may at first be observed only with exertion and crying, but during the first few years of life, the child may become cyanotic even at rest.
   c. Infundibular stenosis may be minimal so that cyanosis never develops ("pink tetralogy").
3. Clubbing of the fingers and toes
4. Squatting (a posture characteristically assumed by children with this defect once they have reached the walking stage)
5. Slow weight gain
6. Dyspnea on exertion
7. Anoxic spells

Diagnostic Evaluation

1. Murmur
   a. Systolic murmur of variable intensity—located along the left sternal border
   b. Diminished pulmonary closure sound
   c. Occasionally, no murmur is audible
   d. Palpable thrill along the left lower sternal border
2. Chest x-ray
   a. Heart size normal
   b. Apex of heart elevated
   c. Pulmonary segment is small and concave ("boot-shaped heart")
   d. Decreased pulmonary vascularity
3. Electrocardiogram—right axis deviation; right ventricular hypertrophy
4. Cardiac catheterization
5. Angiocardiography

Complications

1. Congestive heart failure—may occur in newborn but is uncommon beyond infancy
2. Infectious endocarditis
3. Cerebral vascular accident (due to thrombosis or severe hypoxia)
4. Brain abscess

Treatment

Objective: to improve oxygenation of arterial blood
1. Palliative
   a. Waterston Shunt—anastomosis between the posterior lateral aspect of the ascending aorta and the right pulmonary artery

      b. Blalock-Taussig Shunt—anastomosis between the right subclavian artery and the right pulmonary artery

      c. Potts Procedure—anastomosis between the aorta and the left pulmonary artery

      d. Brock Procedure—closed procedure which achieves infundibular resection or valvulotomy

  2. Total Correction

      a. Removal of shunt if previously performed

      b. With cardiopulmonary bypass, ventricular septal defect is repaired and right ventricular-outflow obstruction is relieved

Treatment and Nursing Management of the Child with a Congenital Heart Defect

Nursing Objectives

A. *To become informed concerning the child's symptomatology and the plan of medical care.*

  1. Discuss with the physician his plan for medical care.

  2. Make a base-line nursing assessment of the child's condition.

      a. Observe and record information relevant to the child's growth and development.

        (1) Motor coordination

        (2) Muscular development

        (3) Emotional maturity

      b. Observe and record the child's level of exercise tolerance.

        (1) Observe the child at play:

           Is play interrupted to rest?

           How does he play as compared with his peers?

           Does he squat during play? (Squatting is a characteristic position a cyanotic child assumes when resting after exertion.)

        (2) Observe infants while feeding.

           Does the infant stop feeding to rest or does he fall asleep during feeding?

      c. Observe the child's skin and mucous membranes for color changes.

        (1) Skin

           Color changes vary from pink, dusky, mottled, to cyanotic.

           Earlobes are good indicators of the degree of oxygen saturation.

           Circumoral cyanosis occurs with oxygen deprivation.

        (2) Mucous membranes

           Lips and tongue indicate color change because they are very vascular areas and contain superficial blood vessels; *mucous membranes are the best places to observe for cyanosis.*

           Nailbeds are good indicators of color change.

      d. Observe for clubbing. (Rounding of the fingers, especially the thumbnails with thickening and shininess of the terminal phalanges—may occur in cyanotic children by 2–3 months of age.)

      e. Observe for chest deformities.

        (1) Visible pulsations

        (2) Left- or right-sided prominence

      f. Palpate the child's pulses.

        (1) Radial or dorsalis pedis is difficult to feel in newborn.

        (2) Femoral pulsations are easily felt in the inguinal region and can be compared with brachial pulsations.

       g. Listen to the child's chest with a stethoscope to become familiar with the murmur or to determine the presence of a murmur not previously heard.

       h. Record vital signs (apical pulse, blood pressure, respirations)

          (1) Have child quiet for base-line vital signs.

          (2) Record which extremity is used for blood pressure measurement.

B. *To relieve the respiratory distress associated with increased pulmonary blood flow or oxygen deprivation.*

    1. Determine the degree of respiratory distress.

       a. Remove any clothing or covers which obscure visualization of the chest.

       b. Count the respirations for 1 full minute.

          (1) Infants—respirations greater than 60 per minute are indicative of respiratory difficulty.

          (2) Young children—respirations greater than 40 per minute are indicative of respiratory difficulty.

          (3) Observe for retractions (drawing in of the soft tissue in the rib interspaces or below the costal margin with each inspiration; may be barely visible, mild or severe).

          (4) Count respirations while child is at rest; if unable to sooth the child, note that he is crying, restless, etc.

          (5) Observe the regularity of the respiratory pattern.

    2. Include specific information in nursing record.

       a. Type and severity of retractions

       b. Number of respirations per minute

       c. Regularity of respirations

       d. Response to oxygen therapy

       e. Response to positioning

       f. Color changes

       g. Irritability or anxiety observed

    3. Position child at 45-degree angle to decrease pressure of the viscera on the diaphragm and increase lung volume.

       a. Infant—place in an infant seat.

       b. Children—elevate head of the bed and support the arms with pillows.

    4. Pin diapers loosely; provide loose fitting pajamas for older children.

    5. Feed slowly allowing frequent rest periods.

       a. Rapid respirations and frequent coughing predispose the child to aspiration.

       b. May require gavage feeding.

       c. Observe for abdominal distention which may increase respiratory difficulty.

    6. Hyperextend the infant's or child's head.

    7. Suction the nose and throat if the child is unable to adequately cough up secretions.

    8. Provide oxygen therapy as indicated.

C. *To relieve the anoxic spells associated with cyanotic types of congenital heart disease (primarily Tetralogy of Fallot).*

    1. Observe for anoxic spells (characterized by increased rate and depth of respiration, increasing cyanosis, progressive limpness and syncope); these occasionally result in convulsions.

    2. Be aware that these attacks frequently occur in the morning after awakening from sleep, during or after crying, during or after defecation, or during or immediately following feeding.

3. Once an attack is recognized, call for assistance and immediately:
    a. Place child in knee-chest position.
    b. Administer oxygen via mask.
    c. Be prepared to administer medications as prescribed.
       Morphine sulfate (0.1–0.2 mg./kg.)
       NaHCO₃ (2 mEq./kg.) to correct acidosis
       Propranolol (0.1–0.2 mg./kg.)
4. Observe child closely following recovery from an attack.

D. *To improve oxygenation so that body functions may be maintained.*
    1. Provide a safe, effective oxygen environment.
    2. Observe the child's response to oxygen therapy.
        a. Improvement of color
        b. Change in rate and character of respiration
        c. Change in anxiety level
    3. Explain to the child how the oxygen will help him and orient him to equipment before it is used on him (e.g., tent, mask).
    4. Observe the child's response while he is being weaned from oxygen.
       Reduce liter flow gradually and observe response after each reduction.
    5. Measures which are directed to relieve respiratory distress will aid in improving oxygenation.

E. *To provide adequate nutritional and fluid intake to maintain the growth and developmental needs of the child.*
    1. Feed slowly in a semierect position; burp infants after each ounce.
    2. Provide small frequent feedings.
    3. Provide foods which have high nutritional value.
    4. Determine the child's likes and dislikes and plan meals with the dietitian, taking into consideration the child's preferences.
    5. Observe the child at mealtime; does a poor appetite represent a lack of interest in food or does the child become fatigued while eating.
    6. Report vomiting and specify the amount, type, relationship to feeding or to medications.
    7. Report diarrhea and specify type and amount.
    8. Maintain adequate hydration in the cyanotic child when he is vomiting, has diarrhea or fever, or is exposed to high environmental temperatures since polycythemia predisposes him to thrombosis.

F. *To reduce the work load of the heart since decreased activity and expenditure of energy will decrease oxygen requirements.*
    1. Organize nursing care to provide periods of uninterrupted rest.
    2. Prevent excessive crying.
        a. Use pacifier.
        b. Hold baby.
        c. Feed when hungry.
        d. Keep baby comfortable.
    3. Avoid discussing the child's condition or the condition of other children in the presence of the child.
    4. Support the child during diagnostic and therapeutic procedures.
        a. Explain to the child what is going to be done in simple terms.
        b. Encourage him to express his fears.

5. Deliver nursing care in a calm, sympathetic, assured manner.
6. Explain to the child the need for rest.
7. Provide diversional activities that require limited expenditure of energy.

G. *To prevent respiratory infection.*
  1. Segregate the child from other children with respiratory infections.
  2. Be alert to the symptoms of infection.
     a. Note fever.
     b. Report stuffy nose, cough etc.
     c. Check skin for rashes.
  3. Practice careful handwashing technique and teach this to the child.
  4. Check with the parents to see that the child's immunization schedule is current.

H. *To explain to the child about his heart condition as early as the child can understand.*
  1. Discuss with the parents the importance of being truthful with the child about his heart condition.
  2. The time to tell the child is generally when the child begins asking questions as to why he visits the doctor so frequently and why the doctor listens to his heart so closely.
  3. The child's questions should be answered truthfully in a simple way.

I. *To encourage the parents and other persons (teachers, peers etc.) to treat the child in as normal a manner as possible.*
  1. Avoid overprotection and overindulgence.
  2. Avoid rejection.
  3. Facilitate performance of the usual developmental tasks within the limits of the child's physiologic state.
       With most congenital cardiac defects it is not necessary to restrict the child's activity; the child will rest when he becomes tired and then resume his play.
  4. Prevent parents from projecting their fears and anxieties onto the child.

J. *To refer the parents to appropriate resources in the community which may relieve the financial burden involved in the treatment of a child with congenital heart disease.*
  1. Crippled Children's Program
  2. Social Service Department of the hospital

K. *To observe for the development of symptoms of congestive heart failure which occurs frequently as a complication of congenital heart disease.*
  1. Be aware of the symptoms of congestive heart failure in the child.
     a. Murmurs (may appear, or the characteristics of previously heard murmur may change)
     b. Retractions (may occur)
     c. Tachypnea (respiratory rate over 60 in infants and over 40 in older children)
     d. Tachycardia (heart rate above 160 in infants and over 100 in older children)
     e. Cyanosis (may occur)
     f. Fatigue (as evidenced by poor feeding in infants)
     g. Gallop heart rhythm
     h. Edema (periorbital edema is observed in infants; older children develop swelling of hands and feet)
     i. Pulmonary rales (may occur)
     j. Irritability

  k. Sweating
  l. Liver enlargement
  m. Splenomegaly
  n. Orthopnea
  o. Neck vein distention (rarely seen in infants)
2. Provide measures to relieve respiratory distress.
  a. Position the infant in an infant seat.
  b. Administer oxygen.
  c. Record the child's response to these measures.
3. Provide the child with adequate rest.
  a. Prevent excessive crying.
  b. Use a pacifier.
  c. Feed when hungry.
  d. Keep baby comfortable.
  e. Organize care to prevent frequent disturbances.
4. Provide adequate nutrition to meet the caloric requirements of the child.
  a. Feed frequently in small amounts.
  b. Feed slowly in a sitting position allowing frequent rest periods.
  c. Supplement the infant's oral feeding with gavage feeding when the infant is unable to take an adequate amount of formula by mouth.
  d. Record the amount of formula taken.
  e. Observe for distention and vomiting following feedings.
5. Observe vital signs and report any significant changes.
6. Administer the medications used in the treatment of congestive heart failure.
  a. *Digoxin*
    (1) Count apical pulse for 1 full minute before administering.
      (a) Be aware of the heart rate at which the physician wants the medication withheld.
      (b) Report vomiting which may occur following administration of digoxin to determine if physician desires dose to be repeated.
      (c) Carefully calculate dosage—digoxin is given to infants and children in very small amounts.
      (d) Observe for the development of premature ventricular contractions when digoxin is initially started; report this to physician.
  b. *Diuretics*
    (1) Weigh infant accurately each day to observe response.
    (2) Maintain a record of intake and output.
    (3) Provide potassium supplement when child is on diuretics for an extended period of time.
7. Practice measures that will serve to prevent infection.
  a. Practice careful handwashing technique.
  b. Avoid exposure to other children with upper respiratory infections, diarrhea etc.
  c. Report temperature elevation, diarrhea, vomiting, upper respiratory symptoms etc. promptly.
8. Prepare the parents for the care of the child at home.
  a. Describe symptoms to be aware of and to be reported.
  b. Teach them how to administer medications.
  c. Explain methods to prevent infection.
  d. Arrange for a community nursing referral if indicated.

L. *To observe for the development of symptoms of infectious endocarditis which may occur as a complication of congenital heart disease.*
  1. Be aware of the symptoms of infectious endocarditis.
     a. Spiking fever   d. Pallor
     b. Petechiae   e. Fatigue
     c. Anorexia
  2. Administer medication used in the treatment of infectious endocarditis.
     a. Administer antibiotics (appropriate for the organism isolated in the blood culture).
     b. Antibiotics are usually administered for 4–6 weeks.
  3. Observe the child's response to treatment.
     a. Observe temperature closely.
     b. Observe for changes in symptoms.
  4. Be aware of the need for infectious endocarditis prophylaxis for selected children undergoing surgery, dental work and laceration repair.

ACUTE RHEUMATIC FEVER

Acute rheumatic fever is a systemic disease characterized by inflammatory lesions of connective tissue and endothelial tissue.

Etiology

  1. The most important factor in the etiology of rheumatic fever is now accepted to be Group A beta-hemolytic streptococcus.
  2. Most first attacks of rheumatic fever are preceded by streptococcal infection at an interval of several days to several weeks.

Altered Physiology

  1. The basic changes consist of exudative and proliferative inflammatory reactions in the mesenchymal supporting tissue of the heart, joints, blood vessels and subcutaneous tissues.
  2. The unique pathologic lesion of rheumatic fever is the Aschoff body.

Clinical Manifestations and Diagnostic Evaluation

No single clinical or laboratory finding is characteristic of rheumatic fever. The diagnosis is based on a combination of manifestations characteristic of this disease and in the absence of other diseases which may mimic it.
     a. For this reason, the Jones Criteria, as established by a committee of the American Heart Association are utilized.
     b. The presence of 2 major criteria, or 1 major and 2 minor criteria indicates a high probability of the presence of rheumatic fever.
A. *Major Manifestations.*
  1. Carditis—manifested by significant murmurs, signs of pericarditis, cardiac enlargement or congestive heart failure.
  2. Polyarthritis—almost always migratory and manifested by swelling, heat, redness and tenderness, or by pain and limitation of motion of 2 or more joints.
  3. Chorea—purposeless, involuntary, rapid movements often associated with muscle weakness.

4. Erythema marginatum—an evanescent, pink rash.
   a. The erythematous areas have pale centers and round or serpiginous (creeping eruption) margins.
   b. They vary greatly in size and occur mainly on the trunk and proximal parts of the extremities, never on the face.
   c. The erythema is transient, migrates from place to place, and may be brought out by the application of heat.
5. Subcutaneous nodules—firm, painless nodules seen or felt over the extensor surface of certain joints, particularly elbows, knees, and wrists, in the occipital region, or over the spinous processes of the thoracic and lumbar vertebrae; the skin overlying them moves freely and is not inflamed.

B. *Minor Manisfestations*
   1. *Clinical*
      a. History of previous rheumatic fever or evidence of pre-existing rheumatic heart disease
      b. Arthralgia—pain in one or more joints without evidence of inflammation, tenderness to touch, or limitation of motion
      c. Fever—temperature in excess of 38°C. (100.4°F).
   2. *Laboratory*
      a. Erythrocyte sedimentation rate—elevated
      b. C-reactive protein—positive
      c. Electrocardiographic changes—mainly P-R interval prolongation

C. *Supporting Evidence of Streptococcal Infection*
   1. Increased titer of streptococcal antibodies
   2. Positive throat culture for Group A streptococci
   3. Recent scarlet fever

D. *Other Clinical Features*
   1. Abdominal pain
   2. Rapid sleeping pulse (tachycardia out of proportion to fever)
   3. Malaise
   4. Anemia
   5. Epistaxis
   6. Precordial pain

Nursing Objectives

A. *To become informed as to the child's symptomatology and the medical plan of care.*
   1. Discuss with the physician his plan for medical treatment.
   2. Make a base-line nursing assessment of the child's condition.
      a. Listen to the child's chest with a stethoscope to become familiar with the murmur or to determine the presence of a murmur not previously heard; listen for a friction rub.
      b. Determine from the child whether he is experiencing any pain or discomfort (also observe the child's facial expression as he moves since children may deny pain thinking they will be able to go home).
      c. Describe the pain as to location, when it occurs, whether there is any heat, swelling redness or tenderness.
      d. Examine the knees, elbows, wrists, occipital region and spine for nodules; describe location.

    e. Determine whether the child has any muscle weakness or rapid, purposeless movements.

    f. Assess the child's emotional status.

    g. Report any significant information to the physician.

B. *To alleviate the child's anxiety about the functioning of his heart, because anxiety utilizes energy and produces fatigue.*

    1. Give the child information about rheumatic fever in terms that he can understand, e.g., "Rheumatic fever is a hard thing to understand because you can't see it. When you scratch yourself, you can see the mark, and you can see the scratch heal. Rheumatic fever is something like that—only you can't see the healing because it happens to the tissue underneath the skin. (And sometimes it happens to the valves in the heart.)"

    2. Continually reinforce the teaching and encourage the child to ask questions.

    3. Assure the child that we know how to treat rheumatic fever.

    4. Communicate information about the child's reactions to all staff members in order to provide consistent information.

C. *To decrease the cardiac workload until the acute inflammatory reaction has subsided.*

    1. Explain to the child the need for rest.

    2. Assure the child that bedrest will be imposed no longer than necessary.

    3. Organize nursing care to provide periods of uninterrupted rest.

    4. Explain to the child what procedures are going to be performed before they are performed.

    5. Assure the child that his needs will be met.

        a. Give the child a bell to call the nurse.

        b. Answer his calls promptly.

D. *To provide frequent and comfortable changes in position to aid in relaxation and to prevent tissue breakdown.*

    1. Elevate the back of the bed and support the arms with pillows when child is dyspneic.

    2. Position the legs in good body alignment—use a footboard.

    3. When the joints are painful, move the child gently, supporting the extremity.

    4. Provide meticulous skin care.

E. *To be aware of the actions and side effects of the specific medications used to suppress the rheumatic inflammatory process.*

    1. *Salicylates*

        a. Observe for gastrointestinal upsets, ringing in the ears, headaches, bleeding, and disturbances in the mental state.

        b. Stimulation of respirations can cause alkalosis through hyperventilation, and acidosis may occur with excessive accumulation of salicylates in the blood.

        c. Administer milk or antacids with salicylates.

        d. Report side effects promptly.

    2. *Steroids*

        a. Prepare the child and his family for the expected side effects of steroid therapy.

          (1) Body appearance may change through rounding facial contour

          (2) Localized fat deposits

          (3) Appearance of acne or excessive hair

          (4) Weight gain with linear markings appearing in the stretched skin

    b. Mental and emotional disturbances may necessitate discontinuance of the medication.

    c. Hypertension and the tendency to accumulate water and sodium within the tissues may result from steroid therapy.

      (1) Provide a low sodium diet.

      (2) Weigh child daily—report sudden weight increases.

    d. Steroids diminish the child's resistance to infection and may mask symptoms of infection.

NURSING ALERT: Do not place a child with an infectious disease in the room with the child with rheumatic fever.

    Restrict visitors and personnel with infectious diseases from contact with the child on steroid therapy.

---

    e. Report side effects promptly.

  3. Report signs of increased rheumatic activity as salicylates or steroids are being tapered.

F. *To assist the child to develop a realistic attitude toward his illness and encourage him to discuss his concerns.*

  1. Help him to realize the restrictions he must face and the fact that progress is slow.

  2. Help him cope with his fears that his playmates may ostracize him or pity him.

  3. Alleviate his anxieties about keeping up with his class and school activities.

    a. Initiate a referral for a hospital-based school teacher to see him on a regular basis.

    b. When this service is not available encourage the parents to contact his teacher who will prepare lesson plans and short assignments for him—encourage the parents to maintain this contact with the teacher.

    c. Plan time each day on a regular basis for the child to complete his assignments.

G. *To provide for diversional activity that will help the child feel a sense of achievement and satisfaction.*

    Initiate some long-term projects.

H. *To help the child to maintain contact with his peers during hospitalization.*

  1. Encourage correspondence.

  2. Maintain telephone contact—if possible.

  3. Place in a room with a child of the same age, sex and interests—preferably a child with a long-term illness.

I. *To begin to prepare for discharge with the parents in time that sufficient adjustments and preparation may be made.*

  1. The child should have a bed of his own and, preferably, a room of his own.

  2. A responsible adult must be in the home to care for him.

  3. Specific information as to:

    a. Specifically what activity is allowed

    b. When to administer medications, correct amounts and specific side effects

    c. Where to obtain the medication

    d. Specific dietary instruction

    e. Specific symptoms to report—

        Pain   Tachycardia (teach to take the pulse)

        Malaise   Tachypnea

        Anorexia   Weight gain

    f. Telephone number of physician or hospital clinic

    g. When to return to clinic

  4. Initiate a community nursing referral—this may be done prior to discharge if a home evaluation is desired.

J. *To initiate specific preventative teaching in order to prevent a recurrence or an additional case of rheumatic fever within the family.*

  1. Have all family members screened for streptococcus by referring them for throat cultures.

  2. All persons with positive cultures should be treated.

  3. Teach the specific symptoms of streptococcal infections.

BIBLIOGRAPHY

Books

Blake, F. G., et al.: Nursing Care of Children, 8th ed. Philadelphia, J. B. Lippincott, 1970.

Davis, E.: Rheumatic Fever. Springfield, Illinois, Charles C Thomas, 1969.

Gasul, B. M., et al.: Heart Disease in Children. Philadelphia, J. B. Lippincott, 1966.

Jude, J. R., et al.: Fundamentals of Cardiopulmonary Resuscitation. Philadelphia, F. A. Davis, 1965.

Krovetz, L. J., et al.: Handbook of Pediatric Cardiology. New York, Harper and Row, 1969.

Markowitz, M., and Gordes, L.: Rheumatic Fever, 2nd ed. (Vol. II in the Series, Major Problems in Clinical Pediatrics). Philadelphia, W. B. Saunders, 1972.

Moss, A. J., et al.: Heart Disease in Infants, Children and Adolescents. Baltimore, Williams and Wilkins, 1968.

Nadas, A., and Fyler, D. C.: Pediatric Cardiology, 3rd ed. Philadelphia, W. B. Saunders, 1972.

Rowe, R., and Mehrizi, A.: The Neonate with Congenital Heart Disease (Vol. V in the Series, Major Problems in Clinical Pediatrics). Philadelphia, W. B. Saunders, 1968.

Articles

Hoffman, J. I.: Ventricular septal defect: indications for therapy in infants. Ped. Clin. N. Amer., *18*:1091, 1971.

Nora, J. J.: Etiologic factors in congenital heart disease. Ped. Clin. N. Amer., *18*:1059, 1971.

Rashkind, W. J.: Transposition of the great arteries. Ped. Clin. N. Amer., *18*:1075, 1971.

Riker, W. L.: Cardiac arrest in infant and children. Ped. Clin. N. Amer., *16*:661, 1969.

Roberts, F. B.: The child with heart disease. Amer. J. Nurs., *72*:1080, June 1972.

Talner, N. S.: Congestive heart failure in the infant: a functional approach. Ped. Clin. N. Amer., *18*:1011, 1971.

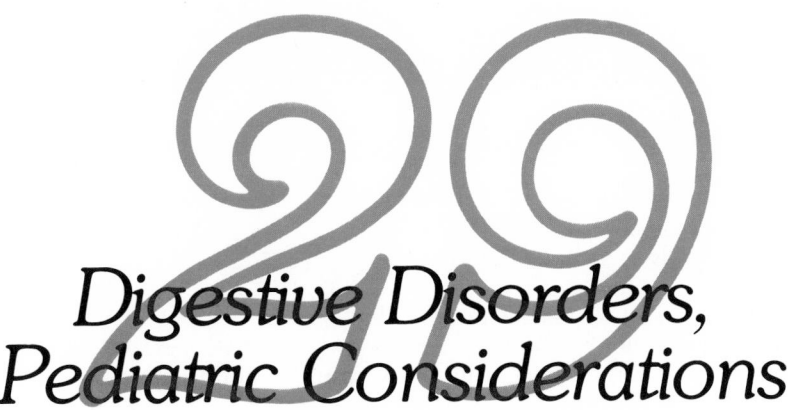

Digestive Disorders, Pediatric Considerations

DENTAL CARIES

Dental caries include loss of tooth structure or the formation of a cavity as a result of bacterial attack, first on the enamel, the hard surface of the tooth, and then progressing inward toward the pulp.

Etiology

A. *Bacteria*
1. Acidogenic organisms—decalcify the hard tissue by producing acids upon the tooth surface.
2. Proteolytic organisms—digest the product of tooth surface (Decalcification thus produces odor and discoloration.)
3. Leptotrichae organisms—form structures on the smooth tooth surface which houses acidogenic organisms

B. *Contributing Factors*
1. Age—most susceptible ages are childhood and adolescence
2. Diet—large intake of simple sugars between meals
3. Familial tendency to decay
4. Lack of oral hygiene
5. Poor state of health (Illness alters the normal bacteriostatic quality of saliva.)

Altered Physiology

As a result of missing teeth or multiple caries, the child may experience many problems.
1. Poor nutrition
   a. Refuses to eat foods that need chewing
   b. Teeth drift and cause malocclusion
2. Faulty speech habits and articulation
   a. Weak jaw muscles
   b. Abnormal alveolar bone development
3. Psychological problems
      Embarrassment by looks and oral odor
4. Oral foci of infection
      Subacute bacterial endocarditis may result in child with congenital heart disease

Clinical Manifestations

1. Decay is acute and rapidly penetrates the tooth in children.
2. Caries occur where food debris collects.
   a. Pits and fissures
   b. Between teeth
   c. At neck of tooth
3. Discoloration of teeth
4. Decay odor
5. Pain, abscess or infection

Nursing Objectives

Hospitalization of a child for treatment of dental caries is likely only when special behavior difficulties are anticipated in treatment, when medical problems complicate dental treatment or when extensive repair is necessary.
(See Preventive Pediatrics, Dental Care, p. 1053.)

A. *To prevent dental caries in all patients.*

B. *To know that there is a direct relationship between incidence of dental caries in children and dental health education or knowledge of parents.*
   1. Assess parental knowledge and use opportunities to teach parents preventive care.
   2. Encourage parental participation with the young child during teeth brushing exercise.

C. *To know the principles of good oral hygiene and practice them when caring for each pediatric patient.*
   1. Encourage mouth rinsing or teeth brushing after eating.
      Brush before bedtime to decrease bacteriogenic activity in the warm, undisturbed mouth during sleep.
   2. Encourage proper brushing of teeth.
      a. Brush crosswise with a soft bristled brush.
      b. Electric tooth brush cleans teeth and stimulates the gingivae.
   3. Supervise brushing in young children. (Dentrifice is not necessary.)

D. *To know the value of good nutrition and its effect in preventing dental caries.*
   1. No in-between meal snacking of refined sugar foods.
      a. Improves appetite at meals.

b. Substitute refined sugars with fresh fruit. (No lollipops between meals; give after meal before brushing.)
2. Discourage a bottle at bedtime or before sleep.
   Residue is left on teeth during long periods of sleep and results in rampant decay.

E. *To know the value of periodic dental examination and preventive measures used to decrease decay.*
   1. Encourage patient and parent to participate in regular dentist visits.
      a. Regular visits for cleaning and checking for decay; repair if necessary.
         First visit is to familiarize the young child with the dentist and equipment.
         (1) Usually age 18–30 months of age
         (2) Should not be when child has toothache
      b. During childhood and adolescence visits are every 3–6 months.
         New decay areas appear suddenly in multiple areas and advances rapidly.
   2. If fluoridation is not supplied in community water, topical application is advisable.
      a. Most effective when applied on newly erupted teeth.
      b. Fluoride makes enamel more resistant to decay as it strengthens calcification of the developing dental tissue.

F. *To keep the adolescent aware of his diet and its effect on dental decay.*
   1. Keep in mind diet fads and peer group pressure.
   2. Have patient keep a dietary record for 1 week. Then evaluate it against an example of a good nutritional menu. Encourage patient to make his own evaluation.

Parental Teaching

1. After assessment of parental knowledge has been made, embark on teaching program. Main areas of concern:
   a. Proper technique of dental hygiene
   b. Value of good nutrition
   c. Value of fluoridation
   d. Importance of visits to the dentist
2. American Dental Association
   211 East Chicago Avenue
   Chicago, Illinois 60611

CLEFT LIP AND PALATE

Cleft lip and palate results when fusion involving the first brachial arch fails to take place during embryonic development.

Etiology

1. Failure of embryonic development—cause not known
2. Hereditary factor

Altered Physiology

1. The lip and palate develop independently; thus any combination of defects can occur.

a. Cleft lip
 (1) Varies from a notch in the lip to complete separation of the lip into the nose
 (2) May be unilateral or bilateral
 b. Isolated cleft palate
 (1) Cleft of uvula
 (2) Cleft of soft palate
 (3) Cleft of both soft and hard palate through roof of mouth
 (4) Unilateral or bilateral
 c. Cleft lip and palate combined
   Any degree of involvement
 d. Submucous cleft
 (1) Muscles of soft palate are not joined
 (2) Not recognized until child talks; cannot be seen at birth
2. Associated problems
 a. Eating
 (1) Suction cannot be created for effective sucking
 (2) Food returns through the nose
 b. Nasal speech
 c. Lack of normal dental function and appearance
 d. Repeated bouts of otitis media with subsequent hearing loss

Clinical Manifestations

Obvious appearance of cleft lip or palate
 a. Incomplete formed lip
 b. Opening in roof of mouth

Nursing Objectives

NEWBORN

A. *To show acceptance of the baby.*
 1. The nurse must maintain her composure and not show shock when handling the infant or child. The manner in which the nurse handles the baby can make a lasting impression on the parents.
 a. The baby with a cleft lip can be unattractive and a shock when first seen.
 b. When showing a newborn baby to parents for the first time, support them by accepting both the baby and the parents' feelings. (Parents may be grieving about the perfect infant they did not have and may harbor ambivalent feelings about this baby.)
 c. Be supportive of parents by reassuring them that reparative surgery can be done with much success.
 (1) The time when reparative surgery is done depends upon the surgeon, the condition of the baby and the degree to which the parents have accepted the baby.
 (2) Lip surgery may be done several hours after birth or when the infant is 2–3 months of age or has gained 4.54 kg. (10 pounds).
 2. Reparative surgery for the palate is done between 18–36 months of age.

B. *To establish and maintain adequate nutrition for growth and development.*
 1. Babies with just a cleft lip may feed well if a regular nipple with enlarged holes is used.

2. With certain cleft lips and palates, the baby is unable to create a vacuum and is thus unable to suck. Several types of nipples and feeding devices are available to make feeding easier.
    a. Regular nipple with enlarged holes
    b. Lamb's nipple
    c. Duckey nipple
    d. Brecht feeder
    e. Rubber tipped asepto syringe or dropper
3. Feed baby in an upright sitting position to decrease possibility of fluid being aspirated or returned through the nose.
    Bubble frequently during feeding as these babies swallow a great deal of air.
4. Advance diet as appropriate for age and needs of the baby.
    Eating often improves when solids are introduced since they are easier for baby to manipulate.

C. *To prevent infection in the child so that surgery will not have to be delayed.*
    1. Avoid patient contact with anyone who has an infection.
    2. Change the baby's position frequently.
    3. Clean the cleft after each feeding with clear water and cotton-tipped applicator.

D. *To assist parents in preparing to take the newborn home from the nursery before lip and palate surgery has been done.*
    1. Prepare mother for home feedings. She should have several days to practice feeding in order to become familiar with the baby's pattern.
        a. Home equipment should be used in the hospital.
        b. Mother should be aware of difficulties with feeding and how to handle them.
            (1) Formula returning through the nose
            (2) Respiratory distress
            (3) Longer time necessary for feeding
        c. Suggest that about a week or so prior to scheduled admission for surgery, mother begin using feeding technique preferred by the surgeon for postoperative feeding.
            (1) Side of spoon
            (2) Rubber-tipped dropper
            (3) Toddler cup
    2. Encourage parents to prepare siblings at home for the arrival of this baby. (Pictures of the new baby might be suggested.)
    3. Initiate a community nurse referral to continue emotional support and teaching program at home.
    4. Offer parents available literature about children with cleft lip and palate.*
    5. Parents should know what plans have been started for surgical treatment.
    6. Social work referral may be indicated.
        a. To listen to mother express her concerns regarding management at home with a handicapped child.
        b. To arrange financial assistance—Crippled Children's Service

* *The Child with a Cleft Palate.* U.S. Department of Health, Education and Welfare, Social and Rehabilitation Service.
Booklets sponsored by Mead Johnson Laboratories, Evansville, Indiana 47721
    Road to Normalcy for the Cleft Lip and Palate Child
    Steps in Habilitation for the Cleft Lip and Palate Child

E. *To be aware of the complexity of long-range care and the importance of the many disciplines involved in the eventual outcome.* The nurse should know all the ramifica-cations and potential problems for this child and his family.

    1. The organization of trained professional people from the many disciplines that become involved include: pediatrician, plastic surgeon, otologist, general dentist, orthodontist, prosthodontist, medical-social worker, nurse, speech therapist and psychologist.

    2. Long-term follow-up and reparative surgery:
       a. Chronic otitis media and hearing loss
       b. Lip, palate and orthodontic repair
       c. Speech therapy
       d. Psychological insult to the child

    3. Financial burden on the family.
       State programs for crippled children can offer relief

    4. Psychological trauma to the family.

F. *To emphasize the importance of the mother's role in caring for the child during out-patient treatment and the many hospitalizations required.*

    Mother can offer a great deal of security to the child when he is subjected to the trauma and frightening experiences of treatment.

PREOPERATIVE CARE OF THE CHILD WITH A CLEFT LIP

A. *To prepare the infant for postoperative care so that it will be familiar to him, less frightening and easier for him to accept after surgery.*

    1. Practice the feeding method to be used as preferred by the surgeon
       a. Rubber-tipped syringe or asepto syringe
       b. Side of spoon

    2. The use of elbow restraints for short periods of time.
       a. Let the child play with them if he is old enough.
       b. Allow mother to become involved in their use.

    3. Help the infant get used to being on his back or propped on his side for long periods of time.

B. *To prepare the mother (parents) as to what to expect when she sees the child post-operatively.*

    1. Explain the use of the Logan bow (a curved metal wire that prevents stress on the suture line) and restraints.

    2. Encourage mother to be with the infant especially when he wakes up from anesthesia to offer him security and comfort.

POSTOPERATIVE CARE OF THE CHILD WITH A CLEFT LIP

A. *To administer good postoperative care based on general principles and to observe for usual postoperative complications.*

B. *To prevent injury to the suture line of the lip.*

    1. Elbow restraints are the most effective way to prevent busy hands from reaching the lip, yet still allow some freedom of movement.
       a. Pad restraint and place it from the axilla to inner aspect of the wrist.
       b. Remove restraints occasionally, one at a time, to exercise the arms.

2. Logan bow or Band-Aid placed cheek-to-cheek across top of lip prevents lateral tension.
    Prevent wetting tape or it will loosen.
3. Prevent baby from crying as crying also increases tension on the suture line.
    a. Encourage mother to hold and cuddle infant.
    b. Keep the infant dry, fed and comfortable.
4. Position infant on his back or propped on his side to keep him from rubbing his lip on the sheets.

C. *To maintain adequate nutrition and fluid intake for weight gain, growth and prevention of dehydration.*
    1. For several days postoperatively feeding will have to be accomplished without tension on the suture line.
        a. Dropper or syringe with a rubber tip
        b. Side of spoon (Never put spoon into the mouth.)
        c. Nasogastric gavage—usually last treatment of choice
    2. Advance slowly to nipple feeding as indicated by physician preference.
        Baby should be able to suck more efficiently with the lip repaired.
    3. Encourage mother to participate as much as possible in the care of the infant. It is good for both infant and mother to continue their relationship.

D. *To keep the suture line clean, to decrease infection and eliminate crust formation which enlarges the resulting scar.* The sutures are removed from 3–14 days after surgery.
    Clean suture line after every feeding.
    a. The cleansing solution used is usually the physician's choice.
        (1) Water
        (2) Hydrogen peroxide
        (3) Saline solution
    b. Gently and frequently wipe with a wet cotton tip applicator.
    c. Gently dry by patting.
        (1) May use antibiotic ointment or petrolatum after drying.
        (2) May be left open to the air.
    d. Water should be given after feeding to clean the mouth of milk.

PREOPERATIVE CARE OF THE CHILD WITH A CLEFT PALATE
    (Repair may require several operations.)

A. *To be familiar with growth and development as well as the emotional and psychological needs of the toddler, 18–24 months old. (This is the age most common for palate repair.)*
    1. Primary objectives for palate repair are to improve speech and dental function.
    2. This toddler age is selected because the anatomical structures involved are still growing.
    3. The toddler finds the hospital strange and frightening. (See p. 1049.)
        a. Encourage mother to stay with the child if possible.
        b. Encourage play.

B. *To prepare the child for postoperative care; if he is familiar with the procedures and routines he will be less frightened and more likely to cooperate.*
    1. Use elbow restraints frequently for short periods of time.
    2. Do not allow the child to suck from a bottle. Hopefully he has been taught to drink from a cup. Feed him in the manner that he will be fed postoperatively.

3. Practice frequent mouth irrigations using the same solution and equipment to be used postoperatively.

Allow the child to handle and become familiar with equipment.

C. *To prevent infection by keeping the child away from anyone with infection.*

D. *To prepare the parents as to what to expect when they see the child postoperatively.*

Include the parents in the preparation of the child. Then, with the parents alone discuss in more depth what to expect.

POSTOPERATIVE CARE OF THE CHILD WITH A CLEFT PALATE

A. *To administer good postoperative care and to observe for possible postoperative complications.*

1. Breathing with a closed palate is different from child's customary way of breathing.
2. Note respiratory effort.

B. *To prevent injury to the suture line in the mouth.*

1. Use elbow restraints.
2. Do not put anything into the mouth.
3. Prevent the child from crying.

C. *To keep the suture line and mouth clean to prevent infection.*

1. Irrigate mouth with normal saline or water.
   a. Direct gentle stream over suture line using ear bulb syringe.
   b. Have child in sitting position with his head forward.
2. Keep mouth moist to promote healing and provide comfort.
3. Rinse mouth after each feeding.

D. *To maintain adequate nutrition for growth and to promote healing.*

1. Diet progresses from clear liquids to full liquids to soft foods
   Soft foods are usually continued for about 1 month after surgery at which time regular diet is started, excluding hard food.
2. Check weight periodically to see if adequate nutrition is being maintained.
3. Feed the child in the manner used preoperatively (Cup, side of spoon or rubber tipped syringe). Never use straw, nipple, plain syringe.

E. *To administer antibiotics as prescribed.*

The mouth and suture line are constantly contaminated.

F. *To provide opportunities for social relationships and play as soon as possible.*

1. While the child must be restrained, he especially needs to have some stimulation and diversional activity.
2. A satisfactory relationship with mother or the nurse can minimize frustration and discomfort from surgery and restraints.

G. *To continue support of parents who have already encountered many frustrations in caring for the child, and to foster continual parental acceptance of the child and his handicap.*

1. Solicit assistance of social worker if appropriate; mother may talk about problems she is having raising a handicapped child.
2. Compliment, sincerely, the parents in the good work they have already done with this child.
3. Help parents understand that this child can live a normal life in the community.

H. *To begin discharge planning and teaching soon after admission so parents can learn how to care for the child at home.*
 1. Continued protection of the mouth.
    a. May need to use elbow restraints.
    b. Child this age will put everything into mouth—restrict this.
    c. No sucking or blowing.
 2. Diet of soft foods will need to be continued.
 3. Infection must be prevented.
    Continue to clean mouth after eating.

Parental Teaching

 1. There are 3 specific periods when parental teaching is vitally important for continual, effective management of the child:
    a. Management of the child with the cleft lip and palate not yet repaired
    b. Preparing for lip or palate surgery.
    c. Preparing for patient's discharge following surgery.
 2. At each time specific instructions need to be given in the following areas:
    a. Good nutrition and feeding techniques
    b. Good oral hygiene
    c. Prevention of injury to operative site
    d. Prevention of infection
    e. Plan for follow-up, especially for surgery
    f. Psychological and social development of child—including speech therapy
 3. Other members of the family must be considered.
    a. The child with a cleft lip or palate should not be thought of as sick, but as a child who has special needs to promote his individual growth and development. But he does not require attention all the time.
    b. The family should be included in his care, but they also must have a life of their own.
    c. The parents need time to themselves.
 4. Help the parents realize that even though rehabilitation of the child is long, drawn out and expensive the child can live a normal life.
    a. Have the parents discuss the child's problem with the school nurse, the teacher and other responsible adults who will have close contact with the child.
    b. Long-range planning should include detailed communication between the family and various disciplines.
       (1) Collaborative effort between disciplines determines the effectiveness of each discipline.
       (2) Parents may need help in understanding the value of each discipline for the future well-being of their child.
           Speech therapy is often 1 area where the value is not completely understood.

ESOPHAGEAL ATRESIA WITH TRACHEO-ESOPHAGEAL FISTULA

Esophageal atresia is a failure of the esophagus to form a continuous passage from the pharynx to the stomach during embryonic development. *Tracheo-esophageal fistula* is the abnormal sinuous connection between the trachea and esophagus.

Etiology

1. Failure of embryonic development
2. Cause unknown in most cases

Altered Physiology

4 types of defect

1. *Type I*—upper and lower segments of esophagus are blind; there is no connection to trachea
2. *Type II*—upper end of esophagus opens into trachea; lower end is blind
3. *Type III*—upper end of esophagus has a blind end; lower end of esophagus connects into trachea by a fistula (most common; discussion will be limited to this type)
   a. Air enters stomach via trachea, fistula and lower part of esophagus
   b. Secretions or oral liquids fill the blind pouch and overflow into larynx and trachea
4. *Type IV*—both upper and lower ends of esophagus open into trachea by a fistula (H-type)

Clinical Manifestations

Appear soon after birth

1. Excessive amount of secretions
   a. Constant drooling
   b. Large amount of secretions from nose
2. Intermittent cyanosis
   Aspiration from overflow from blind pouch
3. Abdominal distention
   Air from trachea passes through fistula into stomach
4. If fed, the infant will respond violently after first or second swallow
   a. Coughs and chokes
   b. Fluid returns through nose and mouth
   c. Cyanosis
   d. Infant struggles
5. Inability to pass catheter through nose or mouth into stomach—tip of catheter will stop at blind pouch, atresia

Diagnostic Evaluation

1. X-ray, flat plate of abdomen and chest—reveals presence of gas in stomach and chest.
2. X-ray with radiopaque catheter or iodized oil via esophageal catheter—catheter tip or iodized oil will show evidence of location of atresia.

Nursing Objectives

PREOPERATIVE

A. *To position baby with head and chest elevated 20–30 degrees to prevent reflux of gastric juices into the tracheobronchial tree.*

B. *To assist in removing nasopharyngeal secretions and support infant's respiration.*
   1. Intermittent nasopharyngeal suctioning or indwelling replogle tube (double lumen tube) or sump tube to maintain constant suction.

   a. Tip of tube is placed at the back of throat or into blind pouch, depending upon site of atresia.
   b. Replogle or sump tube allows air to be drawn in via a second lumen and prevents tube obstruction.
   c. Change indwelling tube as needed and at least every 8–12 hours, alternating nostrils.
 2. Place infant in incubator with high humidity to aid in liquefying secretions and thick mucus.
 3. Administer oxygen as needed.

C. *To administer antibiotics and other medications prescribed.*
   Given to treat or prevent associated pneumonitis.

D. *To monitor parenteral fluids as ordered to prevent dehydration and electrolyte imbalance.* (see p. 1087.)
 1. Supplies water and calories
 2. Cutdown very likely to be performed for easier management in surgery and possible blood transfusion.
 3. The infant does not receive oral feedings.

E. *To observe infant carefully for any change in condition; report immediately.*
   Check vital signs, color, amount of secretions, abdominal distention, respiratory distress.

F. *To prevent infection by using the principles of isolation.*
   Incubator may be used for environmental isolation.

G. *To be available for emergency care or resuscitation.*
   Accompany infant to x-ray or operative room in incubator with portable oxygen and suction equipment.

POSTOPERATIVE CARE

There are 2 types of surgery considered for esophageal atresia with tracheo-esophageal fistula: (1) esophageal anastomosis and fistula division called *primary repair* and (2) palliative surgery using a gastrostomy and cervical esophagostomy temporarily until the infant gains weight so that a bowel transplant or anastomosis can be done (usually the course selected for premature infants). Generally the nursing care is essentially the same for either procedure.

A. *To administer good postoperative care and to observe for signs of possible complications.*

B. *To maintain a patent airway to prevent oxygen starvation, apnea and aspiration of secretions.*
 1. Request physician to mark a suction catheter, indicating how far the catheter can be safely inserted without disturbing the anastomosis.
   a. Suction frequently.
   b. Observe for signs of obstructed airway.
 2. Change infant's position frequently and stimulate him to cry so that he fully expands his lungs.
 3. Continued use of incubator.
   a. For warmth and good observation
   b. Provides humidity to liquefy secretions

    4. Be prepared to function in an emergency.
       a. Have emergency equipment available
         (1) Suction machine, catheter
         (2) Oxygen
         (3) Laryngoscope

C. *To assist in maintaining adequate nutrition to promote healing, growth and development.*
    1. Oral feedings may begin 6–14 days postoperatively following anastomosis.
       a. Feed slowly to allow infant time to swallow.
       b. Use upright sitting position.
       c. Burp frequently.
    2. Gastrostomy feeding
       a. Gastrostomy tube is not clamped between feedings until full feedings are tolerated.
       b. *Allow infant to suck on pacifier during gastrostomy feeding for exercise of jaw, fulfillment of normal sucking desire and to help relax the musculature.*

D. *To care appropriately for cervical esophagostomy.*
    1. Keep the area clean of saliva.
       a. Wash with clear water.
       b. Place an absorbent pad over the area.
    2. As soon as possible allow infant to suck a few milliliters of milk at the same time gastrostomy feeding is being done. Advance to solid foods as appropriate if esophagostomy is retained for a few months.
       a. Encourage sucking and swallowing.
       b. Familiarize infant with food so that when he is able to eat orally, he will be used to it.

E. *To be astutely aware of impending complications of esophageal repair.*
    1. Leak at the anastomosis (development of fistula)
       a. Fever
       b. Pneumothorax
         (1) Severe respiratory distress
         (2) Cyanosis
         (3) Restlessness
         (4) Weak pulses
    2. Stricture at the anastomosis
       a. Difficulty swallowing
       b. Vomiting
    3. Atelectasis or pneumonia
       a. Aspiration
       b. Respiratory distress

F. *To offer the infant emotional support.*
    1. Hold infant for feedings.
    2. Encourage mother to cuddle and love infant.

G. *To encourage parental participation in learning to care for and handle the infant and to foster acceptance of the child by his parents and family.*
    1. Provide opportunities for the parents to learn all aspects of care of their baby.
    2. Initiate a teaching program for the parents early. Offer them available literature and help them become familiar with community resources.

3. Initiate a community nurse referral for continuity of care in the home.
4. Encourage parents to talk about their feelings, fears and concerns.
5. Help to develop a healthy parent-child relationship.
    a. Frequent visiting
    b. Phone calls
    c. Physical contact of child and parents

Parental Teaching

1. Carefully and thoroughly teach all procedures to be done at home.
    Show parents how, then watch return demonstration:
    (1) Gastrostomy feedings and care
    (2) Esophagostomy care with feeding technique
    (3) Suctioning
2. Help parents understand the psychological needs of the infant for sucking, warmth, comfort, stimulation and love. Suggest that activity be appropriate for age.
3. Encourage parents to continue close medical follow-up and help them to understand what they can expect.
    a. Dilatation of esophagus to prevent stricture at the site of the anastomosis.
    b. Raspy cough for 6–24 months
    c. Eating problems
    d. Repeated respiratory tract infection
4. Help parents understand the need for good nutrition and the need to follow the diet regimen suggested by the physician.

CHALASIA

Chalasia is an abnormal, persistent relaxation of the lower end of the esophagus (the cardio-esophageal mechanism) causing vomiting in infants.

Etiology

1. The cause is undetermined in most patients
2. Possible causes:
    a. Neuromuscular imbalance
    b. Cerebral defects
    c. Obstruction at or just below the pylorus

Altered Physiology

Continual relaxation of the cardioesophageal mechanism.
    a. Filling of the esophagus from the stomach with inspiration, producing vomiting
    b. Increased intra-abdominal pressure

Clinical Manifestations

1. Vomiting
    a. Immediately after feeding, especially when infant is placed in prone position
    b. Usually regurgitation rather than projectile vomiting
2. Weight loss or failure to gain weight
3. Dehydration

   4. Onset usually soon after birth
   5. Relief of vomiting with treatment
      a. Thickened formula
      b. Propping in upright position after feeding

Diagnostic Evaluation

   1. Upper G.I. barium x-ray with fluoroscope.
         Barium enters stomach but then is regurgitated back into the esophagus.
   2. Serum studies
      a. Calcium level—may be lowered
      b. Alkalosis—pH greater than 7.45

Nursing Objectives

A. *To assist in treatment of dehydration.*
   1. Monitor intravenous therapy (see p. 1087).
   2. Observe and record accurately urinary output.
      a. Amount, frequency, color and concentration
      b. Specific gravity
   3. Promote good skin care to prevent lesions of dry and delicate tissues.
      a. Change position frequently.
      b. Change soiled diapers often.
      c. Apply lotion and gently rub dry and reddened areas.

B. *To maintain adequate nutrition and to prevent vomiting.*
   1. Thicken formula for each feeding
      a. May use cereal.
      b. Enlarge nipple hole so that formula can be more easily extracted.
   2. Prop infant in upright position after feeding.
      a. May use infant seat or elevate mattress to 80-degree angle.
      b. Use protective devices or straps to prevent infant from slipping.
      c. Keep infant propped 30–60 minutes after feeding.
   3. Handle infant gently, with minimal movement during and after feeding.
   4. Bubble frequently during and at completion of feeding.
   5. Record accurately activity of infant.
      a. Amount of feeding taken; whether retained
      b. Emesis, estimated amount, occurrence in relation to feeding, type
      c. Any change in behavior as a result of feeding technique

C. *To support family, especially mother, and encourage them to participate in care and feeding the infant.*
   1. Mother may be overly concerned about infant and blame herself and feeding technique for infant's condition.
      a. Help mother understand it is not her fault; she is not a "bad mother."
      b. Let her talk about her concerns.
   2. Encourage mother to take an active part in caring for infant—provides a good opportunity to guide mother in correct or preferred methods of handling baby with this condition.

Parental Teaching

1. Plan a program of intensive parental teaching on how to handle and care for infant. Be certain parents understand why this is being done.
   a. Help parents understand that it is not necessary to keep infant in infant seat or propped at all times.
      (1) Bathe or play with infant *prior to feeding*
      (2) Change position about 1 hour after feeding
      (3) During the night after feeding, infant can sleep in upright position
      (4) Expect occasional small amounts of vomiting.
2. Help parents to understand that chalasia is self-limited—symptoms usually disappear within 3 months.

HYPERTROPHIC PYLORIC STENOSIS

Hypertrophic pyloric stenosis is congenital hypertrophy of the muscle of the pylorus, causing vomiting in infants.

Altered Physiology

1. Increase in size of the circular musculature of the pylorus with thickening (size and shape of an olive). The pylorus muscle becomes elongated and thickened and is enlarged about twice the usual size.
2. Then hypertrophy of the pylorus musculature occurs with narrowing of pylorus lumen.
3. Constriction of the lumen of the pyloric canal (at the distal end of the stomach) causes the stomach to become dilated.
4. There is delayed gastric emptying, vomiting after feeding and obstruction.

Clinical Manifestations

Onset is within the first 2 months of life.
1. Vomiting
   a. Occasional, nonprojectile at first
   b. Projectile vomiting, not bile-stained
2. Constipation—decreased stools
3. Loss of weight or failure to gain weight
4. Visible gastric peristaltic waves, left to right
5. Excessive hunger—willingness to eat immediately after vomiting
6. Dehydration
7. Decreased urinary output
8. Palpable pyloric tumor in upper right quadrant of abdomen

Diagnostic Evaluation

1. Tests for metabolic alkalosis—due to loss of hydrochloric acid and potassium from vomiting.
   a. Serum sodium—increases
   b. Serum chloride—decreases
   c. Serum potassium—decreases

        d. Serum pH—increases above 7
        e. Serum CO_2 level—is elevated
    2. Urine becomes alkaline and concentrated—routine urinalysis
    3. Blood hematocrit and hemoglobin—elevated due to hemoconcentration
    4. X-ray examination with barium.
        a. Narrowing of pyloric canal
        b. Delayed gastric emptying time
        c. Enlarged stomach
        d. Increased peristaltic waves

Nursing Objectives

PREOPERATIVE CARE

A. *To assist in restoring hydration and electrolyte balance.*
    1. Intravenous therapy is usually initiated. (See p. 1087.)
        Electrolytes are added to solution for replacement.
    2. Careful observation of output, amount and characteristics.
        a. Urine (Check specific gravity.)
        b. Vomiting
        c. Stools
    3. Accurate daily weight—serves as a guide for calculating need for parenteral fluid.

B. *To prevent or decrease the likelihood of vomiting.*
    1. Patient may be NPO with indwelling nasogastric tube.
        Ensure proper functioning of tube and note drainage.
    2. Oral feedings may be continued.
        a. Feed small, frequent feedings, slowly.
        b. Bubble frequently.
        c. Thickened formula may be ordered.
    3. Proper positioning.
        Prop patient in upright position.
        (1) Elevate head of bed, mattress, or infant seat at a 75- to 80-degree angle.
        (2) Place slightly on right side—to aid in gastric emptying.
        (3) Handle gently and minimally after feeding.

C. *To make accurate observations, frequently, of the infant's condition.*
    1. Dehydration
    2. Vomiting
    3. Stools and urine output
    4. Vital signs

NURSING ALERT: Respiratory rate may be irregular with apnea when patient is in severe alkalosis.

D. *To provide comfort for the infant.*
    1. Mouth care—wet lips
        Let infant suck on pacifier
    2. Physical contact or nearness of the nurse or mother.
    3. Audio or visual stimulation may be soothing.

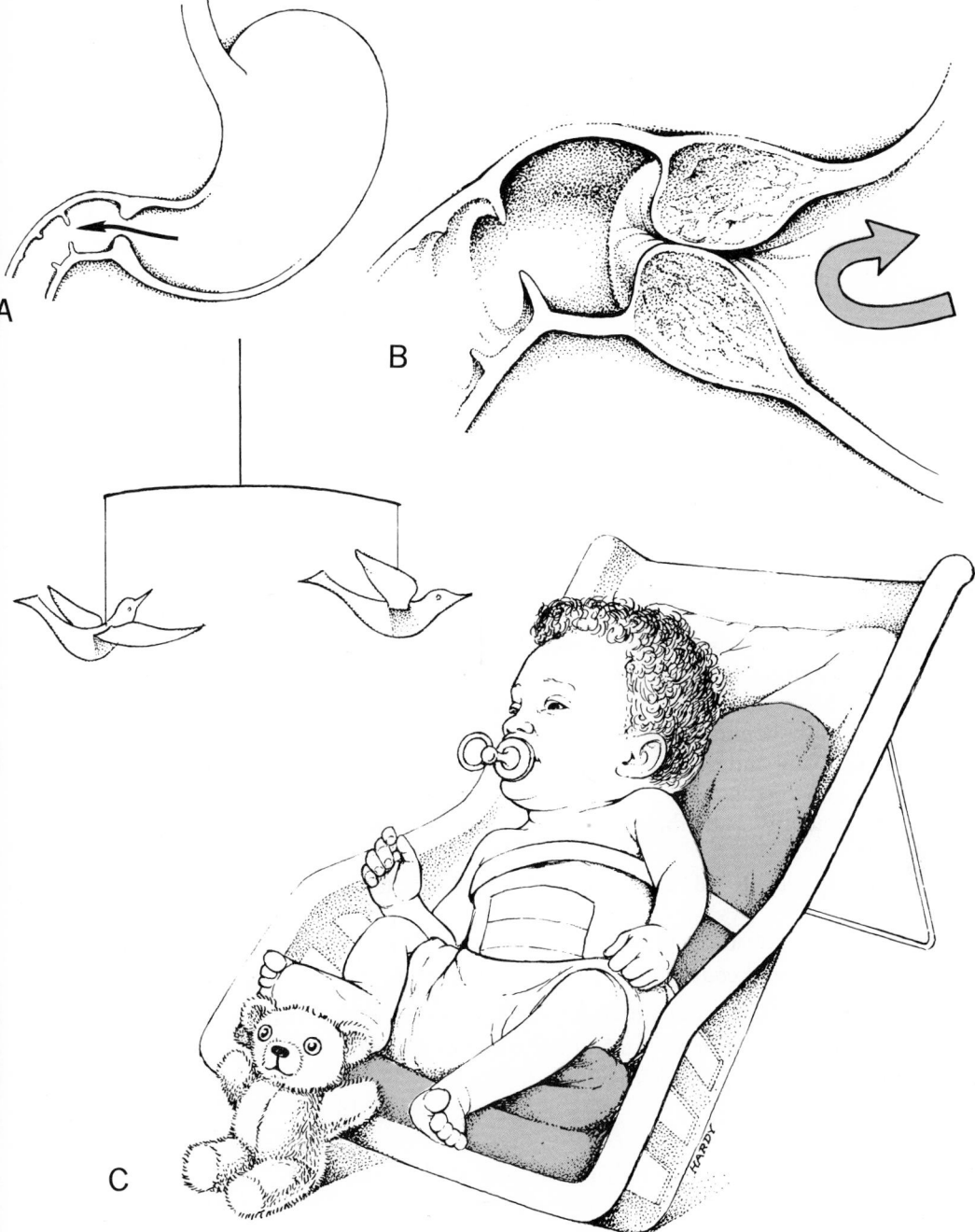

Figure 29-1. Pyloric stenosis. *A.* Normal passage through pyloric sphincter. *B.* Stoppage of flow due to stenotic sphincter. *C.* Postoperative treatment: child propped on right side after feeding to aid gastric emptying.

E. *To support parents who are usually very concerned and worried.*
   1. Mother may feel guilty, i.e., poor feeding technique.
      Help her understand that she did not do anything to cause this deformity.
   2. Prepare parents for surgery of their child.
      a. Be honest with them.
      b. Inform them of the expected postoperative appearance of the infant.
      c. Show them where the operating room and recovery room are located and where to wait during surgery.
   3. Encourage parents to maintain a good relationship with the infant. Allow them to hold infant.
   4. Encourage them to get some rest.
      Mother may be tired and frustrated because of the extensive care she has had to give to the child.

POSTOPERATIVE CARE

A. *To give good postoperative care and to observe for the usual postoperative complications (see p. 1093).*

B. *To monitor parenteral fluids to maintain hydration.*
   1. Intravenous therapy may be continued until adequate oral intake is obtained.

C. *To assist in resuming oral feedings.*
   1. Feeding is usually resumed 2–8 hours after surgery.
      a. Feedings usually start with glucose water and slowly advance to half strength formula or skim milk, to full strength formula and regular diet.
      b. Report any vomiting—amount and characteristics.
      c. Feed slowly and bubble frequently.
      d. Note how feeding is taken and if retained.
      e. The amount of feeding is increased as the time interval between feedings is lengthened.
   2. Continue to elevate infant's head and shoulders after feeding for 45–60 minutes after feeding.
      Place on right side to aid gastric emptying (Fig. 29-1).
   3. Regurgitation may continue for a short period after surgery.

D. *To encourage parents to resume care, especially feeding, of their infant.*
   1. This will help to restore their confidence in caring for their baby.
   2. Provides an opportunity for the nurse to teach.

Parental Teaching

   1. Help parents to understand that surgery has corrected the pyloric stenosis.
      a. Discharge will be from 2–5 days after surgery.
      b. Proper care of the operative site can be done by the mother.
      c. A modified method of feeding technique will be continued at home for only a short period of time.
   2. Since this may be a new mother with her infant under 6 weeks of age she may need help with routine infant care.

CYSTIC FIBROSIS

Cystic Fibrosis is a generalized disorder affecting the exocrine glands so that the substances they secrete are abnormal, affecting primarily pulmonary and gastrointestinal function.

Etiology

1. Underlying cause of the abnormal secretions is unknown.
2. Believed to be hereditary as a recessive trait.

Altered Physiology

1. The secretions of the exocrine glands are thick and sticky rather than thin and slippery.
2. Pulmonary involvement
   a. Thick mucus clogs bronchi and bronchioles
      (1) Lungs overinflate
      (2) Atelectasis results
   b. Associated infection in lungs
   c. Fibrotic changes in the lungs
3. Gastrointestinal involvement
   a. Thick mucus plugs pancreatic ducts
      (1) Prevents pancreatic digestive enzymes from reaching the small intestine; thus, there is abnormality of stools
      (2) Digestion is impaired, especially fats—nutritional failure results
   b. Meconium ileus in infant—bowel obstructed by thick intestinal secretions
   c. Biliary cirrhosis
4. Involvement of sweat glands
   Secretions contain excessive amount of salt

Clinical Manifestations

1. Diagnosis is usually made prior to 6 months of age.
2. Meconium ileus in newborn.
3. Other presenting signs:
   a. Tastes salty when kissed
   b. Cough, wheezing
   c. Failure to gain weight or grow in the presence of a good appetite
   d. Stools are frequent, bulky and foul smelling
   e. Protuberant abdomen—pot belly
   f. Wasted buttocks
   g. Vomiting following coughing
   h. Recurrent pulmonary function

Diagnostic Evaluation

1. Measure of sodium and chloride level in sweat
   Chloride level of more than 60mEq/liter is diagnostic
2. Measure of trypsin concentration in duodenal secretions
   Absence of normal concentration is diagnostic

3. Analysis of digestive enzymes in stool
   Level is lower—used for initial screening for cystic fibrosis
4. Chest x-ray
   a. May be normal initially
   b. Later shows increased areas of infection, overinflation, atelectasis and fibrosis
5. Analysis of stool for steatorrhea

Nursing Objectives

A. *To establish and maintain adequate nutrition to allow for growth and development.*
   1. Diet composed of high calorie, high protein and low fat is usually recommended. (Absorption of food is incomplete.)
   2. Water-soluble vitamins given in 2–3 times the normal dose. (Difficulty in absorption.)
   3. Absent pancreatic enzymes are replaced with extracts of animal pancreas.
      a. Give with each meal.
      b. Mix with small portion of food for infant or small child. *Never mix in formula.*
      c. Offer the older child capsules or tablets.
   4. Salt intake will need to be increased during hot weather or during excessive exercise when sweating increases—to prevent salt depletion and heat prostration.
   5. Use patience when feeding child.
      a. Child may be irritable and fussy.
      b. Breathing may be difficult, coughing and vomiting may be common.

B. *To assist in preventing or treating lung infection and supporting respirations by thinning secretions and clearing them from the respiratory tract.*
   1. Intermittent aerosol therapy.
      a. Usually done prior to postural drainage. (May also be done following drainage.)
      b. Provides small amount of medication in droplet form to penetrate respiratory tract.
      c. Treatment 3–4 times daily.
   2. Mist tent
      a. High humidity loosens secretions.
      b. Used primarily at night or nap time.
   3. Postural drainage
      a. Usually follows aerosol therapy 3–4 times per day.
      b. Treatment ideally done 1 hour after eating to prevent vomiting or discomfort.
      c. Place child in position that gives greatest access to affected lobes of lung and facilitates gravity drainage of mucus from specific lung area.
         (1) Leaning over side of bed.
         (2) Infant may be held in lap.
      d. Clapping with cupped hands and vibrations of 1–2 minutes in each area loosens mucous plugs.
      c. A relaxed patient will cough easier; coughing should be encouraged after postural drainage.
         Suctioning of an infant or young child may be necessary when they will not cough.
   4. Breathing exercises
      Exhaling slowly to increase the duration of exhalation

C. *To understand what medications are given in treatment and why.*
1. Antibiotics
   a. Broad-spectrum for prophylaxis
   b. Specific antibiotics to treat specific organism causing infection
2. Expectorants—to thin bronchial mucous secretions
3. Bronchodilators—to increase width of bronchial tubes allowing free passage of air into lungs

D. *To give meticulous attention and hygiene to the patient.*
1. Provide good skin care and position changes to prevent skin breakdown of malnourished child.
2. See that diaper area is clean to reduce offensive odor from stool and prevent diaper rash.
3. Because child may perspire freely, change clothing as necessary to keep him dry.
4. Mouth care is important since mucus is so frequently present.
5. Shampoo and bathing will provide comfort by removing sticky residue from mist and aerosol therapy.

E. *To aim at supporting the child's emotional, psychological and intellectual needs and development.*
1. Explain each procedure (new or routine), medications, etc. to child in a manner that is appropriate for his age.
2. Allow child to show his frustrations, fears and feelings by talking, complaining or crying.
   a. Support him during these times.
   b. Comfort him by talking to him, holding him.
3. Provide diversional activities appropriate for age, during or in between treatments.
4. Older child may begin to take responsibility for treatments with minimal supervision.

F. *To make and record observations of the child and his condition and behavior which will give information concerning the child's condition.*
1. Characteristics of stools: color, size, consistency, frequency
2. Eating habits
   a. Foods taken or refused
   b. Appetite—good or poor
3. Coughing and description of secretions produced
4. Daily weight to determine weight gain or loss
5. General behavior
   a. Irritable
   b. Cooperative

G. *To encourage parental participation in learning to care for and handle the child and to foster acceptance of the child and his illness by his parents and family.*
1. Provide opportunities for the parents to learn all aspects of care of their child.
2. All the support and help given the parents during hospitalization will make home care easier.

3. Initiate community nurse referral.
   a. Facilitates preparing the home for child's entry, both emotionally and physically.
   b. Can assist family in properly carrying out treatments.
4. Initiate social work referral. The social worker can help parents to better understand their family situation and their feelings about their child and cystic fibrosis.
5. Assist with interpretation of the disease to family and patient. Help them to talk about their feelings and fears.
6. Initiate a teaching program for the child and his family early. Offer them available literature and help them to become familiar with the National Cystic Fibrosis Research Foundation and the nearest chapter.*

Parental Teaching

Education of the parents is important in order that the child's care be continued at home.

1. Parents must have a thorough understanding of the dietary regimen. Help them to know what types of foods the child is allowed to have and those restricted. Talk about ways to make each meal or certain foods attractive.
2. Help parents become thoroughly familiar with the pulmonary therapy regimen.
   Do not rush your explanation; take time to demonstrate and explain procedures. Then allow parents to demonstrate all the treatments to be done at home.
3. Help the family to plan the most normal family pattern of living in relation to treatment of their child.
   Consider the marriage needs of the parents and the needs of other members of the family.
4. Help parents to understand and provide emotional support of their child. Explain that he will experience the usual problems of growing up in conjunction with the problems of cystic fibrosis and hospitalizations.
5. Impress upon the parents the importance of regular medical follow-up care.
   a. Routine immunizations—measles vaccine and influenza given early in infancy.
   b. Continual evaluation and supervision in home management.
   c. New developments through research that may change therapy.
   d. Detection of or prevention of complications.
6. Future in society.
   a. With the medical advancements that have occurred, there is every reason to believe that the child with cystic fibrosis may grow to adulthood, depending upon pulmonary involvement and complications.
   b. Play and school participation depends upon severity of illness.
   c. Have parents discuss the child's problem with the school nurse, teacher, and other responsible adults who have close contact with the child.
   d. Encourage parents to allow the child to participate as well as take additional responsibility in his care and treatments as he gets older.

* National Cystic Fibrosis Research Foundation. 202 E. 44th Street, New York, New York 10017.
  Publications of the National Cystic Fibrosis Research Foundation:
  Your Child and Cystic Fibrosis
  Living with Cystic Fibrosis—a Guide for the Young Adult
  A C/F Child is in Your Class
  Cystic Fibrosis—Most Serious Lung Problem of Children

CELIAC DISEASE

Celiac disease, also called gluten-induced enteropathy, is an inborn error of metabolism characterized by chronic intestinal malabsorption resulting in malnutrition and deficiency symptoms.

Etiology

1. Inborn error of metabolism
2. Trigger mechanisms
   a. Ingestion of wheat or rye glutins
   b. Dietary deficiencies
   c. Chronic infection
   d. Psychologic trauma
3. An allergic reaction

Altered Physiology

1. No specific pathological changes
2. Atrophy of intestinal mucosa
3. Complications of malnutrition
   a. Anemia
   b. Hypoalbuminemia
   c. Osteoporosis
   d. Hypothrombinemia and bleeding
4. Malabsorption—sugar
5. Complications of vitamin or mineral deficiencies

Clinical Manifestations

1. Most common age of diagnosis is 6 months (diagnosis possible up to 6 years)
2. Progressive malnutrition
   a. Flattened buttocks with hanging skin folds
   b. Abdominal distention
   c. Retarded growth and development
   d. Face—round cheeks and plump
3. Stools
   a. Foul odor
   b. Bulky
   c. Greasy
4. Anorexia
5. Chronic or recurrent diarrhea
6. Mood changes—ill humor, irritable, temper, shy

Diagnostic Evaluation

1. Stool examinations
   a. Increase of soaps and fatty acids in stools
   b. % of ingested fat in stool is 75–85%
2. Glucose tolerance test
   a. Oral shows low curve
   b. Intravenous shows normal curve

3. Blood values
   a. Total serum protein is indicative of severity of disease—greater than 5 mg./100 ml. of blood means trouble
   b. Plasma levels of vitamin A after oral ingestion
   c. Hypothrombinemia
4. X-ray examination—osteoporosis is evident
5. Microscopic examination of small intestinal mucosa—atrophy

Complication

Celiac Crisis
1. Constitutes acute medical emergency and a threat to life
2. Results in severe dehydration and acidosis
3. Possible causes
   a. Upper respiratory infection
   b. Vomiting
   c. Large watery stools
4. Signs and symptoms
   a. Drowsiness
   b. Restless sleep
   c. Increased sweating
   d. Extreme cold

Nursing Objectives

A. *To follow explicitly the dietary regimen which has been accurately calculated by the physician to include enough calories for weight gain yet exclude wheat and rye glutins that produce enteropathy.*
   1. Initial diet is high in protein, relatively low in fat and is starch-free.
      a. Milk protein or skim milk is sweetened with sucrose or banana powder.
      b. Infants and young children have a special problem presented by intestinal fat absorption; therefore fat intake is reduced.
   2. Proteins and sugars are added gradually.
      a. Individual foods are added one at a time at several day intervals. Foods included and added are lean meat, cottage cheese, egg white, raw ground apple.
      b. Starchy foods are added to diet last. They include potatoes and bread.
      c. Wheat and rye may not be added to diet for several years.
   3. The child is given nothing by mouth during the initial treatment of celiac crisis or during diagnostic testing.
   4. If the child is ambulatory, take special precautions to ensure that he does not eat restricted foods.
   5. Child may have anorexia—feeding him can be difficult.
      a. Make mealtime pleasant.
      b. Serve small, attractive portions.
      c. Do not force him to eat.
   6. Note carefully child's reaction to food and record the following:
      a. Intake, foods refused.
      b. Appetite.
      c. Change in behavior after eating.

      d. Characteristics of stools

      e. General disposition

  7. New foods may be temporarily eliminated if symptoms increase.

B. *To prevent infection in this child who is malnourished, anemic and very susceptible to respiratory infection, which in turn will increase indigestion.*

  1. Avoid exposing the child to anyone with an infection of any kind.

  2. Child usually perspires freely and has subnormal temperature with cold extremities.

      a. Keep him dry.

      b. Cover lightly when room is cool.

  3. If child remains quiet in bed, change his position frequently.

  4. Promote good hygiene.

C. *To be aware of child's behavior or change in behavior and care for him accordingly.*

  1. Diet and eating have a direct effect on behavior. A hungry child may be irritable.

  2. Behavior is indicative of how the child is feeling.

  3. The child is prone to mood swings from having temper tantrums to being very timid, nervous or unstable.

      a. Allow child to express his feelings freely.

        (1) Older child talks or complains.

        (2) Baby cries and whines.

      b. The nurse must exhibit patience.

      c. Socialize routine procedures.

  4. Chart changes in behavior, especially in relation to eating and diet.

  5. Avoid conflicts or emotionally upsetting situations—may precipitate diarrhea, vomiting and celiac crisis.

D. *To meet the child's emotional and psychological needs and provide diversional activities appropriate for age and severity of disease.*

  1. This child may be withdrawn and indulge in self-play.
     Provide opportunity for play with other children, especially when child begins to feel better.

  2. Frequently, play is more passive than active.
     Activity may be very exhausting.

  3. The toddler may cling to infantile habits for security.
     Allow this behavior; it may disappear as his physical condition improves and he feels better.

  4. The nurse must show the child she understands his mood swings and irritability by being patient with him. He needs a great deal of emotional satisfaction and support.

E. *To support the parents and foster continued parental acceptance of the child, his disease and behavior. Help parents maintain a healthy relationship with their child.*

  1. Encourage parents to visit and care for the child as much as possible. Comforting and holding the child can be very helpful.

  2. Start teaching parents early about the disease and how they should care for the child at home.

      a. Acquaint them with available literature, parent groups and community resources.

      b. Initiate community nurse referral to provide for continued support and teaching at home.

      c. Suggest genetic counseling that may be helpful to parents.

3. Listen to parental concerns and questions.
    a. Give simple, honest answers.
    b. Reinforce what the physician has told them.
4. Allow parents to continue to maintain what other responsibilities they may have outside the hospital. Do not insist they stay at the hospital and attend only to this child.
5. Help parents to understand that after initial rapid weight gain further improvement may be slow.

F. *To be aware of the signs and symptoms of celiac crisis and attend to the child's care according to medical plans.*

Initial treatment.
    a. Replace fluids and electrolytes by parenteral therapy.
    b. Give nothing by mouth, especially if child is vomiting.
    c. Observe the child carefully.

G. *To be familiar with the medications used in treatment of celiac disease and their implications.*

1. Vitamins A and D—not absorbed well
2. Vitamin B complex and vitamin C—if child is receiving antibiotics
3. Iron—if child is anemic
4. Vitamin K—for hypothrombinemia and bleeding
5. Calcium lactate—if milk is not in diet

Parental Teaching

1. Help parents to understand what celiac disease is and how it is controlled by diet.
    a. Provide a specific list of restricted foods as well as foods the child is allowed to eat.
    b. Be certain parents understand the importance of the vitamin regimen.
    c. Help parents understand the importance of continued adherence to diet, even though the child is feeling well, eating well and has normal stools. Advancing diet too rapidly may result in a set-back.
2. Impress upon parents the importance of regular medical follow-up.
    Encourage the parents to seek prompt medical attention should the child have an upper respiratory infection.
3. Encourage parents to practice good hygiene to prevent infection.
    This child is especially prone to infection because of malnutrition and anemia.
4. Help parents to understand that the emotional climate in the home and around the child is vitally important in maintaining the child's medical and physical stability.
    a. Parents must exhibit patience with the child.
    b. Set defined limits of behavior for the child; everyone in the family should know what they are.
    c. Avoid conflicts or any emotional upsets in front of the child.
    d. Social worker may need to become involved if there is domestic disharmony.
    e. Other children and their needs must also be considered in the total family picture.
5. Help parents to understand that the child's physical condition and behavior problems are related to the disease.
    a. Parents may feel guilty or ambivalent toward the child.
    b. Show them how they may avoid becoming overprotective of the child.

DIARRHEA

Diarrhea is an excessive loss of water and electrolytes in repeated passage of unformed stools. It is a symptom of many conditions and may be caused by many diseases.

Etiology
1. Often the cause is difficult to determine.
2. Infectious (intestinal pathogens)
   a. Normal intestinal tract inhabitants act as pathogens in certain circumstances
      (1) Proteus, pseudomonas, streptococcal and staphylococcal groups
      (2) Antibiotic induced
   b. Bacterial infections—*Escherichia coli*
   c. Viral
      (1) From within gastrointestinal tract (gastroenteritis)
      (2) From without the gastrointestinal tract (respiratory)
   d. Fungal
3. Noninfectious factors
   a. Allergy to certain foods
   b. Metabolic disorders
      (1) Celiac disease
      (2) Uremia
      (3) Acidosis
      (4) Secondary to primary cause of diarrhea—disaccharide intolerance
   c. Combination of over-feeding, emotional excitement and fatigue—causes imbalanced proportion of sugar, fat and proteins
   d. Direct irritation of gastrointestinal tract by foods
   e. Inappropriate use of laxatives and purgatives
4. Mechanical disorders
   a. Intussusception
   b. Incomplete small bowel obstruction
5. Congenital anomalies
   Hirschsprung's disease

Altered Physiology
1. The particular etiology of diarrhea does not influence the potentially dangerous cycle of events as much as the severity and duration of diarrhea and the general condition of the child.
2. The effects of diarrhea present more of a threat to infants and young children than to the older child and adult.
   a. Extracellular fluid volume is proportionately larger in infant and young child.
   b. Nutritional reserves are relatively smaller in the young child.
3. Major alterations in physiology
   a. Dehydration—extracellular fluid loss
   b. Electrolyte imbalance
      Potassium—varies
      Chloride—decreases
      Sodium—increases
   c. Acid-base imbalance
      Acidosis
         Serum CO_2 (10 or $>$10mEq./liter)
         Serum pH 7

Clinical Manifestations

A. *Classification of Diarrhea*
  1. Mild diarrhea—hospitalization may not be indicated
  2. Severe diarrhea with gradual onset
  3. Severe diarrhea with sudden onset—incidence of death is high

B. *Symptoms*
  All classifications have similar symptoms, the severity of which is dependent upon severity of diarrhea and time of onset.
  1. Fever—low grade to 41.1°C. (106°F.)
  2. Anorexia
  3. Mild and intermittent to severe vomiting
  4. Stools
     a. Appearance of diarrhea varies from a few hours to 3 days
     b. Loose and fluid in consistency
     c. Color—greenish or yellow-green
     d. May contain mucus, pus or blood
     e. Frequency varies from 2–20 times per day
     f. Expelled with force; may be preceded by pain
  5. Behavior change
     a. Irritable and restless
     b. Weak
     c. Extreme prostration
     d. Stupor and convulsions
     e. Flaccid and pallor
  6. Respirations
     a. Rapid
     b. Hyperneic
  7. Dehydration
     a. Little to extreme loss of subcutaneous fat
     b. Above or below 25% total body weight loss
     c. Urinary output decreases
     d. Poor skin turgor and dry skin
     e. Fontanelles and eyes sunken
     f. Collapse imminent

Diagnostic Evaluation

A. *Studies to establish nature of patient's condition*
  1. Electrolyte status and kidney function
     a. Serum sodium
     b. Serum chloride
     c. Serum potassium
     d. B.U.N.
  2. Acid-base imbalance
     a. Serum pH (acidosis)
     b. Serum CO_2 content or combining power
  3. Plasma volume by hematocrit and hemoglobin
  4. Urinalysis
  5. Stool pH

B. *Studies to determine cause of diarrhea*
1. Bacteriologic cultures of stool
2. Bacteriologic cultures of rectal swab
3. Agglutination studies for pathologic *E. coli*
4. Serological studies for viral pathogens

Nursing Objectives

A. *To monitor intravenous fluid therapy, both amount and rate, which has been appropriately calculated by the physician.*
1. Fluid ordered as maintenance or replacement depending upon degree of patient's dehydration.
2. Fluid is calculated carefully so as not to overload circulatory system.
    a. Check flow rate and amount absorbed hourly and totally.
    b. Check I.V. site for infiltration or improper flow so site can be changed as necessary.
3. Use appropriate protective devices to prevent patient from moving and injuring himself or causing I.V. to malfunction.
4. When preparing solution for therapy, use sterile solution and equipment.
5. Weigh daily to serve as a guide for specific fluid needs and current patient status.

B. *To provide physical comfort for the patient.*
1. If protective devices are used, passive range of motion may help to keep joints from stiffening.
2. While the patient is given nothing by mouth, special mouth care should be administered.
    An infant may find comfort in sucking a pacifier.
    Bubble him frequently to help expel air he has swallowed during sucking.
3. Change position and give good skin care to prevent lesions which may occur due to dehydration.
    Change soiled diapers—acid from stool will cause excoriation.

C. *To make frequent observations and be constantly alert to the patient's condition. Record and report immediately any changes. Careful observations can give clues to improvement or deterioration in the patient's condition and serve as a guide to medical care.*
1. Note and changes in vital signs.
2. Note stool characteristics and number.
    a. Abnormal constituents
    b. Foul odor
3. Activity and level of consciousness are important.
4. Note vomiting—frequency and characteristics.
5. Record urinary output—amount, frequency and characteristics.
6. Use child's behavior to determine how he feels.
    a. Eating and restful sleep indicates he feels fairly good.
    b. Crying or legs drawn up to abdomen usually indicates pain.

D. *To prevent spread of infection by using good handwashing and gown techniques as indicated by hospital policy.*
1. Many hospitals use isolation technique for children admitted with diarrhea until cause is determined. (Infectious pathogens can spread rapidly and easily among infants and young children.)
2. Follow hospital policy as to care of diapers.

E. *To meet the emotional and psychological needs of the patient.*
   1. Hospitalization is frightening, especially when it is sudden as with diarrhea.
   2. Many treatments and procedures are painful—give reassurance to the child during and after them.
      a. Talk to the child.
      b. Hold him and comfort him after the procedure.
      c. Explain to him in language appropriate for his age what is to be done.
   3. Provide some means of pleasant stimulation, entertainment or diversion, especially while he must remain in bed.
      a. Infant—mobile, musical toy
      b. Young child—read to him, something appropriate for age
   4. Comfort him by being physically near.
      a. Petting, stroking
      b. Holding and rocking

F. *To provide and assist in resuming adequate caloric and volume oral intake.*
   1. If diarrhea is mild, oral electrolyte solution may be given.
   2. Fluid is usually advanced slowly from clear liquids, such as gelatin-flavored water, to half-strength formula or skim milk, to regular diet.
   3. As diet is advanced, note any vomiting or increase in stools and report it immediately.

G. *To provide support for the family, especially the mother.*
   1. Reassure the mother that she indeed is not the cause of her child's illness.
   2. Explain procedures and need for treatment in easy to understand language.
      a. Why infant's hair was shaved off his head for an I.V.
      b. Reason for not giving the child anything to eat or drink.
      c. Need for protective devices.
   3. Allow her (parents) to care for and comfort the child as much as possible.
   4. Allow her to leave the hospital and attend to other family members and matters.
        Invite parents to call the hospital when they cannot be there.
   5. Initiate a community nurse referral, especially if other children at home are ill or if home conditions have precipitated the diarrhea.

Parental Teaching

   1. After determining the cause of the diarrhea, it may be necessary to teach proper formula or food preparation, handling and storage.
        It is especially important to be certain that mother knows proper formula and bottle sterilization procedures.
   2. Parents may need help in understanding the symptoms of a sick child.
   3. Help parents understand importance of medical care and general good hygiene.

HIRSCHSPRUNG'S DISEASE

Hirschsprung's disease (congenital aganglionic megacolon) is a congenital absence of the parasympathetic ganglion nerve cells from within the muscle wall of the intestinal tract, usually at the distal end of the colon.

Etiology

   1. Congenital—may show familial pattern
   2. More common in males

Altered Physiology

1. Absence of or reduced number of ganglion cells in the intestinal tract muscle wall, usually the distal end of the colon.
2. No peristalsis occurs in the affected portion of intestine.
   a. This section is usually narrow; therefore no fecal material passes through it.
   b. The intestine above the affected section has an accumulation of fecal material.
3. Proximal to the narrow affected section, the colon is dilated.
   a. Filled with fecal material and gas.
   b. Hypertrophy of muscular coating.
   c. In newborn may see ulceration of mucosa.
4. Abdominal distention and constipation results.

Clinical Manifestations

1. Appearing at birth or within first weeks of life.
   a. No meconium passed
   b. Vomiting—bile-stained or fecal
   c. Abdominal distention
   d. Constipation
   e. Overflow-type diarrhea
   f. Anorexia
   g. Temporary relief of symptoms with enema
2. Older child—symptoms not prominent at birth
   a. History may reveal obstipation at birth
   b. Distention of abdomen—progressive enlarging
   c. Thin abdominal wall—superficial veins are visible
   d. Peristaltic activity observable
   e. Constipation
      (1) Never has fecal soiling
      (2) Relieved temporarily with enema
   f. Stool appears ribbon-like, fluid-like or in pellet–form
   g. Failure to grow
      (1) Loss of subcutaneous fat
      (2) Appears malnourished; perhaps has stunted growth

Diagnostic Evaluation

1. Rectal examination—exhibits absence of fecal material
2. Roentgen examination with barium enema
   a. Narrow segment of intestine proximal to anus
   b. Dilated intestine proximal to narrow segment
3. Rectal biopsy—absence or reduced number of ganglion nerve cells

Nursing Objectives

PREOPERATIVE CARE

A. *To assist in emptying the bowel and preparing it for surgery.*
   1. Give repeated enemas and colonic irrigations.
      a. Procedure for enema in infant is similar to adult, except that less fluid and pressure are used.

b. Chemotherapy agents used to reduce the bacteria flora.
c. Physiologic saline solution should be used for irrigations.
    Tap water may result in large quantities of water being absorbed and in water intoxication.
d. Carefully note return from irrigation and degree of abdominal distention.
e. A continuous rectal tube may be ordered; ensure that it is properly located and remains in place.
f. If enema is not expelled, siphoning may be indicated.
2. Note and record frequency and characteristics of stools. (Obstipation is likely to occur.)
3. Prevent injury to mucosa by taking axillary temperature.

B. *To observe for abdominal distention and its effect on patient's condition.*
1. Note any change in degree of distention before and after irrigation. Chart if location of distention changes, i.e., upper or lower abdomen.
2. Respiratory embarrassment may result from abdominal distention.
    Elevate head and chest of infant by tilting mattress.
3. Note degree of abdominal tenderness.
    a. Legs of infant drawn up
    b. Chest breathing
4. Note color of abdomen and presence of gastric waves.

C. *To establish and maintain adequate nutrition so that growth and weight gain may take place.*
1. Infant may be uncomfortable due to distention and nausea.
2. Offer small, frequent feedings. (Low residue diet will aid in keeping stools soft.)

D. *To properly care for patient when nasogastric tube is used to aid in decreasing abdominal distention.*
1. Note drainage from nasogastric tube and chart characteristics.
2. Check for patency.
    a. Saline irrigations may be ordered.
    b. Carefully record input and output.
    c. Note increasing distention.
3. Give adequate mouth care.
4. Alternate nares when changing nasogastric tube every 24 hours. (Use minimal amount of tape to prevent skin irritation.)

E. *To provide emotional and psychological support needed by the child.*
1. Encourage mother to visit, even for short periods.
2. Irritable child may be calmed with holding and rocking.
3. Provide suitable diversion appropriate for age.

POSTOPERATIVE CARE

One of 2 surgical procedures may be done in treatment of Hirschsprung's disease: (1) primary resection of aganglionic segment or (2) temporary colostomy above the narrowed section; when condition of child is stabilized or weight of 8.17–13.62 kg. (18–30 pounds) is obtained, resection is done and colostomy closed (most common).

A. *To give good postoperative care and to observe for possible postoperative complications (see p. 1093).*

B. *To prevent infection.*
   1. At the site of surgical wound.
      a. Dressing change, using sterile technique.
      b. Prevent contamination from diaper.
         (1) Apply diaper below dressing.
         (2) Change frequently.
      c. Use careful handwashing technique.
      d. Report any redness, swelling or drainage, evisceration or dehiscence immediately.
   2. Of the tracheobronchial tree and lungs.
      a. Frequently suction secretions.
      b. Encourage frequent coughing and deep breathing.
         Allow infant to cry for short periods.
      c. Change position frequently to increase circulation and allow for aeration of all lung areas.

C. *To properly care for colostomy and to understand its purpose.*
   1. Proper functioning of colostomy.
      a. Note drainage from colostomy—characteristics, frequency, fecal material or liquid drainage.
      b. Note abdominal distention.
      c. Measure fluid loss from colostomy as the amount will affect fluid replacement.
   2. Signs of obstruction from peritonitis, paralytic ileus, handling bowel, or swelling.
      a. No output from colostomy
      b. Increased tenderness
      c. Irritability
      d. Vomiting
      e. Increased temperature
   3. Good skin care to prevent breakdown around colostomy.
      a. Change soiled dressing or diaper frequently.
      b. Wash skin with clear water.
      c. Use karaya gum, aluminum paste, Maalox or other means to protect skin from contact with secretions.
      d. Keep area open to air occasionally.

D. *To prevent abdominal distention.*
   1. Nasogastric tube may be used immediately postoperatively.
      a. Check patency (see above).
      b. Watch for increasing abdominal distention.
      c. Measure fluid loss as amount will affect fluid replacement.
   2. Once oral feeding is begun, the nasogastric tube will be removed.
      a. Avoid overfeeding.
      b. Bubble frequently during feeding.
      c. Proper positioning after feeding.

E. *To continue taking axillary temperatures.*
   1. Avoids injury.
   2. Allows for more accurate reading.

F. *To continue to provide emotional support to the patient.* (See p. 1220, diarrhea.)

G. *To help parents understand and accept the child and the disease, as well as all that has happened.*
   1. Even a temporary colostomy can be a difficult procedure to accept and learn to care for.
      a. Support parents when teaching them to care for the colostomy.
      b. Try to help them treat the baby or child as normally as possible.
   2. Encourage parents to talk about their fears and anxieties.
      Anticipating future surgery for resection may be comforting and frightening.
   3. Initiate community nurse referral to help parents care for child at home away from the comfortable situation of the hospital.

Parental Teaching
   1. Begin early to teach thoroughly and carefully what the colostomy is for, how it works, and how to care for it and the child.
      Emphasize the importance of treating the child as normally as possible to prevent behavior problems later.
   2. Encourage close medical follow-up and general good health hygiene.
      a. Nutrition
      b. General growth and development
      c. Immunizations

INTUSSUSCEPTION

Intussusception is the invagination or telescoping of a portion of the intestine into an adjacent, more distal section of the intestine.

Etiology
   1. Not usually known.
      May be due to increased mobility of intestine and hyperperistalsis present in young children.
   2. Possible contributing causes.
      a. Meckel's diverticulum
      b. Polyps, cysts in the bowel
      c. Malrotation of intestines
      d. Acute enteritis
      e. Abdominal injury

Altered Physiology
   1. Mesentery is pulled into intestine when invagination occurs.
   2. Progression to obstruction
      a. Intestine becomes curved, sausage-like—blood supply is cut off.
      b. Bowel begins to swell—hemorrhage may occur.
      c. Complete intestinal obstruction results—necrosis of involved segment.
   3. Classification of location.
      a. *Ileocecal* (most common)—ileum invaginates into ascending colon
      b. *Ileocolic*—ileum invaginates into colon
      c. *Colocolic*—colon invaginates into colon
      d. *Ileo-ileo*—small bowel invaginates into small bowel

Clinical Manifestations

1. Incidence is rare in first month of life.
   a. 4–10 months of age is most common age of onset (50–70%).
   b. 1–2 years of age—frequency of occurrence is high.
2. Onset is sudden.
   a. Paroxysmal abdominal pain
   b. Current jelly-like stools
      (1) Blood and mucus present in stool
      (2) One or more stools with this characteristic
      (3) Presence of bloody mucus on finger following rectal examination
   c. Vomiting
   d. Increasing absence of stools
   e. Increasing abdominal distention and tenderness
   f. Sausage-like mass palpable in abdomen
   g. Dehydration and fever
   h. Shock-like state
      (1) Rapid pulse
      (2) Pale skin
      (3) Marked sweating

Laboratory

X-ray examination
1. Flat plate of abdomen—reveals staircase pattern (invagination appears like stair steps on x-ray)
2. Barium enema—coil-like appearance of bowel

Nursing Principles

PREOPERATIVE CARE

A. *To assist in maintaining or restoring hydration and electrolyte imbalance.* Monitor parenteral fluids. (See p. 1087, I.V. Therapy.)

B. *To prevent vomiting and aspiration.*
   1. Stomach may be deflated by insertion of nasogastric tube.
   2. Maintain patency of nasogastric tube if one is inserted.
      a. Irrigate at frequent intervals.
      b. Note drainage and return from irrigation.
   3. Patient is likely to be N.P.O.
      a. Wet lips and give mouth care.
      b. Give infant pacifier to suck.

C. *To be aware of the patient's condition by frequent observations, thereby contributing to the total care of the patient.*
   1. Respirations are affected because of abdominal distention.
      a. Grunting
      b. Shallow and rapid if patient is in shock-like state
   2. Abdominal distention and unusual appearance of anus—intussuception may look like rectal prolapse.

NURSING ALERT: Take axillary temperatures to prevent injury.

3. Behavior
   a. Irritable—very sensitive to handling (Be gentle!)
   b. Lethargic or unresponsive
   c. Behavior indicative of presence or absence of pain

D. *To prepare the patient for surgery when he is shock-like or febrile.*
   1. Blood or plasma is given to restore circulating blood volume—observe for transfusion reactions.
   2. Observe pulse rate carefully—safe range is below 140/minute.
   3. Reduce temperature—fever increases metabolism and makes oxygenation during anesthesia more complicated.

E. *To offer support to parents during this time of crisis and fear.*
   1. Encourage parents to verbalize their concerns.
   2. Reinforce what the physician has told them.
   3. Encourage them to be with child whenever possible.

POSTOPERATIVE CARE

A. *To give good postoperative care and to observe for possible postoperative complications.* (See p. 1093.)

B. *To be constantly alert for complications arising from surgery for intussusception.*
   1. Fever is usually present.
      a. As a result of absorption of foreign protein
      b. Absorption of bacteria through the damaged intestinal wall
   2. Diarrhea—from exposure to others infected
   3. Shock
   4. Dehydration
   5. Toxicity
   6. Peritonitis

C. *To assist in maintaining stomach decompression until first stool is passed.*
   1. See that indwelling nasogastric tube is functioning properly.
      a. Usually connected to constant intermittent suction.
      b. Note drainage and irrigation returns.
   2. Patient is usually given nothing by mouth.
      Give mouth care.
   3. Note passing of flatus or stool and report—indicates peristalsis has returned to normal activity.
      Oral feedings may start.

D. *To resume gradually full caloric and volume oral intake appropriate for age and weight.*
   1. Oral fluid is usually begun after the first stool, about 4–5 days after surgery.
   2. Feed small amounts frequently.
      a. Start with glucose water or water.
      b. Note and report any abdominal distention or vomiting.

E. *To provide emotional support and meet the psychological needs of the child.* (See p. 1220, Diarrhea.)

F. *To support parents and help them to maintain a good relationship with their child.*
   1. Encourage them to visit and call. Allow parents to become involved in caring for their child.

2. Help parents to understand that recurrence is rare but certain short-term limits must be placed on the child's activity after discharge.

IMPERFORATE ANUS

Imperforate anus is the congenital presence of an intact anal membrane or internal blind pouch of the lower bowel.

Etiology

1. An arrest in embryologic development of the anus, lower rectum and urogenital tract at the 8th week of embryonic life.
2. Cause unknown.

Altered Physiology

1. Lack of normal opening to exterior from lower gastrointestinal tract.
2. Fistula is likely to be formed.
   a. Female—between rectum and vagina or perineum
   b. Male—between rectum and urinary tract, scrotum or perineum
3. Other anomalies likely, especially tracheo-esophageal atresia.

Clinical Manifestations

Usually discovered immediately after birth or within several hours.
1. No anal opening
2. Cannot insert thermometer or small finger into rectum
3. Absence of meconium stool
4. Green-tinged urine—if fistula is present
5. Progressive abdominal distention

Diagnostic Evaluation

X-ray examination
"Upside down" position of infant used to determine distance from rectum to anal dimple

Nursing Objectives

PREOPERATIVE CARE

A. *To assist in maintaining stability in patient's general condition prior to emergency surgery.*
   1. Feedings are usually withheld.
   2. Nasogastric tube may be passed to decompress the stomach.

B. *To observe carefully the infant for any other anomalies or changes in condition.*
   1. Use incubator for better observations.
   2. Observe for stool coming from a fistula.
   3. Note that urine will be green-tinged.
   4. Keep area clean.

POSTOPERATIVE CARE

Depending upon the degree of severity, 1 of 3 surgical procedures will be done: (1) anoplasty, (2) abdominal-perineal pull through, or (3) temporary colostomy with abdominal–perineal pull through at a later time when child is older and larger.

A. *To give good postoperative care and to observe for possible postoperative complications.* (See p. 1093.)

B. *To provide appropriate care for perineal anoplasty.*
    1. Expose perineum to air.
    2. Position baby for easy access to perineum for cleansing and minimal irritation to site.
       a. Place baby on abdomen.
       b. Place baby supine with legs suspended straight up at 90-degree angle to trunk.
    3. Keep perineum meticulously clean to prevent infection and skin irritation.

C. *To provide appropriate care for abdominal–perineal pull through.*
    1. Carry out perineal care as stated above.
    2. Provide proper care of gastrostomy or nasogastric tube used to decompress the gastrointestinal tract until peristalsis returns.
    3. Provide proper care of bladder catheter, if used, and measure accurately urinary output.
    4. Observe carefully for abdominal distention, bleeding from perineum, and respiratory embarrassment.

D. *To provide good colostomy care and prevent skin breakdown.* (See p. 1223, Hirschsprung's disease.)

E. *To maintain adequate nutrition, caloric and fluid intake to prevent dehydration and electrolyte imbalance.*
    1. Oral feeding usually started within hours after an anoplasty.
    2. Oral feedings are usually withheld until peristalsis returns.
    3. Monitor parenteral fluids. (See p. 1087.)

F. *To foster acceptance of the child and his diagnosis by his parents.*
    1. Assure parents that colostomy is temporary.
    2. Encourage parents to become involved in care of the child and to give him the emotional security he needs.
    3. Begin a teaching program early for special care needed at home.
       a. Colostomy care.
       b. Anal dilatation to prevent a stricture at site of anastomosis from scar tissue.
    4. Initiate referral to community nurse, especially if parents are particularly anxious about caring for the child at home.
    5. Encourage parents to talk about their concerns.

Parental Teaching
    1. Careful thorough teaching of special care and procedures to be continued at home—colostomy care, anal dilatation.
    2. Help parents to understand potential problems that may be encountered as a result of imperforate anus as the baby gets older.
       a. Fecal impaction due to lack of sensation to defecate
       b. Future surgery—if primary repair was not done
       c. Toilet training
       d. Inability to control fecal seepage from rectum

BIBLIOGRAPHY

Books

Blake, F. G., et al.: Nursing Care of Children. Philadelphia, J. B. Lippincott, 1970.
Gellis, S. S., and Kagan, B. M.: Current Pediatric Therapy. Philadelphia, W. B. Saunders, 1970.
Latham, H. C., and Heckel, R. V.: Pediatric Nursing. St. Louis, C. V. Mosby, 1972.
Marlow, D.: Textbook of Pediatric Nursing. Philadelphia, W. B. Saunders, 1973.
Nelson, W. E., et al.: Textbook of Pediatrics. Philadelphia, W. B. Saunders, 1969.
Raffensperger, J. G., and Primrose, R. B.: Pediatric Surgery for Nurses. Boston, Little, Brown and Company, 1968.
Your Child and Cystic Fibrosis. New York, National Cystic Fibrosis Research Foundation.
Young, D. G., and Weller, B. F.: Baby Surgery: Nursing Management and Care. Baltimore, University Park Press, 1971.
Shirley, H. C. (ed.): Pediatric Therapy. St. Louis, C. V. Mosby, 1972.

Articles

Cohen, S. J.: Unusual types of espohageal atresia and tracheo-espohageal fistulae. Clin. Ped., 4:271–275, May 1965.
Davis, A. R.: Billy had a tracheo-esophageal fistula. Amer. J. Nurs., 70:326–329, Feb. 1970.
DiSant'Agnese, P. A.: Cystic fibrosis (mucoviscidosis). Amer. Fam. Phys., 7:102–111, March 1973.
Hamilton, J. R.: Diarrhea in infants. Mod. Med., 38:131–139, Sept. 21, 1970.
Johnson, M. E., and Fassett, B. A.: Bronchopulmonary hygiene in cystic fibrosis. Amer. J. Nurs., 69:320–324, Feb. 1969.
Koop, C. E.: The seriously ill or dying child: supporting the patient and the family. Ped. Clin. N. Amer., 16:555–564, August 1969.
Pickett, L. K.: The hospital environment for the pediatric surgical patient. Ped. Clin. N. Amer., 16:531–542, August 1969.

Children with Conditions of the Kidneys, Urinary Tract and Reproductive System

ACUTE GLOMERULONEPHRITIS

Glomerulonephritis is a disorder resulting from an antigen-antibody reaction following an infection in some part of the body. Acute glomerulonephritis is the most common type of nephritis in children.

Etiology

1. Presumed cause
   Antigen-antibody reaction secondary to an infection elsewhere in the body
2. Initial infection
   a. Usually either an upper respiratory or skin infection
   b. Most frequent causative agent
      Group A beta hemolytic streptococcus
   c. Infrequent causative agents
      (1) Pneumococcus
      (2) Staphylococcus
      (3) Streptococcus viridans

Altered Physiology

1. The organisms responsible for nephritis contain antigens similar to those of the basement membrane of the renal glomeruli.
2. Antibodies produced to fight the invading organism also react against the glomerular tissue.
3. The antigen-antibody combination results in an inflammatory reaction in the kidney.
   a. There is proliferation and swelling of the endothelial cells of the glomerular capillary wall.
   b. All of the glomeruli are involved, but the intensity of proliferation varies among them.
4. Changes in the glomerular capillaries allow the passage of blood cells and protein into the glomerular filtrate.
5. General vascular disturbances, including loss of capillary integrity and spasm of arterioles, are secondary to kidney changes and are responsible for much of the symptomatology of the disease.

Incidence

1. Unknown—milder cases are not recognized.
2. More common in males than females.
3. Most common in pre-school and early school age groups.
4. Rare in children under 3 years of age.

Clinical Manifestations

A. *Onset*
   1. Usually 1–3 weeks after the onset of the initiating infection.
   2. May be abrupt and severe or mild and detected only by laboratory measures.

B. *Signs and Symptoms*
   1. Hematuria—usually the first symptom
   2. Malaise
   3. Mild headache
   4. Variable fever
      a. May be high initially
      b. Usually fluctuates at about 37.8°C. (100°F.) for several days
   5. Decreased urine output
   6. Edema
      a. Present in most patients
      b. May appear only as rapid weight gain
      c. May be generalized and influenced by posture
      d. Usually not severe
   7. Hypertension
      a. Present in over 50% of the patients
      b. Rise in blood pressure may be sudden
      c. Usually appears during the first 4–5 days of the illness
   8. Gastrointestinal disturbances, especially anorexia and vomiting
   9. Slight cardiac enlargement

Diagnostic Evaluation

1. Serum complement level—usually reduced
2. Urinalysis
   a. Decreased output—may approach anuria
   b. Microscopic or gross hematuria—urine may have a smoky brown appearance.
   c. High specific gravity
   d. Protein
      (1) Variable
      (2) Usually below 3 gm. per day
   e. White cells—moderate
   f. Granular and cellular casts—especially red cell casts
3. N.P.N. and B.U.N.—usually increased
4. Sedimentation rate—elevated
5. Serum albumin—often slightly depressed
6. Renal function tests—normal in 50% of the patients
7. ASO or antistreptokinase titer—elevated

Prognosis

1. Prognosis is generally good, but variable and is not correlated with the severity of the disease.
2. Approximately 95% of affected children recover completely.
   a. Symptoms usually disappear in 2–3 weeks.
      (1) Blood pressure usually returns to normal by the end of the first week.
      (2) Blood chemistry is usually normal by the end of the second week.
      (3) Urine may remain abnormal for several weeks, especially protein and red cells.
   b. Sedimentation rate may remain elevated for several months:
      Sedimentation rate is a measure of disease progress as it remains elevated for several months in children who develop chronic nephritis.
   c. Exacerbations may occur with acute infections during the recovery phase but usually do not alter the outcome.
3. Approximately 2% of affected children die during the acute phase, usually of the effects of hypertensive encephalopathy or heart failure.
4. Approximately 2% of affected children develop chronic nephritis.

Complications

A. *Hypertensive Encephalopathy*
   1. Manifestations
      a. Restlessness   d. Vomiting
      b. Stupor   e. Severe headache
      c. Convulsions   f. Visual disturbances
   2. Cause—probably ischemia secondary to vasospasm.
   3. No correlation with the degree of renal impairment or fluid retention.
   4. Duration
      a. Usually 1–2 days
      b. Ends spontaneously with decreased blood pressure.

B. *Cardiac Involvement*
   1. Death from acute nephritis is frequently secondary to cardiac failure due to persistent hypertension, hypervolemia and peripheral venoconstriction.

2. Manifestations
   a. Cardiac enlargement
   b. Hypervolemia
   c. Pulmonary edema
   d. Changes in the electrocardiogram
   e. Increased venous pressure
   f. Tachycardia
   g. Gallop rhythm
   h. Dyspnea
3. Duration
   a. Variable
   b. Usually subsides rapidly with the onset of diuresis and the fall in blood pressure.

C. *Uremia*

Manifestations
   a. Evidence of acidosis
   b. Drowsiness
   c. Coma
   d. Stupor
   e. Muscular twitching
   f. Convulsions

D. *Anemia*

Usually caused by hypervolemia rather than a loss of red blood cells in the urine.

Nursing Objectives

A. *To promote healing and prevent disease complications.*
   1. No specific measures have been demonstrated to modify the inflammatory process.
   2. General measures
      a. Maintain bedrest during the acute phase of the illness, at least until gross hematuria has disappeared.
         (1) Organize nursing activities to allow for periods of uninterrupted rest.
         (2) Explain to the child why it is necessary for him to stay in bed. (Bedrest is often interpreted by the child as punishment.)
         (3) Administer sedation if required to keep the child quiet and at rest.
         (4) Provide appropriate diversion for the child's age.
         (5) Place the child's bed in a position where he can watch the activities of the unit and other children.
         (6) Provide alternative means of rest for children who are too young to understand the necessity of remaining in bed. (Such children should be held in a chair.)
         (7) Observe the child closely for fatigue once ambulation is begun.
      b. Protect the child from infection.
         (1) Avoid placing the child in a room with patients who have fevers, upper respiratory infections or any other contagious disease.
         (2) Administer therapeutic doses of antibiotics as ordered by the physician to eradicate existing infection.
            (a) A 10-day course of intramuscular penicillin is often prescribed.
            (b) Points of emphasis.
                Inject the medication into a large muscle.
                Rotate the site of injection.
                Observe the child closely for adverse reactions such as skin rash, urticaria, serum sickness and anaphylaxis.
         (3) Protect the child from chilling or overheating.
         (4) Provide scrupulous daily hygiene, including mouth care. Keep the skin clean and dry.

    c. Provide a diet according to the child's age and the recommendation of his physician.

        (1) A regular diet without added salt is usually prescribed during the acute phase in noncomplicated cases.

        (2) A diet restricted in protein and potassium is necessary for children who demonstrate some degree of renal failure.

        (3) Fluids must be restricted in children with hypertension, edema, congestive failure or renal failure.

        (4) Explain all dietary restrictions to the child and his parents.

        (5) Obtain a careful history of dietary preferences and patterns so that the child's meals can be as acceptable as possible.

        (6) Place a sign indicating dietary restrictions on the child's bed so that anyone approaching him will be aware of his special needs.

        (7) If the child is to be given a restricted amount of fluids, offer small amounts of fluids spaced at regular intervals throughout the day and evening.

            Use a cup of appropriate size for the amount of fluid being offered.

B. *To observe and record disease progress.*

    1. Maintain a complete record of the child's intake and output.

      a. Measure fluids accurately in graduated containers. Do not estimate fluid intake or output.

      b. Place a sign on the child's bed to ensure that no urine is accidentally discarded or intake not recorded.

      c. Total the intake and output every 8 hours.

        (1) Notify the physician if output does not appear adequate.

        (2) In children who are not toilet trained, a fairly accurate record of intake and output can be obtained by weighing diapers before and after voiding.

      d. Record other means of fluid loss such as the number of stools per day, perspiration, etc.

    2. Weigh the child daily.

      a. An increase in weight indicates fluid retention.

      b. Weigh the child on the same scale and at the same time each day.

        (1) It is usually advantageous to weigh the child before breakfast.

        (2) The child should be weighed in a consistent manner with minimal clothing.

    3. Record the blood pressure at frequent intervals.

      a. Refer to the method for determining blood pressure, page 1068.

      b. A diastolic pressure of 100 mm.Hg is an indication of concern and should be reported to the physician immediately.

        Place the child in bed and observe him closely for cerebral changes.

    4. Observe for signs of complications.

      a. Increased blood pressure

      b. Fluid retention or edema

      c. Changes in vital signs, especially increased pulse or respirations

      d. Changes in activity status, especially lethargy, restlessness, stupor or coma

      e. Vomiting

      f. Visual disturbances

      g. Severe headache

      h. Convulsions

    5. Record appearance of each voiding.

      Note the persistence of hematuria or whether the urine appears to be clearing.

C. *To reduce hypertension.*
1. Limit the fluid intake according to the physician's recommendation.
2. Maintain bedrest.
3. Administer antihypertensive drugs as ordered by the physician.
   a. Reserpine is the drug most frequently employed.
      (1) Dosage
         (a) 0.01–0.04 mg./kg. up to 1.2 mg.
         (b) Divide dosage into 1–2 doses/24 hours.
      (2) Route of administration
         (a) Oral, intramuscular or intravenous
         (b) Initial control is usually achieved by intramuscular administration, and the child is later maintained with oral medication.
      (3) Side effects
         Nasal stuffiness, dryness of mouth, diarrhea
   b. Hydralazine (Apresoline) is often combined with reserpine in refractory cases.
      (1) Dosage:
         (a) 0.1 mg./kg. of Apresoline given simultaneously with a dose of reserpine up to 0.07 mg./kg.
         (b) Divide dose into 1–2 doses/24 hours.
      (2) Route of administration
         (a) Intramuscular
         (b) The 2 drugs may be administered together orally to prevent recurrence of hypertension once initial control is established.
      (3) Duration of action
         (a) Effective within ½ hour.
         (b) Effects persist for approximately 12 hours.
      (4) Side effects
         (a) Nausea, vomiting, diarrhea, anorexia
         (b) Headache
         (c) Tachycardia

D. *To provide appropriate nursing care to the child with disease complications.*
1. Encephalopathy
   Refer to the section on care of the child with seizures, page 1339.
2. Congestive heart failure
   Refer to the section on congenital heart disease and care of the child in congestive failure, page 1172.
3. Anemia
   Refer to the section on anemia, page 1159.
4. Renal failure
   a. Maintain strict record of intake and output.
   b. Weigh the child at frequent intervals.
      It may be necessary to weigh the child as often as every 8–12 hours.
   c. Perform all nursing activities as for the care of the child with uncomplicated glomerulonephritis.
   d. Administer fluids as ordered by the physician.
      (1) Fluid intake is usually restricted to equal urinary output plus insensible water loss, (usually between 300–400 ml. per square meter per day).
      (2) Fluid requirements must be recalculated frequently.

These vary with such factors as the child's activity, sweating, vomiting, body temperature, metabolic rate, etc.

(3) Some form of carbohydrate is usually ordered to prevent excessive breakdown of body proteins and to decrease the formation of ketones.

(a) Fluids, such as ginger ale or syrups, should be offered to the child who can tolerate oral fluids.

(b) Glucose solutions may be administered intravenously. (Refer to the procedure for the administration of intravenous fluids, p. 1088.)

e. Have appropriate electrolytes available for administration.

(1) Electrolytes are usually not added to the diet unless indicated by low serum levels or known loss.

Plasma concentrations of sodium, potassium, chloride, and bicarbonate and N.P.N. and B.U.N. must be monitored at frequent intervals.

(2) Replacement of electrolytes is rarely indicated during the oliguric phase.

(3) Potassium intoxication may occur and is usually counteracted by the administration of sodium bicarbonate or a cation exchange resin which exchanges sodium for potassium.

(4) Hypocalcemia requires the administration of calcium.

f. Assist with peritoneal dialysis if this is required. (See Guideline, p. 1237.)

E. *To provide emotional support to the child and his family during hospitalization.*

1. Explain all aspects of the diagnostic tests and treatment in terms that the family can understand.
2. Formulate a nursing care plan which facilitates a consistent approach to the child's care.
3. Allow the child to make some decisions and to participate in his care. He may decide when he wants his bath and should be allowed to make some dietary choices, etc.
4. Maintain discipline. Establish and enforce appropriate limits on the child's behavior.
5. Provide diversion appropriate for the child's age.

Plans should be made for the continued education of the school-aged child.

F. *To prepare the child and his parents for discharge.*

1. Encourage as much family participation as possible during the child's hospitalization.
2. Help the family plan for adaptation of the child's nursing care to the home environment.
   a. Review the medication schedule
   b. Suggest means of implementing sodium restricted diet.
      (1) Provide the family with a list of commercial foods and fluids which are normally high in sodium content.
      (2) Help the parents to plan sample menus.
      (3) Provide suggestions for low sodium cooking and baking.
3. Make certain that the family has an appointment for continued medical supervision.
4. Initiate appropriate referrals.
   a. Community health nurse
   b. Home teaching service

Patient or Parental Teaching

1. Medical explanation of the disease process should be reinforced.
   a. The need for medical evaluation and culture of all sore throats should be emphasized.
   b. The family should be made aware of signs and symptoms of disease recurrence.

2. Tonsillectomy or other oral surgery should not be done for several months after the acute phase of glomerulonephritis.

    If this type of surgery is necessary later, penicillin should be administered before and after the procedure to prevent bacterial spread.

GUIDELINES: *Assisting with Pediatric Peritoneal Dialysis*

Purpose

To correct acidosis, uremia, electrolyte disturbances and water imbalance in the oliguric phase of the illness.

Equipment

Dialysis set including peritoneal catheters and connecting sets
I.V. pole
Dialysis solution
Paracentesis tray

Antiseptic solution
Sterile gloves
Adhesive tape
Dialysis record form

Procedure

Nursing Action	Rationale/Amplification
Preparatory Phase	
1. Explain the procedure to the child and his parents. Emphasize to the parents that the procedure is efficient and well tolerated by children.	1. Helps allay fears.
2. Allow child to handle equipment similar to that which will be used during dialysis.	2. Encourage child to express his fears so you may correct any misconceptions he may have.
3. Have child empty bladder prior to procedure.	
4. Apply protective measures to limit motion.	4. To prevent contamination of sterile field or injury to child. (See p. 1073.)
Performance Phase	
1. Maintain child's position during insertion of needle.	1. To avoid injury.
2. Maintain aseptic technique throughout treatment.	2. To prevent spread of infection.
3. Check the tubing frequently for obstruction or kinks.	3. So that procedure will proceed efficiently.
4. Accurately record the dialysis flow.	
5. Observe the child frequently for: a. Changes in vital signs, including fevers b. Nausea or vomiting c. Difficult respirations d. Local discomforts	5. May indicate complications or untoward reactions to the dialysis.
6. Maintain child's comfort throughout treatment. a. Provide meticulous general hygiene. b. Keep the child clean and dry. c. Change his position at intervals.	
7. Allow parents to visit child during dialysis.	7. Provides a greater sense of security.

Follow-up Phase

1. Remove equipment and store it out of the child's sight.
2. Allow the child to rest.
3. Observe for signs of continued renal failure or peritoneal infection.

NEPHROSIS

Nephrosis refers to a symptom complex characterized by edema, marked proteinuria, hyper-cholesterolemia and hypoalbuminemia. Although there are many types of the disease, lipid nephrosis or so-called minimal disease is the most common in children.

Etiology

1. Unknown.
2. Recurrences and exacerbations are often associated with upper respiratory infections.
3. Possibly represents an auto-immune response to chemical substances or tissue antigens.

Altered Physiology

1. The kidneys appear large, edematous and pale.
2. The cortices are often thickened and the tubules dilated.
3. There is swelling of the foot processes of the epithelial cells lining the basement membrane of the glomeruli.
   a. The extent of swelling usually correlates with the amount of protein that the child is losing in his urine.
   b. Epithelial changes are reversible when the proteinuria disappears, and it is unknown whether they are primary or secondary to the proteinuria.
4. Plasma proteins decrease as proteinuria increases.
5. The colloidal osmotic pressure which holds water in the vascular compartments is reduced by the reduction of serum albumin. This allows flow of fluid from the capillaries into the extracellular space, producing edema.
6. Accumulation of fluid in the interstitial spaces and peritoneal cavity is also increased by an overproduction of aldosterone which causes retention of sodium.
7. There is increased susceptibility to infection because of decreased gamma globulin.
8. Generalized edema is responsible for most of the physical characteristics of the disease, including respiratory distress, gastrointestinal symptoms, umbilical and inguinal hernias, rectal prolapse, decreased ambulation, loss of body tissue, and malnutrition.

Incidence

1. Annually afflicts about 7 children per 100,000 under the age of 9 years.
2. More common in males than in females.
3. Average age at onset—approximately 2½ years.
4. A severe, sometimes familial form of the disease, which is refractory to treatment and fatal, rarely develops in infancy.

Clinical Manifestations

A. *Onset*
   1. Insidious
   2. Edema is often the presenting symptom.
      a. Initially, it is usually slight and inconstant.
      b. It is usually first apparent around the eyes.

B. *Signs and symptoms*
   1. Irritability and depression
   2. Gastrointestinal disturbances including vomiting and diarrhea

3. Anorexia—malnutrition may become severe.
4. Severe, recurrent infections
5. Marked, recurrent edema
   a. Ascites may be severe.
   b. Intense scrotal edema is common.
   c. Peripheral edema is dependent and shifts with the child's position.
   d. Striae may appear on the skin from overstretching.
6. Profound weight gain. The child may actually double his normal weight.
7. Decreased urine output during the edematous phase.
8. Minimal hematuria and hypertension may be present.
9. Pallor—caused by the stretching of skin over the subcutaneous fluid, usually not proportional to the amount of anemia.
10. Nephrotic crisis
    a. Abdominal pain
    b. Fever
    c. Erysipeloid skin eruption possible
    d. Symptoms subside within a few days
    e. Often followed by spontaneous diuresis

Diagnostic Evaluation

1. Urinalysis
   a. Proteinuria—marked
   b. Casts—numerous
   c. Hematuria—absent or transient
2. Renal function tests—variable, often normal
3. Blood
   a. Total serum protein—reduced
   b. Serum albumin—reduced
   c. Total serum globulin—normal or increased
      (1) Alpha and beta fractions—increased
      (2) Gamma fraction—reduced
   d. Amino acid level—decreased
   e. Anemia—absent or slight
   f. Sedimentation rate—elevated
   g. Cholesterol and lipoproteins—increased

Clinical Course and Prognosis

1. Edema becomes severe and generalized, lasting for several weeks to months.
2. Partial or complete remissions occur secondary to spontaneous or induced diuresis.
3. The course of the disease is variable and characterized by recurrent episodes of edema.
4. It is prolonged for varying lengths, usually for at least 18 months.
5. 75–80% of affected children eventually have a complete recovery.
6. Persistent hematuria may be suggestive of progressive glomerular damage, and such patients have the least favorable prognosis.
7. Death may occur from profound sepsis, progressive renal insufficiency or congestive heart failure.

Nursing Objectives

A. *To control progression of the renal lesion.*

Administer steroids as recommended by the physician.
   a. Prednisone is usually the drug of choice.
      (1) Initial dose is usually 30–80 mg./day (divided into 4 doses) depending on the age of the child.

(2) Intermittent steroid therapy is often begun following 4 weeks of continuous treatment.
   (a) The daily steroid dose is then given on the first 3 days of each week and none on the remaining 4.
   (b) The daily steroid dose may also be given on alternate days in a single dose.
(3) Diuresis and reduction of proteinuria are expected within 7–14 weeks.
(4) Intermittent therapy is usually continued for 2 months to a year. (The tendency to relapse is decreased with more prolonged therapy.)
(5) Therapy must be terminated gradually. (Abrupt withdrawal may cause severe rebound of the disease.)

B. *To be aware of the complications of therapy.*
1. Hirsutism
2. Cushinoid appearance of the face
  a. Have a mirror available so that the child can visualize his gradual physical changes.
  b. Explain that these changes are not harmful and are reversible.
3. Gastrointestinal bleeding
  a. Give the medication with milk or an antacid.
  b. Hematest all stools.
4. Decreased resistance to infection
  Observe the child very closely for signs of inflammation or infection as steroids mask these symptoms.
5. Euphoria and excitability
6. Bleeding into the skin or mucous membranes secondary to capillary fragility
7. Excessive appetite and food intake
  Offer small, frequent meals and nutritious between-meal snacks.
8. Sodium retention
  a. Offer a mildly sodium restricted diet.
  b. Do not allow the child to add salt to his food.
9. Hypokalemic alkalosis with convulsions
  a. Give foods high in potassium such as orange juice and bananas.
  b. Potassium chloride may need to be administered.
10. Hypertension
  Obtain blood pressure readings at regular intervals.
11. Atherosclerosis with central nervous system symptoms
12. Increased intracranial pressure
  a. Headache
  b. Diplopia
  c. Convulsions

C. *To protect the child from infection.*
1. Apply measures stated in the section on acute glomerulonephritis, page 1233.
2. Closely observe the child who is on steroids for signs of infection as this medication masks such symptoms.

3. Provide meticulous skin care to the edematous areas of the body.
   a. Bathe the child frequently and apply powder.
      Areas of special concern are the moist parts of the body and edematous male genitalia.
         Support the scrotum with a cotton pad held in place by a T-binder if necessary for the child's comfort.
   b. Position the child so that edematous skin surfaces are not in contact.
      Place a pillow between the child's legs when he is lying on his side, etc.
   c. Irrigate swollen eyes and cleanse the surrounding area several times daily to remove exudate.
      Elevate the child's head to reduce edema.

D. *To control edema.*
   1. Maintain the child on bedrest during periods of severe edema.
      Refer to the section on acute glomerulonephritis, page 1233.
   2. Administer diuretics as recommended by the physician.
      a. Diuretics are occasionally effective, especially early in the course of the disease when steroids may actually aggravate the edema.
      b. Dosage of most frequently used diuretics
         (1) Chlorothiazide: (Diuril)
             20 mg./kg./day in 2 divided doses.
         (2) Spironolactone (Aldactone)
             (a) 1.7–3 mg./kg. weight.
             (b) Often enhances the effect of the thiazides when given simultaneously.
         (3) Ethacrynic acid
             (a) Initial dose—25 mg.
             (b) May be increased by 25 mg. twice a day.
             (c) Effect is also enhanced by the simultaneous administration of Aldactone.
      c. Complications of therapy
         Potassium depletion
             (a) Offer foods high in potassium such as orange juice or bananas.
             (b) Supplemental potassium chloride may be administered orally if the urine output is adequate.

NURSING ALERT: Mercurial diuretics should not be administered intravenously to patients with nephrosis as fatalities have been reported.

---

   3. Assist with abdominal paracentesis when this is required because of marked ascites. (See Guidelines, p. 1243.)

E. *To restore lost plasma and tissue proteins.*
   1. Offer a high protein, high caloric diet.
      a. Salt restriction is generally not necessary, except during periods of edema and hypertension.
      b. Fluid restriction is of little value in controlling edema in nephrosis.
   2. Obtain a complete history of dietary preferences and patterns so that the child's meals can be as acceptable as possible.
   3. Place a sign on the child's bed indicating any dietary restrictions so that anyone approaching him will be aware of his special needs.

4. Offer small amounts of high protein foods at frequent intervals.
   Permit additional amounts of food at the child's discretion.

F. *To observe for disease progress.*
1. Apply nursing measures outlined in objective B in the section on acute glomerulone-phritis, page 1234.
2. Observe the child's entire body at frequent intervals for edema.
   Record areas of transient edema.
3. Record the appearance of each voiding. Especially note:
   a. Presence of hematuria
   b. Cloudiness of urine
   c. Decreased urine output.

G. *To provide emotional support to the child and his family.*
1. Encourage frequent visiting. Allow as much parental participation in the child's care as possible.
2. Allow the child as much activity as he can tolerate.
   a. Bedrest should be enforced during periods of hypertension.
   b. Balance periods of rest, recreation and quiet activities during the convalescent phase.
   c. Allow the child to eat his meals with other children.
3. Encourage the child to verbalize his fears.
   Young children frequently fear abandonment by their parents or loss of body integrity. (The boy who is unable to visualize his penis because of extensive edema may think that he has been castrated and needs reassurance that his body is intact.)

H. *To prepare for the child's discharge.*
1. Begin discharge planning early.
   a. Have the dietitian discuss special diets with the parents. Encourage them to plan sample menus.
   b. Allow the mother to administer the child's medication prior to his discharge.
   c. Provide suggestions regarding activity restriction at home.
2. Provide written discharge instructions concerning:
   a. Diet   d. Administration of medications
   b. Prevention of infection   e. Activity restrictions
   c. Skin care   f. Appointment for continued medical supervision.
3. Initiate a community health nursing referral if necessary for reinforcement of teaching.

Parental Teaching

1. Reinforce medical interpretation of the child's disease. Stress the importance of attention to the details of the child's care and continued medical supervision.
2. Discuss the problem of discipline with the parents. Encourage them to set consistent limits and expectations on their child's behavior.
3. Emphasize the necessity of taking medication according to the prescribed schedule and for an extended period of time. Discuss complications encountered with steroid therapy.

GUIDELINES: *Assisting with Pediatric Abdominal Paracentesis*

Purpose

To withdraw fluid from the peritoneal cavity in order to relieve pressure symptoms and respiratory distress.

Equipment

Sterile equipment

Hypodermic syringe	Suture needles and sutures
Hypodermic and aspiration needles	Forceps
Novocain	Gloves
Scalpel	Towels
Cannula	Graduated receptacle
Trocar	Cotton balls
Rubber tubing	Gauze squares
Needle holder	Abdominal dressing

Nonsterile equipment

Preparation tray	Abdominal binder
Test tubes	Safety pins
Pail for the collection of fluid	

Procedure

Nursing Action	Rationale/Amplification
Preparatory Phase	
1. Explain the procedure to the child in terms he can understand. Stress that he will feel better after the procedure.	1. To allay his fears and assure his cooperation.
2. Have the child void just prior to the procedure.	2. To avoid puncturing the bladder during the procedure.
3. Secure the help of a second person.	3. To observe the child and assist the physician during the procedure.
4. Position the child correctly: a. Place him close to the edge of the examining table. b. Support his back with your body. c. Hold his hands.	
Performance Phase	
1. Maintain the child's position.	1. To avoid injury.
2. Talk to the child frequently and hold his hands. Praise him for his cooperation.	2. To offer emotional support.
3. Observe the child's color and respirations.	3. Symptoms of shock develop if too much fluid is removed.

Follow-up Phase
1. Apply abdominal binder snugly.
2. Place the child in bed.
3. Record the amount and character of the drainage and the child's condition.
4. Observe frequently for signs of shock and note the drainage on the bandages.

URINARY TRACT INFECTION

Urinary tract infection (pyuria) refers to an infection within the urinary system. Either the lower urinary tract (urethra, bladder or the lower portion of the ureters) or the upper urinary tract (upper portion of the ureters or kidney) or both may be involved.

Etiology

1. Causative organisms
   a. Intestinal bacilli are responsible for 75–80% of all cases.
   b. Streptococci and staphylococci cause most of the remainder.
2. Route of entry
   a. Ascent from the exterior (most common)
   b. Circulating blood
3. Contributing causes
   a. Obstruction, usually congenital
   b. Infections elsewhere in the body
      (1) Upper respiratory
      (2) Diarrhea

Altered Physiology

1. Inflammatory changes occur in the affected portions of the urinary tract.
2. Clumps of bacteria may be present.
3. Inflammation results in urinary retention and stasis of urine in the bladder. There may be backflow of urine into the kidneys through the ureters.
4. There are inflammatory changes in the renal pelvis and throughout the kidney when this organ is involved.
5. The kidney may become large and swollen.
6. Scarring of the kidney parenchyma occurs in chronic infection and interferes with kidney function, particularly with the ability to concentrate urine.
7. Eventually, the kidney becomes small, tissue is destroyed and renal function fails.

Incidence

1. More common in infants than in older children.
2. Most prevalent in children from 2 months to 2 years of age.
3. Approximately 5 times more common in females than in males.
4. Most common renal disease in children.

Clinical Manifestations

A. *Onset*

   May be abrupt or gradual.

B. *Signs and symptoms*

1. Fever
   a. May be moderate or severe.
   b. May fluctuate rapidly.
   c. May be accompanied by chills or convulsions.
2. Anorexia and general malaise
3. Urinary frequency, urgency, dysuria
4. Dull or sharp pain in the kidney area
5. Irritability
6. Vomiting
7. Hypertension—may be present in chronic or severe cases.

Diagnostic Evaluation

1. Urinalysis
    a. Pus is present in abnormal amounts.
    b. Casts, especially white cell casts, may be present and are indicative of intrarenal infection.
    c. Pathogenic organisms can be identified.
    d. Hematuria—occurs occasionally.
2. Blood
    a. Leukocytosis
    b. Anemia—associated with chronic cases
3. Urologic Studies
    May reveal abnormalities in the structure or function of the urinary system.

Prognosis

1. Generally good in uncomplicated cases.
2. Persistent infection may occur in patients with obstruction or urinary retention and may lead ultimately to renal failure.
3. There is a tendency for recurrence of both treated and untreated infections.

Nursing Objectives

A. *To obtain a clean urine specimen for examination or culture.*
1. A freshly voided, early morning specimen is most accurate. (This urine is usually acid and concentrated which tends to preserve the formed elements.)
2. Refer to the procedure for the collection of urine specimens, page 1106.
3. Catheterization may be necessary to obtain a sterile specimen in older girls.
    Defer this procedure whenever possible in order to avoid emotional trauma and the accidental introduction of additional bacteria.
4. Obtain a midstream specimen whenever possible.

B. *To eradicate infective organisms.*
1. Administer antibiotics as ordered by the physician.
2. Most frequently used antibiotics:
    a. Sulfisoxazole (Gantrisin)
        (1) Dosage:
            (a) 0.1 to 0.2 gm./kg./day
            (b) Divided into 3 doses
        (2) Side effects and toxic effects
            (a) Nausea and vomiting
            (b) Dizziness, headache, drug fever, dermatitis
            (c) Blood dyscrasias
            (d) Oliguria, crystalluria and anuria—result from precipitation of the drug in the renal tubules.
        (3) Contraindications
            (a) Drug sensitivity.
            (b) Infants under the age of 2–3 months.

NURSING ALERT: Keep the child well hydrated to avoid crystallization of the drug in the renal tubules.

    b. Nitrofurantoin (Furadantin)
      (1) Dosage:
        (a) 50–200 mg./24 hours depending on the weight of the child.
        (b) Divide into 4 equally spaced doses.
      (2) Side effects and toxic effects
        (a) Nausea and vomiting
        (b) Peripheral neuritis
        (c) Hemolytic anemia
        (d) Sensitization
      (3) Contraindications
        (a) Anuria
        (b) Oliguria
        (c) Infants under 1 month of age
      (4) Points of emphasis
        (a) The drug may cause the urine to be amber or brown in color.
        (b) Drug should be administered after meals or with a small amount of food to minimize nausea or vomiting.
        (c) Administration of the drug should be continued for at least 3 days after the urine becomes sterile.
        (d) Prolonged therapy should be closely monitored by clinical and laboratory means and the dosage regulated accordingly.
        (e) Recurrences of infections following the discontinuance of Furadantin may occur more quickly than recurrences following Gantrisin therapy.

C. *To provide for symptomatic relief of the child's discomfort during the febrile period.*
  1. Maintain bedrest.
  2. Administer analgesic and antipyretic drugs as recommended by the physician.
  3. Encourage fluids to reduce the fever and dilute the concentration of the urine. Obtain a complete nursing history regarding the child's fluid preferences and method of taking them.

D. *To observe for progress of disease.*
    Nursing notes should include:
    a. Frequent recording of the child's temperature
    b. Accurate measurement of intake and output
    c. Description of the color and odor of the urine, especially if it is abnormal
    d. Presence of any of the following symptoms
      (1) Frequency of urination
      (2) Burning or pain with voiding
      (3) Enuresis
      (4) Urinary retention
    e. General behavior and activity status of the child
    f. Signs of untoward or toxic effects of drugs
    g. Pain, especially in the kidney area.

E. *To provide emotional support to the child and his parents.*
  1. Reinforce medical explanations of the disease and its therapy.
  2. Explain all diagnostic tests and procedures to the child before they are carried out.
  3. Encourage the verbal child to talk about his experience and how he feels about it. Correct any misconceptions that he may have.

4. Provide an environment that is as close to normal as possible during hospitalization. Include opportunities for the child to play.

F. *To prepare the child and his family for discharge.*

1. Discuss any treatment that will be required at home. Provide written discharge instructions regarding:
   a. Rest
   b. Fluid intake
   c. Administration of medications
   d. Appointment for continued medical supervision
2. Communicate or have the parents communicate with the school nurse if it is necessary for the child to receive medications at school.
3. Complete a community nursing referral if reinforcement of discharge teaching appears necessary.

Parental Teaching

1. Long-term therapy is often prescribed to prevent recurrence of urinary tract infections.
   a. Schedules for prolonged therapy vary from several months to a year.
   b. The infection should not be considered as eradicated until at least 2 negative cultures are obtained at an interval of 4–6 weeks after cessation of therapy.
2. The child should be kept under continued medical surveillance for the possibility of disease recurrence.
   Emphasis should be placed on the fact that even though this disease may have few symptoms, it can lead to very serious, permanent disability.
3. Spread of bacteria from the anal and vaginal areas to the urethra can be minimized in female children by cleansing the perineal area from the urethra back toward the anus.

ABNORMALITIES OF THE GENITOURINARY TRACT WHICH REQUIRE SURGERY

Exstrophy of the Bladder

In *exstrophy of the bladder* the posterior and lateral surfaces of the bladder and urethral outlets are exposed because of failure of the 2 sides of the lower abdomen to unite. The condition allows direct passage of urine to the outside.

Clinical Manifestations

1. Constant dribbling of urine excoriates the skin.
2. Ulceration of the bladder mucosa may occur.
3. There are usually associated defects including separation of the pubic rami, defects of the bowel, epispadias, undescended testes or inguinal hernia in the male and cleft clitoris, separated labia or absent vagina in the female.
4. Affected children walk with a waddling or unsteady gait.

Treatment

1. Transplantation of the ureters to the colon and removal of the bladder. Urine is then passed with stool from the anus.
2. Complete correction with plastic surgery. The child can then void normally.
3. Plastic repair of the bladder, abdominal wall and genitalia.
4. Surgery or braces to correct deformity of the pelvic girdle.

Nursing Management

A. *Preoperative Care.*
  1. Protect the bladder area from trauma and irritation.
     a. Position the infant on his back or side.
     b. Cleanse the area frequently with mild soap and water.
     c. Cover the defect with a sterile gauze to which a bland ointment such as petrolatum has been applied.
     d. Change the gauze covering and the infant's diapers frequently.
  2. Observe the infant closely for signs of infection.
  3. Teach the mother how to cleanse the area and protect the bladder.
     Initiate a community nursing referral if reinforcement of teaching or maternal support appears necessary.
  4. Collect urine specimens by holding the infant over an emesis basin in a position which allows urine to drip into the container.
     A medicine dropper may also be used to collect urine from the opening in the bladder.

B. *Postoperative Care.*
     Teach the child anal sphincter control to prevent seepage of urine.
     a. Expect some soiling of his clothes.
     b. Avoid causing him embarrassment by such accidents.

Patent Urachus

Patent urachus is persistence of the embryonic connection between the umbilicus and the bladder. In many patients only a cyst persists and is located at the upper end of the tract, under the umbilicus.

Clinical Manifestations

1. Urine dribbles from the umbilicus when entire urachus is present.
2. Midline swelling is present in cases of a cyst.
3. Infection of urachal cysts is common.

Treatment

1. Eradication of infection
2. Removal of cysts
3. Surgical obliteration of the patent urachus

Obstructive Lesions of the Lower Urinary Tract

Types of Obstruction

1. Urethral valves
   a. Filamentous valves that obstruct urine flow
   b. Most commonly found in males
2. Congenital narrowing of the urethra
3. Bladder neck obstruction
   Most common site of lower urinary tract obstruction
4. Meatal stricture
5. Severe phimosis (rare)
6. Neuromuscular dysfunction (Refer to the section on spina bifida, p. 1324.)

Clinical Manifestations

Abnormal urination

a. Dysuria
b. Frequency
c. Enuresis
d. Dribbling

e. Decreased forcefulness of urine stream
f. Difficulty starting urine stream
g. Straining during urination
h. Abrupt cessation during urination

Altered Physiology

1. Urinary tract becomes distended proximal to the point of obstruction.
2. The bladder dilates and hypertrophies.
3. Stasis of urine occurs.
4. The ureters become elongated, dilated and tortuous.
5. Hydronephrosis and destruction of kidney tissue inevitably result.

Treatment

1. Eradication and prevention of infection. (See section on urinary tract infection, p. 1245.)
2. Dilation of urethral stenosis or stricture.
3. Surgical relief of the obstruction.

Obstructive Lesions of the Upper Urinary Tract

Types of Obstruction

1. Stricture of a ureter.
2. Congenital absence of 1 ureter.
3. Duplication of the ureter of 1 kidney.
4. Compression of a ureter by an aberrant blood vessel.

Clinical Manifestations

1. Often asymptomatic (There is seldom any problem with voiding.)
2. Vague symptoms such as failure to thrive may be present.
3. Urinary tract infections may be frequent.
4. Hypertension may occur.

Treatment

Same as for obstructions of lower urinary tract.

Hypospadias

Hypospadias is malposition of the urethral opening.

Altered Physiology

A. *Males.*
   1. The urethra opens on the lower surface of the penis, proximal to its usual site.
   2. In severe cases, the urethra may open on the shaft of the penis, at its base or on the perineum.
   3. Frequently associated with congenital chordee in males—cord-like defect which extends from the scrotum up the penis and deflects the penis downward.

B. *Females.*
   The urethra opens into the vagina (rare).

Clinical Manifestations

   1. Inability to void with the penis in the normal elevated position.
   2. Severe forms interfere with the ability to procreate.

Treatment

   Plastic surgery.

Cryptorchidism (Undescended Testis)

Cryptorchidism is the absence of one or both testes from the scrotum. The testes may be located in the abdominal cavity or inguinal canal.

Etiology

   Caused by delayed descent, prevention of descent by some mechanical lesion, or endocrine disorders (rare).

Clinical Manifestations and Altered Physiology

   1. Normal development of secondary sex characteristics.
   2. Degeneration of the sperm-forming cells occurs after puberty because of the higher temperature of the abdomen compared with the normal location in the scrotum. Sterility results.
   3. Emotional disturbances often occur when the child discovers that he is different from his peers.
   4. Associated hernias are found in more than 50% of the patients.

Treatment

   1. Orchiopexy (placement of the testes in the scrotum)
   2. Plastic surgery in patients with an absent testis
   3. Administration of chorionic gonadotropin—has produced descent of the testes in some children (These are probably cases that would have descended spontaneously.)

Nursing Management

A. *Preoperative Care.*
   1. Encourage the child and his parents to express their feelings about the condition. Expect anxieties regarding sterility, homosexuality and perceptions of the child as defective or inadequate.

2. Discuss the condition and surgery frankly and in terms that the child can understand.
   a. Maintain a matter of fact attitude.
   b. Clarify any misconceptions that the child may have.
3. Provide privacy for medical examinations.

B. *Postoperative Care.*
   1. Maintain traction.
      a. A suture is placed in the lower portion of the scrotum and is attached to a rubber band which is fastened to the upper aspect of the inner thigh by a piece of adhesive.
      b. This traction anchors the testis to the scrotum and is removed in approximately 5–7 days.
   2. Prevent contamination of the suture line.
   3. Administer antibiotics as ordered to prevent infection.

Ambiguous Genitalia

Female Pseudohermaphroditism

1. Most common problem of sexual differentiation.
2. A deficiency of hydrocortisone results in adrenocortical hyperplasia and an overproduction of androgens.
3. *Manifestations*—masculinization of the external genitalia in the female infant.
4. *Treatment*
   a. Administration of hydrocortisone in children with adrenal hyperplasia.
   b. Corrective plastic surgery
      This should be undertaken as early in life as possible, before social adjustment becomes a severe problem.

Male Pseudohermaphroditism

TYPE	TREATMENT
1. Normal female genitalia with testes internally.	1. a. Surgical removal of testes. b. Administration of estrogens at puberty. c. Child reared as a girl.
2. Predominantly male genitalia with testes internally.	2. a. Surgical removal of all nonmale structures. b. Child reared as a boy.
3. Ambiguous genitalia due to damaged testes in fetal life.	3. a. Plastic reconstruction. b. Child reared as a boy.

Nursing Management

1. Reinforce medical explanations of the anatomic problems and treatment. Approach the situation matter of factly.
2. Initiate appropriate referrals for family support and counseling. These may include:
   a. Social work
   b. Psychiatry
   c. Community health nursing
   d. Child guidance clinic
   e. Genetic counseling

Care of the Child Requiring Urologic Surgery

Preoperative Care

1. Determine the child's fantasies regarding his illness and hospitalization. Correct any misconceptions that he reveals.
2. Provide an explanation of the anatomy and physiology of the urinary system in terms that the child can understand.
   a. Use a body outline appropriate for the age of the child.
   b. Explain how the child differs from the normal.
      Relate his defect to his symptoms whenever possible.
3. Explain all diagnostic tests prior to their occurrence. These may include: urinalysis, 24-hour urine collections, intravenous and retrograde pyelography, angiography and cystoscopy.
   a. Descriptions should include such information as:
      (1) Preparation required—fasting, enemas, etc.
      (2) Location of the test—operating room, radiology, etc.
      (3) Appearance and attire of personnel
      (4) Positioning
      (5) Anesthesia
      (6) Pain or discomfort
      (7) Expectations following the procedure—diet, rest, urine collections, etc.
   b. Determine the child's understanding of the procedure.
      (1) Ask him simple, direct questions.
      (2) Allow him to perform the procedure on a doll or demonstrate it on a diagram.
4. Explain the surgical procedure.
   a. Explanations should include:
      (1) Preparation required—fasting, enemas, etc.
      (2) Description of the operating room including the appearance of the personnel
      (3) Anesthesia
      (4) Postoperative appearance
         (a) Urinary drainage tubing and collection devices
         (b) Appearance of urine
         (c) Sutures
         (d) Bandages
         (e) Intravenous infusion
   b. Determine the child's understanding of his surgery and reinforce teaching when necessary.
5. Points of emphasis during the preparation:
   a. The child is in no way to blame for his illness.
   b. No other part of the body will be operated on.

Care of the Child Who Has an Ileal Conduit (Ileoloop)

A. *Definition of the Procedure*

   One or both ureters are anastomosed to a segment of ileum which then serves to carry urine to the external body surface of the abdomen.

B. *Preoperative Care.*

   1. Refer to the previous section on the emotional preparation of the child and his family for urologic surgery.

2. Allow the child to try on the ileal conduit apparatus in order to become familiar with it.

    Observe for discomfort and skin reactions to the adhesive or cement.

3. Administer antibiotics as ordered by the physician.
    a. Kanamycin (Kantrex) is a frequently used drug.
        (1) Dosage
            7.5 mg./kg. every 12 hours.
        (2) Adverse effects
            (a) Albuminuria, presence of red or white blood cells, granular casts, or oliguria
            (b) Tinnitus, vertigo, deafness
            (c) Local pain or irritation at the injection site
            (d) Skin rash
            (e) Drug fever
            (f) Headache
        (3) Contraindications
            (a) Damage to 8th cranial nerve
            (b) Known sensitivity to the drug
        (4) Points of emphasis
            The injection should be made deeply into the muscle.

C. *Postoperative Care*

1. Maintain the urinary collection apparatus. (A temporary collection bag is worn in the immediate postoperative period and may be replaced by a permanent appliance once edema in the stoma subsides.)
    a. Cleanse the area around the stoma with mild soap and water and dry it well.
    b. Keep the skin around the stoma completely dry during application of the appliance to insure that it will remain attached.
    c. Place the adhesive plate of the appliance securely around the stoma.
        The opening in the adhesive plate should be such that it fits snugly over the stoma but does not compromise circulation.
    d. Empty the appliance every 2 hours or whenever it contains approximately 100 ml. of fluid. (During the night the appliance may be attached via tubing to a collection bottle.)
    e. Nursing observations related to the appliance
        (1) Leaking around the appliance
        (2) Skin irritation
        (3) Improper fit of the appliance
    f. Points of emphasis
        (1) A properly applied apparatus should remain in place 3–5 days. It needs to be changed only when it begins to leak or becomes uncomfortable.
        (2) It is normal for the urine to contain some mucus and it may be blood tinged.

2. Observe for complications.
    a. Wound infection
    b. Leaking at the site of anastomosis
    c. Peritonitis
    d. Paralytic ileus
    e. Intestinal obstruction
    f. Stenosis of the stoma
    g. Fluid and electrolyte disturbances

D. *Patient or Parental Teaching*
1. Involve the child or his family in his self-care, including application of the urinary appliance as soon as possible.
2. Explain that appliances can be adapted to meet individual patient's needs.
   Some experimentation will probably be necessary before the most suitable equipment can be identified.
3. Adequate fluid intake (approximately 125 ml./kg.) is essential to maintain good urine flow.
4. Two appliances should be available, one in use and the other as a spare.
5. The appliance should be cleaned and aired regularly to avoid odor or crusting.
   a. A few drops of Lysol to a quart of water whitens and deodorizes the bags.
   b. Crusting can be removed by a solution of vinegar and water (approximately 1 cup of vinegar to a quart of water).
   c. A mild soap and warm water should be used to clean the appliance.
6. New appliances should be purchased approximately every 6 months or whenever old ones begin to feel thin or worn out.
7. Activity limitations are usually not necessary unless the child has associated physical problems.
8. Clothing may have to be altered slightly to fit over the pouch of the appliance.

E. *Preparation for Discharge*
1. Provide written information regarding the equipment that the child is using and where to obtain it.
2. Provide at least a 2-week supply of equipment for the family to take home.
   Advise the parents to order new supplies before the old ones are depleted.
3. Initiate appropriate referrals.
   a. Community nursing agency.
   b. Local "ostomy" clubs.

BIBLIOGRAPHY

Books

Becker, E., et al.: Kidney and Urinary Tract Infections. Indianapolis, Eli Lilly and Company, 1971.
Blake, F., et al.: Nursing Care of Children. Philadelphia, J. B. Lippincott, 1970.
Campbell, M., and Harrison, J. H.: Urology. Philadelphia, W. B. Saunders, 1970.
Goettsch, E., and Lyttle, J.: Kidney Disease in the Young. Philadelphia, W. B. Saunders, 1971.
James, J. A.: Renal Disease in Childhood. St. Louis, C. V. Mosby, 1968.
Marlow, D. F.: Textbook of Pediatric Nursing. Philadelphia, W. B. Saunders, 1973.
Nelson, W. (ed.): Textbook of Pediatrics. Philadelphia, W. B. Saunders, 1969.
Petrillo, M., and Sanger, S.: Emotional Care of Hospitalized Children. Philadelphia, J. B. Lippincott, 1972.
Silver, H., et al.: Handbook of Pediatrics. Los Altos, Lange Medical Publications, 1969.

Articles

Brodie, B., and Von Haam, J.: Children born with adrenogenital syndrome. Amer. J. Nurs., 67: 1018, 1967.
Clifton, J.: Collecting 24 hour urine specimens from infants. Amer. J. Nurs., 69:1660, 1969.
Cornfield, D.: Failure to thrive, a clue to renal disease in children. Consultant, 12:97, January 1972.

Cytryn, L., and Cytryn, E., et al.: Psychological implications of cryptorchidism. J. Amer. Acad. Child Psych., *6*:131, 1967.

Froehlich, L.: Care of the infant with exstrophy of the bladder. Nurs. Clin. N. Amer., *2*:573, 1967.

Daily, R. W.: A child confronts kidney disease. J. Pract. Nurs., *21*:34, February 1971.

Downs, A. W., et al.: Bacteriuria and urinary tract infection in infancy and childhood: a review. Nursing Research, *20*:131, March-April 1971.

Holt, J.: A long term study of a child treated for hypospadias. Nurs. Clin. N. Amer., *4*:27–37, March 1969.

Murray, B. S., et al.: The patient has an ileal conduit. Amer. J. Nurs., *71*:1560, August 1971.

McCroy, W. W.: Every infant deserves routine urinalysis. Consultant, *12*:161, May 1972.

McGovern, J. H., et al.: Reimplantation of ureters in children. Hosp. Pract., *6*:64, August 1971.

Riley, H. D.: Pyelonephritis in children: the long-term problem. Hosp. Pract., *7*:141, March 1972.

Agencies

National Kidney Foundation
116 East 27th St.
New York, New York 10016

United Ostomy Association, Inc.
111 Wilshire Boulevard
Los Angeles, California 90017

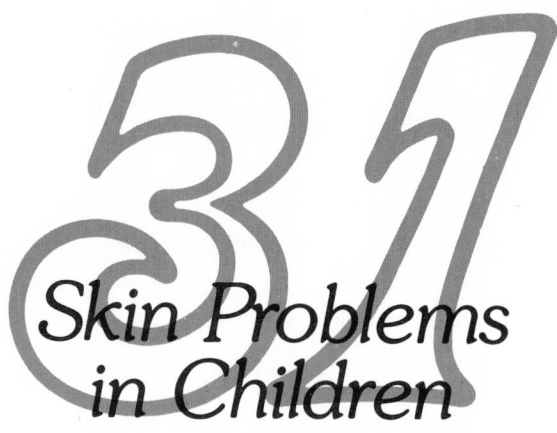

Skin Problems in Children

BURNS IN CHILDREN

Burns are a frequent form of childhood injury. A second degree burn of 10% or more of the body surface in a child younger than 1 year, or a second degree burn of 15% or more of the body surface in a child over 1 year is considered a very serious injury. The effects of burns are not limited to the burn area.

Incidence and Etiology

1. Burns outnumber all other causes of death during infancy, childhood and adolescence; the highest incidence of burns occurs in children under 5 years
2. Causes of burns in children
    a. Burns from hot water
        (1) Child left in tub unsupervised and turns on the hot water tap
        (2) Child placed in tub of hot water that has not been tested
        (3) Spilling of hot coffee, tea, etc. on child
    b. Burns from open flames
        (1) House fires
        (2) Child climbs up to stove and clothing catches fire
    c. Electrical burns
        (1) Child playing with electrical outlets or appliances
        (2) Child playing with extension cords
        (3) Child playing on railroad tracks
    d. Caustic acid or alkali burns
        Child ingests strong household cleaning products

1256

     e. Chemical burns of the skin
         Child plays with gasoline which comes in contact with skin (often the gasoline ignites)
     f. Burns inflicted upon the child as a result of child abuse
     g. Smoke inhalation and burns of the respiratory tract

Altered Physiology

     See section on burns in adults, page 600.

Clinical Manifestations

1. The characteristics of burn wounds are classified as follows:
   a. First-degree burns involve superficial epidermis; the skin is pink or red in appearance and is painful to touch.
   b. Second-degree burns involve the entire epidermis; the skin is red, blistered, moist with exudate and painful to pinprick or touch.
   c. Third-degree burns involve the dermis or underlying fat, muscle or bone; the skin appears white, dry or charred and is painful.
2. Symptoms of shock appear soon after the burn
   a. Rapid pulse   d. Prostration
   b. Subnormal temperature   e. Low blood pressure
   c. Pallor
3. Symptoms of toxemia may develop within 1–2 days after the initial burn
   a. Prostration   e. Vomiting
   b. Fever   f. Edema
   c. Rapid pulse   g. These symptoms may progress to coma and death
   d. Cyanosis
4. Burns of the respiratory tract result in symptoms of upper airway obstruction resulting from acute eczema and inflammation of the glottis, vocal cords and upper trachea.
   a. Rapid breathing
   b. Dyspnea
   c. Stridor
5. Smoke inhalation may cause no initial symptoms other than mild bronchial obstruction during the initial phase following the burn. Within 6–48 hours the child may develop sudden onset of:
   a. Bronchiolitis
   b. Pulmonary edema
   c. Severe airway obstruction

Treatment

Objectives: to maintain circulation.
           to prevent renal failure as well as water infraction intoxication.
           to prevent or treat infection.
           to aim toward early repair of the burn wound.
           to restore the child to the best possible state of physical and psychological functioning.

Calculation of the Burn Area
a. Evans *"rule of nine"* has proved quite inexact when applied to young children.
  (1) During infancy and early childhood the relative surface area of different parts of the body varies with age.
  (2) The younger the child the greater proportion is the surface of the head and the lesser proportion is the size of the legs.
b. *Berkow's table* (below) is used to make allowances for the changes in body surface areas that occur with age.

Variations from Adult Distribution in Infants and Children (in percent)

	Newborn	1 year	5 years	10 years
Head	19	17	13	11
Both thighs	11	13	16	17
Both lower legs	10	10	11	12
Neck	2			
Anterior trunk	13			
Posterior trunk	13	These percentages remain		
Both upper arms	8	constant at all ages.		
Both lower arms	6			
Both hands	5			
Both buttocks	5			
Both feet	7			
Genitals	1			
	100%			

Complications

1. Infection
2. Scarring
3. Contractures
4. Renal failure
5. Psychological trauma

Nursing Objectives

A. *To recognize the symptoms of shock and to know support measures which are initiated to restore and maintain circulation.*
  1. Be alert to the symptoms of shock which occur very shortly after a severe burn.
    a. Tachycardia
    b. Hypothermia
    c. Hypotension
    d. Pallor
    e. Prostration
    f. Shallow respirations
  2. Monitor the administration of intravenous fluid since major burns are followed by a reduction in blood volume due to outflow of plasma into the tissues.
    a. Maintain the administration of plasma.
    b. Maintain the administration of other intravenous fluids once the plasma volume is restored.
  3. Maintain an accurate record of intake and output.
    a. Record time and amount of all fluids given.
    b. Measure urinary output every ½ hour to 1 hour.
      (1) Check specific gravity.
      (2) Report diminishing urinary output.

4. Provide a rich oxygen environment in order to combat anoxia.
   (1) Mask   (3) Intubation may be necessary
   (2) Tent   (4) Tracheostomy may be necessary
5. Provide sedation to relieve pain.
   Sedation must be given in very small amounts to children in order to prevent their depressant effect.
6. Provide a source of heat over the child's bed since additional heat is necessary to maintain body temperature. (Goose neck lamps may be used.)
7. Request laboratory results.
   a. Hematocrit or R.B.C. serves as a rough guide to the adequacy of initial treatment since the loss of plasma results in concentration of red blood cells.
   b. Electrolytes serve as a guide to fluid replacement.
8. Maintain close observation of vital signs in order to continually evaluate the state of peripheral circulation.
   Report immediately any significant changes.

B. *To observe for symptoms of respiratory distress and initiate measures to alleviate distress.*
   1. Be alert for symptoms of respiratory distress.
      a. Dyspnea
      b. Stridor
      c. Rapid respirations
   2. Provide an oxygen source in order to combat anoxia.
   3. Report these symptoms.
   4. Intubation or tracheostomy may be performed.

C. *To provide scrupulous skin care in order to prevent infection and promote healing.*
   1. Burn Treatment
      a. Open method—exposure maintains a dry surface, produces early formation of a protective eschar and predisposes less to infection.
      b. Closed method—burns are kept covered with dressings that have been soaked in a solution, or a topical medicine is applied followed by dressing.
      c. Physicians have their own preference for use of the open or closed method.
   2. Maintain sterility in working with the burn area regardless of whether the open or closed method is used.
   3. The Bradford frame may be used to facilitate skin care.
      a. Provides a method for the collection of urine and feces and maintains cleanliness of the burn areas and dressings.
      b. Contractures may be prevented by maintaining good posture.
      c. Two Bradford frames may be used to change position of the child from back to stomach and vice versa without having to handle the severely burned child.
   4. Position the child and turn frequently.
   5. Apply protective devices to prevent the child from scratching the burn area.
   6. Administer antibiotics as prescribed.

D. *To provide a high protein, high calorie diet in order to provide nutrition necessary for healing and for the growth and developmental needs of the child.*
   1. Determine the child's food preferences.
   2. Offer small amounts of foods that the child prefers.
      a. Offer 4 or 5 very small meals as opposed to 3 large meals.
      b. Offer high protein, high calorie supplements.
      c. Provide vitamin supplements.

E. *To maintain a planned physical therapy program in order to achieve the greatest functional capacity for the child.*
   1. Plan the time each day for the therapy to be carried out.
   2. Utilize play opportunities to help the child accept the program (i.e., tricycle riding may be used as form of exercise).
   3. Allow the child to be ambulatory as soon as he is able to be.

F. *To prepare the child for the many painful and surgical procedures that he must undergo.*
   1. Explain to the child what is going to happen before each procedure.
   2. Explain to the child what will happen before he goes to the operating room, where he will wake up, and who will be there when he does wake up.
   3. Explain and demonstrate what equipment will be used following surgery or other procedures.

G. *To provide emotional support for the child who has been very frightened and traumatized by this painful experience.*
   1. Encourage the child to talk about the way he feels.
      a. The child may feel guilty and think that the burn is punishment for some wrong deed.
      b. Allow the child opportunities at play where he may be able to begin to work out his feelings.
   2. The child will be concerned about his appearance.
      a. Continually inform the child that you love him even though he has a bad burn.
      b. Encourage early contact with other children.
   3. Psychiatric consultation is very frequently necessary in order to assist the child to work out his feelings.
   4. Arrange for services of a school teacher for the school-age child as soon as his condition permits.

H. *To support the parents during this very difficult time.*
   1. Encourage the parents to visit the child often.
   2. Give the parents the opportunity to discuss their feelings.
      Parents frequently feel very guilty because they feel they did not give the child the appropriate supervision he should have had when the accident occurred.
   3. Keep parents informed as to the child's progress.
   4. Attempt to have the parents become actively involved in the child's care.
   5. Psychiatric consultation is frequently required in order to assist parents in coping with their feelings.

INFANTILE AND CHILDHOOD ECZEMA

Infantile and childhood eczema is a term that describes any inflammatory dermatosis that is characterized by erythema, papulovesiculation, oozing, crusting and scaling in various phases of resolution.

Etiology

1. Infantile eczema usually becomes manifest between the 2nd and 6th month.
2. This type of dermatitis is the commonest, earliest manifestation of allergy.
3. The exact allergic etiology is not known. Many infants with eczema have a positive family history of allergy and later develop asthma or hay fever.

4. The following may be triggering factors affecting the day-to-day appearance of the lesions:
   a. Bacterial, viral or fungal infections
   b. Particulate matter and contactant irritants
   c. Inhalants
   d. Foods
   e. Temperature and humidity
   f. Emotional or physical stress
   g. Drugs

Altered Physiology

1. The dermatitis involves the epidermis and the vascular layer of the cutis.
2. The dermatitis goes through a cycle involving areas of erythema, papules, vesicles, wheal reactions and, ultimately, scaling eruption.
3. With superimposed infection, there is exudation, pustulization and crust formation.
4. Various stages of the disease can be present on different parts of the child's body.
5. The disease is subject to remissions and exacerbations.

Clinical Manifestations

1. *Infants*—lesions
   a. Erythematous, papular and weeping lesions
   b. Oozing and crusting of the lesions
   c. Cheeks, face, neck and behind the ears—are the areas most frequently involved
   d. Lesions are more concentrated on the head and body rather than the extremities
2. *Older children*—lesions
   a. Erythematous, papular and weeping lesions
   b. Oozing and crusting of the lesions
   c. The flexor surfaces of the upper and lower extremities in addition to the face and neck are areas frequently involved
   d. As the disease becomes chronic, lichenification (skin becomes leathery and hardened) and hyperpigmentation in the antecubital and popliteal areas of the extremities develop
3. Pruritus—may be mild or severe
4. Excessive scratching may cause restlessness, sleeplessness and irritability
5. Excessive scratching may result in an inflammatory reaction and excoriation, bleeding and subsequent infection
6. The color of lesions is red (may be intense red)

Treatment

1. Patient should avoid the allergen.
2. Control any complicating infection of the skin.
3. Take local measures to improve the condition of the involved skin.

Complications

Infection produced by contamination of the opened epidermis.

Nursing Objectives

A. *To institute measures which prevent the child from scratching himself when he experiences severe itching in order to prevent further irritation and possible infection of the skin.*

1. Apply protective devices to prevent the child from itching and scratching himself.
   a. Any one or combination of the following protective devices may be used (elbow cuff, ankle and wrist restraint, face mask, jacket restraint).
   b. Apply these protective devices only when absolutely necessary—when itching and scratching cannot be controlled by other methods.
   c. Remove protective devices frequently in order to allow free movement.
   d. Apply protective devices securely enough to prevent scratching, yet not so tight as to impair circulation. Check circulation frequently when protective devices are used.
   e. When protective devices are used, the device should be removed at frequent intervals.
      (1) Allow the child to sit on the nurse's or mother's lap.
      (2) Attempt to divert the child's attention by playing with him and reading to him.
      (3) Allow the child to eat his meals free from protective devices; this requires direct supervision.
   f. When the child experiences severe itching and uncontrollable scratching, remove only 1 protective device at a time so that scratching can be controlled.
   g. Anger and frustration are frequently displayed in violent scratching.
      (1) Keep child comfortable and anticipate his needs.
      (2) Provide as much personal contact and supervision as possible.
      (3) Allow play activities that afford the child the opportunity to act out his anger and frustrations.
      (4) Provide infants with a cradle gym and a pacifier.
2. Cotton hand mitts and booties may be applied to prevent the child from scratching himself.
3. Trim fingernails and toenails and keep clean.
4. Provide safe toys that will not be used by the child to scratch himself. (Use soft play things made of hypoallergic material.)
5. Administer prescribed medications.
   a. Sedatives
   b. Antihistamines
   c. The use of local anesthetics to relieve itching is contraindicated due to their potential for skin sensitization.

B. *To provide measures which will improve the condition of the involved skin.*
   1. Bathe the child by the prescribed method.
      a. Water and soap are often irritating.
      b. Starch baths may be used.
      c. Oil may be used if skin is dry and crusted. (Apply oil with a cotton ball.)
      d. While giving the child a bath, keep him from scratching himself. (It may be necessary to maintain protective devices at this time.)
   2. Local care of the skin is aimed at removing the debris and allaying the inflammatory reaction.
      a. Wet soaks of Burrows solution may be applied to the affected areas.
         (1) These soaks are continuous and must be kept wet.
         (2) These bulky, wet dressings may serve to immobilize the child sufficiently that he does not require other protective devices.

    b. Lassar's paste or other hydrophilic preparation may be applied to the affected areas.
      (1) Local medications must be kept on the skin constantly.
      (2) Caution must be exercised to keep ointment out of the child's eyes.
    c. Coal tar preparations are used when the skin becomes dry and relatively free from inflammation.
      (1) All areas being treated are kept covered.
      (2) Each day new ointment is applied.
        (a) Remove all old ointment before applying new ointment.
        (b) Starch bath may be used to remove ointment.
  3. Prevent skin irritation from bed clothing.
    a. Padding may be used.
    b. Heavy plastic covering may be used over the cotton sheets.
  4. Change diapers frequently to prevent skin excoriation.

C. *To promote measures which will prevent contact with dietary and environmental allergies.*
  1. Review the child's chart and question the parents regarding known allergies.
    a. Note the known allergens on the Kardex and place a tag on the head of the bed to indicate that the child has an allergy.
    b. Inform the dietitian as to the child's food allergies.
  2. Avoid substances which have a high potential for sensitization.
    a. Foods such as chocolate, egg and orange juice are to be avoided.
    b. Wool and dust are to be avoided.
  3. Observe the child's reactions when an elimination diet is prescribed.
    a. A minimal diet is ordered.
    b. A new food is added to the diet every 3–5 days during which time the response to that food is observed.
    c. An allergic response occurring during this 3- to 5-day period indicates sensitivity to that food; that particular food is then eliminated from the diet.
    d. If no response is apparent, that food is added to the child's diet.
    e. Another food substance is added and the child is observed for the following 3- to 5-day period, etc.
  4. Provide a substitute for cow's milk when the child is allergic to it.
    a. Goat's milk may be used.
    b. Commercial formulas made from meat or vegetable protein substances are available.

D. *To protect the child from sources of infection.*
  1. Protect the child from exposure to sources of infection known to cause exacerbations and severe infections.
    a. Contact with other children, personnel etc. who have the virus of herpes simplex is to be avoided.

NURSING ALERT: The child should not be vaccinated against smallpox until his skin has been free from eczema for 1 year.

---

    b. The child should not be exposed to individuals who have a fresh vaccine lesion.
  2. When the child is immobilized, his position should be changed frequently to prevent respiratory complications.

E. *To assist the parents in providing for the child's care following hospitalization.*
   1. Explain to the parents the usual cause of the problem.
   2. Demonstrate the application of topical medications and the application of dressings.
   3. Give specific information regarding diet. Emphasize the foods which are allowed rather than foods to be avoided.
   4. Demonstrate the application of protective devices and the precautions in using them.
   5. Encourage the parents to hold and cuddle the child as much as possible to encourage the body contact that is frequently avoided because of protective devices and ointments.
   6. Encourage the parents to discuss their feelings and concerns about the child's illness.
      a. The appearance of the child may be very disturbing to them.
      b. They need to be made to feel adequate in caring for the child at home.

IMPETIGO

Impetigo is an infectious disease affecting the superficial layers of the skin and is characterized by the formation of vesicles, crusts or bullae.

Etiology
   1. Impetigo is caused by staphylococci or streptococci.
   2. Occurs most frequently where personal hygiene is poor.
   3. Occurs most frequently in children under 10 years.

Altered Physiology
   1. Spread by contact—easily conveyed from person to person (using same handkerchief, towels, napkins, pencils, toys, etc.); plastic wading pools in summer where spilled water is replaced and no antiseptic or disinfectant is used.
   2. Any abrasion of skin may serve as portal of entry.

Clinical Manifestations
   1. Incubation period 1–5 days.
   2. Lesion first appears as pink-red macules which quickly change to vesicles which, in turn, enlarge, become pustular, develop crusts and leave temporary superficial erythematous areas.
   3. Face and hands commonly involved, but other parts may be affected—part of the scalp.
   4. Pruritus may occur.

Treatment
   1. No specific therapy.
   2. Ammoniated mercury 3% applied to affected area. Best to remove crusts by applying gauze soaked in boric acid or magnesium sulfate; remove crusts when softened and then apply medication.
   3. The following may be used:
      2% gentian violet
      1:10,000 or 1:15,000 solution of potassium permanganate or bichloride of mercury applied by wet dressings or free application of Mercresin or ointments. (Bacitracin or Neomycin may be used.)

Nursing Objectives

A. *To be aware of the appearance of the characteristic lesion of impetigo.*
   1. Observe the condition of the child's skin upon admission to the hospital.
   2. Report any suspicious appearing lesions.
   3. Record the appearance and location of the lesion.
   4. Initiate appropriate measures to prevent the spread of the infection.
      a. Place the child in a single room.
      b. Maintain medical aseptic technique.
   5. Watch for the development of new lesions.

B. *To provide measures to prevent secondary infections.*
   1. Provide mittens or protective devices to prevent the child from scratching the lesions.
   2. Trim the child's fingernails and toenails.
   3. Maintain cleanliness of fingernails and toenails.

C. *To provide measures to assure the child's comfort until healing has occurred and the child is free from infection.*
   1. Hold child frequently and release from any necessary protective device.
   2. Provide diversional therapy.
   3. Administer medication and treatment to relieve itching—local medications or packs which relieve itching and promote healing may be used.
   4. Provide the child with a diet adequate to meet his growth and development needs.

D. *To practice measures of general health and provide teaching for the child and his parents which will be helpful in preventing spread and further infection.*
   1. General measures to improve personal cleanliness should be encouraged.
   2. Minor wounds should be adequately cleaned and treated.
   3. The child should be isolated if at home.
   4. The child should be kept out of school until the lesions have healed.

RINGWORM OF THE SCALP (Tinea Capitis)

Ringworm of the scalp is a fungal infection of the scalp and hair follicles.

Etiology

   1. Ringworm of the scalp is caused by different species of the *Microsporum* and *Tricophyton fungi.*
   2. Ringworm of the scalp is seen primarily in children before puberty.

Altered Physiology

   1. The fungal infection produces an inflammation of the scalp which causes alopecia and broken hairs.
   2. The lesions of the scalp may have papulovesicular erythematous borders or may appear only as scaling with a few broken hairs.
   3. Kerion, an acute inflammation which produces edema, pustules and granulomatous swelling, may occur.
   4. The infection may be spread through person-to-person contact, as well as through the common use of towels, combs, brushes, hats. Kittens and puppies may be the source of the infection.

Clinical Manifestations

1. The lesions usually develop in the occipital, temporal and parietal areas of the scalp.
2. Pruritus usually occurs in the area.
3. The involved areas of the scalp appear as patches, rounded or oval in outline, covered by scales and lusterless, irregularly broken hairs.
4. Single patches or multiple patches may occur.
5. Systematic manifestations are absent.
6. Evaluation
   a. Wood lamp—a filtered ultraviolet radiation causes microsporon infections to fluoresce with a brilliant, greenish light.
   b. Microscopic evaluation of infected hair follicles—to identify *Trichophyton* which fluoresces poorly under Wood Lamp.

Treatment

1. Griseofulvin—a fungistatic which is administered orally.
2. Duration of treatment is generally guided by periodic use of Wood Lamp or cultures.
3. Topical Whitfield's ointment or salicylanilide ointment may be used in conjunction with Griseofulvin.

Nursing Objectives

A. *To recognize the characteristic lesion of ringworm of the scalp.*
   1. Observe the condition of the hair and scalp, as a part of the routine assessment of the child on admission to the hospital.
   2. Report suspicious appearing lesions.
   3. Record the appearance and location of the lesions.
   4. Initiate appropriate methods to prevent the spread of the infection.
      a. Sterilized stocking caps are placed on the child's head to prevent the spread of infected hair follicles.
         (1) Explain to the child about the infection and why it is necessary for him to wear the cap.
         (2) Explain to other children on the ward why it is necessary for the child to wear the cap in order to prevent their cruel remarks.
         (3) Use creative methods to decorate the cap.
      b. Initiate the appropriate isolation techniques (as per hospital policy).

B. *To be aware of the side effects of the medications used in the treatment of ringworm of the scalp.*
   1. Griseofulvin may produce headache, heartburn, nausea, epigastric discomfort, diarrhea and urticaria.
   2. Record and report to the physician any side effects observed.

C. *To be aware of the case-finding measures to prevent additional cases and to identify the earliest evidence of infection.*
   1. All family contacts should be screened.
   2. The school should be notified so that appropriate case-finding techniques may be initiated.

D. *To teach the child and his family methods to prevent further episodes.*
    1. Teach general hygiene measures—regular shampooing and bathing.
    2. Advise them to avoid the common use of hats, combs, brushes, etc.
    3. Stress the importance of wearing the cap continuously until the infection has been eliminated.

PEDICULOSIS

Pediculosis is the infestation of human beings by lice.

Etiology
    1. Three types of lice affect human beings:
        a. *Pediculosis capitis*—head louse
        b. *Pediculosis corporis*—body louse
        c. *Phthirus pubic*—pubic louse
    2. Each type of louse generally remains in the area designated to its name, but occasionally may be seen in other areas of the body.
    3. The infestation occurs in areas of filth and poverty, where personal cleanliness is neglected, baths infrequently taken, and clothing kept on the body for long periods of time.
    4. Lice are transmitted by personal contact with people harboring them or through contact with articles which temporarily harbor them.

Altered Physiology
    1. The eggs of lice (nits) are attached to the hair or clothing by a sticky substance which hardens. The eggs hatch within 1 week—the lice reach maturity within 1 month and are then capable of reproducing.
    2. The lice on the skin produce itching; the longer the infestation persists, the more severe the skin reaction becomes and the more severe the lesions appear.

Clinical Manifestations
    1. Severe itching in the area affected is the primary symptom of pediculosis; scratch marks will be evident in these areas.
    2. In children, pubic lice are found most frequently in the eyelashes and eyebrows.
    3. Infested scalp areas may become secondarily infected from scratching.
    4. Crusts, pediculi, nits and dirt may combine to cause a foul odor and matted hair.
    5. Body lice may produce minute red lesions.

Treatment
Objective: to eliminate and remove nits and pediculi
           to treat the irritated skin
    1. *Pediculosis capitis* may be treated with gamma benzene hexachloride, benzyl benzoate or crotamiton.
    2. *Pediculosis corporis* may be treated with the above plus chlorophenothane powder.

Nursing Objectives
A. *To maintain technique which will prevent the spread of the infection.*
    Institute measures to carry out medical asepsis.

B. *To perform the treatments prescribed to destroy and eliminate the parasite.*

Observe and record the response to treatment.
   a. Note the change in the degree of discomfort caused by itching.
   b. Observe infected areas for changes in the characteristics of the lesions.
   c. Observe for systemic manifestations of infection.

C. *To provide measures to prevent the child from scratching himself.*
   1. Provide mittens or protective devices to prevent the child from scratching.
   2. Trim fingernails and toenails and keep clean.
   3. Provide the child with diversional therapy to distract him from itching.
   4. Hold the child frequently and release him from the protective devices.

D. *To provide appropriate teaching for the family to prevent recurrent attacks.*

E. *To screen the family for parasitic infection.*

SCABIES

Scabies is a disease of the skin produced by the burrowing action of a parasite resulting in irritation and the formation of vesicles or pustules.

Etiology
   1. Scabies is caused by the *Sarcoptes scabiei.*
   2. Scabies occurs most frequently in areas of poverty, where cleanliness is lacking.
   3. Scabies occurs as a result of direct contact with infected persons or by indirect contact through soiled bed linen, clothing, etc.

Altered Physiology
   1. Both the male and female parasite live upon the skin.
   2. The female parasite burrows into the superficial skin to deposit her eggs.
   3. The burrow is seen most commonly between the fingers but may occur in any natural fold of the skin or in pressure areas.
   4. The burrows may occur in any part of the body of infants and small children and are easily identifiable.
   5. Pruritus occurs, and the scratching of the skin may produce secondary infection.
   6. Inflammation may produce pustules and crusts.

Clinical Manifestations
   1. Itching, particularly at night, is the primary symptom. The itching is usually very severe.
   2. Scratching frequently produces secondary skin infection.
   3. Systemic manifestations are absent, unless they result from the secondary infection. (i.e., fever, leukocytosis).

Treatment
Objective: to destroy the parasite.
             to relieve itching and skin irritation.
A variety of medications are available to be used in irradicating the parasite.

Nursing Objectives
Same as for pediculosis, page 1267.

ORAL THRUSH

Oral thrush is a mycotic stomatitis characterized by the appearance of white plaques on the oral mucous membrane, the gums and the tongue.

Etiology

1. Oral thrush is caused by *Candida albicans*.
2. Oral thrush is most frequently seen in newborns, but may be seen in older infants.
3. Maternal vulvovaginal candidiasis is the primary source of neonatal thrush.
4. The growth of the organisms is favored by:
   - a. Lack of cleanliness
   - b. Malnutrition
   - c. Diabetes
   - d. Antibiotic treatment (destroys normal flora)
   - e. Neoplasms
   - f. Hyperparathyroidism
5. The infection may be acquired from:
   - a. Contaminated hands
   - b. Contaminated feeding equipment
   - c. Contaminated bedding
   - d. Another patient
6. Thrush frequently occurs in children with cleft lip and palate

Altered Physiology

1. Spores lodge between epithelial cells and gradually separate the layers.
2. The infection then spreads to the surface of the mucous membrane.
3. Growth usually begins in several discrete areas of the oral mucous membrane with gradual spreading to the point where a continuous membrane may be formed.

Clinical Manifestations

1. The infant develops small plaques on the oral mucous membrane, tongue or gums; these plaques appear like curds of milk but cannot be wiped out of the mouth.
2. Thrush appears to cause the infant no pain or discomfort.
3. The mouth may be dry.
4. Occasionally, the infant may appear to have some difficulty in swallowing.

Treatment

1. 1–2% aqueous solution of gentian violet swabbed in the mouth may be used.
2. Topical nystatin may be used.

Nursing Objectives

A. *To recognize the appearance of thrush and to be aware of the infant who is particularly susceptible to the development of thrush.*
1. Newborns and infants who have particular susceptibility include:
   - a. Sick, debilitated infants
   - b. Infants who are on antibiotic therapy
   - c. Infants with cleft lip and palate, parathyroidism, neoplasms, etc.
2. Report the appearance of thrush to the physician and record this information on the nursing record.

B. *To practice measures which serve to prevent the development and spread of thrush.*
1. Practice careful handwashing techniques.
2. Practice techniques which assure that nipples, bottles or any object which comes into direct or indirect contact with the infant's mouth is clean.

BIBLIOGRAPHY

Books

Barnett, H. (ed.): Pediatrics, 15th ed. New York, Appleton-Century-Crofts, 1972.

Blake, F. G., et al.: Nursing Care of Children, 8th ed. Philadelphia, J. B. Lippincott, 1970.

Christie, A. B.: Infectious Diseases: Epidemiology and Clinical Practice. London, E. & S. Livingston, Ltd., 1969.

Fontana, V.: Practical Management of the Allergic Child. New York, Appleton-Century-Crofts, 1969.

Nelson, W., et al. (eds.): Textbook of Pediatrics, 9th ed. Philadelphia, W. B. Saunders, 1969.

Ramsey, A., et al.: Infectious Diseases. London, William Heinemann Medical Books, Ltd., 1967.

Top, F., and Wehrle, P. F. (eds.): Communicable and Infectious Diseases, 7th ed. St. Louis, C. V. Mosby, 1972.

Articles

Bamford, H.: Burns in children. AORN J., *13*:56, 1971.

Bernstein, N. R., et al.: Nurse adaptation to treating severely burned children. Hospital Topics, *49*:6, 1971.

Caudia, S. M.: TLC and sulfamylon for burned children. Amer. J. Nurs., *69*:755–757, April 1969.

Faulkner, B. L.: From first base to home plate (burns). Amer. J. Nurs., *71*:2331–2333, Dec. 1971.

Fontana, V.: Lasting relief in childhood eczema. Consultant, *12*:30, 1972.

Lund, C. C., and Browder, N. C.: Estimation of areas of burns. Surg. Gyn., Obst., *79*:352, 1944.

Margolius, F.: Burned children: infections and nursing care. Nurs. Clin. N. Amer., *5*:131, 1970.

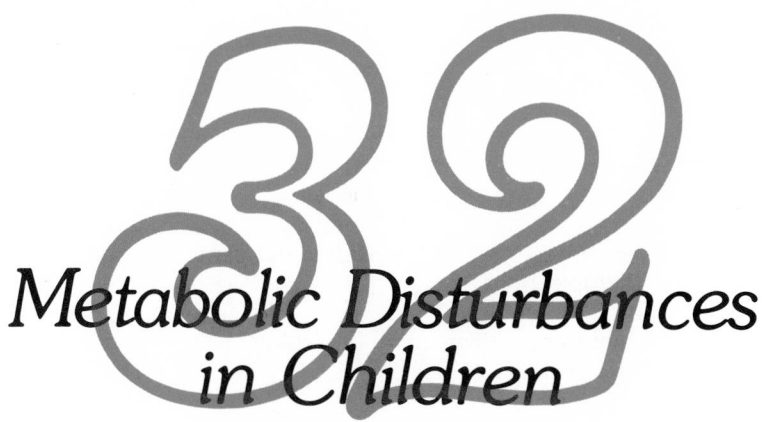

JUVENILE DIABETES MELLITUS

Diabetes mellitus is a disorder of carbohydrate metabolism resulting in high serum levels of glucose and the spilling of glucose in the urine. The disease is also associated with abnormal metabolism of fat and protein.

Etiology

1. An hereditary disease
2. Thought to be recessive in character
3. Parents of juvenile diabetics may be heterozygous for the disease

Altered Physiology

1. The pancreas produces an insufficient amount of insulin.
2. The body is unable to oxidize glucose properly.
3. Protein and fat are oxidized at abnormal rates.
4. Hyperglycemia results from the deficient oxidation of glucose and the inability of tissues to use glucose as fuel.
5. Glycosuria results when the serum level of glucose exceeds the renal threshold.
6. Diuresis is initiated and may progress to dehydration and impaired renal function.
7. Ketones accumulate in the blood when fat is oxidized at abnormal rates.
8. Ketones are excreted in the urine.
9. This leads to acidosis and may progress to diabetic coma.

Clinical Manifestations

1. Rapid onset (usually over a period of a few weeks)
2. Major symptoms
   a. Increased thirst
   b. Increased appetite
   c. Increased urination
   d. Wasting
   e. Easy fatigability

3. Minor symptoms
    a. Skin infections
    b. Dry skin
4. Diabetic acidosis
    a. Precomatose state

   Drowsiness   Nausea
   Dryness of skin   Vomiting
   Cherry red lips   Abdominal pain
   Increased respirations

    b. Comatose state

   Extreme hyperpnea, (Kussmaul breathing)   Rapid, weak pulse
   Soft, sunken eyeballs   Decreased temperature
   Rigid abdomen   Decreased blood pressure

Complications

1. Gangrene
2. Stunting of growth
3. Failure to develop secondary sex characteristics
4. Cataracts, arteriosclerosis and other degenerative vascular changes

Nursing Objectives

A. *To recognize signs of diabetic acidosis (see clinical manifestations) and provide supportive care to the child should this develop.*
    1. Beware of common causes of diabetic acidosis
        a. Untreated diabetes
        b. Inadequate insulin coverage
        c. Failure to adhere to the prescribed diet
        d. Chronic or repeated infections
    2. Apply the principles of nursing care of the comatose child. (See nursing the unconscious patient, p. 728.)
    3. Maintain intravenous therapy. (See I.V. procedure, p. 1087.)
        a. Be prepared to administer intravenous sodium bicarbonate.
        b. Have intravenous glucose available should the child suddenly become hypoglycemic.
    4. Be prepared to administer relatively large quantities of regular insulin.
        a. This may be 1½ units per kg. of weight initially.
        b. Subsequent dosage depends on the degree of ketosis and repeated blood glucose levels.
    5. Insert a nasogastric tube to relieve abdominal distention and prevent vomiting.
    6. Monitor urine output exactly.
       Test urinary sugar and acetone of each specimen.
    7. Provide emotional support to the child and his family.
        a. Respond immediately to the child's needs for physical comfort.
        b. Discuss the child's treatment plan and expected response with his parents to alleviate their anxiety.
    8. Reinstitute oral feedings when the child is sufficiently responsive and the acidosis has disappeared as evidenced by absence of acetone in the urine.
        a. This is usually after 12–16 hours of parenteral therapy.
        b. Begin with a low fat, liquid diet.

    c. Offer quantities of tea, fruit juice or milk to replace the large amount of potassium lost during the acute phase of acidosis.

    d. Observe closely for signs of insulin shock or recurrent acidosis once oral feedings are reinstituted.

  9. Begin a teaching program with the child as soon as possible to allay his worries concerning his physical status, prognosis and treatment.

B. *To provide a diet adequate for the child's normal growth and development and sufficient to satisfy his appetite.*

  1. The diet is restricted in carbohydrate and is usually based on the exchange method as recommended by the American Diabetes Association.

  2. Specific requirements are that the diet supply sufficient caloric intake for activity and growth, protein for growth, and the required vitamins and minerals.

  3. Determine the child's usual dietary habits so that adherence to his controlled diet will be easier.

  4. Allow the child normal activity while hospitalized so that the observed result of his dietary control will be valid.

  5. Allow the child to eat with other diabetic children (if available).

  6. Make certain that the child adheres to his prescribed diet.

  7. Make appropriate substitutions if necessary because of food preferences, etc.

  8. Include the child and his parents in his meal planning as soon as possible.

C. *To administer insulin in an amount adequate to maintain the child's approximate glycemic equilibrium.*

  1. The dose and kind of insulin is estimated from the results of fractional testing of the urine for sugar and acetone.

  2. Be aware of the major types of insulin and their effect (Table 32-1).

TABLE 32-1. TYPES OF INSULIN AND THEIR EFFECTS

TYPE OF INSULIN	ACTIVITY (Hours)		
	Onset	Maximal	Duration
Regular insulin	½–1	2–4	5–8
Semi-Lente insulin	½–¾	4–8	12–18
NPH insulin	½–2	8–12	24–30
Lente insulin	1–2	12–18	26–32

  3. Always administer insulin subcutaneously and not too near the skin.

  4. Develop a systematic plan for injections which emphasizes rotation of sites. In this way, it is possible to use each extremity for several weeks.

    a. Start the injections at the inner and upper corner of the area to be used. Each succeeding injection is made 1¼ cm. (½ inch) below the preceding one.

    b. When each vertical line is completed, the site should be moved outward 1¼ cm. at the upper level.

    c. This pattern should be followed until that extremity is exhausted and another is then utilized in the same manner.

    d. The upper arms and thighs are the most acceptable sites for injection in children, but the buttocks or abdomen may also be used.

  5. Observe the skin closely for signs of irritation. Avoid the injection site for several weeks if signs of local irritation are observed.

6. Observe the skin for a rash indicating an allergic reaction to the insulin.
7. Be aware of factors which vary the need for and utilization of insulin, particularly exercise and infection.
   a. Exercise
      (1) Tends to lower the blood sugar level.
      (2) Encourage normal activity, regulated in amount and time.
   b. Infection
      (1) Increases the child's insulin requirement.
      (2) Be alert for signs of infection.
8. Be alert for signs of insulin shock.
   a. Common causes
      (1) Overdose of insulin
      (2) Reduction in diet or exercise without a reduction in insulin
   b. Symptoms
      (1) Sudden hunger   (6) Dilated pupils
      (2) Weakness   (7) Tremors
      (3) Restlessness   (8) Dizziness
      (4) Pallor   (9) Unconsciousness
      (5) Sweating
   c. Be prepared to give orange juice or other food containing readily available simple sugars.
   d. Have glucose available for intravenous injection or glycogen available for intramuscular injection.

D. *To test the child's urine regularly for sugar and acetone in order to determine the effectiveness of treatment.*
   1. Collect urine specimens 4 times daily, before each meal and before bed.
      a. Because analysis is more accurate if the second voided specimen is used, have the child void from ½–1 hour before each of the specimens to be tested is obtained.
      b. Discard the first specimen and test the second.
      c. Since obtaining specimens from young children may be difficult, it may be preferable to test the urine with each voiding.
   2. Record the results of urine testing accurately.
      a. Use a form so that the information will be clear and readily available.
      b. Help the child to understand about controlling his disease by teaching him to record urine test results on the form.

E. *To prevent infection.*
   1. Bathe daily.
   2. Maintain meticulous skin care through frequent ambulation of the child, application of body lotion, etc.
   3. Keep fingernails and toenails clean and well trimmed.
   4. Provide prompt treatment for any violations of the skin (bruises, abrasions, lacerations, etc.).

F. *To foster acceptance on the part of the child that he is a normal, healthy person and able to compete with his peers.*
   1. Include the child and his parents in the treatment plan at its earliest stages.
   2. Emphasize that daily management of his disease can become as routine as matters of personal hygiene.

3. Permit and encourage the development of the child's natural talents. Do not allow him to use his disease as a crutch.
4. Allow the child independence in his care as soon as possible, but provide the necessary direction.
5. Initiate a teaching program for the child and his parents early. Offer them available literature.
6. Invite parents to join a group of parents of diabetic children if such a group is available in the area.
7. Initiate a community nursing referral if the parents or the child appear exceptionally apprehensive or unsure of themselves.

Patient or Parental Teaching

Patient teaching is one of the most important aspects in the nursing care of the diabetic child. It is essential in the following areas:
1. Recognition of the signs of insulin shock and diabetic acidosis and knowledge of their treatment.
2. The influence of exercise on the body's requirement for insulin.
   Encourage moderate exercise regularly every day.
3. Prevention of infection
   a. Give frequent baths.
   b. Attend to regular body hygiene with special attention to foot care.
   c. Report any breaks in the skin. Treat them promptly.
   d. Report infections promptly to the physician.
   e. Discard shoes and replace as the child outgrows them.
   f. Dress the child appropriately for the weather.
   g. Keep the child away from people with upper respiratory or other infections.
   h. See that child receives regular dental check-ups and maintenance.
   i. Follow routine immunizations according to the recommended schedule.
4. Urine testing
   a. Demonstrate the procedure.
   b. Have the child and his parent demonstrate to the nurse.
   c. Allow the child to do the procedure under supervision until his accuracy is certain.
   d. Encourage the child to assume responsibility for his own urine testing.
   e. Help the child to develop an easy method of recording urine results.
5. Administration of insulin
   a. Both the child and his parents should be taught how to do this procedure and what effects the various forms of insulin have.
   b. Explain the procedure simply and demonstrate.
   c. Have the parent and the child practice insulin administration using an orange or similar object.
   d. Allow the parent and child to practice by injecting normal saline into the nurse.
   e. Have the parent inject his child under supervision.
   f. Have the child inject himself.
      (1) Most children over the age of 7 can be taught to give insulin to themselves.
      (2) Generally, the earlier this responsibility is given to the child, the easier it is for him.
   g. Carefully check the dosage measured by the child and his parent until certain of their accuracy.

    h. Complete a community nursing referral for assistance with this procedure at home if indicated.

6. Maintenance and sterilization of insulin equipment
    a. The use of disposable equipment should be encouraged because it is easier and safer.
    b. Nondisposable syringes and needles must be sterilized before each injection in the following manner:
      (1) Remove the plunger from the barrel of the syringe.
      (2) Place them both into a strainer along with the needle.
      (3) Place the strainer in a saucepan of water and boil for 5 minutes.
        If the family does not have a strainer, the syringe parts and needle should be wrapped in gauze before being placed in water.
      (4) Reassemble the syringe being careful to touch only the outside of the syringe and the knob of the plunger.
      (5) Slip the needle onto the syringe with a twisting motion, being careful to touch only the hub of the needle, never its point.
      (6) Work the plunger back and forth several times to force out any water that remains in it.
      (7) A community nursing referral may also be indicated to assist the family with this procedure until they feel comfortable doing it.

7. Diet
    a. Review the prescribed diet with the family.
    b. Discuss acceptable modifications of exchanges.
    c. Allow the child to manage his own diet as early as possible.
    d. Emphasize that the diet is based on normal household foods. The purchase of special, dietetic and expensive foods is usually not necessary.
    e. Stress that food labels must be scrutinized. A label of "dietetic" or "low-calorie" does not necessarily mean that the food is acceptable for the child.

8. Precautionary measures
    a. Have the child carry with him an identifying card which states that he has diabetes and includes his name, address, phone number and his physician's name and phone number.
    b. See that the child has orange juice, a lump of sugar or a bar of candy available in case of insulin reaction.
    c. Have the family discuss the child's disease with the school nurse and with other responsible adults who are in close contact with the child (teachers, scout leaders, etc.).

DIABETES INSIPIDUS

Diabetes insipidus is a disorder of water metabolism caused by a deficiency of vasopressin, the antidiuretic hormone (ADH) secreted by the posterior pituitary.

Etiology

1. Deficient secretion of vasopressin (antidiuretic hormone)
    a. Idiopathic
    b. Lesions of the posterior pituitary or hypothalamus
      (1) Tumors
      (2) Infections
      (3) Trauma

2. Failure of the renal tubules to respond to vasopressin (nephrogenic diabetes insipidus)
   a. Hereditary (dominant) disease
   b. More common in males

Altered Physiology

1. Vasopressin normally acts on the distal tubules and collecting ducts of the kidney to facilitate reabsorption of water.
2. Pathology of the pituitary or hypothalamus results in a deficiency of vasopressin.
3. The kidney is unable to produce a concentrated urine without sufficient vasopressin.
4. Nephrogenic diabetes insipidus
   a. Vasopressin secretion is normal.
   b. The renal tubules do not respond to vasopressin.
   c. The kidney is unable to produce a concentrated urine.

Clinical Manifestations

1. Onset—usually sudden
2. Symptoms
   a. Depends on the age of the child and his primary lesion
   b. Universal symptoms
      (1) Polydipsia (excessive thirst)
      (2) Polyuria (excessive urine output)
      (3) Inability to concentrate urine
   c. Symptoms in infants
      (1) Excessive crying (Quieted with water rather than additional milk)
      (2) Hyperthermia
      (3) Vomiting
      (4) Constipation
      (5) Rapid weight loss
      (6) Dehydration
      (7) Growth failure
   d. Symptoms in older children
      (1) Excessive thirst
         (a) Interferes with play and sleep
         (b) Anorexia
         (c) Pale and dry skin
         (d) Enuresis

Nursing Objectives

A. *To prevent dehydration and restore electrolyte balance.*
   1. Nursing actions when the disorder is caused by a deficiency of vasopressin.
      a. Pitressin tannate in oil is the preparation of choice for replacement therapy.
         (1) Dosage
            (a) Regulated by trial for each child.
            (b) Usual dose is 0.3–2.0 ml. every 2–4 days.
         (2) Route of administration
            (a) Intramuscular
            (b) Never intravenously
         (3) Special precautions
            (a) Careful attention must be given to adequate suspension of the pitressin tannate in oil.
            (b) Inject the medication with a 2.5-cm. (1-inch) No. 20–22 gauge needle.
            (c) Inject the medication deeply into the muscle.

(d) Establish a pattern of systematic rotation of injection sites.

(e) Used with caution in patients with vascular disease or epilepsy.

   b. Pitressin may also be administered as a nose spray or drops.

  2. Nursing actions when the disorder is caused by failure of the kidney to respond to vasopressin.

    a. Administration of pitressin is ineffective.

      These children already produce a sufficient quantity of vasopressin.

    b. Offer relatively large quantities of fluids at frequent intervals.

B. *To observe and record the child's response to therapy.*

  1. Intake and output

    a. Total the intake and output record every 8 hours.

    b. Record the urine specific gravity of each voiding.

  2. Temperature

    Be alert for the development of fever

  3. Skin turgor

    Decreased skin turgor is sign of dehydration

  4. Color

  5. Appetite

    Record the child's intake accurately with each meal.

C. *To participate in laboratory tests for diabetes insipidus.*

  1. Test to differentiate diabetes insipidus from psychogenic polydipsia and polyuria.

    a. Hydrate the child.

    b. Withhold fluids and food for 6 hours.

    c. Collect a urine sample and test it for specific gravity.

    d. The specific gravity will not rise above 1.008 if the child has diabetes insipidus.

  2. The pitressin and hypertonic saline tests.

    a. Explain the test to the child and his parents

      (1) Purpose of the test

        To establish the diagnosis and the specific variety of the disorder.

      (2) Procedure

        (a) Start an I.V. of 5% dextrose.

        (b) Collect urine samples initially and every 20 minutes for 1 hour.
Record volume and specific gravity with each voiding.

        (c) Change the I.V. solution to 2.5% saline once water diuresis has reached a steady state.

        (d) Collect, measure and test urine samples for specific gravity at the onset and twice more at 20-minute intervals.

        (e) Inject vasopressin I.V. and restart the 5% dextrose infusion simultaneously.
Dose of vasopressin is calculated by the physician.

        (f) Collect and assay urine as before for 1 hour.

    b. Maintain the appropriate intravenous infusion. (See procedure for the administration of intravenous fluids, p. 1087.)

    c. Collect the urine specimens.

      (1) Attempt to collect the urine on schedule.

(2) Record carefully:
    (a) Time of the collection
    (b) Type of infusion running at the time of collection
    (c) Volume of urine
    (d) Specific gravity of urine

D. *To provide emotional support to the family.*

Prognosis depends on the underlying condition.
1. Hereditary and idiopathic types
    Favorable with adequate treatment.
2. Trauma
    Spontaneous recovery often occurs.
3. Tumor
    a. Varies with the site of the lesion and type of tumor.
    b. Needs of the family accentuated by many problems including surgery and facing the death of the child.

HYPOTHYROIDISM

Hypothyroidism is an endocrine disease resulting from deficient production of thyroid hormone. It may be either congenital (cretinism) or acquired (juvenile hypothyroidism).

Etiology

A. *Congenital*
1. Embryonic defect with partial or complete absence of the thyroid gland
2. Destruction of fetal thyroid as a result of antigen-antibody reaction
3. Defect in the synthesis of thyroid hormone
    Nonendemic goiterous cretinism
4. Ingestion of medications during pregnancy
    a. Propylthiouracil
    b. Methimazole
    c. Iodides
5. Iodide deficiency
    Endemic cretinism

B. *Acquired*
1. Hypoplasia of the thyroid gland
2. Partial defect of thyroid hormone
3. Disease
    a. Autoimmune disease
    b. Cancer
    c. Infection
4. Thyroidectomy
5. Medications
    a. Iodides
    b. Cobalt
    c. Propylthiouracil
6. Iodine deficiency
7. Unknown

Clinical Manifestations

1. Approximately 3 times more common in females than males.
2. Severity of clinical findings depends on the age at onset.

3. Early signs and symptoms (several days or weeks after birth).
   a. Prolonged physiological jaundice
   b. Nasal obstruction and stuffiness
   c. Feeding difficulties
   d. Hoarse cry
   e. Decreased intestinal activity—constipation
   f. Poor muscle tone—umbilical hernia
   g. Physical and mental sluggishness
   h. Subnormal temperature
   i. General appearance
      (1) Skin—dry, thick, scaly, coarse, cool and pale
      (2) Facial characteristics
         (a) Bridge of nose—flat, broad and undeveloped
         (b) Eyes—widely spaced with swollen eyelids
         (c) Anterior fontanelle widely open
         (d) Tongue—thick and protruding
      (3) Hair—frequently excessive, dry, coarse, and brittle
      (4) Skeletal
         (a) Short, thick neck
         (b) Broad hands
         (c) Short fingers
4. Later signs and symptoms
   a. Poor muscle tone
      (1) Protuberant abdomen
      (2) Lumbar lordosis
   b. Delayed dentition
      Teeth decay easily
   c. Delayed skeletal development
      (1) Short stature
      (2) Retarded bone age
      (3) Infantile skeletal proportions
         (a) Large head
         (b) Short extremities
   d. Slow motor and mental development
      (1) Late sitting, standing, walking, talking
      (2) Late attaining normal milestones
      (3) Subnormal intelligence
   e. Retarded sexual development

Diagnostic Evaluation

1. X-ray—shows retarded bone age
2. Cholesterol level—elevated
3. Basal metabolic rate—low
4. Plasma bound iodine—low
5. Radioactive iodine uptake—low
6. Alkaline phosphatase—reduced
7. Creatinine—elevated
8. Urinary creatinine excretion—increased

Prognosis

1. Depends on the child's age at onset and the effectiveness of his therapy
2. If untreated—mentally deficient dwarf results
3. When treated:
   a. Normal physical growth and development
   b. Mental development unpredictable (usually remains somewhat retarded)

Altered Physiology

Same as in the adult. (See section on hypothyroidism, p. 626.)

Nursing Objectives

A. *To administer dessicated thyroid as replacement therapy for the deficient hormone.*
  1. Dosage
     a. Initially very low.
     b. Gradually increased to the maximum amount which the child can tolerate without producing signs of toxicity.
  2. Route of administration
     a. Always administer dessicated thyroid by the oral route.
     b. The tablet may be crushed and mixed with fruit for infants.
  3. Special precautions
     a. The total daily requirement is given as a single dose.
     b. Administer the medication at the same time each day.
  4. Observe for toxic effects.
     a. Excitability   d. Diarrhea
     b. Tachycardia   e. Fever
     c. Cramps   f. Vomiting

B. *To provide a complete, well-balanced diet.*
  1. Special problems related to nutrition
     a. Anemia
        (1) Increases the child's need for iron.
        (2) Include high quantities of meat, fish, poultry, eggs, enriched breads and cereals in the child's diet.
     b. Increased skeletal development
        (1) Increases the need for additional vitamin D.
        (2) Encourage the child to drink 3–4 glasses of milk daily.
     c. Constipation
        Provide foods which are high in roughage such as raw fruits and vegetables.
  2. Determine the child's dietary preferences and use this information to plan his menus. Include the child in menu planning when this is possible.

C. *To prevent tooth decay.*
  1. Provide mouth care after each meal.
  2. Discourage the intake of sweets, gum, soda, etc.

D. *To provide support to the parents of a mentally defective child.* (See section on mental retardation, p. 1356.)

Patient or Parental Teaching

A. *Medication*
  1. Give the medication conscientiously at the same time every day.
  2. Adjust the dosage (by the physician) to the needs of each individual child.
     a. Regular medical follow-up and frequent re-evaluation are essential.
     b. Dose may have to be increased during puberty and the reproductive period.

3. The medication must be continued throughout life.
4. Allow the parent to administer the medication during the child's hospitalization so that she will be confident of the procedure.

B. *Diet*
   1. Discuss the importance of a well-balanced diet.
   2. Suggest sample menus. These should be economical and based on the family's normal dietary patterns.
   3. Refer the family to an appropriate social service if they are unable to afford sufficient food.
   4. Assist the mother of an infant with techniques of feeding.

C. *Dental Care*
   1. Teach the child correct techniques for brushing his teeth.
      Stress that he should follow this procedure after each meal.
   2. Encourage regular (every 6 months) evaluations by a dentist.
      Refer the family to a dental clinic if necessary.

HYPERTHYROIDISM

Hyperthyroidism is an endocrine disease resulting from an excessive secretion of thyroid hormone. It is frequently characterized by an enlarged thyroid gland (goiter) and prominent eyeballs (exophthalmus).

Etiology

1. Unknown
2. Possible precipitating factors
   a. Infection   c. Autoimmune response
   b. Psychic trauma   d. Heredity

Clinical Manifestations

1. Rare and less severe in children as compared to adults.
2. Incidence is 6 times higher in females than males.
3. Onset is usually between 10–15 years of age (usually gradual onset).
4. Signs and symptoms
   a. Enlarged thyroid gland (goiter)   g. Skin
   b. Exophthalmus   Warm
   c. Nervousness and motor hyperactivity   Moist
      (1) Inability to sit still   Flushed
      (2) Decreased attention span   h. Muscular weakness and fatigue
      (3) Mood shifts   i. Tachycardia, palpitation and dyspnea
             Irritable   j. Increased systolic blood pressure
             Excitable   Increased pulse pressure
             Cries easily   k. Accelerated growth rate
   d. Increased appetite and food intake   l. Delayed sexual maturation
   e. Weight loss or no weight gain   Amenorrhea is common in females
   f. Increased urinary excretion   m. Thyroid "crisis" or "storm" (very rare
                                                  in children)

Diagnostic Evaluation

1. Radioactive iodine uptake—rapid
2. Plasma-bound iodine—high
3. Basal metabolic rate—increased
4. Glucose tolerance—decreased
5. Cholesterol—low
6. Urinary creatinine excretion—elevated

Altered Physiology

Same as in the adult. (See section on hyperthyroidism, p. 627.)

Nursing Objectives

Nursing care of the child with hyperthyroidism is similar to that of the adult (see section on hyperthyroidism). The following objectives are of special importance in pediatrics:

A. *To avoid excitement.*
   1. Provide a quiet environment.
      a. Avoid assigning the child to a large ward or room with several other patients.
      b. Limit the number of playmates that the child has at any one time.
      c. Maintain a fairly constant schedule of daily activities.
      d. Sedate if necessary.
         (1) Barbiturates or tranquilizers are the drugs of choice.
         (2) Sedation may be especially beneficial at bedtime.
   2. Encourage quiet rather than strenuous activities.
      Interest the child in diversionary activities which do not require lengthy mental concentration.
   3. Maintain constant but gentle discipline.

B. *To provide a diet high in protein, calories and vitamins.*
   1. Offer between-meal snacks such as milk shakes.
   2. Vitamin supplements may be necessary.

C. *To administer propylthiouracil or methimazole.*
   1. Dose
      a. Dosage must be individually regulated for each child.
      b. It is essential to space the dose at regular intervals (every 6–8 hours) throughout a 24-hour period.
         Each dose is fully effective for only a few hours.
   2. Observe for clinical response.
      a. Disappearance of symptoms including enlargement of the thyroid gland.
      b. Usually apparent in 2–3 weeks.
      c. Exophthalmus may not reverse, but it should not advance.
   3. Observe for toxic effects.
      a. Fever
      b. Mild, sometimes purpuric, papular rash
      c. Headache
      d. Nausea, abdominal cramps, diarrhea
      e. Pain and stiffness in joints, especially hands and wrists
   4. Observe for relapse when the drug is discontinued.
      a. Usually discontinued slowly after 1–2 years of administration.
      b. Relapse usually occurs within 6 months of discontinuing the drug.
      c. Treatment usually continued throughout early adolescence in pubertal children.

D. *To demonstrate understanding of the child's physical and emotional problems.*
 1. The disease frequently has its onset during adolescence when the child is very concerned with his body image.
 2. Encourage the child to talk about his disease and how he feels about it.
  Correct misinformation and misinterpretations as necessary.
 3. Assist the adolescent girl to apply make-up which can significantly reduce the obviousness of her exophthalmus.
 4. Discuss the child's disease and treatment with his parents and teachers so that their demands and expectations will be realistic.

Patient or Parental Teaching

A. *Medication*
 1. Allow the parent to administer the child's medication under supervision during his hospitalization to ensure accuracy after discharge.
 2. Points of emphasis
  a. The medication must be administered in the exact amount that was ordered.
  b. Daily administration of the drug at regular intervals is essential.
  c. The child must be observed for signs and symptoms of drug toxicity.

B. *Medical supervision*
  Close medical follow-up is necessary in order to evaluate the child's progress and regulate his drug dosage.

C. *Suggested source material*
 1. *Books for the diabetic patient and his family*
  Dolger, H., and Seeman, B.: How to Live With Diabetes. New York, W. W. Norton and Company, 1965.
  Fischer, A. E., and Horstmann, D. L.: A Handbook for the Young Diabetic. New York, Intercontinental Medical Book Corporation, 1964.
  Ferguson, M. P.: An Introduction to Diabetes for the Young Child. Springfield, Illinois, Charles C Thomas, 1972.
  Rogers, F. L., and Leverton, R. M.: Your Diabetes and How to Live With It. Lincoln, University of Nebraska Press, 1961.
  Rosenthal, H., and Rosenthal, J.: Diabetic Care in Pictures. Philadelphia, J. B. Lippincott Company, 1968.
  Schmitt, G. F.: Diabetes for Diabetics. Miami, Diabetes Press of America, 1968.
 2. *Teaching aids and other information*
  American Diabetes Association (18 East 48th St., New York, New York 10017) Facts About Diabetes.
  British Diabetic Association (152 Harley St., London) Diabetes in Childhood and Adolescence.
  Eli Lilly and Company (Indianapolis, Indiana, 46206) A Guide for the Diabetic.
  E. R. Squibb and Sons (745 Fifth Ave., New York, New York) A Handbook for Diabetics.
  Upjohn Company (Kalamazoo, Michigan 49001) Calorie Control for You. You and Diabetes.
  U.S. Department of Health, Education and Welfare (Government Printing Office, Washington, D.C. 20402) Are You Related To A Diabetic? Diabetes Mellitus, A Guide for Nurses.

BIBLIOGRAPHY

Books

American Diabetes Association: Learning About Diabetes. New York, American Diabetes Association Inc., 1969.

Blake, F., et al.: Nursing Care of Children. Philadelphia, J. B. Lippincott, 1970.

Dolger, H., and Seeman, B.: How To Live With Diabetes. New York, Pyramid Books, 1968.

Gardner, L. (ed.): Endocrine and Genetic Diseases of Childhood. Philadelphia, W. B. Saunders, 1969.

Gillis, S. S., and Kagan, B. M. (eds.): Current Pediatric Therapy. Philadelphia, W. B. Saunders, 1970.

Marlow, D. R.: Textbook of Pediatric Nursing. Philadelphia, W. B. Saunders, 1973.

Nelson, W., et al.: Textbook of Pediatrics. Philadelphia, W. B. Saunders, 1969.

Rosenthal, H., and Rosenthal, J.: Diabetic Care in Pictures. Philadelphia, J. B. Lippincott, 1968.

Silver, H., et al.: Handbook of Pediatrics. Los Altos, California, Lange Medical Publications, 1971.

Steiner, M. M.: Clinical Approach to Endocrine Problems in Children. St. Louis, C. V. Mosby, 1970.

Articles

Huang, S. H.: Nursing assessment in planning care for a diabetic patient. Nurs. Clin. N. Amer., 6:135–143, March 1971.

Watkins, J. D.: Nursing assessment of the patient's management of diabetes mellitus. Diabetes Consultation and Education Service, ANA Clinical Sessions, pp. 23–29, 1970.

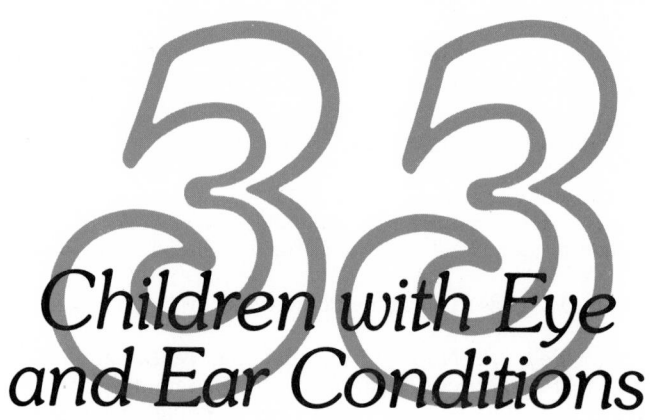

Children with Eye and Ear Conditions

1. Conditions of the Eye

THE BLIND CHILD

Impaired vision (blindness) refers to insufficient or inadequate vision in varying degrees, which prevents a person from being able to perform the ordinary activities of daily living.

Etiology

1. Familial factors
   Genetic determination
2. Prenatal or intrauterine factors
   a. Rubella
   b. Toxoplasmosis
   c. Syphilis
3. Perinatal factors
   a. Prematurity
   b. Oxygen poisoning—retrolental fibroplasia
   c. Infections
4. Postnatal factors
   a. Injury or trauma
   b. Infections
   c. Inflammatory disease

Altered Physiology

1. Defective visual fields
2. Impaired color vision
3. Decreased visual acuity
4. No vision—or a small percent of vision (may have light perception)

Clinical Manifestations

A. *Infant*
   1. No eye-to-eye contact, especially with mother
   2. Abnormal eye movements
   3. Does not follow objects at 2 months of age
   4. Failure to locate distant objects at 6–12 months of age
   5. Mother senses "something is wrong"

B. *Older Child*
   1. Squinting, frequent blinking
   2. Bumping into things
   3. Awkward gait
   4. Holding work too close to eyes; sitting too close to television
   5. Doing poorly at school

Diagnostic Evaluation

   1. Legal definition—visual acuity 20/200 or less with correction
   2. Tunnel vision—peripheral field of vision has an angular distance not greater than 20 degrees

Treatment

   1. Surgical repair of defect
   2. Glasses
   3. Special training
      a. Language development and acquisition
      b. Mobility-perceptual motor training

Nursing Objectives

The nurse may become involved with the blind child in the hospital in 2 critical situations: (1) before diagnosis has been made when she may detect a visual loss, usually in an infant, and (2) after diagnosis has been made when giving nursing care to the hospitalized blind child.

DETECTION AND EARLY CARE OF THE BLIND CHILD AFTER DIAGNOSIS

A. *To be familiar with the normal pattern of visual development and to be able to recognize deviations as well as manifestations of visual impairment.*
   1. Knowing the stages of growth and development can be helpful in recognizing or suspecting visual impairment or blindness in the individual child.
   2. The appreciation of vision by the infant begins at about 3 months of age; before this he recognizes dark and light.
   3. Be alert to and assess the child's response to visual stimulation.
      a. Does the infant follow the human face or bright object with his eyes according to development stage?
      b. Does the infant reach for objects?
      c. Does the 9- to 12-month-old child move around?

B. *To be familiar with the causes of visual impairment and blindness in order to recognize from the history whether or not the child is in a high-risk stage.*
   1. Neonatal and perinatal factors
      a. Prematurity
      b. Oxygen therapy
      c. Infections
   2. Past infections—inflammatory diseases

C. *To record observations and report any suspicious behavior by the infant or child indicating visual impairment.*
   1. Early diagnosis is the key to successful habilitation and optimal development of the child's capabilities.
   2. The complication of complete withdrawal of the child can be avoided by early diagnosis and proper stimulation and emotional support.

D. *To be familiar with the community resources and the professional team to be involved in habilitation of the visually impaired or blind child.*
   Several types of school programs are available to the child, depending upon his confidence and coping abilities.
      a. Residential schools
         (1) Used when nothing is available in the local community.
         (2) Preferred when the home care of the child would be detrimental to his progress.
      b. Day schools for the blind (attends school during day but lives at home)
      c. Public school where blind child is integrated with sighted child (have special training in braille)
      d. Vocational rehabilitation programs (training for some occupation)

E. *To work with physician and parents in helping the child master certain developmental tasks thus aiding the child in achieving his fullest potential.* Parents need help in recognizing the clues the child presents indicating his need and readiness for new learning experiences. The child must also learn in his own natural way.
   1. Communication between mother and child
      Mother must learn techniques of touching and handling and talking to the child.
   2. The child must be allowed and encouraged to use his hands for exploring his world.
      a. Give child objects of different shapes, sizes and textures.
      b. Allow child to finger-feed himself at about 10 months of age.
   3. The child needs to learn to become mobile.
      Mother's voice can encourage child to move toward her.
   4. The child needs much help in learning to talk.
      a. Expose the child to sounds that have a specific function—cleaning equipment, dishes
      b. Mother should talk a great deal to the child.
   5. The child needs social exposure to his peers.
      Nursery school can be very helpful.

F. *To foster continual acceptance of the child by his parents and provide support for them.*
   1. Evaluate the parents' state and offer them reassurance and explanations.
      a. Parental acceptance and a healthy home atmosphere are vitally important in helping the visually impaired or blind child accept and adjust to his limitations.
      b. The child can sense his parents' approval or disapproval and the degree to which they love and accept him.

2. Help parents to understand and accept their responsibilities in the care of their child. Indicate that they should:
   a. Provide proper stimulation for the child to learn that which is ordinarily learned through vision.
   b. Avoid being overprotective of the child.
   c. Accept the child as an individual with unique needs, without undue emphasis on his handicap.
3. Help parents understand how they can develop the child's skills in interpreting information through the senses of hearing, touch, smell and taste.
   a. Hearing
      (1) Help child to determine distance by ringing a bell.
      (2) Familiarize him with appliances, birds, voices.
   b. Touch
      Allow child to handle different textured material.
   c. Smell
      Acquaint child with flowers, perfume, kitchen odors.
   d. Taste
      Help child distinguish different kitchen substances.
   e. Memory
      Have child practice retelling stories, his telephone number, address, etc.
4. Initiate referral to the public health or community nurse who can make home visits to reinforce and interpret what mother has heard from the physician and to encourage mother in her efforts.
5. Encourage parents to discuss their feelings about caring for a handicapped child at home.
      Initiate a social worker referral. (The social worker can help parents deal with their feelings.)
6. Help parents understand the problems the child faces and will face as he gets older.
   a. Child will probably be delayed in development—first recognized about 2 years of age.
   b. Training may be more difficult, especially self-feeding and toileting.
   c. Child will be unable to conceptualize—words about color, motion, shape are vague; thus learning experiences are different.
   d. Blindisms—habits or mannerisms of blind children
      (1) Eye-rubbing, rocking, body turning and hand-waving
      (2) These are normal and disappear as the child becomes more confident and competent in managing himself and his world
   e. Child must cope with growing up as well as being blind.
7. Encourage parents to write for literature on blindness.*

G. *To evaluate how well the child who was once able to see accepts visual impairment, as far as his physical abilities and psychologic dependence are concerned.*
   1. A serious impairment in relationships with people can result when the child is unable to express his innermost sentiments.
   2. Allow the child to express his feelings, especially of fear and anger. Talk, play and certain activities help the child express these feelings.

* American Foundation for the Blind, Inc.   National Society for the Prevention of Blindness, Inc.
  15 West 16th Street   79 Madison Avenue
  New York, New York 10011   New York, New York 10016

HOSPITAL CARE OF THE VISUALLY IMPAIRED OR BLIND CHILD

Many of the important areas discussed above must be considered when caring for the child in the hospital situation. In addition, emphasis must be placed on the following objectives:

A. *To interview the parents at the time of admission to learn as much as possible about the child and his care and activities at home.*
  1. Be aware of the child's schedule and activities during the day. Know what activities he can or cannot do, and what he likes to do.
  2. Become familiar with how he is oriented to his new surroundings.
     a. How much does he ambulate?
     b. What precautions are necessary?
  3. Be aware of how parents comfort and discipline the child.
       How does he comfort himself or seek security?
  4. What special care or treatment must be continued while the child is hospitalized?
  5. Share this information with nursing staff in a nursing care plan so continuity of care from home to hospital can minimize fear and frustration in the child.

B. *To attend to the child's needs according to the medical problem that required his hospitalization.*

C. *To plan and provide for the appropriate type of play, activities program and stimulation for the child.*
  1. Assess the child's level of growth and development and use the information obtained from parents.
  2. Allow the child as much independence as possible in his care, but provide guidance as necessary.
       Orient the ambulatory child thoroughly to his room and surroundings.
  3. Encourage the development of the child's abilities. Avoid overprotecting him.
  4. Provide activities that will increase his learning and give him pleasure (talking records).

D. *To meet the psychological and emotional needs of the visually impaired or blind child for protection and security against harm.*
  1. The nurse should always speak to the child prior to touching him so as not to frighten or startle him.
  2. Always use a warm and gentle touch.
  3. Explain strange sounds that may be frightening.
  4. Plan frequent nurse-patient interactions to increase the child's sense of security.
  5. Place items he needs and uses within his reach.
       Familiar items that give the child security should also be close to him.

E. *To avoid overemphasizing the child's handicap and to be unobtrusive about meeting his needs.*
       Allow the child to explore and learn about his new environment and the hospital.

F. *To provide continual parental support.*
  1. Encourage parents to become involved in the care of their child to help maintain or develop a healthy parent-child relationship.
  2. Encourage parents to talk about their fears and feelings concerning this child. Help them relax.
       Parents can be invaluable in increasing the security and decreasing the fear the child may have as a result of being in a strange place.

3. Discuss realistically long-term and short-term planning for the child, i.e., educational opportunities.
   a. Encourage parents to tell teachers and adults responsible for his care about his special needs.
   b. Avoid overemphasis on educational achievements.
4. Help parents understand that discipline, order and consistency are necessary in the child's environment to give him security.
5. Emphasize that the parents' role is to give this child love and physical care as well as to stimulate and influence him so he may have a satisfactory mental, social and emotional growth.
6. Help parents see that other members of the family must also be considered.
   a. Their handicapped child does need special attention, but he does not need all the attention all the time.
   b. Other members of the family should be included in his care, but they also have a life of their own and need as much attention from parents as they would have if the handicapped child were not present in the family.
   c. Parents need time to themselves. They should be encouraged to go out alone together and to give time to their marriage.
7. Help parents realize that even though habilitation of their blind child is long, drawn out and expensive, the child may be able to live a normal life in the community.
   a. Are parents aware of and accept the short- and long-term goals?
   b. Many blind people are successful as technicians and professionals.

EYE DEFECTS REQUIRING SURGERY

Eye defects requiring surgery are (1) structural manifestations of the eye present at birth or (2) acquired conditions of the eye. They can be extraocular or intraocular conditions.

Etiology

1. Congenital
   a. Hereditary tendencies
   b. Birth injury
   c. Innervational factors
   d. Intrauterine influences
2. Disease
   a. Metabolic
   b. Infection
3. Trauma to the eye

Strabismus

Strabismus is the inability to balance the extraocular muscles; thus the eyes cannot function together at the same time.

Altered Physiology

The visual axis of only 1 eye goes to the object being observed. Person appears to be looking in 2 directions at once.

Clinical Manifestations

1. Deviations of the eye (constant or intermittent)
2. Squinting
3. Closing 1 eye to see
4. Tilting head
5. Stumbling or clumsy behavior
6. Inaccuracy in picking up objects
7. Double vision

Complications

1. Amblyopia ex anopsia—poor vision in eye not used
2. Emotional problems resulting from cosmetic aspect of deformity

Treatment

1. Corrective glasses
2. Orthoptics
   a. Therapeutic eye exercises
   b. Patching nondiverging eye
3. Surgery
   Lengthening or shortening of extraocular structures

Cataract

Cataract is an opacification or milk-white appearance of the eye lens.

Altered Physiology

Inability of light to pass through the clouded lens in adequate amounts—loss of vision as lens becomes more opaque.

Clinical Manifestations

1. Gradual diminution of visual acuity
2. Strabismus
3. Nystagmus
4. Gray opacities of lens

Diagnostic Evaluation

Ophthalmoscopic examination reveals an opaque area which appears black.

Treatment

1. Medication—dilation of pupil with mydriatic eye drops
2. Surgery
   a. Optical iridectomy
   b. Discission—breaking up of lens cortex and nucleus and aspiration
   c. Removal of lens or capsule

Complications

Following surgery for congenital cataract:
1. Retinal detachment several years later
2. Average vision only 20/70
3. Need for glasses for light refraction

Trauma

Trauma is injury to the globe, adnexa and surrounding tissue of the eye as a result of blunt objects (baseball, rock) striking the eye area, or sharp items (scissors, knife) penetrating the eye area.

Altered Physiology

A. *Blunt Injury*
   1. Subconjunctival hemorrhage and suffusion of blood into eyelid
   2. Secondary hemorrhage days after injury
      a. Accumulation of blood in anterior chamber and blocking of overflow channels
      b. Rapid rise of intraocular pressure
   3. Retinal detachment

B. *Penetrating Injury*
   1. Loss of aqueous fluid
   2. Bleeding into anterior chamber

Complications

Sympathetic ophthalmia—inflammation of the uninjured eye probably due to an allergic reaction of pigment released from injured eye. This can lead to retinal detachment and atrophy of the eyeball.

Nursing Management of the Child Undergoing Eye Surgery

Nursing Objectives

PREOPERATIVE CARE

A. *To help the child and his parents to know and understand what the surgery entails. (Explanations should be appropriate for the age of the child.)*
   1. Take a trip to the operating and recovery rooms, if the child is not on bedrest due to trauma.
   2. Practice applying eye patches for short frequent periods.
      a. Allow the child to handle the equipment to be used.
      b. Explain that the patches will only be temporary.
   3. Help the child become familiar with the protection devices if they are to be used postoperatively.
   4. Discuss and practice postoperative exercises if feasible.
   5. Relieve child's fears about pain by telling him that there will be only a little pain as if something is in the eye.

B. *To assess the child and his needs according to age and specifically to his eye problem.*
   1. Does the child have the ability to read or watch television?
   2. Does the child wear glasses and when?
      Help him to learn to protect his glasses when not in use.

C. *To provide as much comfort and reassurance to the child as possible to diminish his fears especially concerning hospitalization and impending surgery.*
   1. Room assignment can be significant.
      a. A quiet room with subdued lighting can be more comfortable for trauma patients.
      b. Placement in a room with other children (without infection) may be comforting for elective surgery patients.
   2. Allow the child to have familiar tactile and auditory stimulating objects around him.

POSTOPERATIVE CARE

A. *To administer good postoperative care and to observe for possible postoperative complications. (See p. 1093.)*

Most eye surgery in children is performed under general anesthesia.

B. *To prevent the child from pulling off the dressing and causing injury or contamination.*
   1. Sedation may be warranted until the child becomes accustomed to having his eye continually bandaged.
   2. Protective devices may be used only if necessary.
      Rest during the immediate postoperative period is necessary and a child struggling because of restraints can defeat their intended purpose.
   3. Diet should be increased slowly to prevent vomiting and possible injury to the eye due to increased pressure.

C. *To provide emotional and psychological reassurance and support to the child who is anxious because his eyes are bandaged preventing him from seeing.*
   1. Encourage parents to be with child, especially when he is waking up from anesthesia. If parents are not able to do this, someone should.
      a. Sit with child, stroke him and speak gently and softly to him.
      b. Let him hold a familiar object.
      c. Hold him if there are no contraindications to his being lifted and held.
   2. Always speak to child before touching him so as not to startle him.
      Explain what is going to be done to him before doing it.
   3. Tell the child what foods are on his tray.
      Allow him to finger feed himself.
   4. Explain sounds. (Sounds in the world without sight can be very frightening.)
   5. Reassure child that patches will be removed soon and he will be able to see again (if he is going to see).
   6. Provide appropriate diversional activities for the child.
      a. Read him stories.
      b. Provide radio or phonograph.
      c. Talk with him.

D. *To administer appropriate eye medications and change dressing as ordered.*
   1. First dressing change is usually done by physician.
      a. Strabismus—dressing removed day after surgery.
      b. Cataract—dressing may stay in place 4–6 days after surgery.
   2. Be familiar with types of eye medications used.
      a. Mydriatic—used for eye examination to dilate pupil and paralyze muscles of accommodation.
      b. Miotic—constricts pupil and decreases increased intraocular pressure in early glaucoma.
      c. Anti-inflammatory drugs.
      d. Antibiotics.
   3. Be familiar with the principles of instilling eye medications (drops, ointments and irrigations).
      a. Have room darkened—light may be uncomfortable.
      b. Try to gain the confidence and cooperation of the child and reassure him by talking to him during the procedure.

    c. Assistance may be necessary to stabilize child's head and prevent injury.

    d. Irrigate from inner canthus outward.

    e. To instill drops, pull lower lid down and drop medication onto conjunctiva from dropper parallel to lid.

    f. Do not force lid open.

    g. Avoid contaminating dressing.

    h. Always wash hands before and after contact with the eye for any procedure.

E. *To involve parents and child in preparation for discharge.*

    1. Teach parents how to instill eye medications.

    2. Postoperative orthoptic exercises or glasses may be necessary.
    Help parents and child understand the value and importance of the exercises or glasses.

    3. Encourage parents to contact the school nurse and other adults responsible for child's care to explain special exercises or specific care for the child.

    4. Encourage follow-up as advised by the physician.

Parental Teaching

Help parents understand what was wrong with the child, what was done to help correct the problem and what the parental responsibilities are in continuing any recommended therapy with the child.

Be certain parents understand what special care is to be done and how it is to be accomplished.

2. *Conditions of the Ear*

OTITIS MEDIA

Otitis media is an infection of the middle ear.

Etiology

1. Bacteriologic
   a. Pneumococci
   b. Beta hemolytic streptococci

2. Secondary
   a. Cold
   b. Measles
   c. Scarlet fever

Altered Physiology

1. Obstruction of the eustachian tube by swelling of mucous membranes.
   a. Air exchange does not take place between the pharynx and middle ear.
   b. Obstruction impedes drainage of secretions to the nasopharynx.

2. Secretions and bacteria become trapped in the middle ear.
   Bacteria multiply rapidly in that environment.

3. Fluid and exudate replace air in the middle ear.
   a. Eardrum bulges.
   b. Tympanic membrane may rupture.

Clinical Manifestations

1. History of cold for several days
2. Fever
3. Older child
   a. Pain in affected ear
   b. Blurred hearing
   c. Headache
   d. Vomiting
4. Infant
   a. May rub ear
   b. Anorexia
   c. Turns head from side to side
   d. Diarrhea

Diagnostic Evaluation

1. Examination will reveal bulging of eardrum and lack of normal luster; ruptured drum may be obscured by secretions.
2. Culture and sensitivity of drainage from ruptured drum in order to select appropriate antibiotic therapy.

Complications

From untreated or ineffective treatment of acute otitis media
1. Chronic otitis media
2. Mastoiditis
3. Septicemia
4. Meningitis and brain damage
5. Chronic otitis media with perforated eardrum may lead to impaired hearing or deafness

Nursing Objectives

A. *To administer medications and treatments as prescribed.*
1. Give appropriate antibiotics according to sensitivity of organisms.
   Usual course of treatment is 10 days.
2. Instill nose drops and decongestant.
   May help to shrink mucous membranes and allow drainage from obstructed eustachian tube.
3. Give ear irrigations and instill glycerine or oil for relief of pain.
   a. Child may need to be held, or "mummy" restraint used.
   b. For child under 3 years old—pull auricle down and back.
   c. For child over 3 years old—pull auricle up and back.
   d. Position child so the affected ear is up—allows fluid to run onto the eardrum.

B. *To prevent mixed infection and reduce the chances of complications arising from present infection.*
1. Always wash hands prior to any treatment or contact with the ear.
2. Change position of the child as appropriate.
   a. Position affected ear up to instill medications or to irrigate ear.
   b. Position affected ear down to facilitate drainage when child is resting.

3. Clean any exudate present from myringotomy or perforated drum.
   Prevents excoriation from drainage.

C. *To provide physical comfort for the child while continuing therapy.*

1. Local heat
   a. Use hot water bottle containing water not over 63°C. (145°F.).
   b. Place child on side, with affected ear on top of bottle to facilitate drainage.
2. A mild analgesic may be necessary if child is restless and indicates pain.
3. Myringotomy may be done in cases where there is severe pain.
   Small incision of the tympanic membrane to relieve pressure and prevent a jagged opening from a spontaneous rupture.
4. Encourage fluid intake to help maintain hydration since the child may have a fever.

D. *To observe for signs of complications and report them.*

1. Mastoiditis
   a. Pain behind affected ear
   b. Increasing irritability
   c. Onset or increase of fever
   d. Tenderness, redness and swelling over mastoid area

2. Meningitis
   a. Sudden onset of high fever
   b. Stiffness of neck
   c. Irritability
   d. Headache
   e. Lethargy

3. Chronic otitis media with perforation of tympanic membrane
   Usually not observed until follow-up care by physician

E. *To provide emotional and psychological support appropriate for child's age and degree of illness.*

1. Encourage child to participate in diversional activities.
2. Reassure child
   a. Talk to him gently.
   b. Allow child to express his feelings, fears and frustrations by talking, playing and drawing.
   c. Hold and rock the younger child.
3. Encourage parental visits and involvement in the child's care.

F. *To help the parents understand that prevention of recurring otitis media is vitally important for the future well-being of the child.*

1. Explain the value of preventing and treating the common cold.
2. Removal of hypertrophied and infected adenoid tissue may be necessary at a later date at the recommendation of the physician.
3. Explain that the child may have decreased hearing for several weeks following this episode of illness.
4. Help parents learn what signs indicate recurrent otitis media and the need for immediate medical intervention. Prompt treatment can prevent permanent hearing loss.

THE CHILD WITH IMPAIRED HEARING

Impaired hearing occurs when the average hearing loss in speech frequencies is 70 decibels or 80 decibels or less and the child does not learn to talk in the normal way.

Etiology

1. Unknown
2. Familial factors
3. Prenatal or intrauterine factors
   a. Rubella
   b. Preeclampsia or eclampsia
   c. Drugs
4. Perinatal factors
   a. Prematurity
   b. Anoxia at birth
   c. Hyperbilirubinemia
5. Postnatal factors
   a. Oxytoxic drugs
   b. Acquired disorders of the central nervous system
   c. Acute infections
   d. Injury

Altered Physiology

A. Conductive hearing loss
   1. Impairment in the mechanism of conducting sound waves to the cochlea
      a. Blockage of sound waves from outer ear, external canal or middle ear (lack of loudness)
      b. Tympanic membrane damage and scarring
      c. Dislocation or disturbance of tiny ossicular bones in the middle ear
   2. Often recognized in the school-age child

B. Sensorineural
      Malfunction of inner ear apparatus or 8th cranial nerve
      a. Lack of loudness
      b. Distorted sounds due to defect of cochlea or neural pathways to temporal lobe of the brain
      c. Problems with discrimination of sound

Clinical Manifestations

A. *Infant*
   1. Little or no interest in sounds of his environment
      a. Does not blink at loud noise
      b. No response to musical toy or mother's voice
   2. Lack of or minimal vocalization
      a. Does not coo or gurgle
      b. May not smile
   3. Lack of neonatal reflex to noise 1–2 meters (3–6 feet) away

B. *Toddlers*
   1. Little or no vocalization
      a. Sounds produced poorly
      b. Uses gestures to express needs
   2. Little interest in environmental sounds
      a. Does not respond to name, doorbell or telephone

C. *Pre-school and School-age Child*
  1. Behavioral disturbances
     a. Intense, constant activity
     b. Temper tantrums
     c. Inattentiveness
     d. Slow learner
  2. May show abrupt change in social or communicative behavior

Diagnostic Evaluation

  1. Otolaryngologic examination (inspection of external ear and tympanic membrane)—to rule out involvement of conductive apparatus
  2. Audiologic examination—to establish the extent of hearing loss and to determine type of hearing aid needed
     a. Observation of child's response to sounds calibrated for intensity and frequency
     b. Objective measuring techniques of hearing loss, i.e., cortical audiometry

Complications

  1. In childhood when there is a hearing disorder, there is a delay of speech and language, thus a loss of contact between the individual, his peers and his environment.
  2. Biologic, behavioral and social complications may result when there is a breakdown of the normal communicative process.
  3. The seriousness of the total problem depends upon the nature and extent of auditory involvement and upon the age of onset and length of time before the hearing problem is detected.

Treatment

  1. Conductive hearing loss
     a. Surgical correction of defect
     b. Hearing aid
  2. Sensorineural hearing loss
     a. Hearing aid
     b. Special training
        (1) Language acquisition
        (2) Auditory training
        (3) Speech therapy
        (4) Perceptual motor training

Nursing Objectives

The nurse may become involved with the child with impaired hearing in the hospital in 2 situations: (1) before diagnosis has been made when she may detect a hearing loss and (2) after diagnosis has been made when giving nursing care to the hospitalized child.

DETECTION AND EARLY CARE AFTER DIAGNOSIS

A. *To be familiar with the normal pattern of language and learning development* and the manifestations of hearing loss in the infant and child.*
  1. Knowing the stages of growth and development can be helpful in recognizing and suspecting hearing impairment in the individual child.

---

* See Bibliography, Deweese and Saunders.

2. Be alert to and assess the child's response to auditory stimulation.
   a. Does infant stop activity and listen to vocal sounds?
   b. Does the child respond to his name?
   c. Does the child have unusual visual alertness at age 1 year?
3. The critical period of learning or language development is from birth to 16 months.

B. *To be familiar with the causes of hearing impairment and recognize from the history if the child may be in a high-risk area.*
   1. Past infections
      a. Mumps
      b. Meningitis
      c. Otitis media
      d. Trauma
   2. Neonatal problems
      a. Erythroblastosis fetalis
      b. Prematurity
      c. Birth trauma
      d. Hypoxia

C. *To record observations and report to physician any suspicious behavior by the infant or child that indicates possible hearing loss.*

   Early diagnosis is the key to successful habilitation and optimal development of the capabilities of the child.
   a. After 16 months of age, habilitation is more difficult.
   b. If hearing loss occurs after the time of critical language development, rehabilitation is less difficult as the groundwork for verbal communication has been established.

      Impulse for learning spontaneous speech reaches its peak during the first 3–4 years of life.

D. *To be familiar with community resources and the professional team involved in habilitation.*
   1. Each child must be treated as an individual.
   2. Knowing general philosophies and training techniques of the involved resource can be helpful.

      Help child to capitalize on assets and minimize limitations.

E. *To be familiar with the guidelines and techniques of educating a child with impaired hearing.*
   1. The main mode of communication for the child with impaired hearing is visual, supplemented by auditory clues.
      a. Educational task is to develop the child's understanding and expression of language.
      b. Speech can be learned through a multisensory approach, using visual, tactile, kinesthetic and auditory stimulation.
   2. The child with a less severe hearing loss uses auditory stimulation, supplemented by visual clues, as his main mode of communication.

      Educational task is to develop adequate speech and language and the best use of residual hearing.

F. *To foster continual parental acceptance of the child and provide support for them.*
   1. Invite parents to become involved in the care of their hospitalized child as much as possible.

2. Help parents understand the problems the child faces and will face as he gets older.
   a. Child may not be able to participate in activities where sounds and verbal commands are used.
   b. Often the referral agency will become very involved in this area.
3. Help parents become aware of their importance in the success of the habilitation of the child.
   The child needs the warmth and security of a family setting.
4. Help parents understand what can be accomplished in their child's education to enable him to be a contributing member of society.
5. Stress the importance of close follow-up by the specialists caring for the child.
6. Help shape healthy parental attitudes about their child and guide them through this difficult time.
   a. Prevent denial.
   b. Parents need sympathetic understanding during the time of diagnosis and immediately following when they are bewildered and grieving.
   c. Parental attitudes may be the primary factor in determining the success or failure of the child's progress.
7. Encourage parents to write for literature from appropriate agencies.*

CARE OF THE HOSPITALIZED CHILD WHO HAS A HEARING LOSS

A. *To interview the parents at the time of admission to learn as much as possible about the child and his activities at home.*
   1. What is the child's way of communicating his needs? How do parents communicate with the child?
   2. Be aware of the child's schedule and activities at home.
      Know what activities he can or cannot do and what he likes to do.
   3. Be aware of how parents discipline child and how they comfort him.
   4. Does the child wear a hearing aid? When? Any special exercises or training that needs to be continued?
   5. Share this information with nursing staff in the nursing care plan to assure continuity of care from home to hospital and to minimize fear and frustration in the child.

B. *To attend to the child's needs according to the medical or surgical problem that required his hospitalization.*

C. *To plan and provide for the appropriate type of play program and stimulation for the child.*
   1. Assess the child's level of development and growth and use information provided by parents.
   2. Allow the child as much independence as possible in his care, but provide guidance as necessary—prevent boredom.
   3. Encourage the development of the child's abilities.

* Alexander Graham Bell Association for the Deaf, 1537 35th Street, N.W., Washington, D.C. 20007
American Hearing Society, 919 18th Street, N.W. Washington, D.C. 20006
John Tracy Clinic Correspondence Course (aid in speech and hearing therapy), John Tracy Clinic, 806 West Adams Boulevard, Los Angeles, California 90007

D. *To meet the emotional needs of the child with impaired hearing for closeness and belonging.*
   1. Place the child in a room with a friendly, outgoing child.
   2. Plan frequent nurse-patient interactions.
      a. Gentle touch
      b. Games or activities he enjoys
   3. Encourage parents, especially mother, to take an active part in his care, thus decreasing fear of desertion.

E. *To offer continual parental support.*
   1. Help parents to think of their child as a child first, then as a child with special needs.
   2. Emphasize their importance in the habilitation of their child. Point out the value of the home environment in his development.
      a. Talk about the daily routines.
      b. Talk about mother's role in stimulating the child's interest in sounds and speech.
      c. Encourage the use of hearing aids and the learning program set up by specialists in hearing problems in children.
      d. Residential placement may be considered when local facilities are nonexistent or when the home environment would be detrimental to the child's progress.
   3. Encourage parents to talk about their fears, frustrations and feelings in caring for the child at home.
      Initiate a social worker referral, if a social worker is not already involved from the special training center.
   4. Other members of the family must be considered.
      a. This child does need special handling, but he does not need all the attention all the time.
      b. Other members of the family should be included in his care, but they also have a life of their own and need as much parental attention as they would receive if this child were not present in the family.
      c. Parents need time to themselves. They should be encouraged to go out alone together and to give time to their marriage.
   5. Help the parents realize that even though habilitation of their child is long, drawnout and expensive, the child may be able to live a somewhat normal life in the community.
      a. Are parents aware of and accept the short-term and long-term goals?
      b. Is the child receiving special training in a local facility, if available?

BIBLIOGRAPHY

1. Conditions of the Eye

Books

Bishop, V. E.: Teaching the Visually Limited Child. Springfield, Illinois, Charles C Thomas, 1972.
Blake, F. G., et al.: Nursing Care of Children. Philadelphia, J. B. Lippincott, 1970.
Green, M., and Haggerty, R. (eds.): Ambulatory Pediatrics. Philadelphia, W. B. Saunders, 1968.
Latham, H. C., and Heckel, R. V.: Pediatric Nursing. St. Louis, C. V. Mosby, 1972.
Lowenfeld, B.: Our Blind Children. Springfield, Illinois, Charles C Thomas, 1971.
Marlow, D.: Textbook of Pediatric Nursing. Philadelphia, W. B. Saunders, 1973.

Nelson, W. E.: Textbook of Pediatrics. Philadelphia, W. B. Saunders, 1969.
Raffensperger, J. G., and Primrose, R. B.: Pediatric Surgery for Nurses. Boston, Little, Brown and Company, 1968.
The Eye in Childhood. The Ophthalmologic Staff of the Hospital for Sick Children, Toronto. Chicago, Year Book Medical Publishers, Inc., 1967.

Articles

Bean, M. A.: Camp lighthouse. Amer. J. Nurs., 72:950–953, May 1972.
Chodil, J., and Williams, B.: The concept of sensory deprivation. Nurs. Clin. N. Amer., 5:453–465, Sept. 1970.
Condl, E. D.: Ophthalmic nursing: the gentle touch. Nurs. Clin. N. Amer., 5:467–476, Sept. 1970.
Cullin, I. C.: Techniques for teaching patients with sensory defects. Nurs. Clin. N. Amer., 5:527–538, Sept. 1970.
Gillman, A. E.: Handicap and cognition: the assumption that visual deprivation affects the infant's rate of motor development. Selected papers from the Sixth Annual Conference, American Association for Child Care in Hospitals. May 19–22, 1971. Cleveland, American Association for Child Care in Hospitals, 1972.

2. Conditions of the Ear

Books

Blake, F. G., et al.: Nursing Care of Children. Philadelphia, J. B. Lippincott, 1970.
Deweese, D. O., and Saunders, W. H. (eds.): Textbook of Otolaryngology. St. Louis, C. V. Mosby, 1973.
Ewing, Sir Alexander, and Ewing, Lady Ethel: Hearing-impaired Children Under Five: A Guide for Parents and Teachers. Washington, D.C., the Volta Bureau, 1971.
Gustafson, S. R., and Coursin, D. B.: The Pediatric Patient—1966. Philadelphia, J. B. Lippincott, 1966.
Green, M., and Haggerty, R. (eds.): Ambulatory Pediatrics. Philadelphia, W. B. Saunders, 1968.
Gellis, S., and Kagan, B. M.: Current Pediatric Therapy. Philadelphia, W. B. Saunders, 1970.
Latham, H. C., and Heckel, R. V.: Pediatric Nursing. St. Louis, C. V. Mosby, 1972.
Learning to Talk. U. S. Department of Health, Education and Welfare, Public Health Service, National Institute of Health, No. 1970 0-387-794.
Marlow, D.: Textbook of Pediatric Nursing. Philadelphia, W. B. Saunders, 1973.
Nelson, W. E.: Textbook of Pediatrics. Philadelphia, W. B. Saunders, 1969.

Articles

Chodil, J., and Williams, B.: The concept of sensory deprivation. Nurs. Clin. N. Amer., 5:453–465, Sept. 1970.
Conover, M., and Cober, J.: Understanding and caring for the hearing impaired. Nurs. Clin. N. Amer., 5:497–506, Sept. 1970.
Horton, K. B.: Home demonstration teaching for parents of very young deaf children. Volta Review, 70:97–104, 1968.
Knox, L. L., and McConnell, F.: Helping parents to help deaf infants. Children, 15:183–187, 1968.
Linnell, C., Long, Sister Victoria, and Proehl, J.: The hearing-impaired infant. Nurs. Clin. N. Amer., 5:507–515, Sept. 1970.
McConnell, F.: A new approach to the management of childhood deafness. Ped. Clin. N. Amer., 17:347–362, May 1970.
Patterson, M. E., and Linthicum, F. H., Jr.: Congenital hearing impairment. Otolaryn. Clin. N. Amer., 3:201–220, June 1970.
Payne, P. O., and Payne, R. L.: Behavior manifestations of children with hearing loss. Amer. J. Nurs., 70:1718–1719, Aug. 1970.

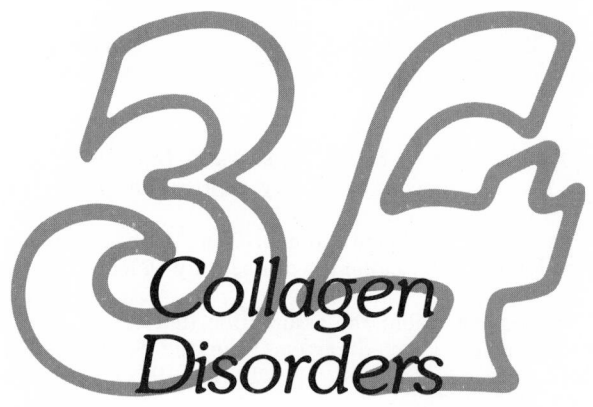

Collagen Disorders

SYSTEMIC LUPUS ERYTHEMATOSUS

Systemic lupus erythematosus is a disease of the connective tissue with vascular and perivascular fibrinoid changes that may involve any organ or system.

Incidence and Etiology

1. Girls are affected more frequently than boys.
2. The cause is not known, but it is felt to be related to an immunopathologic aberration, giving rise to a heightened reactivity to diverse antigenic stimuli.

Altered Physiology

1. Connective tissue in different organs develops nonspecific aberrations such as fibrinoid change in collagen and cellular infiltration, either in the walls of small blood vessels or elsewhere.
2. Alteration of collagen and subendothelial thickening of small blood vessels obstruct the flow of blood. These changes may be widespread or limited in distribution.

Clinical Manifestations

1. The onset is occasionally abrupt with the development of:
   a. Fever
   b. Weight loss
   c. Hepatomegaly
   d. Splenomegaly
   e. Lymphadenopathy
   f. Malar erythema which usually spreads over bridge of nose (Butterfly rash may consist only of an erythematous blush or scaly erythematous papules; rash may be photosensitive.)

g. Indications of system involvement
  (1) Renal disease—proteinuria
  (2) Cardiomegaly
  (3) Central nervous system signs
    (a) Behavioral disturbances
    (b) Convulsions
    (c) Coma
2. The onset is usually insidious.
  a. Joint symptoms
    (1) Large joints usually affected with pain, swelling and occasionally redness
    (2) Joint symptoms come and go
  b. Systemic reactions
    (1) Weakness   (4) Loss of weight
    (2) Anorexia   (5) Fever
    (3) Malaise
  c. Symmetrical bilateral malar erythema
    (1) Patchy erythema may occur
    (2) Purpura may be observed
  d. Lupus glomerulitis may be present in varying degree of severity
    (1) Hematuria
    (2) Proteinuria
  e. Splenomegaly
  f. Hepatomegaly
  g. Inguinal, cervical and axillary lymphadenopathy
  h. Myocarditis with striking cardiomegaly
  i. Central nervous system involvement

Treatment

Steroid therapy is frequently utilized to suppress symptoms and to prevent progression when there is systemic involvement.

Nursing Objectives

A. *To discuss with the child (if age is appropriate) and the parents their understanding of the illness.*
  1. Determine what information has been given to them by the physician.
  2. Support them in accepting this illness as a long-term illness, with exacerbations and remissions.
B. *To assist the child in developing a realistic attitude about his illness, and assist him in expressing his feelings about his illness.*
  1. Provide the child with the opportunity to openly discuss his feelings about illness when he is able to verbalize these feelings.
  2. Provide the child with the opportunity to express his feelings utilizing play as a method.
  3. Arrange for a visiting teacher so that the child may have the opportunity to continue his education.
  4. Encourage the child to continue contact with his peers (i.e., telephone, letter writing, etc.).
  5. Allow the child to make some decisions and become involved in planning his own care.

C. *To observe closely for the development of symptoms which may be indicative of the development of complications.*
   1. Observe for the development of renal symptoms.
      a. Record intake and output.
      b. Record specific gravity.
      c. Observe the color and characteristics of urine.
      d. Observe for the development of edema.
   2. Report to the physician any abnormal findings.
D. *To teach the parents the information that is necessary to care for the child at home.*
   1. Prevent direct exposure to the sun; if exposure to the sun cannot be avoided, a sunscreen lotion should be used.
   2. Make the parents aware of the side effects of any medications being administered at home.
   3. Provide measures that will be helpful in preventing infection.
      a. Avoid exposure to individuals with infections.
      b. Practice general measures of personal hygiene.
      c. Provide a well-balanced diet.
E. *To be aware of the action and side effects of medications used in the treatment of systemic lupus erythematosus.*
   Steroids and salicylates (See section on Rheumatic Fever, p. 1186.)

JUVENILE RHEUMATOID ARTHRITIS
(Still's Disease)

Juvenile rheumatoid arthritis is a chronic systemic disease, involving a wide spectrum of manifestations. Arthritis is most characteristic, although there is wide variation in the pattern of joint involvement. Systemic manifestations may be present and may be more obvious than the arthritis.

Etiology
1. The etiology of juvenile rheumatoid arthritis is unknown.
2. Onset of the disease often becomes manifest after physical trauma to a joint or following an acute systemic infection. No direct causative relationship to such events has been demonstrated.
3. It has been proposed that the disease results from infection with an organism such as mycoplasma or virus. It has also been proposed that the disease represents a hypersensitivity or autoimmune response to unknown stimuli.

Altered Physiology
1. In early stages one or many joints show signs of inflammation.
2. The inflammation is initially localized in a joint capsule, primarily in the synovium. The tissue becomes thickened from congestion and edema.
3. A characteristic inflammatory response develops in the form of a synovial proliferation which invades the interior of the joint.

4. The inflammatory tissue extends into the interior of the joint along the surface of the articular cartilage to which it may be adherent, so that it deprives the cartilage of nutrition.
5. By starvation and invasion, this inflammatory tissue slowly destroys the articular cartilage.
6. Synovial tissue eventually frees the joint space leading to narrowing, fibrous ankylosis and bony fusion.
7. Growth centers next to inflamed joints may undergo either premature epiphyseal closure or accelerated epiphyseal growth.
8. Tendons and tendon sheaths may develop inflammatory changes similar to the synovial tissues.
9. Inflammation of muscle may occur.
10. Rheumatoid nodules are uncommon in children.

Clinical Manifestations

A. *Joints* (changes may occur with or without systemic symptoms)
1. Symptoms may develop gradually with gradual development of stiffness, swelling and impaired motion of a joint or joints.
2. Symptoms may develop rapidly with sudden appearance of symptomatic arthritis in one or more joints.
3. Knees, ankles, feet, wrists or fingers are usually involved initially.
4. Joints are swollen and warm.
5. Pain and stiffness of joint may appear before objective changes develop.
6. Limitation of motion of inflamed joints occurs.
7. Characteristic posture is one of guarding joints from movement; an anxious pained expression (with polyarthritis) is common.
8. Stiffness of joints following periods of inactivity occurs.
9. Atrophy and weakness of muscles near the affected joints may develop.
10. Skin over inflamed joints may be pigmented.
11. Chronically affected joints may become dislocated, deformed or fused.
12. Subcutaneous nodules may appear over pressure points (knees, elbows, etc.).
13. Condition may ultimately affect any joint in the body (knees, ankles, wrists, feet, fingers, toes, shoulders, elbows, neck, jaw, hips and sacroiliac joints are frequently involved).
14. Small, deformed feet result from foot involvement in early childhood.
15. Micrognathia (unusually small lower jaw), as a result of temporomandibular arthritis, is one hallmark of juvenile rheumatoid arthritis.
16. Spindling or fusiform changes of the fingers may occur.

B. *Systemic characteristics*
1. Irritability, anorexia and malaise may result.
2. Fever—daily spikes up to 41°C. (105.8°F.) may occur.
3. Rash consisting of small, discrete, pink macules with pale centers occurs on trunk and extremities.
4. Hepatosplenomegaly
5. Generalized lymphadenopathy
6. Anemia

C. *Inflammation of the eye* (unilateral or bilateral)

Child may have no early symptoms. If symptoms occur late, child may develop irreversible eye damage including scarring and adhesions of the iris and cataracts.

1. Redness
2. Pain
3. Photophobia
4. Decreased visual acuity
5. Nonreactive pupil

D. *Generalized growth retardation*

1. During periods of remission, growth spurts may occur.
2. Treatment with long-term steroid therapy may also contribute to growth failure.

Diagnostic Evaluation

1. Elevated sedimentation rate
2. Leukocytosis
3. High total serum proteins
4. Positive creatine protein
5. Low reticulocyte count
6. Possible alteration in serum proteins (increased alpha and gamma; decreased albumin)
7. Changes in bone, demonstrated by x-ray

Treatment

Objectives: to preserve good joint function.
to support the emotional outlook of the child and his family.

1. Although this is a disease that is painful and of long duration, the outlook for remission is good.
2. There is no specific cure.

Complications

1. Bony deformities
2. Psychological reactions to this chronic illness

Nursing Objectives

A. *To discuss with the parents and the child what they know about the disease and what they expect from treatment.*

1. The need to treat the illness optimistically should be discussed with both the child and his family.
2. The child and his family must understand the treatment since this is a chronic disease and has an unpredictable course.

B. *To plan a program of physical therapy in order to improve motion and muscular strength about the affected joints.*

1. The parents and the child are instructed in the exercises.
2. Night splints for the wrists and knees may aid in correcting or in preventing deformity.
3. A hot tub bath prior to the exercises may make the exercises less painful.
4. Full range of motion exercises should be performed every day.
5. Orthopedic surgery may be required to correct some deformities.

C. *To administer medications which are utilized to suppress inflammation of the joints.*

See Salicylates and Steroids, under Rheumatic Fever, page 1186.

D. *To provide the child with the freedom to engage in as much activity as he is a*
   tolerate.
   1. Children will limit their own activity.
   2. Those activities that produce overtiring or joint pain should be avoided.
   3. The child should attend school regularly and participate in regular school acti
   4. Encourage the child to be as self-sufficient as possible.
   5. Allow the child to make some decisions himself (i.e., when he prefers to
      exercises).
E. *To encourage parents to report any eye symptoms that the child may develop.*
   Report any decrease in visual acuity (symptom of eye involvement and m
   treated early).

BIBLIOGRAPHY

Books

Barnett, H. L. (ed.): Pediatrics, 15th ed. New York, Appleton-Century-Crofts, 1972.
Blake, F. G., et al.: Nursing Care of Children, 8th ed. Philadelphia, J. B. Lippincott, 1970.
Brewer, E. J.: Juvenile Rheumatoid Arthritis (Vol. VI in the Series, Major Problems in C
   Pediatrics). Philadelphia, W. B. Saunders, 1970.
Nelson, W., et al.: Textbook of Pediatrics, 9th ed. Philadelphia, W. B. Saunders, 1969.

Articles

Brewer, E. J.: Rheumatoid arthritis in childhood. Amer. J. Nurs., 65:66, 1965.
Limbeck, G. A.: Juvenile rheumatoid arthritis. Amer. Fam. Phys., 1:88–97, May 1970.

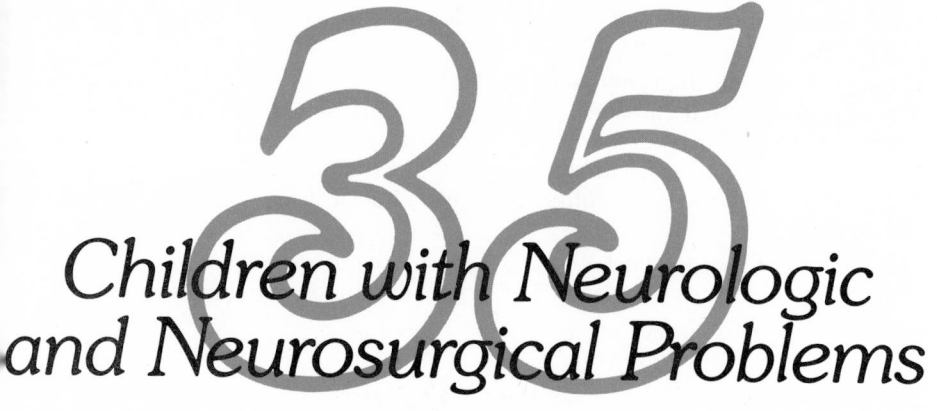

Children with Neurologic and Neurosurgical Problems

CEREBRAL PALSY

al palsy is a comprehensive diagnostic term used to designate a group of nonprogres-
sorders resulting from malfunction of the motor centers and pathways of the brain.
haracterized by paralysis, weakness, incoordination and ataxia. Cerebral palsy is a
l, incurable condition which is the greatest cause of crippling of children in the
States.

gy

natal Factors

Maternal anoxia
Maternal bleeding
Rh of ABO incompatibility
X-ray radiation to the mother

5. Maternal rubella infection
6. Toxoplasmosis
7. Cytomegalic inclusion disease

al Factors

Anoxia from any cause
a. Anesthetic and analgesic drugs administered to the mother may cause anoxia to
   the infant brain
b. Prolonged labor
c. Premature separation of the placenta
Cerebral trauma during delivery
Hyperbilirubinemia due to blood group incompatibility

C. *Postnatal Factors*
1. Trauma—brain contusion or hemorrhage
2. Infections
    a. Meningitis
    b. Encephalitis
3. Anoxia
4. Lead poisoning
5. Progressive causes for brain damage such as neoplasm, hydrocephalus or degenerative disease are not accepted as cerebral palsy.

Incidence

Approximately 100–600 cases per 100,000 children

Clinical Manifestations

A. *Early Signs*
1. Asymmetry in motion or contour
2. Listlessness or irritability
3. Twitching
4. Stiffness or convulsions
5. Difficulty feeding, sucking or swallowing
6. Vomiting
7. Excessive or feeble crying
8. Cyanosis or pallor
9. Long, thin infants, who are slow to gain weight

B. *Later Signs*
1. Failure to follow normal pattern of motor development
2. Persistence of infantile reflexes
3. Weakness
4. Apparent preference for one hand before 12–15 months
5. Delayed or defective speech
6. Evidence of mental retardation

C. *Factors Influencing Symptoms and Degree of Involvement*
(Ranges from very mild to severe)
1. Extent and location of cerebral lesion
2. Age at which interruption of brain development occurred.
    Intellectual, language and social skills which were acquired before damage can usually be retained.
3. Status of reflex patterns

Types of Cerebral Palsy

A. *Spastic Type*
1. 60% of those afflicted are of this type.
2. Signs
    a. Fixed postures, often opisthotonus or maintained partial tonic neck responses.
    b. Arms—fist is usually clenched, forearm flexed and upper arm pressed against the chest.
    c. Legs—scissoring (child crosses his legs and points his toes)

B. *Athetotic Type*
    1. Types of athetosis:
        a. Rotary (most common)   d. Shudder types
        b. Tremorlike (rare in children)   e. Tension
        c. Dystonic (atonia or hypotonia)   f. Nontension
    2. Often found as mixed types
    3. Signs
        a. Hypotonia—abnormally decreased tonicity or strength
        b. Incoordination
        c. Bizarre, purposeless movements and grimaces
    4. May not be detected until the second year of life

C. *Rigidity—Dystonias*
    Signs
        a. Rigid postural attitudes
        b. Usually slow moving

D. *Ataxias*
    Signs—loss of balance

E. *Topographical Classification*
    1. Monoplegia—involving only one limb   3. Triplegia
    2. Hemiplegia   4. Quadriplegia

Diagnostic Evaluation

Common associated findings:
    1. Convulsions (approximately 25%)   3. Visual defect
    2. Mental retardation (at least 50%)   4. Hearing deficiency

Prognosis

Factors influencing the prognosis
    1. Extent of the manifestations
    2. Existence of associated defects, especially mental retardation
    3. The family's ability to use their own and community resources

Altered Physiology

A. *Spastic Type*
    1. Defect in the cortical motor area or pyramidal tract causes abnormally strong tonus of certain muscle groups.
    2. Attempts to move a joint causes muscles to contract and block the motion.
        Permanent contractures develop without muscle training.

B. *Athetotic Type*
    Lesions of the extrapyramidal tract and basal ganglia cause involuntary, incoordinated, uncontrollable movements of muscle groups.

C. *Rigidity—Dystonias*
    Muscles remain in a state of semicontraction and resist movement.

D. *Ataxia*
    Disturbances of balance result from cerebellar involvement.

Nursing Objectives

A. *To maintain a safe environment for the child.*
1. Respiratory distress may result from involvement of the chest or abdominal muscles.
   a. Have a suction machine available to aspirate mucus.
   b. Position the child so that he is most comfortable and can breathe with the least exertion.
2. Ataxic children are especially subject to falls.
   Require these children to wear helmets to protect against head injury.
3. Maintain seizure precautions for children who are subject to convulsions.
4. Select toys which are safe.

B. *To maintain adequate nourishment.*
1. Maintain a pleasant environment, free from distractions.
   a. Provide a comfortable chair.
   b. Serve the child alone, initially.
      After he begins to master the task of eating, he may enjoy eating with other children.
   c. Do not attempt feedings if the child is very fatigued.
2. Feed the child slowly and carefully. Patience is essential.
   a. These children have difficulty sucking and swallowing because they cannot control the muscles of their throat.
   b. They often vomit because of a hyperactive gag reflex.
   c. Offer foods which the child likes.
   d. Cut solid foods into small pieces.
   e. Place the food back on the tongue for ease in swallowing.
3. Encourage independence, but do not force the child.
   a. Find the eating position in which the child can do the most for himself.
   b. Allow the child to hold the spoon even if he has to be fed with another one.
   c. Stand behind the child and reach over his shoulder to guide the spoon from the plate to his mouth.
   d. Serve foods that stick to the spoon such as peanut butter, thick applesauce, mashed potato, etc.
   e. Encourage finger foods that the child can handle alone.
   f. Provide appropriate special equipment for the child to feed himself.
      (1) Spoon and fork with special handles
      (2) Plate and glass holders, etc.
      (3) Feeding chair
   g. Disregard "messy" eating
      (1) Place newspapers around the feeding chair.
      (2) Use a large plastic bib or towel to protect the child's clothes.

C. *To provide adequate relaxation.*
1. This is especially important as children with cerebral palsy are under constant strain even when attempting to perform simple acts.
2. Provide for frequent rest periods with little stimuli.
   a. Avoid exciting events before rest or bedtime.
   b. Organize nursing activities to prevent unnecessary interruptions.
3. Administer tranquilizing agents if ordered by the physician.
4. Avoid stress and frustration during the child's program of physical therapy.

5. Teach him specific techniques of relaxation.
6. Play:
   a. Games and toys should be chosen which have educational value but will not frustrate the child or cause excessive excitement.
   b. Toys must be safe.
   c. The child should be allowed to play in groups with other children on the nursing unit.

D. *To prevent contractures and eliminate unwanted movements.*
   1. Carry out appropriate exercises under the direction of the physical therapist.
   2. Use appropriate appliances to facilitate muscle control and improve body functioning.
      a. Splints
      b. Casts
      c. Braces
   3. Encourage active motions of functional use.
   4. Use play (games, peg boards, puzzles, etc.) as techniques to improve coordination.

E. *To allow the child to progress to his maximum potential.*
   1. Be alert for associated defects which could be corrected.
      a. Vision
         (1) Squinting
         (2) Failure to follow objects
         (3) Bringing things very close to his face
      b. Hearing
      c. Speech
   2. Communicate with all of the disciplines involved with the child's management. Formulate a consistent nursing care plan which is well coordinated with the plans and goals of related disciplines and meets the needs of the *entire* child and his family.
   3. Maintain ego support.
      a. Structure the child's activities so that failures are kept to a minimum. Set realistic short-term goals which progress toward a long-term goal of maximum independence.
      b. Provide appropriate praise for the child's successes and understanding of his failures.

F. *To assist parents to plan for the long-term care of their child.*
   1. Encourage them to care for the child during his hospitalization so that they will feel secure to meet his daily physical needs (feeding, exercises, braces, etc.).
   2. Introduce them to members of the health team who will be involved with the child's care and management.
      a. Physicians   e. Occupational therapist
      b. Social worker   f. Speech therapist
      c. Psychologist or psychiatrist   g. Nurses
      d. Physical therapist
   3. Provide the parents with appropriate literature and reading material. Encourage their questions and provide them with the information they need.
   4. Assist them to appraise the child's assets so that they may capitalize on these positive features.
      a. Early recognition of the extent of the child's handicap and realistic direction for obtainable goals are essential.

      b. Help the parents to recognize immediate needs and identify short-term goals which can be integrated into the long-range plan.

  5. Encourage parents to express their feelings about the child and his diagnosis and help them to deal with these feelings.

      Prolonged feelings of rejection, guilt and grief should not be allowed to exist. The services of a social worker or psychiatrist may be necessary.

  6. Have a social worker discuss with them the financial aspects of the child's care, assess their ability to pay for needed services and make appropriate referrals for financial assistance.

      Special equipment that the child may require is not necessarily expensive but can be easily adapted from materials available in the home.

  7. Assist parents to interpret the child's diagnosis and needs to other family members, teachers and friends.

  8. Initiate appropriate referrals.
      a. Community agencies for crippled children
      b. Community health nurse
      c. Day care centers
      d. Clinics
      e. Local branch of the United Cerebral Palsy Association
      f. Parent groups

G. *To be familiar with nursing activities associated with the hospitalization of the child previously diagnosed as having cerebral palsy.*

  1. Obtain a thorough history from the mother regarding the child's usual home routines.

      a. Feeding   d. Stage of growth and development
      b. Sleeping   e. Play
      c. Physical therapy   f. Special interests, security objects, etc.

  2. Allow the child's parents to participate in the child's care if they desire and if it is medically feasible.

  3. Ask the parents to bring to the hospital any special devices or equipment which the child uses in his daily activities.

  4. Utilize the information and equipment obtained to formulate a nursing plan which provides for continuity of care from home to hospital.

Parental Teaching

  1. Instruct parent in all areas of the child's physical care.

  2. The child needs regular medical and dental evaluations.

      a. It is important that the child receives his childhood immunizations.

      b. He should be taken to the dentist every 6 months starting at the age of 2 years.

      c. He may require some adaptations of his toothbrush in order to use it effectively.

         (1) The handle can be built up with sponge or a more sophisticated enlarging device.

         (2) Brushes with specially bent handles are available.

  3. The child needs to be helped to establish capabilities that a normal child develops naturally.

      Therapy and activities of daily living must be in accord with the child's developmental level, both physical and mental.

  4. The child needs discipline in order to feel secure and relaxed.

      a. He should have realistic limits set within which he can function successfully.

      b. Parents should be firm but not rejecting.

5. The child should be allowed as normal an environment as possible.
   a. He should be allowed to play with other children.
   b. He should be allowed to play away from home.
      (1) Nursery school
      (2) Camp
      (3) Play groups and recreational organizations
      (4) Proper identification is essential.
           The child should wear a medical-alert bracelet.
   c. He needs the joy of achieving realistic expectations.
      (1) Muscular control
      (2) Educational attainments
          (a) Education must be adapted to individual potentials.
          (b) Learning is difficult even for those children with normal mentality because of their physical handicaps.
   d. He should not have all of his problems solved for him but should receive the necessary help in seeking his own solutions so that he can advance to more complex experiences.
   e. Every bit of independence possible should be encouraged, even for children confined to bed or wheelchairs.
6. The child needs to be helped to face reality and to accept himself objectively.
   a. Foundation for this ability is laid down in the toddler period.
   b. Success in this area is impossible if his parents are unable to accept the situation and deal with it.
   c. Additional help is usually required to face the responsibilities of maturation and adulthood.
      (1) Vocational counseling should be available to older school-age children and adolescents.
      (2) The child may need help to make the special adjustments necessitated by his condition.
          (a) Prolonged support from others
          (b) Adaptation of his sexual role
          (c) Emancipation from his family

HYDROCEPHALUS

Hydrocephalus is a condition of imbalance between the production of cerebrospinal fluid and its absorption, via the surface of the brain, into the circulatory system. It is characterized by an abnormal increase in cerebrospinal fluid volume within the intracranial cavity and enlargement of the child's head.

Etiology

1. Failure in the absorption system—cause unknown
2. Excessive production of cerebrospinal fluid—cause unknown
3. Obstruction in the system between the source of cerebrospinal fluid and the area of its reabsorption (the obstruction may be partial, intermittent or complete.)
   a. The majority of cases are of this type.
   b. Causes
      (1) Developmental defects

        (a) Atresia, stenosis or absence of one or more of the intraventricular communications

        (b) Failure of the cisterna magna to form

        (c) Failure of cleavage of the pia arachnoid

    (2) Inflammatory reactions with resulting adhesions

    (3) Neoplasms

    (4) Hemorrhage

    (5) Unknown

Incidence

Approximately 1 out of 500 children demonstrates some form of this condition.

Types of Hydrocephalus

A. *Internal Hydrocephalus*

    1. Noncommunicating Hydrocephalus

        An obstruction is located within or at the outlets of the ventricular system, preventing any or all of the cerebrospinal fluid from leaving the ventricles and entering the subarachnoid space.

    2. Communicating Hydrocephalus

        a. There is free communication between the ventricles and the spinal theca.

        b. The obstruction is located in the subarachnoid cisternae at the base of the brain or within the subarachnoid space.

B. *External Hydrocephalus*

    1. Rare

    2. Secondary to pre-existing internal hydrocephalus

    3. Excessive fluid accumulates outside the cerebrum rather than within the ventricles.

    4. Cause

        Rupture of the arachnoid membrane which allows the cerebrospinal fluid to flow into the subdural space.

Altered Physiology

1. The ventricular system is greatly distended.
2. The increased ventricular pressure results in thinning of the cerebral cortex and cranial bones, especially in the frontal, parietal and temporal areas.

    Mental retardation is an associated finding secondary to cerebral compression.
3. The floor of the third ventricle commonly bulges downward, compresses the optic nerves, dilates the sella turcica, and often compresses the hypophysis cerebri.
4. The basal ganglia, brain stem and cerebellum remain relatively normal but compressed.
5. The choroid plexus is usually atrophied to some degree.

Clinical Manifestations

(May be rapid or slow and steadily advancing or remittent)

1. Macrocephaly

    a. Head is normal or only slightly enlarged at birth.

    b. Abnormal rate of enlargement is most frequently noted within 2–3 months after birth.

    c. Increase in size is vertical, lateral and anteroposterior.

    2. Tense, widened fontanelles
    3. Sutures often palpably separated
    4. Signs of increased intracranial pressure

       a. Restlessness and irritability
       b. High pitched or shrill cry
       c. Vomiting
       d. Disturbances in vital signs
          (1) Increased blood pressure
          (2) Decreased pulse
          (3) Decreased and irregular respirations

       e. Headache
       f. Convulsions (possible)
       g. Lethargy
       h. Stupor
       i. Coma

    5. Alteration in muscle tone of the extremities
    6. Rigidity of extremities, especially legs
    7. Hyperactive reflexes
    8. Incontinence
    9. Later physical signs
       a. Forehead becomes prominent.
       b. Eyebrows and eyelids are drawn upward, exposing the sclera above the iris.
       c. "Sunset" eyes result from depression of the orbital plate.
       d. Strabismus, nystagmus and optic atrophy occur.
       e. Infant cannot gaze upward.
       f. Scalp is shiny with prominent scalp veins.
       g. The infant has difficulty holding his head up.
       h. Percussion of the skull produces a typical "cracked pot" sound (Macewen's Sign) because of increased fluid and decreased brain tissue.
       i. Physical and mental development lag.

Diagnostic Evaluation

A. *X-ray Findings*
    1. Widening of the fontanelles and sutures
    2. Erosion of intracranial bone
    3. Soft tissue swelling in the region of the anterior fontanelle

B. *Dye Tests* (indigo carmine or phenolsulfonphthalein tests)
    1. Complete block
       Dye injected into the lateral ventricle fails to appear in the lumbar spinal fluid within 20 minutes. (Normal appearance time is 2–12 minutes.)
    2. Obstruction of the surface subarachnoid pathway distal to the cisterna magna
       a. Normal appearance time in the lumbar spinal fluid—2½ minutes
       b. Less than 15% excretion in the urine in 2 hours
    3. Block in the ventricular system, aqueduct or cisterna magna
       a. No appearance in the lumbar spinal fluid
       b. Less than 15% excretion in the urine in 2 hours

C. *Pneumoencephalogram*
    1. Shows dilated ventricles.
    2. May reveal extent of the brain damage and the location of the block.

D. *Ventriculography*
    Abnormalities are visualized in the ventricular system or the subarachnoid spaces.

E. *Combined ventricular and lumbar puncture with pressure measurements*
1. Determines whether there is free communication between the ventricles and the lumbar subarachnoid space.
2. Estimates the thickness of the brain cortex.

Prognosis

1. Spontaneous arrest sometimes occurs as a result of natural compensatory mechanisms or rupture of the ventricle into the subarachnoid space.
2. Postmeningitic hydrocephalus might also undergo spontaneous remission following gradual disappearance of adhesions.
3. Approximately two-thirds of patients will die at an early age without surgery.
4. With surgery, probably no more than 15% or 20% will be normally competitive both physically and mentally. Correction will not restore damaged or destroyed brain tissue.

Surgical Treatment

A. *General Procedure*

A tube with a one-way valve is inserted surgically to lead fluid from the brain directly into the bloodstream or into some other body cavity.

B. *Purpose*

To reduce the volume of the cerebrospinal fluid within the ventricles.

C. *Specific Surgical Procedures*
1. *Ventriculovenous Shunt*
   a. A tube is passed from the dilated lateral ventricle through a burr hole in the parietal region of the skull.
   b. It is then passed under the skin behind the ear and into a vein down to a point where it discharges into the right atrium or superior vena cava.
   c. The tube passes at one point through a one-way pressure sensitive system.
   d. The valve or valves close to prevent reflux of blood into the ventricle and open as ventricular pressure rises, allowing fluid to pass from the ventricle into the bloodstream.
   e. Complications
      (1) Need for revision of shunt occurs in almost 40% of the cases.
      (2) Septicemia with persistent bacterial growth on the valve.
      (3) Multiple pulmonary thromboses with pulmonary hypertension and congestive heart failure occurring in later years.
2. *Ventriculoperitoneal Shunt*
   a. Diverts cerebrospinal fluid from a lateral ventricle or the spinal subarachnoid space to the peritoneal cavity.
   b. A tube is passed from the lateral ventricle through an occipital burr hole subcutaneously through the posterior aspect of neck and paraspinal region to the peritoneal cavity through a small incision in the right lower quadrant.
   c. This procedure is not as effective as the ventriculoureteral shunt but allows sparing of the kidney.
   d. The procedure is usually used when brief, temporary shunting is necessary.

3. *Ventriculoureteral or Ventriculoureterostomy*
   a. Diverts cerebrospinal fluid from lateral ventricle to the ureter.
   b. One kidney is removed.
   c. A tube is placed from the lateral ventricle out through a burr hole in the low occipitotemporal region, subcutaneously down through the posterior aspect of neck and paraspinal region to a point just below the 12th rib.
   d. It is then tunneled through paraspinal muscles and inserted into the free ureter.
   e. Must be revised as child grows.
4. *Spinoureterostomy*
   a. Diverts cerebrospinal fluid from lumbar spinal subarachnoid space to the ureter.
   b. One kidney is removed.
   c. A tube is passed from the lumbar subarachnoid space through the paraspinal muscles to the free ureter.
   d. This procedure is most successful with communicating types of hydrocephalus.
   e. Not affected by growth.
5. *Ventriculopleural Shunt*
   a. Diverts cerebrospinal fluid from a lateral ventricle to the pleural cavity.
   b. A tube is passed from the ventricle through a subcutaneous tunnel to the right posterior thorax in the region of the 5th or 6th rib.

Preoperative Nursing Objectives

A. *To observe the progress of the disease.*
   1. Measure and record the head circumference daily.
      a. Record the greatest circumference each time.
      b. Measure the head at approximately the same time each day.
      c. Use a centimeter measure for greatest accuracy.
   2. Observe and record the size and fullness of the anterior fontanelle.
   3. Observe for evidence of increased intracranial pressure.
      a. Irritability or lethargy
      b. High pitched cry
      c. Vomiting
      d. Change in body temperature
      e. Changes in vital signs
         (1) Increased blood pressure (increased systolic blood pressure, increased pulse pressure)
         (2) Decreased pulse
         (3) Decreased or irregular respirations
      f. Convulsions
      g. Change in level of consciousness
   4. Changes in appearance
      a. Increased head size
      b. Prominent forehead
      c. "Sunset" eyes
      d. Opisthotonic positioning

B. *To provide adequate nutrition.*
   1. Feeding is often a problem as the child may be listless, anorectic and prone to vomiting.
   2. Complete nursing care and treatments before feeding so that the child will not be disturbed after feeding.

3. Hold the child in a semisitting position for feeding.

   The nurse's arm should be rested on a pad placed over the arm of the chair or on the mattress of the crib if the child's head is heavy.

4. Offer small, frequent feedings.

5. Allow ample time for bubbling.

6. Place the child on his side with his head elevated after feeding to prevent aspiration.

C. *To provide supportive nursing care.*

1. Prevent pressure sores and the development of contractures.
   a. Place the child on a sponge rubber or lamb's wool pad or an alternating-pressure mattress to keep his weight evenly distributed.
   b. Keep the scalp clean and dry.
   c. Turn the child's head frequently; change his position every 2 hours.
      (1) When turning the child, rotate his head and body together to prevent strain on the neck.
      (2) A firm pillow may be placed under the head and shoulders for further support when lifting the child.
   d. Provide meticulous skin care to all parts of the body.
      Observe the skin for evidence of pressure sores.
   e. Give passive range of motion exercises to the extremities, especially the legs.

2. Keep the eyes moistened if the child is unable to close his eyelids normally.
   This prevents corneal ulcerations and infections.

3. Provide for the child's emotional needs of love and affection.
   a. Hold and cuddle the infant as much as possible.
   b. Play with the child according to his mental development.

D. *To assist with diagnostic procedures.*

1. Be familiar with the procedure which is being performed. (See diagnostic tests.)

2. Explain the procedure to the child and his parents at their levels of comprehension.
   a. Make certain that they understand what will happen before and after as well as during the procedure.
   b. Play is frequently helpful for explaining the procedure to a young child.

3. Administer a sedative as ordered by the physician.
   a. Any sedative should be given at the exact prescribed time.
   b. Nursing activities must be organized so that the child is permitted to rest after administration of the medications.
   c. Observe the child for signs of reaction to the sedative such as depressed respirations.

4. Apply protective measures to limit motion as necessary. (See section on pediatric procedures, p. 1073; restraints, and positioning for a lumbar puncture, p. 1109.)

5. Observe the child closely following the procedure for:
   a. Leaking of cerebrospinal fluid from the sites of subdural or ventricular taps
      These tap holes should be covered with a small piece of gauze or cotton saturated with collodion.
   b. Reactions to the sedative, especially respiratory depression
   c. Changes in vital signs indicative of shock
   d. Signs of increased intracranial pressure which may occur if air has been injected into the ventricles.

E. *To provide emotional support to the parents.*
    1. Encourage the parents to visit and allow them to participate in the child's care as much as possible.
    2. Encourage the parents to talk about the child's problem and how they feel about it.
    3. Provide parents with appropriate information concerning the defect. Answer their questions directly and honestly. Correct any misconceptions that they may have such as fear that the child's head may burst.

Postoperative Nursing Objectives

A. *To provide immediate, supportive nursing care.*
    1. Take the infant's temperature, pulse, respiration and blood pressure every 15 minutes until he is fully reactive and then every 1 to 2 hours.
    2. Avoid hypo- or hyperthermia.
        a. Provide appropriate blankets or covers as indicated by body temperature.
        b. An isolette or warming cradle may be used for an infant.
        c. An older child may profit from use of the hypothermia blanket.
        d. Administer a tepid sponge bath or medication as ordered for temperature elevation (See procedure for tepid sponge bath p. 1339.)
    3. Aspirate mucus from the nose and throat as necessary to prevent respiratory difficulty.
    4. Turn the child every 2 hours.
    5. Use a nasogastric tube if necessary for abdominal distention.
        a. This is most frequently used when a ventriculoperitoneal shunt has been performed.
        b. Measure the drainage and record the amount and color.
    6. Give frequent mouth care to prevent dryness of the mucous membranes.
    7. Observe for pallor or mottled condition of the skin, coldness or clamminess of the body and decreased level of consciousness.
    8. Administer prophylactic antibiotics as ordered by the physician.

B. *To allow for optimal draining of cerebrospinal fluid through the shunt.*
        Record observations of the bulging or tenseness of the fontanelle as a guide for positioning the child.
        Position the child according to the physician's order.
        (1) To decrease the rate of drainage if indicated by a depressed fontanelle, the child is placed flat in bed or with his head slightly lowered.
        (2) To promote drainage if indicated by a tense fontanelle, the child is placed flat in bed or with his head slightly elevated.

C. *To prevent the development of decubitus ulcers of the skin overlying the valve in patients with ventriculovenous shunt.*
    1. Place cotton behind and over the ears under the head dressing.
    2. Avoid positioning the child on the area of the valve or the incision until the wound is well healed.

D. *To maintain fluid and electrolyte balance.*
    1. This is especially important when a spinoureterostomy or ventriculoureterostomy has been performed as sodium and chloride lost by drainage of the cerebrospinal fluid into the bladder must be replaced daily in order to prevent peripheral vascular collapse and death.

2. Accurately measure and record total fluid intake and output.

An external collecting device rather than an indwelling catheter should be used to measure urine output whenever possible as this reduces the danger of an infection ascending from the bladder to the spinal canal. (See procedure for urine collection p. 1106.)

Elevate the head of the bed slightly if the infant's condition permits to prevent backflow of urine.

3. Administer intravenous fluids as ordered. (See procedure, p. 1087.)

4. Begin oral feedings once the child is fully recovered from the anesthetic and displays interest.

    a. Begin with small amounts of 5% dextrose, water and saline.

    b. When the child resumes normal feedings, add salt to his formula or milk in the amount ordered by the physician (usually one-half teaspoon) to replace that lost through a ureteral shunt.

        A total daily replacement dose of 2–4 gm. of sodium or ammonium chloride is usually required.

    c. Introduce solid foods suitable to the child's age.

    d. Encourage a high protein diet.

E. *To observe for signs of complications such as increased intracranial pressure, dehydration, intracranial infection or septicemia.*

1. Vomiting
2. Tenseness or bulging of the anterior fontanelle
3. Irritability
4. Muscular rigidity
5. Opisthotonus
6. Convulsions or signs of paralysis
7. Alterations in the state of consciousness
8. Fever (temperature normally fluctuates during the first 24 hours after surgery)
9. Purulent drainage from the incision
10. Sunken fontanelle (Without additional signs of dehydration, this may only indicate a successful shunt.)
11. Diminished skin turgor and dryness of the mucous membranes

F. *To provide continued emotional support to the parents.*

1. Begin discharge planning early. (See parental teaching.)
2. Accompany all instructions with reassurance necessary to prevent the parents from becoming anxious or fearful about assuming the care of the child.

    Relay the success that other mothers have had in dealing with similar infants.

3. Encourage the parents to treat the child as normally as possible, providing him with appropriate toys and love.
4. Help the parents with problems of assisting siblings and grandparents to deal with the child's needs.
5. Initiate appropriate referrals.

    a. Social worker
    b. Community health nurse
    c. Parent groups
    d. Community agencies
    e. Specialty clinics and schools

Parental Teaching

1. Parents should be given complete explanations of the disease, the surgery and the changes that the surgery produced.
2. Physical nursing care
    a. Special attention should be directed toward specific techniques of supportive nursing care, for example:
       (1) Turning   (3) Play
       (2) Skin care   (4) Exercises to strengthen the child's muscles.
    b. Feeding techniques and patterns
       Special emphasis should be placed on the importance of adding salt to the formula if this is required.
3. Symptoms of increased intracranial pressure, recurrent hydrocephalus and dehydration: Parents must be taught not only to recognize these complications, but to report them immediately to the physician.
4. Illnesses which cause vomiting and diarrhea or prevent an adequate fluid intake are a great threat to the child who has had a shunt procedure. The mother should be instructed regarding:
    a. Prevention of such illnesses.
    b. Early recognition of warning symptoms.
    c. Necessity of seeking immediate medical care so that the child can receive intravenous therapy to replace fluid and salt loss.
5. The child's emotional needs should be stressed. Parents should be encouraged to treat the child as normal as much as possible.
6. Refer to the sections on mental retardation for additional areas of parent teaching.

SPINA BIFIDA

Spina bifida refers to a malformation of the spine in which the posterior portion of the laminae of the vertebrae fails to close. Several types of spina bifida are recognized of which the following 3 are most common (Fig. 35-1):

Spina bifida occulta, in which the defect is only in the vertebrae. The spinal cord and meninges are normal.

Meningocele, in which the cord membranes protrude through the opening in the spinal canal forming a cyst filled with cerebrospinal fluid and covered with skin.

Meningomyelocele, in which both the spinal cord and the cord membranes protrude through the defect in the bony rings of the spinal canal.

Etiology

1. Unknown
2. Involves an arrest in the orderly formation of the vertebral arches which occurs between the 4th and 6th week of embryogenesis.
3. May be the result of interacting chemical, hereditary and ecological factors.

Incidence

1. Most common developmental defect of the central nervous system.
    a. Occurs in approximately 1 in every 1000 newborns, but may occur in as many as 3 per 1000.
    b. Approximately 11,000 children are born with this defect each year.

2. More common in females and may be more severe than in males.
3. Risk is highest in the first child and beyond the 6th pregnancy.
4. More common in white than nonwhite population.
5. Often accompanies other congenital malformations.

Altered Physiology

A. *Spina Bifida Occulta*
1. The bony defect may range from a very thin slit separating one lamina from the spinous process to a complete absence of the spines and laminae.
2. A thin fibrous membrane sometimes covers the defect.
3. The spinal cord and its meninges may be connected with a fistulous tract extending to and opening on the surface of the skin.

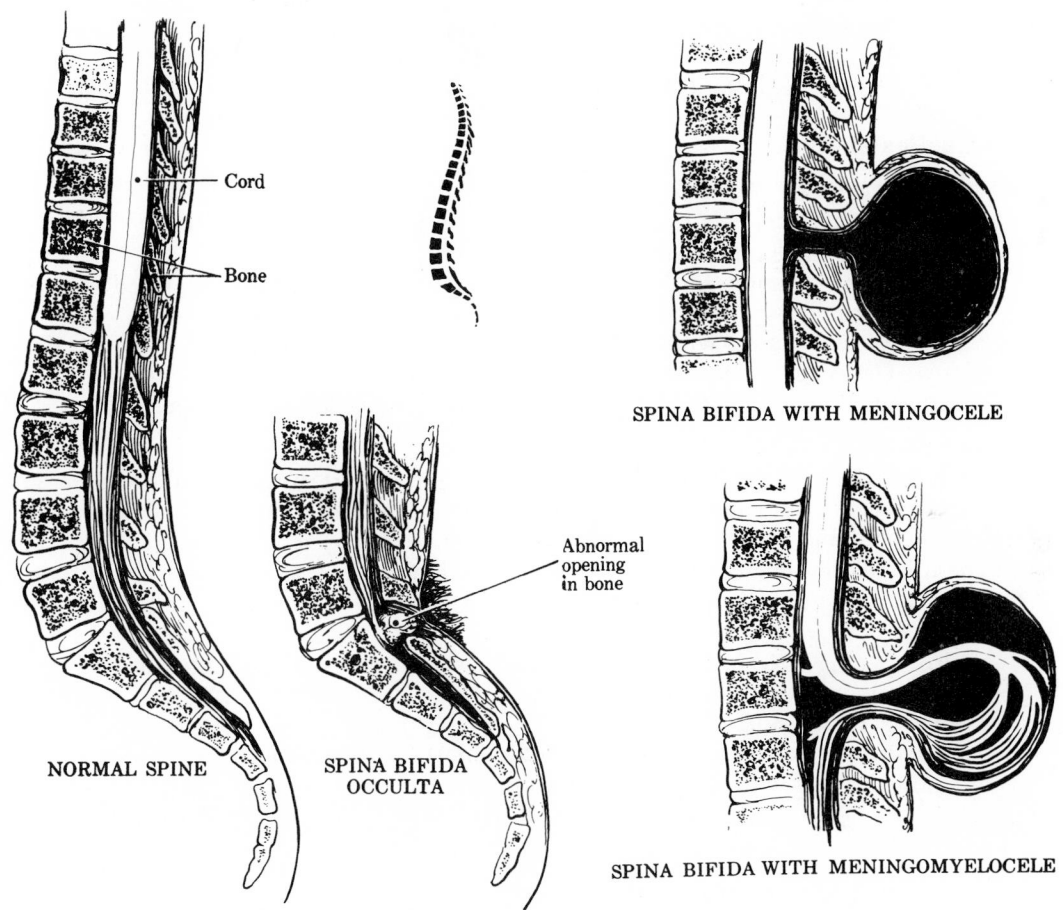

Cord

Bone

SPINA BIFIDA WITH MENINGOCELE

Abnormal opening in bone

NORMAL SPINE

SPINA BIFIDA OCCULTA

SPINA BIFIDA WITH MENINGOMYELOCELE

Figure 35-1. Spina bifida. (From Spina Bifida: Hope Through Research. PHS Pub. No. 1023, Health Information Series No. 103, 1970.)

B. *Meningocele and Meningomyelocele*
   1. The external cystic sac is usually in communication with the subarachnoid space.
   2. There is usually increased pressure of the cerebrospinal fluid.
   3. This causes the sac to increase in size, its wall becoming thinner.
   4. Enlargement continues and leads to spontaneous rupture of the sac or ulcerative perforations secondary to poor blood supply.
   5. The infant may develop meningitis.
   6. Additional pathology associated with meningomyelocele
      a. There is a deficiency in the number of lower motor units resulting in weakness or paralysis of the lower extremities.
      b. Electromyographic studies reveal varying degrees of muscle denervation.
      c. The central canal of myelon above the site of the defect may be markedly distended with resultant neural destruction.
      d. Arnold-Chiari malformation
         (1) Associated malformation of the brain stem and downward displacement of the cerebellar tonsils and the fourth ventricle.
         (2) Causes a block in the lower part of the ventricular system.
         (3) Occurs in almost 65% of patients with meningomyelocele.

Clinical Manifestations

A. *Spina Bifida Occulta*
   1. Most common type. May occur in as many as 25% of normal children.
   2. Most patients have no symptoms.
      a. May have a dimple in the skin or a growth of hair over the malformed vertebra.
      b. No externally visible sac.
      c. May be associated with motor weakness or disorders of sphincter control.
         These symptoms and orthopedic complaints may appear later in life.
   3. Treatment is not required unless neurologic abnormalities show progression.

B. *Meningocele*
   1. An external cystic defect can be seen in the spinal cord, usually in the center line.
      a. The sac is composed only of meninges and filled with cerebrospinal fluid.
      b. The cord and nerve roots are usually normal.
   2. There is seldom evidence of weakness of the legs or lack of sphincter control.
   3. Surgical correction is necessary to prevent rupture of the sac and subsequent infection.
   4. Hydrocephalus may be an associated finding and may be aggravated after surgery for a meningocele.
      a. Occurs in about 9% of patients.
      b. Usually not associated with the Arnold-Chiari malformation.
   5. Prognosis is good with surgical correction.

C. *Meningomyelocele*
   1. A round bulge resembling a meningocele is located usually in the lumbosacral region.
   2. The sac contains both the spinal cord and the cord membranes.
   3. Most common type of open spinal defect.
      Occurs 4–5 times more frequently than other types.

4. Associated Clinical Problems
    a. Motor Function
        (1) Feet may be deformed, or there may be additional vertebral deformities.
        (2) Joints of ankles, knees, or hips may be immobile.
        (3) Variable degrees of weakness present in the lower extremities.
        (4) Spontaneous and induced movements are decreased or absent.
        (5) The nature and degree of involvement depend largely on the location of the lesion.
    b. Sensory Function
        (1) Sensation is usually absent below the level of the defect.
        (2) Ulcerations of the skin are common.
    c. Impaired functioning of the autonomic nervous system below the level of the defect
        (1) Skin is dry and cool.
        (2) Sweating ability is impaired.
    d. Urinary and bowel problems
        (1) Inefficient bladder causes constant urinary dribbling.
        (2) There is stasis of urine and repeated urinary tract infections.
        (3) This leads to lower urinary tract damage and dilatation of the ureters.
        (4) There is frequently upper urinary tract damage and renal destruction.
        (5) Fecal incontinence or retention is caused by poor innervation of the anal sphincter and bowel musculature.
    e. Hydrocephalus
        (1) Occurs in 65% of patients.
        (2) Usually associated with the Arnold-Chiari malformation.
        (3) Usually develops within the first 6 weeks of life.

Complications

1. Hydrocephalus
2. Meningitis
    a. Caused by bacterial contamination of the spinal fluid.
    b. Occurs in approximately 15% of infants with meningocele or meningomyelocele.

Prognosis

1. Guarded except in patients with spina bifida occulta.
2. Depends on the extent of spinal cord involvement.
    a. Only ⅓ of patients with meningocele and meningomyelocele do not have their life significantly hampered.
    b. Prognosis is better with simple meningocele than with meningomyelocele.
    c. Prognosis is poor with associated hydrocephalus.
3. Surgery early in life can either correct or arrest the condition so that other complications do not occur.
    New surgical techniques on the bladder, rectum or spinal cord may be beneficial.
4. Deaths before the age of 2 years are most frequently due to effects on the brain and spinal cord.
5. Deaths after the age of 2 years are usually the result of chronic renal failure.

Surgical Treatment

A. *Procedure*

   Laminectomy and exploration of the spinal cord in the area of the defect.

B. *Purpose*

   1. To prevent further deterioration of neural function.
      Surgery cannot be expected to improve existing neurologic deficits.
   2. To minimize the danger of rupture and infection.
   3. To improve cosmetic effect.

C. *Indications*

   1. Progressively increasing neural deficit or orthopedic deformity.
   2. Extensive vertebral arch defect.
   3. Myelographic demonstration of spinal cord abnormality.

Preoperative Nursing Objectives

A. *To prevent leakage of cerebrospinal fluid or rupture of the meningocele sac.*

   1. Position the infant on its abdomen or support on its side.
      a. Avoid placing the infant on its back as this would cause pressure on the sac.
      b. Apply protective devices to limit movement if necessary to maintain the infant in correct position. (See procedure for protective devices, p. 1073.)
      c. A Bradford frame may be used to facilitate positioning. (See procedure for the use of the Bradford frame, p. 1115.)
      d. A doughnut-shaped sterile padding may be placed around the sac.
      e. Check the position of the infant at least every hour.
   2. Do not place a diaper or other covering directly over the sac.
   3. Observe the sac frequently for evidence of irritation or leakage of cerebrospinal fluid.

B. *To prevent infection.*

   1. Infection of the sac
      a. This is most commonly caused by contamination by urine and feces.
      b. Keep the buttocks and genitalia scrupulously clean.
         (1) The buttocks may be exposed to the air most of the day and to a heat lamp for 15–20 minutes, 2 or 3 times during the day.
         (2) A silicone cream should be used to provide a protective coating over the skin.
      c. Do not diaper the infant if the meningocele is in the lower portion of the spine.
      d. Keep the infant's head higher than his buttocks.
      e. Utilize a divided Bradford frame to allow urine and feces to drain away from the body.
      f. A piece of plastic sheeting may be taped over the defect to shield it from feces.
      g. A sterile gauze or towel or a sterile, moistened dressing covered with a sterile towel may be applied according to the physician's preference.
         When this is used, it should be changed frequently to keep the area free of exudate and to maintain sterility.
   2. Infection of the bladder and urinary tract
      a. This is frequently caused by stasis of urine.
      b. Apply pressure to the bladder if urine is being retained.

       (1) Apply firm, gentle pressure beginning in the umbilical area and progressing under the symphysis pubis toward the anus.

       (2) This practice should be repeated every 2 hours during the day and at least once at night.

C. *To prevent deformities and ulcerations of the lower extremities.*

  1. Support the infant's ankles with foam rubber pads or a diaper roll so that his toes do not rest on the bed.

  2. Place foam rubber pads covered with soft cloth or a diaper roll between the legs to prevent pressure on the skin of the ankles and knees.

  3. Change the infant's position frequently from abdomen to side.

  4. Provide meticulous skin care.

      Mild ointments may be used to prevent chafing of the skin.

  5. Provide passive range of motion exercises for those muscles and joints which the infant does not use spontaneously.

D. *To provide normal infant stimulation.*

  1. Hold the infant in normal feeding position with elbow rotated in order to avoid touching the sac.

  2. The infant may also be fed while positioned on his side on the nurse's lap.

  3. Stop the feeding frequently so that the baby can rest and air can be expelled.

    a. These infants cannot be bubbled like normal babies.

    b. Small, frequent feedings may be necessary.

  4. Provide the infant with appropriate toys such as a bright mobile or musical toy.

E. *To observe for signs of complications.*

  1. Hydrocephalus

    a. Irritability   d. Tense fontanelle

    b. Feeding difficulty or decreased appetite   e. Temperature fluctuations

    c. Increased head circumference   f. Decreased alertness

  2. Infection

    a. Oozing of fluid or pus from the meningocele sac

    b. Fever

    c. Irritability or listlessness

    d. Convulsions

    e. Concentrated or foul-smelling urine

F. *To record evidence of disease progress. Nursing record should include:*

  1. Frequent vital signs   5. Evidence of urine retention or fecal impaction

  2. Behavior of the infant   6. Daily head circumference

  3. Activity of the legs   7. Evidence of complications

  4. Degree of continence

G. *To provide initial emotional support to the family.*

  1. Encourage parents to talk about their child and how they feel about the defect.

  2. Provide them with basic information about the condition. Answer their questions simply and directly.

  3. Encourage (but do not force) them to become involved with the child's care from the beginning.

    a. Demonstrate techniques for holding and feeding the child, etc.

    b. Emphasize what is *normal* and *well* about their infant.

4. Provide the parents with as much valid information as possible on which to base their decision about surgery to repair the infant's defect.

Support their decision for or against surgery.

Postoperative Nursing Objectives

A. *To prevent postoperative complications.*
   1. Shock
      a. Keep the infant warm by placing him in an isolette or infant warmer.
      b. *Keep the infant's head slightly lower than his spine for a few postoperative days.* This maintains spinal fluid pressure in the brain and lessens pressure at the operative site.
   2. Respiratory Problems
      a. Periodically turn the infant from his abdomen to side.
      b. Have oxygen available if necessary.
      c. Report abdominal distention which may interfere with breathing and feeding.
   3. Nutritional Problems
      a. The infant may be fed intravenously for several days, or may be gavage fed if he is unable to take oral feedings. (See procedures for intravenous therapy and gavage feeding, pp. 1087 and 1080.)
      b. Apply previously stated principles when bottle feeding the infant (p. 1079).
   4. Infection
      a. Keep the surgical dressing clean and dry.
      b. Observe the dressing frequently for drainage.
      c. Apply previously stated principles to prevent infection (p. 1328).
      d. Administer antibiotics as ordered by the physician.
   5. Nursing Observations

      Record the following:

      a. Frequent measurements of temperature, pulse and respirations
      b. Color
      c. Evidence of abdominal distention
      d. Condition of the dressing
      e. Evidence of infection
      f. Degree of continence
      g. Behavior of the infant
      h. Evidence of hydrocephalus

B. *To continue nursing activities as listed under objectives of preoperative nursing care.*

C. *To provide continued emotional support to the family.*
   1. Encourage their continued participation in the infant's care.
   2. Complete appropriate referrals. These may include:
      a. Community health nurse
      b. Social worker
      c. Multidisciplinary clinic for birth defects
      d. Parent groups for children with spina bifida
      e. Voluntary agencies
      f. Physical therapist
      g. Occupational therapist
      h. Nursery schools
   3. Foster a goal of helping the child to become as independent as possible.
      a. Emphasize habilitation which makes use of the normal parts of the body and minimizes the disabilities.

  b. Help the child in his orientation to reality.
  c. Focus on immediate planning in the areas of walking, speech, bowel and bladder management and formal education.
  4. Begin a comprehensive teaching program early. See Parental Teaching (below).
  5. Provide support for dealing with the usual problems of a newborn baby.
       Answer questions related to formula, bath, problems of growth and development, discipline, etc.

D. *To foster the development of the child's maximum potential later in life.*
  1. Develop a nursing care plan early which is well coordinated with the plans of other disciplines.
     a. Orthopedics
        (1) Surgery is often necessary to correct deformities.
        (2) Braces, crutches, corrective shoes or other supportive devices are usually ordered.
        (3) See sections on dislocated hip, page 1374, and orthopedic procedures, page 1111.
     b. Urology
        (1) Surgery to separate the bladder and distal ureters from the upper urinary tract is often necessary to prevent hydronephrosis.
        (2) This must be closely coordinated with the orthopedic management as casts and braces may interfere with the placement of urinary collection devices.
        (3) See section on genitourinary surgery, page 1247.
     c. Neurosurgery
     d. Physical Therapy
        (1) Exercise should be initiated early to foster development of the arms, encourage head control and strengthen the muscles above the defect.
        (2) Passive range of motion exercises should be done with the infant's legs.
        (3) Special positioning to prevent or correct existing deformities is usually done.

Parental Teaching

A. *Techniques of Physical Care*
  1. Safe methods of holding the infant
  2. Techniques of feeding
  3. Care of the incision
  4. Provision of adequate elimination
     a. Application of pressure to express urine to reduce the volume of residual urine
        Stress the importance of carrying out this procedure about every 2 hours during the day to help establish a routine for voiding later in life.
     b. Care of ureterostomies if present
     c. Care of indwelling catheters if their use is necessary
     d. Administration of antibacterial drugs if ordered to decrease the incidence of renal infection
     e. Administration of glycerin suppositories or pediatric enemas if needed to prevent impaction.
        Stress the importance of establishing at an early time the routine times for defecation.
  5. Physical Therapy
     Exercises

6. Skin Care
   a. General measures for avoiding pressure sores, such as frequent position changes
   b. Perineal Care
      (1) Frequent diaper changes
      (2) Careful laundering of diapers
      (3) Application of protective ointments
   c. Prevention of ulcerations
      (1) Avoid extremes of temperature.
      (2) Bath water should be lukewarm, not hot.
   d. Daily inspection of the skin for reddened areas, bruises, etc.
7. Method for checking the shunt if one is present

B. *Signs of Complications*
   1. Hydrocephalus or signs of obstruction in the ventricular shunt
   2. Infection, especially meningitis or urinary tract infection

C. *Maintenance of Good General Health*
   1. Infections must be treated immediately.
   2. Diet
      a. Obesity should be prevented as this puts added stress on the underdeveloped parts of the child's body.
      b. Fluid intake of at least 2 ounces/lb. is necessary to maintain good urinary flow and prevent urinary tract infection.
      c. Foods which keep the feces of normal or slightly firm consistency should be encouraged since this minimizes the possibility of involuntary defecation.
      d. Gas-producing foods or those which cause diarrhea should be avoided.
   3. Other sensory defects such as vision or hearing deficits should be corrected as soon as possible.
   4. A proper balance must be maintained between activities of physical therapy and play and relaxation.
   5. The child will require frequent evaluations by specialists:
      a. Pediatricians   d. Neurologists
      b. Urologists   e. Physical therapists
      c. Orthopedists

D. *Clothing*
   1. Loose fitting clothes are most practical and safe.
   2. Socks should fit the feet well. Thin, cotton socks are probably best.
      a. Large socks will wrinkle and cause pressure on the toes or heel.
      b. Small socks may squeeze the leg and cause skin breakdown.
      c. Tight, elastic socks are also constricting.
   3. Fabrics which hold body heat should be avoided.
         These materials may cause unnecessary perspiration and cause skin breakdown.

E. *Family life*
   1. The child should be treated as any other member of the family whenever possible.
   2. He should be praised when he does well and disciplined when he does wrong.
   3. He should be included in family decisions and activities.
   4. Other family members should be allowed to assist in the handicapped child's care.
   5. Dwelling on the medical details of the child's care should be avoided.
   6. Any talent or ability which may give the child a feeling of accomplishment should be developed.

BACTERIAL MENINGITIS

Bacterial meningitis is an inflammation of the meninges which follows the invasion of the spinal fluid by a bacterial agent.

Etiology
1. The proportion of cases due to a specific organism varies from year to year; there is also considerable geographic difference.
2. The specific organisms causing bacterial meningitis in different childhood age groups include:
   a. Newborn Period
      Escherichia coli and other gram negative organisms
      Haemophilus influenzae
      Listeria monocytogenes
      Hemolytic streptococci
      Hemolytic staphylococci
      D. pneumococci
   b. Older infants and children
      Haemophilus influenzae—occurs most frequently in children 2–7 years and occurs most frequently in the fall and early winter.
      Pneumococci
      Meningococci—occurs in epidemics every 8–10 years and occurs most frequently in early spring.
   c. Meningitis is usually related to 1 specific agent, although 2 or more organisms may occur simultaneously. This mixed bacterial meningitis occurs most frequently in young infants.

Altered Physiology
1. Bacterial meningitis is almost always preceded by a febrile upper respiratory infection.
2. Bacteria in the circulating blood then invade the spinal fluid.
3. Bacterial meningitis may occur as an extension of a local bacterial infection such as otitis media, mastoiditis or sinusitis.
4. Purulent bacterial material impairs circulation of the cerebrospinal fluid.
5. Cerebral edema results from impaired circulation.

Clinical Manifestations
1. The onset of bacterial meningitis is usually abrupt with the following manifestations:
   a. Newborn period

      Vomiting
      Poor feeding, or refusal to feed
      Fever or hypothermia
      Periods of apnea or cyanosis
      Diarrhea
      Jaundice

      Lethargy
      Jitteriness
      Bulging fontanelles
      Convulsions
      Sudden enlargement of the
      　head (over 24 hours)

   b. Infants up to 2 years

      Fever
      Vomiting, often projectile
      Drowsiness and irritability
      Jitteriness
      Bulging fontanelle

      Convulsions
      Pain and resistance to neck flexion
      Hyperesthesia
      Vacant stare
      High pitched cry

    c. Over 2 years

      Fever   Pain and resistance to neck flexion

      Vomiting, often projectile   Headache

      Drowsiness and irritability   Photophobia

2. The severity of the meningeal infection and the cerebral involvement are closely related to the rapidity with which the symptoms develop. The child may progress from convulsions to stupor and coma within a short period.

3. Petechiae or purpura may develop.
   a. Have no characteristic distribution.
   b. Most often associated with a meningococcal infection.

Diagnostic Evaluation

Cerebrospinal fluid

a. High cell count

b. Polymorphonuclear cells

c. Low sugar

d. Elevated protein (may be normal)

e. Gram stain and cultures positive— to identify the specific organism

Treatment

1. Identification of the organism
2. Intravenous administration of the appropriate antimicrobial agents to promote rapid destruction of the bacteria and to suppress the emergence of resistant strains.
3. Recognition and treatment of hyponatremia
4. Appropriate prophylactic treatment provided for contacts when indicated

Complications

1. Seizures
2. Water intoxication
3. Subdural effusion
4. Hydrocephalus
5. Cerebral palsy

Nursing Objectives

A. *To practice measures which will prevent the transmission of infection in the nursery.*

1. Practice careful handwashing technique and serve as a model of good technique.
2. Personnel with infection should avoid contact with infants.
   a. Seek medical care for infection (Cultures should be taken.)
   b. Remain out of the nursery.
   c. Wear a mask when it is necessary to enter the nursery.
3. Teach parents and other persons entering the nursery proper handwashing and gown technique.
4. Maintain sterile technique when procedures demanding this technique are performed.
5. Promote general cleanliness of the nursery environment.

B. *To observe infants for the vague symptoms which appear early in the course of meningeal irritation.*

1. Observe for the following:
   a. Lethargy, decreased activity and loss of muscle tone
   b. Poor feeding or refusal to feed
   c. Loss of weight

2. Be consistent in planning for the care of infants to provide a means whereby these early symptoms may be detected.
   a. Accurate charting of the infant's previous behavior.
   b. Assigning the same nurse to care for an infant on successive days.
3. Report to the physician the symptoms observed.

C. *To observe for episodes of apnea and initiate measures to stimulate respiration.*
   1. Observe the infant closely for apnea or have the infant placed on a respiratory monitor.
   2. Stimulate infant when apnea does occur.
      a. Slap on feet and provide more vigorous stimulation if necessary.
      b. When spontaneous respiration does not occur within 15 to 30 seconds apply hand resuscitator or mouth-to-mouth resuscitation. (See section on resuscitation.)
   3. Report frequent periods of apnea to physician.
   4. Record length of apnea episode and response to stimulation on nursing record.

D. *To observe the child for convulsive activity which may occur with sepsis.*
   1. Observe the infant for any twitching or convulsive activity.
   2. Report immediately any twitching or convulsive activity.
      a. Remain with infant.
      b. Suction mouth and nose if infant has secretions or vomitus in his mouth.
      c. Turn head to side.
      d. Protect infant from banging against side of isolette or incubator.
      e. Provide oxygen if cyanosis or respiratory distress occurs.
      f. Administer any medication prescribed to control the convulsions.
   3. Record the length of the convulsion, the type, the parts of the body involved, the infant's general appearance before and following the convulsion, and response to any therapy given.

E. *To provide for the nutritional needs of the infant in order to provide for caloric needs.*
   1. During the acute phase of the illness, the infant may not be able to take or tolerate feedings.
      a. Monitor the administration of intravenous fluids.
      b. Provide for the sucking needs of the infant by providing a pacifier.
      c. Gavage feedings may be given to the infant. (See section on feeding methods, p. 1080.
   2. Initiate oral feedings or formula as soon as the infant's condition improves.
      a. Begin by offering small feedings and observe for following responses:
         (1) Vomiting
         (2) Abdominal distention
         (3) Infant's interest in feeding and ability to suck
         (4) If the infant tires with feeding
      b. Supplement oral feedings with gavage feedings if necessary.
      c. Gradually increase amount of feeding.
      d. Resume regular feeding schedule based on infant's ability to tolerate it.
   3. Hold the infant for feedings as soon as his condition warrants it.

F. *To provide measures to maintain the infant's temperature within normal range.*
   1. Take infant's temperature at hourly intervals.
   2. Adjust the incubator temperature to maintain infant's temperature between 36–36.5°C. (97 and 98°F.).

3. When infant is placed in an open crib, maintain temperature and cover the infant appropriately.
4. Report hypothermia or hyperthermia.

G. *To administer the prescribed antibiotic therapy to control the infection.*
   1. Administer the prescribed medications.
      a. Be aware of the action and side effects of the specific medications.
      b. Be aware of the route by which the medication is excreted.
      c. Be aware of drug incompatibilities and interactions.
   2. Observe the infant's apparent response to therapy.
      a. Note child's activity, feeding behavior and weight.
      b. Observe for the development of new symptoms.

H. *To provide for the emotional needs of the infant.*
   1. Place bright colorful objects in the crib or isolette.
   2. Talk gently and quietly while caring for the infant.
   3. Touch and gently stroke the infant.
   4. Encourage the parents to visit and allow them to hold the infant as soon as possible.

I. *To involve the parents in the infant's care in the hospital and prepare them for the infant's discharge.*
   1. Encourage parents to visit the infant.
      a. Allow them to hold and feed the baby.
      b. Answer questions they may have regarding the infant's progress and care.
      c. Provide them with an opportunity to explain their concerns.
   2. Discuss symptoms they should watch for as signs of possible complications.
   3. Give specific instruction regarding medications to be given at home.

CONVULSIVE DISORDERS

Convulsive disorder is a term used to encompass a number of varieties of episodic disturbances of brain function. Convulsions should not be regarded as one specific disease, but as a symptom of an underlying disorder. They are relatively common in children, being more prevalent during the first 2 years than at any other time in life. They may be classified as acute or chronic.

Acute Convulsions

Acute convulsions refer to nonrecurrent seizures.

Etiology

A. *Febrile Convulsions*
   1. Acute extracranial infections
   2. High environmental temperatures

B. *Intracranial Infections*
   1. Meningitis
   2. Encephalitis
   3. Cerebral abscess

C. *Intracranial Hemorrhage*
   1. Birth trauma
   2. Hemorrhagic disease
   3. Sickle cell disease
   4. Rupture of defective blood vessels

D. *Toxic*
   1. Convulsant drugs
   2. Lead encephalopathy
   3. Uremia

E. *Anoxic*
1. Prolonged anoxia at birth
2. Sudden severe asphyxia

F. *Metabolic*
1. Acute hypocalcemic tetany
2. Alkalosis
3. PKU (phenylketonuria)
4. Hypoglycemic states

G. *Acute Cerebral Edema*

H. *Brain Tumor*

Altered Physiology

1. Brain cells become overactive and discharge in a sudden, violent, disorderly manner.
2. This paroxysmal burst of electrical energy spreads to adjacent areas or may jump to distant areas of the central nervous system.
3. A seizure results.

Clinical Manifestations

A. *General Features*
1. Clinical signs and symptoms—similar to the grand mal seizures of epilepsy. (See p. 1341.)
2. Electroencephalogram
   a. Similar to that found during and after a grand mal seizure.
   b. Abnormality of the EEG does not persist.
3. Prognosis
   a. Depends on eradication and control of the underlying disease.
   b. Less favorable if the convulsion is prolonged or if a second seizure occurs before the child has recovered from the first.

B. *Febrile Convulsions*
1. Incidence
   a. Occurs in approximately 6–8% of all children.
   b. Usually occurs after the first 6 months but within the first 2–3 years of life.
   c. Rare after age 6–8 years.
   d. Males are more often affected than females.
   e. There may be an increased susceptibility in some families.
2. Clinical signs and symptoms—similar to the grand mal seizures of epilepsy.
3. Electroencephalogram
   a. Similar to that found during and after a grand mal seizure.
   b. Abnormality frequently persists for as long as a week after the seizure.
4. Prognosis
   a. Single febrile seizure
      Excellent prognosis for complete recovery.
   b. Multiple febrile seizures
      (1) High probability that the child will develop chronic epilepsy. (Approximately 25% of epileptic children have a history of febrile seizures.)
      (2) Factors predisposing to the development of chronic epilepsy in children with febrile seizures
         (a) Five febrile convulsions within a 1-year period.
         (b) A convulsion that lasts for over an hour.
         (c) Persistent electroencephalographic abnormalities

Chemotherapy

A. *Antipyretic Drugs*
  1. Acetaminophen (Tempra or Tylenol)
     a. Dosage
        (1) Under 1 year (60 mg.)
        (2) 1–3 years (60–120 mg.)
        (3) 3–6 years (120 mg.)
        (4) 6–12 years (240 mg.)
        (5) Maximum dose (3.6 gm./24 hours)
     b. Side Effects
        (1) Nausea and vomiting
        (2) Skin eruption
        (3) Weakness
        (4) Decreased pulse and respiration
        (5) Allergic symptoms
     c. Advantage
        Less overall toxicity than the salicylates
  2. Acetylsalicylic Acid (aspirin)
     a. Dosage
        65 mg./kg./24 hours in divided doses every 4–6 hours.
     b. Side effects
        Are rare in small doses but may occur as a matter of personal idiosyncracy.
        (1) Nausea, vomiting and diarrhea
        (2) Excessive sweating
        (3) Ringing in ears
        (4) Disturbances in hearing and vision
        (5) Skin eruption and other allergic reactions
        (6) Increased bleeding tendency
        (7) Depression and coma

B. *Anticonvulsant Drug*
  Sodium phenobarbital
     a. Dosage
        (1) 3 mg./kg.
        (2) Average doses
             6 months of age (60 mg.)
             2–3 years of age (120 mg.)
             Maximum single dose (200 mg.)
        (3) Dose may be repeated if seizure is not controlled within 15 minutes.
             One half of the original dose should be administered if the convulsion is partially controlled.
     b. Route
        (1) Intramuscular
        (2) May be given *slowly* intravenously in dilute solution
        (3) Oral
     c. Contraindications
        (1) Severe hepatic or renal dysfunction
        (2) Hypersensitivity to barbiturates
     d. Untoward effects (rare)
        (1) Excitement
        (2) Drowsiness
        (3) Dermatitis
        (4) Gastrointestinal symptoms
        (5) Vertigo
     e. Toxic effects (rare)
        Respiratory, circulatory or renal depression

Nursing Objectives

A. *To control the seizures.*

1. Reduce fever by any of the following nursing measures or by a combination of these measures:
    a. Give a tepid sponge bath.
       (1) Place a rubber or plastic sheet and blanket under the patient with the blanket next to the patient.
       (2) Place a warm water bottle at the child's feet to prevent chilling.
       (3) Place moist cloths over the superficial blood vessels in the axillae and the groins.
       (4) Slowly stroke the extremities with long soothing strokes of the washcloth.
          (a) Stroke the arms from the neck to the axilla and down to the palms of the hand.
          (b) Stroke the legs from the groin to the feet.
       (5) Use gentle friction to bring the blood to the surface.
       (6) Change the water as often as necessary to maintain a water temperature of 24–27°C. (75–80°F.).
       (7) Continue this procedure until temperature is adequately reduced or more drastic measures are ordered.
       (8) Observe the child for chilling or change in his general condition.
       (9) Pat dry with a towel.
       (10) Cover the child with a sheet and allow him to rest for one-half hour.
       (11) After this interval, take the vital signs again.
       (12) Point of emphasis:
              Avoid using alcohol since it may reduce temperature too rapidly, thereby stimulating another convulsive episode.
       (13) Secure the child's cooperation during the procedure.
          (a) A small infant may be held during the sponging.
          (b) Allow the child or his parent to participate in the procedure.
          (c) Discontinue sponging if the child is extremely upset and uncooperative.
    b. Utilize the hypothermia blanket (often the method of choice for older children).
    c. Administer medications as ordered.

B. *To observe the child for recurrent seizures.*

1. Place the child where he can be watched closely.
2. Take the vital signs frequently especially if the child is febrile.
3. Check the child frequently. Report:
    a. Behavior changes   c. Restlessness
    b. Irritability   d. Listlessness

C. *To protect the child from injury during a convulsive episode.*

1. Preventive Measures
    a. Remove hard toys from the bed.
    b. Keep a padded tongue blade immediately available to put between the child's teeth to prevent him from biting his tongue.
    c. Pad the sides of the crib.
    d. Have a suction machine available to remove secretions during a seizure.
    e. Have an emergency oxygen source in the room in case of sudden respiratory difficulty.

2. Emergency Actions
   a. Clear the area around the child if he is not in bed.
   b. Do not restrain him.
   c. Loosen the clothing around his neck.
   d. Insert the tongue blade carefully to prevent injury to the child's mouth.
      (1) Do not force his mouth open.
      (2) Do not force anything between his teeth.
   e. Turn the child on his side so that saliva can flow out of his mouth.
   f. Suction the child and administer oxygen as necessary.
   g. Place him in bed after the seizure if he is not already there.

D. *To record the convulsion accurately. Include the following:*
   1. Behavior before the convulsion
   2. Types of movements observed
      a. Tonic
         (1) Body becomes stiff.
         (2) Muscles in a state of constant contraction
      b. Clonic
            Twitching, jerking motions
   3. Time convulsion began and ended
   4. Site where twitching or contraction began
   5. Areas of the body involved
   6. Movements of the eyes and changes in pupil size
   7. Incontinence
   8. Amount of perspiration
   9. Respiratory changes
   10. Color
   11. Foaming at the mouth or vomiting
   12. Apparent degree of consciousness during the seizure
   13. Behavior after the seizure
       a. Degree of memory for recent events   d. Paralysis or weakness
       b. Types of speech   e. Sleeping after the attack
       c. Coordination

E. *To provide emotional support to the parents.*
   1. Remain calm and efficient if the child has a seizure in the presence of his parents.
   2. Encourage parents to acknowledge their fears.
   3. Provide them with realistic, reassuring information.
      a. A convulsion does not necessarily imply that the underlying disease is a serious one.
      b. A convulsion is equivalent to a "chill" experienced by adults under similar conditions.
      c. Children rarely die in seizures.
      d. Approximately 7% of infants have a convulsion at some point, but few suffer brain damage.
      e. The prognosis depends on the cause of the convulsion.
         (1) A single febrile seizure is not indicative of later chronic epilepsy.

(2) Children who have the tendency to develop febrile convulsions usually lose it as they grow older.

(3) Occasional, brief convulsions have no adverse effects on the child's ultimate development.

Parental Teaching

Stress the following points:

1. Emergency management of seizures
2. Prompt administration of antipyretic measures is necessary whenever the child is febrile.
   a. Immediate medical evaluation is indicated as soon as the child develops fever.
   b. Prophylactic phenobarbital may be prescribed during a febrile episode.

Epilepsy

Epilepsy is a recurrent convulsive disorder marked by sudden and periodic lapses of consciousness and distinctive disturbances in the electrical discharges within the brain.

Etiology

A. *Idiopathic*

B. *Organic*
   1. Trauma
   2. Hemorrhage
   3. Anoxia
   4. Infection
   5. Toxic Reactions
   6. Degenerative Diseases
      a. Idiopathic atrophy
      b. Intracranial neurofibromatosis

   7. Congenital
      a. Cerebral aplasia
      b. Vascular anomalies
   8. Parasitic brain disease

C. *Sensory*
   1. Light
   2. Sound
   3. Reading
   4. Self-induced

Altered Physiology

Same as in acute convulsions. (See p. 1337.)

Types of Epilepsy

1. Aura
2. Grand mal
3. Petit mal

4. Focal
5. Infantile myoclonic seizures

Clinical Manifestations

A. *Aura*
   1. Small, localized seizures. Sometimes precede grand mal seizures and act as a warning.
   2. The child cannot explain them but knows they exist.
   3. May include vague symptoms such as irritability, headache, gastrointestinal disturbances or mental dullness.
   4. The interval between the aura and grand mal seizure is usually short, but it may be an hour or more than a day.

B. *Grand Mal*
   1. Onset
      a. Onset is abrupt.
      b. May occur at night.
      c. An aura occurs in about ⅓ of epileptic children prior to a grand mal seizure.
   2. Tonic spasm
      a. The child's entire body becomes stiff.
      b. He usually loses consciousness.
      c. The face may become pale and distorted.
      d. His eyes are frequently fixed in one position.
      e. His back may be arched with his head held backward or to one side.
      f. His arms are usually flexed and his hands clenched.
      g. The child may be incontinent and may bite his tongue or cheek. (This occurs because of sudden forceful contraction of his jaw and abdominal muscles.)
      h. He is often unable to swallow his saliva.
      i. Breathing is ineffective and cyanosis results if spasm includes the muscles of respiration.
      j. The pulse may become weak and irregular.
   3. Clonic phase
      a. Characterized by twitching movements which follow the tonic state.
      b. Usually start in one place and become generalized, including the muscles of the face.
   4. Duration
      a. Varies.
      b. Usually, convulsions cease after a few minutes and consciousness returns.
   5. Postconvulsive state of child
      a. Usually is sleepy or exhausted.
      b. May complain of headache.
      c. May appear to be in a dazed state.
      d. Often performs relatively automatic tasks without being able to recall the episode.
   6. Secondary symptomatology
      a. Less common in children than in adults.
      b. Represents the patient's response over a long period of time to the injurious attitudes of other people toward the child and his diagnosis.
   7. EEG
      a. Definite abnormalities can be demonstrated in the interval between seizures.
         (1) Random spike discharges
         (2) Diffuse high-voltage slow waves
         (3) Pattern not consistent with the child's chronologic age
      b. Multiple high-voltage spike discharges are demonstrated during the seizure.
      c. Asymmetries between the 2 hemispheres and diffuse slowing are observed after the seizure.

C. *Petit Mal*
   1. Onset—rarely appears before 3 years of age.
   2. Clinical signs
      a. Loss of contact with the environment for a few brief seconds:
         (1) The child may appear to be staring or daydreaming.

(2) If reading or writing, the child will suddenly discontinue the activity and resume it when the seizure has ended.

b. Minor manifestations include rolling of the eyes, nodding of the head and slight quivering of the trunk and limb muscles.

3. Duration—usually less than 30 seconds.
4. Frequency—varies from 1 or 2 per month to several hundred each day.
5. Postconvulsive state
   a. Child appears normal.
   b. Is not aware of having had a convulsion.
6. EEG
   Has characteristic spike and wave pattern during the seizure.

D. *Focal Seizures*

1. Psychomotor
   a. Clinical signs
      (1) Child undertakes purposeful but inappropriate motor acts.
      (2) Child may pick at his clothes with his hands.
      (3) He may make chewing movements with his mouth or perform other complicated actions.
      (4) The young child may emit a shrill cry or attempt to run for help.
      (5) There is usually a gradual loss of postural tone.
      (6) May have circumoral pallor.
   b. Duration—brief, usually about 1 minute.
   c. Postconvulsive state—the child may be confused after an attack but has no memory of what happened.
   d. EEG—normal except at the time of the seizure.

2. Focal Motor (Jacksonian seizures)
   a. Clinical signs
      (1) Sudden jerking movements occur in a particular area of the body such as the face, arms or tongue (less often the leg or foot).
      (2) Seizure begins in one area of the body and spreads to adjacent areas on the same side in a fixed progression.
      (3) Consciousness may or may not be disturbed.
   b. Prognosis
      Seizures may become more extensive as the child matures, leading to grand mal seizures.

3. Focal sensory (rare in children)
   Sensations occur, such as numbness, tingling and coldness in the part of the body controlled by the area of the brain cell overactivity.

E. *Infantile Myoclonic Seizures*

1. Onset—before 2 years of age.
2. Clinical signs
   Mass myoclonus commonly manifested in sudden dropping of the head and flexion of the arms.
3. Frequency—usually recur several hundred times each day.
4. EEG—random high-voltage slow waves and spikes suggestive of a diffuse, disorganized state.

5. Prognosis
   a. Usually, seizures disappear spontaneously after 4 years of age.
   b. Subsequent grand mal seizures may develop.
   c. Mental retardation usually accompanies this disorder.

Prognosis

1. General prognosis depends on coexisting mental retardation, organic disorders and the medical management.
   a. Medically treated seizures
      (1) Spontaneous cessation of seizures may occur.
          Drugs may be gradually discontinued when the child has been free from attacks for an extensive period and his EEG pattern has reverted to normal.
      (2) Seizures seldom occur even during participation in athletic activities.
   b. Nontreated epilepsy
      Seizures tend to become more numerous.
2. Mental Development
   a. Convulsive episodes themselves do not usually cause irreversible brain damage.
   b. Epileptic children with normal mentality can be expected to maintain it with proper control of seizures.
      Children with petit mal and essentially normal EEG patterns generally have a more favorable prognosis for normal mentality than do children with grand mal or psychomotor seizures.

Chemotherapy

A. *General Principles Related to the Administration of Medications*
   1. A drug level is desired which will prevent attacks without producing drowsiness or unsteadiness.
   2. Accurate timing is essential to prevent seizures.
      This is especially true when there is a tendency for the child to have convulsions at a certain period each day.
   3. Enteric coated tablets which have a delayed effect should be used for children who are prone to attacks during sleep.
   4. Most anticonvulsants are available in liquid form as well as in capsules or tablets. Tablets can be crushed and given to infants and small children in coke syrup or applesauce.
   5. It may take several months to find the best combination of medications and the best dosages of each to control the child's seizures.

B. *Common Drugs Used for the Control of Epilepsy in Children*
   1. Phenobarbital
      a. Dose
         (1) 6 mg./kg./24 hours
         (2) Usually divided into 3 doses
         (3) Maximum doses
             Under 3 years (30 mg. 3 times daily)
             3–6 years (65 mg. 3 times daily)
             Over 6 years (0.1 gm. 3 times daily)

    b. Route
      (1) Oral
      (2) Rectal
    c. Indications and advantages
      (1) Drug of choice for initial trial
      (2) One of the safest anticonvulsant drugs
      (3) Relatively inexpensive
    d. Untoward effects
      (1) Excitement   (4) Vertigo
      (2) Rash   (5) Aggravated psychomotor seizures
      (3) Gastrointestinal symptoms   (6) Drowsiness
    e. Toxic effects (rare)
        Respiratory, circulatory or renal depression
    f. Contraindications
      (1) Severe hepatic or renal dysfunction
      (2) Hypersensitivity
2. Diphenylhydantoin (Dilantin)
    a. Dose
      (1) 3–8 mg./kg./24 hours
      (2) Usually divided into 2 doses but may be given as a single dose
      (3) Doses above 8 mg./kg. may result in toxic symptoms
    b. Route—oral
    c. Indications and advantages
      (1) Does not produce excessive drowsiness
      (2) Safest drug for the management of psychomotor epilepsy
      (3) Often used with phenobarbital
    d. Untoward effects
      (1) May accentuate petit mal seizures
      (2) Hypertrophy of the gums
        Daily gum massage is an important aspect of nursing care for a patient taking Dilantin.
    e. Toxic effects (rare)
      (1) Ataxia   (5) Vomiting
      (2) Paralytic manifestations   (6) Skin rash
      (3) Mild psychoses   (7) Blood dyscrasias
      (4) Tremor of the hands
3. Ethosuximide (Zarontin)
    a. Dose
      (1) Initial
        Under 6 years (250 mg./24 hours)
        Over 6 years (250 mg. twice a day)
      (2) Continuing
        Increase by 250 mg. as needed every 4–7 days
    b. Route—oral
    c. Indications and advantages
      (1) Used for petit mal seizures
      (2) Occurrence of blood dyscrasia is less common following administration of Zarontin than with trimethadione (Tridione)—the other medication frequently used to control petit mal seizures.

  d. Untoward effects
   (1) Drowsiness
   (2) May increase grand mal seizures
   (3) Dermatitis
   (4) Gastrointestinal symptoms
   (5) Headache
   (6) Dizziness
   (7) Swelling of the tongue
   (8) Hiccough
  e. Toxic effects
   (1) Blood dyscrasias
   (2) Psychiatric symptoms
  f. Contraindications
    Hepatic or renal disease

Nursing Objectives

A. *To control the seizures.*

  Administer medications as ordered.

B. *To minimize anxiety during the child's hospitalization.*

  1. Rationale

   The therapeutic value of anticonvulsant drugs is decreased if the child has more anxiety than he can handle.

  2. Explain the diagnostic and treatment plan to the child in a manner that he can understand.

   a. The use of play is very effective in explaining things to younger children and allowing them to express their feelings.

   b. The older child should be encouraged to ask questions and talk about his experience.

  3. Allow the child as much normal activity as possible.

   Allow him to be dressed if desired.

  4. If the child does have a seizure, stay with him and remain calm.

   a. Stay with the child after a convulsion and reassure him and his parents that he is all right.

   b. Maintain a quiet environment if the child has had a long convulsive episode.

  5. Provide diversion appropriate for the child's age.

   Play equipment should be such that it will not cause injury during a seizure.

  6. Avoid unnecessary stimulation.

C. *To observe the child for recurrent seizures.*

  Nursing activities are the same as for the child with acute convulsions. (See p. 1339.)

D. *To protect the child from injury during a convulsive episode.*

  Nursing activities are the same as for the child with acute convulsions. (See p. 1339.)

E. *To accurately record the seizures.*

  Nursing activities are the same as for the child with acute convulsions. (See p. 1340.)

F. *To provide emotional support to the child's parents.*

  1. Describe completely any examinations, evaluations, treatments that the child is receiving.

   a. EEG
   b. Pneumoencephalogram
   c. Blood studies
   d. Medications

  2. Provide information regarding the disease itself.

   a. Orientation should be a continuing process.

  b. Too much information at one time is undesirable.
  c. Points of emphasis:
   (1) Epilepsy is *not* contagious, is seldom dangerous and does *not* indicate insanity or mental retardation.
   (2) Most children with epilepsy have infrequent seizures or are able to control their convulsions completely.
   (3) The child may have normal intelligence and can live a useful and productive life.
   (4) The child's medication should in no way influence his mental ability or personality or cause him to become a drug addict.
   (5) It is impossible to predict accurately the possibility of the convulsive disorder appearing in siblings or offspring of the affected child.
  d. Refer the family to appropriate community resources and services.
   (1) Social worker   (4) Psychiatrist
   (2) Community health nurse (5) Parent groups
   (3) School nurse   (6) Voluntary agencies
  e. Provide the parents with appropriate literature.
 3. Observe the parent-child reaction for evidence of rejection or overprotection. Offer reassurance and praise for achievements in dealing with the child's problem.
 4. Prepare parents for the fact that it may take several months of regulating drug dosages before adequate control is obtained.

Parental Teaching

 1. The child should have as normal an environment as possible.
  a. Attendance at a regular school with healthy children should be encouraged.
   (1) Contact should be made with the school nurse who can help the child's teacher understand his disease, emergency treatment of seizures, etc.
   (2) Child should be allowed to participate in organizations and outside activities with limited restrictions.
    (a) Each child must be treated individually; the kind of activity depends on the degree of control.
    (b) Responsible adults should be made aware of the child's disease.
   (3) Child should not be made to feel that he can never be left alone.
   (4) He needs to be disciplined as a normal child.
    He should not gain attention directly or indirectly by having seizures.
 2. The child should be given appropriate information regarding his diagnosis and treatment. He is less confident of his body and his control over it and therefore less confident of himself.
  a. He should be included in conferences with the physician.
  b. He needs an opportunity to ask questions which should be answered honestly.
  c. He should be aware of his restrictions and helped to deal with them.
  d. He should gradually be given responsibility for taking his own medications faithfully.
 3. The older child and adolescent should be helped to achieve independence.
  a. He should be given the opportunity for privacy to discuss his diagnosis with his physician.
  b. He should be allowed to use his own judgment in his daily activities.

   c. He should be helped to develop realistic educational and career goals.
     (1) The assistance of a social worker or psychiatrist may be invaluable during this period.
     (2) Genetic counseling may be indicated in some cases.
       (a) People with epilepsy can marry and have children.
       (b) There is no proof that epilepsy is hereditary although there may be a tendency to transmit a low convulsive threshold.
       (c) The decision to marry must be based on the individual's own feelings of security and self-confidence and his ability to assume the responsibility of marriage.
   d. Any fantasies that "there is nothing wrong with me" or refusal to take medications must be dealt with immediately.

4. Factors which may precipitate a convulsive episode should be avoided.
   a. The seizures should be treated matter-of-factly. A calm reassuring attitude is essential during and after a seizure.
     The attitude of adults when the child has a seizure influences the attitude of other children toward him.
   b. The child should be kept in optimal physical condition with special attention to the status of his teeth and eyes and to the prevention of infection.
   c. Excessive fatigue, overhydration and hyperventilation should be avoided.
   d. Irregular, fluctuating schedules are detrimental. A routine of daily living should be encouraged.

5. Medical care and supervision to control convulsions are essential.
   Routine immunizations are often postponed and then started with only a fraction of the usual dose, especially in children with febrile convulsions.

6. Instructions regarding medical and nursing home care should be stressed.
   a. Administration of medications
   b. Emergency care during a seizure
   c. Observations
     (1) Signs of impending seizure
     (2) Behavior during and after the seizure
   d. Diet
     (1) Ketogenic diets are no longer widely used.
     (2) Fluids should be restricted as overhydration may predispose the child to a convulsive episode.

SUBDURAL HEMATOMA

Subdural hematoma refers to an accumulation of fluid, blood and its degradation products within the subdural space. It may be acute, subacute or chronic.

Etiology

1. Direct or transmitted trauma to the head
   a. Birth trauma
   b. Accidental causes
   c. Purposeful violence such as in the battered child syndrome (see p. 1390)
2. Meningitis

Incidence of Chronic Subdural Hematoma

1. Greatest between 2–4 months of age
2. Less common after age 14–16 months
3. More common in males than females

Altered Physiology

1. Trauma to the head causes tearing of the delicate subdural veins, resulting in small hemorrhages into the subdural space.
2. As the blood breaks down, there is an increased capillary permeability and effusion of blood cells and protein into the subdural space.
3. The breakdown products of blood stimulate the growth of connective tissue and capillaries largely from the dura.
4. A membrane is formed which usually extends frontally and laterally over the hemispheres, surrounding the clot.
5. Fluid accumulates within the membrane and increases the width of the subdural space.
6. Further hemorrhages occur.
7. The lesion enlarges, expanding the skull and, if unrelieved, ultimately causes cerebral atrophy or death from compression and herniation.
8. The lesion may arrest spontaneously at any point.
9. Further bleeding may occur into an already existing sac and may increase symptoms.
10. In long-standing subdural hematoma, the fluid may disappear leaving a constricting membrane which prevents normal brain growth.

Clinical Manifestations

A. *Acute*

Rapid onset of signs of increased intracranial pressure, usually following trauma. (See p. 1323.)

B. *Chronic*

1. Onset
   a. Insidious
   b. Early symptoms apparently unrelated to the central nervous system
2. Infants
   a. Early signs
      (1) Anorexia
      (2) Difficulty feeding
      (3) Vomiting
      (4) Irritability
      (5) Low grade fever
      (6) Failure to gain weight
   b. Later signs
      (1) Enlargement of the head
      (2) Bulging and pulsation of the anterior fontanelle
      (3) Tight, glossy scalp with dilated scalp veins
      (4) Retinal hemorrhages
      (5) Strabismus, pupillary inequality, ocular palsies (rare)
      (6) Hyperactive reflexes
      (7) Retarded motor development

3. Older children
    a. Early signs:
        (1) Lethargy
        (2) Anorexia
        (3) Symptoms of increased intracranial pressure
            (a) Vomiting   (d) Decreased pulse
            (b) Irritability   (e) Decreased or irregular respirations
            (c) Increased blood pressure   (f) Headache
    b. Later signs (may occur immediately if bleeding takes place rapidly)
        (1) Convulsions
        (2) Coma

Diagnostic Evaluation

1. Complete blood count—anemia of blood loss; low serum protein level
2. X-ray—sutural separation in infants
3. Transillumination of the skull in infants—increased
4. Lumbar puncture—spinal fluid is often under increased pressure. May contain red blood cells, a slight excess of white cells and increased protein.
5. Bilateral subdural taps—fluid of any sort in excess of 1–2 ml. or with a protein content significantly higher than that of the cerebrospinal fluid obtained at the same time.
6. Electroencephalogram—frequently abnormal
7. Carotid angiography—shows filling defect

Complications

1. Mental retardation
2. Ocular abnormalities
3. Paralysis

Prognosis

1. Generally excellent with treatment.
2. Complete recovery is expected in more than 50% of the patients, depending on the condition of the brain at the time of surgery.

Treatment

1. Daily subdural taps to remove the abnormal fluid
    a. In infants, the needle can be inserted through the fontanelle or suture line.
    b. In older children, burr holes into the skull are necessary before the needle can be inserted.
    c. This may be the only treatment required if the fluid disappears entirely and a membrane is not present.
2. Frontoparietal burr holes
    a. Usually done after 7–10 days of daily subdural taps.
    b. Necessary to determine the presence of a membrane.
3. Craniotomy
    a. Is necessary in order to remove a membrane if it has formed.
    b. Subdural taps may continue to be necessary in the postoperative period as all of the membrane can seldom be removed.

  c. Usually necessary in older children.

  d. Craniotomies are performed at intervals of several days in patients with bilateral hematoma.

 4. Subdural–pleural shunt may be indicated.

Nursing Objectives

A. *To provide adequate nutrition.*

  Apply principles stated in the section on hydrocephalus, page 1320.

B. *To prevent pressure sores.*

 1. Place the child on a sponge rubber or lamb's wool pad.

 2. Change the child's position every 2 hours.

 3. Provide meticulous skin care.

  Observe skin for evidence of breakdown.

C. *To avoid additional increase in intracranial pressure.*

 1. Maintain a quiet environment.

 2. Avoid sudden changes in position.

 3. Organize nursing activities to allow for long periods of uninterrupted rest.

 4. Administer suppositories or enemas as needed to prevent straining during a bowel movement.

D. *To provide for the child's emotional needs.*

 1. Hold and cuddle the infant as much as possible according to his condition.

 2. Provide diversion according to the child's age.

  a. Infants—mobiles or musical toys

  b. Older children—quiet games, reading, etc.

E. *To assist with subdural taps.*

 1. Wrap the infant or young child in a mummy restraint. (See procedure on protective devices to limit motion, p. 1073.)

 2. Hold the child securely to avoid injury caused by sudden movement.

 3. Observe the child frequently after the procedure for:

  a. Shock

  b. Drainage from the site of the tap

   (1) Note whether this is serous drainage or frank blood.

   (2) Reinforce the dressing to prevent contamination of the wound.

   (3) Cotton balls or sterile gauze soaked in collodion are usually used to seal off the area of the tap.

F. *To observe for evidence of disease progress. Nurse's record should contain information relating to:*

 1. General behavior—irritability, lethargy, etc.

  It is important to obtain a thorough history from the child's parents regarding his normal behavior and level of functioning so that abnormalities can be more easily recognized.

 2. Appetite and feeding difficulties, including vomiting.

 3. Signs of increased intracranial pressure

  a. Vital signs should be taken frequently.

  b. Be alert for:

   (1) Increased systolic blood pressure

   (2) Increased pulse pressure

(3) Decreased pulse or irregularities

(4) Changes in respiratory rate or difficulty breathing.

4. State of consciousness
5. Pupillary changes, especially dilated pupil
6. Convulsions
7. Motor function

    The ability to grasp should be checked and compared bilaterally in older children.

G. *To observe for signs of complications.*

1. Infection
    a. Record temperature frequently.
    b. Report purulent drainage from the site of the subdural tap.
2. Recurrent bleeding

    Note rapid changes in vital signs indicating shock or increased intracranial pressure.

3. Paralysis

H. *To provide supportive care to the child in a coma.*

1. Prevent pressure sores.
2. Prevent contractures.
    a. Apply passive range of motion exercises to all extremities.
    b. Place pillows appropriately to support the child's body in good alignment.
    c. Use a footboard for the older child.
3. Keep the child's eyes well lubricated to prevent corneal damage.
4. Suction the child as necessary to remove secretions in the mouth and nasopharynx.
5. Provide frequent mouth care.
6. Administer suppositories or enemas as necessary to prevent fecal incontinence.
7. Administer intravenous fluids accurately to avoid danger of rapidly increasing intracranial pressure.

I. *To care for the child with a craniotomy.*

    See section on the postoperative care of the child with a brain tumor, page 1397.

J. *To provide emotional support to the parents.*

1. Encourage as much parental participation in the child's care as possible.
2. Reassure the parents that the prognosis is favorable with adequate treatment.
3. Avoid blaming the parents for the child's injury.
    a. Attempt to alleviate their guilt feelings if present.
    b. Refer the parents to a social worker or psychiatrist if this problem is severe.

Parental Teaching

Reinforce explanations in the following areas:

1. The condition
2. The causes of the child's specific symptoms
3. The need and rationale for treatment
4. Postoperative and recovery expectations
5. Signs of recurrent bleeding

BIBLIOGRAPHY

Books

Abnormalities of the Central Nervous System: Nursing Education Service #14. Columbus, Ohio, Ross Laboratories, Department of Nursing Service, 1964.

Buist, C. A., and Schulman, J. L.: Toys and Games for Educationally Handicapped Children. Springfield, Illinois, Charles C Thomas, 1969.

Carlson, B., and Gingland, D.: Play Activities for the Retarded Child. New York, National Recreation Association, 1961.

Cruickshank, W. M.: The Brain Injured Child in Home, School and Community. Syracuse, Syracuse University Press, 1967.

Gordon, S., and Galob, R. (eds.): Recreation and Socialization for the Brain Injured Child. East Orange, New Jersey Association for Brain Injured Children, 1967.

Grossman, F. K.: Brothers and Sisters of Retarded Children: An Exploratory Study. Syracuse, Syracuse University Press, 1962.

Haynes, U.: A Developmental Approach to Casefinding With Special Reference to Cerebral Palsy, Mental Retardation and Related Disorders. U. S. Department of Health, Education and Welfare, Maternal and Child Health Service, Pub. No. 2017, 1969.

Livingston, S.: Comprehensive Management of Epilepsy in Infancy, Childhood and Adolescence. Springfield, Illinois, Charles C Thomas, 1972.

Menolascino, F. J. (ed.): Psychiatric Aspects of the Diagnosis and Treatment of Mental Retardation. Seattle, Special Child Publications, Inc., 1971.

Millichap, J. G.: Febrile Convulsions. New York, Macmillan, 1968.

Petrillo, M., and Sangar, S.: Emotional Care of Hospitalized Children. Philadelphia, J. B. Lippincott, 1972.

Phillips, I. (ed.): Prevention and Treatment of Mental Retardation. New York, Basic Books Inc., 1966.

Schaffer, A. J.: Diseases of the Newborn. Philadelphia, W. B. Saunders, 1971.

Stock, C.: Learning Tasks; A Handbook for Programming Developmental Disabilities. Boulder, Colorado, Pruett Publishing Co., 1972.

The Care of the Retarded Child: Therapy and Prognosis, Proceedings of the Seventh Arthur Parmalee Sr. Child Development Institute, U. S. Department of Health, Education and Welfare, Social and Rehabilitation Service, Children's Bureau, Pub. No. 417, 1969.

The Child With Central Nervous System Deficit: A Report of Two Symposiums. U. S. Department of Health, Education and Welfare, Pub. No. 2181, 1971.

The Child With Cerebral Palsy. Children's Bureau Folder No. 34. Office of Child Development, Health, Education and Welfare Building So. Washington, D.C., Rev. 1971.

Wolf, J. M., and Anderson, R. M.: The Multiply Handicapped Child. Springfield, Illinois, Charles C Thomas, 1969.

Articles

Avery, G. B., et al.: Meningomyelocele and hydrocephalus. Clinical Proceedings. Children's Hospital of the D.C., 26:135–152, May 1970.

Bonine, G.: The myelodysplastic child—Hospital–home care. Amer. J. Nurs., 69:541, March 1969.

Boyle, J.: Learning experience in helping parents get what they want. Children, 17:126, July-August 1970.

Cortazzo, A. D., et al.: Innovations to improve care in an institution for the mentally retarded. Children, 18:149–154, July-August 1971.

Diamond, F.: A play center for developmentally handicapped infants. Children, 18:174–178, Sept.-Oct. 1971.

Flax, N., and Peters, E.: Retarded children at camp with normal children. Children, 16:232, Nov.-Dec. 1969.

Freeman, R. D.: Emotional reactions of handicapped children. Rehab. Lit., 28:274–281, Sept. 1967.

Garrett, B.: Foster family services for mentally retarded children. Children, 17:228, Nov.-Dec. 1970.

Hamilton, E.: Developments in techniques for ambulation for spina-bifida children. J. Canad. Physiother. Assoc., 24:17–19, Feb. 1972.

Hill, M., et al.: The myelodysplastic child—bowel and bladder control. Amer. J. Nurs., 69:545–550, March 1969.

Hillsman, G., and O'Grady, D.: Helping adolescents with mental retardation. Children Today, 1:2–6, May-June 1972.

Hoffman, E. P.: The problems of spina bifida and cranium bifidum. Clin. Ped., 4:709–716, Dec. 1965.

Kessler, J., et al.: Reactions in young, mildly retarded children. Children, 16:2, Jan.-Feb. 1969.

Kugel, R.: Combatting retardation in infants with Down's syndrome. Children, 17:188, Sept.-Oct. 1970.

Mamula, R. A.: The use of developmental plans for mentally retarded children in foster family care. Children, 18:65–68, March-April 1971.

Maxwell, J. C.: Home care for the retarded child. Nurs. Outlook, 19:112–114, Feb. 1971.

Mrozinski, C. M.: Complications encountered in the course of shunt therapy for hydrocephalus in children. J. Neurosurg. Nurs., 2:41–61, Dec. 1970.

Noble, M. A.: Nursing's concern for the mentally retarded is overdue. Nurs. Forum, 9:192, 1970.

Olshansky, S.: Chronic sorrow: a response to having a mentally defective child. Social Casework, 43:190–193, 1962.

Paine, R. S.: Hydrocephalus. Ped. Clin. N. Amer., 14:779, 1967.

Parriott, S.: Music as therapy. Amer. J. Nurs., 69:1723, Aug. 1969.

Patterson, R.: Toward a theory of mental retardation nursing. An educational model. Amer. J. Nurs., 70:531, March 1970.

Pothier, P. C.: Therapeutic handling of the severely handicapped child. Amer. J. Nurs., 71:321–324, Feb. 1971.

Reeves, K.: Children's reactions to head injuries. Amer. J. Nurs., 70:108, Jan. 1970.

Snolock, M. A.: The nurse's role in rehabilitation of the handicapped child. Nurs. Clin. N. Amer., 5:411, Sept. 1970.

Waechter, E.: The birth of an exceptional child. Nurs. Forum, 9:202, 1970.

Governmental Agencies

Maternal and Child Health Service, Department of Health, Education and Welfare, 5600 Fisher's Lane, Rockville, Maryland 20852

National Institute of Neurological Diseases and Stroke, National Institutes of Health, Bethesda, Maryland 20014

Office of Child Development, Children's Bureau, U. S. Department of Health, Education and Welfare, Washington, D.C. 20013

Social and Rehabilitation Service, U. S. Department of Health, Education and Welfare, Washington, D.C. 20001

Voluntary Agencies

American Eugenics Society, 230 Park Ave., N.Y., N.Y. 10017

Association for the Aid of Crippled Children, 345 E. 46th St., N.Y., N.Y. 10017

Child Study Association of America, 9 E. 89th St., N.Y., N.Y. 10028

Epilepsy Foundation of America, Suite 1116, 733 15th St., N.W., Washington, D.C. 20005

Family Service Association of America, 44 E. 23rd St., N.Y., N.Y. 10010

Joseph P. Kennedy Jr. Foundation, Room 3021, 200 Park Avenue, N.Y., N.Y. 10017

National Association for Retarded Children, Inc., 2709 Ave. E. East, Arlington, Texas 76011

National Easter Seal Society for Crippled Children and Adults, 2023 West Ogden Avenue, Chicago, Illinois 60612

National Foundation—March of Dimes, 800 Second Avenue, N.Y., N.Y. 10017

National Recreation Association, Consulting Service on Recreation for the Ill and Handicapped, 8 West 8th St., N.Y., N.Y. 10011

Public Affairs Committee Inc., 381 Park Ave. So., N.Y., N.Y. 10015

United Cerebral Palsy Association, Inc., 66 East 34th St., N.Y., N.Y. 10016

Patient and Parent Education

Allegra, J. W.: A guide for parents of children receiving special education. Rehab. Lit., *30*:269–270, Sept. 1969.

Bruce, M., and Veigh, G.: A Practical Manual for the Parents of Children With Myelomeningocele. Pittsburgh, Pennsylvania, Home for Crippled Children, Feb. 1972.

Dittman, L. L.: The Mentally Retarded Child at Home, A Manual for Parents. U.S. Department of Health, Education and Welfare, Children's Bureau, Pub. No. 374, 1959.

Egg-Benes, M.: When a Child is Different: A Basic Guide for Parents and Friends of Mentally Retarded Children. New York, John Day Co., 1964.

Feeding the Child With a Handicap. U. S. Department of Health, Education and Welfare, Public Health Service, Pub. No. 2091, 1970.

Finnie, N. R.: Handling the Young Cerebral Palsied Child at Home. New York, E. P. Dutton and Co., 1970.

French, E. L., and Scott, J. C.: How You Can Help Your Retarded Child: A Manual for Parents. Philadelphia, J. B. Lippincott, 1967.

Frey, M.: ABC's for parents: aids to management of the slow child at home. Rehab. Lit., *26*:270–272, Sept. 1965.

Gardner, R. A.: The Child's Book About Brain Injury. New York, Association for Brain Injured Children, 1966.

Litter, J.: Mine for Keeps. Boston, Little, Brown and Company, 1962.

Shere, M. O.: Speech and Language Training for the Cerebral Palsied Child At Home. Danville, Illinois, Interstate Printers and Publishers, Inc., 1964.

Swinyard, C. A.: The Child With Spina Bifida. New York, Association for the Aid of Crippled Children, 1971.

Thompson, M.: Recreation for the Homebound Person With Cerebral Palsy. New York, United Cerebral Palsy Associations, Inc., 1970.

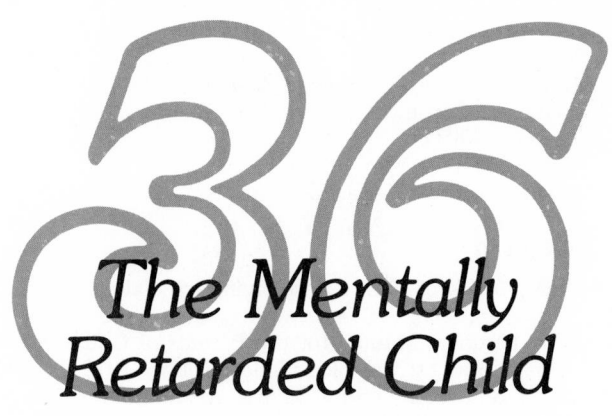

The Mentally Retarded Child

Mental Retardation   1356
Down's Syndrome   1362

MENTAL RETARDATION

Mental retardation is not a single disease entity, but a term used to refer to a complex of symptoms. It is characterized by impaired intelligence from early childhood and inadequate mental development throughout the growth period which limits the child's ability to adapt to his environment. Mental retardation is a cause of lifetime disability.

Etiology

A. *General*
  1. Congenital lack of brain cells
  2. Later destruction of cells originally present

B. *Prenatal Factors*
  1. Heredity
  2. Fetal irradiation
  3. Infection—maternal or fetal
  4. Kernicterus due to Rh of ABO incompatibility
  5. Anoxia
  6. Cranial anomalies
     a. Hydrocephalus
     b. Craniosynostosis
  7. Chromosomal abnormalities
  8. Disorders of metabolism

C. *Natal Factors*
  1. Anoxia
     a. Maternal
     b. Placental
     c. Respiratory obstruction
  2. Breech delivery with delay in delivery of the head
  3. Cerebral injury
     a. Trauma
     b. Cephalopelvic disproportion
     c. Precipitate delivery
     d. Prematurity
  4. Infection
  5. Intracranial hemorrhage

D. *Postnatal Factors*

1. Central nervous system infection
2. Brain injury or hemorrhage
3. Cerebral degenerative disease
4. Anoxia
5. Toxic encephalopathy—lead poisoning
6. Postimmunization encephalopathy
   a. Pertussis
   b. Smallpox
7. Vascular disorders

E. *Unknown*

1. No identifiable organic or biologic cause for 65–75% of retarded children
2. Probably caused by sociocultural or environmental deprivation or poverty
3. Generally, these children are more mildly retarded than children with associated organic and physical defects

Incidence

1. Approximately 3–4% (more than 126,000) of children born annually in the United States will at some time in their life be classified as mentally retarded.
2. Slightly more frequent in males than in females.
3. An increased birth rate, decrease in infant deaths and longer life span have caused a rise in the total number of persons classified as mentally retarded.

Classification

A. *Mildly retarded* (educable)

1. I.Q. between 51 and 75.
2. Able to reach a mental age of 8–12 years.
3. Often able to function fairly well in the home and community.
4. Has ability for self-support with some supervision.

B. *Moderately retarded* (trainable)

1. I.Q. between 21 and 50.
2. Able to reach a mental age of 3–7 years.
3. May have some earning power but needs more supervision and protection.

C. *Severely retarded*

1. I.Q. between 0 and 20.
2. Able to reach a mental age of 0–2 years.
3. Usually remains completely dependent on others for care, but may be able to contribute partially to self-maintenance.

D. *Profoundly retarded*

1. Gross retardation with minimal capacity for functioning in the sensorimotor areas.
2. May achieve very limited self-care.
3. Needs nursing care for daily needs.

Clinical Manifestations

A. *Developmental*

1. Neuromuscular coordination does not develop consistently at a normal rate.
2. Does not achieve normal developmental milestones for his age.
   a. Infant
      (1) Fails to learn to suck.

        (2) Slow to sit, stand and walk.

        (3) Behaves very placidly.

   b. Toddler

        (1) Slow in learning to feed self and in toilet training.

        (2) Drooling is common.

B. *Educational*

   1. Unable to profit from experience and instruction.

   2. Disease is usually recognized between the ages of 6–16 years (during the school years) when the child is expected to understand abstract concepts.

C. *Social*

   Fails to achieve social standards of maturation at successive age levels.

D. *Physical*

   1. Approximately 75% of retarded individuals have no obvious physical stigma.

   2. These children have a greater percentage of sensory defects, language disorders, neuromuscular impairment, seizures and physical anomalies than the general population.

Diagnostic Evaluation

   1. Abnormalities are identified in the areas of:

     a. Intelligence   c. Social adjustment

     b. Emotional reactions   d. Adaptive behavior

   2. The diagnosis is extremely difficult and is most reliable when the determination is made by a comprehensive team which offers medical, psychological, social and educational examinations.

     Care must be taken to insure that no child is mislabeled as mentally retarded.

Prognosis

   1. Factors which influence the prognosis

     a. Degree of retardation

     b. Existence of additional, physical defects

     c. Family and community resources available to help the child to use his mental resources

   2. Factors which favor improvement in intelligence

     a. Modification of the environment to eliminate stress and deprivation

     b. Improvement in learning opportunities

     c. Increased social acceptance

     d. Early intervention

   3. The prognosis is best in the mildly retarded child without a coexistent physical defect.

Nursing Objectives

A. *To assist parents to adjust to the diagnosis.*

   1. Explain that the emotional health of the retarded child depends on the parents' good emotional health.

   2. Encourage both parents to talk about the diagnosis and how they feel about it.

     a. Expect attitudes of guilt and denial, feelings of hostility, shame and self-pity and thoughts that the child may be a great burden.

The parents' reaction will be individually determined by such factors as: their own situation, their previous life experiences and their individual makeup.

    b. Express sympathetic understanding of the family's problems and acceptance of their attitudes.

Reassure them that most parents react to the diagnosis with intense grief and sorrow.

    c. Help parents to develop a fundamental understanding of what has happened to their child and what this means in terms of his future development.

      (1) Clarify and support medical speculations regarding the cause of the retardation.

        (a) Genetic counseling is indicated, especially in familial types of retardation.

        (b) Answer parental questions sensitively but directly.

        (c) Provide simple explanations in terms they can understand.

        (d) Avoid vague generalities, such as "the child is slow," and demoralizing words, such as "moron" or "imbecile."

      (2) Provide as much specific information as possible.

Parents have the right to know what diagnostic tests have been done, what positive or negative conclusions have been made, what uncertainties remain and what general prognosis can be made.

    d. Provide privacy for discussions.

    e. Provide time for the parents to comprehend the extent of their problem and mobilize their resources to work on its solution.

Offer counseling at a slow pace, one step at a time.

3. Initiate a referral to a social worker or psychiatrist who may assist the family to deal with their immediate reactions and plan for the child's long-term care.

Most parents need some source of continuous support in learning how to live with a problem they may never be able to accept.

4. Involve both parents in the child's care so that they may gain a realistic concept of his ability.

    a. Point out the child's areas of strengths and weaknesses and show how these can be considered in his management.

    b. Emphasize the *well* part of the child and that he has the same needs as a normal child for love and security.

5. Assure the family that their child has had the benefit of the best diagnostic procedures and any treatment that is indicated.

6. Include the family as soon as possible with other members of the health team in planning for the child's future care.

    a. The plan should be based on the degree of the child's retardation, the reaction of the family to the diagnosis and the available community resources.

    b. The family should be supported in the decisions they make.

    c. The family should be guided to make decisions for the child's care which will allow for maximum utilization of his capabilities.

7. Discuss with parents their plans for dealing with the siblings of the retarded child.

    a. Adequate explanations and information should be given to siblings early to avoid their misconceptions later.

    b. Siblings often need help in explaining the retarded child's abnormality to their friends.

    c. Warn parents to guard against intense sibling rivalry caused by children feeling neglected because of the amount of time the mother devotes to the retarded child.

  8. Refer the family to appropriate community resources for assistance with problems of daily management and the development, and implementation of long-term plans.

a. Community nursing agencies	g. Volunteer organizations
b. Day care centers	h. Specialized diagnostic facilities
c. Foster grandparent programs	i. Recreational programs
d. Nursery groups	j. Vocational training
e. Special schools	k. Residential institutions
f. Parent groups	l. National associations*

B. *To provide mental and motor stimulation.*

  1. Play is an essential part of the child's care.
    Select toys on the basis of the child's mental *not* chronological age.

  2. Expose the child to a variety of materials and toys which stimulate all of his senses.
    a. Equipment such as rocking chairs, musical instruments, record players, blocks, art materials and simple picture books are indispensable.
    b. Toys should be accessible for the child to use when he desires.

  3. An occupational therapist may be able to provide invaluable guidance in this area.

C. *To teach the child basic skills with the long-range goal of developing independent behavior at the highest level possible according to the child's potential mentality.*

  1. Determine the child's care plan according to his individual areas of strengths and weaknesses and coordinate it with the plans of the related health professionals.

  2. Because a retarded child has a limited attention span, present a smaller amount of material to him at a slower rate and over a longer period of time than to a normal child.

  3. Provide organized, consistent and repetitive experiences.

  4. Employ techniques of positive reinforcement.
    a. Give rewards for positive responses so that the probability of recurrence of that response will be strengthened.
      Rewards should be given consistently and immediately after the approved response.
    b. Do not reward unacceptable behaviors.

  5. Break complex behaviors down into small steps which the child can easily achieve.
    a. This is very important in the areas of feeding, dressing and toilet training.
    b. Do not expect the child to transfer learning from one situation to another.

  6. Base expectations for the child on his mental ability, *not* on his chronological age.

  7. Maintain a relaxed learning environment.

D. *To reduce destructive behavior and encourage that which is socially acceptable.*

  1. Establish a routine of daily living so that the child knows precisely what is expected of him.

  2. Employ consistent discipline.
    a. Use language that the child understands so that he can comprehend his misdeed.
    b. When punishment is necessary, it should follow the misdeed immediately.

* American Association on Mental Deficiency, 5201 Connecticut Avenue, N.W., Washington, D.C. 20015
National Association for Retarded Children, Inc., 420 Lexington Avenue, New York, N.Y. 10017

E. *To prepare the mentally retarded individual so that he may cope successfully (within his potentiality) with the problems and adjustments of adult life.*
1. Help parents identify areas of home responsibilities which may be delegated to the retarded child.
2. In the child's early learning activities, provide habits which are essential to his later vocational life.
   a. Getting to places on time
   b. Cooperating
   c. Focusing and holding attention on the task at hand
   d. Establishing acceptable interpersonal relationships
   e. Accepting failure and mistakes
3. All teaching should educate the child to be happy and efficient in his social relationships.
   His early education should tie into later social and vocational programs.
4. The child should be helped to develop a set of attitudes and behaviors which will motivate him to work.
5. Attainable occupational goals should be identified early in the child's educational experience.

F. *To be aware of nursing activities associated with hospitalization of a child previously diagnosed as mentally retarded.*
1. Apply all of the previously outlined principles.
2. Obtain a thorough nursing history from the parent regarding the child's usual home routines.
   a. Feeding
   b. Sleeping
   c. Toilet habits
   d. Learning activities
   e. Play
3. Utilize the information obtained to develop a nursing care plan which provides for continuity of care from home to hospital in order to maintain the child's security and minimize his regression.
   Counsel the mother that some regression can be anticipated even in normal children who require hospitalization.
4. Encourage as much parental participation as possible in the child's care.

Parental Teaching

1. The child may require even more medical check-ups and advice than the normal person. Regular dental care is also essential.
   a. The child is often more susceptible to infections.
   b. He may feed poorly.
   c. He may be underweight or overweight.
   d. He may have poor motor coordination.
   e. He often has speech and language problems.
2. Secondary handicaps such as visual or hearing problems should be treated immediately.
3. Parents need to be helped to recognize their child's methods of communicating so that they can respond to his needs.
4. Parents should be assisted to identify learning readiness in their child in order to help him achieve his maximum level of development without subjecting him to unnecessary experiences of failure and frustration.

5. Practical, tangible suggestions relative to everyday living should be offered to the parents.
   a. Selection of toys
   b. Techniques of feeding
   c. Patterns for toilet training
6. The child should have the opportunity of participating in social, religious and recreational activities.
   a. Organizations should be selected in which the probability of success is the highest.
   b. The parent should discuss the situation with the group leader and the leader should have an opportunity to meet the child so that both child and leader can assess each other.
   c. A responsible member of the group may be assigned to act as a "big brother" until the child is comfortable in the situation.
7. Parents need to know that they are important as people. They need to lead normal lives. They need to be taught that they are not their child's only resource, but that others care and are willing to help. They need to be assisted to let their child go forth.

DOWN'S SYNDROME

Down's Syndrome is a chromosomal abnormality involving an extra chromosome (number 21), resulting in a typical picture in physical appearance and mental retardation.

Etiology

A. *Trisomy 21*
   1. The abnormality is an error in cell division.
      a. Both number 21 chromosomes in the pair migrate to one daughter cell during miosis instead of just one of the pair.
      b. 47 chromosomes are present in the new individual rather than the normal 46.
      c. There are 3 number 21 chromosomes, thus extra genetic material.
   2. Occurrence is associated with advanced maternal age
      a. Risk is increased after maternal age of 35.
      b. Occurrence in the same set of parents is rare, but dependent upon maternal age.
   3. This form of Down's syndrome is not inherited.

B. *Translocation*
   1. Chromosome number 21 attaches to another chromosome, usually number 15.
   2. This abnormal attachment occurs in the parent.
      a. Parent passes on to the offspring an extra dose of chromosome 21, plus a normal chromosome 21.
      b. The child with this type of Down's syndrome has 46 chromosomes.
   3. This form of Down's syndrome is inherited.

Altered Physiology

1. The normal person, without Down's syndrome, has 46 chromosomes, 23 pairs.
   a. One pair of chromosomes is sex determining.
   b. 22 pairs of chromosomes are non-sex determining and are called autosomes.

2. The individual with Down's syndrome has an extra chromosome, number 21. He carries extra genetic material.
3. Abnormalities that are present at birth occurred during fetal growth.
   a. Normal fetal growth has been interfered with.
   b. This interference affects mainly the heart, brain, eyes, hands and general growth.

Clinical Manifestations

1. Physical stigmata recognized at birth
   a. Marked hypotonia and floppiness
   b. Joint hyperextension
   c. Tendency to keep mouth open with tongue protruding
   d. Brachycephaly with relatively flat occiput
   e. Eyes slant upward and outward with internal epicanthal folds
   f. Excess skin on back of neck
   g. Flattened nasal bridge and flat facial profile
   h. Small ears, often incompletely developed
   i. Spade-like hands; there is inward curving of distal phalanx of fifth finger; simian crease
   j. Short, broad feet; there is a wide separation between first and second toe (plantar furrow)
   k. Male genitalia are small
2. Complications most likely to be present at birth
   a. Congenital cardiac defects, especially atrial septal defect
   b. Duodenal stenosis and other intestinal obstruction
3. Later findings in the child (up to 1 year of age)
   a. Slow intellectual development (I.Q. 20–75, mean 50)
   b. Slow motor development

Complications

1. Recurrent infection of upper respiratory tract
2. Skin infections
3. Complications secondary to physical anomalies present at birth

Diagnostic Evaluation

Chromosomal analysis (keryotyping) will show how the third chromosome, number 21, is attached to another autosome in translocation or nondisjunction.

Nursing Objectives

NEWBORN

A. *To establish and maintain adequate nutrition to allow for growth and development.*
   1. The diet is calculated according to infant's needs.
   2. Due to poor muscle tone and protruding tongue, the infant may be a poor eater with a weak and ineffective suck.
      a. Provide the appropriate nipple so that minimal sucking effort is needed to feed.
      b. Allow adequate time for feeding. Do not allow the infant to become overly tired.
      c. Note and report poor eating and insufficient suck.

B. *To observe carefully for any signs of physical complications that may occur with Down's syndrome. Record and report them immediately.*
1. Intestinal obstruction (duodenal stenosis)
   a. Observe for abdominal distention and its association with feeding.
   b. Note vomiting—what is vomited and when.
      (1) Bile-stained emesis indicates lower tract obstruction.
      (2) Partially digested milk indicates upper tract obstruction.
   c. Note absence of stools.
2. Congenital cardiac defect
   a. When taking vital signs, note any irregularity of the heart rate. Murmurs may not be evident to the untrained ear. Note any respiratory distress or labored respirations.
   b. Note any cyanosis and when it occurs—with crying, feeding, or all the time.
   c. Be particularly alert to the infant tiring easily during feeding.

C. *To provide a safe environment for the infant.*
1. Infant is usually very floppy due to poor muscle tone. When handling the infant, support him well with a firm grasp.
2. Position infant in such a manner that if vomiting should occur he will not aspirate.
   a. If he is on his abdomen, be certain that he can turn his head to the side.
   b. Prop him with a diaper roll so that position will be maintained.
   c. This infant is not usually very active, thus his position will need to be changed frequently.

D. *To provide proper stimulation according to the child's age.*
1. Be aware that this infant needs stimulation from the very start to begin to help him develop to his potential. Develop a plan of stimulation so that your activity and actions have a purposeful goal.
2. Hold and fondle infant, especially during feeding.
3. When the infant is awake, the adult face in his visual field is good stimulation and should interest him for a few seconds.
4. The gentle sound of talking or music can provide a pleasant auditory experience. The infant should stop activity and listen.

E. *To encourage parental participation in caring for and handling the infant and to foster acceptance of the child by his parents and family.*
1. Provide opportunities for the parents to learn all aspects of caring for their baby.
2. All the support and help given the parents during hospitalization will make home care easier.
3. Initiate community nurse referral. A community nurse can be helpful to the family in planning home care.
4. Initiate social work referral. The social worker can help parents to better understand their family situation and their feelings about their child.
5. Help parents to understand the reason genetic counseling is important. Guide them in seeking proper counseling.
6. Invite parents to join a group of parents who have children with Down's syndrome.
7. Emphasize the infant's need for love, affection, consideration and individual attention.

THE OLDER CHILD

The older child with Down's syndrome is usually admitted to the hospital because of some medical complication such as an acute respiratory infection.

A. *To interview the parents thoroughly at the time of admission to learn as much as possible about the child and his activities at home.*
   1. What is the child's vocabulary? What words or sounds does he use for elimination, certain foods, etc.?
   2. Be aware of the child's schedule and activities at home.
      a. This patient usually functions better in a familiar environment. He may react adversely to the new situation.
      b. Know what activities the child can or cannot do and what he likes to do.
   3. Be familiar with the child's eating habits and pattern.
      a. Give him foods he likes and avoid foods he dislikes.
      b. Adjust his mealtimes to those he is used to as much as possible and know at which mealtime he eats best.
   4. Be aware of how parents discipline the child.
   5. Share this information with nursing staff to assure continuity of care from home to hospital to minimize fear and frustration in the child.
   6. Plan the child's day according to what he is used to as much as possible.

B. *To attend to the child's needs according to the medical problem that required his hospitalization.*

C. *To provide a safe environment for the child according to his needs.*
   1. This can best be judged by observing the child and by obtaining information during the parental interview.
   2. If possible, use the type of bed the child is familiar with.
   3. Remove any objects which might be injurious to the child should he play with them.

D. *To plan and provide for the appropriate type of play program and stimulation for the child.*
   1. Assess the child's level of growth and development and consider this in the plan.
   2. Do not try to teach the child new or different things as he may react adversely to the newness.
   3. Allow the child as much independence as possible in his care, but provide guidance as necessary.
   4. Permit the development of the child's abilities. Minimize frustrating situations.

E. *To foster continual parental acceptance of the child and provide support for them.*
   1. Invite parents to care for their child as much as they can. Rooming-in may be advisable.
   2. Help the parents to understand why the child behaves as he does.
   3. Encourage the parents to talk about their feelings or problems they have with the child.
   4. Initiate a teaching program for the child and his parents early. Offer them available literature and help them to become familiar with community resources.
   5. Allow parents to continue to maintain what other responsibilities they may have outside the hospital, i.e., other children, work.
      Do not insist they stay at the hospital and attend only to this child.

Parental Teaching

Parent teaching is one very important aspect in the nursing care of a child with Down's syndrome, especially in the following areas:

1. The influence of environment on the child's behavior, growth and development.
   a. Encourage the whole family to be included in child's care.
   b. The child will usually be lovable and quiet, affectionate and socially responsive if he is loved and if individual attention is given to his specific needs.
   c. Patience and understanding must be developed by parents and family.
2. The child learns best in the play situation.
   a. The child is slower at learning and will require more time to learn each new skill.
   b. The child tends to mimic, which results later in learning.
   c. He may have a sensitivity to rhythmic stimulation and usually likes music.
3. Provide a safe environment.
   Because he may be less sensitive to heat, cold and pain, attention should be directed toward eliminating these hazards.
4. Help parents understand that in spite of signs of slow mental growth, the child can make steady progress.
   a. The child needs a great deal of repetition in all areas of learning.
   b. He usually has a good memory, can acquire a fairly large vocabulary and can learn to spell. Arithmetic may be more difficult for him.
   c. Speech may lag behind walking by 1–2 years. He may encounter trouble in pronouncing certain words. Stammering may occur if the child is under pressure.
   d. Parents need help in learning to recognize the child's readiness to learn these skills.
5. The child's motor development is slow.
   a. Encourage motor coordination. It will take time for the child to learn to sit. At age 5 or 6 years, he may still walk like a 2 year old.
   b. The child's liking for music and sense of rhythm can be used to help develop motor coordination.
   c. He may always have trouble with fine motor skills.
   d. Encourage child to do as much for himself as he can.
6. Precautionary measures should be taken.
   a. Discuss the importance of good nutrition for growth. Supply available literature for a balanced diet appropriate for age.
   b. Obtain prompt treatment for any medical problems that may occur. This child is particularly prone to infection. Good nutrition, proper exercise, appropriate dress and good general hygiene can help prevent infection.
   c. The child with Down's syndrome needs discipline. Limits need to be set so he knows what he can or cannot do.
7. Other members of the family must be considered.
   a. The child should not be thought of as a sick child, but as a child who needs special handling to promote his individual growth and development. But he does not need all the attention all the time.
   b. The family should be included in his care, but they also must have a life of their own and as much parental attention as they would receive if the child were not present in the family.

c. Parents need time to themselves. They should be encouraged to go out alone together and to give time to their marriage.

8. Future in society
   a. The child with Down's syndrome should go to school. He learns by copying. Have parents discuss the child's problem with the school nurse, the teacher and other adults who have close contact with the child.
   b. Help parents understand that the child may be able to contribute to society. Girls can learn routine housework. Boys can learn gardening or farming. They can run errands, learn to obey traffic rules and ride buses.
   c. Help parents to discuss their feelings or plans regarding continued home care or placement in an institution.

BIBLIOGRAPHY

Books

Cooke, R. E. (ed.): The Biologic Basis of Pediatric Practice. New York, McGraw-Hill, 1968.
Gellis, S. S., and Kagan, B. M.: Current Pediatric Therapy. Philadelphia, W. B. Saunders, 1970.
Knamm, E. R.: Families of Mongoloid Children. U. S. Department of Health, Education and Welfare, Social and Rehabilitation Service, Children's Bureau, 1969.
Smith, D. W.: Recognizable Patterns of Human Malformations. Philadelphia, W. B. Saunders, 1970.
Smith, D. W., and Wilson, A. A.: The Child with Down's Syndrome. Philadelphia, W. B. Saunders, 1973.

Article

Mori, M.: My child has Down's syndrome. Amer. J. Nurs., 73:1386–1387, Aug. 1973.

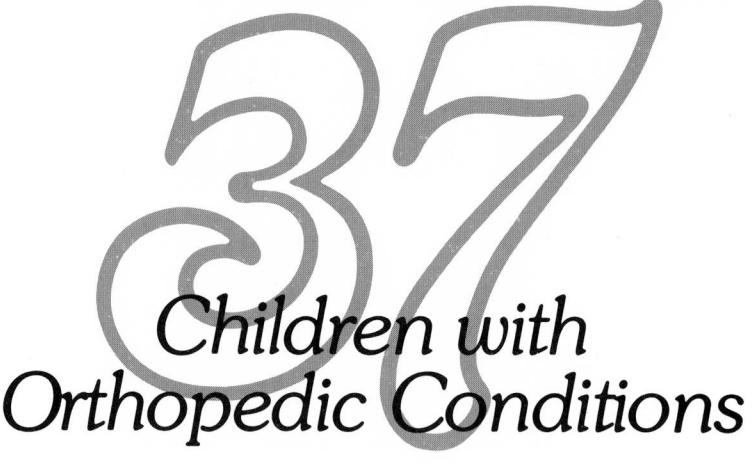

Children with
Orthopedic Conditions

FRACTURES

Generally, nursing care of the child with a fracture is similar to that of an adult. The child is usually hospitalized only for application of a cast (see procedure for cast care, p. 1117) or to be placed in traction (see procedure for traction, p. 1110). The nurse should be aware of the following principles concerning fractures in pediatrics.

General Considerations

1. Bones do not fracture as easily in children as adults.
   Bones are softer and more pliable.
2. Greenstick fractures in normal bones are unique to children.
   a. The bone breaks at one cortex and bends at the other.
   b. There is no complete loss of bony continuity.
   c. The younger the child, the more likely he is to sustain a greenstick fracture.
   d. The radius or ulna, clavicle or long bone in the hand are most likely to sustain a greenstick fracture.
3. Comminuted fractures are less common in pediatrics.
4. Injuries of the epiphyseal plate are unique to children.
   a. The epiphyseal plate is weaker than normal tendons, ligaments or joint capsule.
   b. Injury resulting in a torn ligament or dislocation in the adult is more likely to produce a separation of the epiphysis in a child.
   c. The lower radial epiphysis is more frequently separated than any other.
5. Fractures in pediatrics heal more readily than those in adults.
   a. The younger the child, the more rapidly the fracture unites.
   b. The thick periosteum and abundant blood supply make nonunion rare.

6. End-to-end apposition of fracture surfaces is not essential in pediatrics.
   a. The long bones may be allowed to unite with side-to-side apposition in children up to 11–12 years of age.
   b. Subsequent moulding will produce a normal bone by the end of growth.
7. Following injury, the limbs in children are likely to swell much more rapidly and the swelling to disappear more quickly than in an adult.
8. Function is usually restored rapidly and sometimes spontaneously following injury in children.

Common Fractures in Children

Fracture of the Clavicle

A. *Treatment*
1. Immobilization with a figure-of-eight bandage.
2. Complete fixation by supporting the limb in a triangular sling suspended from the opposite shoulder.
   Necessary in complete fractures with overriding of the fragments.

B. *Healing Time*
   Usually 3 weeks.

Fracture of the Neck of the Humerus

A. *Treatment*
1. Minimal displacement
   Collar and cuff sling
2. Considerable displacement
   a. Reduction under anesthesia
   b. Immobilization by a collar and cuff sling and strapping of the upper arm to the chest
   c. Light traction may be necessary in cases where adduction of the arm to the side causes redisplacement of the bone fragments
      (1) Traction is applied so that the shoulder is flexed forward, slightly abducted and medially rotated.
      (2) After 3 weeks, immobilization may be continued by a collar and cuff sling or a shoulder spica.

B. *Healing Time*
1. Minimal displacement—3–4 weeks
2. Considerable displacement—4–5 weeks

Fracture of the Shaft of the Humerus

A. *Treatment*
1. Immobilization with a U-slab of plaster applied directly to the inner and outer surfaces of the upper arm
2. Fixation completed by a collar and cuff sling

B. *Healing Time*
1. Younger children—4 weeks
2. Older children—6 weeks

Supracondylar Fracture of the Humerus

A. *Treatment*
    1. Undisplaced
        a. Collar and cuff sling are used under the clothes with the elbow flexed 20–30 degrees above a right angle.
        b. After 3 weeks the sling may be placed outside the clothes.
        c. Mobilization of the elbow is begun as soon as the elbow has become painless and spasm of the elbow flexors has disappeared.
    2. Displaced
        a. Usually requires reduction under general anesthesia.
        b. The arm may be placed in an overhead suspension apparatus to reduce edema.
        c. Immobilization by a collar and cuff sling with the elbow flexed a little above the right angle.

B. *Healing Time*
    May take several months for complete restoration of function.

Fracture of the Lower End of the Radius and Ulna

A. *Treatment*
    1. Angulation below 25 degrees
        a. No reduction required.
        b. Radius only
            Plaster cast from just below the elbow to the metacarpal heads.
        c. Radius and ulna
            Full-arm plaster cast.
    2. Angulation above 25 degrees
        a. Manipulation under anesthesia
        b. Full-arm plaster cast

B. *Healing Time*
    1. Angulation below 25 degrees—2–3 weeks
    2. Angulation above 25 degrees—4–5 weeks

Fracture Separation of the Lower Radial Epiphysis

A. *Treatment*
    1. Forearm slab of plaster from just below the elbow to the metacarpal heads applied to the posterior and radial aspects of the forearm and wrist.
    2. Full-arm plaster may be required.

B. *Healing Time*
    3–4 weeks

Fracture of the Proximal and Middle Phalanges

A. *Treatment*
    1. Aluminum finger splints
    2. Splintage of the adjoining finger

B. *Healing Time*
    1. 2–3 weeks
    2. Up to 5 weeks

Femoral Shaft Fracture

A. *Treatment*
   1. Manipulative reduction under anesthesia
   2. Maintenance of reduction by traction
   3. Open reduction of fracture is seldom required in children
   4. Traction may be removed after 3–4 weeks and a spica cast applied to allow the child to return home.

B. *Healing Time*
   1. Under 5 years—5 weeks
   2. 4–12 years—6–7 weeks
   3. 12–15 years—8–10 weeks

Fracture of the Tibia or Fibula

A. *Treatment*
   1. Plaster cast from the groin to the toes
   2. Weight bearing allowed usually after the second week
   3. Nonunion is rare in children

B. *Healing Time*
   1. Young child (not walking)—3 weeks
   2. Older child—5 weeks

OSTEOMYELITIS

Osteomyelitis is an inflammatory process which may involve all parts of a bone.

Etiology

   1. Pathogenic bacteria commonly associated with osteomyelitis
      a. *Staphylococcus aureus*—responsible for the majority of cases (up to 90%)
      b. Streptococcal organisms
      c. *Escherichia coli*
      d. Salmonella
      e. *Neisseria gonorrhoeae*
   2. Identifiable primary lesions
      a. Furunculosis
      b. Impetigo
      c. Vaccinations
      d. Infected chicken-pox
      e. Burns
   3. Preconditions favoring development of osteomyelitis in children
      a. Bone regions that have suffered trauma
      b. Bone that suffers from low oxygen tension of sickle cell anemia

Altered Physiology

   1. Infection starts in the soft, medullary tissues.
   2. This causes hyperemia, changes in the capillary permeability and edema of the tissue.
   3. Granulocytic leukocytes infiltrate the area and are destroyed by bacteria, liberating a proteolytic enzyme which causes tissue necrosis.

4. The inflammatory reaction causes thrombosis of vessels, producing irregular areas of bone ischemia.
5. Pus forms and spreads toward the diaphysis and extends through the cortex of the bone.
6. A subperiosteal abscess is formed with elevation of the periosteum.
7. There is further interference of blood supply to the bone shaft.
   a. Vascular supply may remain sufficient to maintain life of bone tissue:
      (1) New bone is created.
      (2) Bone healing occurs.
   b. Vascular supply may be diminished below that which is necessary to maintain life of bone tissue.
      (1) Bone dies and becomes inert.
          Small pieces of dead bone may be completely destroyed by granulation tissue from contiguous living tissue.
      (2) Large pieces of dead bone cannot be completely destroyed.
          (a) Central residual remains as a sequestrum composed of cancellous or cortical bone or a combination.
          (b) New bone is laid down beneath the elevated periosteum and tends to form an encasement (involucrum) around the sequestrum.
          (c) The involucrum is punctured by numerous channels through which pus may escape from the inside.
          (d) Pockets of infection are walled off in which organisms can lie dormant for long periods of time.
          (e) Chronic sinuses are formed which eventually reach the surface and drain.
          (f) Drainage continues until infection quiets once more.
              Channels become plugged up with granulations and remain closed until the pressure of the pus builds up and causes the sinuses to reopen or reach the surface via new channels (chronic osteomyelitis).
          (g) Complete healing takes place only when all of the dead bone has been destroyed, discharged or excised.

Incidence

1. Most frequently occurs between 5–14 years of age.
2. Twice as frequent in males as in females.

Clinical Manifestations

A. *Onset*
   1. Usually abrupt.
   2. May be altered when osteomyelitis follows an infection which has been treated by antibiotics.

B. *Initial Symptoms*
   1. Fever   3. Pain—localized tenderness in the bone at the metaphysis
   2. Malaise

C. *Later Symptoms*
   1. Swelling and redness over the affected bone
   2. Weakness
   3. Irritability
   4. Generalized signs of sepsis
D. *Common Sites of Infection in Children*
   1. Large, cylindrical bones of the extremities
      a. Femur
      b. Tibia
      c. Humerus
      d. Radius
   2. Primary focus is usually in the metaphysis of a bone at the end of the area of most rapid growth.
      a. Knee region
      b. Lower end of the femur
      c. Upper end of the tibia

Diagnostic Evaluation

   1. Leukocytosis
   2. Blood culture—usually positive
   3. X-ray data
      a. Progressive findings
         (1) Periosteal reaction
         (2) Areas of radiolucency secondary to bone destruction
         (3) Evidence of the formation of involucrum (reactive, living bone)
      b. Progress of the disease not seen on x-ray for at least 5 days in small children; as long as 8–10 days in older children.

Prognosis

   1. Mortality rate markedly improved with the advent of modern antimicrobial agents.
   2. Depends on early institution of appropriate therapy and adequate continuation.

Nursing Management

Generally, nursing activities for the care of the child with osteomyelitis are the same as for the adult. The following considerations are important.
   1. Intravenous administration of antibiotics must often be continued for several weeks. This is usually difficult, especially in a young child. A cut-down should be considered. (See procedure for the administration of intravenous fluid, p. 1087.)
      A constant infusion pump should be used as the rate of flow is usually slow.
   2. It is important for the child to assume as many of his normal activities as possible.
      a. He can usually be dressed, even during hospitalization.
      b. Plans should be made for his continuing education.
      c. Liberal visiting by family and friends should be encouraged.
   3. A community health nursing referral should be considered especially for children requiring dressing changes, immobilization in a splint, or appliances such as crutches.
   4. Parents often feel guilty if they did not recognize early signs of the disease. They should be helped to express their feelings and deal with them. A referral to social service may be indicated.

CONGENITAL DISLOCATION OF THE HIP

Congenital dislocation of the hip refers to a malposition of the head of the femur in the acetabulum. The head of the femur is usually dislocated posterosuperiorly. Dislocation may be either partial or complete.

Etiology

1. Unknown
2. Possible causes
    a. Abnormal development of the joint caused by:
        (1) Fetal position
        (2) Genetic factors
    b. Abnormal relaxation of the capsule and ligaments of the joint caused by hormonal factors

Altered Physiology

1. Acetabulum tends to be shallow and extremely oblique.
2. Head of the femur tends to be smaller than normal.
3. Ossification centers are delayed in appearance.

Incidence

More common in female infants than in males.

Clinical Manifestations

Clinical signs (may not be observed until 1–2 months of age)

1. Asymmetry of the gluteal folds
2. Limited ability to abduct the leg
    a. Abduction on the affected side is limited to no more than 45 degrees when the infant is lying on his back with his knees and hips flexed.
    b. Audible click is heard when abduction is forced.
3. Trendelenburg's sign
    Pelvis drops on the normal side if the child stands on his abnormal leg.
4. Shortening of the affected leg
5. Delayed walking
6. Limp
    a. Trunk dips when the child puts weight on his involved leg.
    b. Waddling gait is observed in children with bilateral dislocation.

Diagnostic Evaluation

X-ray data

1. Upper end of the femur does not point into the acetabulum.
2. Poor development of the acetabulum.

Prognosis

1. Depends on the age of the child when the condition is diagnosed.
2. Delay in diagnosis prolongs treatment and may preclude formation of a normal hip.

Nursing Objectives

Generally, nursing care of the child with congenital dislocation of the hip is provided in a convalescent hospital or by the mother at home. Nursing activities encountered in the general hospital are those related to the child's care after application of a hip spica cast which is used to hold the hip in abduction and to enlarge and deepen the socket.

A. *To observe for complications resulting from pressure of the cast.*
    1. Impaired circulation to the toes
       a. Discoloration or cyanosis   d. Edema
       b. Impaired movement   e. Temperature change
       c. Loss of sensation
    2. Complaints of pain or pressure in any area where the cast fits closely over the body

B. *To prevent urine and feces from soiling the cast.*
    1. Offer the bedpan frequently.
       a. Elevate the child's head slightly higher than his feet.
       b. Place a sheet of plastic under the front and back edges of the cast opening for the buttocks and genitalia.
       c. Slip the fracture pan beneath the buttocks.
       d. Allow the ends of the plastic strips to hang into the pan.
    2. Place the child who is not toilet trained on a Bradford frame.
       a. See procedure for care of the child on a Bradford frame, page 1115.
       b. Line the edges of the cast with waterproof material such as plastic or cellophane.
    3. Keep the perineum clean.
       a. Wash the skin under the edge of the cast whenever necessary.
       b. Dry it thoroughly.
       c. Change diapers immediately after they become soiled.
    4. Wash the cast with a damp cloth immediately if it should become soiled.
       A solution of zephiran chloride 1:750 may be used sparingly to eliminate odor-causing bacteria.

C. *To prevent the skin around the edge of the cast from becoming excoriated.*
    1. Smooth the edges of the cast and petal it with waterproof adhesive tape.
       a. This prevents flakes of plaster from breaking off and slipping under the cast.
       b. It also facilitates cleansing of the cast.

D. *To maintain correct position of the cast.*
    1. Keep the child as still as possible to promote healing of the area.
    2. Support the contour of the cast with pillows.
       Allow heel to extend beyond pillow to avoid decubitus ulcers.

E. *To prevent the development of pressure sores or hypostatic pneumonia.*
    1. Turn the child every 4 hours unless contraindicated.
    2. Provide passive or active exercise of the unaffected joints several times daily.
    3. Provide exercise for the lungs.
       a. Blow bottles
       b. Inflating balloons
       c. Blowing soap bubbles

F. *To provide as normal an environment as possible.*
    1. Place the child on a cart or a stretcher so that he may leave his room.
       The child may be taken outdoors if the weather is suitable.
    2. Allow the child to be dressed. (Wide, flared pants are especially suitable.)
    3. Encourage contact with peers.

   4. Provide for play activities.
      a. Provide the young child with large toys which he cannot put into his cast.
      b. Television is a good method of diversion if used with discretion.
      c. Older children often enjoy checkers, sewing, art work, building models, etc.
   5. Provide for education.
      a. Refer the child to a visiting teacher service.
      b. Provide for study time during each day.
G. *To evaluate the home situation for the feasibility of home care.*
   Consider:
   1. The child's place in the family and the number of siblings
   2. Additional needs of the parents, such as pursuing their vocations
   3. Physical set-up of the home
      a. Number of stairs
      b. Sleeping arrangement (type of bed, etc.)
   4. Financial situation
   5. Ability of the family to keep follow-up appointments
H. *To assist the family to care for the child after discharge.*
   1. Initiate the appropriate referrals.
      a. Community health nurse   c. Home tutoring service
      b. Social service agency   d. Physical therapy
   2. Begin teaching early. (See below.)

Patient or Parental Teaching

   1. The parent must be instructed in all of the above aspects of the child's care.
      a. Teach only a few aspects of care each day.
      b. Have the parent participate in the child's care until she is capable of providing total nursing care under supervision.
   2. The need for regular medical evaluations should be emphasized.

LEGG-CALVÉ-PERTHES DISEASE (Coxa Plana)

Legg-Calvé-Perthes disease is an aseptic necrosis of the capital femoral epiphysis secondary to ischemia.

Etiology

   Unknown

Incidence

   Males between the ages of 4–10 years of age are most frequently affected.

Clinical Manifestations
(May be intermittent initially)

   1. Synovitis causing limp and pain in the hip
   2. Referred pain to the knee, front of the thigh and the groin
   3. Limited abduction and rotation of the hip

4. Mild to moderate muscle spasm
5. Involvement is infrequently bilateral

Diagnostic Evaluation

X-ray data
1. Flattened, fragmented femoral head
2. Widening of the neck of the femur
3. Increase in the joint space

Prognosis

Depends on the age of the child at the onset and the amount of involvement demonstrated on x-ray.

Younger children are more prone to complete recovery without permanent, residual deformity.

Altered Physiology*

A. *Stage I (Aseptic Necrosis)*
1. Femoral head becomes necrotic.
   Opacity of the epiphysis apparent on x-ray.
2. Slight widening of the joint space occurs.
3. Swelling of the soft tissues around the hip occurs.

B. *Stage II (Revascularization)*
1. Epiphysis becomes mottled and fragmented.
2. Density of the femoral head increases.
3. Epiphysis may show some flattening in the vertical direction.

C. *Stage III (Reossification)*
1. The head of the femur gradually reforms.
2. Nucleus of the epiphysis breaks up into a number of fragments with cyst-like spaces between them.
3. New bone starts to develop at the medial and lateral edges of the epiphysis which becomes widened.
4. Dead bone is removed and is replaced with new bone which gradually spreads to heal the lesion.

D. *Stage IV (Postrecovery Period)*
1. Without treatment
   a. Head of the femur flattens and becomes mushroom shaped.
   b. Incongruity between the head of the femur and the acetabulum persists.
   c. Degenerative changes develop later in life.
2. Complete recovery
   a. Head of the femur remains spherical.
   b. Acetabulum appears normal.
   c. Width of the neck of the femur is normal.

* Each stage lasts approximately 9 months to 1 year.

Nursing Objectives

Generally, the child with Legg-Calvé-Perthes disease is hospitalized to avoid weight-bearing on his affected extremity. This is usually accomplished by complete bedrest with or without traction or by immobilization of the hip by surgery, casts or braces. Because treatment is necessary for an extensive period, it is usually continued at a convalescent facility or in the home. Nursing objectives are essentially the same as for the child with a dislocated hip (see p. 1374). The following points of emphasis must be considered.

A. *To evaluate the home very carefully and provide guidance to the family regarding the child's home care.*
  1. The family should be made aware of convalescent facilities as an alternative to home care.
     They should be helped to make the decision between these alternatives and should be supported in their decision.
  2. A firm mattress and bedboard are necessary.
  3. Appropriate referrals may include:
     a. Community health nurse   d. Physical therapy
     b. Social service   e. Occupational therapy
     c. Home teacher

B. *To enable the child to participate in as many normal activities of life as possible because recovery may take from 2 to 5 years.*
  1. Plans must be made for continuing education.
  2. Diversion is an extremely important consideration.

C. *To provide emotional support to the child and his family because of the long-term nature of the illness.*
  1. Provide the family with frequent opportunities to express their feelings and concerns.
     Techniques of therapeutic play should be used with the child.
  2. Point out even small indications of the recovery process.
     Allow the child and his parents to view his x-rays.
  3. Introduce the family to other families with similarly affected children if available.

Patient and Parental Education

  1. General techniques of home nursing
     a. Bathing and skin care
     b. Maintenance of good muscle tone, proper body alignment and prevention of contractures
     c. Provision for elimination
     d. Nutritional considerations
     e. Bedmaking
  2. Pathology of the disease and rationale of treatment
     a. Reinforce medical explanations and clarify interpretations as necessary.
     b. Allow the child and his parents to view his own x-rays to increase his knowledge of the disease.
     c. Emphasize that complete recovery can occur only with prolonged avoidance of weight-bearing on the affected extremity.
  3. Necessity of regular medical follow-up for evaluation of the child's progress.

BIBLIOGRAPHY

Books

Aegerter, E. M., and Kirkpatrick, J. A.: Orthopedic Diseases. Philadelphia, W. B. Saunders, 1968.

Blake, F., et al.: Nursing Care of Children. Philadelphia, J. B. Lippincott, 1970.

Ferguson, A. B.: Orthopedic Surgery in Infancy and Childhood, 3rd ed. Baltimore, Williams and Wilkins, 1968.

Marlow, D. R.: Textbook of Pediatric Nursing. Philadelphia, W. B. Saunders, 1973.

Nelson, W., et al.: Textbook of Pediatrics. Philadelphia, W. B. Saunders, 1969.

Powell, M.: Orthopedic Nursing, 5th ed. Baltimore, Williams and Wilkins, 1968.

Sharrard, W. J. W.: Pediatric Orthopedics and Fractures. Oxford, Blackwell Scientific Publications, 1971.

Silver, H. K., et al.: Handbook of Pediatrics. Los Altos, Lange Medical Publications, 1971.

Article

Lane, P.: A mother's confession—home care of a toddler in a spica cast: what it is really like. Amer. J. Nurs., 71:2142–2143, Nov. 1971.

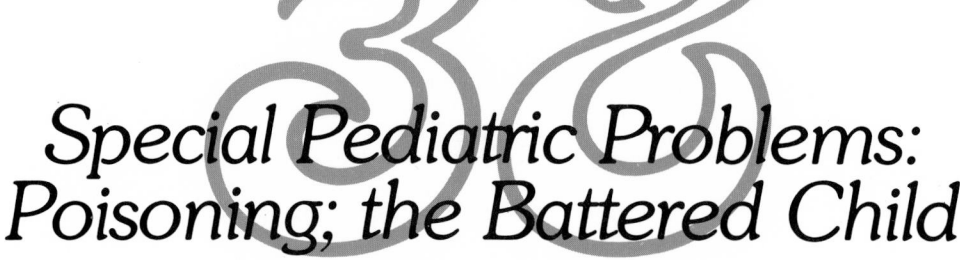

Special Pediatric Problems: Poisoning; the Battered Child

POISONING

Ingested Poisons

Poisoning by ingestion refers to the oral intake of a harmful substance which, even in a small amount, can damage tissues, disturb bodily functions and cause possible death. In the pediatric population, poisoning is often caused by the ingestion of medications, lye and household cleaners, and spoiled food.

Etiology

1. Improper or dangerous storage
2. Poor lighting
3. Human factors
   a. Failure to read label properly
   b. Failure to return poison to its proper place
   c. Failure to recognize the material as poisonous

Clinical Manifestations

1. Gastrointestinal symptoms (common in metallic, acid, alkali and bacterial poisonings)
   a. Anorexia
   b. Abdominal pain
   c. Nausea
   d. Vomiting
   e. Diarrhea
2. Central nervous system symptoms
   a. Convulsions—common in poisoning due to ingestion of central nervous system stimulants such as camphor and strychnine.
   b. Coma—common in poisoning due to ingestion of central nervous system depressants such as alcohol, atropine, chloral hydrate, barbiturates.

     c. Dilated pupils—common in poisoning due to atropine, nicotine, cocaine, ephedrine.

     d. Pinpoint pupils—common in poisoning due to opiates.

  3. Skin symptoms

     a. Lesions of the mucous membranes of the mouth—alkali poisonings

     b. Cyanosis and dyspnea—cyanide and strychnine poisoning

Diagnostic Evaluation

Analysis reveals presence of toxic substances in:

  1. Blood   3. Gastric washings

  2. Urine   4. Vomitus

Nursing Objectives

A. *To identify the poison.*

  1. Instruct parents to save vomitus, unswallowed liquid or pills and the container and bring them to the hospital as aids in identifying the poison.

  2. Call the nearest poison control center or toxicology section of the medical examiner's office to identify the toxic ingredient and obtain recommendations for emergency treatment.

  3. Save vomitus and urine output for analysis once the child reaches the hospital.

B. *To remove the poison from the body.*

  1. Induce vomiting.

     a. Administer 15 ml. of ipecac syrup.

     b. Stimulate posterior pharynx with finger.

     c. Do not induce vomiting if:

       (1) Child is convulsing, semiconscious or comatose

       (2) Poison is known to be acid, alkali, kerosene or gasoline

  2. Gastric lavage (see p. 923).

     a. Use the largest sized tube that can be passed orally.

     b. Place the child's head lower than his stomach.

     c. Lavage with small, repeated introductions and withdrawals of tap water.

     d. Do not leave large amount of water in the child's stomach.

     e. Follow lavage with a cathartic to hasten removal of the poison from the gastrointestinal tract.

     f. Be aware of the dangers associated with lavage.

       (1) Esophageal perforation may occur in corrosive poisoning.

       (2) Convulsions may result from stimulation in strychnine ingestion.

       (3) Aspiration and pneumonia may result from improper lavage technique in kerosene ingestion.

C. *To administer an antidote to the poison.*

  1. An antidote may either react with the poison to prevent its absorption or counteract the effects of the poison after its absorption.

  2. Not all poisons have specific antidotes.

  3. Information regarding appropriate antidotes for specific poisons is available through all poison control centers and many pediatric textbooks.

    Antidotes for the most common poisons should be listed in the emergency room of the hospital.

4. Effectiveness of the antidote usually depends on the amount of time which elapses between the ingestion and administration of the antidote.

5. Universal antidote
   2 parts powdered charcoal (burned toast)
   1 part milk of magnesia
   1 part tannic acid (strong tea)

D. *To observe the child for progression of symptoms and to provide supportive care should these develop.*

   1. Central Nervous System Involvement
      a. Observe for:
         Restlessness, confusion, delirium, convulsions, lethargy, stupor, coma
      b. Administer sedation with caution to avoid depression and masking of symptoms.
      c. Avoid excessive manipulation of the child.
      d. See nursing care of the child with seizures, page 1339.
      e. See nursing care of the unconscious patient, page 728.

   2. Respiratory Involvement
      a. Observe for:
         Respiratory depression, obstruction, pulmonary edema, pneumonia, tachypnea
      b. Have an artificial airway available.
      c. Be prepared to administer oxygen and provide artificial respiration.
      d. Other nursing concerns.
         (1) Nursing care of the child on a respirator.
         (2) Procedures for administration of oxygen, page 1094.
         (3) Procedure for cardiopulmonary resuscitation, page 1097.

   3. Cardiovascular Involvement
      a. Observe for:
         Peripheral circulatory collapse, disturbances of heart rate and rhythm, cardiac failure
      b. Maintain intravenous therapy of saline and glucose solution, plasma or blood.
         See procedure for the administration of intravenous fluids, page 1087.
      c. Be prepared for cardiac arrest.
         See procedure for cardiopulmonary resuscitation, page 1097.

   4. Gastrointestinal Involvement
      a. Observe for:
         Nausea, pain, abdominal distention, and difficulty swallowing
      b. Maintain intravenous therapy to replace water and electrolyte loss.
         See procedure for intravenous therapy, page 1087.
      c. Offer a diet which is easily swallowed and digested.
         (1) Begin with clear liquid.
         (2) Progress to full liquids, soft foods and then a regular diet as the child's condition improves.

   5. Kidney Involvement
      a. Observe the child for decreased urine output.
         Record urine output exactly.
      b. Observe for hypertension.
      c. Insert indwelling catheter if necessary for urinary retention.
      d. Administer appropriate amounts of fluids and electrolytes.
      e. See nursing care of the child with renal failure, page 1233.

6. General Considerations
   a. Maintain adequate caloric, fluid and vitamin intake.
      Oral fluids are preferable if they can be retained.
   b. Avoid hypo- or hyperthermia.
      (1) Control of body temperature is impaired in many types of poisoning.
      (2) Monitor the child's temperature frequently.
   c. Observe closely for infection.
      (1) This is especially important in kerosene or other hydrocarbon ingestions which cause chemical pneumonitis.
      (2) Isolate the patient from other children, especially those with respiratory infections.
      (3) Administer antibiotics as ordered by the physician.

E. *To provide emotional support for the child and his family.*
   1. Remain calm and efficient while working rapidly.
   2. Discourage anxious parents from handling, caressing and overstimulating their child.
   3. Counsel parents who often feel guilty about the accident.
      a. Encourage parents to talk about the poisoning.
      b. Emphasize how their quick action in getting treatment for their child has helped.
      c. Discuss ways that they can be supportive to their child during his hospitalization.
      d. Do not allow prolonged periods of self-incrimination to continue.
         Refer the parents to a social worker or psychiatrist for assistance in resolving these feelings if necessary.
   4. Involve the young child in therapeutic play to determine how he views the situation.
      a. The child often sees nursing measures as punishments for his misdeed involving the poisoning.
      b. Explain the child's treatment and correct his misinterpretations in a manner appropriate for his age.

Patient and Parental Teaching

A. *Prevention*
   1. Information concerning poison prevention should be available on any hospital pediatric unit.
      a. Many free booklets are available through insurance companies, drug companies, etc.
      b. Teaching may be done with any parent regardless of the reason for the child's hospitalization.
   2. General Precautions
      a. Keep medicines and poisons out of the reach of children.
      b. Provide locked storage for highly toxic substances.
      c. Do not store poisons in the same area as foods.
      d. Be certain all containers are properly marked and labeled. Keep medicines, drugs and household chemicals in their original containers.
      e. Do not discard poisonous substances in receptacles where children can reach them.
      f. Teach children not to taste or eat unfamiliar substances.
      g. Medications
         (1) Clean out medicine cabinets periodically.
            (a) Dispose of old medications in containers out of the reach of children.
            (b) Prescription medications should be discarded when the illness for which they were prescribed has run its course.

          (2) Read all labels carefully before each use.
            (a) Follow exact directions on the label.
            (b) Never take a drug from an unlabeled bottle.
          (3) Don't give medicines prescribed for one child to another child.
          (4) Never refer to drugs as candy or bribe children with such inducements.
          (5) Never give or take medications in the dark.
    h. Never puncture or burn aerosol containers.
    i. Store lawn and garden pesticides in a separate place under lock and key outside of the house.
    j. Keep a 30-ml. (1-ounce) bottle of ipecac syrup and a can of activated charcoal available in the home.
    k. Keep a list of emergency phone numbers including the poison control center, physician's number, nearest hospital and ambulance service.

B. *Emergency Actions*
    1. Read the label on the ingested product or call physician, hospital or poison control center for instructions regarding treatment of the poisoning.
    2. Dilute the poison by giving water (1–2 glassfuls).
    3. Make the child vomit if so directed. *Do not induce vomiting if:*
       a. Child is unconscious or convulsive
       b. Ingested poison was a strong corrosive such as lye, drain cleaner, etc.
       c. Ingested poison contains gasoline, kerosene or other petroleum distillates
       d. *Directions for making the child vomit:*
          (1) Administer 1 tablespoon of ipecac syrup with at least 1 cup of water.
          (2) If vomiting does not occur in 20 minutes this dose may be repeated once only.
          (3) Vomiting may also be induced by tickling the back of the throat with a spoon handle or other blunt instrument.
    4. Transport the child promptly to the nearest medical facility.
       a. Wrap the child in a blanket to prevent chilling.
       b. Bring the container and any vomitus or urine to the hospital with the child.
    5. If transportation to a medical facility is impossible:
       a. Continue to induce vomiting until clear.
       b. Administer milk or the universal antidote between vomiting episodes.
    6. Avoid excessive manipulation of the child.
    7. Act promptly but calmly.

Lead Poisoning

Lead poisoning (plumbism) is a relatively common disease in young children which results from the consumption of lead in some form. Each year it causes the death of many children and leaves others with chronic neurological handicaps or mental retardation.

Etiology

    1. Ingestion of substances containing lead
       a. Paint and plaster from repainted walls, windowsills, furniture, toys
       b. Lead toys
       c. Oil paints
       d. Industrial crayons
       e. Lead nipple shields
       f. Water from lead pipes
       g. Fruit covered with insecticides
       h. Face powders

2. Inhalation of fumes containing lead (less common cause in children)
   a. Motor fuel
   b. Burning storage batteries
   c. Dust containing lead salts

Altered Physiology

1. Lead salts are absorbed by the blood from the respiratory tract or intestines.
2. A large portion of the absorbed lead enters the portal circulation and is excreted by the liver.
3. Lead that reaches the systemic circulation is deposited in bone and soft tissues.
   a. Brain—edema, vascular damage, destruction of brain cells
   b. Peripheral nerves
      (1) Lead is slowly transferred from soft tissues to bone.
      (2) Deposited in insoluble form with calcium.
      (3) Causes increased thickness and density of long bones.
      (4) Decalcification is associated with the release of lead from bone.
4. Affects the surface of the red blood cell, increasing its fragility and reducing its half-life.

Epidemiological Factors

1. Slums are high risk areas because of old, deteriorating housing.
2. Pica (a tendency to eat dirt and plaster) is a common precondition.
   a. Poisoning associated with pica is a chronic process.
   b. Clinical manifestations appear after 3–6 months of fairly steady lead ingestion.

Incidence

1. Highest in children between 1–6 years of age
2. High in Blacks and Puerto Ricans
3. No significant difference in sex
4. High among siblings
5. Symptomatic lead poisoning usually occurs in the summer months
6. Recurrence rate is high

Clinical Manifestations

1. Gastrointestinal symptoms
   a. Vomiting
   b. Vague abdominal pain
   c. Colic
   d. Constipation
   e. Loss of appetite
   f. Weight loss
2. Central nervous system symptoms (common in children)
   a. Falling, clumsiness, loss of coordination
   b. Irritability
   c. Peripheral neuritis
   d. Convulsions with or without local paralysis
   e. Drowsiness, coma
3. Hematological symptoms
   a. Anemia
   b. Pallor

    4. Cardiovascular symptoms
      a. Hypertension
      b. Bradycardia
    5. Symptoms depend on the amount of lead in the soft tissues and blood:
      a. Onset is insidious.
      b. Usually progresses from mild to severe manifestations as the lead slowly accumulates.
      c. Infants and toddlers may present severe manifestations initially.
      d. Symptoms may be intermittent for several months.

Diagnostic Evaluation

    1. Increased urinary excretion
    2. Increased serum levels (a finger stick technique is available for determining serum lead levels.)
    3. Urinary excretion of coproporphyrin
    4. Cerebrospinal fluid under pressure (in patients with lead encephalopathy)
    5. Glycosuria
    6. Elevated lead level in hair

Prognosis

    1. Generally poor especially in children with central nervous system involvement.
    2. Residual effects on the nervous system are permanent and progressive.
      a. Late symptoms of mental retardation may appear 3–9 years after treatment.
      b. Specific intellectual defect may interfere with the child's progress at school.

Nursing Objectives

A. *To collect a urine specimen as a diagnostic tool.*

    A 24-hour specimen is more accurate than a single voided specimen. (See section on specimen collection.)

B. *To prevent absorption of lead.*

    1. Offer relatively large quantities of milk.
      a. Promotes the formation of insoluble, poorly absorbed lead salts in the intestines.
      b. Hastens the deposit of lead in bone.
    2. Make certain that all sources of lead are removed from the child's environment.

C. *To increase urinary excretion of lead.*

    1. Administer EDTA (ethylenediamine tetra-acetic acid)
      a. Action—combines with lead to form a nontoxic compound which is excreted in the urine.
      b. Route of administration
        (1) Intramuscular injection is the preferred route in children.
        (2) Rapid intravenous infusion may be lethal by suddenly increasing intracranial pressure in patients with cerebral edema.
      c. Dosage
        (1) Should not exceed 1 gm./15 kg./day.
        (2) Administered in divided doses every 8–12 hours.
        (3) Usually administered for 5 days.

(4) A second course of therapy may be necessary after an interval of 2 days if signs and symptoms of lead poisoning persist or serum level remains elevated.
   d. Untoward reactions
      (1) Rash, vomiting, tetany, lethargy, shock
      (2) Usually appear with intravenous rather than intramuscular administration of EDTA
   e. Toxic reactions—renal toxicity
      (1) Do not administer EDTA to dehydrated patients.
      (2) Avoid overhydration during therapy.
      (3) Check urine daily for protein and blood.
   f. Special precautions
      (1) Minimize the pain at the injection site.
         (a) Add enough procaine to give a concentration of 0.5% procaine to each injection.
             1 ml. of 1% procaine may be added to each ml. of concentrated EDTA.
             Crystalline procaine may be used to reduce the volume of injection.
         (b) Inject the medication deeply into the muscle.
         (c) Establish a pattern for the rotation of injection sites.
         (d) Record the site of each injection.
         (e) Apply warm compresses or allow the child to soak in a warm bath to alleviate muscular soreness.
2. Administer BAL (dimercaprol)
   a. Action—removes lead from the tissues by forming stable, relatively nontoxic compounds.
   b. Route—intramuscular
   c. Dosage
      2.5 mg./kg. every 4 hours for 5 days.
      Administer with EDTA at a separate site.
   d. Observe for untoward effects.
      (1) Symptoms begin within 10–15 minutes after injection of BAL and subside within 1–2 hours.
      (2) Symptoms
             Increased lacrimation, salivation, sweating
             Nausea and vomiting
             Headache
             Pain in teeth
             Burning sensation of lips, mouth, throat
             Sensation of constriction of chest, tachycardia
             Muscular aching
             Fever
   e. Observe for toxic reaction
      Check urine daily for protein and abnormalities of urinary sediment.

D. *To increase the deposition of lead in the bones.*
   1. Offer relatively large quantities of milk.
   2. Observe for electrolyte imbalance. (Acidosis inhibits lead deposition in bones.)
   3. Observe for and treat infection—interferes with lead deposition in bones.

E. *To provide supportive care to the child with encephalopathy.*
   1. Observe for:
      a. Rising blood pressure
      b. Papilledema
      c. Slow pulse
      d. Convulsions
      e. Unconsciousness
   2. See section on pediatric neurological problems, page 1339.
   3. Plan nursing care around periods when medications must be given.

F. *To prevent re-exposure of the child to lead.*
   1. Instruct parents regarding the seriousness of repeated exposure to lead.
   2. Initiate a referral to a community health nurse to determine if exposure to lead is continuing.
   3. Advise parents to require landlord to remove lead paint from the walls.
      a. Refer to the housing authority.
      b. Do not allow the child in the home while lead paint is being removed. Place the child temporarily in a convalescent home or foster home if necessary.
   4. Refer the family for additional social or psychiatric casework if indicated to reduce the psychological or cultural factors which result in pica in the child.

G. *To participate in the prevention of lead poisoning.*
   1. Provide literature in clinics, waiting rooms, etc., stressing the hazards of lead, sources of lead, methods of lead poisoning, signs of lead intoxication, etc.
   2. Inquire regarding pica in all children under 6 years of age.
   3. Screen sibling of known cases immediately.
   4. Screen all children from high-risk areas.

Patient or Parental Teaching

Parent education is an extremely important part of the nursing care of a child with lead poisoning. It should include the following points of emphasis:
   1. Long-term medical follow-up is essential.
      a. Residual lead is liberated gradually after treatment.
         (1) May result in the renewal of symptoms.
         (2) May increase serum iron to a dangerous level.
         (3) Additional damage to the central nervous system may become apparent for several months (after discharge from the hospital).
      b. Acute infections must be recognized and treated promptly. (These may reactivate the disease.)
   2. Re-exposure to lead must be prevented.
   3. Siblings and playmates should be screened for lead poisoning.
   4. Literature stressing the causes and prevention of lead poisoning should be provided.

Poison Control Centers

Purpose

   1. To provide information on a 24-hour basis to the physician and the general public regarding ingestion of the myriad of household products and medicines available to children.
      a. Ingredients
      b. Toxicity
      c. Expected signs and symptoms

      d. Recommended treatment
        (1) Whether or not medical treatment is necessary
        (2) First-aid instructions such as the use of an emetic or dilution
  2. To establish a program of prevention of childhood poisonings.
      a. Foster awareness among both medical and nonmedical professions
      b. Stimulate federal and state legislation

History and Present Status

  1. Initiated as a pilot project in Chicago by the Illinois Chapter of the Academy of Pediatrics in 1953.
  2. Presently there are nearly 600 centers in the United States. (A directory of poison control centers is available.*)
  3. The National Clearinghouse for Poison Control Centers was established by the Public Health Service in 1956 in order to coordinate the activities of the various poison control centers.

Operation of the Centers

  1. Autonomous organizations developed by local hospitals or paramedical groups in cooperation with state health departments.
  2. Location
      a. Most are located in hospitals.
      b. Some are located in health departments.
  3. Financial support—usually from the hospital in which it resides.
  4. Resources
      a. Index card files of household products and medicines
      b. Textbooks on poisoning, plant toxicity, pharmacology, etc.
      c. Lists of consultants for unusual poisonings

Functions of the National Clearinghouse

  1. Coordinates activities of each individual center.
  2. Supplies index card file system concerning the toxicity of trade name products. (Supplements and revises card files every 1–2 months.)
  3. Publishes a bimonthly bulletin on current poisoning topics.
  4. Compiles statistical data and tabulates reports of the experiences of all of the centers.

Future of Poison Control Centers

  1. Creation of centralized, regional centers from already existing centers
      a. Responsible for smaller centers which will handle the less complex cases
      b. Provides information, toxicological evaluation and educational resources to the local center
  2. Location dictated by population and need
  3. Centralization of finances from federal and state sources
  4. Close cooperation and coordination with medical centers
      Provides continued training of medical and paramedical personnel
  5. Extension of activities to include:
      a. Injury control   c. Suicides
      b. Other accidents   d. Drug abuse

* *Directory of Poison Control Centers* (FDA Publication #72-7001). U. S. Department of Health, Education and Welfare, Food and Drug Administration, Bureau of Product Safety, Division of Hazardous Substances and Poison Control, Washington, D.C., 1971.

THE BATTERED CHILD
(Child Abuse)

Child abuse is nonaccidental physical attack or physical injury, including minimal as well as fatal injury, inflicted upon children by persons caring for them.

Etiology

Child abuse is not a uniform phenomenon with one set of causal factors, but a multi-dimensional phenomenon. The phenomenon may be related to:
  a. Psychopathology of the abuser
  b. Cultural, social and economic factors

Factors Relating to Child Abuse

1. Incidents of child abuse may develop as a result of disciplinary action taken by the abuser who responds in uncontrolled anger to real or perceived misconduct of the child.
2. Incidents of child abuse may develop from a general attitude of resentment or rejection on the part of the abuser toward the child.
3. Atypical child behavior (e.g., hyperactivity) may provoke the abuser. This may be child-initiated or child-provoked abuse.
4. Incidents of child abuse may develop out of a quarrel between the caretakers. The child may come to the aid of one parent, may just happen to be in the midst of the quarrel, or may object to the quarrel.
5. The abuser may be a stern, authoritarian disciplinarian.
6. The abuser may be under a great deal of stress due to life circumstances (debt, poverty, illness) and resort to child abuse.
7. The abuser may be intoxicated with alcohol or drugs at the time of the abuse.
8. Child abuse frequently occurs while the mother is out of the home and the child is left in the care of a babysitter or boyfriend.
9. Lack of early mothering is related to later child abuse.

Clinical Manifestations

A. Physical characteristics utilized as an index of suspicion.
  1. Child usually under 3 years of age.
  2. General health of the child indicates neglect (diaper rash, poor hygiene, malnutrition)
  3. Characteristic distribution of fractures (many different parts of body)
  4. Disproportionate amount of soft tissue injury
  5. Evidence that injuries occurred at different times (healed and new fractures, resolving and fresh bruises)
  6. Cause of recent trauma in question
  7. History of similar episodes in past
  8. No new lesions occurring during the child's hospitalization

B. Injuries or types of abuse that may occur.
  1. Bruises, welts (most common)
  2. Abrasions, contusions, lacerations (most common)
  3. Wounds, cuts, punctures
  4. Burns (cigarette, radiator, etc.), scalding

5. Bone fractures (including skull)
6. Sprains, dislocations
7. Subdural hemorrhage or hematoma
8. Brain damage
9. Internal injuries
10. Poisoning
11. Malnutrition (deliberately inflicted)
12. Freezing, exposure

Nursing Objectives

A. *To inspect every child's body upon admission to the hospital for evidence of abuse.*
  1. Describe on nursing record all bruises, lacerations, etc. as to location and state of healing.
  2. Discuss with the physician the case of any child suspected of being abused. (Every state and territory has child abuse legislation and provides a mechanism for the reporting and investigation of cases of real and suspected child abuse.)

B. *To observe and record pertinent information regarding the parent-child relationship.*
  1. Do the parents visit the child?
  2. How does the parent respond to the child Does he talk to him, touch him, hold him, play with him?
  3. How does the child react to the parent? Is he excited when the parent arrives? Does he appear frightened and withdrawn? Does he cry when the parent leaves?

C. *To foster a trusting relationship with the child who may be fearful of adults.*
  1. Assign 1 nurse to care for the child over a period of time.
  2. Make no theatening moves toward the child.
  3. Touch the child gently.
  4. Provide nonthreatening physical contact (hold the child frequently and cuddle him, etc.).
  5. Enlist the cooperation of volunteers to provide additional mothering.
  6. Provide appropriate opportunities for play.

D. *To foster a relationship with the parents that will encourage them to accept guidance and help in dealing with the problem.*
  1. Assume a nonjudgmental attitude which is neither punitive nor threatening.
  2. Refrain from questioning regarding the incident of abuse. (The suspected abuser will be interviewed by the physician, the social worker, and the authority who investigates the case.)

E. *To teach the parents about normal growth and development. (See section on Growth and Development, p. 1033–1047.)*
  1. Give specific information and examples as to what type of behavior to expect at the various stages of development.
  2. Give specific information as to how to deal with this behavior.

F. *To teach the parents how to use discipline without resorting to physical force.*
  1. Discipline must be consistent.
  2. Rewards may be used for acceptable behavior (e.g., a trip to the zoo, staying up later than usual for a special TV show, a special treat).
  3. Rewards are withheld for unacceptable behavior.

G. *To support the parent and the child when a decision is made to have the child removed from the home.*
   1. The decision is made for the safety and protection of the child.
   2. The parents are afforded the opportunity to have counselling to help them learn to deal with their problem.

H. *To be aware of the child who has the potential for being abused and provide antici-patory guidance.*
   1. The premature infant, the hyperactive child, the chronically ill child, the retarded child, the child who takes a great deal of time and confines the mother to the home has the potential for being abused.
   2. *Encourage early participation of mother (parents) in the care of the child during hospitalization.*
   3. Prepare the mother for the fact that the child does require a great deal of care, but encourage her to find outlets for her frustrations.
   4. Provide her with the name and telephone number of someone at the hospital to whom she can look for help (e.g., social worker).
   5. Intiate a community nursing referral.

BIBLIOGRAPHY

Books

Blake, F., et al.: Nursing Care of Children. Philadelphia, J. B. Lippincott, 1970.
Facts About Lead and Pediatrics. New York, Lead Industries Assoc. Inc., 1969.
Gil, D. G.: Violence Against Children. Cambridge, Massachusetts, Harvard University Press, 1970.
Helfer, R. E., and Kempe, C. H. (eds.): Helping the Battered Child and His Family. Philadelphia, J. B. Lippincott, 1972.
Lead Poisoning in Children. U. S. Department of Health, Education and Welfare, Social and Reha-bilitation Service, Children's Bureau. Publication No. 452, 1967.
Marlow, D. R.: Textbook of Pediatric Nursing. Philadelphia, W. B. Saunders, 1973.
Nelson, W., et al.: Textbook of Pediatrics. Philadelphia, W. B. Saunders, 1969.
Silver, H., et al.: Handbook of Pediatrics. Los Altos, California, Lange Medical Publications, 1971.
Silver, W., and Rodrigues, T. R.: Lead intoxication *In* Gellis, S. S., and Kagan, B. M. (eds.): Cur-rent Pediatric Therapy. Philadelphia, W. B. Saunders, 1971.

Articles

Coleman, A., and Alpert, J. (eds.): Poisoning in children. Ped. Clin. N. Amer., *17*: (no. 3), August 1970.
Holland, W.: Deadly walls: a report on the control of childhood lead-based paint poisoning, a pro-gram of the Bureau of Community Environmental Management. HSMHA World, Jan.-Feb. 1972.
Lin-Fu, J. S.: Childhood lead poisoning, an eradicable disease. Children, *17*:2–9, Jan.-Feb. 1970.
Lonsdale, D., and Evarts, C. M.: Guide to the battered child syndrome. Hosp. Med., 8:8–23, March 1972.
Sachs, H. K., et al.: Ambulatory treatment of lead poisoning: report of 1155 cases. Pediatrics, *46*: 389, 1970.

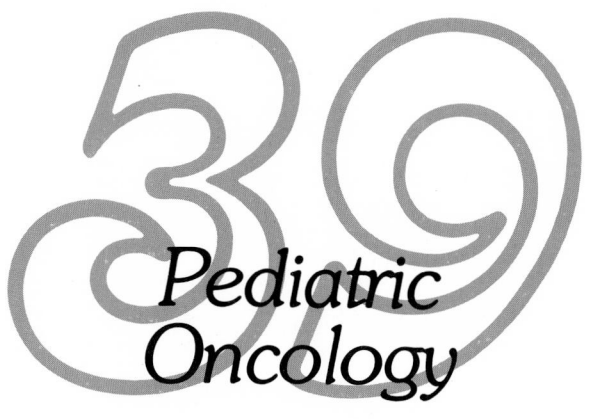

Pediatric Oncology

BRAIN TUMORS IN CHILDREN

Brain tumors are expanding lesions within the skull and account for 10 to 15% of the malignant tumors which occur in children.

Etiology

The etiology of brain tumors is unknown.

Clinical Manifestations

1. Signs and symptoms produced by increased intracranial pressure caused by a blocking of the flow of cerebrospinal fluid.
   a. Headache
      (1) May occur at any time, but usually is more severe in early morning hours.
      (2) May be intermittent and disappear for days or weeks—this may be due to a yield of the sutures.
   b. Vomiting
      (1) May be projectile.
      (2) May be unaccompanied by nausea.
      (3) May occur at any time, but frequently occurs at early morning hours.
   c. Slow cerebration
      (1) Child answers questions after a considerable delay.
      (2) Child appears to talk slowly.
      (3) Child responds to any stimulus in a slow manner.
   d. Sixth cranial nerve palsy
      (1) Diplopia
      (2) Blurred vision

    e. Personality changes
       (1) Irritability
       (2) Apathy
       (3) Disturbances in sleep and eating patterns
    f. Sudden enlargement of the head circumference
    g. Alterations of consciousness
    h. Bulging fontanelles
    i. Tilting of head
    j. Opisthotonus tonic seizures and stupor
    k. Papilledema
  2. Signs produced by the direct, local effect of the tumor
    a. Infratentorial
       (1) Ataxia
       (2) Nystagmus
       (3) Signs of increased intracranial pressure
    b. Supratentorial
       (1) Contralateral hemiparesis   (4) Loss of peripheral vision
       (2) Spasticity   (5) Progressive difficulty with speech
       (3) Seizures

Cerebellar Astrocytoma

Cerebellar astrocytoma is a slow growing, often cystic type of tumor of the cerebellum.

Etiology

  1. Cerebellar astrocytomas account for 25% of brain tumors in children.
  2. The peak incidence occurs at 5–8 years of age.

Altered Physiology

The tumor produces slowly increasing intracranial pressure.

Clinical Manifestations

The signs and symptoms develop slowly.
  1. Increased intracranial pressure   3. Nystagmus
  2. Ataxia, predominating or confined to one side.   4. Head tilt

Diagnostic Evaluation

  1. Skull x-ray—shows spread of cranial sutures.
  2. Ventriculography—may demonstrate tumor and hydrocephalus.
  3. Brachial angiography—may demonstrate hydrocephalus, abnormal vascular patterns and herniation.
  4. Brain scan—usually difficult to demonstrate this tumor.

Treatment

Surgical removal—the tumor can usually be removed with little sequelae.

Prognosis

The prognosis is good if the tumor is completely removed.

Medulloblastoma

Medulloblastoma is a rapid growing tumor of the cerebellum.

Incidence

The peak incidence occurs at 3–5 years.

Altered Physiology

1. The tumor grows rapidly and produces evidence of increased intracranial pressure progressing over a period of weeks.
2. As the tumor grows, it seeds along the subarachnoid space.

Clinical Manifestations

The signs and symptoms develop rapidly.

1. Increased intracranial pressure
2. Ataxia
3. Nystagmus
4. Obstructive hydrocephalus
5. Loss of tendon reflexes
6. Root pain
7. Paresthesias
8. Cranial nerve involvement

Diagnostic Evaluation

1. Skull x-ray—spread of cranial sutures will be visualized.
2. Ventriculography—may demonstrate tumor.
3. Brachial angiography—may demonstrate hydrocephalus, abnormal vascular patterns.
4. Brain scan—may demonstrate tumor.

Treatment

1. Surgical—complete removal rarely possible
2. Radiation therapy and chemotherapy

Prognosis

Prognosis is grave

Brain Stem Glioma

Brain stem glioma is a tumor of the brain stem.

Incidence

1. Brain stem gliomas occur almost exclusively in children.
2. The peak age at onset is 6–7 years.

Altered Physiology

This type of tumor, through its growth, interferes early with the function of cranial nerve nuclei, pyramidal tracts and cerebellar pathways.

Clinical Manifestations

1. Onset of neurologic signs and symptoms is usually insidious.
2. Increased intracranial pressure occurs late in the illness.
3. Palsy of extraocular muscles—causes strabismus.
4. Weakness, atrophy and fasciculations of the tongue occur.
5. Swallowing difficulties are noted.
6. Hemiplegia occurs.

Diagnostic Evaluation

Pneumoencephalogram visualizes the tumor.

Treatment

1. Surgical removal is not possible; a shunt procedure may relieve intracranial pressure.
2. Radiotherapy.

Nursing Care of the Child with a Brain Tumor

Nursing Objectives

A. *To make pertinent nursing observations which may be of value in helping to locate or determine the extent of involvement of the tumor.*
   1. Observations which may be of value in localizing the tumor:
      a. Change in nature of the pulse
         (1) Lowering pulse rate (particularly irregular pulse)
         (2) Widening pulse pressure
      b. Change in body temperature
      c. Lowering of the respiratory rate
   2. Observe for the following symptoms:
      a. Convulsion
         Give exact details as to activity prior to convulsion, type of convulsion, areas of body affected, length, behavior during convulsion
      b. Headache
         (1) Location—describe location if child can give this information (sometimes difficult)
         (2) Lethargy
         (3) Fecal or urinary incontinence
         (4) Visual disturbances
         (5) Muscular weakness
         (6) Pain
         (7) Vital signs including pupillary reaction
B. *To provide the parents with emotional support during the very stressful preoperative period.*
   1. Allow them to ask questions and encourage them to discuss their fears and concerns.
   2. The manner in which nursing care is delivered to the child is a method of providing support.
      Assume a gentle, concerned attitude toward both parents and child.
   3. Prepare the parents for what to expect following surgery.

C. *To prepare the child for the surgery giving him all the necessary information regarding what equipment will be used, where he will wake up, who will be there and where his parents will be.*
   1. Prepare the child for having his head shaved.
   2. Prepare the child for the large bandage on his head.

D. *To provide an adequate diet for the child preoperatively.*
   Refeed the child when he vomits. (Vomiting is usually not associated with nausea.)

E. *To provide supportive postoperative care for the child, paying special attention to the following considerations.*
   1. Carefully regulate fluid administration in order to prevent increased intracranial pressure.
   2. Move the child carefully and slowly, being particularly careful to move the head in line with the body.
   3. Maintain the position of the bed as specified.
   4. Check the dressing for bleeding and for drainage of cerebrospinal fluid.
   5. Irrigate the eyes frequently when severe edema of the face and eyes occurs.
   6. Provide measures to reduce the body temperature since hyperthermia frequently results from disturbance of the heat regulating system due to intracranial edema or bleeding.
      a. Place child on a thermal regulating blanket.
      b. Give tepid sponge baths.
   7. Provide gavage feeding if the child is unable to eat. (See p. 1080.)

F. *To make provisions for play activities as the child recuperates.*
   1. Allow the child to meet and play with other children.
   2. Provide the child with quiet play activities when it is necessary to encourage rest.
   3. Allow child to assume greater participation in his own care as his condition improves.

WILMS' TUMOR

Wilms' tumor is a malignant renal tumor.

Etiology
   1. The etiology of Wilms' tumor is not known.
   2. The tumor occurs most frequently between the ages of 4 months and 8 years of age, with an average being 5 years.

Altered Physiology
   1. The tumor is most often encapsulated.
   2. The tumor causes a dislocation of the pelvis of the kidney, either upward or downward, depending on the exact location of the tumor.
   3. The tumor growth will eventually interfere with kidney function.

Clinical Manifestations
   1. A firm, abdominal mass is usually the presenting sign; it may be on either side of the abdomen or flank. (Is frequently observed by the parents.)

2. Abdominal pain, which is related to rapid growth of the tumor may occur. As tumor enlarges, pressure symptoms cause constipation, vomiting, abdominal distress and dyspnea, weight loss, pallor and anorexia, pain, hematuria and increased blood pressure.
3. Fever
4. Hypertension
5. Hematuria (possible)

Diagnostic Evaluation

Intravenous urogram will demonstrate a renal mass.

Treatment

1. Nephrectomy
2. Radiation therapy
3. Chemotherapy

Complications

Metastasis—by direct infiltration to omentum and peritoneal cavity through venous extension or through lymphatic channels to any organ.

Nursing Objectives

A. *To support the family and the child at the time the diagnosis is made.*
   1. Discuss with the physician what specific information has been given to the parents.
   2. Provide the parents with the opportunity to express their concerns.
   3. Provide the parents with a place where they may have some privacy when they wish to be alone.
   4. Convey a compassionate attitude to the parents in talking with them, and assure them that their child's needs will be met.
B. *To explain to the child and his parents the elements of preoperative and postoperative care.*
   1. Plan a teaching program for the child that will include diagnostic tests, preoperative care and postoperative care.
   2. Involve the parents in the teaching plan and encourage them to support the child at this time.
   3. Provide preoperative and postoperative care. (See section on postoperative nursing care of children, p. 1093.)
C. *To exercise caution preoperatively in the manipulation of the child in order to prevent trauma to the abdomen.*
   1. Bathe the child carefully, avoiding manipulation of the abdomen.
   2. Hold the child carefully in order to prevent abdominal pressure.
   3. Communicate this information to all staff members.
D. *To prepare the child and the family for the possible side effects of chemotherapeutic agents and radiation therapy, and provide symptomatic nursing care when these side effects occur.*
   1. Side effects of chemotherapeutic agents. (See section on Leukemia, p. 1400–1402.)

2. Side effects of radiation therapy
   a. Nausea
   b. Vomiting
   c. Diarrhea
   d. Anorexia
   e. Skin irritation
   f. Lethargy

E. *To provide diversional therapy for the child.*
   1. Provide the child with the opportunity for play as his condition permits.
   2. Arrange for a visiting teacher when the child is of school age and his condition warrants this activity.

F. *To provide supportive care appropriate for the dying child when the tumor metastasizes and the child's condition deteriorates.* See section on The Dying Child, page 1404.

ACUTE LYMPHOCYTIC LEUKEMIA

Acute lymphocytic leukemia is a hematopoietic malignancy occurring primarily in children. It is characterized by the accumulation of abnormal cells in the bone marrow and peripheral blood, by tissue invasion by these cells, and by bone marrow failure.

Etiology

1. The exact etiology of acute leukemia is unknown.
2. Physical, chemical, and infectious agents, as well as genetic factors and chromosomal abnormalities are felt to be related in some patients.
3. The peak incidence of acute lymphocytic leukemia occurs at 3 to 4 years of age.

Altered Physiology

1. Acute lymphocytic leukemia results from the growth of an abnormal type of non-granular, fragile leukocyte in the blood-forming tissues, particularly in the bone marrow, spleen and lymph nodes.
2. The abnormal cell has little cytoplasm and a round, homogenous nucleus which resembles that of a lymphoblast.
3. Normal bone marrow elements may be displaced or replaced in this type of leukemia.
4. The changes in the blood and bone marrow result from the accumulation of leukemic cells and from the deficiency of normal cells. The bone marrow is hyperplastic with a uniform appearance due to the presence of sheets of leukemic cells.

Clinical Manifestations

A. *Onset*

The onset of acute lymphocytic leukemia is almost always acute and is seldom preceded by preleukemic manifestations. Symptoms are generally of short duration and usually not present for more than 2–3 months when the diagnosis is made.

B. *Presenting Symptoms*
   1. Fatigability
   2. General malaise
   3. Persistent fever of unknown cause
   4. Recurrent infection
   5. Prolonged bleeding following simple surgical procedures (e.g., dental extractions and tonsillectomy)

     6. Enlarged lymph nodes
     7. Abdominal pain due to organomegaly

C. *Rare Symptoms*
     1. Bone pain
     2. Arthralgia

D. *Causes of Primary Manifestations*
     1. Anemia   4. Bone and joint disease
     2. Infection   5. Local tissue invasion
     3. Hemorrhage

Diagnostic Evaluation

A. *Physical Findings*
     1. Pallor   3. Purpura
     2. Petechiae

B. *Laboratory Evaluation*
     1. Leukocyte count—increased, often to 100,000 or more (may be normal or low)
     2. Granulocyte count—decreased
     3. Platelet count—decreased
     4. Bone marrow—infiltrated with abnormal cells which resemble those in the circulating blood except they are less mature. The normal bone marrow elements are reduced in number or almost completely replaced
     5. X-ray—may demonstrate mediastinal lymphadenopathy

Complications

     1. Hemorrhage—usually due to thrombocytopenia
     2. Infection—most frequently occurs in the lungs, gastrointestinal tract or skin
     3. Intracerebral leukemia
     4. Meningeal leukemia
     5. Peripheral nerve involvement
     6. Urate nephropathy

Treatment

Objectives: to rapidly eliminate the manifestations of the disease.
              to restore normal bone marrow function while avoiding cerebral, renal and other complications.

A. *Chemotherapy*
     1. Has significantly altered natural course of the disease.
     2. May possibly reverse temporarily the disease process and increase the duration of life.

B. *Folic Acid Antagonists*—these agents interfere with folic acid metabolism
     Amethopterin (methotrexate)
          a. May be administered orally, intravenously or intrathecally
          b. Toxic effects
               (1) Ulceration of oral mucosa
              (2) Bone marrow suppression

      (3) Ulceration of the gastrointestinal tract producing nausea, vomiting, diarrhea and abdominal pain

      (4) Short-term therapy may produce transient abnormalities of liver function

      (5) Long-term therapy may cause irreversible hepatic fibrosis

C. *Adrenal Corticosteroids*—exact mechanism of action on leukemic cells is unknown but they are capable of inducing lympholysis of normal lymphocytes and involution of lymphoid tissue

    Prednisone

    a. Administered orally

    b. Toxic effects

      (1) Electrolyte imbalances   (4) Hyperglycemia

      (2) Cushinoid features   (5) Hypertension

      (3) Obesity   (6) Osteoporosis

D. *Purine Antagonists*—inhibit various steps in purine biosynthesis

    6-mercaptopurine

    a. Administered orally or parenterally

    b. Toxic effects

      (1) Bone marrow suppression   (3) Liver toxicity

      (2) Nausea and vomiting   (4) Possible oral ulceration

E. *Pyrimidine Antagonists*—interfere with DNA synthesis

    Arabenosyl Cytosin

    a. Administered by slow intravenous infusion

    b. Toxic effects

      (1) Bone marrow suppression

      (2) Nausea and vomiting

      (3) Alopecia and liver toxicity (rare)

F. *Alkylating Agents*

    Cyclophosphamide (Cytoxan)

    a. Administered orally

    b. Toxic effects

      (1) Bone marrow suppression   (3) Alopecia

      (2) Nausea and vomiting   (4) Hemorrhagic cystitis (rare)

G. *Periwinkle Alkaloids*

    Vincristine—exact mechanism of action is unknown but this drug arrests cell division in metaphase

    a. Administered intravenously

    b. Toxic effects

      (1) Minimal toxic effects if administered no more than 3 times a week

      (2) Prolonged administration

         (a) General muscle weakness   (f) Alopecia

         (b) Interosseous wasting   (g) Neurotic pain

         (c) Footdrop   (h) Jaw pain after injection

         (d) Ptosis   (i) Constipation

         (e) Ophthalmoplegia (paralysis of eye muscles)   (j) Abdominal pain

H. *Antibiotics*

Daunorubicin (rubidomycin, daunomycin)—inhibits DNA-dependent RNA synthesis
    a. Administered intravenously
    b. Toxic effects
        (1) Bone marrow suppression   (3) Alopecia
        (2) Stomatitis   (4) Nausea and vomiting

I. *Combination Chemotherapy*
  1. Since the various types of antileukemic agents act independently on the leukemic process, resistance to one agent does not indicate resistance to another agent.
  2. Some combinations of antileukemic agents are felt to have a synergistic rather than an additive effect.
  3. The following combinations of antileukemic agents have produced remissions in children and are frequently used.
    a. Vincristine and prednisone
    b. Prednisone and 6-mercaptopurine
    c. Amethopterin and 6-mercaptopurine
    d. Vincristine, amethopterin, 6-mercaptopurine and prednisone

Nursing Objectives

A. *To provide emotional support to the parents when the diagnosis of leukemia is made known to them.*
  1. Be available to the parents when they feel that they want to discuss their feelings.
  2. Kindness, concern, consideration and sincerity toward the child and his parents help to serve as a source of consolation.
  3. Contact the family's clergyman or the hospital chaplain if the parents desire this.
  4. Utilize the services of a social worker (if available) in helping the family work out their feelings.
  5. Avoid discussing life expectancy in terms of the time element—offer the hope that therapy will be effective and will prolong life.
  6. Allow the parents to participate in the child's care so that they will feel that they are actually doing something for the child. This also helps the family feel more secure if they plan to take the child home to care for him.

B. *To give skillful, supportive care in the early stages of treatment and to sustain life until antileukemic agents have had a chance to become effective.*
  1. Provide adequate hydration.
    a. Maintain parenteral fluid administration.
    b. Offer small amounts of oral fluids if tolerated.
    c. Record and report vomiting if this occurs.
  2. Observe renal function carefully.
    a. Measure and record urinary output.
    b. Check specific gravity.
    c. Observe the urine for any evidence of gross bleeding.
  3. Provide a high nutritional diet if the child can tolerate it.
    a. Determine the child's likes and dislikes.
    b. Offer small, frequent meals.
    c. Offer supplemental feedings which are high in calories and protein.

4. Protect the child from sources of infection.
   a. Family, friends, personnel and other patients who have infections should not be visiting or caring for the child.
   b. Do not place a child with an infection in the room with a child with leukemia.
   c. Reverse isolation procedure may be utilized (a protective technique that provides the child with protection from those people with whom he has contact—gowns and masks are worn by any person with whom the child has contact).
      Explain to both the child and his parents the purpose of this protective technique.
   d. Observe the child closely and be alert to signs of impending infection.
      (1) Observe any area of broken skin or mucous membrane for signs of infection.
      (2) Report any febrile incidents.

C. *To be alert for the symptoms of hemorrhage which may occur when the platelet count is diminished or may appear as side effects of antileukemic therapy.*
   1. Record vital signs and report any changes which may be indicative of hemorrhage.
      a. Tachycardia
      b. Lowered blood pressure
      c. Pallor
      d. Diaphoresis
      e. Increasing anxiety and restlessness
   2. Give careful oral hygiene since the gums and mucous membranes of the mouth bleed easily.
      a. Do not use a toothbrush.
      b. Clean the mouth and teeth with a moistened cotton swab.
      c. Use a nonirritating rinse for the mouth (i.e., hydrogen peroxide).
      d. Apply petroleum jelly to cracked, dry lips.
   3. Observe for gastrointestinal bleeding.
      a. Hematemesis.
      b. Tarry stools or blood-stained stools.
   4. Move and turn the child gently since hemiarthrosis may occur and cause movement to be very painful.
      a. Handle child in a gentle manner.
      b. Turn frequently to prevent bedsores.
      c. Place the child in proper body alignment, in a position comfortable for him.
      d. Allow child to be out of bed in a chair if this position is more comfortable for him.

D. *To prepare the child and his family for the possible side effects of the antileukemic agents he is receiving.*
   Explain to the child that the medicine is to help him to feel better, but when he first begins to take the medicine he may feel more sick. By explaining this prior to the development of symptoms, the child will be more trusting and less frightened.

E. *To be aware of the chemotherapeutic agents and the side effects of these agents which are capable of inducing remissions in children with acute leukemia.*

F. *To prepare the child and his family for frequent returns to the hospital for specific diagnostic tests, transfusions and flare-ups requiring hospital care.*
   1. It is preferable that the child return to the same nursing unit each time a readmission is necessary.
   2. Be sympathetic toward the child and tell him that you, too, feel badly that he must come back to the hospital.

THE DYING CHILD

Nursing Objectives

A. *To work out one's own feelings about death and to develop a philosophy which enables the nurse to be a source of support to the dying child and his family.*
   1. Become familiar with literature in the area of death and dying and use as a resource in planning and developing nursing care.
   2. Recognize that the goal is to assist the child and his family to cope with this pain and grief in such a way that the experience will promote growth rather than destroy family integrity and emotional well-being of the family.

B. *To understand the meaning of illness and death to the child at the various stages of growth and development and to utilize this information in planning and implementing care.*
   1. Child up to 3 years
      a. At this stage the child cannot comprehend the relationship of life to death since he has not developed the concept of infinite time.
      b. The child fears separation from protecting and comforting adults.
   2. Preschool-age Child
      a. At this stage the child has no real understanding of the meaning of death; he feels safe and secure with his parents.
      b. The child may interpret his illness as a type of punishment for real or imagined wrongdoing.
      c. The child may interpret the separation that occurs with hospitalization as punishment; the painful tests and procedures that he is subjected to support this idea.
      d. The child may become depressed because he is not able to correct these wrong-doings and regain the grace of adults.
      e. The child functions on the basis of day-to-day reality.
   3. School-age Child
      a. The child at this age sees death as the cessation of life; he understands that he is alive and that he can become "not alive"; he fears dying.
      b. The child differentiates death from sleep. Unlike sleep, the horror of death is in pain, progressive mutilation and mystery.
      c. The child learns the meaning of death from his own personal experiences.
         Pets
         Death of family members, political figures etc.
      d. Television and movies have contributed to his concepts of death and understanding of the meaning of illness.
         Develops more knowledge in the meaning of diagnosis
         Death may occur violently
   4. Adolescent
      a. The adolescent comprehends the permanence of death much as the adult does.
      b. He wants to live—he sees death as impeding the goals he is striving for: independence, success, achievement, physical improvement and self image.
      c. He fears death before fulfillment.
      d. The adolescent may become depressed and resentful because of bodily changes which may occur, dependency, and the loss of his social environment.
      e. The adolescent may feel isolated and rejected since his own adolescent friends may withdraw when faced with his impending death.

f. The adolescent may express rage, bitterness and resentment. He especially resents the fact that he is fated to die.

C. *To utilize the knowledge about children's interpretation of the meaning of death at the various stages of growth and development in talking to the child about his illness and in answering questions concerning death.*

  1. It is important that the child's questions be answered simply, but truthfully and based on his particular level of understanding.

  2. The following responses have been suggested by Eassom in *The Dying Child* and may be useful as a guide.

    a. Preschool-age Child

      (1) When the child at this age is comfortable enough to ask questions about his illness, he should be told what he asks. When death is anticipated at some future time and the child asks "Am I going to die?" a response might be, "We will all die someday, but you are not going to die today or tomorrow."

      (2) When death is imminent and the child asks, "Am I going to die?" the response might be, "Yes, you are going to die but we will take care of you and stay with you."

      (3) The parents should be allowed to stay with the child to provide him with protection and support.

      (4) When the child asks "Will it hurt?" the response should be truthful and factual. Death may be described as a form of sleep—a sleep where he will be secure in the love of those around him. (Some children may fear sleep as the result of this type of explanation.)

      (5) Parents can express to the child the fact that they do not want him to go and that they will miss him very much; they feel sad too that they are going to be separated.

    b. School-age Child

      (1) Responses to the school-age child's questions about death should be answered truthfully. The child looks for support from those he trusts.

      (2) The school-age child should be given a simple explanation of his diagnosis and its meaning; he should also receive an explanation of all treatments and procedures.

      (3) The child should be given no specific time in terms of days or months since each individual and each illness is different.

      (4) When the school-age child asks "Am I going to die?" and death is inevitable, he should be told the truth. The school-age child does have the emotional ability to look to his parents and those he trusts for comfort and support.

      (5) The school-age child believes in God and his parents. He should be allowed to die in the comfort and security of his family.

      (6) The school-age child knows death means final separation and he knows what he will miss. He must be allowed to mourn this loss as he dies. He may be sad and bitter and demonstrate aggressive behavior. He must be allowed the opportunity to verbalize this if he is able to.

    c. Adolescent

      (1) The adolescent should be given an explanation of his illness and all necessary treatment procedures.

      (2) The adolescent feels deprived and reasonably resentful regarding his illness because he wants to live and reach fulfillment.

(3) As death approaches the adolescent becomes emotionally closer to his family.

(4) The adolescent should be allowed to maintain his emotional defenses—he may deny absolutely. The adolescent will indicate by his questions what kind of answer he wants.

(5) If the adolescent states "I am not going to die" he is pleading for support. Be truthful and state "No, you are not going to die right now."

(6) The adolescent may ask "How long do I have to live?" He is able to face reality more directly and can tolerate more direct answers. No absolute time should be given since that absolutely blocks all hope. If an adolescent has what is felt to be a prognosis of approximately 3 months, the response might be "People with an illness like yours may die in 3 to 6 months, but some may live much longer."

(7) The bitterness and resentment of the fact that he is fated to die may interrupt necessary procedures and treatments. This behavior must be appropriately handled.

D. *To confer with the parents regarding feelings about discussing the illness with the child, and give them information which will be helpful in allowing them to play a more supportive role.*

1. Determine what information they have given the child about his illness, and how the child related to this information.

2. Determine what specific questions the child has asked about his illness, and how the parents have responded.

3. Discuss with the parents how children of various age levels interpret the meaning of death, and offer suggestions as to how children's questions regarding death may be answered.

E. *To assist the parents in dealing with their adaptation to their child's illness and anticipated death.*

1. Develop a plan of care that includes the following approach.
   a. The primary responsibility for communicating with the parents should be designated to one nurse.
   b. Information regarding the parents concerns, etc. should be communicated to all staff members.

2. Recognize the various stages that the parents will go through during the child's illness.

F. *To perform the nursing measures which provide the child with both physical and emotional care during illness.*

1. Provide physical care that makes the child as comfortable as possible.
   Deliver care in a calm, assured, gentle manner.

2. Talk to the child and answer his questions truthfully.

3. Provide an atmosphere that offers the child the greatest security (e.g., room with another child, room near nurse's station, etc.).

4. Provide opportunities for play therapy as the child's condition permits.

G. *To encourage the parents to spend as much time as possible with the child and allow the opportunity to participate in the child's care.*

1. Allow the parents to bathe the child and to do procedures within their ability and desire—this allows the parents the feeling that they are doing something for their child.

2. Provide the parents with the opportunity to feel free to learn how to take care of the child, and assure them that he will be cared for in their absence.

3. Provide the parents with a place to stay and be comfortable. They should be told where they can find privacy when they want to be alone.

H. *To utilize the additional services and resources available in planning the care for the child and his family as indicated.*

1. Social worker
2. Psychiatrist
3. Clergyman
4. Community health nurse
5. Parent groups

BIBLIOGRAPHY

Books

Barnett, H. L. (ed.): Pediatrics, 15th ed. New York, Appleton-Century-Crofts, 1972.

Bauchard, R., and Owens, N.: Nursing Care of the Cancer Patient, 2nd ed. St. Louis, C. V. Mosby, 1972.

Blake, F. G., et al.: Nursing Care of Children, 8th ed. Philadelphia, J. B. Lippincott, 1970.

Eassom, W. M.: The Dying Child. Springfield, Illinois, Charles C Thomas, 1970.

Hamovitch, M.: The Parent and the Fatally Ill Child. Los Angeles, California, Delmar Publishing Company, 1968.

Kübler-Ross, E.: On Death and Dying. New York, Macmillan, 1969.

Matson, D. D.: Neurosurgery of Infancy and Childhood, 2nd ed. Springfield, Illinois, Charles C Thomas, 1969.

Mauer, A. M.: Pediatric Hematology. New York, McGraw-Hill, 1969.

Petrillo, M., and Sanger, S.: Emotional Care of the Hospitalized Child. Philadelphia, J. B. Lippincott, 1972.

Smith, C. H., and Miller, D.: Blood Diseases in Infancy and Childhood, 3rd ed. St. Louis, C. V. Mosby, 1972.

Solnit, A. J., and Green, A.: The Pediatric Management of the Dying Child, Part II: The Child's Reaction to the Fear of Dying. *In* Solnit, A. J., and Provenco, S. A. (eds.): Modern Perspectives in Child Development. New York, International Universities Press, 1963.

Articles

Bredlurd, D. J.: A nurse's look at children's questions about death. AMA Clinical Sessions, 1970.

Crosby, M. H.: Control systems in children with lymphoblastic leukemia. Nurs. Clin. N. Amer., 6:407, 1971.

Freeman, J. M.: Wilms' tumor. Nurs. Mirror, 134:18, 1972.

Goldfogel, L.: Working with the parents of a dying child. Amer. J. Nurs., 70:1675, 1970.

Koop, C. E.: The severely ill or dying child: supporting the patient and the family. Ped. Clin. N. Amer., 16:555, 1969.

Lampkin, B. C., et al.: Treatment of acute leukemia. Ped. Clin. N. Amer., 19:1123, Nov. 1972.

Pratt, C. B.: Management of malignant solid tumors in children. Ped. Clin. N. Amer., 19:1141, Nov. 1972.

Svoboda, E. H.: Wilms' tumor and neuroblastoma: the child under treatment. Amer. J. Nurs., 68:532, 1968.

Swenson, O., and Brenner, R.: Aggressive approach to the treatment of Wilms' tumor. Annals. Surg., 166:4, 1967.

Waechter, E. H.: Children's awareness of fatal illness. Amer. J. Nurs., 71:1168, 1971.

Whitmore, W. F.: Wilms' tumor and neuroblastoma. Amer. J. Nurs., 68:527, 1968.

APPENDIX I

Laboratory Tests

TABLE ABBREVIATIONS

gm. = gram
μg. = microgram
$\mu\mu$g. = micromicrogram
ng. = nanogram
pg. = picogram

mm. = millimeter
cu.mm. = cubic millimeter

mU. = milliunit
μU. = microunit
mEq. = milliequivalent

μ = micron or micrometer
cuμ = cubic microns

I.U. = international unit
L. = liter

NORMAL VALUES—HEMATOLOGY

Determination	Normal Value	Clinical Significance
A$_2$ hemoglobin	1.90–3.86%	Increased in certain types of thalassemia
Bleeding time	30 sec.–6 min.	Prolonged in purpura hemorrhagica, where platelets are reduced, and in chloroform and phosphorus poisoning
Clotting time	5–10 min.	Prolonged in hemorrhagic disease and in various coagulation factor deficiencies
Factor V assay	75–125%	Pro-accelerin factor
Factor VIII assay (antihemophiliac factor)	50–200%	Deficient in classical hemophilia

* Laboratory values vary according to the methology used.

NORMAL VALUES—HEMATOLOGY *(Continued)*

Determination	Normal Values	Clinical Significance
Clotting time (*cont.*)		
Factor IX assay (plasma thromboplastin component)	75–125%	Deficient in Christmas disease (pseudohemophilia)
Factor X (Stuart factor)	75–125%	Stuart clotting defect
Fibrinogen	0.2–0.4 gm./100 ml.	Increased in pregnancy, pneumonia, infections accompanied by leukocytosis, and nephrosis. Decreased in acute yellow atrophy of liver, cirrhosis, typhoid fever, chloroform poisoning, abruptio placentae
Fibrinolysins (whole blood clot lysis time)	No lysis in 24 hrs.	Increased activity associated with massive hemorrhage, extensive surgery, and transfusion reactions
Partial thromboplastin time (cephalin time)	35–45 sec.	Prolonged in factor VIII, IX, and X deficiency
Prothrombin consumption	Over 25 sec.	Impaired in factor VIII, IX, and X deficiency
Prothrombin time	70–100% of control	Prolonged in factor X deficiency and other hemorhagic diseases, and in cirrhosis, hepatitis, and acute toxic necrosis of the liver
Erythrocyte count	Male: 4,600,000– 6,200,000 per cu. mm. Female: 4,200,000– 5,400,000 per cu. mm.	Increased in severe diarrhea and dehydration, polycythemia rubra vera, secondary polycythemia, acute poisoning, pulmonary fibrosis, and Ayerza disease. Decreased in all anemias, leukemia, and after hemorrhage, when blood volume has been restored
Erythrocyte indices		
Mean corpuscular volume (MCV)	80–94 (cu. microns)	Increased in macrocytic anemias, decreased in microcytic anemia
Mean corpuscular hemoglobin (MCH)	27–32 μμg. per cell	Increased in macrocytic anemias, decreased in microcytic anemia
Mean corpuscular hemoglobin concentration (MCHC)	33–38%	Decreased in severe hypochromic anemia
Reticulocytes	0.5–1.5% of red cells	Increased with any condition stimulating increase bone marrow activity, i.e., infection, blood loss (acute and chronic), following iron therapy in iron deficiency anemia, polycythemia rubra vera. Decreased with any condition depressing bone marrow activity, acute leukemia, late stage of severe anemias
Erythrocyte sedimentation rate	Male: 0–9 mm./hr. Female: 0–20 mm./hr.	Increased in tissue destruction, whether inflammatory or degenerative, and during menstruation, pregnancy, and in acute febrile diseases

NORMAL VALUES—HEMATOLOGY *(Continued)*

Determination	Normal Values	Clinical Significance
Hematocrit	Male: 42–50% Female: 40–48%	Decreased in severe anemias, anemia of pregnancy, acute massive blood loss. Increased in erythrocytosis of any cause, and in dehydration or hemoconcentration associated with shock
Hemoglobin	Male: 13–16 gm./100 ml. Female: 12–14 gm./100 ml.	Decreased in various anemias, pregnancy, severe or prolonged hemorrhage, and with excessive fluid intake. Increased in polycythemia, chronic obstructive pulmonary diseases, failure of oxygenation because of congestive heart failure, and normally, in people living at high altitudes
Hemoglobin F	Less than 2%	Increased in infants and children, in thalassemia and many anemias
Leukocyte alkaline phosphatase	Score of 40–100	Decreased in chronic myelocytic leukemia and chronic lymphocytic leukemia. Increased in nonleukemic leukocytosis and myeloproliferative diseases
Leukocyte count	Total: 5,000–10,000 cu. mm.	Elevated in acute infectious diseases—predominately in the neutrophilic fraction with bacterial diseases, and in the lymphocytic and monocytic fractions in viral diseases. Eosinophils elevated in collagen diseases, allergy, intestinal parasitosis. Elevated in acute leukemia, following menstruation, and following surgery or trauma. Depressed in aplastic anemia, agranulocytosis, and by toxic agents, such as chemotherapeutic agents used in treating malignancy
Neutrophils	60–70%	
Eosinophils	1–4%	
Basophils	0–0.5%	
Lymphocytes	20–30%	
Monocytes	2–6%	
Osmotic fragility of red cells	Increase if hemolysis occurs in over 0.5% NaCl. Decrease if hemolysis is incomplete in 0.3% NaCl	Increased in congenital spherocytosis, idiopathic acquired hemolytic anemia, isoimmune hemolytic disease, ABO hemolytic disease of newborn. Decreased in sickle-cell anemia, thalassemia
Platelet count	200,000–350,000 per cu. mm.	Increased with chronic granulocytic leukemia, hemoconcentration. Decreased in thrombocytopenic purpura, acute leukemia, aplastic anemia, and during cancer chemotherapy

NORMAL BLOOD OR SERUM VALUES

Determination	Normal Adult Values	Clinical Significance (Increased)	(Decreased)
Acetoacetate and acetone	0.3–2.0 mg./100 ml.	Diabetic acidosis Fasting Toxemia of pregnancy Carbohydrate-free diet High-fat diet	
Aldolase	3–8 units/ml.	Hepatic necrosis Granulocytic leukemia Myocardial infarction Skeletal muscle disease	

NORMAL BLOOD OR SERUM VALUES *(Continued)*

Determination	Normal Adult Values	Clinical Significance (Increased)	(Decreased)
Alpha amino nitrogen	3.0–5.5 mg./100 ml.	Phosphorus, arsenic, chloroform, carbon tetrachloride poisoning Infectious hepatitis Eclampsia	Pneumococcal pneumonia Administration of anterior pituitary extracts Administration of insulin
Alpha-1-antitrypsin	200–400 mg./100 ml.	Early inflammatory processes Pneumonia Abscess formations Arthritis	Chronic lung disease
Alpha-1-fetoprotein	Absent	Primary carcinoma of liver	
Alpha-hydroxybutyric dehydrogenase	0–140 I.U./L.	Myocardial infarction Granulocytic leukemia Hemolytic anemias Muscular dystrophy	
Ammonia	50–170 µg./100 ml.*	Severe liver disease Hepatic decompensation	
Amylase	80–150 units/ml.	Acute pancreatitis Mumps Duodenal ulcer Carcinoma of head of pancreas Prolonged elevation with pseudocyst of pancreas	Chronic pancreatitis Pancreatic fibrosis and atrophy Cirrhosis of liver Acute alcoholism Toxemias of pregnancy
Ascorbic acid	0.4–1.5 mg./100 ml.		Rheumatic fever Collagen diseases Deficient vitamin C intake Renal and hepatic disease Congestive heart failure
Bilirubin	Total: 0.1–1.0 mg./100 ml. Direct: 0.1–0.2 mg./100 ml. Indirect: 0.1–0.8 mg./100 ml.	Hemolytic anemia (indirect) Biliary obstruction Hepatocellular damage Pernicious anemia Hemolytic disease of newborn Eclampsia	
Bromsulfophthalein (BSP)	Less than 5% retention in 45 min.	Acute hepatic diseases	
Calcium	8.5–10.5 mg./100 ml.	Tumor or hyperplasia of parathyroid Hyperparathyroidism Hypervitaminosis D Multiple myeloma Nephritis with uremia	Hypoparathyroidism Diarrhea Celiac disease Rickets Osteomalacia Malnutrition Nephrosis After parathyroidectomy

* Whole blood

NORMAL BLOOD OR SERUM VALUES *(Continued)*

Determination	Normal Adult Values	Clinical Significance (Increased)	(Decreased)
CO_2 content	Adults: 24–32 mEq./L. Infants: 20–26 mEq./L.	Tetany Respiratory disease Intestinal obstruction Vomiting	Acidosis Nephritis Eclampsia Diarrhea Anesthesia
Carotene, Beta	100–300 µg./100 ml.	Carotenemia Hypothyroidism Diabetes Hyperlipemia	Malabsorption syndromes Hepatic disease Dietary deficiencies
Cephalin flocculation	Negative to 1+	Severe liver disease Atypical viral pneumonia Malaria Lues Infectious mononucleosis Congestive heart failure	
Ceruloplasmin	0.14–0.57 O.D. units	Pregnancy Myocardial infarction Hepatic cirrhosis	Wilson's disease (hepato- lenticular degeneration)
Chloride	95–105 mEq./L.	Nephritis Urinary obstruction Cardiac decompensation Anemia Ether anesthesia	Diabetes Diarrhea Vomiting Pneumonia Heavy metal poisoning Cushing's syndrome Burns Intestinal obstruction Febrile conditions
Cholesterol	150–270 mg./100 ml.	Lipemia Obstructive jaundice Diabetes Hypothyroidism	Pernicious anemia Hemolytic jaundice Hyperthyroidism Severe infection Terminal states of debilitating disease
Cholesterol esters	65–70% of total		The esterified fraction decreases in liver disease
Cholinesterase	Plasma: 1.15–1.65 units Red cells: 0.65–1.0 units	Nephrosis Exercise	Nerve gas intoxication (greater effect on red cell activity) Insecticides, organic phosphates (greater effect on plasma activity)
Complement, Human C_3	90–150 mg./100 ml.		Acute glomerulonephritis Disseminated lupus erythematosis with renal involvement
Congo red	60–100% retained in bloodstream		Deposits of amyloid in tissue absorb congo red. In amyloid disease, less than 40% of the dye will remain in the plasma. In severe cases, less than 10% is retained

NORMAL BLOOD OR SERUM VALUES *(Continued)*

Determination	Normal Adult Values	Clinical Significance (Increased)	(Decreased)
Copper	Males: 97–130 µg./ 100 ml. Females: 105–140 µg./ 100 ml.	Cirrhosis of liver Pregnancy	Wilson's disease
Cortisol	8:00 A.M.: 5–26 µg./ 100 ml. 4:00 P.M.: 1.5–15 µg./ 100 ml.	Stress: infectious disease, surgery, burns, etc. Pregnancy Cushing's syndrome Pancreatitis Eclampsia	Addison's disease Anterior pituitary hypofunction
Creatine phosphokinase (CPK)	Male: 0–20 I.U./L. Female: 0–14 I.U./L.	Myocardial infarction Skeletal muscle diseases	
Creatine	3–7 mg./100 ml.	Biliary obstruction Pregnancy Nephritis Renal destruction Trauma to muscle Pseudohypertrophic muscular dystrophy	
Creatinine	1–2 mg./100 ml.	Nephritis Chronic renal disease	
Cryoglobulin	Zero	Multiple myeloma Chronic lymphocytic leukemia Lymphosarcoma Systemic lupus erythematosus Rheumatoid arthritis Subacute bacterial endocarditis Some malignancies	
Fatty acids	Total: 250–390 mg./ 100 ml.	Diabetes Anemia Nephrosis Hypothyroidism Nephritis	Hyperthyroidism
Fibrinogen*	0.1–0.4 gm./100 ml.	Pneumonia Acute infections Pregnancy Nephrosis Carcinoma	Cirrhosis Acute toxic necrosis of liver Anemia Typhoid fever Chloroform or phosphorus poisoning Abruptio placentae
Folic acid	Greater than 3 ng./ml.		Megaloblastic anemias of infancy and pregnancy Inadequate diets Liver disease Malabsorption syndrome Severe hemolytic anemia

* Plasma

NORMAL BLOOD OR SERUM VALUES *(Continued)*

Determination	Normal Adult Values	Clinical Significance	
		(Increased)	(Decreased)
Follicle stimulating hormone	Men: 3–12 mU./ml. Women: luteal & follic 5–15 mU./ml. Ovulatory: approximately 60 mU./ml. Postmenopause: 40–70 mU./ml.	Menopause and primary ovarian failure	Pituitary failure
Gamma glutamyl transpeptidase	Men: less than 45 I.U./L. Women: less than 30 I.U./L.	Hepatobiliary disease Anicteric alcoholics Drug therapy damage	
Glucose	65–110 mg./100 ml.	Diabetes Nephritis Hyperthyroidism Early hyperpituitarism Cerebral lesions Infections Pregnancy Uremia	Hyperinsulinism Hypothyroidism Late hyperpituitarism Pernicious vomiting Addison's disease Extensive hepatic damage
Glucose-6-phosphate dehydrogenase	1.86–2.90 I.U./ml. RBC		Drug induced hemolytic anemia Hemolytic disease of newborn
Haptoglobin	50–200 mg./100 ml.	Pregnancy Estrogen therapy Chronic infections Various inflammatory conditions Tissue destruction or necrosis	Newborn Hemolytic anemia Hemolytic blood transfusion reaction
Icterus index	1–6 units	Biliary obstruction Hemolytic anemias	Secondary anemias
Immunoglobulin A	80–200 mg./100 ml. (In children the normals are lower and vary with age)	Gamma A myeloma	Ataxia telangiectasis Agammaglobulinemia Hypogammaglobulinemia, transient Dysgammaglobulinemia Protein-losing enteropathies
Immunoglobulin D	3 mg./100 ml.	Gamma D myeloma	
Immunoglobulin G	800–1500 mg./100 ml.	Gamma G myeloma Cirrhosis of the liver	Agammaglobulinemia, congenital or acquired Hypogammaglobulinemia, transient Dysgammaglobulinemia Protein-losing enteropathies
Immunoglobulin M	40–120 mg./100 ml.	Waldenstrom's macroglobulinemia Parasitic diseases	Agammaglobulinemia Hypogammaglobulinemia Dysgammaglobulinemia Protein-losing enteropathies

NORMAL BLOOD OR SERUM VALUES *(Continued)*

Determination	Normal Adult Values	Clinical Significance (Increased)	(Decreased)
Insulin	4–24 µU./ml.	Insulinoma Acromegaly	Diabetes mellitus
Iodine, protein-bound	4.0–8.0 µg./100 ml.	Hyperthyroidism	Hypothyroidism
Iron	65–150 µg./100 ml.	Pernicious anemia Aplastic anemia Hemolytic anemia Hepatitis Hemochromatosis	Iron deficiency anemia
Iron binding capacity	150–225 µg./100 ml.	Iron deficiency anemia	Chronic infectious diseases
Isocitric dehydrogenase	50–180 units	Hepatitis, cirrhosis Obstructive jaundice Metastatic carcinoma to the liver Megaloblastic anemia	
Lactic acid*	6–16 mg./100 ml.	Increased muscular activity Congestive heart failure Hemorrhage Shock	
Lactic dehydrogenase (LDH)	90–200 mU./ml.	Untreated pernicious anemia Myocardial infarction Pulmonary infarction Liver disease	
Lactic dehydrogenase isoenzymes Total lactic dehydrogenase Isoenzyme fraction 1 Isoenzyme fraction 2 Isoenzyme fraction 3 Isoenzyme fraction 4 Isoenzyme fraction 5	90–200 mU./ml. 15–30% 22–50% 15–30% 0–15% 0–15%	Isoenzyme fraction 1 and 2 are increased in myocardial infarction Isoenzyme fraction 5 is increased in liver disease	
Leucine aminopeptidase	1–3 micromoles/hr./ml.	Liver or biliary tract diseases Pancreatic disease Metastatic carcinoma of liver and pancreas Biliary obstruction	
Lipase	0.2–1.5 units/ml.	Acute and chronic pancreatitis Biliary obstruction Cirrhosis Hepatitis Peptic ulcer	
Total lipids	400–1000 mg./100 ml.	Hypothyroidism Diabetes Nephrosis Glomerulonephritis	Hyperthyroidism

* Whole blood

NORMAL BLOOD OR SERUM VALUES *(Continued)*

Determination	Normal Adult Values	Clinical Significance (Increased)	(Decreased)

Lipoprotein phenotype

SUMMARY OF FINDINGS IN THE PRIMARY HYPERLIPOPROTEINEMIAS

| TYPE | APPEAR- ANCE | TRIGLYC- ERIDE | CHOLES- TEROL | LIPOPROTEIN STAINING | | | | SECONDARY CAUSES |
				BETA	PRE-BETA	ALPHA	CHYLOMI- CRONS	
Normal	Clear	Normal	Normal	Moderate	Zero to Moderate	Moderate	Weak	
I	Creamy	Markedly increased	Normal to moderately increased	Weak	Weak	Weak	Markedly increased	Dysglobulinemia
II	Clear	Normal to slightly increased	Slightly to markedly increased	Strong	Zero to strong	Moderate	Weak	Hypothyroidism, myeloma, hepatic disease, nephrotic syndrome, macroglobulinemia, and high dietary cholesterol
III	Clear, cloudy or milky	Increased	Increased	Broad intense band	Extends into beta	Moderate	Weak	
IV	Clear, cloudy or milky	Slightly to markedly increased	Normal to slightly increased	Weak to moderate	Moderate to strong	Weak to moderate	Weak	Hypothyroidism, diabetes mellitus, pancreatitis, glycogen storage diseases, nephrotic syndrome, myeloma, pregnancy and oral contraceptives
V	Cloudy to creamy	Markedly increased	Increased	Weak	Moderate	Weak	Strong	Diabetes mellitus, pancreatitis and alcoholism

Types I and II are fat induced; III and IV are carbohydrate induced; type V is fat and carbohydrate induced

Lithium	Usual maintenance level: 0.5–1.0 mEq./L.		
Magnesium	1.8–2.2 mEq./L.	Ingestion of epsom salts Parathyroidectomy	Chronic alcoholism Toxemia of pregnancy Severe renal disease
Nonprotein nitrogen	20–35 mg./100 ml.	Acute nephritis Polycystic kidneys Obstructive uropathy Peritonitis Congestive heart failure Pregnancy	
Osmolality	285–295 milliosmoles/kg.		Inappropriate secretion of antidiuretic hormone
Oxygen saturation, arterial*	96–100%	Polycythemia Anhydremia	Anemia Cardiac decompensation Chronic obstructive pulmonary disease
pCO_2*	35–45 mm. Hg	Respiratory acidosis Metabolic alkalosis	Respiratory alkalosis Metabolic acidosis
pH*	7.35–7.45	Vomiting Hyperpnea Fever Intestinal obstruction	Uremia Diabetic acidosis Hemorrhage Nephritis

* Whole blood

NORMAL BLOOD OR SERUM VALUES *(Continued)*

Determination	Normal Adult Values	Clinical Significance (Increased)	(Decreased)
pO_2*	75–100 mm. Hg	Directly related to oxygen saturation	
Pepsinogen	200–425 units/ml.		Conditions which decrease gastric acidity Pernicious anemia Achlorhydria
Phenylalanine	0–2 mg./100 ml.	Phenylketonuria Oasthouse urine disease	
Phosphatase, acid	0–2 units/ml. (Shinowara-Jones-Reinhart units)	Carcinoma of prostate Advanced Paget's disease Hyperparathyroidism	
Phosphatase, alkaline	4–17 King-Amstrong units/ml.	Conditions reflecting increased osteoblastic activity of bone Rickets Hyperparathyroidism Liver disease	
Phospholipids	125–300 mg./100 ml.	Diabetes Nephritis	
Phosphorus, inorganic	3.0–4.5 mg./100 ml.	Chronic nephritis Hypoparathyroidism	Hyperparathyroidism
Potassium	3.5–5.0 mEq./L.	Addison's disease Oliguria Anuria Tissue breakdown or hemolysis	Diabetic acidosis Diarrhea Vomiting
Protein, total	6–8 gm./100 ml.	Hemoconcentration Shock	Malnutrition Hemorrhage
Albumin	3.5–5 gm./100 ml.	Multiple myeloma (globulin fraction)	Loss of plasma from burns Proteinuria
Globulin	1.5–3 gm./100 ml.	Chronic infections (globulin)	
Paper electrophoresis Albumin Alpha 1 globulin Alpha 2 globulin Beta globulin Gamma globulin	% of total proteins 45–60% 2.7–6.1% 7.7–16.2% 10–17% 8.7–27%	Liver disease (globulin)	
Pyruvic Acid*	0.3–0.7 mg./100 ml.	Diabetes Severe thiamine deficiency Acute phase of some infections, possibly secondary to increased glycogenolysis and glycolysis	

* Whole blood

NORMAL BLOOD OR SERUM VALUES *(Continued)*

Determination	Normal Adult Values	Clinical Significance (Increased)	(Decreased)
Renin	Recumbent: 0.07–0.75 ng./ml./hr. Upright: 0.30–2.04 ng./ml./hr.	Renovascular hypertension Malignant hypertension Untreated Addison's disease Primary salt-losing nephropathy Low salt diet Diuretic therapy Hemorrhage	Frank primary aldosteronism Increased salt intake Salt-retaining steroid therapy Antidiuretic hormone therapy Blood transfusion
Sodium	135–145 mEq./L.	Hemoconcentration Nephritis Pyloric obstruction	Alkali deficit Addison's disease Myxedema
Sulfate	0.5–1.5 mg./100 ml.	Nephritis Nitrogen retention	
Testosterone	Adult males: 400–1200 ng./100 ml. Adult females: 30–150 ng./100 ml.	Females: Polycystic ovary Virilizing tumors	Males: Orchidectomy for neoplastic disease of the prostate or breast Estrogen therapy Klinefelter's syndrome Hypopituitarism Hypogonadism Hepatic cirrhosis
T_3 uptake	25–35%	Hyperthyroidism TBG deficiency Androgens and anabolic steroids	Hypothyroidism Pregnancy TBG excess Estrogens and antiovulatory drugs
Thyroxine (Murphy-Pattee) method	5.8–11.8 µg./100 ml.	Hyperthyroidism Pregnancy TBG excess Estrogens & antiovulatory drugs	Hypothyroidism TBG deficiency Androgens & anabolic steroids
Thyroid stimulating hormone (TSH)	Less than 23 mU./ml.	Primary hypothyroidism	
Thymol turbidity	1–4.5 units/ml.	Liver disease Infectious diseases with antibody production	
Transaminase (SGOT)	15–45 units/ml.	Myocardial infarction Skeletal muscle disease Liver disease	
Transaminase (SGPT)	5–36 units/ml.	Same conditions as SGOT, but increase is more marked in liver disease than SGOT	
Tyrosine	1.36–3.6 mg./100 ml.	Hyperthyrodism Tyrosinosis	

NORMAL BLOOD OR SERUM VALUES *(Continued)*

		Clinical Significance	
Determination	**Normal Adult Values**	**(Increased)**	**(Decreased)**
Urea nitrogen	10–20 mg./100 ml.	Acute glomerulonephritis Obstructive uropathy Mercury poisoning Nephrotic syndrome	Severe hepatic failure Pregnancy
Uric acid	1–6 mg./100 ml.	Gouty arthritis Acute leukemia Lymphomas treated by chemotherapy Toxemia of pregnancy	
Vitamin A	15–60 µg./100 ml.	Hypervitaminosis A	Vitamin A deficiency Celiac disease Sprue Obstructive jaundice Cystic fibrosis Giardiasis Parenchymal hepatic disease
Vitamin B_{12}	300–1000 pg./ml.	Hepatic cell damage and in association with the myeloproliferative disorders (The highest levels are encountered in myeloid leukemia)	Strict vegetarianism Alcoholism Pernicious anemia Total or partial gastrectomy Ileal resection Sprue and celiac disease Fish tapeworm infestation
Zinc	55–150 µg./100 ml.	Hyperthermia	Alcoholic cirrhosis Pernicious anemia Leukemia Severe atherosclerosis
Zinc turbidity	2–12 units/ml.	Same clinical significance as thymol turbidity	

NORMAL VALUES—URINE CHEMISTRY

		Clinical Significance	
Determination	**Normal Value**	**(Increased)**	**(Decreased)**
Acetone and acetoacetate	Zero	Uncontrolled diabetes mellitus Starvation	
Acid mucopolysaccharides	Negative	Hurler's syndrome Marfan's syndrome Morquio-Ulrich disease	
Aldosterone	2–26 µg./24 hrs.	Primary aldosteronism (adrenocortical tumor) Secondary aldosteronism Salt depletion Potassium loading ACTH in large doses Cardiac failure Cirrhosis with ascites formation Nephrosis Pregnancy	

NORMAL VALUES—URINE CHEMISTRY *(Continued)*

Determination	Normal Value	Clinical Significance (Increased)	(Decreased)
Alpha amino nitrogen	64–199 mg./24 hrs.	Leukemia Diabetes Phenylketonuria Other metabolic diseases	

Ammonia	20–70 mEq./L.
	0.6 gm./L.
		Diabetes mellitus
		Pernicious vomiting
		Cirrhosis and other
		  destructive diseases of
		  the liver	

Bile melanin	Zero	Advanced melanoma Ochronosis	
Calcium	Less than 150 mg./24 hrs.	Hyperparathyroidism	

Catecholamines	Epinephrine: less than 10
	  µg./24 hrs.
	Norepinephrine: less than
	  100 µg./24 hrs.
		Pheochromocytoma	

Chorionic gonadotropin	Zero	Pregnancy Chorionepithelioma Hydatidiform mole	
Copper	0–100 µg./24 hrs.	Wilson's disease Cirrhosis of liver	
Coproporphyrin	50–200 µg./24 hrs.	Poliomyelitis Lead poisoning	
Creatine	Less than 100 mg./24 hrs.	Muscular dystrophy Fever Carcinoma of liver Pregnancy	
Creatinine	1–2 gm./24 hrs.	Typhoid fever Salmonella infections Tetanus	Muscular atrophy Anemia Advanced degeneration of kidneys Leukemia
Chlorides	9 gm./L (as NaCl)		
Bile melanin	Zero	Advanced melanoma Ochronosis	

Creatinine clearance	150–180 L./24 hrs./1.73
	  sq. M. of body surface
			Measures glomerular
			  filtration rate
			Renal diseases

Cystine	8–86 mg./24 hrs.	Cystinuria	
Delta amino- levulinic acid	0.00–0.54 mg./100 ml.	Lead poisoning Porphyria hepatica Hepatitis Hepatic carcinoma	

NORMAL VALUES—URINE CHEMISTRY *(Continued)*

Determination	Normal Value	Clinical Significance (Increased)	(Decreased)
Estriol (placental)	Week of Pregnancy 16 20 24 28 32 36 40	Estriol values to 3 mg./24 hrs. 1–9 4–12 5–17 6–22 8–32 9–37	Decreased values occur with fetal distress of many conditions, including preeclampsia, placental insufficiency and poorly controlled diabetes mellitus
Estrogens, total	Female: Onset of menstruation: 4–25 µg./24 hr. Ovulation peak: 28–99 µg./24 hr. Luteal peak: 22–105 µg./24 hr. Menopausal women: 1.4–19.6 µg./24 hr. Male: 5–18 µg./24 hrs.	Hyperestrogenism due to gonadal or adrenal neoplasm	Primary or secondary amenorrhea
Etiocholanolone	Male: 1.9–6.0 mg./24 hrs. Female: 0.5–4.0 mg./ 24 hrs.	Adrenogenital syndrome Idiopathic hirsutism	
Glucose	Zero	Diabetes mellitus Pituitary disorders Intracranial pressure Lesion in floor of 4th ventricle	
Hemoglobin and myoglobin	Zero	Extensive burns Transfusion of incompatible blood Myoglobin increased in severe crushing injuries to muscle	
Homogentisic acid	Zero	Alkaptonuria Ochronosis	
17–hydroxycorticosteroids	2–10 mg./24 hrs.	Cushing's syndrome	Addison's disease Anterior pituitary hypofunction
5–Hydroxyindoleacetic acid	Zero	Malignant carcinoid syndrome	
17–ketosteroids, alpha beta fractionation	Alpha concentration 85% or more	Adrenal carcinomas (in beta fraction)	

NORMAL VALUES—URINE CHEMISTRY *(Continued)*

Determination	Normal Value	Clinical Significance (Increased)	(Decreased)
17–ketosteroids, total	Male: 10–22 mg./24 hrs. Female: 6–16 mg./24 hrs. Up to 1 yr.: Less than 1 mg./24 hrs. 1–4 yrs.: Less than 2 mg./24 hrs. 5–8 yrs.: Less than 3 mg./24 hrs. 9–12 yrs.: 3–10 mg./24 hrs. 13–16 yrs.: 5–12 mg./24 hrs.	Interstitial cell tumor of testes Simple hirsutism, occasionally Adrenal hyperplasia Cushing's syndrome Adrenal cancer, virilism Arrhenoblastoma	Thyrotoxicosis Female hypogonadism Diabetes mellitus Hypertension Debilitating disease of mild to moderate severity Eunuchoidism Addison's disease Panhypopituitarism Myxedema Nephrosis
Lead	120 μg. or less/24 hrs.	Lead poisoning	
Metanephrines, total	Less than 1.3 mg./24 hrs.	Pheochromocytoma	
Phenolphthalein (PSP)	At least 25% excreted in 15 min., 40% by 30 min., and 60% by 120 min.		Delayed in renal diseases Low in nephritis, cystitis, pyelonephritis, congestive heart failure
Phenylpyruvic acid	Zero	Phenylketonuria	Primarily measures of renal tubular function
Phosphorus, inorganic	Average 1 gm./24 hrs. Varies with intake	Fever Nervous exhaustion Tuberculosis Rickets Chronic lead poisoning	Acute infections Nephritis Chlorosis Pregnancy
Pituitary gonadotropin	Males: 6–24 mouse units/24 hrs. Females: 5–40 mouse units/24 hrs.	Seminoma Teratoma of testis Pregnancy Menopause	
Porphobilinogen	Zero	Acute porphyria Liver disease	
Pregnanediol	Proliferative phase: 0.5–1.5 mg./24 hrs. Luteal phase: 2–7 mg./24 hrs. Menopause: 0.2–1.0 mg./24 hrs.	Corpus luteum cysts When placental tissue remains in the uterus following parturition Some cases of adrenal-cortical tumors	Placental dysfunction Threatened abortion Intrauterine death
Pregnanetriol	0–4 mg./24 hrs.	Congenital adrenal androgenic hyperplasia	
Protein	Up to 100 mg./24 hrs.	Nephritis Cardiac failure Mercury poisoning Bence-Jones protein in multiple myeloma Febrile states Hematuria Amyloidosis	

NORMAL VALUES—URINE CHEMISTRY *(Continued)*

Determination	Normal Value	Clinical Significance (Increased)	(Decreased)
Titratable acidity	20–40 mEq./24 hrs.	Metabolic acidosis	Metabolic alkalosis
Urea clearance	Over 40 ml. blood cleared of urea/min., or greater than 60%		Renal diseases
Urobilinogen	Up to 4 mg./24 hrs.	Liver and biliary tract disease Hen．olytic anemias	Complete or nearly complete biliary obstruction Diarrhea Renal insufficiency
Uroporphyrins	Zero	Porphyria	
Vanilmandelic acid	0.7–6.8 mg./24 hrs.	Pheochromocytoma	
D-Xylose absorption	5-hr. excretion of 16–33% of test dose		Malabsorption syndromes
Urea	25–35 gm./24 hrs.	Excessive protein catabolism	Impaired kidney function
Uric acid	0.6–1 gm./24 hrs. as urate	Gout (see blood uric acid)	Nephritis (see blood uric acid)

NORMAL VALUES—CEREBROSPINAL FLUID

Determination	Normal Value	Clinical Significance (Increased)	(Decreased)
Cell count	0–5 mononuclear cells/ cu. mm.	Bacterial meningitis Neurosyphilis Anterior poliomyelitis Encephalitis lethargica	
Chloride	100–130 mEq./L.	Uremia	Acute generalized meningitis Tubercular meningitis
Colloidal gold	0000000000	Acute meningitis Neurosyphilis	
Glucose	50–75 mg./100 ml.	Diabetes mellitus Diabetic coma Epidemic encephalitis Uremia	Acute meningitides Tuberculous meningitis Insulin shock
Protein Lumbar Cisternal Ventricular	15–45 mg./100 ml. 15–25 mg./100 ml. 5–15 mg./100 ml.	Acute meningitides Tubercular meningitis Neurosyphilis Poliomyelitis Guillain-Barré syndrome	

MISCELLANEOUS VALUES

Toxicology Determination	Normal Value	Clinical Significance	
Barbiturate	Zero	Coma level approximately 11 mg./100 ml. for phenobarbital; most other compounds 1.5 mg./100 ml.	
Bromide	Zero	Toxic level = 17 mEq./L.	
Carbon monoxide	0–2%	Symptoms with over 20% saturation	
Dilantin	Zero	Therapeutic level = 1–11 mg./100 ml.	
Ethanol	0–0.05%	Maximal level allowable by courts = 0.15% 0.3–0.4% = marked intoxication 0.4–0.5% = alcoholic stupor	
Methanol	Zero	May be fatal in concentrations as low as 10 mg./100 ml.	
Salicylate	Zero	Therapeutic level = 20–25 mg./100 ml. Toxic level = over 30 mg./100 ml.	
Sulfonamide	Zero	Therapeutic levels: Sulfadiazine Sulfaguanidine Sulfamerazine Sulfanilamide	8–15 mg./100 ml. 3–5 mg./100 ml. 10–15 mg./100 ml. 10–15 mg./100 ml.
Gastric Analysis		**(Increased)**	**(Decreased)**
Free HCl	0–30 mEq./L.	Neuroses	Pernicious anemia
Total acidity	15–45 mEq./L.	Peptic ulcer	Gastric carcinoma
Combined acid	10–15 mEq./L.	Zollinger-Ellison syndrome	Chronic atrophic gastritis Decreases normally with age

APPENDIX II

Conversion Tables

METRIC UNITS AND SYMBOLS

Quantity	Unit	Symbol	Equivalent
Length	millimeter	mm.	1000 mm. = 1 m.
	centimeter	cm.	100 cm. = 1 m.
	decimeter	dm.	10 dm. = 1 m.
	meter	m.	1000 m. = 1 km.
Volume	cubic centimeter	cc. or cm.^{3}	$1000 \left\{ \begin{array}{l} \text{cc. or cm.}^3 \\ \text{ml.} \end{array} \right. = 1$ dm.^{3} or 1 liter
	milliliter	ml.	
	cu. decimeter	dm.^{3}	$1000 \left\{ \begin{array}{l} \text{dm.}^3 \\ 1 \end{array} \right. = 1$ m.^{3}
	liter	L.	
Mass	microgram	μg.	1000 μg. = 1 mg.
	milligram	mg.	1000 mg. = 1 g.
	gram	g.	1000 g. = 1 kg.
	kilogram	kg.	1000 kg. = 1 metric ton (t)

TABLE OF METRIC AND APOTHECARIES' SYSTEMS*

(Approved *approximate* dose equivalents are enclosed in parentheses. Use *exact* equivalents in calculations.)

Conversion Factors

METRIC	APOTHECARIES	METRIC	APOTHECARIES
1 milligram (mg.)	$\frac{1}{64}$ grain	3.888 cubic centimeters or grams	1 dram (4 cc. or grams)
64.79 milligrams	1 grain (65 mg.)	31.103 cubic centimeters or grams	1 ounce (30 cc. or grams)
1 gram	15.43 grains (15 grains)	473.167 cubic centimeters	1 pint (500 cc.)
1 cubic centimeter (cc.)	16 minims		

WEIGHTS

METRIC	APOTHECARIES	METRIC	APOTHECARIES
0.0001 gram—0.1 mg.	$\frac{1}{640}$ grain ($\frac{1}{600}$ grain)	0.057 gram —57 mg.	$\frac{7}{8}$ grain
0.0002 gram—0.2 mg.	$\frac{1}{320}$ grain ($\frac{1}{300}$ grain)	0.06 gram —60 mg.	$\frac{9}{10}$ grain (1 grain)
0.0003 gram—0.3 mg.	$\frac{1}{210}$ grain ($\frac{1}{200}$ grain)	0.065 gram —65 mg.	1 grain (60 mg.)
0.0004 gram—0.4 mg.	$\frac{1}{150}$ grain	0.07 gram —70 mg.	$1\frac{1}{20}$ grains
0.0005 gram—0.5 mg.	$\frac{1}{120}$ grain	0.08 gram —80 mg.	$1\frac{1}{5}$ grains
0.0006 gram—0.6 mg.	$\frac{1}{100}$ grain	0.09 gram —90 mg.	$1\frac{1}{3}$ grains
0.0007 gram—0.7 mg.	$\frac{1}{90}$ grain	0.097 gram —97 mg.	$1\frac{1}{2}$ grains (0.1 gram)
0.0008 gram—0.8 mg.	$\frac{1}{80}$ grain	0.12 gram —120 mg.	2 grains
0.0009 gram—0.9 mg.	$\frac{1}{75}$ grain	0.2 gram —200 mg.	3 grains
0.001 gram—1 mg.	$\frac{1}{64}$ grain ($\frac{1}{60}$ grain)	0.24 gram —240 mg.	4 grains (0.25 gram)
0.0011 gram—1.1 mg.	$\frac{1}{60}$ grain	0.3 gram —300 mg.	$4\frac{1}{2}$ grains
0.0013 gram—1.3 mg.	$\frac{1}{50}$ grain (1.2 mg.)	0.33 gram —330 mg.	5 grains (0.3 gram)
0.0014 gram—1.4 mg.	$\frac{1}{48}$ grain	0.4 gram —400 mg.	6 grains
0.0016 gram—1.6 mg.	$\frac{1}{40}$ grain (1.5 mg.)	0.45 gram —450 mg.	7 grains
0.0018 gram—1.8 mg.	$\frac{1}{36}$ grain	0.5 gram —500 mg.	$7\frac{1}{2}$ grains
0.0020 gram—2 mg.	$\frac{1}{32}$ grain ($\frac{1}{30}$ grain)	0.53 gram —530 mg.	8 grains
0.0022 gram—2.2 mg.	$\frac{1}{30}$ grain	0.6 gram —600 mg.	9 grains
0.0026 gram—2.6 mg.	$\frac{1}{25}$ grain	0.65 gram —650 mg.	10 grains (0.6 gram)
0.003 gram—3 mg.	$\frac{1}{20}$ grain	0.73 gram —730 mg.	11 grains
0.004 gram—4 mg.	$\frac{1}{16}$ grain ($\frac{1}{15}$ grain)	0.80 gram —800 mg.	12 grains (0.75 gram)
0.005 gram—5 mg.	$\frac{1}{12}$ grain	0.86 gram —860 mg.	13 grains
0.006 gram—6 mg.	$\frac{1}{10}$ grain	0.93 gram —930 mg.	14 grains
0.007 gram—7 mg.	$\frac{1}{9}$ grain	1. gram —1000 mg.	15 grains
0.008 gram—8 mg.	$\frac{1}{8}$ grain	1.06 grams—1060 mg.	16 grains
0.009 gram—9 mg.	$\frac{1}{7}$ grain	1.13 grams—1130 mg.	17 grains
0.01 gram—10 mg.	$\frac{1}{6}$ grain	1.18 grams—1180 mg.	18 grains
0.013 gram—13 mg.	$\frac{1}{5}$ grain (12 mg.)	1.26 grams—1260 mg.	19 grains
0.016 gram—16 mg.	$\frac{1}{4}$ grain (15 mg.)	1.30 grams—1300 mg.	20 grains
0.02 gram—20 mg.	$\frac{1}{3}$ grain	1.50 grams—1500 mg.	22 grains
0.025 gram—25 mg.	$\frac{3}{8}$ grain	2 grams—2000 mg.	30 grains ($\frac{1}{2}$ dram)
0.03 gram—30 mg.	$\frac{2}{5}$ grain ($\frac{1}{2}$ grain)	4 grams	1 dram (60 grains)
0.032 gram—32 mg.	$\frac{1}{2}$ grain (30 mg.)	5 grams	75 grains
0.04 gram—40 mg.	$\frac{3}{5}$ grain ($\frac{2}{3}$ grain)	8 grams	2 drams (7.5 grams)
0.043 gram—43 mg.	$\frac{2}{3}$ grain (40 mg.)	10 grams	$2\frac{1}{2}$ drams
0.05 gram—50 mg.	$\frac{3}{4}$ grain	15 grams	4 drams
		30 grams	1 ounce

LIQUID MEASURES**

METRIC	APOTHECARIES	METRIC	APOTHECARIES
0.03 cubic centimeter	$\frac{1}{2}$ minim	8 cubic centimeters	2 fluid drams
0.05 cubic centimeter	$\frac{3}{4}$ minim	10 cubic centimeters	$2\frac{1}{2}$ fluid drams
0.06 cubic centimeter	1 minim	15 cubic centimeters	4 fluid drams
0.1 cubic centimeter	$1\frac{1}{2}$ minims	20 cubic centimeters	$5\frac{1}{2}$ fluid drams
0.2 cubic centimeter	3 minims	25 cubic centimeters	$\frac{5}{6}$ fluid ounce
0.25 cubic centimeter	4 minims	30 cubic centimeters	1 fluid ounce
0.3 cubic centimeter	5 minims	50 cubic centimeters	$1\frac{3}{4}$ fluid ounces
0.5 cubic centimeter	8 minims	60 cubic centimeters	2 fluid ounces
0.6 cubic centimeter	10 minims	100 cubic centimeters	$3\frac{1}{2}$ fluid ounces
0.75 cubic centimeter	12 minims	120 cubic centimeters	4 fluid ounces
1 cubic centimeter	15 minims	200 cubic centimeters	7 fluid ounces
2 cubic centimeters	30 minims	250 cubic centimeters	8 fluid ounces
3 cubic centimeters	45 minims	360 cubic centimeters	12 fluid ounces
4 cubic centimeters	1 fluid dram	500 cubic centimeters	1 pint
5 cubic centimeters	$1\frac{1}{4}$ fluid drams	1000 cubic centimeters	1 quart

* (From Culver, V. M.: Modern Bedside Nursing. Philadelphia, W. B. Saunders, 1969.)

** Note: A cubic centimeter (cc.) is the approximate equivalent of a milliliter (ml.). The terms are used interchangeably in general medicine.

24-HOUR CLOCK

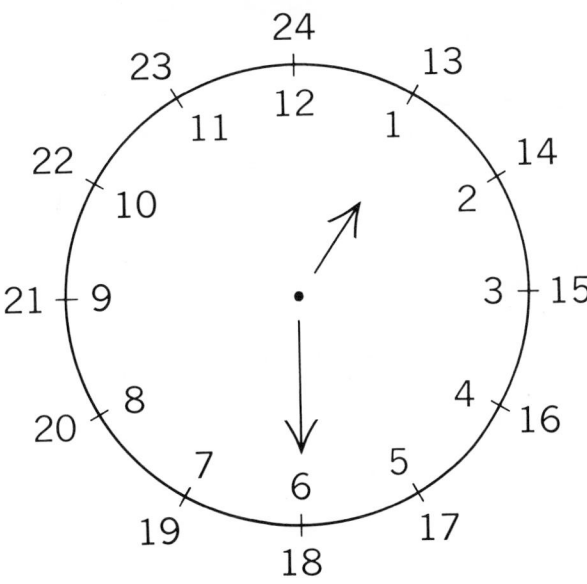

From midnight to noon — 12-hour time $\Big\}$ identical
24-hour time

From noon to midnight — Add 12 to P.M. time = 24-hour time

12-hour Time		**24-hour Time**
12:00 midnight		24:00
12:01 A.M.		00:01
12:59 A.M.		00:59
1:00 A.M.		01:00
12:00 noon		12:00
12:01 P.M.		12:01
1:00 P.M.		13:00
5:30 P.M.		17:30
10:08 P.M.		22:08
12:00 midnight		24:00

A useful clock to avoid confusion about A.M. and P.M. designations.

NOMOGRAM FOR ESTIMATING SURFACE AREA OF INFANTS AND YOUNG CHILDREN

HEIGHT		SURFACE AREA	WEIGHT	
feet	centimeters	in square meters	pounds	kilograms

To determine the surface area of the patient draw a straight line between the point representing his height on the left vertical scale to the point representing his weight on the right vertical scale. The point at which this line intersects the middle vertical scale represents the patient's surface area in square meters. (Courtesy, Abbott Laboratories.)

NOMOGRAM FOR ESTIMATING SURFACE AREA OF OLDER CHILDREN AND ADULTS

HEIGHT		SURFACE AREA	WEIGHT	
feet	centimeters	in square meters	pounds	kilograms

HEIGHT
- 7' — 220, 215, 210
- 10" — 210
- 8" — 205
- 6" — 200
- 4" — 195, 190
- 2" — 190
- 6' — 185, 180
- 10" — 175
- 8" — 170
- 6" — 165
- 4" — 160
- 2" — 155
- 5' — 150
- 10" — 145
- 8" — 140
- 6" — 135
- 4" — 130
- 2" — 125
- 4' — 120
- 10" — 115
- 8" — 110
- 6" — 105
- 4" — 100
- 2" — 95
- 3' — 90
- 10" — 85
- 8" — 80
- 6" — 75

SURFACE AREA (in square meters)
3.00, 2.90, 2.80, 2.70, 2.60, 2.50, 2.40, 2.30, 2.20, 2.10, 2.00, 1.95, 1.90, 1.85, 1.80, 1.75, 1.70, 1.65, 1.60, 1.55, 1.50, 1.45, 1.40, 1.35, 1.30, 1.25, 1.20, 1.15, 1.10, 1.05, 1.00, .95, .90, .85, .80, .75, .70, .65, .60

WEIGHT (pounds / kilograms)
- 440 / 200
- 420 / 190
- 400 / 180
- 380 / 170
- 360 / 160
- 340 / 150
- 320 / 140
- 300 /
- 290 / 130
- 280 /
- 270 / 120
- 260 /
- 250 /
- 240 / 110
- 230 /
- 220 / 100
- 210 / 95
- 200 / 90
- 190 / 85
- 180 / 80
- 170 /
- 160 / 75
- 150 / 70
- 140 / 65
- 130 / 60
- 120 / 55
- 110 / 50
- 100 / 45
- 90 / 40
- 80 / 35
- 70 / 30
- 60 / 25
- 50 /
- 20

(Courtesy, Abbott Laboratories.)

CELSIUS (Centigrade) and FAHRENHEIT TEMPERATURES

Centigrade (Celsius)	Fahrenheit
0	32
36.0	96.8
36.5	97.7
37.0	98.6
37.5	99.5
38.0	100.4
38.5	101.3
39.0	102.2
39.5	103.1
40.0	104.0
40.5	104.9
41.0	105.8
41.5	106.7
42.0	107.6

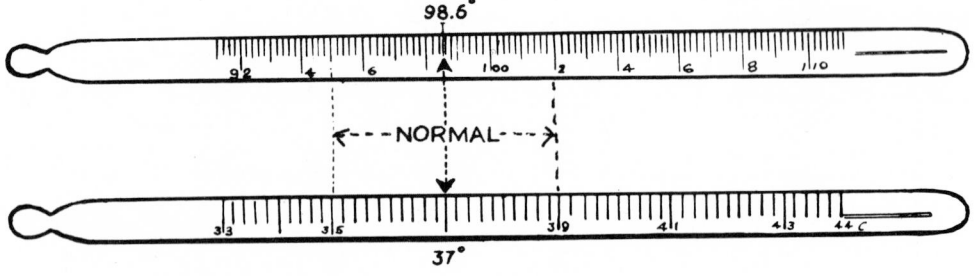

FAHRENHEIT

CENTIGRADE

To convert degrees F. to degrees C.
    Subtract 32, then multiply by 5/9

To convert degrees C. to degrees F.
    Multiply by 9/5, then add 32

COMPARATIVE SCALES OF MEASURES, WEIGHTS AND TEMPERATURES*

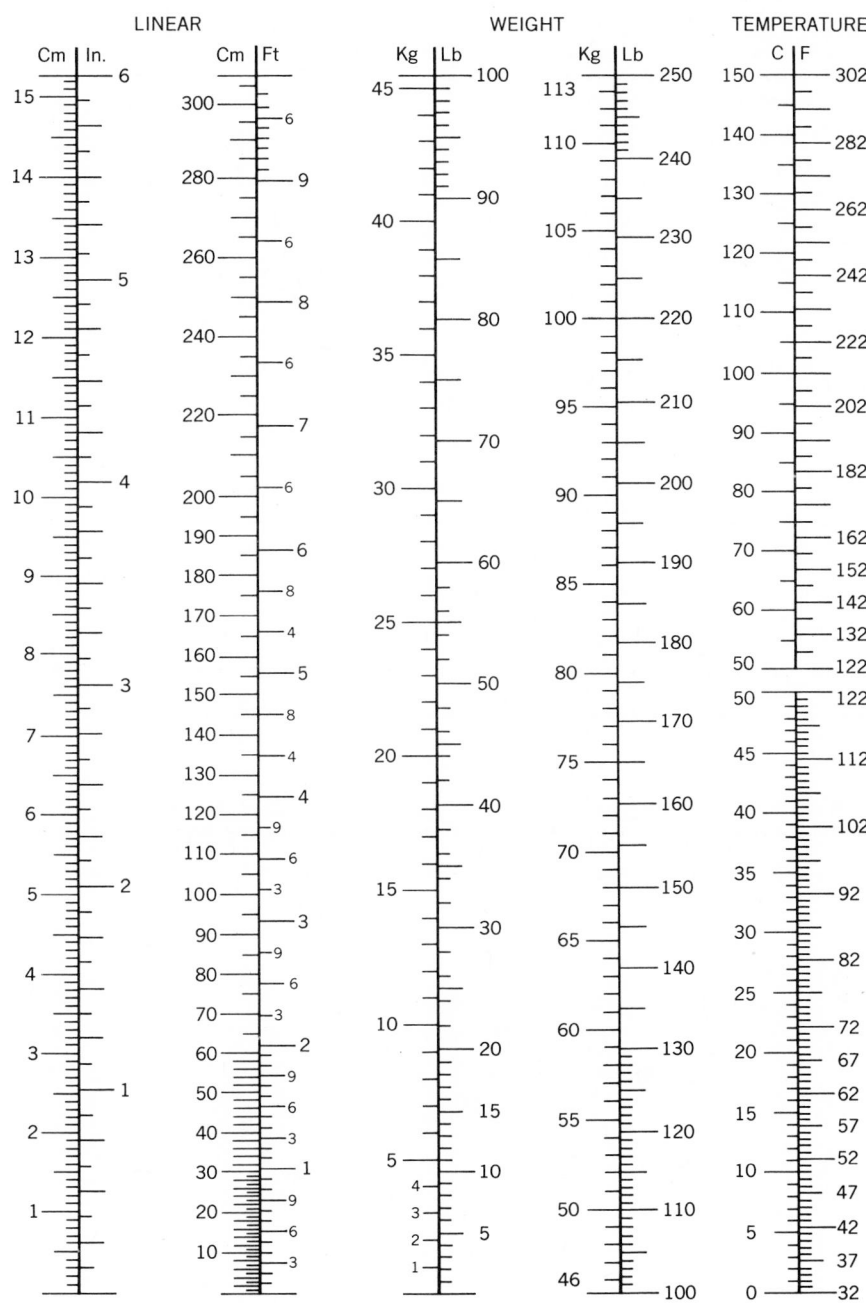

LINEAR   WEIGHT   TEMPERATURE

* 2.5 cm = 1 in.   1 kg. = 2.2 lb.

RECOMMENDED DAILY DIETARY ALLOWANCES

FOOD AND NUTRITION BOARD, NATIONAL ACADEMY OF SCIENCES—
NATIONAL RESEARCH COUNCIL
RECOMMENDED DAILY DIETARY ALLOWANCES,[a] Revised 1968
Designed for the maintenance of good nutrition of practically all healthy people in the U.S.A.

	AGE[b] (years) From – Up to	WEIGHT (kg)	(lbs)	HEIGHT cm	(in.)	kcal	PROTEIN (gm)	Fat-Soluble Vitamins VITAMIN A ACTIVITY (IU)	VITAMIN D (IU)	VITAMIN E ACTIVITY (IU)
Infants	0 – 1/6	4	9	55	22	kg × 120	kg × 2.2[e]	1,500	400	5
	1/6 – 1/2	7	15	63	25	kg × 110	kg × 2.0[e]	1,500	400	5
	1/2 – 1	9	20	72	28	kg × 100	kg × 1.8[e]	1,500	400	5
Children	1 – 2	12	26	81	32	1,100	25	2,000	400	10
	2 – 3	14	31	91	36	1,250	25	2,000	400	10
	3 – 4	16	35	100	39	1,400	30	2,500	400	10
	4 – 6	19	42	110	43	1,600	30	2,500	400	10
	6 – 8	23	51	121	48	2,000	35	3,500	400	15
	8 – 10	28	62	131	52	2,200	40	3,500	400	15
Males	10 – 12	35	77	140	55	2,500	45	4,500	400	20
	12 – 14	43	95	151	59	2,700	50	5,000	400	20
	14 – 18	59	130	170	67	3,000	60	5,000	400	25
	18 – 22	67	147	175	69	2,800	60	5,000	400	30
	22 – 35	70	154	175	69	2,800	65	5,000	—	30
	35 – 55	70	154	173	68	2,600	65	5,000	—	30
	55 – 75+	70	154	171	67	2,400	65	5,000	—	30
Females	10 – 12	35	77	142	56	2,250	50	4,500	400	20
	12 – 14	44	97	154	61	2,300	50	5,000	400	20
	14 – 16	52	114	157	62	2,400	55	5,000	400	25
	16 – 18	54	119	160	63	2,300	55	5,000	400	25
	18 – 22	58	128	163	64	2,000	55	5,000	400	25
	22 – 35	58	128	163	64	2,000	55	5,000	—	25
	35 – 55	58	128	160	63	1,850	55	5,000	—	25
	55 – 75+	58	128	157	62	1,700	55	5,000	—	25
Pregnancy						+200	65	6,000	400	30
Lactation						+1,000	75	8,000	400	30

[a] The allowance levels are intended to cover individual variations among most normal persons as they live in the United States under usual environmental stresses. The recommended allowances can be attained with a variety of common foods, providing other nutrients for which human requirements have been less well defined. See text for more-detailed discussion of allowances and of nutrients not tabulated.

[b] Entries on lines for age range 22–35 years represent the reference man and woman at age 22. All other entries represent allowances for the midpoint of the specified age range.

Water-Soluble Vitamins							Minerals				
ASCORBIC ACID (mg)	FOLACIN c (mg)	NIACIN (mg EQUIV) d	RIBOFLAVIN (mg)	THIAMIN (mg)	VITAMIN B_6 (mg)	VITAMIN B_{12} (μg)	CALCIUM (g)	PHOSPHORUS (g)	IODINE (μg)	IRON (mg)	MAGNESIUM (mg)
35	0.05	5	0.4	0.2	0.2	1.0	0.4	0.2	25	6	40
35	0.05	7	0.5	0.4	0.3	1.5	0.5	0.4	40	10	60
35	0.1	8	0.6	0.5	0.4	2.0	0.6	0.5	45	15	70
40	0.1	8	0.6	0.6	0.5	2.0	0.7	0.7	55	15	100
40	0.2	8	0.7	0.6	0.6	2.5	0.8	0.8	60	15	150
40	0.2	9	0.8	0.7	0.7	3	0.8	0.8	70	10	200
40	0.2	11	0.9	0.8	0.9	4	0.8	0.8	80	10	200
40	0.2	13	1.1	1.0	1.0	4	0.9	0.9	100	10	250
40	0.3	15	1.2	1.1	1.2	5	1.0	1.0	110	10	250
40	0.4	17	1.3	1.3	1.4	5	1.2	1.2	125	10	300
45	0.4	18	1.4	1.4	1.6	5	1.4	1.4	135	18	350
55	0.4	20	1.5	1.5	1.8	5	1.4	1.4	150	18	400
60	0.4	18	1.6	1.4	2.0	5	0.8	0.8	140	10	400
60	0.4	18	1.7	1.4	2.0	5	0.8	0.8	140	10	350
60	0.4	17	1.7	1.3	2.0	5	0.8	0.8	125	10	350
60	0.4	14	1.7	1.2	2.0	6	0.8	0.8	110	10	350
40	0.4	15	1.3	1.1	1.4	5	1.2	1.2	110	18	300
45	0.4	15	1.4	1.2	1.6	5	1.3	1.3	115	18	350
50	0.4	16	1.4	1.2	1.8	5	1.3	1.3	120	18	350
50	0.4	15	1.5	1.2	2.0	5	1.3	1.3	115	18	350
55	0.4	13	1.5	1.0	2.0	5	0.8	0.8	100	18	350
55	0.4	13	1.5	1.0	2.0	5	0.8	0.8	100	18	300
55	0.4	13	1.5	1.0	2.0	5	0.8	0.8	90	18	300
55	0.4	13	1.5	1.0	2.0	6	0.8	0.8	80	10	300
60	0.8	15	1.8	+0.1	2.5	8	+0.4	+0.4	125	18	450
60	0.5	20	2.0	+0.5	2.5	6	+0.5	+0.5	150	18	450

[c] The folacin allowances refer to dietary sources as determined by *Lactobacillus casei* assay. Pure forms of folacin may be effective in doses less than ¼ of the RDA.

[d] Niacin equivalents include dietary sources of the vitamin itself plus 1 mg equivalent for each 60 mg of dietary tryptophan.

[e] Assumes protein equivalent to human milk (p. 1432). For proteins not 100 percent utilized factors should be increased proportionately.

(Recommended Dietary Allowances, Pub. No. 1694, The Food and Nutrition Board, National Academy of Sciences—National Research Council, Washington, D.C.)

Index